Systemic Lupus Erythematosus

Dedication

To Cathy, Donna, Alice, Thomas, Luz, Betty, Leosha
and all who fight lupus from dawn to dusk.
We promise to do better.

Systemic Lupus Erythematosus
Basic, Applied and Clinical Aspects

Edited by

George C. Tsokos
Harvard Medical School, Boston, MA, USA

AMSTERDAM • BOSTON • HEIDELBERG • LONDON • NEW YORK • OXFORD • PARIS
SAN DIEGO • SAN FRANCISCO • SINGAPORE • SYDNEY • TOKYO

Academic Press is an imprint of Elsevier

Academic Press is an imprint of Elsevier
125 London Wall, London EC2Y 5AS, UK
525 B Street, Suite 1800, San Diego, CA 92101-4495, USA
225 Wyman Street, Waltham, MA 02451, USA
The Boulevard, Langford Lane, Kidlington, Oxford OX5 1GB, UK

Notices
Knowledge and best practice in this field are constantly changing. As new research and experience broaden our understanding, changes in research methods, professional practices, or medical treatment may become necessary.

Practitioners and researchers must always rely on their own experience and knowledge in evaluating and using any information, methods, compounds, or experiments described herein. In using such information or methods they should be mindful of their own safety and the safety of others, including parties for whom they have a professional responsibility.

To the fullest extent of the law, neither the Publisher nor the authors, contributors, or editors, assume any liability for any injury and/or damage to persons or property as a matter of products liability, negligence or otherwise, or from any use or operation of any methods, products, instructions, or ideas contained in the material herein.

ISBN: 978-0-12-801917-7

British Library Cataloguing-in-Publication Data
A catalogue record for this book is available from the British Library

Library of Congress Cataloging-in-Publication Data
A catalog record for this book is available from the Library of Congress

For information on all Academic Press publications
visit our website at http://store.elsevier.com/

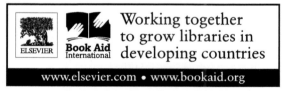

Working together
to grow libraries in
developing countries

www.elsevier.com • www.bookaid.org

Typeset by TNQ Books and Journals
www.tnq.co.in

Printed and bound in the United States of America

Contents

32. Genes and Genetics of Murine Systemic Lupus Erythematosus

Dwight H. Kono and Argyrios N. Theofilopoulos

Part III
Mechanisms of Tissue Damage

33. Mechanisms of Renal Damage in Systemic Lupus Erythematosus

Shu Man Fu, Chao Dai, Hongyang Wang, Sun-Sang J. Sung and Felicia Gaskin

34. Mechanisms of Vascular Damage in Systemic Lupus Erythematosus

Sarfaraz A. Hasni and Mariana J. Kaplan

35. The Mechanism of Skin Damage

Xin Huang, Haijing Wu, Christopher Chang and Qianjin Lu

36. Pathogenesis of Tissue Injury in the Brain in Patients with Systemic Lupus Erythematosus

Bruce T. Volpe

52. Incomplete Lupus

George Stojan

53. Childhood-Onset Systemic Lupus Erythematosus

Mindy S. Lo

54. Drug-Induced Lupus

Mary Anne Dooley

55. Vasculitis in Lupus

Anisur Rahman

Part V
Antiphospholipid Syndrome

56. Pathogenesis of Antiphospholipid Syndrome

Olga Amengual and Tatsuya Atsumi

57. Antibodies and Diagnostic Tests in Antiphospholipid Syndrome

*Cecilia Beatrice Chighizola, Maria Orietta Borghi
and Pier Luigi Meroni*

58. Clinical Manifestations

Miyuki Bohgaki and Takao Koike

Part VI
Treatment of the Disease

59. Nonsteroidal Anti-inflammatory Drugs in Systemic Lupus Erythematosus

Robert G. Lahita and Chengqun Shao

60. Value of Antimalarial Drugs in the Treatment of Lupus

Ziv Paz

61. Systemic Glucocorticoids

Zahi Touma and Murray B. Urowitz

62. Cytotoxic-Immunosuppressive Drug Treatment

Eleni A. Frangou, George Bertsias and Dimitrios T. Boumpas

63. Treatment of Antiphospholipid Syndrome

Savino Sciascia and Munther Khamashta

64. New Treatments for Systemic Lupus Erythematosus

Vasileios C. Kyttaris

65. Management Lessons from Clinical Trials of Kidney Disease in Systemic Lupus Erythematosus

Brad H. Rovin and Isabelle Ayoub

66. Repositioning Drugs for Systemic Lupus Erythematosus

Amrie C. Grammer, Matthew M. Ryals, Michelle D. Catalina and Peter E. Lipsky

List of Contributors

Nancy Agmon-Levin The Zabludowicz Center for Autoimmune Diseases Sheba Medical Center, Sackler Faculty of Medicine, Tel-Aviv University, Tel Aviv, Israel

Graciela S. Alarcón Department of Medicine, Division of Clinical Immunology and Rheumatology, School of Medicine, The University of Alabama at Birmingham, Birmingham, AL, USA

Olga Amengual Division of Rheumatology, Endocrinology and Nephrology, Hokkaido University Graduate School of Medicine, Sapporo, Japan

Stacy P. Ardoin Ohio State University, Columbus, OH, USA

John P. Atkinson Division of Rheumatology, Department of Medicine, Washington University School of Medicine, Saint Louis, MO, USA

Tatsuya Atsumi Division of Rheumatology, Endocrinology and Nephrology, Hokkaido University Graduate School of Medicine, Sapporo, Japan

Isabelle Ayoub Division of Nephrology, Ohio State University Wexner Medical Center, Columbus, OH, USA

Bonnie L. Bermas Brigham and Women's Hospital, Boston, MA, USA

Sasha Bernatsky McGill University Health Centre, Montreal, QC, Canada

George Bertsias Rheumatology, Clinical Immunology and Allergy Medical School, University of Crete Heraklion, Heraklion, Greece

Patrick Blanco University of Bordeaux, CIRID, UMR/CNRS, Bordeaux, France; CHU de Bordeaux, Bordeaux, France

Miyuki Bohgaki NTT Sapporo Medical Center, Sapporo Hokkaido, Japan

Gisela Bonsmann Department of Dermatology, University of Muenster, Muenster, Germany

Maria Orietta Borghi Immunology Research Laboratory, IRCCS Istituto Auxologico Italiano, Milan, Italy; Department of Clinical Sciences and Community Health, University of Milan, Milan, Italy

Dimitrios T. Boumpas Rheumatology and Clinical Immunology, 4th Department of Medicine, Medical School, University of Athens and Biomedical Research Foundation of the Academy of Athens, Athens, Greece

Rebecka Bourn Arthritis and Clinical Immunology, Oklahoma Medical Research Foundation, Oklahoma City, OK, USA

Jill P. Buyon Division of Rheumatology, New York University School of Medicine, New York City, NY, USA

Roberto Caricchio Department of Medicine, Section of Rheumatology and Department of Microbiology and Immunology, Temple University School of Medicine, Philadelphia, PA, USA

Michelle D. Catalina AMPEL BioSolutions, University of Virginia Research Park, Charlottesville, VA, USA

Edward K.L. Chan Department of Oral Biology, University of Florida, Gainesville, FL, USA

Christopher Chang Division of Rheumatology, Allergy and Clinical Immunology, University of California at Davis, Davis, CA, USA

Sandra Chartrand Hôpital Maisonneuve-Rosemont affiliated to Université de Montréal, Montréal, QC, Canada

Cecilia Beatrice Chighizola Immunology Research Laboratory, IRCCS Istituto Auxologico Italiano, Milan, Italy; Department of Clinical Sciences and Community Health, University of Milan, Milan, Italy

Ann E. Clarke Division of Rheumatology, Department of Medicine, University of Calgary, Calgary, AB, Canada

José C. Crispín Department of Immunology and Rheumatology, Instituto Nacional de Ciencias Médicas y Nutrición Salvador Zubirán, Mexico City, Mexico

Chao Dai Division of Rheumatology, Department of Medicine, University of Virginia, Charlottesville, VA, USA; Center for Immunity, Inflammation, and Regenerative Medicine, Department of Medicine, University of Virginia, Charlottesville, VA, USA

Erika M. Damato Birmingham Midland Eye Centre, City Hospital, Birmingham, UK

Yun Deng Division of Rheumatology, Department of Medicine, David Geffen School of Medicine, University of California, Los Angeles, Los Angeles, CA, USA

Alastair K.O. Denniston Department of Ophthalmology, University Hospitals Birmingham NHS Foundation Trust, Birmingham, UK; Academic Unit of Ophthalmology, University of Birmingham, Birmingham, UK

Amy Devlin Beth Israel Deaconess Medical Center, Division of Rheumatology, Boston, MA, USA

Betty Diamond Autoimmune & Musculoskeletal Disease Center, Feinstein Institute for Medical Research, North Shore LIJ Health System, Manhasset, NY, USA

Mary Anne Dooley Dooley Rheumatology, Chapel Hill, NC, USA

Jefte M. Drijvers Ragon Institute of MGH, MIT and Harvard, Cambridge, MA, USA

Roland M. du Bois Imperial College, London, UK

Yong Du Department of Biomedical Engineering, University of Houston, Houston, TX, USA

T. Ernandez Service of Nephrology, University Hospital of Geneva, Switzerland

Concetta Ferretti Department of Medicine, University of California Los Angeles, Los Angeles, CA, USA

Aryeh Fischer University of Colorado School of Medicine, Aurora, CO, USA

Samantha Fisher Department of Dermatology, University of Florida, Gainesville, FL, USA

Eleni A. Frangou Biomedical Research Foundation of the Academy of Athens, Athens, Greece

Marvin J. Fritzler Department of Biochemistry and Molecular Biology, Cumming School of Medicine, University of Calgary, Calgary, AB, Canada

Richard Furie North Shore LIJ Division of Rheumatology, Great Neck, NY, USA; Hofstra North Shore LIJ School of Medicine, Hofstra University, Hempstead, NY, USA

Shu Man Fu Division of Rheumatology, Department of Medicine, University of Virginia, Charlottesville, VA, USA; Center for Immunity, Inflammation, and Regenerative Medicine, Department of Medicine, University of Virginia, Charlottesville, VA, USA; Department of Microbiology, Immunology, and Cancer Biology, School of Medicine, University of Virginia, Charlottesville, VA, USA

Felicia Gaskin Department of Psychiatry and Neurobehavioral Sciences, School of Medicine, University of Virginia, Charlottesville, VA, USA

Gary S. Gilkeson Medical Research Service, Ralph H. Johnson VA Medical Center, Charleston, SC, USA; Department of Medicine, Division of Rheumatology, Medical University of South Carolina, Charleston, SC, USA

Dafna Gladman University of Toronto, Toronto, ON, Canada

Rosalind Ramsey Goldman North-western University Feinberg School of Medicine, Chicago, IL, USA

Luis A. González-Naranjo Division of Rheumatology, Department of Internal Medicine, School of Medicine, Universidad de Antioquia, Medellín, Colombia

Caroline Gordon Department of Rheumatology, City Hospital, Sandwell and West Birmingham Hospitals NHS Trust, Birmingham, UK; Rheumatology Research Group, College of Medical and Dental Sciences, University of Birmingham, Edgbaston, Birmingham, UK

Amrie C. Grammer AMPEL BioSolutions, University of Virginia Research Park, Charlottesville, VA, USA

Eric L. Greidinger Division of Rheumatology, Miami VAMC, University of Miami Miller School of Medicine, Miami, FL, USA

Niklas Hagberg Section of Rheumatology, Department of Medical Sciences, Uppsala University, Uppsala, Sweden

John G. Hanly Dalhousie University, Halifax, Nova Scotia, Canada; Nova Scotia Health Authority, Halifax, Nova Scotia, Canada

James E. Hansen Department of Therapeutic Radiology, Yale School of Medicine, New Haven, CT, USA

Shuhong Han Division of Rheumatology & Clinical Immunology, University of Florida, Gainesville, FL, USA

Sarfaraz A. Hasni National Institute of Arthritis and Musculoskeletal and Skin Diseases, National Institutes of Health, Bethesda, MD, USA

Christian M. Hedrich Children's Hospital Dresden, Pediatric Rheumatology and Immunology Section, University Medical Center Carl Gustav Carus, TU Dresden, Dresden, Germany

Diane Horowitz North Shore LIJ Division of Rheumatology, Great Neck, NY, USA; Hofstra North Shore LIJ School of Medicine, Hofstra University, Hempstead, NY, USA

Xin Huang Department of Dermatology, Hunan Key Laboratory of Medical Epigenomics, Second Xiangya Hospital, Central South University, Changsha, Hunan, China

Peter M. Izmirly Division of Rheumatology, New York University School of Medicine, New York City, NY, USA

Clément Jacquemin University of Bordeaux, CIRID, UMR/CNRS, Bordeaux, France; CHU de Bordeaux, Bordeaux, France

Judith James Arthritis and Clinical Immunology, Oklahoma Medical Research Foundation, Oklahoma City, OK, USA; Departments of Medicine and Pathology, Oklahoma Clinical and Translational Science Institute, University of Oklahoma Health Sciences Center, Oklahoma City, OK, USA

Wael N. Jarjour Ohio State University, Columbus, OH, USA

Mariana J. Kaplan National Institute of Arthritis and Musculoskeletal and Skin Diseases, National Institutes of Health, Bethesda, MD, USA

Munther Khamashta Division of Women's Health, Graham Hughes Lupus Research Laboratory, Lupus Research Unit, The Rayne Institute, King's College, London, UK; Louise Coote Lupus Unit, Guy's and St Thomas' NHS Foundation Trust, St Thomas' Hospital, London, UK

Takao Koike NTT Sapporo Medical Center, Sapporo Hokkaido, Japan; Department of Medicine II, Hokkaido University Graduate School of Medicine, Sapporo Hokkaido, Japan

Dwight H. Kono Department of Immunology and Microbial Science, The Scripps Research Institute, La Jolla, CA, USA

Christine Konya Division of Rheumatology & Lupus Center, BIDMC, Harvard Medical School, Boston, MA, USA

Annegret Kuhn Interdisciplinary Center for Clinical Trials (IZKS), University Medical Center Mainz, Mainz, Germany; Division of Immunogenetics, Tumor Immunology Program, German Cancer Research Center (DKFZ), Heidelberg, Germany

Vasileios C. Kyttaris Division of Rheumatology, Beth Israel Deaconess Medical Center, Harvard Medical School, Boston, MA, USA

Antonio La Cava Department of Medicine, University of California Los Angeles, Los Angeles, CA, USA

Robert G. Lahita Newark Beth Israel Medical Center, Newark, NJ, USA; Rutgers New Jersey Medical School, Newark, NJ, USA

Aysche Landmann Division of Immunogenetics, Tumor Immunology Program, German Cancer Research Center (DKFZ), Heidelberg, Germany

Peter E. Lipsky AMPEL BioSolutions, University of Virginia Research Park, Charlottesville, VA, USA

Mindy S. Lo Boston Children's Hospital, Harvard Medical School, Boston, MA, USA

Qianjin Lu Department of Dermatology, Hunan Key Laboratory of Medical Epigenomics, Second Xiangya Hospital, Central South University, Changsha, Hunan, China

Mary Mahieu Northwestern University Feinberg School of Medicine, Chicago, IL, USA

Susan Malkiel Autoimmune & Musculoskeletal Disease Center, Feinstein Institute for Medical Research, North Shore LIJ Health System, Manhasset, NY, USA

Susan Manzi Department of Medicine, Lupus Center of Excellence, Allegheny Health Network, Pittsburgh, PA, USA

Galina Marder North Shore LIJ Division of Rheumatology, Great Neck, NY, USA; Hofstra North Shore LIJ School of Medicine, Hofstra University, Hempstead, NY, USA

T.N. Mayadas Department of Pathology, Brigham and Women's Hospital and Harvard Medical School, Boston, USA

Terry K. Means Center for Immunology and Inflammatory Diseases and Division of Rheumatology, Allergy, and Immunology, Massachusetts General Hospital and Harvard Medical School, Charlestown, MA, USA

Pier Luigi Meroni Immunology Research Laboratory, IRCCS Istituto Auxologico Italiano, Milan, Italy; Department of Clinical Sciences and Community Health, University of Milan, Milan, Italy; Division of Rheumatology, Istituto Ortopedico Gaetano Pini, Milan, Italy

Joan T. Merrill Clinical Pharmacology Research Program, Oklahoma Medical Research Foundation, University of Oklahoma, OK, USA

Chandra Mohan Department of Biomedical Engineering, University of Houston, Houston, TX, USA

Chi Chiu Mok Department of Medicine, Tuen Mun Hospital, New Territories, Hong Kong

Vaishali R. Moulton Division of Rheumatology, Department of Medicine, Beth Israel Deaconess Medical Center, Harvard Medical School, Boston, MA, USA

Philip I. Murray Academic Unit of Ophthalmology, University of Birmingham, City Hospital, Birmingham, UK

Jim C. Oates Medical Research Service, Ralph H. Johnson VA Medical Center, Charleston, SC, USA; Department of Medicine, Division of Rheumatology, Medical University of South Carolina, Charleston, SC, USA

Ziv Paz Division of Rheumatology & Lupus Center, BIDMC, Harvard Medical School, Boston, MA, USA

William F. Pendergraft III University of North Carolina Kidney Center, Chapel Hill, NC, USA

Andras Perl Division of Rheumatology, Department of Medicine, College of Medicine, Upstate Medical University, State University of New York, Syracuse, NY, USA; Department of Microbiology and Immunology, College of Medicine, Upstate Medical University, State University of New York, Syracuse, NY, USA

Shiv Pillai Ragon Institute of MGH, MIT and Harvard, Cambridge, MA, USA

Guillermo J. Pons-Estel Department of Autoimmune Diseases, Institut Clinic de Medicina I Dermatologia, Hospital Clinic, Barcelona, Catalonia, Spain

Bo Qu Shanghai Institute of Rheumatology, Renji Hospital, Shanghai Jiao Tong University School of Medicine, Shanghai, China

Anisur Rahman Division of Medicine, University College London, London, UK

Rosalind Ramsey-Goldman Northwestern University Feinberg School of Medicine, Chicago, IL, USA

Westley H. Reeves Division of Rheumatology & Clinical Immunology, University of Florida, Gainesville, FL, USA

Noé Rodríguez-Rodríguez Department of Medicine, Division of Rheumatology, Beth Israel Deaconess Medical Center, Harvard Medical School, Boston, MA, USA; Department of Immunology, Universidad Complutense de Madrid, Madrid, Spain

Lars Rönnblom Section of Rheumatology, Department of Medical Sciences, Uppsala University, Uppsala, Sweden

Florencia Rosetti Department of Immunology and Rheumatology, Instituto Nacional de Ciencias Médicas y Nutrición Salvador Zubirán, Mexico City, Mexico

Brad H. Rovin Division of Nephrology, Ohio State University Wexner Medical Center, Columbus, OH, USA

Matthew M. Ryals AMPEL BioSolutions, University of Virginia Research Park, Charlottesville, VA, USA

G. Saggu Department of Pathology, Brigham and Women's Hospital and Harvard Medical School, Boston, USA

Lisa R. Sammaritano Hospital for Special Surgery, New York, NY, USA

Minoru Satoh Department of Clinical Nursing, University of Occupational and Environmental Health, Japan, Kitakyushu, Fukuoka, Japan; Department of Medicine, University of Florida, Gainesville, FL, USA; Department of Pathology, Immunology, and Laboratory Medicine, University of Florida, Gainesville, FL, USA

Amr H. Sawalha Division of Rheumatology, Department of Internal Medicine, University of Michigan, Ann Arbor, MI, USA; Center for Computational Medicine and Bioinformatics, University of Michigan, Ann Arbor, MI, USA

Amit Saxena Division of Rheumatology, New York University School of Medicine, New York City, NY, USA

Savino Sciascia Division of Women's Health, Graham Hughes Lupus Research Laboratory, Lupus Research Unit, The Rayne Institute, King's College, London, UK; Centro di Ricerche di Immunologia Clinica ed Immunopatologia e Documentazione su Malattie Rare (CMID), Università di Torino, Torino, Italy; Louise Coote Lupus Unit, Guy's and St Thomas' NHS Foundation Trust, St Thomas' Hospital, London, UK

Syahrul Shaharir Department of Rheumatology, City Hospital, Sandwell and West Birmingham Hospitals NHS Trust, Birmingham, UK; Department of Internal Medicine, National University of Malaysia Medical Centre, Cheras, Kuala Lumpur, Malaysia

Chengqun Shao Newark Beth Israel Medical Center, Newark, NJ, USA

Nan Shen Shanghai Institute of Rheumatology, Renji Hospital, Shanghai Jiao Tong University School of Medicine, Shanghai, China; Institute of Health Sciences, Shanghai Institutes for Biological Sciences (SIBS) & Shanghai Jiao Tong University School of Medicine (SJTUSM), Chinese Academy of Sciences (CAS), Shanghai, China; Division of Rheumatology, The Center for Autoimmune Genomics and Etiology (CAGE), Cincinnati Children's Hospital Medical Center, Cincinnati, OH, USA

Robert Shmerling Beth Israel Deaconess Medical Center, Division of Rheumatology, Boston, MA, USA

Yehuda Shoenfeld The Zabludowicz Center for Autoimmune Diseases Sheba Medical Center, Sackler Faculty of Medicine, Tel-Aviv University, Tel Aviv, Israel; Incumbent of the Laura Schwarz-Kipp Chair for Research of Autoimmune Diseases, Sackler Faculty of Medicine, Tel-Aviv University, Tel Aviv, Israel

Stepan Shumyak Division of Rheumatology & Clinical Immunology, University of Florida, Gainesville, FL, USA

Samantha Slight-Webb Arthritis and Clinical Immunology, Oklahoma Medical Research Foundation, Oklahoma City, OK, USA

Isaac Ely Stillman Beth Israel Deaconess Medical Center, Boston, MA, USA

George Stojan Harvard Medical School, Division of Rheumatology, Beth Israel Deaconess Medical Center, Boston, MA, USA

Sun-Sang J. Sung Division of Rheumatology, Department of Medicine, University of Virginia, Charlottesville, VA, USA; Center for Immunity, Inflammation, and Regenerative Medicine, Department of Medicine, University of Virginia, Charlottesville, VA, USA

Argyrios N. Theofilopoulos Department of Immunology and Microbial Science, The Scripps Research Institute, La Jolla, CA, USA

Donald E. Thomas Jr. Department of Medicine, Uniformed Services University of the Health Sciences, Bethesda, MD, USA; Arthritis and Pain Associates of Prince Georges County, Greenbelt, MD, USA

Hiromi Tissera McGill University Health Centre, Montreal, QC, Canada

Zahi Touma University of Toronto Lupus Clinic, Toronto Western Hospital, Centre for Prognosis Studies in the Rheumatic Diseases, Toronto, ON, Canada; Department of Internal Medicine, Division of Rheumatology, University of Toronto, Toronto, ON, Canada

Betty P. Tsao Division of Rheumatology, Department of Medicine, David Geffen School of Medicine, University of California, Los Angeles, Los Angeles, CA, USA

Manuel F. Ugarte-Gil Servicio de Reumatología, Hospital Nacional Guillermo Almenara Irigoyen, EsSalud, Lima, Peru; Universidad Científica del Sur, Lima, Peru

Murray B. Urowitz University of Toronto Lupus Clinic, Toronto Western Hospital, Centre for Prognosis Studies in the Rheumatic Diseases, Toronto, ON, Canada; Department of Internal Medicine, Division of Rheumatology, University of Toronto, Toronto, ON, Canada; Toronto Western Research Institute, Toronto, ON, Canada

Bruce T. Volpe Biomedical Sciences, Feinstein Institute for Medical Research, Hofstra North Shore LIJ School of Medicine, Manhasset, NY, USA

Hongyang Wang Division of Rheumatology, Department of Medicine, University of Virginia, Charlottesville, VA, USA; Department of Microbiology, Immunology, and Cancer Biology, School of Medicine, University of Virginia, Charlottesville, VA, USA

Mark H. Wener Departments of Laboratory Medicine & Medicine, University of Washington, Seattle, WA, USA

Haijing Wu Department of Dermatology, Hunan Key Laboratory of Medical Epigenomics, Second Xiangya Hospital, Central South University, Changsha, Hunan, China

Yuan Xu Division of Rheumatology & Clinical Immunology, University of Florida, Gainesville, FL, USA

Lijun Yang Department of Pathology, Immunology, & Laboratory Medicine, University of Florida, Gainesville, FL, USA

C. Yung Yu Center for Molecular and Human Genetics, The Research Institute at Nationwide Children's Hospital and Department of Pediatrics, The Ohio State University, Columbus, OH, USA

Haoyang Zhuang Division of Rheumatology & Clinical Immunology, University of Florida, Gainesville, FL, USA

Introduction

As long as we consider systemic lupus erythematosus one disease and we see one clinical trial after another fail, we can offer the people who suffer only qualified hope and encouragement. There is no doubt that we understand the disease better now than we did 50 years ago but we still use the same immunosuppressive and cytotoxic drugs, albeit more wisely.

We have enlisted additional players to the processes that lead to the expression of the disease as we have followed new advances in the fields of immunology, inflammation, cell and molecular biology, and genomics. Yet we have not made much-needed advances in delineating the relative contribution of each mechanism to the expression of disease in each individual. It has become increasingly clear that cellular and molecular pathways may contribute to immunopathology at different degrees in each patient. There is no doubt that the biologics that have been tested in each trial do exactly what they were designed to do (deplete a cell, neutralize a cytokine or block a receptor, and so on) but if given indiscriminately to every lupus patient, the statistically recorded benefit may not rise to significant levels. There is no doubt that lupus cries out for individualized medicine and that herding everybody under the 11 American College of Rheumatology criteria misses the fact that each person with lupus "employs" individual pathways to express the same set of clinical manifestations.

We have also been slow in identifying the molecular and cellular mechanisms that are involved in the expression of injury in each affected organ. Even if the autoimmune response is responsible for instigating tissue injury it is now better understood that autoimmunity and organ damage do not go hand-in-hand. Attempts to reverse injurious processes in organs should prove of clinical value. We understand that molecules (cell surface receptors, kinases, phosphatases, and others) that are found to be abnormally expressed in lupus and claimed to contribute to disease pathology are usually expressed by additional cells in the body and if inhibited across the board will invariably bring about unwanted side effects. This argument mandates the consideration of targeted delivery of drugs and biologics to maximize clinical efficacy and minimize side effects.

This book has taken a different approach in presenting the readers with state-of-the-art authoritative information on current topics of lupus. In order to minimize the load to the contributors we have presented a rather large (66) number of chapters, after parsing out topics. Each contributor was asked to present available information in a critical, authoritative manner in shorter text and a limited (around 50) number of references selected critically. There is no doubt that readers will recognize shortcomings. I invite all possible feedback to improve the next edition.

While planning the book, we had in mind the increasing number of scientists, care givers, disease activists, clinical trial planners, and industry officers who enter the battle against lupus. I believe that the organization of the book will facilitate information retrieval and useful synthesis.

The 66 chapters are organized in six sections. The first introduces the history, epidemiology, diagnosis, and the efforts to develop biomarkers for the disease. In the second section (pathogenesis) 24 players are presented including various cells, antibodies, inflammation mediators, and processes. In the third section (mechanisms of tissue damage) elements and processes involved in the development of organ injury are presented synthetically. In the fourth the clinical manifestations of the disease are presented in 19 chapters. Special space was allotted to chapter 41, which presents the pathology of lupus nephritis. My friend Isaac Stillman understands the pathology of lupus nephritis in a way that very few do and I believe we should have a clear understanding of the pathology before we commit our patients to intense treatment with cytotoxic drugs. The fifth section is dedicated to the antiphospholipid syndrome and the sixth to the treatment of the disease. Besides the required chapters on the drugs used, a chapter on the lessons we have learned from clinical trials is included, along with a chapter on the efforts to repurpose existing drugs to treat lupus.

This book exists because of the encouragement and excitement of Linda Versteeg-Buschman of Elsevier whom I thank warmly through these lines. Halima Williams has provided unwavering support of the highest quality throughout the solicitation, collection, and editing phases of the chapters. She made my job easy and joyful.

George C. Tsokos
Harvard Medical School

Part I

Epidemiology and Diagnosis

Chapter 1

History of Systemic Lupus Erythematosus

Christine Konya, Ziv Paz

Division of Rheumatology & Lupus Center, BIDMC, Harvard Medical School, Boston, MA, USA

Declare the past, diagnose the present, foretell the future.

Hippocrates

When we interview and treat patients who were diagnosed with systemic lupus erythematosus (SLE), read their posts in social networks, follow their support groups and forums, we see how their hope brings them together. They find comfort in sharing their stories. The story of each SLE patient is different, but not only because the patients are different. The disease affects every single patient in distinct ways and changes its nature over time. The many faces of this disease make its history so unique and fascinating. Systemic lupus erythematosus is one of the most complex autoimmune systemic diseases. Its cause remains unknown and our treatment options are still limited, despite the fact that SLE has been recognized as a defined clinical entity for more than 100 years.

Hippocrates was thought to be the first to describe the cutaneous manifestations of SLE, calling it *herpes esthiomenos* (gnawing dermatosis).[1,2] It is not completely clear when the word *lupus* became synonyms with the disease. However, records indicate that it may have been Hebernus, the archbishop of Tours, France, in 855 AD, who was the first to use the word "lupus" to describe the disease in his writing: "The Miracles of Saint Martin." He mentions the bishop of Liège who was suffering from a severely consuming disease called *lupus* in the common tongue, and was miraculously cured after spending time in the shrine of Saint Martin in Tours.[3] Later, Paracelsus, a fifteenth century Swiss German renaissance physician who was known for his astute observations, considered SLE to be a skin disease with "greater blood supply" and recommended treatment with bloodletting, which was the treatment of most conditions in those days. He used the term "lupus" to define the cutaneous manifestations of the disease or, by his own words, "a hungry wolf eating flesh."[3]

Rudolph Virchow (1821–1902) was the first to review systematically the history of SLE. In his writings, Virchow mentioned a reference from the old German book *Margerita Medicine*, published in 1502 by the German physician Johann Trollat von Vochenberg. In this reference, von Vochenberg

suggested the use of caprifolin to treat the conditions of cancer and wolf, or as quoted (translated from German): "*for the wolf and for cancer, caprifolin (honeysuckle).*" Rudolf Virchow quoted even an older text dating back to the end of the thirteenth century and referred to Roger de Palma, from the school of Salerno: "Sometimes lupus arises in the thighs and the lower legs (and is) distinguished from cancer from the symptoms mentioned above."[4] In the middle ages, the term "lupus" was used to describe ulcerative or necrotizing skin diseases as it reminded the describers of the bite of a wolf. Superstitious people at that time related these skin conditions to the bite of a werewolf given the grotesque appearance of the ulcerative skin disease.[5,6]

Robert Willan (1757–1808) and his student Thomas Bateman were British dermatologists who used the term "lupus" to describe a destructive skin disease preferentially affecting the face and the nose.[7] In the mid-nineteenth century, the French dermatologist Laurent Theodore Biett used the term "erythema centrifugum" to describe these skin lesions.[2,8] The current name of the disease, lupus erythematosus, was given in 1833 by Biett's student Pierre Louis Cazenave, who called it "*lupus érythèmateux* or lupus erythematosus." Cazenave was also the first to describe other aspects of the disease. He appreciated the predilection to young females, the painless nature of the facial lesions, and other features of the disease. His exact words are still relevant today and many times used by rheumatologists to describe examination findings:

"In some circumstances (lupus) manifests itself at first as a violet rubefaction on part of the face, and mainly on the nose, which at the same time is rather swollen: over many months the color rises little by little; the surface becomes animated; a small ulcer forms and on top of it, a scab, which then thickens and covers the ulcer, which becomes progressively deeper. Lastly, the skin may get thinner in imperceptible stages and adopt the appearance of a scar, without there being tubercles or ulcers, and without displaying worse injuries than a livid color and, from time to time, a light and barely perceptible peeling."[9]

Ferdinand von Hebra used the phrase "butterfly rash" to describe Cazenave's skin findings of lupus erythematosus.[10] In 1872 at the Vienna School of Medicine, Moritz Kaposi, Hebra's son-in-law, was the first one who appreciated the systemic features of "lupus erythematosus" including lymphadenopathy, fever, and arthritis. Kaposi was also the one who coined the term "discoid lupus" to describe a specific form of cutaneous involvement. Even though cutaneous tuberculosis was a prevalent condition in these days, Kaposi believed that discoid lupus erythematosus was a separate entity, even though this notion was argued by others. Kaposi also used the term "disseminated lupus erythematosus" to describe widespread cutaneous involvement.[11]

Sir William Osler (1849–1919) was the first to use the phrase "systemic lupus erythematosus." Osler diagnosed 29 patients who presented with erythema and visceral injuries as SLE. Many of these cases correspond to our current descriptions of lupus erythematosus, even though there were no official criteria at that time. Osler also recognized that SLE can affect the kidneys, lungs, and the heart.[12] At the beginning of the twentieth century, Jonathan Hutchinson described the photosensitivity of the lupus skin rash.[13,14] In 1923, Emanuel Libman and Benjamin Sacks identified four cases of noninfectious endocarditis, of which three patients displayed cutaneous injuries of SLE. Later, it was confirmed that the endocarditis of Libman-Sacks could occur even without the cutaneous involvement.[15,16]

This was the beginning of the modern era of SLE, and the way we clinically diagnose the disease today has not changed much since. However, even though the physical findings of the disease were known at that time, they were not specific. The diagnosis of SLE was still challenging due to a lack of objective diagnostic tests. Extensive research began to improve our understanding of the underlying pathophysiology of SLE and to identify objective diagnostic and prognostic markers.

In 1948, Malcolm Hargraves, a hematologist from the Mayo Clinic, and his colleague Robert Morton described lupus erythematosus (LE) cells. Hargraves identified LE cells seen in the bone marrow of 25 patients with confirmed or suspected diagnosis of SLE. LE cells are neutrophils or macrophages that have phagocytized denatured nuclear material of another cell. Even though initially they were thought to be specific for SLE, these cells were later found in other connective tissue diseases and other medical conditions. Moreover, the cells were not present in many cases of SLE.[17]

In 1967, George Friou found that serum sampled from patients with SLE contains immunoglobulins against DNA.[18] He named these "antinuclear factors," and they were called by their current name: antinuclear antibodies (ANA). ANA is still the most sensitive test for the diagnosis of SLE and is counted as one of the classification criteria of SLE by the American College of Rheumatology. Since then, many more antibodies have been described. Few of these antibodies were shown to be very specific for the diagnosis of SLE (e.g., anti-Smith, anti-double stranded DNA) while other antibodies were shown to be associated with specific disease entities (e.g. anti-Ro and subacute cutaneous lupus).

Diagnostic capabilities improved dramatically during the mid-twentieth century, but treatment options were limited because of the partial understanding of the disease pathophysiology and also due to its versatile nature. In 1894, Payne described the benefits of using quinine in the treatment of SLE. Only decades after, chloroquine and hydroxychloroquine therapies became the cornerstone of SLE treatment.[19] Philip S. Hench demonstrated the high effectivity of ACTH and cortisone in rheumatoid arthritis and later on in SLE, and he received the Nobel Prize in 1950 for these discoveries.[20]

Unfortunately, the majority of the current treatments are still not specific and are associated with significant adverse effects. This started to change in 2011 when the U.S. Food and Drug Administration approved belimumab, a human monoclonal antibody that inhibits B-cell activating factor, for treatment of SLE. Even though belimumab has marginal effect, its approval opened a new era and currently many other biologic agents and small molecules are being investigated in murine models and clinical trials.

We now have our own story to share with our patients. Even though we did not reach the epilogue yet, there is hope. Active and exciting research holds promise for new treatment options and for better understanding of this disease. Indeed, this is a story of a fascinating disease.

REFERENCES

1. Lahita RG. *Systemic lupus erythematosus.* New York: John Wiley and Sons; 1987.
2. Smith CD, Cyr M. The history of lupus erythematosus, from Hippocrates to Osler. *Rheum Dis Clin North Am* 1988;**14**:1–14.
3. Donald Jr ET. *The lupus encyclopedia: a comprehensive guide for patients and families.* Johns Hopkins University Press; 2014.
4. Virchow R. Historische notizen uber lupus. *Arch F Pathol Anat u Physiol u F Kin Med* 1865;**32**:139–43.
5. Blotzer JW. Systemic lupus erythematosus, I: historical aspects. *Md State Med J* 1983;**32**:439–41.
6. Fatovic-Ferencic S, Holubar K. Early history and iconography of lupus erythematosus. *Clin Dermatol* 2004;**22**:100–4.
7. Bateman TA. *Practical synopsis of cutaneous diseases, according to the arrangements of Dr. Willan.* 8th ed. London: Longman, Rees, Orme, Brown, Green and Longman; 1936.
8. Biett M. *Cutaneous diseases.* Philadelphia: Lea & Carey; 1857.
9. Cazenave PLA, Schedel HE. *Manual of the diseases of the skin. Burgess (trans).* London: Henry Renshaw; 1852.
10. Hebra F. [Adams F, Trans.]. *On diseases of the skin including the exanthemata,* vol. 1. London: The New Sydenham Society; 1866.
11. Kaposi M. Lupus vulgaris. [Tay W, Trans.]. In: Hebra FKM, editor. *On diseases of the skin including the exanthemata,* Vol. 7. London: The New Sydenham Society; 1875.
12. Osler W. On the visceral manifestations of the erythema group of skin diseases. *Am J Med Sci* 1904;**127**:1–23.

13. Hutchinson J. Lupus erythematosus. *Med Times Gaz* 1879;**1**:1–3.

14. Hutchinson J. On lupus and its treatment. *Br Med J* 1880;**1**:650–2.

15. Libman E, Sacks B. A hitherto undescribed form of valvular and mural endocarditis. *Trans Ass Am Phys* 1924;**38**:46–61.

16. Belote GH, Ratner HS. The so-called Libman-Sacks syndrome: its relation to dermatology. *Arch Dermatol Syphilol* 1936;**33**:642–64.

17. Hargraves MM. Discovery of the LE cell and its morphology. *Mayo Clin Proc* 1969;**44**:579–99.

18. Friou GJ. Antinuclear Antibodies: diagnostic significance and methods. *Arthritis Rheum* 1967;**10**:151–9.

19. Payne JF. A post-graduate lecture on lupus erythematosus. *Clin J* 1894;**4**:223.

20. Hench PS. The reversibility of certain rheumatic and non-rheumatic conditions by the use of cortisone or of the pituitary adrenocorticotrophic hormone. *Ann Intern Med* 1952;**36**:1–38.

Chapter 2

The Patient

Donald E. Thomas Jr.[1,2]

[1]Department of Medicine, Uniformed Services University of the Health Sciences, Bethesda, MD, USA; [2]Arthritis and Pain Associates of Prince Georges County, Greenbelt, MD, USA

Any idiot can prescribe antibiotics to treat an ear infection, but that's not what makes you a good physician.

Dr Levana Sinai in Vital Conversations: Improving Communications between Doctors and Patients[1]

Health care providers are usually good at keeping up with the pathophysiology, diagnosis, and management of diseases. Yet, we typically spend little time learning how to optimally communicate with patients. In fact, many of us never receive formal training in this subject. This chapter of the book will provide you with important tools for taking care of patients who have systemic lupus erythematosus (SLE). I guarantee that if you put all of these measures to work in your own practice, you will take better care of your patients. For further reading, I recommend *Vital Conversations* by Dennis Rosen, MD.[1] His book is an easy read, packed with a wealth of practical information.

IMPROVE THE INTERACTIONS WITH YOUR PATIENTS

Here are some concrete steps you can take to improve your interactions with your patients.

Do Not Make Your Patient Wait

One of the biggest complaints that patients have about their physician visits is long wait times.[2] We must remember that our patient's time is just as valuable as our own. We cannot control some problems, such as needing to answer important physician phone calls, having to wait on insurance referrals, or needing to spend a longer amount of time on a particularly ill patient. However, we do have control over other potential causes of running behind.

I recommend not overbooking your appointments. Some physicians will double-book patients in the same time slot, feeling that some patients may cancel that day or just to ensure that their work time is kept busy. However, I am not at all a fan of this practice, which I believe is disrespectful of the patient's time.

I also reschedule patients who run significantly late for their appointment if it will end up causing other patients scheduled after them to be seen later. I feel it is not fair to the other patients to still see the late patient. In these situations, I will see the late patient toward the end of the clinic, or at least get their laboratory work, refill their medications, and reschedule them to see me as soon as possible.

If you are running behind due to something out of your control, make sure that someone on your staff informs the patient of the delay. Then, when you enter the room and greet the patient, make sure to apologize and even explain why you are running behind. These simple measures let the patients know that you respect them and truly value their time.

Smile as You Enter the Patient's Room

Smiling as you enter the room can help set the stage for the rest of the encounter. A smile as you enter the room lets your patient know that you are glad to be there, that the patient is important, and that you are eager to help. It is not uncommon to have to give bad news to patients who have lupus, such as a new onset of nephritis or worsening of a known manifestation. Initially smiling is important, even when you know that you need to give bad news. If you begin the encounter on a positive note, your patient will feel more comfortable, and this can help decrease any pre-existing anxiety. As you enter the conversation where you need to discuss bad test results, then your body language and speech can change appropriately.

Exhibit a Visible Show of Hand Washing

One of my most vivid memories of being a patient was when I had an appointment with a surgeon in preparation for surgery. I clearly heard him wash his hands outside my examination room. Then, when he examined me, I

Systemic Lupus Erythematosus. http://dx.doi.org/10.1016/B978-0-12-801917-7.00002-4

smelled the aroma of soap on his hands. The involvement of several senses, hearing him wash as well as smelling the soap made a strong impression and made me believe that cleanliness was important to him. This caused me to automatically have confidence in him. I have read and heard criticisms from patients regarding their health care providers not washing their hands. By consciously showing our patients that we wash our hands, we can automatically increase their trust in us.

This is not simply a mere performance to please patients; apparently, they have good reason to question our cleanliness. Studies show that health care providers have dismally low rates of hand washing before and after contact with our patients.[3] Infections continue to be among the top three causes of death in patients who have SLE,[4] and hand washing is an important measure in decreasing the transmission of infections to patients. It is also important to remember to wash your hands immediately after the encounter with your patient in order to not transfer organisms that you may pick up from examining your patient onto door knobs and other objects in the office or hospital.

Shake Hands

After greeting your patient with a smile and washing your hands, shake the patient's hand. This immediately adds a welcoming gesture to your patient and provides that first human touch to the encounter. Shaking hands allows you to immediately connect nonverbally with the patient and, along with the smile, sets the stage for a positive, open experience. Shaking the patient's hand at the end of the encounter also helps to "seal the deal" regarding what was discussed and what the plan for management is.

Acknowledge and Greet Others in the Room

I will never forget the time that I accompanied my grandfather to an appointment with his ophthalmologist. The doctor never acknowledged my presence in the room the entire visit. I was there to help my grandfather understand what the doctor said and to communicate back to our family regarding his condition. I felt uncomfortable the entire visit as the doctor rushed through the examination. At the end of the encounter, I introduced myself at what seemed to be the first opportune time, and the doctor still barely spoke to me as he rushed out of the room. If he had acknowledged me initially and found out I was the physician grandson, I would have felt more included in the visit and the doctor may have explained things to me more thoroughly in medical terminology so that I could then discuss the findings in layperson's terms with my grandfather and family. If you acknowledge other people in the examination room, including children, it creates a more positive environment for everyone involved.

Sit Down When You Talk to Your Patients

A randomized controlled trial performed at the University of Kansas showed that when health care providers sat while talking to their patients, the patients perceived that the provider spent more time with them compared to when providers stood. It appears that we can at least give the impression of spending more time by sitting compared to standing. In addition, the patients reported a more positive interaction and a better understanding of their condition compared to when the provider would stand.[5] Sitting down also places you at eye level or lower. This provides a less intimidating and more approachable position. It lets patients know that you are not in a rush, you have time for them, and that you are committed to listening. Also make sure that your examination rooms have enough chairs and stools to accommodate visitors and you.

Body Position

Not only should you be sitting while you converse with your patient, but you should also make sure to face the patient squarely and make direct eye contact. Lean toward the patient in a relaxed posture in order to let him or her know that you are truly interested. You want the patient to know that he or she is indeed the center of your attention. Body position is also important if you are rounding with a group of other health care providers. The senior person of the group should try to sit during the encounter and face the patient. Before talking about the patient with the group, it is polite to ask permission first, and then make sure to angle your body in such a way that you address the group as well as your patient. Turning your back on the patient while you speak can appear demeaning and can even provoke anxiety.

Ask Open-Ended Questions

When rushed for time, it can become a bad habit to ask questions that only require a yes-or-no answer (closed-ended questions). However, this makes it more difficult for the patient to truly communicate. A patient with lupus often has fears or concerns that should be addressed. If you only ask closed-ended questions, it is difficult for the patient to open up. However, if you train yourself to ask open-ended questions (e.g., "Why are you here today, and how can I help you?"), you immediately show sincere concern and allow patients to bring up issues that are important to them. Our predetermined agenda for the meeting may be very different than what the patient wishes and needs.

You may often review other doctors' and hospital records on your patients with SLE. If you have reviewed records, it can be helpful to say something to the effect of, "I have reviewed the records from _____, and I understand you were _____. However, I'd like to hear from you, in your own words, why you are here today and how I can help you." This shows that you care enough about the patient to have taken time to read over the records beforehand, but that you are also interested in the patient's concerns.

Provide a Mechanism for Your Patient to Set the Agenda

At each patient visit, we usually have our own agenda. This typically revolves around assessing lupus disease activity and making changes in management aimed at achieving our goals of clinical quiescence and preventing complications of treatment and of the disease. However, we must allow our patients to have input regarding the visit agenda as well. Our patients usually will have questions about their care that are important to them. It can be difficult for them to remember these concerns in the midst of the appointment.

In my office, we have found that an easy way of encouraging our patients to express additional concerns is by including a question on the patient's intake paperwork that asks, "What questions do you have for your doctor today?" This allows our patients to list questions before the visit during a relaxed time period. We feel that this simple addition to our patients' intake paperwork adds considerable value to their appointment.

Speak in Nonmedical Terms

One of the most important aspects of the visit is to ensure that patients comprehend their medical condition and your instructions. If patients do not understand, then they will not be compliant with your recommendations. You should speak in nonmedical terms and avoid medical jargon so that the patient can fully understand you. It is important to tell patients their diagnoses and problems using the proper medical terms, but make sure to also write them down so that the patient can see these terms in print. Then, define the terms in easy-to-understand language. This is especially important in a disease such as lupus, where the test results and complications can be so confusing.

In addition, write down your instructions and ask the patient to repeat what he or she is to do. Studies show that most patients do not understand what is discussed by their doctors and what their instructions are after their visits. One study showed that 72% of patients could not name their medications, and another 63% did not understand what the medications were even for.[6] Patients can feel shame, anxiety, or be overwhelmed with information, preventing them from knowing what their doctor tells them. This can keep them from asking their doctor for clarification. If you ask your patients to repeat your instructions, then you can be assured that they understand you. If not, then you can adjust how you explain your instructions in a more easily understood manner.

Be Honest and Compassionate

You are only human and are bound to make mistakes. Hopefully, you challenge yourself to constantly improve over time to prevent these mistakes from recurring. When physicians or their staff cause a medical mistake, it is important to deal with this mistake directly and honestly. Studies show that admitting to mistakes helps significantly in preventing anger and even litigation.[7]

I especially like the approach of Harvard-affiliated hospitals, which recommends three elements in addressing medical errors: take responsibility, apologize, and then discuss preventative measures with the patient or the family.[8] I have found this approach to be very helpful with anything in my office that does not go well. For example, if a patient states that she had great difficulty contacting me and left unanswered messages, I will acknowledge the problem as well as voice how frustrating it had to be for her. I will apologize for it occurring and then discuss my plan for looking into the matter with my office manager to ensure that this does not recur in the future. This approach shows the patient that I care about her and want to improve and supply the best care possible. Admitting to mistakes can be uncomfortable, but it is the right thing to do. This is much better than hiding them and allows us to learn from our mistakes and improve over time.

Few things can be more difficult for a patient who is dealing with an illness than to be confronted by a health care provider who appears uncaring or distant. Learning to be compassionate and empathetic is a skill that all physicians need to strive for. In fact, 95% of patients state that bedside manner is one of the most important factors in choosing a physician.[9] I have found one of the best methods for achieving compassion and empathy is by treating every patient as if he or she were one of my most beloved relatives. I like to think about how I would want a physician to talk to and approach that relative, or myself, in the same situation.

Always Examine Your Patient

Of course, you should perform a physical examination on patients with SLE regularly. Picking up the pulmonary crackles of early interstitial lung disease, hearing the loud P2 sound of early pulmonary hypertension, noting periungual erythema, or observing painless palatal ulcers may provide insights to active disease. Do not forget to examine the concha of the outer ear; it is an area commonly involved in discoid lupus that is easily missed.

Although physical examinations are not clinically necessary at every encounter, it is important to note that the simple laying on of hands during the examination can provide immense meaning to our patient beyond what we feel is clinically needed. Many patients will assume that a proper visit is not complete without an examination. I have heard patients complain that another doctor did not do a good job because he did not examine them at each visit, and that they did not feel confident in the physician. Even a quick auscultation of the lungs and heart can impart a big sense of confidence.

End the Visit with, "Do You Have Any Other Concerns or Questions?"

Most of us dread hearing, "Oh, by the way doctor, I also have been having this other problem," just as we are heading out the door. It can then be difficult not to appear hurried as you try to quickly address this last-minute issue. However, if you ask this question at the end of the visit, you will mentally prepare yourself to address any other concerns in a more thoughtful and unrushed manner. Some patients may have concerns that they may be ashamed or embarrassed about. If you offer one last chance to ask, it can show that you truly care.

Consulting in the Hospital

All of the above recommendations also apply when you have been consulted upon in a hospital setting. I have heard from my own family members about how upset they were when they received a bill from the hospital charging them for visits from doctors who they never even remembered seeing or interacting with. One study found that 85% of patients admitted to the hospital could not even name the physician taking care of them.[10] I myself have been in situations where health care providers have entered my stall in the emergency room (where I was a patient), asked me some quick questions, yet never introduced themselves or stated why they were even there. These abrupt, anonymous encounters make the experience less than satisfactory. It is important to make every patient visit a positive one by following the above recommendations. Even if it is a consultation that you know will end up not requiring your continued help, make sure to introduce yourself, write down your name, explain why the admitting physician asked for your assistance and explain your assessment. Make sure to discuss your role in the patient's care. This will let patients know why it is important that you see them and will provide value to your consultation on their cases.

IMPROVING COMPLIANCE

Dr C. Everett Koop, a former Surgeon General of the United States of America, said, "Drugs won't work in patients who don't take them."[11] Unfortunately, this is a common occurrence in patients with SLE. Studies show that only 50% of patients take their hydroxychloroquine regularly. The evidence is even worse for immunosuppressant medications.[12]

I find that my SLE patients' compliance with therapies, such as using sunscreen and taking vitamin D supplements regularly, can be challenging.

You should ask your patients at each visit how often they forget to take their medications. Only 50% of patients voluntarily admit to medication nonadherence on their own.[13] I prefer to ask, "How often do you forget to take [name of medication]?" rather than, "Do you take your medicines regularly?" The former implies that I understand that it is impossible to take medicines 100% of the time and allows my patient to give a more honest answer. The latter is more apt to get a less-than-honest "yes" for an answer.

One of the most important tools in improving compliance is education. If your patient understands why you recommend a particular treatment (e.g., how sunscreen prevents ultraviolet damage to skin cells, therefore decreasing immune system overactivity; how low vitamin D levels increase lupus disease activity), he or she will be more likely to abide by your recommendations. It is also important to investigate other potential barriers. Some patients may have difficulty affording their medicines, pills may be too large or cause side effects, or the patient may be so busy that he or she keeps forgetting to take them. Once the reasons for noncompliance are identified, you can address the problems with practical solutions.

It is important to also ask your patients about stressors that may be interfering with good health. The more you know about your patients' lifestyles, the more insight you can have into how they deal with their disease. If you do not understand their difficulties, it can be easy to make statements that are insensitive and unrealistic. For example, telling a young woman with SLE complaining of fatigue to "just go home and rest," when she is a single parent of two young children and works a full-time job, would not be a reasonable recommendation.

COMMON PITFALLS

There are several scenarios that deserve special mention. The first I would like to address is the patient who is referred to a rheumatologist because of positive autoantibodies (e.g., RNP or SSA antibodies) yet does not have other evidence of a systemic disease. We now know that autoantibodies can show up many years before SLE becomes apparent.[14] When you see this patient in your clinic who is positive for autoantibodies but not much else, I would recommend discussing how these antibodies could possibly not represent any disease at all, but that they can sometimes be a sign that something, such as SLE, may develop in the future. Educate the patient about the symptoms of systemic autoimmune disorders along with instructions to contact and see you as soon as possible if any develop. You should also see the patient on a regular basis, such as every 6–12 months, for a history, physical examination, and laboratory testing. If this patient does develop SLE and you diagnose it at an early stage, you may be able to help prevent unnecessary suffering and permanent organ damage through early intervention.

Today, antinuclear antibody (ANA)-negative lupus is rare when ANA is tested using immunofluorescence. However, there has become widespread use of less sensitive methods of ANA detection using solid-phase assays, which can result in negative ANAs in patients with SLE. This can result in missing the diagnosis of SLE. In patients who have problems that can be caused by lupus, it is imperative to ensure that an ANA is performed by immunofluorescence in order to prevent these diagnostic mistakes and delays in proper management.[15]

Another problem occurs when antibodies become negative with treatment. We typically encounter this when a patient must leave their rheumatologist and see a new one. We now realize that up to 20% of SLE patients become ANA negative on treatment.[16] This, of course, presents a problem when the new rheumatologist does initial laboratory work on his new SLE patient who is under excellent control. Having normal laboratory results can prevent the doctor from confirming the diagnosis. It is of paramount importance to take the extra steps of obtaining old records, biopsies, and laboratory results to confirm the diagnosis and continue proper treatment.

DISABILITY

Unfortunately, SLE can be severe in many patients, preventing them from continuing in their line of work.[17,18] As physicians, few of us are trained in how to deal with disability. Applying for and obtaining disability can be very difficult and frustrating for patients. There are some simple habits that we can get into as physicians that can greatly simplify the process. In fact, these habits can also make our jobs as the physician much easier in the disability process. If you enact the following suggestions, your progress notes on your patient can often suffice in the support of disability, possibly eliminating the need for you to write extensive letters or filling out a lot of paperwork.

It is important to clearly designate how your patient was diagnosed with SLE. I recommend documenting the manifestations and laboratory abnormalities of your patient's SLE on each progress note. I am in this habit primarily because it reminds me of the clinical aspects to pay particular attention to in my patients at each visit. I will then add any new manifestations to this list as they occur over time. From a disability standpoint, this habit makes it easier for reviewing officials to ascertain if a proper diagnosis was made rather than having to sift through mounds of medical paperwork.

The US Social Security Administration (SSA) lists SLE in Section 14.02 of its "Blue Book" as one of its listed conditions. It states that a person with SLE needs to have two of the following in order to be disabled: severe fatigue, fevers, malaise, and involuntary weight loss. These are common problems in our patients, yet it is easy for us to forget to document them. Therefore, do not forget to also include these in your list of lupus manifestations. Make sure to include malaise for most patients. Mosby's medical dictionary defines malaise as "a vague uneasy feeling of body weakness, distress, or discomfort."[19] The SSA also requires involvement of at least two organ systems, one of which must be of at least moderate severity.

Simply having SLE is not sufficient for getting disability. The SSA requires that lupus must cause severe limitations in the person's activities of daily living, social functioning, or in "completing tasks in a timely manner due to deficiencies in concentration, persistence, or pace" in order to be considered disabled.[20] On your office visit intake sheet, ask your patients about what difficulties they have at home or work due to their condition. If any difficulties are occurring, add this information to your clinic note. This should suffice for documenting how lupus may or may not limit a patient's daily activities. We do this regularly in our office; it is an easy and useful habit. It is also important to include in your note that the condition, SLE, is permanent and lifelong as these are also required to disability.

(This section was written after a consultation with Sharon Christie, Esq, a disability attorney in Baltimore, MD.)

PATIENT EDUCATION

Today, patients have more access to patient education than ever before, thanks to the internet. Unfortunately, much of what patients encounter online is incorrect. Therefore, it is up to physicians to lead them in the right direction. SLE is complex and requires patients to do much more than take medications. Proper treatment includes using sunscreen regularly, avoiding substances that can worsen lupus, eating a proper diet, getting proper vaccinations to prevent infections, and taking vitamin D regularly (often lifelong) if deficient. Due to this long list of recommendations, I have come up with a list that I call "The Lupus Secrets" that I hand out to all my patients. It is a checklist of what patients should be doing regularly in order to ensure good health with their lupus. A copy of my "Lupus Secrets" is provided at the end of this chapter.[21] I encourage you to consider making copies of this list and giving it to your patients as well.

In addition, some accurate patient resources that I recommend are provided here.

Books

The Lupus Encyclopedia: A comprehensive guide for patients and families, by Donald Thomas, Johns Hopkins University Press, 2014.

The Lupus Book: A guide for patients and their families, 5th edition, by Daniel Wallace, Oxford University Press, 2013.

Lupus Q&A Revised and Updated, 3rd edition: Everything you need to know, by Robert Lahita and Robert Phillips, Avery Trade, 2014.

Online

The Lupus Encyclopedia: http://www.facebook.com/LupusEncyclopedia

The Lupus Foundation of America: http://www.lupus.org

Molly's Fund Fighting Lupus: http://www.mollys-fund.org

Lupus Patient Advocacy Groups

The Lupus Foundation of America, 800-558-0121, www.lupus.org

Molly's Fund Fighting Lupus, 503-775-3497, www.mollysfund.org

International Lupus Groups: http://www.lupus.org/resources/international-resources

THE LUPUS SECRETS

1. Avoid sulfa antibiotics (Septra and Bactrim); include them in your allergy list.
2. Keep a personal record of your laboratories, biopsy results, X-rays, and doctors' notes (especially those that established your diagnosis of SLE).
3. See a rheumatologist or other lupus specialist regularly, commonly every 3 months, even if you feel great. Kidney inflammation occurs in around 40% of SLE patients and doctors can identify it at early stages when it is easy to treat.
4. Take 81 mg of aspirin a day if you are at increased risk for heart attacks or strokes or if you are positive for antiphospholipid antibodies (check with your doctor first).
5. Get 8 h of quality sleep daily. (Get a list of sleep hygiene recommendations from your doctor if sleep is a problem.)
6. Tell your doctor if you feel depressed or down in the dumps, especially if you have thoughts about hurting yourself.
7. If you have problems with dryness, ask your doctor if you could have Sjögren's syndrome. Treatment is important and available.
8. Keep blood pressure consistently <140/90 mm/Hg; or <130/80 mm/Hg if you have had a heart attack or stroke, or have chronic kidney disease.
9. Keep cholesterol normal (check with your doctor).
10. Do not smoke cigarettes. Smoking causes lupus to be more active, keeps hydroxychloroquine from working, increases strokes and heart attacks (which are the most common causes of death in lupus patients), increases the risk for lung cancer (which occurs more commonly in lupus patients), and causes broken bones from osteoporosis.
11. If unable to stop smoking on your own, go to www.smokefree.gov or call 1-800-QUIT-NOW.
12. Exercise regularly. If you are uncertain how to exercise safely with your medical condition, ask your doctor for a physical therapy referral to learn how.
13. Maintain normal weight. If you have trouble, ask your doctor for recommendations.
14. If you get a fever, call/see your primary care doctor ASAP in order to make sure you do not have an infection.
15. Get an influenza vaccination yearly in the fall.
16. Get the Pneumovax and Prevnar PCV-13 pneumonia vaccines if you are on medicines that lower your immune system.
17. Keep up to date on all vaccinations to prevent infections (ask your doctors).
18. Have cancer screening tests done regularly (e.g., breast, cervical, colon, prostate, etc.).
19. Consider getting the human papilloma virus (HPV) vaccine (Gardasil) series to prevent HPV-associated cancers if you are less than 26 years old.
20. Get adequate calcium (ask your doctor how much).
21. If you are on any stomach acid-lowering medicines, consider taking calcium citrate, which may be better absorbed than other forms.
22. Get adequate vitamin D. If you are vitamin D deficient, you may need vitamin D supplements for the rest of your life.
23. If you take steroids (such as prednisone) regularly, make sure you are taking a medicine to prevent osteoporosis if it is appropriate; check with your doctor.
24. If you take steroids regularly, consider wearing a medical alert bracelet.
25. Take your medications regularly.
26. Take a completed medication list or a bag of all your medicines to every doctor's visit.
27. Take hydroxychloroquine or chloroquine regularly as one of your medications if prescribed by your doctor.
28. Make sure to see your eye doctor regularly for eye exams on your hydroxychloroquine.
29. Use an Amsler grid monthly when taking hydroxychloroquine or chloroquine. You can get one from your eye doctor, or download one from www.amslergrid.org.
30. Use sunscreen every day, and regularly avoid UV light.
31. Avoid alfalfa and mung bean sprouts, which can cause lupus to get worse.
32. Eat a well-balanced diet with plenty of fruits and vegetables.
33. Include fish, walnuts, and flax seed rich in omega-3 fatty acids in your diet. These may decrease inflammation in lupus.
34. Learn how to decrease stress in your life. (Stress can make lupus worse).
35. Do not take Echinacea (supplement promoted to treat colds) as it can worsen lupus.

36. Consider taking DHEA to help your lupus if approved by your rheumatologist.
37. Do not get pregnant until cleared by your rheumatologist.
38. If you are anti-SSA or anti-SSB positive and get pregnant, alert your obstetrician so you can get fetal heart monitoring beginning at 16 to 18 weeks of pregnancy.
39. If you get pregnant, see your rheumatologist more often to monitor your lupus closely.
40. Ensure your work environment is conducive for your SLE. If you feel that you need work accommodations, learn more from the Job Accommodation Network at www.askjan.org and 800-526-7234.
41. Continue to educate yourself about lupus; consider joining a lupus educational organization such as The Lupus Foundation of America at www.lupus.org or 800-558-0121.
42. Every day, tell yourself it is going to be a good day, that there is a lot in your power to do well, and remember that knowledge is power.

REFERENCES

1. Rosen D. *Vital conversations: improving communication between doctors and patients*. New York: Columbia University Press; 2014.
2. Feddock CA, Bailey PD, Griffith CH, Lineberry MJ, Wilson JF. Is time spent with the physician associated with parent dissatisfaction due to long waiting times? *Eval Health Prof* 2010;**33**(2):216–25.
3. Alex-Hart BA, Opara PI. Observed hand washing practices among health workers in two critical paediatrics wards of a specialist hospital. *Am J Infect Dis* 2014;**10**(2):95–9.
4. Telles RW, Lanna CCD, Souza FL, Rodrigues LA, Reis RCP, Ribeiro AL. Causes and predictors of death in Brazilian lupus patients. *Rheumatol Int* 2013;**33**(2):467–73.
5. Swayden KJ, Anderson KK, Connelly LM, Moran JS, McMahon JK, Arnold PM. Effect of sitting vs standing on perception of provider time at bedside: a pilot study. *Patient Educ Couns* 2012;**86**(2):166–71.
6. Makaryus AN, Friedman EA. Patients' understanding of their treatment plans and diagnosis at discharge. *Mayo Clin Proc* 2005;**80**:991–4.
7. Glauser J. For medical errors, honesty is the best policy: the anger that often motivates litigation was diminished and settlements decreased when physicians and hospitals admitted to their mistakes. *Emergen Med* 2002;**24**(6):24–5.
8. Full Disclosure Working Group. *When things go wrong: responding to adverse events. A consensus statement of the Harvard Hospitals.* Massachusetts: Massachusetts Coalition for the Prevention of Medical Errors; March 2006. 37 p.
9. American Board of Medical Specialties. *Facts about the 2008 ABMS Consumer Survey: how Americans choose their doctors.* http://www.abms.org/media/1319/abms_2010_consumer_survey_fact_sheet.pdf.
10. Makaryus AN, Friedman EA. Does your patient know your name? an approach to enhancing patients' awareness of their caretaker's name. *J Healthc Qual* 2005;**27**(4):53–6.
11. Osterberg L, Blaschke T. Adherence to medication. *New Engl J Med* 2005;**5**:487–97.
12. Koneru S, Kocharla L, Higgins GC, Ware A, Passo M, Farhey Y, et al. Adherence to medications in systemic lupus erythematosus. *J Clin Rheumatol* 2008;**14**(4):195–201.
13. Tarn DM, Mattimore TJ, Bell DS, Kravitz RL, Wenger NS. Provider views about responsibility for medication adherence and content of physician–older patient discussions. *J Am Geriatr Soc* 2012;**6**:1019–26.
14. Arbuckle MR, McClain MT, Rubertone MV, Scofield RH, Dennis GJ, James JA, et al. Development of autoantibodies before the clinical onset of systemic lupus erythematosus. *New Engl J Med* 2003;**349**:1526–33.
15. Committee on Rheumatologic Care. *Position statement: methodology for testing for antinuclear antibodies.* American College of Rheumatology; 2011.
16. Merrill JT. Reply to: the rarity of antinuclear antibody negativity in systemic lupus erythematosus: comment on the article by Merrill et al (original comment by Major GAC). *Arthritis Rheum* 2011;**63**(4):1158. http://dx.doi.org/10.1002/art.30226.
17. Lim SS, Agan M, Drenlard CM. Impact of systemic lupus erythematosus organ damage on unemployment or disability from a population-based cohort. *Arthritis Res Ther* 2012;**14**(Suppl. 3):A13.
18. Ekblom-Kullberg S, Kautiainen H, Alha P, Leirisalo-Repo M, Julkunen H. Education, employment, absenteeism, and work disability in women with systemic lupus erythematosus. *Scand J Rheumatol Online* October 29, 2014;**44**(2).
19. *Mosby's medical dictionary.* 7th ed. St. Louis, MO: Mosby Elsevier; 2006. Malaise; p. 1138.
20. Social Security. *Medical/Professional Relations: Disability Under Social Security. 14.02 Systemic lupus erythematosus.* http://www.ssa.gov/disability/professionals/bluebook/14.00-Immune-Adult.htm#14_02; 2015 [accessed 10.10.15].
21. Thomas D. *The lupus encyclopedia: a comprehensive guide for patients and families.* Baltimore: The Johns Hopkins University Press; 2014. 788–790.

Chapter 3

Epidemiology

Manuel F. Ugarte-Gil[1,2], Guillermo J. Pons-Estel[3], Graciela S. Alarcón[4]

[1]Servicio de Reumatología, Hospital Nacional Guillermo Almenara Irigoyen, EsSalud, Lima, Peru; [2]Universidad Científica del Sur, Lima, Peru;
[3]Department of Autoimmune Diseases, Institut Clinic de Medicina I Dermatologia, Hospital Clinic, Barcelona, Catalonia, Spain; [4]Department of
Medicine, Division of Clinical Immunology and Rheumatology, School of Medicine, The University of Alabama at Birmingham, Birmingham, AL, USA

SUMMARY

Systemic lupus erythematosus (SLE) is a disease distributed worldwide that occurs in both genders and across racial/ethnic and age groups; however, higher rates are observed in adults, women, and non-Caucasians. Genetic, environmental, sociodemographic, and methodological issues are responsible for these differences and for the variable course and outcome of the disease. Non-Caucasians may have more severe disease with a higher risk for early mortality and damage accrual. Males also may have a more severe disease; however, a negative impact of male gender on lupus outcomes has not been firmly established. Childhood onset is associated with a more severe disease; however, it is not associated with higher damage or diminished survival. Finally, late-onset lupus is associated with a mild disease but with higher damage accrual and a diminished survival.

INTRODUCTION

Systemic lupus erythematosus (SLE) is a complex multisystemic autoimmune disease characterized by a wide spectrum of clinical manifestations, overabundant immunological and laboratory abnormalities, and a variable course and outcome. Descriptive, observational, and experimental studies and a few population-based ones have used classification criteria to include patients with similar clinical and laboratory abnormalities and are the basis for the epidemiological data currently available.

In 1982, the American College of Rheumatology (ACR) developed and validated classification criteria to consistently define SLE for research and epidemiological surveillance; these criteria were updated but never validated in 1997 and are used for case definition currently. In 2012, the Systemic Lupus International Collaborating Clinics (SLICC) group revised these criteria, establishing a more precise and clinically relevant set; in fact, clinical relevance and sensitivity increased but not specificity.[1] These criteria allow the inclusion of patients with biopsy-proven nephritis in the presence of autoimmunity markers [antinuclear antibodies (ANA) and/or anti-dsDNA antibodies]. By including alopecia and other neurological manifestations and by separating acute and chronic cutaneous lupus manifestations, improved clinical relevance has been attained.

INCIDENCE AND PREVALENCE

Using, for the most part, the ACR criteria (1982 or 1997) to classify patients, the overall incidence rates for SLE have varied around the globe from approximately ≤1 to 23 per 100,000 person-years,[2,3] whereas prevalence rates have ranged from 6,5 to 150 per 100,000.[4,5] Detailed data on the incidence and prevalence of SLE around the world from 1975 to 2000[6] and from 2000 onwards have been published.[2–4,7–12] Herein, we will describe the most salient studies.

There is no consensus related to temporal changes of SLE incidence and prevalence rates. Uramoto et al. demonstrated, in a US population-based study, that the disease has more than tripled in the past 40 years,[13] which likely reflects not only an actual increase in disease occurrence but a more accurate case ascertainment, the inclusion of milder cases, and the use of ANA testing. However, a UK cohort study using a clinical practice research datalink has shown a decline of 1.8% in SLE annual incidence while its prevalence increased from 64.9 per 100,000 in 1999 to 97.04 in 2012.[7]

The wide variations in the SLE incidence and prevalence rates most likely represent differences in patient characteristics such as age, gender, ethnic/racial group, geographic region, national origin, socioeconomic status (SES), and environmental exposures. However, differences in case ascertainment (self-reported, physician diagnosed, inclusion of serology), study type, and time when the study was conducted may also explain these differences.

Distribution According to Gender

SLE is more frequent in women, with a female-to-male ratio of 9:1. In the US Nationwide Medicaid claims data showed that the incidence and prevalence was six times higher among women (30.5 and 192.2, respectively) than among men (4.9 and 31.8, respectively).[2] Nevertheless, prevalence and incidence rates tend to be similar before puberty but diverge sharply thereafter, with a maximum ratio difference during the childbearing years until approximately the seventh decade of life, where rates again become similar.[8,14] Importantly, the peak incidence/prevalence rates among women occur approximately 10–20 years earlier than in men.

Hormones (primarily estrogens), candidate risk genes for SLE in the X chromosome (which are crucial in determining sex hormone levels), and some immunologically relevant genes (interferon-related and CD40 ligand) probably explain the preponderance of lupus among women.[15]

Distribution According to Age

SLE can develop at any age, although disease onset for most patients occurs between ages 20 and 55 years. Childhood-onset lupus (cSLE) occurs most consistently around ages 11–12 and represents 10–20% of SLE cases. On the contrary, late-onset lupus (occurring at age ≥50) represents 15% of all cases.

Age of onset is influenced by patient characteristics, with ethnicity having a major impact. The mean age of onset in Canadian Aboriginals is 34, followed by 33 for Caucasians, 30 for Afro-Caribbeans, and 25 for Asians. In Latin America, Caucasians represent the patients with the oldest age at onset, followed by Mestizos (mixed European and Amerindian background) and African-Latin Americans.

Finally, incidence and prevalence rates are considerably lower in cSLE. The annual incidence rate of cSLE (<16 years) has been reported to be less than 1 per 100,000 persons in studies from Europe and North America,[16] while higher figures have been reported in China.[17]

Distribution According to Ethnic/Racial Group

Large differences in incidence and prevalence rates as a function of ethnic/racial group are known to occur in SLE, with, by and large, non-Caucasians experiencing higher rates than Caucasians. In the US Medicaid population, the overall incidence/prevalence rates according to ethnicity are 31.2/223.4 in African Americans, 30.0/165.7 in Native Americans, 22.1/126.6 in US Hispanics, 16.7/175.1 in Asians, and 18.0/111.6 in Caucasians.[2] Studies of Aboriginal Australians have shown that this group has the highest worldwide incidence rates with prevalence rates almost twice higher than in Caucasians.[18,19]

No population-based study has yet defined the prevalence and incidence of lupus in Mestizos (Caucasian and Amerindian background) and other ethnic/racial groups in Latin American. However, on the basis of data from the GLADEL (*Grupo Latinoamericano de Estudio de Lupus*) cohort, it has been inferred that SLE in Mestizos and African Latin Americans presents at younger age and with higher frequency and greater severity than in Caucasians.[20]

Distribution Around the World

SLE occurs worldwide. It seems to be infrequent on the African continent but surprisingly common in African descendants (Afro-Caribbean, African-American, and Afro-Latin-American) around the world. The *prevalence gradient* hypothesis suggests that genetic admixture, environmental exposures, disease severity, low survival, and competing causes of death may explain these differences. Furthermore, no reliable prevalence data from western Africa are available to date. Such rates have been assumed based on data from immigrant women to the UK, which reveal a prevalence of SLE three times higher among them compared to Caucasians, albeit not as high as in patients of Afro-Caribbean origin.[21]

Several environmental factors may influence SLE rates around the globe. For example, in a study performed in China, a number of factors such as rural residency, the type of food and water ingested, sun exposure, infections (hepatitis B), physical activity, negative life events, and reproductive milestones were associated with higher SLE occurrence.[10] Finally, a low socioeconomic status (SES) has been associated with higher prevalence (but not incidence) rates in the US Medicaid study (167.9 per 100,000).[2]

FACTORS THAT AFFECT THE COURSE OF SLE

Several factors can affect the presentation and course of SLE. The most important are ethnicity/race, gender, age at onset, and SES factors.

Impact of Race/Ethnicity

Given that ethnicity is not merely a biological but a social and cultural construct, the impact of race/ethnicity-genetic and SES factors may be hard to disentangle. Genetic ancestry has been associated with phenotypic differences among SLE patients; Amerindian and African ancestry are associated with a higher risk for kidney involvement.[22,23] Among European descendants, Southern European ancestry is associated with a higher risk of renal involvement and of autoantibody production but a lower risk of discoid rash and photosensitivity. Western European ancestry is associated with an increased risk of serositis and auto-antibody production, whereas Ashkenazi Jewish ancestry was protective against neurologic manifestations.[24]

In addition, acute onset is more frequent in US Hispanics and African descendants than in Caucasians.[25] Caucasians present cutaneous manifestations more frequently than US Hispanic, Mestizo, African descendant, or Asian patients[20,26,27] but discoid rash occurs more frequently in African descendants.[20,26,27] Arthritis and serositis occur less frequently in Asians[26,28] and pericarditis occurs more frequently in African descendants.[20] General manifestations occur less frequently in Asians and Canadian Aboriginals than in Caucasians and African descendants.[26]

Fever and weight loss occur less frequently in Latin America Mestizos than in Caucasians and African descendants.[20] Hematologic manifestations occur more frequently in Caucasians than Asians,[28] whereas lymphopenia occurs less frequently in Caucasians than in Mestizos or African descendants.[20] Cutaneous vasculitis and mononeuritis multiplex are more frequent in Canadian Aboriginals.[26]

Kidney involvement, one of the most worrisome SLE manifestations, occurs more frequently among US Hispanics, Mestizo, African descendants, and Asians.[20,26,27] Furthermore, US Hispanics and African descendants have a high risk of developing end-stage renal disease than Caucasians[22,29] and developing hypertension,[20] contributing to poor renal outcomes among them. Furthermore, the response to treatment in patients with lupus nephritis differs by ethnic group; for example, Hispanic patients respond better to mycophenolate mofetil than to cyclophosphamide, but Caucasians do not.[30]

Anti-DNA antibodies are more frequent in Mestizos,[20] US Hispanics,[31] and African-Americans,[31] compared to Caucasians, particularly those of Northern European ancestry.[24] Furthermore, anti ribonucleoprotein (RNP) antibodies occur more frequently among African descendants.[32]

US Hispanics and African descendants also experience higher levels of disease activity, which also tends to decline at a slower pace than in Caucasians.[33,34] In terms of damage, US Hispanics, Asians, and African descendants tend to accrue more damage.[35,36] However, Asians from the SLICC cohort accrued less new damage compared to European Caucasians.[36] As to the type of damage, renal damage occurs more frequently in US Hispanics, African descendants, and Asians than in Caucasians,[27,35,37] integument and diabetes in African descendants,[27,35] ocular damage in US Hispanics and Caucasians[27]; gastrointestinal damage and malignancy in Caucasians[27]; cardiovascular damage occurs less frequently in Asians.[37] However, SES factors like health insurance,[20,38] education level,[20,35] poverty,[35] level of helplessness,[38] and abnormal illness behaviors[35,38] also impact these intermediate outcomes and could explain, at least in part, the impact of ethnic group in the course of SLE.

Impact of Gender

Gender also affects the clinical phenotype of lupus. Men tend to have more severe manifestations than women, such as renal disease,[39,40] hematologic involvement,[39,40] and serositis[41] and women tend to have mild manifestations such as arthritis/arthralgia,[39,40,42] photosensitivity,[39,40] malar rash,[40,41] oral ulcers,[40,41] alopecia,[39,40,42] and Raynaud's phenomenon more frequently than men.[39–42] Finally, a lower prevalence of anti-Ro[41,42] and a higher prevalence of anti-Sm,[40] anti-ds-DNA,[40] Coombs positivity,[40] and low C3[39,40] have been reported in male SLE patients.

In addition, male patients present a higher frequency of thrombosis,[40] including antiphospholipid antibodies,[39,40,43] antiphospholipid syndrome, and hypertension.[39,40]

The association between damage and gender is still controversial. In LUMINA,[43] both were found to be associated, but this has not been corroborated in other studies.[39,41,42] However, the association of male gender with certain damage items (e.g., seizures, myocardial infarction, angina, thrombosis, and kidney involvement) has been described in the Hopkins Lupus cohort.[40] Kidney damage and cardiovascular damage have been found to be associated with male gender in Asians[42] and Latin Americans, respectively.[39] Whether these gender differences are due to a higher genetic load among men is controversial.[44,45]

Impact of Age

cSLE is associated with a higher frequency of severe manifestations, such as renal involvement,[46,47] seizures,[47] hematologic involvement (including leucopenia,[46] hemolytic anemia,[46,47] and thrombocytopenia[47]) but a lower frequency of sicca symptoms,[47] Raynaud's phenomenon[47] and pleuritis[47] as compared to adult-onset SLE. Also, cSLE is associated with a higher frequency of anti-DNA and anticardiolipin antibodies and a lower frequency of rheumatoid factor.[48]

Patients with cSLE show significantly higher levels of disease activity.[48] However, the impact of childhood onset on damage accrual is still controversial.[48] Given that the SLICC/ACR damage index includes several items that occur frequently in older populations but does not include those that specifically occur in children, such as growth and physical maturation, the impact of lupus in children may have been underestimated. In addition, a higher genetic load for SLE has been found in African descendant cSLE patients but not in Caucasians.[46]

There are differences in the clinical manifestations of late- and adult-onset SLE. Late onset is associated with less severe manifestations such as sicca syndrome,[49] pulmonary involvement,[49] and serositis[49] and lower frequency of nephritis,[46,50–52] particularly proliferative nephritis,[51] malar rash,[51] and arthritis.[51] Also, late-onset SLE patients have lower frequencies of low complement levels,[49,51,52] positive anti-DNA antibodies,[46,52] and anti-Sm antibodies,[46,50] but a higher frequency of positive rheumatoid factor.[51] Finally, late-onset patients experience lower levels of disease activity,[50,52] but higher levels of damage than those with adult-onset disease.[50]

MORTALITY AND SURVIVAL IN SLE

Survival in SLE has steadily improved during the past 60 years, with 5-year survival increasing from around 50% in the 1950s to around 95% in the 2000s.[53] Data of selected survival studies are shown in Table 1. Earlier diagnosis and a better disease and disease-related comorbidities management probably explain the improved survival rates. Nevertheless, the standardized mortality ratio (SMR) for SLE is almost three times higher than for the general population.[54]

TABLE 1 Selected Cumulative Probability of Survival in Patients with Systemic Lupus Erythematosus (1981–2014)[a]

Author	Country	N	Ethnic Group (%)					Publication Date	Survival (%)			
			C	Af	H	As	O		5-y	10-y	15-y	20-y
USA and Canada												
Wallace et al.[65]	USA	609	79	6	7	7		1981	88	79	74	
Ginzler et al.[66]	USA	1103	58	32	5	3		1982	77	71		69
Abu-Shakra et al.[56]	Canada	665	86	7	0	7	2	1995	93	85	79	68
Kasitanon et al.[60]	USA	1378	56	49	5			2006	95	91	85	78
Europe												
Cervera et al.[67,68]	Europe	1000	97	2			1	2003	95	92		
Ruiz-Irastorza et al.[57]	Spain	202	100					2004	95	91	86	69
Voss et al.[69]	Denmark	215	94				6	2013	94	87	73	
Pamuk et al.[70]	Turkey	428						2013	96	92	89	
Latin America												
Pons-Estel et al.[20]	Latin America	1480	41	13	44		2	¶	94			
Asia												
Kasitanon et al.[71]	Thailand	349				100		2002	84	75		
Mok et al.[63]	Hong Kong	285				100		2005	92	83	80	
Funauchi et al.[72]	Japan	101				100		2007	94	88		
Wu G et al.[73]	China	665				100		2014	91	80		77
Arabic Region												
Al Arfaj et al.[74]	Saudi Arabia	624				2	98	2009	98	97		
Africa												
Houman et al.[75]	Tunisia	100					100	2004	86			

N, Population; C, Caucasian; Af, African descendant; H, Hispanic; As, Asian; O, Other; 5-y, Five-year survival; 10-y, Ten-year survival; 15-y, Fifteen-year survival; 20-y, Twenty-year survival; ¶, Unpublished data.
[a]These data are, by and large, not from inception cohorts; therefore, a survival effect bias cannot be ruled out.

Cardiovascular disease, infections, and renal disease are the most common causes of death among SLE patients.[54] Although overall cancer-associated mortality does not seem to be increased in patients with lupus, mortality related to hematologic neoplasms, including non-Hodgkin lymphoma and lung cancer, are.[55] SMR is influenced by age, whereby it is higher in younger patients (19.2 in SLE patients between 16 and 24 years), thus reflecting the more severe disease these patients experience. In older patients, comorbidities rather than disease activity account for their increased SMR.[55]

Older age at diagnosis[56–58] has been associated with higher mortality rates in lupus. With the exception of the Duke cohort,[59] ethnicity is not associated with mortality after adjusting for SES.[60] SES factors (education,[20] poverty[59] and lack of or inadequate health insurance[20,58]) could partially explain the different survival rates in Caucasians and non-Caucasians.

As to disease-related factors, higher levels of disease activity, both at diagnosis[56] and over time,[61] higher damage accrual,[61–63] hematologic disorders[63] (including thrombocytopenia[56,64] and hemolytic anemia[60]), neurological,[58] lung,[56] and kidney[56,57] involvement have been associated with an increased mortality in SLE. The concomitant presence of either the antiphospholipid syndrome or coronary artery disease has also been associated with a higher mortality rate.[57,61,62]

Within the treatments commonly used in lupus, high doses of glucocorticoids[64] and immunosuppressive drugs,[61] including cyclophosphamide[62] have been associated with higher mortality rates, reflecting both a more severe disease among these patients but also the adverse effects of these treatments. Otherwise, antimalarials have been repeatedly shown to prolong survival in patients with SLE[61]; this effect is probably time dependent.[58]

REFERENCES

1. Petri M, Orbai AM, Alarcon GS, Gordon C, Merrill JT, Fortin PR, et al. Derivation and validation of the systemic lupus international collaborating clinics classification criteria for systemic lupus erythematosus. *Arthritis Rheum* 2012;**64**(8):2677–86.
2. Feldman CH, Hiraki LT, Liu J, Fischer MA, Solomon DH, Alarcon GS, et al. Epidemiology and sociodemographics of systemic lupus erythematosus and lupus nephritis among US adults with Medicaid coverage, 2000–2004. *Arthritis Rheum* 2013;**65**(3):753–63.
3. Nasonov E, Soloviev S, Davidson JE, Lila A, Ivanova R, Togizbayev G, et al. The prevalence and incidence of systemic lupus erythematosus (SLE) in selected cities from three Commonwealth of Independent States countries (the Russian Federation, Ukraine and Kazakhstan). *Lupus* 2014;**23**(2):213–9.
4. Chakravarty EF, Bush TM, Manzi S, Clarke AE, Ward MM. Prevalence of adult systemic lupus erythematosus in California and Pennsylvania in 2000: estimates obtained using hospitalization data. *Arthritis Rheum* 2007;**56**(6):2092–4.
5. Hochberg MC. Prevalence of systemic lupus erythematosus in England and Wales, 1981–2. *Ann Rheum Dis* 1987;**46**(9):664–6.
6. Pons-Estel GJ, Alarcon GS, Scofield L, Reinlib L, Cooper GS. Understanding the epidemiology and progression of systemic lupus erythematosus. *Semin Arthritis Rheum* 2010;**39**(4):257–68.
7. Rees F, Doherty M, Grainge M, Davenport G, Lanyon P, Zhang W. The incidence and prevalence of systemic lupus erythematosus in the UK, 1999–2012. *Ann Rheum Dis* 2014 Sep 19. Epub ahead of print.
8. Brinks R, Fischer-Betz R, Sander O, Richter J, Chehab G, Schneider M. Age-specific prevalence of diagnosed systemic lupus erythematosus in Germany 2002 and projection to 2030. *Lupus* 2014;**23**(13):1407–11.
9. Somers EC, Marder W, Cagnoli P, Lewis EE, DeGuire P, Gordon C, et al. Population-based incidence and prevalence of systemic lupus erythematosus: the Michigan Lupus Epidemiology and Surveillance program. *Arthritis Rheumatol* 2014;**66**(2):369–78.
10. Zou YF, Feng CC, Zhu JM, Tao JH, Chen GM, Ye QL, et al. Prevalence of systemic lupus erythematosus and risk factors in rural areas of Anhui Province. *Rheumatol Int* 2014;**34**(3):347–56.
11. Pelaez-Ballestas I, Sanin LH, Moreno-Montoya J, Alvarez-Nemegyei J, Burgos-Vargas R, Garza-Elizondo M, et al. Epidemiology of the rheumatic diseases in Mexico. A study of 5 regions based on the COPCORD methodology. *J Rheumatol Suppl* 2011;**86**:3–8.
12. Lim SS, Bayakly AR, Helmick CG, Gordon C, Easley KA, Drenkard C. The incidence and prevalence of systemic lupus erythematosus, 2002–2004: the Georgia Lupus Registry. *Arthritis Rheumatol* 2014;**66**(2):357–68.
13. Uramoto KM, Michet Jr CJ, Thumboo J, Sunku J, O'Fallon WM, Gabriel SE. Trends in the incidence and mortality of systemic lupus erythematosus, 1950-1992. *Arthritis Rheum* 1999;**42**(1):46–50.
14. Somers EC, Thomas SL, Smeeth L, Schoonen WM, Hall AJ. Incidence of systemic lupus erythematosus in the United Kingdom, 1990–1999. *Arthritis Rheum* 2007;**57**(4):612–8.
15. Lu LJ, Wallace DJ, Ishimori ML, Scofield RH, Weisman MH. Review: male systemic lupus erythematosus: a review of sex disparities in this disease. *Lupus* 2010;**19**(2):119–29.
16. Huemer C, Huemer M, Dorner T, Falger J, Schacherl H, Bernecker M, et al. Incidence of pediatric rheumatic diseases in a regional population in Austria. *J Rheumatol* 2001;**28**(9):2116–9.
17. Huang JL, Yao TC, See LC. Prevalence of pediatric systemic lupus erythematosus and juvenile chronic arthritis in a Chinese population: a nation-wide prospective population-based study in Taiwan. *Clin Exp Rheumatol* 2004;**22**(6):776–80.
18. Anstey NM, Bastian I, Dunckley H, Currie BJ. Systemic lupus erythematosus in Australian aborigines: high prevalence, morbidity and mortality. *Aust NZ J Med* 1993;**23**(6):646–51.
19. Bossingham D. Systemic lupus erythematosus in the far north of Queensland. *Lupus* 2003;**12**(4):327–31.
20. Pons-Estel BA, Catoggio LJ, Cardiel MH, Soriano ER, Gentiletti S, Villa AR, et al. The GLADEL multinational Latin American prospective inception cohort of 1214 patients with systemic lupus erythematosus: ethnic and disease heterogeneity among "Hispanics". *Med Baltim* 2004;**83**(1):1–17.
21. Molokhia M, McKeigue PM, Cuadrado M, Hughes G. Systemic lupus erythematosus in migrants from west Africa compared with Afro-Caribbean people in the UK. *Lancet* 2001;**357**(9266):1414–5.
22. Alarcon GS, Bastian HM, Beasley TM, Roseman JM, Tan FK, Fessler BJ, et al. Systemic lupus erythematosus in a multi-ethnic cohort (LUMINA) XXXII: [corrected] contributions of admixture and socioeconomic status to renal involvement. *Lupus* 2006;**15**(1):26–31.

23. Sanchez E, Rasmussen A, Riba L, Acevedo-Vasquez E, Kelly JA, Langefeld CD, et al. Impact of genetic ancestry and sociodemographic status on the clinical expression of systemic lupus erythematosus in American Indian-European populations. *Arthritis Rheum* 2012;**64**(11):3687–94.

24. Richman IB, Chung SA, Taylor KE, Kosoy R, Tian C, Ortmann WA, et al. European population substructure correlates with systemic lupus erythematosus endophenotypes in North Americans of European descent. *Genes Immun* 2010;**11**(6):515–21.

25. Bertoli AM, Vila LM, Reveille JD, Alarcon GS. Systemic lupus erythaematosus in a multiethnic US cohort (LUMINA) LIII: disease expression and outcome in acute onset lupus. *Ann Rheum Dis* 2008;**67**(4):500–4.

26. Peschken CA, Katz SJ, Silverman E, Pope JE, Fortin PR, Pineau C, et al. The 1000 Canadian faces of lupus: determinants of disease outcome in a large multiethnic cohort. *J Rheumatol* 2009;**36**(6):1200–8.

27. Alarcon GS, McGwin Jr G, Petri M, Reveille JD, Ramsey-Goldman R, Kimberly RP. Baseline characteristics of a multiethnic lupus cohort: PROFILE. *Lupus* 2002;**11**(2):95–101.

28. Thumboo J, Uramoto K, O'Fallon WM, Fong KY, Boey ML, Feng PH, et al. A comparative study of the clinical manifestations of systemic lupus erythematosus in Caucasians in Rochester, Minnesota, and Chinese in Singapore, from 1980 to 1992. *Arthritis Rheum* 2001;**45**(6):494–500.

29. Alarcon GS, McGwin Jr G, Petri M, Ramsey-Goldman R, Fessler BJ, Vila LM, et al. Time to renal disease and end-stage renal disease in PROFILE: a multiethnic lupus cohort. *PLoS Med* 2006;**3**(10):e396.

30. Appel GB, Contreras G, Dooley MA, Ginzler EM, Isenberg D, Jayne D, et al. Mycophenolate mofetil versus cyclophosphamide for induction treatment of lupus nephritis. *J Am Soc Nephrol* 2009;**20**(5):1103–12.

31. Alarcon GS, Friedman AW, Straaton KV, Moulds JM, Lisse J, Bastian HM, et al. Systemic lupus erythematosus in three ethnic groups: III. A comparison of characteristics early in the natural history of the LUMINA cohort. LUpus in MInority populations: NAture vs Nurture. *Lupus* 1999;**8**(3):197–209.

32. Ko K, Franek BS, Marion M, Kaufman KM, Langefeld CD, Harley JB, et al. Genetic ancestry, serum interferon-alpha activity, and autoantibodies in systemic lupus erythematosus. *J Rheumatol* 2012;**39**(6):1238–40.

33. Alarcon GS, Calvo-Alen J, McGwin Jr G, Uribe AG, Toloza SM, Roseman JM, et al. Systemic lupus erythematosus in a multiethnic cohort: LUMINA XXXV. Predictive factors of high disease activity over time. *Ann Rheum Dis* 2006;**65**(9):1168–74.

34. Zhang J, Gonzalez LA, Roseman JM, Vila LM, Reveille JD, Alarcon GS. Predictors of the rate of change in disease activity over time in LUMINA, a multiethnic US cohort of patients with systemic lupus erythematosus: LUMINA LXX. *Lupus* 2010;**19**(6):727–33.

35. Alarcon GS, McGwin Jr G, Bartolucci AA, Roseman J, Lisse J, Fessler BJ, et al. Systemic lupus erythematosus in three ethnic groups. IX. Differences in damage accrual. *Arthritis Rheum* 2001;**44**(12):2797–806.

36. Bruce IN, O'Keeffe AG, Farewell V, Hanly JG, Manzi S, Su L, et al. Factors associated with damage accrual in patients with systemic lupus erythematosus: results from the Systemic Lupus International Collaborating Clinics (SLICC) Inception Cohort. *Ann Rheum Dis* 2015;**74**(9):1706–13.

37. Kuan WP, Li EK, Tam LS. Lupus organ damage: what is damaged in Asian patients? *Lupus* 2010;**19**(12):1436–41.

38. Alarcon GS, Roseman J, Bartolucci AA, Friedman AW, Moulds JM, Goel N, et al. Systemic lupus erythematosus in three ethnic groups: II. Features predictive of disease activity early in its course. LUMINA Study Group. Lupus in minority populations, nature versus nurture. *Arthritis Rheum* 1998;**41**(7):1173–80.

39. Garcia MA, Marcos JC, Marcos AI, Pons-Estel BA, Wojdyla D, Arturi A, et al. Male systemic lupus erythematosus in a Latin-American inception cohort of 1214 patients. *Lupus* 2005;**14**(12):938–46.

40. Tan TC, Fang H, Magder LS, Petri MA. Differences between male and female systemic lupus erythematosus in a multiethnic population. *J Rheumatol* 2012;**39**(4):759–69.

41. Voulgari PV, Katsimbri P, Alamanos Y, Drosos AA. Gender and age differences in systemic lupus erythematosus. A study of 489 Greek patients with a review of the literature. *Lupus* 2002;**11**(11):722–9.

42. Mok CC, Lau CS, Chan TM, Wong RW. Clinical characteristics and outcome of southern Chinese males with systemic lupus erythematosus. *Lupus* 1999;**8**(3):188–96.

43. Andrade RM, Alarcon GS, Fernandez M, Apte M, Vila LM, Reveille JD. Accelerated damage accrual among men with systemic lupus erythematosus: XLIV. Results from a multiethnic US cohort. *Arthritis Rheum* 2007;**56**(2):622–30.

44. Alonso-Perez E, Suarez-Gestal M, Calaza M, Blanco FJ, Suarez A, Santos MJ, et al. Lack of replication of higher genetic risk load in men than in women with systemic lupus erythematosus. *Arthritis Res Ther* 2014;**16**(3):R128.

45. Hughes T, Adler A, Merrill JT, Kelly JA, Kaufman KM, Williams A, et al. Analysis of autosomal genes reveals gene-sex interactions and higher total genetic risk in men with systemic lupus erythematosus. *Ann Rheum Dis* 2012;**71**(5):694–9.

46. Webb R, Kelly JA, Somers EC, Hughes T, Kaufman KM, Sanchez E, et al. Early disease onset is predicted by a higher genetic risk for lupus and is associated with a more severe phenotype in lupus patients. *Ann Rheum Dis* 2011;**70**(1):151–6.

47. Livingston B, Bonner A, Pope J. Differences in clinical manifestations between childhood-onset lupus and adult-onset lupus: a meta-analysis. *Lupus* 2011;**20**(13):1345–55.

48. Livingston B, Bonner A, Pope J. Differences in autoantibody profiles and disease activity and damage scores between childhood- and adult-onset systemic lupus erythematosus: a meta-analysis. *Semin Arthritis Rheum* 2012;**42**(3):271–80.

49. Ward MM, Polisson RP. A meta-analysis of the clinical manifestations of older-onset systemic lupus erythematosus. *Arthritis Rheum* 1989;**32**(10):1226–32.

50. Bertoli AM, Alarcon GS, Calvo-Alen J, Fernandez M, Vila LM, Reveille JD. Systemic lupus erythematosus in a multiethnic US cohort. XXXIII. Clinical [corrected] features, course, and outcome in patients with late-onset disease. *Arthritis Rheum* 2006;**54**(5):1580–7.

51. Boddaert J, Huong DL, Amoura Z, Wechsler B, Godeau P, Piette JC. Late-onset systemic lupus erythematosus: a personal series of 47 patients and pooled analysis of 714 cases in the literature. *Med Baltim* 2004;**83**(6):348–59.

52. Formiga F, Moga I, Pac M, Mitjavila F, Rivera A, Pujol R. Mild presentation of systemic lupus erythematosus in elderly patients assessed by SLEDAI. SLE Disease Activity Index. *Lupus* 1999;**8**(6):462–5.

53. Mak A, Cheung MW, Chiew HJ, Liu Y, Ho RC. Global trend of survival and damage of systemic lupus erythematosus: meta-analysis and meta-regression of observational studies from the 1950s to 2000s. *Semin Arthritis Rheum* 2012;**41**(6):830–9.

54. Yurkovich M, Vostretsova K, Chen W, Avina-Zubieta JA. Overall and cause-specific mortality in patients with systemic lupus erythematosus: a meta-analysis of observational studies. *Arthritis Care Res* 2014;**66**(4):608–16.

55. Bernatsky S, Boivin JF, Joseph L, Manzi S, Ginzler E, Gladman DD, et al. Mortality in systemic lupus erythematosus. *Arthritis Rheum* 2006;**54**(8):2550–7.

56. Abu-Shakra M, Urowitz MB, Gladman DD, Gough J. Mortality studies in systemic lupus erythematosus. Results from a single center. II. Predictor variables for mortality. *J Rheumatology* 1995;**22**(7):1265–70.
57. Ruiz-Irastorza G, Egurbide MV, Ugalde J, Aguirre C. High impact of antiphospholipid syndrome on irreversible organ damage and survival of patients with systemic lupus erythematosus. *Arch Intern Med* 2004;**164**(1):77–82.
58. Shinjo SK, Bonfa E, Wojdyla D, Borba EF, Ramirez LA, Scherbarth HR, et al. Antimalarial treatment may have a time-dependent effect on lupus survival: data from a multinational Latin American inception cohort. *Arthritis Rheum* 2010;**62**(3):855–62.
59. Studenski S, Allen NB, Caldwell DS, Rice JR, Polisson RP. Survival in systemic lupus erythematosus. A multivariate analysis of demographic factors. *Arthritis Rheum* 1987;**30**(12):1326–32.
60. Kasitanon N, Magder LS, Petri M. Predictors of survival in systemic lupus erythematosus. *Med Baltim* 2006;**85**(3):147–56.
61. Urowitz MB, Gladman DD, Tom BD, Ibanez D, Farewell VT. Changing patterns in mortality and disease outcomes for patients with systemic lupus erythematosus. *J Rheumatology* 2008;**35**(11):2152–8.
62. Telles RW, Lanna CC, Souza FL, Rodrigues LA, Reis RC, Ribeiro AL. Causes and predictors of death in Brazilian lupus patients. *Rheumatol Int* 2013;**33**(2):467–73.
63. Mok CC, Mak A, Chu WP, To CH, Wong SN. Long-term survival of southern Chinese patients with systemic lupus erythematosus: a prospective study of all age-groups. *Med Baltim* 2005;**84**(4):218–24.
64. Mok CC, Lee KW, Ho CT, Lau CS, Wong RW. A prospective study of survival and prognostic indicators of systemic lupus erythematosus in a southern Chinese population. *Rheumatol Oxf* 2000;**39**(4):399–406.
65. Wallace DJ, Podell T, Weiner J, Klinenberg JR, Forouzesh S, Dubois EL. Systemic lupus erythematosus–survival patterns. Experience with 609 patients. *JAMA J Am Med Assoc* 1981;**245**(9):934–8.
66. Ginzler EM, Diamond HS, Weiner M, Schlesinger M, Fries JF, Wasner C, et al. A multicenter study of outcome in systemic lupus erythematosus. I. Entry variables as predictors of prognosis. *Arthritis Rheum* 1982;**25**(6):601–11.
67. Cervera R, Khamashta MA, Font J, Sebastiani GD, Gil A, Lavilla P, et al. Morbidity and mortality in systemic lupus erythematosus during a 5-year period. A multicenter prospective study of 1000 patients. European Working Party on Systemic Lupus Erythematosus. *Med Baltim* 1999;**78**(3):167–75.
68. Cervera R, Khamashta MA, Font J, Sebastiani GD, Gil A, Lavilla P, et al. Morbidity and mortality in systemic lupus erythematosus during a 10-year period: a comparison of early and late manifestations in a cohort of 1000 patients. *Med Baltim* 2003;**82**(5):299–308.
69. Voss A, Laustrup H, Hjelmborg J, Junker P. Survival in systemic lupus erythematosus, 1995–2010. A prospective study in a Danish community. *Lupus* 2013;**22**(11):1185–91.
70. Pamuk ON, Akbay FG, Donmez S, Yilmaz N, Calayir GB, Yavuz S. The clinical manifestations and survival of systemic lupus erythematosus patients in Turkey: report from two centers. *Lupus* 2013;**22**(13):1416–24.
71. Kasitanon N, Louthrenoo W, Sukitawut W, Vichainun R. Causes of death and prognostic factors in Thai patients with systemic lupus erythematosus. *Asian Pac J allergy Immunol/Launched by Allergy Immunol Soc Thail* 2002;**20**(2):85–91.
72. Funauchi M, Shimadzu H, Tamaki C, Yamagata T, Nozaki Y, Sugiyama M, et al. Survival study by organ disorders in 306 Japanese patients with systemic lupus erythematosus: results from a single center. *Rheumatol Int* 2007;**27**(3):243–9.
73. Wu G, Jia X, Gao D, Zhao Z. Survival rates and risk factors for mortality in systemic lupus erythematosus patients in a Chinese center. *Clin Rheumatol* 2014;**33**(7):947–53.
74. Al Arfaj AS, Khalil N. Clinical and immunological manifestations in 624 SLE patients in Saudi Arabia. *Lupus* 2009;**18**(5):465–73.
75. Houman MH, Smiti-Khanfir M, Ben Ghorbell I, Miled M. Systemic lupus erythematosus in Tunisia: demographic and clinical analysis of 100 patients. *Lupus* 2004;**13**(3):204–11.

Chapter 4

Measuring Disease Activity

Joan T. Merrill

Clinical Pharmacology Research Program, Oklahoma Medical Research Foundation, University of Oklahoma, OK, USA

SUMMARY

Clinical trials for systemic lupus erythematosus (SLE) currently depend on outcome measures that were originally developed for epidemiological or outcomes research and never optimized to discriminate treatment effects. Because these systems were devised to encompass simultaneous assessment of multiple organs, their interpretation can be complicated, requiring specialized training. Not surprisingly, there has been minimal adaptation of these disease activity scales in clinical practice, leaving clinicians without practical or reproducible methods for tracking progress, justifying treatment approvals, or documenting quality assurance. This chapter focuses on two of the most widely used SLE measures, the Systemic Lupus Erythematosus Disease Activity Index (SLEDAI) and the British Isles Lupus Assessment Group (BILAG) index. Definitions and scoring rules for these instruments were originally conceived through expert consensus, followed by formal validation studies to test reliability of their use over time and between clinicians. Both the SLEDAI and BILAG have demonstrated reliability, relevance, and sensitivity to change in disease severity. However, when these mature, well-validated instruments began to be applied in registrational trials of investigational treatments, significant pitfalls were recognized. Subsequent accommodations in how the instruments are applied to study endpoints has led to more interpretable results in some recent trials, but continue to illuminate ongoing obstacles to successful treatment development, and to the ability, in clinic, to accurately track progress in this complex patient population. The solution may lie in the development of a measure that is not first keyed to expert ideas, then later tested for validity, but is originally scaled to live patient outcomes in the clinic to discriminate real-world, clinically significant disease changes from minor fluctuations.

A number of indices have been used for several decades to evaluate systemic lupus erythematosus (SLE) disease activity for epidemiological or outcomes research. This chapter focuses on two of the most widely used systems, the Systemic Lupus Erythematosus Disease Activity Index (SLEDAI), which currently has several very similar (but not quite identical) versions,[1] and the British Isles Lupus Assessment Group (BILAG) index, which has evolved over several iterations vetted by a working group in the United Kingdom.[2]

The methods originally followed to create these scales involved group consensus meetings of clinicians where definitions and scoring rules were developed, followed by formal validation studies in which consistency of scoring was compared to expert opinion. Validation programs were taken very seriously in the community of clinical lupus investigators, and the instruments underwent repeated refinements and retesting over time, resulting in the newest models, which have been widely applied to clinical trials: the SELENA SLEDAI, the SLEDAI 2K, and the BILAG 2004.[1,2]

During this process, these tools have repeatedly demonstrated interobserver and intraobserver validity, face validity, and sensitivity to change in disease states.[3–9] However, when the mature instruments began to be used in registrational treatment trials—a task that they were not designed for—critical pitfalls were recognized in this application.[10–13] Analysis of these snares led to the development of novel, combined applications of the instruments,[14,15] and a degree of improvement in discriminatory capacity appears to be reported for some trials.[16,17] Nevertheless, the limited treatment effects that are discernable even with improved juxtapositioning of the instruments continue to underscore a serious evidence gap, leaving uncertainty in its wake as to whether the investigational treatments are failing or whether the outcome measures are failing. Importantly, endpoints are needed that discriminate between clinically significant and insignificant change, either by optimizing detection of the difference in a group receiving an effective treatment or by minimizing false-positive (or minimal) responses in patients treated with background therapies plus placebo. The current instruments were not developed, nor have they been widely critiqued with this critical goal in mind.

Importantly, because the original invention of the instruments was by theoretical construct and only later tested against clinical outcomes, the construction of the instruments

Systemic Lupus Erythematosus. http://dx.doi.org/10.1016/B978-0-12-801917-7.00004-8

themselves was never adapted by real-world scaling. No measure has yet been purposefully designed, optimized, or revised using changes in disease of actual lupus patients as the template for increments of change. Perhaps it should not be surprising that the current measures still seem to fall short in clinical trials of an enormously complicated multisystem illness, because it remains unknown how to optimally discriminate between mild, moderate, and severe disease, or how to best construct increments of clinically significant improvement or worsening.

The BILAG index ranks symptoms first by separating them into organs and then by assigning a grade to each organ based on the highest ranking symptom within that structure. The final grade is influenced by the intensity of symptoms, with a link between how disease severity is gaged and intent to change therapy. This is interesting in that the design is to effectively mirror the thought process of clinicians. The SLEDAI charts the presence or absence of symptoms, but it does not have the same level of complexity as the BILAG. Each active symptom receives a single score, regardless of severity. The assignment of the SLEDAI point scale was developed by consensus on the usual importance (in "most" patients) of a given manifestation. Thus, a major weakness of the SLEDAI is an inability to distinguish severely affected patients from those who meet minimal criteria with the same symptom.

Although the SLEDAI was not designed to separately evaluate each different organ, it can be used that way, and it may have an advantage over the BILAG by its capacity to separate the assessment of multiple features within one organ. This is especially valuable in the mucocutaneous system, where—when all signs and symptoms assigned by the BILAG organ category are lumped together—multiple signs or symptoms commonly occur at the same time, rendering all but one of them (one with the highest severity rating) impotent in increasing the score. Both the BILAG and SLEDAI can be useful in clinical trials, but an understanding of their relative strengths and weaknesses are important in designing outcome measures.

Originally, the BILAG instrument assessed a patient's condition during the month prior to and up until the date of a given evaluation, and the SLEDAI only evaluated disease activity back to 10 days before the visit. Most studies now use both instruments to assess back one month, and that has been validated for the SLEDAI 2K.[18] Some studies have tried to use the BILAG Index or SLEDAI to capture all activity between tri-monthly visits,[19] but this approach has obvious pitfalls. There may have been multiple disease levels within that time, interim changes in therapy are more common, and memory for mild or moderate flares can be deceptive over a 3-month period. Importantly, the 3-month assessment has never been validated against monthly assessments to determine how accurate or inaccurate it might be.

The BILAG Index originally included eight organ systems.[20] Scoring was, and still is, based on the principle of

intention to treat, using the following ratings: (A) "Action," meaning severe disease that requires urgent, disease-modifying therapy; (B) "Beware," meaning moderate disease that demands close attention and, perhaps, modest therapy changes (C) *Content*, meaning mild, improving, or static disease requiring no treatment or only symptomatic therapy and (D) Absence of symptoms or laboratory abnormalities.

Ratings are given for each organ system based on the assessor's evaluation of the patient's clinical condition in the month leading up to the day of evaluation compared to the previous month.

BILAG 2004[6] was updated in order to address pitfalls in the original instrument that were discovered during its use in clinical trials, and also to include two additional organ systems that, although they involve relatively rare manifestations of lupus, would be important to record when they become active—the gastrointestinal and ophthalmic systems. The BILAG 2004 has been formally validated[7,8] and reliability was demonstrated by calculating intraclass correlation coefficients, which showed good agreement between physicians in the constitutional, mucocutaneous, neurological, cardiorespiratory, renal, ophthalmic, and hematological systems. The musculoskeletal system, however, did not score as well. It is possible that this particular issue is related to a new definition for arthritis, which requires a decreased range of motion in an affected joint. There may be some confusion among physicians about how literally to take this definition (e.g., it is unclear whether to count decreased range of motion due to pain) or whether decreased passive range of motion needs to be demonstrated objectively at the clinic visit.

The BILAG-2004 instrument retains the intent to treat principle of the original BILAG index. However, given the many reasons why patients may not actually receive a change of treatment when the degree of symptoms would usually justify this, the index now clearly specifies the difference between "intention" to treat and an actual change being made. For example, perhaps a new treatment was started a few weeks ago that takes time to achieve full effect, perhaps a patient refuses new or increased medications, or perhaps there are toxicity issues that, when weighted against the degree of risk or discomfort from a flare, mandate a delay in treatment increase. In all of these situations, there might not be an actual change in treatment at the visit, but the BILAG instructions have clarified that the degree of symptoms should still be scored according to the treatment that would have been considered in most circumstances.

The BILAG-2004 modified and/or elaborated definitions for disease severity categories. For comparable statistical comparison with other numerically based indices, the following weights are now recommended for assigning numerical scores to the four severity categories: A (severe disease) = 12; B (moderate disease) = 8; C (mild disease) = 1; and D or E (no activity) = 0. Because there are nine organ systems, each receiving a score of A, B, C, D, or E (the latter referring to organs in which there are no current symptoms, nor any in the past), the cumulative total disease activity score could theoretically range from 0 to 108, although patients with severe disease in more than two or three organ systems are likely to be critically ill. In practice, scores greater than 30 are rare.

A weakness of the BILAG Index, which is not shared by the SLEDAI, was mentioned above. If there is more than one manifestation within an organ system, only one (of the highest scoring features) counts. For example, if there are two active signs or symptoms within an organ and each could, by themselves engendering an A (severe) score, only one A is credited to the final organ score. Therefore, cumulative manifestations in an individual organ are lumped together. As another example, one could not differentiate a patient with one B (moderate) manifestation from a patient with 2 B and 1 C-qualifying manifestations when these occur within a single organ. Both situations simply render one B score for that organ.

The BILAG 2004 is sensitive to change,[9] which underscores its practical potential in longitudinal epidemiological studies and clinical trials. In a prospective multicenter study of 1761 assessments from 347 SLE patients, both composite and individual organ scores were examined. Regression models tested sensitivity to change of disease and change of therapy in consecutive visits. Not surprisingly, greater change in disease activity had better predictive power. A change in cumulative index scores was associated with changes in therapy, but this trend was less pronounced when evaluating individual organ scores. Not all A or B scores were accompanied by actual changes in treatment, even in the hands of these experts, justifying the decision to avoid making the intent-to-treat guideline proscriptive as opposed to using it as a landmark in the thought process determining severity. Despite these important individual exceptions, the association of changes in disease score with altered therapy remains strong, as confirmed by a more recent paper using an analysis of receiver operating characteristic (ROC) curves to demonstrate therapy changes longitudinally that were commensurate with degrees of worsening or improvement.[21]

The SLEDAI was developed at the University of Toronto.[3] Initially, an expert panel of physicians rated the importance, in their opinion, of a spectrum of variables in defining SLE activity. Using the highest-rated variables, patient case descriptions were written and rheumatologists were asked to rank the severity of disease in each case. Regression models were applied to derive consensus weights for each variable in contributing to lupus activity as had been ranked by this group. Real patients were then used in a study comparing the scoring of this measure with the physician's global assessment. The resulting index is a straightforward, one-page form with 24 items, each with a brief definition provided on the form. Scoring is easy to master because it is calculated by a simple cumulative sum

of the predetermined weights for each item. Items that were considered by experts to usually be severe when occurring in most patients were given higher weights. In theory, possible total scores could vary from zero to 105, but it is rare in actual practice for a patient to score higher than 20. Although the SLEDAI avoids the pitfall in the BILAG of subsuming all manifestations within an organ into one score, the SLEDAI cannot distinguish partial improvement or worsening of symptoms. Furthermore, some disorders such as thrombocytopenia, which is usually a benign condition, receive a low score whenever it occurs, even in the rare cases when it is life-threatening. Similarly, mild arthritis receives the same score as severe arthritis, and mild rash receives the same score as severe rash.

Two modifications of the original SLEDAI are in wide use. The Safety of Estrogens in Lupus Erythematosus-National Assessment (SELENA)-SLEDAI was adapted from the SLEDAI for use in studies of exogenous hormone safety in women with SLE.[22,23] The main purpose in its development was to provide clarifications to some descriptors of the original SLEDAI. Scleritis and episcleritis were added to the visual disturbance definition. Pleurisy and pericarditis scoring no longer required objective proof, such as electrocardiogram or echocardiogram evidence. Several definitions were changed to ensure that ongoing disease activity would count, not just worsening activity. The only exception to this was the proteinuria descriptor, which retained the requirement of the original SLEDAI that it must be substantially worsening in order to score. This was unfortunate because proteinuria that is unchanged or minimally improving after a month would suddenly seem to disappear. The second SLEDAI modification, the SLEDAI-2K,[24] was devised by the original SLEDAI group in Toronto. It is similar to the SELENA-SLEDAI but not identical. The major advantage of it is that the definition for proteinuria was simplified to count any proteinuria >500 mg per 24 h as long as it could be attributed to active lupus disease.

The SLEDAI-2K was validated against the original SLEDAI in prediction of mortality and in the scoring of global disease activity in a study of 960 Toronto patients. Both versions predicted mortality equally well (p = 0.0001).[24] The subsequent study that validated the use of the SLEDAI-2K for monthly assessments found almost complete agreement between the 10-day and 30-day assessments.[18] This outcome suggests that it may be unusual to have a symptom present within 1 month of a clinical visit and then have complete resolution by 10 days before that visit. However, in an international year-long trial of 800 or 900 patients, this could potentially occur often enough to miss transient disease flares if using only the 10-day version.

Despite a long list of theoretically promising treatments that have been in development for lupus over several decades, so far only one, belimumab, demonstrated efficacy in two pivotal trials, gaining widespread regulatory approval and availability to patients.[16,17] However, differences between treatment and placebo response rates, even in these trials, were modest. Attempts to explain the disappointing results of most clinical trials in lupus have pointed, at least in part, to pitfalls in clinical outcome measures.[10–13] Various recommendations have been endorsed by SLE trialists, EULAR, ACR, OMERACT and the U.S. Food and Drug Administration,[10–13,25–31] with general agreement that ideal endpoints should simultaneously identify improvement and worsening if they occur in different organs, as well as discern acute lupus disease activity from chronic damage and from changes related to other causes. Many have endorsed a proposal by the OMERACT group that patient-reported outcomes should be given a prominent role in endpoints.[28,29]

All of these conditions could not be met using either the SLEDAI or the BILAG index alone. Both instruments have been modified over time to avoid confusing damage with disease activity, and, as summarized in Table 1, each has strengths and weaknesses. Patient-reported outcomes are not included in either instrument and must currently be evaluated separately in trials, with measurement milestones constructed so that they cannot be directly compared with those of the clinician. The BILAG can be problematic because, as mentioned before, different symptoms within one organ are not captured additively in its organ-based scoring system, and gradations between mild, moderate, and severe disease are restricted by limited threshold definitions. The SLEDAI cannot detect either worsening in previously active symptoms or concurrent improvement and worsening in different organs; however, a newer version, called the SRI-50 has been adapted so that a given descriptor or symptom will decrease by half of its score when there is 50% or greater improvement.[32,33] The high threshold for 50% improvement and the consistency of directional scoring are likely to be quite useful, but the accuracy of this expanded SLEDAI at picking up relative degrees of improvement from patient to patient is necessarily limited by the restrictiveness of the original scoring system in assigning a set value to each active manifestation regardless of the original severity. For example a≥50% improvement from four modestly active tender and swollen joints decreases the score by 2 points because all arthritis at baseline is scored 4 points regardless of severity. In a different patient, a much >50% improvement from a severe, painful, burning, scarring discoid rash to a very mild inconsequential rash (without complete resolution) decreases the score by only 1 point because all rashes at baseline receive 2 points, regardless of severity.

TABLE 1 Comparison of BILAG and SLEDAI

	SLEDAI	SLEDAI Pitfalls	BILAG	BILAG Pitfalls
Basis of score	Consensus of experts on the most common severity of a given symptom	Very mild rash scores 2 points. Extremely severe rash scores 2 points. A patient with mild arthritis in 2 small joints gets 4 points and a patient with severe, weeping discoid rash on 30% of the body surface area receives 2 points	Actual current severity can influence score, but this advantage is limited a little by incremental thresholds for scoring	Significant arthritis in one joint is a moderate "B" score. If this worsens to 12 joints but does not impair activities of daily life, it remains a "B" score. If it does interefere with ADL, it will increase to a severe "A" score
Type of score	Each symptom listed is scored separately	Some important SLE symptoms are missing and never counted (e.g., hemolytic anemia, interstitial lung disease, myocarditis, gastrointestinal serositis, severe constitutional symptoms such as weight loss or lymphadenopathy)	Scores for individual features are summed into a single score for each organ system, but only the most severe feature is counted, additional symptoms do not add to the score	A patient with moderate rash, moderate cutaneous vasculitis, and mild oral ulcers receives the same score (a moderate "B" score) as one with only a mild rash that meets threshold definition for "B"
Landmark of score	Disease Activity over the past 10 days or past month	Changes in symptoms during the month is not accounted for	Disease Activity over the past month	Adjusts for changes in symptoms over the month
Ease of scoring and interpretation	Relatively easy	Certain rules and definitions remain critically important and are sometimes overlooked by those who do not take training	Relatively difficult	Once mastered, the BILAG index is easy to perform and interpret and with training, its less likely important caveats are overlooked

Both the SLEDAI and the BILAG are known to fall short when used as single endpoints in trials.[34–36] This has led to the use of composite endpoints of improvement. The composite SLE Responder Index (SRI) was developed[14] based on a post-hoc analysis of data from a failed phase II study of belimumab, and the BILAG-based Composite Lupus Assessment (BICLA)[15] was developed for Phase II studies of epratuzumab. These compound measures are similar to each other by requiring improvement on one instrument (the SLEDAI or BILAG, respectively) coupled to no worsening by other measures. Direct comparison of BICLA and SRI has been addressed only by preliminary studies,[27,37] but each index is known to have significant shortfalls, based largely on their use of SLEDAI or BILAG to define improvement. The SRI, which uses the SLEDAI to measure improvement, cannot capture partial response in a given feature, requires a near total remission in at least one symptom, and cannot differentiate between resolution of only one symptom and resolution of all symptoms. The BICLA (using BILAG to rate improvement) requires only partial improvement as the increment of response, but some response must be present in all organs active at baseline, so that one relatively minor feature that does not improve can negate major response in one or several different symptoms.[27]

Both compound endpoints also incorporate imperfect definitions for disease worsening, missing some clinically significant flares, and allowing minor fluctuations in disease to overrule a clinically meaningful response. Attempts to devise more accurate flare indices have also fallen short. The classic SELENA-SLEDAI Flare Index was originally developed specifically for the Safety of Estrogens in Lupus Erythematosus National Assessment (SELENA) study,[22,23] with the aim of very sensitively capturing flares of all types as well as distinguishing severe flares. Mild and moderate flares are not discriminated at all with this instrument—an important limitation in assessing drug efficacy—as is the tiny incremental threshold separating moderate from severe flares.[38] A novel organ-based instrument to rate mild, moderate, and severe flares has been proposed by the SELENA study group (revised SELENA Flare index).[39] This instrument has rare use in clinical trials and its validation process was impeded by a poor performance in a comparative study with a new BILAG-based flare index, which itself rendered only imperfect agreement with expert clinician consensus when evaluating the degree of flare in clinic patients.[39]

The disappointing results of the BILAG flare index could be due to the inability to identify flares in multiple symptoms within an organ.[11] The SELENA index may be inhibited by proscriptive rules requiring certain medication changes that are not always given in practice.[11] Finally, the restrictive threshold definitions in both instruments appear to confuse the degree of disease severity with the degree of worsening so that a small incremental change can be rated as a severe flare if it does cross the threshold, whereas a major worsening might be rated as a moderate flare if it falls slightly short of that threshold.

In summary, the outcomes of lupus treatment trials have been difficult to interpret because of pitfalls in the design of instruments used to measure improvement and worsening. What is lacking in the current state of the art is a simple, scaleable instrument that can accurately measure improvement or worsening on an organ-specific or global level, and can be used to derive either a continuous endpoint (mean or median change) or dichotomous endpoint (percent of patients who achieve a certain degree of change). Table 2 summarizes features that could be addressed in a differential manner for different clinical trial designs by an instrument scaled to real-world outcomes, where there is a natural tension between sensitivity to change and the height of the bar defining improvement.

The Lupus Foundation of America Rapid Evaluation of Activity in Lupus (LFA REAL) system has been tested in preliminary form in patients in two clinics.[40] Although still early in development and yet to be validated, the concept of this instrument is simple and potentially versatile. Based

TABLE 2 Discriminating an Effective Treatment from Placebo in Trials: Shaded Areas May Indicate Optimal Trial Designs

Features of Outcome Measure	Sensitive to Change/Low Bar for Efficacy	Less Sensitive to Change/High Bar for Efficacy
Impact of more aggressive background and rescue treatments	Placebo group response may be as high as treatment group	Placebo group less likely to meet response criteria than with low bar for efficacy and active treatment group more likely to respond to a high bar with sustaining background treatment on board
Impact of less aggressive background and rescue treatments	Placebo group less likely to respond than with more aggressive background treatment, response in active treatment group would increase with low bar for efficacy versus a high bar	Placebo group responses should be fully minimized here, but response in active treatment group will also be decreased with a high bar for efficacy

on a series of additive, organ-specific linear scales, the LFA REAL might, due to the ease of scoring, be used effectively both in international clinical trials and in busy clinical practices. Unlike any previous instrument, it is being designed to include certain scales to directly compare some aspects of a clinician's assessment with those of the patient.

With measurements obtained along a sensitive, continuous scale, outcome increments could be directly scaled for dichotomous endpoints directly derived from changes in disease of real-world lupus patients. Different degrees of discrimination could be tested for discriminatory capacity optimized for different trial designs. This addresses two critical gaps in evidence: (1) Although endpoints in use for lupus today have been tested on live patients after they were created, none was originally scaled into meaningful increments of clinical change by using the evaluation of real-world patients or by incorporating patient-reported endpoints. (2) Different increments of improvement are likely to be optimal for different trial types. In trials designed to allow aggressive background treatments, dichotomous increments that are less sensitive to change will raise the threshold for response and decrease the chances of placebo group response rates. In trials with limited background medications, placebo group responses will already, by design, be decreased, and response rates to an effective treatment can be optimally separated with a more sensitive increment.

Using a real-world scaleable instrument, it should be possible to derive an evidence base to determine optimal increments of change suitable for these different trial designs.

Despite the fact that the current standard of care for lupus is universally acknowledged to be inadequate, clinical trials in lupus have been failing, creating a bottleneck in new treatment development. A major gap in evidence required to improve the interpretability of lupus trials is represented by the following variables that need to be determined: (1) Optimal increments of change reflecting clinically meaningful improvement, (2) Appropriate increments of change delineating mild, moderate, and severe flares, and (3) Increments of change determining appropriate sensitive versus stringent endpoints for different trial designs. Current outcome measures were validated in real-world clinics but their cutoffs for waxing or waning disease were based on educated opinion and never scaled to real patients. The proposed development of the LFA REAL system could potentially address this evidence gap.

REFERENCES

1. Thanou A, Merrill JT. Top 10 things to know about lupus activity measures. *Curr Rheumatol Rep* 2013;**15**:334–6.
2. Yee CS, Farewell V, Isenberg DA, Griffiths B, Teh LS, Bruce IN, et al. The BILAG-2004 index is sensitive to change for assessment of SLE disease activity. *Rheumatology (Oxford)* 2009;**48**:691–5.
3. Gladman DD, Goldsmith CH, Urowitz MB, Bacon PA, Bombardier C, Isenberg D, et al. Crosscultural validation and reliability of three disease activity indices in systemic lupus erythematosus. *J Rheumatol* 1992;**19**:608–11.
4. Gladman DD, Goldsmith CH, Urowitz MB, Bacon PA, Bombardier C, Isenberg D, et al. Sensitivity to change of three SLE disease activity indices: international validation. *J Rheumatol* 1994;**21**:14568–71.
5. Yee CS, Farewell V, Isenberg DA, Prabu A, Sokoll K, Teh LS, et al. Revised British Isles Lupus Assessment Group 2004 index: a reliable tool for assessment of systemic lupus erythematosus activity. *Arthritis Rheum* 2006;**54**:3300–5.
6. Isenberg DA, Rahman A, Allen E, Farewell V, Akil M, Bruce IN, et al. BILAG 2004. Development and initial validation of an updated version of the British Isles Lupus Assessment Group's disease activity index for patients with systemic lupus erythematosus. *Rheumatology (Oxford)* 2005;**44**:902–6.
7. Yee CS, Farewell V, Isenberg DA, Rahman A, Teh LS, Griffiths B, et al. British Isles Lupus Assessment Group 2004 index is valid for assessment of disease activity in systemic lupus erythematosus. *Arthritis Rheum* 2007;**56**:4113–9.
8. Yee CS, Farewell V, Isenberg DA, Griffiths B, Teh LS, Bruce IN, et al. The BILAG-2004 index is sensitive to change for assessment of SLE disease activity. *Rheumatology (Oxford)* 2009;**48**:691–5.
9. Buyon JP, Petri MA, Kim MY, Kalunian KC, Grossman J, Hahn BH, et al. The effect of combined estrogen and progesterone hormone replacement on disease activity in systemic lupus erythematosus: a randomized trial. *Ann Intern Med* 2005;**142**:953–62.
10. Bruce IN, Gordon C, Merrill JT, Isenberg D. Clinical trials in lupus: what have we learned so far? *Rheumatology (Oxford)* 2010;**49**(6):1025–7.
11. Thanou A, Chakravarty E, James JA, Merrill JT. How should lupus flares be measured? Deconstruction of the safety of estrogen in lupus erythematosus national assessment-systemic lupus erythematosus disease activity index flare index. *Rheumatology (Oxford)* 2014;**53**:2175–81.
12. Thanou A, Merrill JT. Treatment of systemic lupus erythematosus: new therapeutic avenues and blind alleys. *Nat Rev Rheumatol* 2014;**10**:23–34.
13. Steinman L, Merrill JT, McInnes IB, Peakman M. Optimization of current and future therapy for autoimmune diseases. *Nat Med* 2012;**18**:59–65.
14. Furie RA, Petri MA, Wallace DJ, Ginzler EM, Merrill JT, Stohl W, et al. Novel evidence-based systemic lupus erythematosus responder index. *Arthritis Rheum* 2009;**61**(9):1143–51.
15. Wallace D, Strand V, Furie R, Petri M, Kalunian K, Pike M, et al. Evaluation of treatment success in systemic lupus erythematosus clinical trials: development of the british isles lupus assessment group-based composite lupus assessment endpoint. *Arthritis Rheum* 2011;**63**(Suppl. 10):S894.
16. Navarra SV, Guzmán RM, Gallacher AE, Hall S, Levy RA, BLISS-52 Study Group, et al. Efficacy and safety of belimumab in patients with active systemic lupus erythematosus: a randomised, placebo-controlled, phase 3 trial. *Lancet* 2011;**377**(9767):721–31.
17. Furie R, Petri M, Zamani O, Cervera R, Wallace DJ, BLISS-76 Study Group, et al. A phase III, randomized, placebo-controlled study of belimumab, a monoclonal antibody that inhibits B lymphocyte stimulator, in patients with systemic lupus erythematosus. *Arthritis Rheum* 2011;**63**(12):3918–30.
18. Touma Z, Gladman DD, Ibanez D, Urowitz MB. SLEDAI-2K Responder Index 50 captures 50% improvement in disease activity over 10 years. *Lupus* 2012;**21**(12):1305–11.

19. Ginzler EM, Wallace DJ, Merrill JT, Furie RA, Stohl W, LBSL02/99 Study Group, et al. Disease control and safety of belimumab plus standard therapy over 7 years in patients with systemic lupus erythematosus. *J Rheumatol* 2014;**41**(2):300–9.

20. Hay EM, Bacon PA, Gordon C, Isenberg DA, Maddison P, Snaith ML, et al. The BILAG index: a reliable and valid instrument for measuring clinical disease activity in systemic lupus erythematosus. *Q J Med* 1993;**86**(7):447–58.

21. Yee CS, Gordon C, Isenberg DA, Griffiths B, Teh LS, Bruce IN, et al. The BILAG-2004 systems tally–a novel way of representing the BILAG-2004 index scores longitudinally. *Rheumatology (Oxford)* 2012;**51**(11):2099–105.

22. Petri M, Kim MY, Kalunian KC, Grossman J, Hahn BH, Sammaritano LR, et al. Combined oral contraceptives in women with systemic lupus erythematosus. *N Eng J Med* 2005;**15**(353):2550–8.

23. Buyon JP, Petri MA, Kim MY, Kalunian KC, Grossman J, Hahn BH, et al. The effect of combined estrogen and progesterone hormone replacement therapy on disease activity in systemic lupus erythematosus: a randomized trial. *Ann Intern Med* 2005;**142**(12 Pt 1):953–62.

24. Gladman DD, Ibanez D, Urowitz MB. Systemic lupus erythematosus disease activity index 2000. *J Rheumatol* 2002;**29**:288–91.

25. Merrill JT, Buyon JP. Connective tissue diseases: what does the death of Riquent hold for the future of SLE? *Nat Rev Rheumatol* 2009;**5**(6):306–7.

26. Merrill JT, Erkan D, Buyon JP. Challenges in bringing the bench to bedside in drug development for SLE. *Nat Rev Drug Discov* 2004;**3**(12):1036–46.

27. Thanou A, Chakravarty E, James JA, Merrill JT. Which outcome measures in SLE clinical trials best reflect medical judgment? *Lupus Sci Med* 2014;**1**(1):e000005.

28. Gordon C, Bertsias G, Ioannidis PA, Boletis J, et al. EULAR points to consider for conducting clinical trials in systemic lupus erythematosus. *Ann Rheum Dis* 2009;**68**:470–6.

29. Smolen JS, Strand V, Cardiel M, Edworthy S, Furst D, Gladman D, et al. Randomized clinical trials and longitudinal observational studies in systemic lupus erythematosus: consensus on a preliminary core set of outcome domains. *J Rheumatol* 1999;**26**(2):504–7.

30. *Guidance for industry systemic lupus erythematosus developing medical products for treatment.* US Dept of Health and Human Services Food and Drug Administration; June 2010. http://www.fda.gov/downloads/drugs/guidancecomplianceregulatoryinformation/guidances/ucm072063.pdf.

31. American College of Rheumatology Ad Hoc Committee on systemic lupus erythematosus clinical trials: measures of overall disease activity. *Arthritis Rheum* 2004;**50**:3418–26.

32. Touma Z, Gladman DD, Ibañez D, Taghavi-Zadeh S, Urowitz MB. Systemic Lupus Erythematosus Disease Activity Index 2000 Responder Index-50 enhances the ability of SLE Responder Index to identify responders in clinical trials. *J Rheumatol* 2011;**38**(11):2395–9.

33. Touma Z, Urowitz MB, Taghavi-Zadeh S, Ibañez D, Gladman DD. Systemic lupus erythematosus disease activity Index 2000 Responder Index 50: sensitivity to response at 6 and 12 months. *Rheumatology (Oxford)* 2012;**51**(10):1814–9.

34. Wallace DJ, Stohl W, Furie RA, Lisse JR, McKay JD, Merrill JT, et al. A phase II, randomized, double-blind, placebo-controlled, dose-ranging study of belimumab in patients with active systemic lupus erythematosus. *Arthritis Rheum* 2009;**61**:1168–78.

35. Merrill JT, Neuwelt CM, Wallace DJ, Shanahan JC, Latinis KM, Oates JC, et al. Efficacy and safety of rituximab in patients with moderately-to-severely active systemic lupus erythematosus (SLE): results from the randomized, double-blind phase II/III study EXPLORER. *Arthritis Rheum* 2010;**62**:222–33.

36. Merrill JT, Burgos-Vargas R, Westhovens R, Chalmers A, D'Cruz D, Wallace DJ, et al. The efficacy and safety of abatacept in patients with non-life-threatening manifestations of SLE: results of a 12-month exploratory study. *Arthritis Rheum* 2010;**62**:3077–87.

37. Petri M, Pike MC, Kelley L, Kilgallen B, Gordon C. Systemic lupus erythematosus responder Index assessment of responders in EMBLEM, a phase IIb study in patients with moderate to severe systemic lupus erythematosus. *Arthritis Rheum* 2011;**63**(Suppl. 10):S548.

38. Ruperto N, Hanrahan LM, Alarcon GS, Belmont HM, Brey RL, Brunetta P, et al. International consensus for a definition of disease flare in lupus. *Lupus* 2011;**20**(5):453–62.

39. Isenberg DA, Allen E, Farewell V, D'Cruz D, Alarcon GS, Aranow C, et al. An assessment of disease flare in patients with systemic lupus erythematosus: a comparison of BILAG 2004 and the flare version of SELENA. *Ann Rheum Dis* 2011;**70**(1):54–9.

40. Askanase A, Li X, Pong A, Shum K, Kamp S, Carthen F, et al. Preliminary test of the LFA rapid evaluation of activity in lupus (LFA-REAL™): a more efficient outcome measure correlates with validated instruments. Lupus Sci Med, in press.

Chapter 5

Disease Development and Outcomes

Mary Mahieu[1], Dafna Gladman[2], Rosalind Ramsey-Goldman[1]

[1]*Northwestern University Feinberg School of Medicine, Chicago, IL, USA;* [2]*University of Toronto, Toronto, ON, Canada*

HISTORICAL PERSPECTIVE

Systemic lupus erythematosus (SLE) is a disease of exacerbations and remissions with variable course and prognosis. There were no criteria to classify SLE before the early 1970s, and no standardized method to evaluate disease activity, flares, or remissions existed until the 1980s. SLE patients had a poor prognosis with a 5-year survival rate of only 55% in 1955.[1] Corticosteroid treatment was introduced in 1948, the same year the lupus erythematosus (LE) cell test for SLE was discovered.[2] In the following decades, antimetabolite and cytotoxic therapy for lupus nephritis became available. These early milestones facilitated the earlier diagnosis and treatment of SLE.

Approximately 10 years after the discovery of the LE cell test, the introduction of fluorescent antinuclear antibody (ANA) testing led to a new emphasis on laboratory diagnosis of SLE through ANA determination. A positive ANA test was initially thought to be synonymous with active disease.[3] It was later recognized that a positive ANA, especially at low titers, has high sensitivity but low specificity for SLE. An estimated 32 million persons in the United States have a positive ANA,[4] and one-third of persons with autoimmune thyroid disease are ANA-positive.[5] The description of anti-DNA antibodies and lowered serum complement levels allowed more precise and earlier detection of SLE disease onset and flares.[6] The American College of Rheumatology (ACR) subsequently developed SLE classification criteria that included more autoantibody systems.[7] These criteria, while not intended to replace clinical judgment in diagnosing SLE, provided a framework for considering a diagnosis of SLE.

In the 1970s, it was noted that some patients with clinical features of SLE were ANA-negative.[8] Case series of ANA-negative patients suggest a higher frequency of photosensitive rash and milder renal and central nervous system (CNS) disease than ANA-positive patients. Disease manifestations and course in patients with undetectable ANA may otherwise be typical of classical SLE. Many of these patients have measurable autoantibodies to extractable nuclear antigens, especially anti-SSA/Ro and anti-SSB/La.[8]

ANA-negative disease among persons with complement deficiency is also well described.[9]

Another group of patients with "latent" or "incomplete" lupus has been identified. These patients present with suggestive symptoms but lack key clinical features of classic SLE.[10] For example, incomplete lupus patients will exhibit one or two of the ACR classification criteria plus other nonspecific clinical characteristics, such as fever, fatigue, headache, lymphadenopathy, or neuropathy. Laboratory abnormalities may also exist, including hypergammaglobulinemia, increased erythrocyte sedimentation rate, or depressed complement. Only a minority of these patients (approximately 20%) will develop classic SLE, and the presence of anti-DNA, oral ulcers, and proteinuria or cellular casts are independent predictors of developing definite lupus.[11] Patients with incomplete lupus often have a milder disease course.

Two subsets of SLE patients with discordant clinical symptoms and serologic profile have been described. First, patients may have serologically active and clinically quiescent (SACQ) disease. In the Toronto Lupus Clinic cohort, 6.1% of patients remained serologically active but without clinical activity for 3 years on average.[12] These patients took less steroids and immunosuppressants, and they accrued less damage compared to matched controls.[12,13] Thus, active surveillance without treatment during a SACQ period may be appropriate. In contrast, patients may have clinically active and serologically quiescent (CASQ) disease, with severe lupus manifestations requiring aggressive treatment despite a lack of serologic markers.[14] Knowing whether a patient is concordant or discordant with clinical symptoms and serology will facilitate optimal disease monitoring and clinical care.

CLINICAL MANIFESTATIONS

SLE is characterized by multiorgan involvement, a wide spectrum of manifestations, and an unpredictable clinical course (Box 5.1). The dynamic nature of the disease with intermittent signs and symptoms can make the diagnosis particularly challenging. Other diseases with multisystem

Systemic Lupus Erythematosus. http://dx.doi.org/10.1016/B978-0-12-801917-7.00005-X

Box 5.1 Spectrum of Disease Manifestations in SLE

- Constitutional: Fever, weight loss, lymphadenopathy, fatigue.
- Mucocutaneous: Photosensitivity, acute lupus rash (e.g., malar, bullous), subacute cutaneous lupus rash, chronic lupus rash (e.g., discoid, panniculitis), oral or nasal ulcers, alopecia.
- Musculoskeletal: Arthralgia, arthritis, tendonitis, myalgia, myositis.
- Cardiopulmonary: Pleurisy, pericarditis, myocarditis, endocarditis, inflammatory lung disease.
- Peripheral vascular: Raynaud phenomenon, vasculitis, thrombophlebitis.

- Renal: Proteinuria, hematuria, renal insufficiency, hypertension, nephritis on renal biopsy.
- Hematologic: Hemolytic anemia, leukopenia, lymphopenia, thrombocytopenia.
- Neurologic: Cognitive impairment, acute confusional state, seizure, stroke, aseptic meningitis, transverse myelitis, peripheral neuropathy, unremitting headache (unresponsive to narcotics).
- Gastrointestinal: Serositis, bowel ischemia, pancreatitis, hepatitis.
- Immunologic: Presence of ANA, anti-DNA, anti-Smith, anticardiolipin, lupus anticoagulant, false-positive serologic test for syphilis, positive Coombs test, low complement.

---

involvement may mimic SLE. An extended observation period is often necessary before making a definite diagnosis.

Skin disease and arthritis are common manifestations, but any organ system may be involved in variable combinations. SLE may have diverse clinical presentations such as rash, arthritis, pleurisy, proteinuria, Raynaud phenomenon, seizures, or fever of unknown origin. The diagnosis will only be recognized with a high index of suspicion, a careful history and physical examination, and appropriate laboratory confirmation.

Neuropsychiatric dysfunction and renal disease are two critical SLE manifestations. The spectrum of neuropsychiatric abnormalities potentially related to SLE is broad, including seizure, stroke, cognitive impairment, or myelopathy.[15] Lupus renal disease also has variable expression, histopathology, and clinical course. Virtually all persons with SLE display some degree of glomerular pathology by renal biopsy, but only 50% have clinically apparent disease. Early detection of lupus nephritis is crucial, because early intervention may prevent or delay progression to end-stage renal disease.

Constitutional complaints such as fever, overwhelming fatigue, and weight loss are frequent but nonspecific manifestations of SLE. The presence of these symptoms does not aid in diagnosing disease or recognizing disease flare because they are just as likely to result from other medical problems, such as infection or fibromyalgia (see Chapter 37 for further discussion).

ASSESSMENT OF DISEASE ACTIVITY

A number of validated instruments have been developed to measure disease activity, which should be assessed at every visit (see Chapter 4 for a full discussion.) The clinician must distinguish whether signs and symptoms are attributable to active lupus, chronic damage, comorbidity, or drug toxicity.

Some commonly-used disease activity indices are the SLE Disease Activity Index revised in 2000 (SLEDAI-2K), the Systemic Lupus Activity Measure (SLAM), the European

Consensus Lupus Activity Measurement (ECLAM), and the British Isles Lupus Assessment Group index (BILAG).[16,17] The BILAG index takes into account changes in disease activity compared to the prior assessment. However, the BILAG may be cumbersome to complete in a busy practice setting. SLAM is frequently utilized in observational studies, but a disadvantage is scoring based on patient-led reporting of symptoms. SLEDAI, ECLAM, and BILAG have all been employed in clinical trials. Composite disease activity indices have also been used in clinical trials, including the SLEDAI-based SLE Responder Index (SRI) and S2K-RI-50 version and the BILAG-based Combined Lupus Assessment (BICLA).[16,18]

Other indices are used to identify the presence of disease flare. The Safety of Estrogens in Lupus Erythematosus National Assessment-SLEDAI (SELENA-SLEDAI) Flare Index (SFI) was developed for clinical trials to distinguish the presence of mild, moderate, or severe flare. Minimally important differences for changes in SLEDAI-2K or BILAG scores have been proposed to indicate flare.[16]

DISEASE DAMAGE

Damage from recurrent disease activity and treatment also impact the health status of SLE patients (Box 5.2). The Systemic Lupus International Collaborating Clinics (SLICC) group, in conjunction with the ACR, developed a damage index for SLE. The SLICC/ACR Damage Index (SDI) measures damage accrual from disease onset and is scored irrespective of attribution to SLE.[19] The SDI has been validated and used in numerous studies. SDI scores also predict mortality.[20,21] The damage index is an important outcome measure for evaluating the prognosis and long-term effects of SLE disease activity and treatment.

Damage accumulates during the first 5 years after diagnosis of SLE despite decreasing disease activity.[22] Older age at disease onset, longer disease duration, male sex, and degree of disease activity at presentation and over time

Box 5.2 Spectrum of Disease Damage in SLE

- Musculoskeletal damage, including deformity from inflammatory joint disease and avascular necrosis, commonly results in loss of functional status.
- Cardiovascular complications occur late in disease but earlier than in the general population.
- Lupus nephritis is the most serious complication with potential for disease damage.

- Neuropsychiatric problems typically occur early in disease course and may be difficult to diagnose or attribute to SLE.
- Up to 50% of patients will be ill with at least one serious infection.
- A small association between SLE and malignancy exists, primarily with an increased risk of non-Hodgkin lymphoma.

all contribute to disease damage.[23] Certain ethnic groups, including African, Chinese, and Hispanic patients, are at higher risk for damage accrual.[21,23] Poverty is also independently associated with disease damage and mortality.[24] Organ-specific disease is prognostic, with the most damage accrual from renal and neuropsychiatric lupus.[23] Finally, HCQ use is protective against disease damage, while corticosteroids and immunosuppressant treatment correlate with damage accumulation.[23] These data on medications must be interpreted cautiously because escalation of treatment is also indicative of more active disease.

Major areas of disease damage include cardiovascular, renal, CNS, musculoskeletal, osteoporosis, infection, and malignancy.

Cardiovascular disease: Fatal and nonfatal cardiovascular events, including myocardial infarction and stroke, are increasingly reported in longitudinal lupus cohorts. Rates of traditional cardiovascular disease risk factors such as smoking, obesity, hypertension, hypercholesterolemia, and diabetes mellitus are similar in SLE compared to the general population.[25] However, myocardial infarction and stroke rates are increased in SLE, even after adjusting for the effect of traditional cardiovascular disease risk factors.[26] SLE appears to be a risk factor for the development of accelerated atherosclerosis.

Renal complications: Lupus nephritis is an important determinant of morbidity and mortality in SLE patients. Clinically relevant kidney disease occurs in about half of patients. Up to 17% of these patients develop renal failure requiring dialysis or transplantation.[27] Lupus nephritis tends to develop early in the disease course, but it can newly develop even late after diagnosis.[28]

Neuropsychiatric dysfunction: Neuropsychiatric complications occur in 13–24% of SLE patients and usually present early in the disease course. Manifestations can be characterized by chronicity (acute or chronic) and localization (central or peripheral; focal or diffuse).[15] Diffuse cerebral dysfunction presents with an affective disorder, psychosis, or coma. Myelopathy is an example of focal involvement. Headache is commonly reported in SLE patients, although rarely is it directly attributable to active SLE. Recurrent involvement of the CNS may result in organic brain syndrome and dementia.

Musculoskeletal complications: Nearly every patient with SLE will have musculoskeletal complaints during the disease course. Synovitis and tendon damage lead to joint deformity. Osteonecrosis is a complication of active SLE or treatment that often necessitates joint replacement surgery.[29] Osteoporosis is a late complication, with an estimated prevalence near 20%. Risk factors for osteoporosis include high disease activity, vitamin D deficiency from sun avoidance, early menopause from use of cytotoxic therapy, and corticosteroid use.

Infections: At least 50% of patients have one or more serious infections during the course of their disease. The spectrum of infections is related to disease severity, treatment, and endemic organisms.[30]

Malignancy: Persons with SLE are at increased risk of cancer compared to the general population. In one multicenter cohort study, SLE patients had an increased risk of hematologic malignancy and cancer of the vulva, lung, and thyroid.[31,32] The mechanism of this risk is unknown. One hypothesis is that the immune dysregulation inherent in the pathogenesis of SLE increases susceptibility to cancer. However, disease activity has failed to correlate with development of lymphoma in that cohort.[32] Impaired tumor surveillance from corticosteroids and immunosuppressants is another proposed mechanism. There was a suggestion of increased lymphoma in cyclophosphamide or high cumulative steroid treatments. No increased risk related to prior immunosuppressant use was found.[32]

PATIENT-REPORTED OUTCOMES

A patient-reported outcome (PRO) refers to an assessment of a patient's health condition that comes directly from the individual (see Chapter 6 for further discussion). PROs are increasingly recognized as an important aspect of clinical practice and clinical trials. Many PRO instruments evaluate both global outcomes and specific quality-of-life domains. Examples of generic PRO instruments employed in SLE studies are the Short-Form 36 (SF-36) and EuroQol 5-dimension. Domains assessed by PRO tools include fatigue (e.g., Fatigue Severity Scale), pain (e.g., McGill Pain Scale), depression (e.g., Hospital Anxiety and Depression Scale), and work productivity (Work Productivity and Activity

Impairment Questionnaire:Lupus).[33] There is also interest in using the Patient-Reported Outcome Measures Information System (PROMIS) instruments in SLE assessment.[34]

A variety of SLE-specific PRO tools have been developed to assess important SLE experiences that may be underemphasized or missed by generic tools, such as fatigue, pain, and emotional well-being.[33] Examples of lupus-specific instruments include the Lupus Quality of Life (LupusQoL) and the Lupus Patient-Reported Outcome (LupusPRO). In one study, LupusQoL was equivalent to the generic SF-36 for measuring quality of life over time.[35]

MORTALITY

Patient survival has improved in recent decades, and SLE is now considered to be a chronic disease. In the 1950s, only 50% of patients survived for 2 years. More recent international cohorts identified 5- and 10-year survival rates of 80–90% and 70–90%, respectively, for SLE patients in Europe,[36] Pakistan,[37] and the Asia–Pacific region,[38] including China[39,40] and Thailand.[41] The 4-year survival in a Latin American cohort was 95%.[42]

Treatment advances, including the widespread use of dialysis, corticosteroids, immunosuppressive agents, improved antihypertensive therapy, and advancements in vaccinations and antibiotic therapy to mitigate infection, have improved survival. Earlier diagnosis and inclusion of milder cases in studies from recent decades have also led to the appearance of increased survival. However, a full understanding for this survival trend remains unclear. A prospective cohort study from Toronto demonstrated improved survival over a 36-year period, but disease-related variables (adjusted for mean SLEDAI, SDI, coronary artery disease, and osteonecrosis) only partially explained this trend.[43] Most importantly, SLE patients still have a 2–3 times higher mortality than the general population.[31,43]

CAUSES OF DEATH

Death in SLE patients can be caused by disease activity, damage, treatment, or comorbidities. The mortality trend is bimodal in SLE. Death within 5 years of diagnosis most commonly results from infection and disease activity, such as CNS vasculitis or acute renal disease.[31,39] Cardiovascular disease, other organ failure (especially renal), and possibly malignancy are major late causes of death.[31,37–40] Treatment for SLE may result in fatal complications such as fulminant infection or peptic ulcer disease with bowel perforation.

Certain aspects of SLE itself affect prognosis, including time between symptom onset and diagnosis and changes in disease expression over time. Disease activity and damage are other critical prognostic factors. Higher SLEDAI score at diagnosis[39] and higher SDI score one year after diagnosis[40] are independent predictors of mortality. Specific organ manifestations also impact mortality. Renal involvement is

especially crucial,[37,41] with the LUMINA (Lupus in Minorities, Nature vs. Nurture) study determining that renal damage is the most important predictor of mortality within the SDI.[44] Hematologic abnormalities, serositis, infection, and CNS disease also correlate with increased mortality.[37,40,41]

Other factors that influence mortality are not directly related to the disease process, including race/ethnicity, SES, sex, and age:

Race/Ethnicity: Important geographic and racial/ethnic differences in SLE mortality have been reported. In the SLICC cohort, the standardized mortality rate was nearly twice as high for blacks with SLE compared to whites.[31] SLE survival rates are also lower in Australian Aborigines[38] and Pakistanis[37] than in Europeans and Chinese. In the United States, the incidence and prevalence of SLE is higher in blacks, Native Americans, and Alaskan natives than in whites. The frequency of end-stage renal disease is also higher in blacks than in Native Americans or whites.[45–47] Genetic differences that influence disease course and mortality likely exist between racial/ethnic groups, but it is difficult to separate these from economic and environmental confounders.

Socioeconomic status (SES): SES influences disease outcome in a complex interplay with race/ethnicity. Poverty is associated with ethnic minority status in the United States and other countries, and some have argued that poverty is a more important determinant of SLE-related mortality than race/ethnicity.[48] The LUMINA study showed that Hispanics and African-Americans have the highest SLE mortality, but this difference was not significant when statistical models adjusted for poverty.[48] Similarly, lupus nephritis prevalence is higher among all racial/ethnic minority groups than Whites in the United States, but the prevalence is highest in regions with the lowest SES.[49] SES also impacts access to care. Public health insured patients travel farther to see a physician for SLE care than private insured patients.[50] Lower education and medical insurance type, considered surrogate markers of SES, were also associated with increased mortality in a Latin American cohort.[42]

Sex: SLE is more common in women, but men tend to have accelerated and more severe damage.[51] Whether men have higher mortality than women due to SLE remains controversial. In the SLICC cohort, females had a higher standardized mortality ratio than males.[31] However, male sex was associated with increased mortality in other United States and Chinese cohorts.[39,52]

Age: Reports are also conflicting as to whether age at disease onset impacts mortality. Onset of disease in the pediatric age group has been associated with worse prognosis, with an increased risk of lupus nephritis and mortality in juvenile-onset compared to adult-onset SLE.[53] However, an older age at diagnosis of adult SLE is associated with greater organ damage and predicts mortality.[39,54]

TREATMENT GUIDELINES AND QUALITY INDICATORS

As awareness of the association between disease damage accumulation and increased mortality has grown, there has been a movement toward developing SLE treatment guidelines. These guidelines aim to provide a framework for achieving disease remission, preventing disease damage, and improving quality of life. Recommendations for the treatment of lupus nephritis and neuropsychiatric lupus have been published,[55,56] and a "treat-to-target" approach for management of lupus has been proposed.[57]

A set of quality indicators has been established to assess the quality of care that SLE patients receive from health care providers.[58,59] These quality indicators range from counseling on sun avoidance to reproductive issues. Subsequent investigations revealed that achievement of some quality indicators was poor, with important disparities in care. Most patients were counseled about sun avoidance, but only 29% reported an assessment of cardiovascular risk factors. Racial/ethnic minorities and low-income patients were less likely to receive the recommended health care. Factors associated with the health care system (including type of insurance) were primary determinants of performance on quality measures.[60]

CONCLUSIONS

Outcomes in SLE patients have changed over the years. Decreased survival was initially from disease activity. Medical treatment advances have led to improved survival, but SLE patients still have a three times higher risk of death than the general population. The trend toward improved survival is also counterbalanced by accrual of organ damage. Physicians must adequately address disease activity and minimize disease damage. Inclusion of patient-reported outcomes in the assessment of disease control has also become a priority. Clinicians should be aware of SLE treatment guidelines and quality indicators to guide management of SLE, with the goals of mitigating disease damage and improving patient outcomes.

REFERENCES

1. Merrell M, Shulman LE. Determination of prognosis in Chronic disease, illustrated by systemic lupus erythematosus. *J chronic Dis* 1955;**1**(1):12–32.
2. Hargraves MM, Richmond H, Morton R. Presentation of two bone marrow elements; the tart cell and the L.E. cell. *Proc Staff Meet Mayo Clin* 1948;**23**(2):25–8.
3. Notman DD, Kurata N, Tan EM. Profiles of antinuclear antibodies in systemic rheumatic diseases. *Ann Intern Med* 1975;**83**(4):464–9.
4. Satoh M, Chan EK, Ho LA, Rose KM, Parks CG, Cohn RD, et al. Prevalence and sociodemographic correlates of antinuclear antibodies in the United States. *Arthritis Rheum* 2012;**64**(7):2319–27.
5. Tektonidou MG, Anapliotou M, Vlachoyiannopoulos P, Moutsopoulos HM. Presence of systemic autoimmune disorders in patients with autoimmune thyroid diseases. *Ann Rheum Dis* 2004;**63**(9):1159–61.
6. Schur PH, Sandson J. Immunologic factors and clinical activity in systemic lupus erythematosus. *N Engl J Med* 1968;**278**(10):533–8.
7. Hochberg MC. Updating the American College of Rheumatology revised criteria for the classification of systemic lupus erythematosus. *Arthritis Rheum* 1997;**40**(9):1725.
8. Gladman DD, Chalmers A, Urowitz MB. Systemic lupus erythematosus with negative LE cells and antinuclear factor. *J Rheumatol* 1978;**5**(2):142–7.
9. Vandersteen PR, Provost TT, Jordon RE, McDuffie FC. C2 deficient systemic lupus erythematosus: its association with anti-Ro (SSA) antibodies. *Arch Dermatol* 1982;**118**(8):584–7.
10. Swaak AJ, van de Brink H, Smeenk RJ, Manger K, Kalden JR, Tosi S, et al. Incomplete lupus erythematosus: results of a multicentre study under the supervision of the EULAR Standing Committee on International Clinical Studies Including Therapeutic Trials (ESCISIT). *Rheumatol Oxf Engl* 2001;**40**(1):89–94.
11. Al Daabil M, Massarotti EM, Fine A, Tsao H, Ho P, Schur PH, et al. Development of SLE among "potential SLE" patients seen in consultation: long-term follow-up. *Int J Clin Pract* 2014;**68**(12):1508–13.
12. Steiman AJ, Gladman DD, Ibanez D, Urowitz MB. Prolonged serologically active clinically quiescent systemic lupus erythematosus: frequency and outcome. *J Rheumatol* 2010;**37**(9):1822–7.
13. Steiman AJ, Gladman DD, Ibanez D, Urowitz MB. Outcomes in patients with systemic lupus erythematosus with and without a prolonged serologically active clinically quiescent period. *Arthritis Care Res* 2012;**64**(4):511–8.
14. Gladman DD, Hirani N, Ibanez D, Urowitz MB. Clinically active serologically quiescent systemic lupus erythematosus. *J Rheumatol* 2003;**30**(9):1960–2.
15. ACR Ad Hoc Committee on Neuropsychiatric Lupus Nomenclature. The American College of Rheumatology. *Arthritis Rheum* 1999;**42**(4):599–608.
16. Nuttall A, Isenberg DA. Assessment of disease activity, damage and quality of life in systemic lupus erythematosus: new aspects. *Best Pract Res Clin Rheumatol* 2013;**27**(3):309–18.
17. Romero-Diaz J, Isenberg D, Ramsey-Goldman R. Measures of adult systemic lupus erythematosus: updated version of British Isles Lupus Assessment Group (BILAG 2004), European Consensus Lupus Activity Measurements (ECLAM), Systemic Lupus Activity Measure, Revised (SLAM-R), Systemic Lupus Activity Questionnaire for population studies (SLAQ), Systemic Lupus Erythematosus Disease Activity Index 2000 (SLEDAI-2K), and Systemic Lupus International Collaborating Clinics/American college of Rheumatology Damage Index (SDI). *Arthritis Care Res* 2011;**63**(Suppl 11):S37–46.
18. Touma Z, Gladman DD, Ibanez D, Taghavi-Zadeh S, Urowitz MB. Systemic Lupus Erythematosus Disease Activity Index 2000 Responder Index-50 enhances the ability of SLE Responder Index to identify responders in clinical trials. *J Rheumatol* 2011;**38**(11):2395–9.
19. Gladman D, Ginzler E, Goldsmith C, Fortin P, Liang M, Urowitz M, et al. The development and initial validation of the Systemic Lupus International Collaborating Clinics/American College of Rheumatology damage index for systemic lupus erythematosus. *Arthritis Rheum* 1996;**39**(3):363–9.
20. Urowitz MB, Gladman DD. Measures of disease activity and damage in SLE. *Bailliere's Clin Rheumatol* 1998;**12**(3):405–13.
21. Bruce IN, O'Keeffe AG, Farewell V, Hanly JG, Manzi S, Su L, et al. Factors associated with damage accrual in patients with systemic lupus erythematosus: results from the Systemic Lupus International Collaborating Clinics (SLICC) Inception Cohort. *Ann Rheum Dis* 2014;**74**(9):1706–13.

22. Urowitz MB, Gladman DD, Ibanez D, Fortin PR, Bae SC, Gordon C, et al. Evolution of disease burden over five years in a multicenter inception systemic lupus erythematosus cohort. *Arthritis Care Res* 2012;**64**(1):132–7.

23. Sutton EJ, Davidson JE, Bruce IN. The systemic lupus international collaborating clinics (SLICC) damage index: a systematic literature review. *Semin Arthritis Rheum* 2013;**43**(3):352–61.

24. Alarcon GS, McGwin Jr G, Bastian HM, Roseman J, Lisse J, Fessler BJ, et al. Systemic lupus erythematosus in three ethnic groups. VII [correction of VIII]. Predictors of early mortality in the LUMINA cohort. LUMINA Study Group. *Arthritis Rheum* 2001;**45**(2):191–202.

25. Manzi S, Meilahn EN, Rairie JE, Conte CG, Medsger Jr TA, Jansen-McWilliams L, et al. Age-specific incidence rates of myocardial infarction and angina in women with systemic lupus erythematosus: comparison with the Framingham Study. *Am J Epidemiol* 1997;**145**(5):408–15.

26. Esdaile JM, Abrahamowicz M, Grodzicky T, Li Y, Panaritis C, du Berger R, et al. Traditional Framingham risk factors fail to fully account for accelerated atherosclerosis in systemic lupus erythematosus. *Arthritis Rheum* 2001;**44**(10):2331–7.

27. Adler M, Chambers S, Edwards C, Neild G, Isenberg D. An assessment of renal failure in an SLE cohort with special reference to ethnicity, over a 25-year period. *Rheumatol Oxf Engl* 2006;**45**(9):1144–7.

28. Peschken CA, Esdaile JM. Systemic lupus erythematosus in North American Indians: a population based study. *J Rheumatol* 2000;**27**(8):1884–91.

29. Zhu KK, Xu WD, Pan HF, Zhang M, Ni J, Ge FY, et al. The risk factors of avascular necrosis in patients with systemic lupus erythematosus: a meta-analysis. *Inflammation* 2014;**37**(5):1852–64.

30. Gladman DD, Hussain F, Ibanez D, Urowitz MB. The nature and outcome of infection in systemic lupus erythematosus. *Lupus* 2002;**11**(4):234–9.

31. Bernatsky S, Boivin JF, Joseph L, Manzi S, Ginzler E, Gladman DD, et al. Mortality in systemic lupus erythematosus. *Arthritis Rheum* 2006;**54**(8):2550–7.

32. Bernatsky S, Ramsey-Goldman R, Joseph L, Boivin JF, Costenbader KH, Urowitz MB, et al. Lymphoma risk in systemic lupus: effects of disease activity versus treatment. *Ann Rheum Dis* 2014;**73**(1):138–42.

33. Holloway L, Humphrey L, Heron L, Pilling C, Kitchen H, Hojbjerre L, et al. Patient-reported outcome measures for systemic lupus erythematosus clinical trials: a review of content validity, face validity and psychometric performance. *Health Qual Life Outcomes* 2014;**12**(1):116.

34. Ow YL, Thumboo J, Cella D, Cheung YB, Yong Fong K, Wee HL. Domains of health-related quality of life important and relevant to multiethnic English-speaking Asian systemic lupus erythematosus patients: a focus group study. *Arthritis Care Res* 2011;**63**(6):899–908.

35. Touma Z, Gladman DD, Ibanez D, Urowitz MB. Is there an advantage over SF-36 with a quality of life measure that is specific to systemic lupus erythematosus? *J Rheumatol* 2011;**38**(9):1898–905.

36. Manger K, Manger B, Repp R, Geisselbrecht M, Geiger A, Pfahlberg A, et al. Definition of risk factors for death, end stage renal disease, and thromboembolic events in a monocentric cohort of 338 patients with systemic lupus erythematosus. *Ann Rheum Dis* 2002;**61**(12):1065–70.

37. Rabbani MA, Habib HB, Islam M, Ahmad B, Majid S, Saeed W, et al. Survival analysis and prognostic indicators of systemic lupus erythematosus in Pakistani patients. *Lupus* 2009;**18**(9):848–55.

38. Jakes RW, Bae SC, Louthrenoo W, Mok CC, Navarra SV, Kwon N. Systematic review of the epidemiology of systemic lupus erythematosus in the Asia-Pacific region: prevalence, incidence, clinical features, and mortality. *Arthritis Care Res* 2012;**64**(2):159–68.

39. Wu G, Jia X, Gao D, Zhao Z. Survival rates and risk factors for mortality in systemic lupus erythematosus patients in a Chinese center. *Clin Rheumatol* 2014;**33**(7):947–53.

40. Mok CC, Mak A, Chu WP, To CH, Wong SN. Long-term survival of southern Chinese patients with systemic lupus erythematosus: a prospective study of all age-groups. *Medicine* 2005;**84**(4):218–24.

41. Kasitanon N, Louthrenoo W, Sukitawut W, Vichainun R. Causes of death and prognostic factors in Thai patients with systemic lupus erythematosus. *Asian Pac J Allergy Immunol* 2002;**20**(2):85–91.

42. Pons-Estel BA, Catoggio LJ, Cardiel MH, Soriano ER, Gentiletti S, Villa AR, et al. The GLADEL multinational Latin American prospective inception cohort of 1214 patients with systemic lupus erythematosus: ethnic and disease heterogeneity among "Hispanics". *Medicine* 2004;**83**(1):1–17.

43. Urowitz MB, Gladman DD, Tom BD, Ibanez D, Farewell VT. Changing patterns in mortality and disease outcomes for patients with systemic lupus erythematosus. *J Rheumatol* 2008;**35**(11):2152–8.

44. Danila MI, Pons-Estel GJ, Zhang J, Vila LM, Reveille JD, Alarcon GS. Renal damage is the most important predictor of mortality within the damage index: data from LUMINA LXIV, a multiethnic US cohort. *Rheumatol Oxf Engl* 2009;**48**(5):542–5.

45. Somers EC, Marder W, Cagnoli P, Lewis EE, DeGuire P, Gordon C, et al. Population-based incidence and prevalence of systemic lupus erythematosus: the Michigan Lupus Epidemiology and Surveillance program. *Arthritis Rheumatol* 2014;**66**(2):369–78.

46. Lim SS, Bayakly AR, Helmick CG, Gordon C, Easley KA, Drenkard C. The incidence and prevalence of systemic lupus erythematosus, 2002–2004: the Georgia Lupus Registry. *Arthritis Rheumatol* 2014;**66**(2):357–68.

47. Ferucci ED, Johnston JM, Gaddy JR, Sumner L, Posever JO, Choromanski TL, et al. Prevalence and incidence of systemic lupus erythematosus in a population-based registry of American Indian and Alaska Native people, 2007–2009. *Arthritis Rheumatol* 2014;**66**(9):2494–502.

48. Fernandez M, Alarcon GS, Calvo-Alen J, Andrade R, McGwin Jr G, Vila LM, et al. A multiethnic, multicenter cohort of patients with systemic lupus erythematosus (SLE) as a model for the study of ethnic disparities in SLE. *Arthritis Rheum* 2007;**57**(4):576–84.

49. Feldman CH, Hiraki LT, Liu J, Fischer MA, Solomon DH, Alarcon GS, et al. Epidemiology and sociodemographics of systemic lupus erythematosus and lupus nephritis among US adults with Medicaid coverage, 2000–2004. *Arthritis Rheum* 2013;**65**(3):753–63.

50. Gillis JZ, Yazdany J, Trupin L, Julian L, Panopalis P, Criswell LA, et al. Medicaid and access to care among persons with systemic lupus erythematosus. *Arthritis Rheum* 2007;**57**(4):601–7.

51. Andrade RM, Alarcon GS, Fernandez M, Apte M, Vila LM, Reveille JD. Accelerated damage accrual among men with systemic lupus erythematosus: XLIV. Results from a multiethnic US cohort. *Arthritis Rheum* 2007;**56**(2):622–30.

52. Tan TC, Fang H, Magder LS, Petri MA. Differences between male and female systemic lupus erythematosus in a multiethnic population. *J Rheumatol* 2012;**39**(4):759–69.

53. Amaral B, Murphy G, Ioannou Y, Isenberg DA. A comparison of the outcome of adolescent and adult-onset systemic lupus erythematosus. *Rheumatol Oxf Engl* 2014;**53**(6):1130–5.

54. Maddison P, Farewell V, Isenberg D, Aranow C, Bae SC, Barr S, et al. The rate and pattern of organ damage in late onset systemic lupus erythematosus. *J Rheumatol* 2002;**29**(5):913–7.

55. Hahn BH, McMahon MA, Wilkinson A, Wallace WD, Daikh DI, Fitzgerald JD, et al. American College of Rheumatology guidelines for screening, treatment, and management of lupus nephritis. *Arthritis Care Res* 2012;**64**(6):797–808.

56. Bertsias GK, Ioannidis JP, Aringer M, Bollen E, Bombardieri S, Bruce IN, et al. EULAR recommendations for the management of systemic lupus erythematosus with neuropsychiatric manifestations: report of a task force of the EULAR standing committee for clinical affairs. *Ann Rheum Dis* 2010;**69**(12):2074–82.

57. van Vollenhoven RF, Mosca M, Bertsias G, Isenberg D, Kuhn A, Lerstrom K, et al. Treat-to-target in systemic lupus erythematosus: recommendations from an international task force. *Ann Rheum Dis* 2014;**73**(6):958–67.

58. Yazdany J, Panopalis P, Gillis JZ, Schmajuk G, MacLean CH, Wofsy D, et al. A quality indicator set for systemic lupus erythematosus. *Arthritis Rheum* 2009;**61**(3):370–7.

59. Gillis JZ, Panopalis P, Schmajuk G, Ramsey-Goldman R, Yazdany J. Systematic review of the literature informing the systemic lupus erythematosus indicators project: reproductive health care quality indicators. *Arthritis Care Res* 2011;**63**(1):17–30.

60. Yazdany J, Trupin L, Tonner C, Dudley RA, Zell J, Panopalis P, et al. Quality of care in systemic lupus erythematosus: application of quality measures to understand gaps in care. *J Gen Intern Med* 2012;**27**(10):1326–33.

Chapter 6

Socioeconomic Aspects of Systemic Lupus Erythematosus

Luis A. González-Naranjo[1], Manuel F. Ugarte-Gil[2,3], Graciela S. Alarcón[4]

[1]Division of Rheumatology, Department of Internal Medicine, School of Medicine, Universidad de Antioquia, Medellín, Colombia;

[2]Servicio de Reumatología, Hospital Nacional Guillermo Almenara Irigoyen, EsSalud, Lima, Peru; [3]Universidad Científica del Sur, Lima, Peru;

[4]Department of Medicine, Division of Clinical Immunology and Rheumatology, School of Medicine, The University of Alabama at Birmingham, Birmingham, AL, USA

SUMMARY

Lower socioeconomic status (SES) can affect systemic lupus erythematosus (SLE) outcomes by several possible mechanisms, such as inadequate access to quality care services, communication barriers, and malnutrition. SES should be systematically measured at the individual level (education, income, and occupation), as well as at the household and neighborhood levels. Lower SES has been associated with higher disease activity, mainly over the disease course, higher damage accrual, mortality, and disability. Furthermore, outcome differences between Caucasians and non-Caucasians are partially explained by socioeconomic factors. The association between non-Caucasian ethnicities and lower SES makes genetic and environmental risks difficult to disentangle.

DEFINITION AND MEASURES OF SOCIOECONOMIC STATUS

Socioeconomic status (SES) includes resource- and prestige-based measures, which can be measured at three levels (individual, household, and neighborhood) and at different points in the lifespan (e.g., infancy, childhood, adolescence, and adult). Resource-based measures include assets such as income, wealth, and educational credentials; prestige-based measures refer to the individual's rank in the social hierarchy.[1]

SES can be assessed through individual measures (education level, income, occupation)[2–4] and through composite measures that combine them to provide an overall SES level index.[3] The choice of SES measure(s) should relate to the research question and proposed mechanism linking SES to the outcome being investigated, but this is rarely done.[2,4]

PROBLEMS WITH MEASURING SES IN HEALTH RESEARCH

Measuring SES in health studies has some problems that could affect research findings. Thus, some critiques have emerged[4]:

- *Education and income are not interchangeable*. Education level is frequently used as a proxy for income or overall SES. When education and income are available, researchers may hesitate to use both because of possible colinearity; the correlation between these measures, however, does not justify this action.[4]
- *Inadequacy of occupational status measurements*. Measurements of occupational status may lack accuracy, particularly when dealing with manual and nonmanual work categories. More meaningful classifications are needed to obtain information on how occupation may affect health.[4]
- *Past socioeconomic experiences*. Childhood SES may influence health independently of adult SES,[4–6] but this is rarely considered.
- *Neighborhood socioeconomic conditions*. The place of residence is related to social position and ethnicity. People's health is influenced by their neighborhood's socioeconomic characteristics above and beyond her or his own individual-level SES.[4] However, few health studies measure neighborhood-level along with individual-level SES measures.
- *Variability over time of the SES variables*. No feature of SES is completely reliable or stable over time. The most stable measure of SES is the level of education because most patients have completed schooling prior to disease onset, and this level cannot decline.[7]

Systemic Lupus Erythematosus. http://dx.doi.org/10.1016/B978-0-12-801917-7.00006-1

IMPACT OF SES ON SYSTEMIC LUPUS ERYTHEMATOSUS OUTCOMES

Diverse studies have studied the relationship between SES and systemic lupus erythematosus (SLE) features/outcomes, including disease activity,[7–13] organ damage,[14–18] lupus nephritis (LN),[19–26] and mortality.[27–29] Most of these studies found poorer outcomes among those with lower SES.

DISEASE ACTIVITY

The relationship between lower SES and greater disease activity and even poorer mental health has been reported in SLE.[7–13] This may relate to inadequate access to quality care or the patients being unaware of an impending flare. Communication barriers compromise a patient's understanding of his or her disease, its complications, and medication adherence. Lower SES may also be associated with high disease activity due inadequate nutrition.[8] Conversely, individuals with higher education and private insurance or Medicare were more likely to be above poverty levels and having less active disease at SLE diagnosis.[7] In turn, high disease activity contributes to lower SES because of disability, missed work, and decreased earning potential.[25]

In many areas of the world, and particularly in the United States, ethnic minorities characteristically have poorer SES than the Caucasian majority,[30] probably due to their poor literacy levels, inadequate health-related knowledge and beliefs, inadequate social support, limited access to health care, missed appointments and treatment nonadherence, discrepant perception of disease activity by patient and physician, lower education level, and limited language proficiency.[31]

In the LUMINA (Lupus in Minorities: Nature versus Nurture) study, a multiethnic longitudinal outcome of disease activity was higher among ethnic minorities (African-Americans and Hispanics from Texas), who had a lower SES than the Caucasian majority.[9,10,32] Noteworthy, data from the LUMINA cohort demonstrated the importance of genetic factors contributing to disease activity at disease onset while socioeconomic, behavioral, and psychological variables exerted a more important role on disease activity over the disease course.[9,10,32]

The contribution of neighborhood SES to SLE outcomes, over and above the contribution of individual-level SES, was assessed in the Lupus Outcomes Study. In this study, lower individual SES, measured by education, household income, or poverty status, was associated with greater disease activity (measured by the Systemic Lupus Activity Questionnaire), poorer physical functioning, and greater depressive symptomatology. Neighborhood-level SES was reflective of the individual's SES, but it did not reach statistical significance in adjusted analyses for SLE disease activity.[12]

The influence of place of residence (i.e., rural vs urban) in SLE was addressed in the multi-ethnic Latin American cohort (GLADEL, *Grupo Latino Americano De Estudio del Lupus*). Patients residing in rural areas were more frequently Mestizo, of lower SES and educational level, and had inadequate medical insurance, more active disease at diagnosis, and renal disease over time even after adjusting for pertinent variables. These data suggest that rural Latin American residents may have inadequate access to specialized care and to social services; consequently, they present to the rheumatologist only when the disease is evident and active.[33] In the same cohort, Mestizos and African Latin Americans had lower SES, fewer years of formal education, and less accessibility to medical care than Caucasians—variables that were associated with higher levels of disease activity.[13]

DAMAGE ACCRUAL

Poverty and lack of education have been linked to the accrual of damage.[13–18] In LUMINA, factors associated with damage accrual were Hispanic ethnicity, older age, poverty, lack of health insurance, acute disease onset, ACR criteria number and disease activity at diagnosis, maximum glucocorticoid dose, higher helplessness levels, poor social support, and having HLA-DRB1*01. Hispanics may have accrued more damage due to ethnic-related differences in health care.[14]

On the other hand, in a Canadian multiethnic cohort (Caucasians 62%, Asians (19%), Afro-Caribbean (9%), and Aboriginal (5%)) older age, longer disease duration, prednisone and cyclophosphamide treatment, higher disease activity, and low income (despite equal access to health insurance) but no ethnicity were significant predictors of damage accrual.[17]

In the population-based case-control Carolina Lupus Study of recently diagnosed SLE patients, the association between sociodemographic variables and total and organ specific damage measures was examined. African-American ethnicity and lower income were associated with total damage scores and with higher renal, cardiovascular, musculoskeletal, skin damage and diabetes.[18]

The relationship between SES, race, psychosocial factors, and damage was studied in the United Kingdom. Non-Caucasian patients with longer disease duration, lower education level, and higher disease activity were more likely to develop organ damage. In addition, patients with lower education level were more likely to be not working due to their lupus.[15] Finally, in the GLADEL cohort, damage was associated with medium SES and inadequate medical coverage; urban residence was protective.[13]

DISABILITY

Work disability has important effects on an individual and his or her family, and this is particularly true in diseases with early onset, like SLE. Work disability among SLE patients ranges between 15% and 50%, in patients with 3–15 years of follow-up.[34] Work disability increased during the follow-up, being 15% 5-years after diagnosis, and 36%, 51%, and 63% 10-, 15-, and 20-years after diagnosis.[35] In addition to disease activity and damage,[34] disability has been associated with several features, including African-American ethnicity,[36] poverty,[37] lower education level,[15,35,36,38] and lower local employment rate.[38] Furthermore, jobs with increased physical or psychosocial demands and low job control are associated with a higher risk of work disability,[35] lower job tenure,[39] and decision latitude,[40] suggesting that less educated and skilled patients are even at higher risk for disability.

MORTALITY

Survival in SLE patients has improved over the last 60 years; however, survival among Caucasians is still higher than among non-Caucasians.[41] Furthermore, the difference between mortality in Caucasian and African-American patients is even higher than for all-cause mortality in the United States.[42] Similar results were found for Asians compared to Caucasians.[43] Noteworthy, with the exception of Duke's cohort,[44] ethnicity is not associated with mortality after adjusting for socioeconomic factors such as educational level,[13] poverty,[27,29,44] and health insurance.[13,29] Genetic and environmental risk are difficult to disentangle because some associations are common[26]; however, it is important to point out that among US patients with lupus nephritis, including those with end-stage renal disease, Hispanics and Asians had lower mortality rates than Caucasians.[45,46] Several hypotheses have been proposed; however, a definitive explanation about this paradox is still missing.

CONCLUSIONS

Lower SES is associated with high SLE disease activity because these patients may not have access to quality care for SLE, be aware that certain symptoms indicate an SLE flare, have inadequate transportation to clinic visits, and lack resources—all contributing to poor medication adherence and inadequate nutrition. Damage accrual has been shown to be higher among patients with lower SES than among those with higher SES. Work disability is associated with lower education level, lower SES, and jobs with higher physical and/or mental demands. Non-Caucasian patients have a higher mortality rate; however, this seems to be related mainly to socioeconomic factors, such as poverty and lower level of education.

REFERENCES

1. Krieger N, Williams DR, Moss NE. Measuring social class in US public health research: concepts, methodologies, and guidelines. *Annu Rev Public Health* 1997;**18**:341–78.
2. Galobardes B, Shaw M, Lawlor DA, Lynch JW, Davey Smith G. Indicators of socioeconomic position (part 1). *J Epidemiol Community Health* 2006;**60**(1):7–12.
3. Galobardes B, Shaw M, Lawlor DA, Lynch JW, Davey Smith G. Indicators of socioeconomic position (part 2). *J Epidemiol Community Health* 2006;**60**(2):95–101.
4. Braveman PA, Cubbin C, Egerter S, Chideya S, Marchi KS, Metzler M, et al. Socioeconomic status in health research: one size does not fit all. *JAMA* 2005;**294**(22):2879–88.
5. Rahkonen O, Lahelma E, Huuhka M. Past or present? Childhood living conditions and current socioeconomic status as determinants of adult health. *Soc Sci Med* 1997;**44**(3):327–36.
6. Lynch JW, Kaplan GA, Salonen JT. Why do poor people behave poorly? Variation in adult health behaviours and psychosocial characteristics by stages of the socioeconomic lifecourse. *Soc Sci Med* 1997;**44**(6):809–19.
7. Karlson EW, Daltroy LH, Lew RA, Wright EA, Partridge AJ, Roberts WN, et al. The independence and stability of socioeconomic predictors of morbidity in systemic lupus erythematosus. *Arthritis Rheum* 1995;**38**(2):267–73.
8. Karlson EW, Daltroy LH, Lew RA, Wright EA, Partridge AJ, Fossel AH, et al. The relationship of socioeconomic status, race, and modifiable risk factors to outcomes in patients with systemic lupus erythematosus. *Arthritis Rheum* 1997;**40**(1):47–56.
9. Alarcon GS, Roseman J, Bartolucci AA, Friedman AW, Moulds JM, Goel N, et al. Systemic lupus erythematosus in three ethnic groups: II. Features predictive of disease activity early in its course. LUMINA Study Group. Lupus in minority populations, nature versus nurture. *Arthritis Rheum* 1998;**41**(7):1173–80.
10. Alarcon GS, Calvo-Alen J, McGwin Jr G, Uribe AG, Toloza SM, Roseman JM, et al. Systemic lupus erythematosus in a multiethnic cohort: LUMINA XXXV. Predictive factors of high disease activity over time. *Ann Rheum Dis* 2006;**65**(9):1168–74.
11. Alarcon GS, McGwin Jr G, Sanchez ML, Bastian HM, Fessler BJ, Friedman AW, et al. Systemic lupus erythematosus in three ethnic groups. XIV. Poverty, wealth, and their influence on disease activity. *Arthritis Rheum* 2004;**51**(1):73–7.
12. Trupin L, Tonner MC, Yazdany J, Julian LJ, Criswell LA, Katz PP, et al. The role of neighborhood and individual socioeconomic status in outcomes of systemic lupus erythematosus. *J Rheumatol* 2008;**35**(9):1782–8.
13. Pons-Estel BA, Catoggio LJ, Cardiel MH, Soriano ER, Gentiletti S, Villa AR, et al. The GLADEL multinational Latin American prospective inception cohort of 1,214 patients with systemic lupus erythematosus: ethnic and disease heterogeneity among "Hispanics". *Medicine* 2004;**83**(1):1–17.
14. Alarcon GS, McGwin Jr G, Bartolucci AA, Roseman J, Lisse J, Fessler BJ, et al. Systemic lupus erythematosus in three ethnic groups. IX. Differences in damage accrual. *Arthritis Rheum* 2001;**44**(12):2797–806.
15. Sutcliffe N, Clarke AE, Gordon C, Farewell V, Isenberg DA. The association of socio-economic status, race, psychosocial factors and outcome in patients with systemic lupus erythematosus. *Rheumatology* 1999;**38**(11):1130–7.

16. Lotstein DS, Ward MM, Bush TM, Lambert RE, van Vollenhoven R, Neuwelt CM. Socioeconomic status and health in women with systemic lupus erythematosus. *J Rheumatol* 1998;**25**(9):1720–9.

17. Peschken CA, Katz SJ, Silverman E, Pope JE, Fortin PR, Pineau C, et al. The 1000 Canadian faces of lupus: determinants of disease outcome in a large multiethnic cohort. *J Rheumatol* 2009;**36**(6): 1200–8.

18. Cooper GS, Treadwell EL, St Clair EW, Gilkeson GS, Dooley MA. Sociodemographic associations with early disease damage in patients with systemic lupus erythematosus. *Arthritis Rheum* 2007;**57**(6):993–9.

19. Feldman CH, Hiraki LT, Liu J, Fischer MA, Solomon DH, Alarcon GS, et al. Epidemiology and sociodemographics of systemic lupus erythematosus and lupus nephritis among US adults with Medicaid coverage, 2000-2004. *Arthritis Rheum* 2013;**65**(3):753–63.

20. Bastian HM, Roseman JM, McGwin Jr G, Alarcon GS, Friedman AW, Fessler BJ, et al. Systemic lupus erythematosus in three ethnic groups. XII. Risk factors for lupus nephritis after diagnosis. *Lupus* 2002;**11**(3):152–60.

21. Costenbader KH, Desai A, Alarcon GS, Hiraki LT, Shaykevich T, Brookhart MA, et al. Trends in the incidence, demographics, and outcomes of end-stage renal disease due to lupus nephritis in the US from 1995 to 2006. *Arthritis Rheum* 2011;**63**(6):1681–8.

22. Ward MM. Access to care and the incidence of endstage renal disease due to systemic lupus erythematosus. *J Rheumatol* 2010;**37**(6):1158–63.

23. Alarcon GS, Bastian HM, Beasley TM, Roseman JM, Tan FK, Fessler BJ, et al. Systemic lupus erythematosus in a multi-ethnic cohort (LUMINA) XXXII: [corrected] contributions of admixture and socioeconomic status to renal involvement. *Lupus* 2006;**15**(1):26–31.

24. Barr RG, Seliger S, Appel GB, Zuniga R, D'Agati V, Salmon J, et al. Prognosis in proliferative lupus nephritis: the role of socio-economic status and race/ethnicity. *Nephrol Dial Transpl* 2003;**18**(10):2039–46.

25. Petri M, Perez-Gutthann S, Longenecker JC, Hochberg M. Morbidity of systemic lupus erythematosus: role of race and socioeconomic status. *Am J Med* 1991;**91**(4):345–53.

26. Sanchez E, Rasmussen A, Riba L, Acevedo-Vasquez E, Kelly JA, Langefeld CD, et al. Impact of genetic ancestry and sociodemographic status on the clinical expression of systemic lupus erythematosus in American Indian-European populations. *Arthritis Rheum* 2012;**64**(11):3687–94.

27. Kasitanon N, Magder LS, Petri M. Predictors of survival in systemic lupus erythematosus. *Medicine* 2006;**85**(3):147–56.

28. Krishnan E. Hospitalization and mortality of patients with systemic lupus erythematosus. *J Rheumatol* 2006;**33**(9):1770–4.

29. Ward MM, Pyun E, Studenski S. Long-term survival in systemic lupus erythematosus. Patient characteristics associated with poorer outcomes. *Arthritis Rheum* 1995;**38**(2):274–83.

30. Gonzalez LA, Toloza SM, Alarcon GS. Impact of race and ethnicity in the course and outcome of systemic lupus erythematosus. *Rheum Dis Clin North Am* 2014;**40**(3):433–54. vii–viii.

31. Uribe AG, Alarcon GS. Ethnic disparities in patients with systemic lupus erythematosus. *Curr Rheumatol Rep* 2003;**5**(5):364–9.

32. Reveille JD, Moulds JM, Ahn C, Friedman AW, Baethge B, Roseman J, et al. Systemic lupus erythematosus in three ethnic groups: I. The effects of HLA class II, C4, and CR1 alleles, socioeconomic factors, and ethnicity at disease onset. LUMINA Study Group. Lupus in minority populations, nature versus nurture. *Arthritis Rheum* 1998;**41**(7):1161–72.

33. Pons-Estel GJ, Saurit V, Alarcon GS, Hachuel L, Boggio G, Wojdyla D, et al. The impact of rural residency on the expression and outcome of systemic lupus erythematosus: data from a multiethnic Latin American cohort. *Lupus* 2012;**21**(13):1397–404.

34. Scofield L, Reinlib L, Alarcon GS, Cooper GS. Employment and disability issues in systemic lupus erythematosus: a review. *Arthritis Rheum* 2008;**59**(10):1475–9.

35. Yelin E, Trupin L, Katz P, Criswell L, Yazdany J, Gillis J, et al. Work dynamics among persons with systemic lupus erythematosus. *Arthritis Rheum* 2007;**57**(1):56–63.

36. Utset TO, Baskaran A, Segal BM, Trupin L, Ogale S, Herberich E, et al. Work disability, lost productivity and associated risk factors in patients diagnosed with systemic lupus erythematosus. *Lupus Sci Med* 2015;**2**(1):e000058.

37. Bertoli AM, Fernandez M, Alarcon GS, Vila LM, Reveille JD. Systemic lupus erythematosus in a multiethnic US cohort LUMINA (XLI): factors predictive of self-reported work disability. *Ann Rheum Dis* 2007;**66**(1):12–7.

38. Mau W, Listing J, Huscher D, Zeidler H, Zink A. Employment across chronic inflammatory rheumatic diseases and comparison with the general population. *J Rheumatol* 2005;**32**(4):721–8.

39. Yelin E, Tonner C, Kim SC, Katz JN, Ayanian JZ, Brookhart MA, et al. Sociodemographic, disease, health system, and contextual factors affecting the initiation of biologic agents in rheumatoid arthritis: a longitudinal study. *Arthritis Care Res (Hoboken)* 2014;**66**(7):980–9.

40. Al Dhanhani AM, Gignac MA, Beaton DE, Su J, Fortin PR. Work factors are associated with workplace activity limitations in systemic lupus erythematosus. *Rheumatology* 2014;**53**(11):2044–52.

41. Ippolito A, Petri M. An update on mortality in systemic lupus erythematosus. *Clin Exp Rheumatol* 2008;**26**(5 Suppl. 51):S72–9.

42. Krishnan E, Hubert HB. Ethnicity and mortality from systemic lupus erythematosus in the US. *Ann Rheum Dis* 2006;**65**(11):1500–5.

43. Kaslow RA. High rate of death caused by systemic lupus erythematosus among US residents of Asian descent. *Arthritis Rheum* 1982;**25**(4):414–8.

44. Studenski S, Allen NB, Caldwell DS, Rice JR, Polisson RP. Survival in systemic lupus erythematosus. A multivariate analysis of demographic factors. *Arthritis Rheum* 1987;**30**(12):1326–32.

45. Gomez-Puerta JA, Barbhaiya M, Guan H, Feldman CH, Alarcon GS, Costenbader KH. Racial/Ethnic variation in all-cause mortality among United States medicaid recipients with systemic lupus erythematosus: a Hispanic and asian paradox. *Arthritis Rheumatol* 2015;**67**(3):752–60.

46. Gomez-Puerta JA, Feldman CH, Alarcon GS, Guan H, Winkelmayer WC, Costenbader KH. Racial and ethnic differences in mortality and cardiovascular events among patients with end-stage renal disease due to lupus nephritis. *Arthritis Care Res (Hoboken)* 2015.

Chapter 7

Biomarkers in Systemic Lupus Erythematosus

Stacy P. Ardoin, Wael N. Jarjour

Ohio State University, Columbus, OH, USA

INTRODUCTION

Systemic lupus erythematosus (SLE) management remains challenging for several reasons: the remarkable heterogeneity in clinical presentation, the unpredictable disease course and treatment response, and the difficulty of early flare detection. A robust biomarker repertoire is needed, including diagnostic biomarkers that predict SLE in patients with ambiguous presentations, activity biomarkers that examine SLE disease activity and differentiate SLE flares from other disease processes, biomarkers detecting specific organ involvement, theranostics biomarkers predicting treatment response, and those identifying susceptibility to develop SLE.

BIOMARKER DEFINITION AND VALIDATION

The National Institute of Health (NIH) Biomarkers Definitions Working Group defines biomarkers as "a characteristic that is objectively measured and evaluated as an indicator of normal biological processes, pathogenic processes, or pharmacologic responses to a therapeutic intervention."[1] Biomarkers include genetic, biologic, biochemical, molecular, or imaging tests. Ideal biomarkers sensitively and accurately respond to changes in disease state; are pathophysiologically relevant, minimally invasive, simple, and cost effective enough for routine clinical practice; and are not impacted by comorbid conditions.

Phases of biomarker development are outlined in Table 1[1] and several (but not all, due to space constraints) proposed SLE biomarkers will be discussed in this chapter (see Table 2). Most of these biomarkers have been studied only in small patient populations or are limited to cross-sectional observations; however, biomarker vetting requires validation in large, multicenter studies. Biomarker detection methods include hypothesis-driven and "unbiased" approaches. With a hypothesis-driven approach, individual biomarkers are tested based upon biological plausibility and preliminary data. In unbiased approaches, samples from SLE patients are assessed for multiple markers simultaneously and analyzed to detect those that are differentially expressed, for example, during disease activity.

BIOMARKERS FOR DIAGNOSIS OF SLE

SLE diagnosis currently relies upon a combination of clinical features and laboratory tests. Classification criteria that incorporate clinical and laboratory findings identify patients for clinical trials and basic science investigations but have significant limitations when utilized in clinical practice.[2] Biomarkers widely used for SLE diagnosis include antinuclear antibodies (ANAs), anti-Smith antibodies, antibodies to double stranded DNA (anti-dsDNA), and levels of complement components C3, C4, CH50. ANAs are highly sensitive but lack specificity and have very little positive predictive value for SLE.[2,3] In contrast, anti-dsDNA and anti-Smith antibodies have high specificity for SLE but poor sensitivity.[4,5] Other autoantibodies including anti-SSA (or anti-Ro), anti-SSB (or anti-La), and anti-ribonuclear protein (RNP) antibodies widely used in evaluating patients with suspected SLE are not reliable to differentiate SLE from other autoimmune disorders. Furthermore, the methodology of autoantibody measurement is not standardized, which impacts sensitivity and specificity.[3,4,6]

Cell-Bound Complement Activation Products

Because complement activation is critical in SLE pathogenesis but soluble complement proteins (C3 and C4) are imperfect biomarkers, cell-bound complement proteins have been studied as diagnostic biomarkers. Compared to healthy controls and patients with non-SLE inflammatory disease, SLE patients have higher levels of erythrocyte-bound C4d (72% sensitivity and 79% specificity in differentiating SLE from other inflammatory diseases, 81% sensitivity and 91% specificity in differentiating SLE from healthy patients).[7] SLE patients have higher levels

Systemic Lupus Erythematosus. http://dx.doi.org/10.1016/B978-0-12-801917-7.00007-3

TABLE 1 Phases of Biomarker Discovery

Preclinical discovery	Discover potential biomarkers in tissues, body fluids in animal and human studies.
Assay development	Develop clinically useful assay and test in existing samples of patients with and without disease.
Retrospective study	Test biomarker in previously collected samples to assess sensitivity and specificity for detecting disease state.
Prospective study	Study biomarker prospectively in population to identify sensitivity, specificity, positive and negative predictive values.
Disease control	Determine the impact of the biomarker on screening for disease, influencing treatment and outcomes.

TABLE 2 Potential Biomarkers in SLE

Candidate Biomarker	Potential Utility in SLE
Cell-bound complement activation proteins:	
Erythrocyte-bound C4d	Diagnosis
Reticulocyte-bound C4d	Diagnosis, disease activity
Platelet-bound C4d	Diagnosis, stroke risk
Lymphocyte-bound C4d	Diagnosis
Interferon (IFN)-α and IFN-α-inducible genes:	
Lymphocyte antigen 6 complex–locus E (LY6E) Oligoadenylate synthetase 1 (OAS1) Oligoadenylate synehetise-like (OASL) IFN-Υ-inducible protein (IP-10) Myxovirus resistance 1 (MX1) Sialic acid binding Ig-like lectin-1 (SIGLEC-1) IFN-α-inducible protein 27, 44 (IFI27, IFI44) IFN-induced protein with tetratricopeptide repeats 1 (IFIT-1) IFN-stimulated gene 15 (ISG15)	Diagnosis, disease activity
T-cell gene expression assays	
Cytokines: IL2, IL10, IL21, IL23A, IFNγ, and BAFF Cell surface receptors: CD40L, CD44, CD70, ICAM1, Notch1, CTLA4, TNFRSF4, PDCD1, ITGAM, and LY9 Transcription factors: CREB1, CREMa, FOXp3, GATA3, NFATC2, and RELA Signaling molecules: protein kinases (ERK, PRKAR1B, PRKAR2B, PRKCD, PRKCQ, ROCK1) and protein phosphatases (PPP2CA, PPP2CB)	Diagnosis
B-lymphocyte stimulating factor (BLys)/B-cell activating factor (BAFF)	Disease activity
CD27^{high} plasma cells	Disease activity
CD44+ T cells	Disease activity
Antibodies to complement C1q (anti-C1q)	Lupus nephritis
Monocyte chemoattractant protein-1 (MCP-1)	Lupus nephritis
Neutrophil gelatniase-associated lipocalin (NGAL)	Lupus nephritis
Hepcidin-25	Lupus nephritis
Urinary TWEAK	Lupus nephritis
Urinary/serum microRNAs	Lupus nephritis
Urinary "protein signature"	
Transferrin α-1-Acid glycoprotein Ceruloplasmin Lipocalin-type prostaglandin-D-synthase	Lupus nephritis

TABLE 2 Potential Biomarkers in SLE—cont'd

Candidate Biomarker	Potential Utility in SLE
Anti-NMDA receptor antibody	CNS lupus
Antiribosomal P antibody	CNS lupus
High cardiovascular risk panel:	
Total cholesterol, triglycerides, low density lipoprotein (LDL), high density lipoprotein (HDL) Pro-inflammatory HDL High sensitivity C-reactive protein Leptin Adiponectin Apolipoprotein A-1 Soluble TWEAK	Carotid artery plaque

of reticulocyte, platelet, and lymphocyte-bound C4d.[7–9] Platelet-bound C4d was found only in 18% of SLE patients but had near 100% specificity.[10] In a multicenter, cross-sectional study, a panel incorporating ANA, anti-dsDNA, anti-mutated citrullinated vimentin antibody, erythrocyte, and platelet-bound C4d identified SLE with sensitivity of 80% and specificity of 87%.[11]

Interferon-α and Interferon-α-Inducible Genes

Enthusiasm for interferon-α (IFN-α) as an SLE diagnostic biomarker stems from studies identifying an IFN-α signature and differential expression of several polymorphisms of IFN-inducible genes in the peripheral blood cells of SLE patients.[12–14] However, other autoimmune disorders and infections also demonstrate heightened IFN-α expression, raising concerns about specificity in SLE. Most studies have focused on IFN-α as it relates to SLE disease activity (discussed later) and few upon IFN-α as a diagnostic marker. This was examined in 69 SLE and 42 connective tissue disease controls and 26 normal controls. A panel of five IFN-α-inducible genes (Table 2) were significantly increased in SLE. A panel of three of these genes comprising a modified IFN score or LY6E level alone had 70–80% specificity and 70–80% sensitivity for SLE.[15]

T-Cell Gene Expression Assays

T cells are critical in SLE pathogenesis and T-cell regulation is aberrant in SLE.[16] To address whether T-cell gene expression could serve as a diagnostic marker in SLE, a 40-gene T-cell gene expression panel (including genes coding for cytokines, cell surface receptors, transcription factors, protein kinase, and protein phosphatases; Table 2) was studied in a cohort of 65 SLE patients. It identified SLE patients versus rheumatoid arthritis (RA) patients and healthy controls with 91% sensitivity and 37% specificity, with positive predictive value of 79% and negative predictive value of 63%.[17]

BIOMARKERS FOR MEASURING SLE DISEASE ACTIVITY

For over 50 years, anti-dsDNA, C3, and C4 have been the most widely used biomarkers for SLE disease activity. While useful in individual patients, their inconsistency is problematic. In addition, erythrocyte sedimentation rate and C-reactive protein are nonspecific and often affected by comorbidities.

Cell-bound Complement Activation Proteins

Given reticulocytes' brief 48-h life span, reticulocyte-bound C4d was investigated as an SLE disease activity biomarker. In a 5-year longitudinal study of 157 patients with SLE, 290 patients with other diseases, and 256 healthy controls, erythrocyte-bound C4d was independently associated with SLE disease activity after controlling for C3, C4, and anti-dsDNA, suggesting potential utility as a disease activity biomarker.[18]

Interferon-α and Interferon-α-Inducible Genes

Several cross-sectional studies have established a relationship between SLE disease activity and IFN-α and its transcriptional signature,[12,19–22] and a monoclonal antibody targeting IFN-α in SLE is in clinical trials.[23] However, longitudinal studies have not shown robust data for IFN-α as an SLE disease activity biomarker. In a 66 SLE patient cohort, with 11 followed longitudinally, a panel of three IFN-α-responsive genes (IFI27, OAS3, and IFI44) was associated with SLE disease activity in cross-sectional analysis but not in longitudinal analysis.[24] Similarly, in 94 SLE patients, a panel of five IFN-α-responsive genes (LY6E, OAS1, IFIT, ISG15, and MX1) was preferentially expressed in active SLE in cross-sectional analysis, but it did not correlate with disease activity over time.[25] In a study comparing three IFN system biomarkers (IFN-α, IP-10, SIGLEC-1) to C3, C4, and anti-dsDNA in detecting SLE disease activity, SIGLEC-1 alone showed 86% sensitivity in detecting active SLE.[26]

B-Lymphocyte Stimulating Factor/B-Cell Activating Factor

B-cell lymphocyte activating factor (BLyS), also known as B-cell activating factor (BAFF, a member of the tumor necrosis factor (TNF) ligand superfamily), is expressed on monocytes, macrophages, monocyte-derived dendritic cells, and neutrophils.[27,28] Belimumab, an anti-BLyS monoclonal antibody, has been approved by the U.S. Food and Drug Administration for SLE treatment.[29] Circulating BLyS levels are elevated in 30% of SLE patients and correlate with anti-dsDNA levels and disease activity in cross-sectional studies.[30,31] However, longitudinal studies have shown mixed results. In a 68 SLE patient cohort, BLyS levels varied over time but did not significantly correlate with disease activity. Similarly, in 42 SLE patients, BLyS levels were higher in SLE compared to RA patients and controls but did not correlate significantly with disease activity over time.[33] In a multicenter study of 245 SLE patients, circulating BLyS levels were independently associated with anti-dsDNA levels and higher BLyS levels at a prior visit predicted higher disease activity at a subsequent visit.[34]

CD27[high] Plasma Cells

SLE is characterized by B-cell hyperactivity. The CD27 molecule, a member of the TNF receptor superfamily, is expressed on B and T lymphocytes.[35] Naïve B cells lack CD27 expression, while antigen-experienced lymphocytes are either CD27+ memory B cells or CD27[high] plasma cells. In cross-sectional studies, an increased number and frequency of CD27[high] plasma cells were identified in the peripheral blood of patients with active SLE compared to inactive SLE and correlated with disease activity and anti-dsDNA levels.[36–38] However, CD27[high] populations in SLE have yet to be studied in a multicenter, longitudinal fashion.

CD44+ T Cells

T-cell infiltration is an important mediator of tissue inflammation and end organ damage in SLE. T cells expressing CD44 bind with high affinity to hyaluronic acid and may facilitate T-cell migration and adherence to inflamed tissue, thereby increasing risk for SLE disease activity and damage. T-cell expression of CD44 isoforms was analyzed in a multicenter, cross-sectional study of 72 SLE patients.[39] CD4+ and CD8+ T-cell expression of CD44 isoforms CD44v3 and CD44v6 was significantly higher in patients compared to healthy controls. Expression of CD44v3 (on total T cells, CD4+ and CD8+ T cells) and CD44v6 (on total T cells and CD4+ T cells) correlated with SLEDAI scores. In addition, both anti-dsDNA antibodies and lupus nephritis (LN) were associated with expression of CD44v6 in T-cell populations.[39]

BIOMARKERS TO DETECT SPECIFIC ORGAN INVOLVEMENT

Lupus Nephritis Biomarkers

Because up to 75% of patients with SLE will develop LN in their lifetimes, early and accurate detection of LN is critically important. Traditional LN biomarkers include urinalysis, measurements of renal function (blood urea nitrogen, serum creatinine, glomerular filtration rate), serum albumin, C3, C4, and anti-dsDNA antibodies. Unfortunately, levels of C3, C4, and anti-dsDNA antibodies have low sensitivity and specificity for detecting LN flares. Fewer than 25% of SLE patients with low C3/C4 or elevated anti-dsDNA have an LN flare. About 50% of LN flares are preceded by a decline in C3/C4 or increase in anti-dsDNA antibodies. Renal biopsy is the gold standard, but it is invasive and subject to sampling error. Thus, reliable, noninvasive biomarkers are needed to improve LN detection and management.

While serum biomarkers are generally more stable, they are more likely to represent systemic response than specific organ response. Urine biomarkers may allow more direct assessment of disease activity in the kidney. However, challenges of urinary biomarkers include contamination of urine from bacteria and squamous epithelial cells.[40]

Antibodies to Complement C1q

Antibodies to complement protein C1q (anti-C1q) have been proposed as an LN biomarker. C1q facilitates clearance of immune complexes, and up to 88% of individuals homozygously deficient for C1q develop SLE (30% of these develop LN).[41] In cross-sectional studies, serum C1q levels are low in active SLE and are associated with anti-C1q antibodies; however, results have shown poor sensitivity for SLE diagnosis.[42] In longitudinal studies, anti-C1q antibodies detected LN similarly to traditional biomarkers C3, C4, and anti-dsDNA antibody.[43] Anti-C1q levels increased 4–6 months prior to clinically detected LN flares and became significantly different from baseline about 2 months prior to flare.[44] A positive predictive value for detection of LN of 50–71% has been reported for anti-C1q antibody.[43]

Monocyte Chemoattractant Protein-1

Monocyte chemoattractant protein-1 (MCP-1) is a chemokine that functions as a leukocyte chemotactic factor. Urinary MCP-1 (uMCP-1) levels are higher in LN flares compared to healthy controls, patients with active or inactive non-renal SLE, and patients with stable LN. In addition to detecting LN flares, uMCP-1 correlated with flare severity, proliferative renal histology, and was not influenced by type of immunosuppression. Furthermore, in a small longitudinal cohort, uMCP increased 2–4 months before a renal flare, suggesting uMCP-1 as a predictive biomarker for nephritis flare.[44] Challenges of uMCP-1 as an LN biomarker include the fact that MCP-1 is involved in fibrotic response, is associated with scarring on renal biopsy, and thus may not be specific for renal inflammation.

Neutrophil Gelatinase-Associated Lipocalin

Neutrophil gelatinase-associated lipocalin (NGAL) is an antibacterial protein expressed in neutrophils, epithelial, and renal tubular cells that binds bacterial siderophores and sequesters iron. Its exact role in renal and SLE pathophysiology is not known. NGAL messenger RNA (mRNA) expression is increased in loops of Henle and collecting ducts in acute kidney injury and has a protective effect on renal tubules in experimental models of acute kidney injury. Urinary NGAL (uNGAL) is used as a biomarker for ischemic kidney damage in children undergoing cardiac surgery. In a longitudinal pediatric SLE cohort, uNGAL levels increased 3–6 months prior to clinically diagnosed LN flare.[45] Using renal BILAG, uNGAL showed sensitivity of 82% and specificity of 82%, positive predictive value of 61%, and negative predictive value of 93% for LN flare. Urinary NGAL was higher in patients with diffuse proliferative versus membranous LN.[46] In adults, uNGAL showed specificity of 92% with low sensitivity of 50% for detecting LN.[47] Because uNGAL is elevated in non-lupus renal injury, it is not specific for lupus.[45]

Urinary TWEAK

TNF-like weak inducer of apoptosis (TWEAK) is a cytokine involved in chronic inflammation and apoptosis induction. Urinary TWEAK (uTWEAK) is hypothesized to reflect renal injury.[48] In a cross-sectional, multicenter cohort of 78 LN patients, uTWEAK discriminated LN patients from nonnephritis SLE patients with a sensitivity of 50% and specificity of 90%.[49] In longitudinal analysis of 13 LN patients, uTWEAK increased prior to flare, peaked during renal flare, and decreased after flare. Levels of uTWEAK were significantly different 4 and 6 months before and after renal flare.[49]

MicroRNAs

MicroRNAs (miRNAs) are short, noncoding RNA sequences that regulate gene expression by inducing mRNA degradation or blocking protein translation. Several studies suggest that miRNA plays a role in SLE pathogenesis.[50] In LN biopsies, several miRNA are differentially expressed in active LN compared to nonrenal SLE, inactive LN, or healthy controls. In a cross-sectional study of 365 SLE patients who were compared to patients with non-SLE autoimmune disease and healthy controls, circulating miRNA-142-3p, miR-181a, miR106a, miR-17, miR20a, and miR-92a were differentially expressed in LN; results were validated in two independent cohorts.[51]

Transferrin, α-1-Acid-Glycoprotein, Ceruloplasmin, Lipocalin-Type Prostaglandin D-Synthase

In a pediatric SLE cohort, surface-enhanced laser desorption/ionization laser time-of-flight mass spectrometry (SELDI-TOF) identified a urinary protein signature including transferrin (TF), α-1-acid-glycoprotein (AAG), ceruloplasmin (CP), and lipocalin-type prostaglandin D-synthase (L-PGDS) for active LN.[46] Although the role of these proteins in renal disease and SLE is unknown, they were elevated in the urine of SLE patients with active LN compared to those with nonrenal SLE. In a prospective study, many of these proteins increased significantly 3 months before renal flare. TF increased only in the patients who developed LN flares, while AAG increased in patients with flares but also in those with stable or improving LN. Urinary L-PGDS increased both in patients with renal flares but also in those with active but stable LN.[45,46,52]

Hepcidin

In a cohort of SLE patients followed at 2-month intervals, urinary protein expression detected by SELDI-TOF identified that the 20 and 25 amino acid isoforms of hepcidin correlated with renal flare.[53] Urinary hepcidin-20 increased significantly 4 months before LN flare and normalized by 4 months of treatment. Hepcidin-25 decreased at renal flare and returned to baseline after treatment. While its role in SLE pathophysiology remains unknown, hepcidin is an iron-regulatory hormone involved in the pathogenesis of anemia of chronic disease and is upregulated by proinflammatory cytokines, TNF-α and IL-6. Hepcidin has also been identified in renal interstitial leukocytes in biopsies of SLE patients with active nephritis.[53,54]

Central Nervous System Biomarkers

Neuropsychiatric SLE (NPSLE) is common, with a highly variable described prevalence (30–80%), and it remains a diagnostic dilemma. The American College of Rheumatology Classification Criteria for NPSLE recognizes 19 case definitions for heterogeneous manifestations including headache, cognitive dysfunction, cerebritis, and stroke. Traditional NPSLE biomarkers include cerebrospinal fluid (CSF) protein, cell count, and oligoclonal bands, as well as central nervous system (CNS) magnetic resonance imaging (MRI).[55]

Anti-NMDA Receptor Antibody

N-Methyl-D-aspartate (NMDA, also known as NR2) receptors are expressed throughout the brain and bind the excitatory neurotransmitter, glutamate. In animal models, circulating anti-NMDA antibodies enter the CSF when the blood–brain barrier is disrupted, bind NMDA receptors in the brain (particularly in the hippocampus), and correlate with cognitive dysfunction and depression.[56] In humans, anti-NMDA antibodies cross-react with dsDNA, but the sensitivity and specificity of anti-NMDA receptor antibodies in detecting NPSLE has not been established.[57] In a prospective study, an increase in anti-NMDA antibodies did not predict development of NPSLE or cognitive decline over a 5-year follow-up period.[58]

Antiribosomal P Antibody

The 60S subunit of ribosomes contains three highly conserved phosphoproteins—P0 (38 kDa), P1 (19 kDa), and P2 (17 kDa)—which are the targets of antiribosomal P antibodies, and their biological function is not known. Several small studies have suggested a relationship between antiribosomal P antibody and NPSLE, particularly psychosis.[59–61] An inception cohort of more than 100 SLE patients found that antiribosomal P antibody predicted development of lupus psychosis.[58,61] However, a meta-analysis including over 1500 SLE patients suggested that antiribosomal P antibody is a poor biomarker for diagnosis of NPSLE.[62]

Antiphospholipid Antibodies

Antiphospholipid antibodies are clearly linked to increased risk of stroke.[58] The association between antiphospholipid antibodies and other CNS manifestations of SLE is not as clear. Cross-sectional studies assessing the relationship between chorea and cognitive impairment have shown mixed results.[63–65]

Platelet-Bound C4d

In a cohort of 356 SLE patients, platelet-bound C4d levels were associated with all-cause mortality and ischemic stroke, even after adjustment for age and presence of antiphospholipid antibodies.[66] In addition, elevated platelet-bound C4d was associated with stroke severity.[8]

Cardiovascular System Biomarkers

Cardiovascular (CV) disease, particularly atherosclerosis and its complications, is a major cause of morbidity and mortality in SLE. There is an unmet need for biomarkers that could identify patients with subclinical atherosclerosis who may benefit from aggressive prevention strategies. A recent multicenter, longitudinal study assessed whether a panel of CV biomarkers (PREDICTS profile, see Table 2) predicted baseline or incident carotid plaque in 210 women with SLE and 100 sex and age-matched healthy controls.[67] A high risk profile, defined by presence of ≥3 biomarkers (or ≥1 biomarker with diabetes history) predicted incident carotid plaque with 81% sensitivity and 79% specificity and had positive predictive value of 40% with negative predictive value of 95%.[67] A high risk PREDICTS profile increased the odds of carotid plaque by 38-fold in SLE patients and correlated with progression of carotid intima medial thickening.[67] These promising results need to be validated in other SLE populations.

GENETIC SUSCEPTIBILITY AND THERANOSTICS

Numerous genetic markers are associated with increased or reduced risk of SLE. As discussed in Chapter X, SLE genetics are quite complex and there is no single causative gene. The current model proposes that individual genetic contributions cumulatively either enhance or reduce the threshold of autoimmune activation. A discussion of SLE genetics is beyond the scope of this chapter, but several genes associated with increased risk of SLE are listed in Table 3.

The field of theranostics is in its infancy as it relates to SLE, but there are significant opportunities for the

TABLE 3 Candidate Genes That Increase Susceptibility to Systemic Lupus Erythematosus

Immune System Component	Candidate Genes
Apoptosis, DNA breakdown, debris clearance	FCGR2B, ACP5, TREX1, DNASE1, DNASE1L3, ATG5
Type 1 interferon and toll-like receptor signaling	TLR7, IRF5, IRF7/PHRF1, IRF8, IRAK1, IFIH1, TYK2, PRDM1, Stat4, TREX1, ACP5
Nuclear factor κB signaling	IRAK1, TNFA1P3, TNIP1, UBE2L3, SLC15A4, PRKCB
Immune complex processing	C1Q, C1R/C1S, C2, C4A/B, FCGR2A/B, FCGR3A/B
Neutrophil/monocyte function	ITGAM, ICAMS, FCGR2B, FCGR3A/B, IL20, IRF8
B-cell function	FCGR2B, BLK, LYN, BANK1, PRDM1, ETS1, IKZF1, AFF1, RASGRP3, IL10, IL21, NCF2, PRKCB, HLA-DR2, HLA-DR3, MSH5, IRF8
T-cell function	PTPN22, TNFS4, CD44, ETS1, IL10, IL21, TYK2, STAT4, PRDM1, AFF1, IZKF1, HLA-DR2, HLA-DR3

Adapted from: Rullo OJ, Tsao BP. *Ann Rheum Dis* 2013;**72S**:56–61.

development of markers that can help stratify patients for clinical trials and ultimately be used for patient care.

CONCLUSIONS

The quest for SLE biomarkers continues. Most of the biomarkers discussed in this chapter require further validation in large, multicenter studies prior to considering their routine use in clinical practice or clinical trials. SLE complexity and the need for multiple biomarkers to improve prediction, diagnosis, detection, and monitoring of SLE points to the necessity of collaborative efforts focusing on systems biology and mathematical modeling in order to understand how potential biomarkers can be ideally developed and in order to avoid so-called biomarker fatigue. Despite the challenges of biomarker development, it is critically important to strive for the development and validation of novel, reliable, noninvasive, and cost-effective SLE biomarkers reflective of lupus pathogenesis to allow accurate diagnosis, timely and appropriate therapy, evaluation of therapies in clinical trials, and ultimately improved outcomes for SLE patients.

REFERENCES

1. Biomarkers Definitions Working Group. Biomarkers and surrogate endpoints: preferred definitions and conceptual framework. *Clin Pharmacol Ther* March 2001;**69**(3):89–95.
2. Hochberg MC. Updating the American College of Rheumatology revised criteria for the classification of systemic lupus erythematosus. *Arthritis Rheum* September 1997;**40**(9):1725.
3. Mariz HA, Sato EI, Barbosa SH, Rodrigues SH, Dellavance A, Andrade LE. Pattern on the antinuclear antibody-HEp-2 test is a critical parameter for discriminating antinuclear antibody-positive healthy individuals and patients with autoimmune rheumatic diseases. *Arthritis Rheum* January 2011;**63**(1):191–200.
4. Tzioufas AG, Terzoglou C, Stavropoulos ED, Athanasiadou S, Moutsopoulos HM. Determination of anti-ds-DNA antibodies by three different methods: comparison of sensitivity, specificity and correlation with lupus activity index (LAI). *Clin Rheumatol* June 1990;**9**(2):186–92.
5. Carmona-Fernandes D, Santos MJ, Canhao H, Fonseca JE. Anti-ribosomal P protein IgG autoantibodies in patients with systemic lupus erythematosus: diagnostic performance and clinical profile. *BMC Med* April 4, 2013;**11**:98. http://dx.doi.org/10.1186/1741-7015-11-98.
6. Hanly JG, Thompson K, McCurdy G, Fougere L, Theriault C, Wilton K. Measurement of autoantibodies using multiplex methodology in patients with systemic lupus erythematosus. *J Immunol Methods* January 31, 2010;**352**(1–2):147–52.
7. Manzi S, Navratil JS, Ruffing MJ, Liu CC, Danchenko N, Nilson SE, et al. Measurement of erythrocyte C4d and complement receptor 1 in systemic lupus erythematosus. *Arthritis Rheum* November 2004;**50**(11):3596–604.
8. Mehta N, Uchino K, Fakhran S, Sattar MA, Branstetter 4th BF, Au K, et al. Platelet C4d is associated with acute ischemic stroke and stroke severity. *Stroke* December 2008;**39**(12):3236–41.
9. Liu CC, Ahearn JM, Manzi S. Complement as a source of biomarkers in systemic lupus erythematosus: past, present, and future. *Curr Rheumatol Rep* April 2004;**6**(2):85–8.
10. Navratil JS, Manzi S, Kao AH, Krishnaswami S, Liu CC, Ruffing MJ, et al. Platelet C4d is highly specific for systemic lupus erythematosus. *Arthritis Rheum* February 2006;**54**(2):670–4.
11. Kalunian KC, Chatham WW, Massarotti EM, Reyes-Thomas J, Harris C, Furie RA, et al. Measurement of cell-bound complement activation products enhances diagnostic performance in systemic lupus erythematosus. *Arthritis Rheum* December 2012;**64**(12):4040–7.
12. Bennett L, Palucka AK, Arce E, Cantrell V, Borvak J, Banchereau J, et al. Interferon and granulopoiesis signatures in systemic lupus erythematosus blood. *J Exp Med* March 17, 2003;**197**(6):711–23.
13. Obermoser G, Pascual V. The interferon-alpha signature of systemic lupus erythematosus. *Lupus* August 2010;**19**(9):1012–9.
14. Crow MK, Kirou KA. Interferon-induced versus chemokine transcripts as lupus biomarkers. *Arthritis Res Ther* 2008;**10**(6):126.
15. Feng X, Huang J, Liu Y, Xiao L, Wang D, Hua B, et al. Identification of interferon-inducible genes as diagnostic biomarker for systemic lupus erythematosus. *Clin Rheumatol* October 26, 2014.
16. Tsokos GC. Systemic lupus erythematosus. *N Engl J Med* December 1, 2011;**365**(22):2110–21.
17. Grammatikos AP, Kyttaris VC, Kis-Toth K, Fitzgerald LM, Devlin A, Finnell MD, et al. A T cell gene expression panel for the diagnosis and monitoring of disease activity in patients with systemic lupus erythematosus. *Clin Immunol* February 2014;**150**(2):192–200.
18. Kao AH, Navratil JS, Ruffing MJ, Liu CC, Hawkins D, McKinnon KM, et al. Erythrocyte C3d and C4d for monitoring disease activity in systemic lupus erythematosus. *Arthritis Rheum* March 2010;**62**(3):837–44.
19. Liu CC, Manzi S, Ahearn JM. Biomarkers for systemic lupus erythematosus: a review and perspective. *Curr Opin Rheumatol* September 2005;**17**(5):543–9.
20. Kirou KA, Lee C, George S, Louca K, Papagiannis IG, Peterson MG, et al. Coordinate overexpression of interferon-alpha-induced genes in systemic lupus erythematosus. *Arthritis Rheum* December 2004;**50**(12):3958–67.
21. Blanco P, Palucka AK, Gill M, Pascual V, Banchereau J. Induction of dendritic cell differentiation by IFN-alpha in systemic lupus erythematosus. *Science* November 16, 2001;**294**(5546):1540–3.
22. Niewold TB, Kelly JA, Kariuki SN, Franek BS, Kumar AA, Kaufman KM, et al. IRF5 haplotypes demonstrate diverse serological associations which predict serum interferon alpha activity and explain the majority of the genetic association with systemic lupus erythematosus. *Ann Rheum Dis* March 2012;**71**(3):463–8.
23. Petri M, Wallace DJ, Spindler A, Chindalore V, Kalunian K, Mysler E, et al. Sifalimumab, a human anti-interferon-alpha monoclonal antibody, in systemic lupus erythematosus: a phase I randomized, controlled, dose-escalation study. *Arthritis Rheum* April 2013;**65**(4):1011–21.
24. Petri M, Singh S, Tesfasyone H, Dedrick R, Fry K, Lal P, et al. Longitudinal expression of type I interferon responsive genes in systemic lupus erythematosus. *Lupus* October 2009;**18**(11):980–9.
25. Landolt-Marticorena C, Bonventi G, Lubovich A, Ferguson C, Unnithan T, Su J, et al. Lack of association between the interferon-alpha signature and longitudinal changes in disease activity in systemic lupus erythematosus. *Ann Rheum Dis* September 2009;**68**(9):1440–6.
26. Rose T, Grutzkau A, Hirseland H, Huscher D, Dahnrich C, Dzionek A, et al. IFNalpha and its response proteins, IP-10 and SIGLEC-1, are biomarkers of disease activity in systemic lupus erythematosus. *Ann Rheum Dis* October 2013;**72**(10):1639–45.

27. Nardelli B, Belvedere O, Roschke V, Moore PA, Olsen HS, Migone TS, et al. Synthesis and release of B-lymphocyte stimulator from myeloid cells. *Blood* January 1, 2001;**97**(1):198–204.

28. Moore PA, Belvedere O, Orr A, Pieri K, LaFleur DW, Feng P, et al. BLyS: member of the tumor necrosis factor family and B lymphocyte stimulator. *Science* July 9, 1999;**285**(5425):260–3.

29. Wallace DJ, Stohl W, Furie RA, Lisse JR, McKay JD, Merrill JT, et al. A phase II, randomized, double-blind, placebo-controlled, dose-ranging study of belimumab in patients with active systemic lupus erythematosus. *Arthritis Rheum* September 15, 2009;**61**(9):1168–78.

30. Pers JO, Daridon C, Devauchelle V, Jousse S, Saraux A, Jamin C, et al. BAFF overexpression is associated with autoantibody production in autoimmune diseases. *Ann N Y Acad Sci* June 2005;**1050**:34–9.

31. Cheema GS, Roschke V, Hilbert DM, Stohl W. Elevated serum B lymphocyte stimulator levels in patients with systemic immune-based rheumatic diseases. *Arthritis Rheum* June 2001;**44**(6):1313–9.

32. Stohl W, Metyas S, Tan SM, Cheema GS, Oamar B, Xu D, et al. B lymphocyte stimulator overexpression in patients with systemic lupus erythematosus: longitudinal observations. *Arthritis Rheum* December 2003;**48**(12):3475–86.

33. Becker-Merok A, Nikolaisen C, Nossent HC. B-lymphocyte activating factor in systemic lupus erythematosus and rheumatoid arthritis in relation to autoantibody levels, disease measures and time. *Lupus* 2006;**15**(9):570–6.

34. Petri M, Stohl W, Chatham W, McCune WJ, Chevrier M, Ryel J, et al. Association of plasma B lymphocyte stimulator levels and disease activity in systemic lupus erythematosus. *Arthritis Rheum* August 2008;**58**(8):2453–9.

35. Jacobi AM, Odendahl M, Reiter K, Bruns A, Burmester GR, Radbruch A, et al. Correlation between circulating CD27high plasma cells and disease activity in patients with systemic lupus erythematosus. *Arthritis Rheum* May 2003;**48**(5):1332–42.

36. Yang DH, Chang DM, Lai JH, Lin FH, Chen CH. Significantly higher percentage of circulating CD27(high) plasma cells in systemic lupus erythematosus patients with infection than with disease flare-up. *Yonsei Med J* November 2010;**51**(6):924–31.

37. Jacobi AM, Mei H, Hoyer BF, Mumtaz IM, Thiele K, Radbruch A, et al. HLA-DRhigh/CD27high plasmablasts indicate active disease in patients with systemic lupus erythematosus. *Ann Rheum Dis* January 2010;**69**(1):305–8.

38. Dorner T, Lipsky PE. Correlation of circulating CD27high plasma cells and disease activity in systemic lupus erythematosus. *Lupus* 2004;**13**(5):283–9.

39. Crispin JC, Keenan BT, Finnell MD, Bermas BL, Schur P, Massarotti E, et al. Expression of CD44 variant isoforms CD44v3 and CD44v6 is increased on T cells from patients with systemic lupus erythematosus and is correlated with disease activity. *Arthritis Rheum* May 2010;**62**(5):1431–7.

40. Rovin BH, Birmingham DJ, Nagaraja HN, Yu CY, Hebert LA. Biomarker discovery in human SLE nephritis. *Bull NYU Hosp Jt Dis* 2007;**65**(3):187–93.

41. Truedsson L, Bengtsson AA, Sturfelt G. Complement deficiencies and systemic lupus erythematosus. *Autoimmunity* December 2007;**40**(8):560–6.

42. Orbai AM, Truedsson L, Sturfelt G, Nived O, Fang H, Alarcon G, et al. Anti-C1q antibodies in systemic lupus erythematosus. *Lupus* August 14, 2014.

43. Yin Y, Wu X, Shan G, Zhang X. Diagnostic value of serum anti-C1q antibodies in patients with lupus nephritis: a meta-analysis. *Lupus* September 2012;**21**(10):1088–97.

44. Rovin BH, Zhang X. Biomarkers for lupus nephritis: the quest continues. *Clin J Am Soc Nephrol* November 2009;**4**(11):1858–65.

45. Suzuki M, Wiers KM, Klein-Gitelman MS, Haines KA, Olson J, Onel KB, et al. Neutrophil gelatinase-associated lipocalin as a biomarker of disease activity in pediatric lupus nephritis. *Pediatr Nephrol* March 2008;**23**(3):403–12.

46. Brunner HI, Bennett MR, Mina R, Suzuki M, Petri M, Kiani AN, et al. Association of noninvasively measured renal protein biomarkers with histologic features of lupus nephritis. *Arthritis Rheum* August 2012;**64**(8):2687–97.

47. Yang CC, Hsieh SC, Li KJ, Wu CH, Lu MC, Tsai CY, et al. Urinary neutrophil gelatinase-associated lipocalin is a potential biomarker for renal damage in patients with systemic lupus erythematosus. *J Biomed Biotechnol* 2012;**2012**:759313.

48. Schwartz N, Su L, Burkly LC, Mackay M, Aranow C, Kollaros M, et al. Urinary TWEAK and the activity of lupus nephritis. *J Autoimmun* December 2006;**27**(4):242–50.

49. Schwartz N, Rubinstein T, Burkly LC, Collins CE, Blanco I, Su L, et al. Urinary TWEAK as a biomarker of lupus nephritis: a multicenter cohort study. *Arthritis Res Ther* 2009;**11**(5):R143.

50. Shen N, Liang D, Tang Y, de Vries N, Tak PP. MicroRNAs–novel regulators of systemic lupus erythematosus pathogenesis. *Nat Rev Rheumatol* December 2012;**8**(12):701–9.

51. Carlsen AL, Schetter AJ, Nielsen CT, Lood C, Knudsen S, Voss A, et al. Circulating microRNA expression profiles associated with systemic lupus erythematosus. *Arthritis Rheum* May 2013;**65**(5):1324–34.

52. Suzuki M, Wiers K, Brooks EB, Greis KD, Haines K, Klein-Gitelman MS, et al. Initial validation of a novel protein biomarker panel for active pediatric lupus nephritis. *Pediatr Res* May 2009;**65**(5):530–6.

53. Zhang X, Jin M, Wu H, Nadasdy T, Nadasdy G, Harris N, et al. Biomarkers of lupus nephritis determined by serial urine proteomics. *Kidney Int* September 2008;**74**(6):799–807.

54. Zhang X, Nagaraja HN, Nadasdy T, Song H, McKinley A, Prosek J, et al. A composite urine biomarker reflects interstitial inflammation in lupus nephritis kidney biopsies. *Kidney Int* February 2012; **81**(4):401–6.

55. Sanna G, Bertolaccini ML, Cuadrado MJ, Laing H, Khamashta MA, Mathieu A, et al. Neuropsychiatric manifestations in systemic lupus erythematosus: prevalence and association with antiphospholipid antibodies. *J Rheumatol* May 2003;**30**(5):985–92.

56. Kowal C, Diamond B. Aspects of CNS lupus: mouse models of anti-NMDA receptor antibody mediated reactivity. *Methods Mol Biol* 2012;**900**:181–206.

57. DeGiorgio LA, Konstantinov KN, Lee SC, Hardin JA, Volpe BT, Diamond B. A subset of lupus anti-DNA antibodies cross-reacts with the NR2 glutamate receptor in systemic lupus erythematosus. *Nat Med* November 2001;**7**(11):1189–93.

58. Hanly JG, Urowitz MB, Su L, Bae SC, Gordon C, Clarke A, et al. Autoantibodies as biomarkers for the prediction of neuropsychiatric events in systemic lupus erythematosus. *Ann Rheum Dis* October 2011;**70**(10):1726–32.

59. Briani C, Lucchetta M, Ghirardello A, Toffanin E, Zampieri S, Ruggero S, et al. Neurolupus is associated with anti-ribosomal P protein antibodies: an inception cohort study. *J Autoimmun* March 2009;**32**(2):79–84.

60. Fragoso-Loyo H, Cabiedes J, Orozco-Narvaez A, Davila-Maldonado L, Atisha-Fregoso Y, Diamond B, et al. Serum and cerebrospinal fluid autoantibodies in patients with neuropsychiatric lupus erythematosus. Implications for diagnosis and pathogenesis. *PLoS One* October 6, 2008;**3**(10):e3347.

61. Hanly JG, Urowitz MB, Siannis F, Farewell V, Gordon C, Bae SC, et al. Autoantibodies and neuropsychiatric events at the time of systemic lupus erythematosus diagnosis: results from an international inception cohort study. *Arthritis Rheum* March 2008;**58**(3):843–53.

62. Karassa FB, Afeltra A, Ambrozic A, Chang DM, De Keyser F, Doria A, et al. Accuracy of anti-ribosomal P protein antibody testing for the diagnosis of neuropsychiatric systemic lupus erythematosus: an international meta-analysis. *Arthritis Rheum* January 2006;**54**(1):312–24.

63. Avcin T, Benseler SM, Tyrrell PN, Cucnik S, Silverman ED. A followup study of antiphospholipid antibodies and associated neuropsychiatric manifestations in 137 children with systemic lupus erythematosus. *Arthritis Rheum* February 15, 2008;**59**(2):206–13.

64. Borowoy AM, Pope JE, Silverman E, Fortin PR, Pineau C, Smith CD, et al. Neuropsychiatric lupus: the prevalence and autoantibody associations depend on the definition: results from the 1000 faces of lupus cohort. *Semin Arthritis Rheum* October 2012;**42**(2):179–85.

65. Orzechowski NM, Wolanskyj AP, Ahlskog JE, Kumar N, Moder KG. Antiphospholipid antibody-associated chorea. *J Rheumatol* November 2008;**35**(11):2165–70.

66. Kao AH, McBurney CA, Sattar A, Lertratanakul A, Wilson NL, Rutman S, et al. Relation of platelet C4d with all-cause mortality and ischemic stroke in patients with systemic lupus erythematosus. *Transl Stroke Res* August 2014;**5**(4):510–8.

67. McMahon M, Skaggs BJ, Grossman JM, Sahakian L, Fitzgerald J, Wong WK, et al. A panel of biomarkers is associated with increased risk of the presence and progression of atherosclerosis in women with systemic lupus erythematosus. *Arthritis Rheumatol* January 2014;**66**(1):130–9.

Part II

Pathogenesis

Chapter 8

Overview of the Pathogenesis of Systemic Lupus Erythematosus

Concetta Ferretti, Antonio La Cava

Department of Medicine, University of California Los Angeles, Los Angeles, CA, USA

GENETIC PREDISPOSITION

Due to its complex and only partly understood etiology,[1] systemic lupus erythematosus (SLE) has been labeled "the cruel mystery" by the Lupus Foundation of America. SLE is a polygenic disorder that can appear in individuals without a family history of the disease, yet siblings of affected individuals are much more likely to develop SLE, and monozygotic twins present a tenfold higher risk than dizygotic twins.[2] This suggests that genetics play a key role in the predisposition to developing SLE, as discussed in Chapters 10 and 32.

As a disease with polygenic inheritance, affected individuals in SLE can inherit multiple predisposing genes that, alone, would not predict the illness (with notable exceptions such as C1q deficiency).[3] In this context, certain genetic variants and pathological mechanisms in SLE can be common with other autoimmune disorders such as type 1 diabetes, rheumatoid arthritis, and multiple sclerosis.[3] Additionally, genetic heterogeneity among humans may at times defy in part the expected frequency due to stochastic variations, possibly because of an evolutionary advantage that could positively select certain genotypes rather than others. These aspects create grounds for genetic predisposition, on which the presence of additive or cumulative factors ultimately promote the development of the disease. For example, certain infectious agents might facilitate certain initial steps in the disease pathogenesis, as discussed in Chapter 22, or provide selective pressure, as suggested by the SLE-associated single nucleotide polymorphism (SNP) in *FCGR2B* in Asians and Africans that also associate with a reduced susceptibility to malaria infection.[3] Other risk loci for SLE (*PTPN22*, *TNFSF4*, *ITGAM*, *BLK*) also show an evidence for positive selection by evolutionary advantage under adverse conditions (e.g., infection),[3] leading to the consideration that certain genes involved in handling infection could possibly play a relevant role in the pathogenesis of autoimmune diseases, including SLE.

In any case, the identification of risk alleles in SLE has been facilitated by SNP genotyping and genome-wide association studies (GWAS) that have both identified risk loci and confirmed previously described associations with defined alleles.[4] To date, more than 60 genetic regions have been recognized as robustly associated with SLE,[3] as discussed in Chapters 10 and 32. These regions can be grouped according to function into immunological pathways (including uptake and processing of antigen), clearance of immune complexes (ICs), cell signaling, and innate and adaptive immune responses.[5] GWAS have also unveiled genes involved in immune cell regulation and DNA epigenetic modifications, although the roles of some genes have not yet been fully characterized (Table 1).

In general, however, the identification of SLE-associated loci through genetic discovery represents only an initial step in the process of understanding the underlying mechanisms of disease, considering that the assessment of the effects of structural variations and their link with clinical features and phenotypes in SLE require mechanistic studies that can definitely link the role of specific gene products to the pathogenesis of the disease. Moreover, it is not always possible to understand how certain polymorphisms can influence the pathogenesis of SLE because of the gene–gene interactions, which can be additive or epistatic ones (the latter mechanism being proposed for human leukocyte antigen (*HLA*) and *CTLA4*, *ITGAM* and *IRF5*, *STAT4* and *IRF5*, *BLK* and *TNFSF4*).[5] Yet frequently, the gene polymorphisms associated with SLE are recognized as influential on defined processes that are relevant to the pathogenesis of the disease, such as when they are involved in the modulation of key immunological and hematological mechanisms (e.g., *STAT4*, *HLA*, *ITGAM*, and *IRF5*).[4] Polymorphisms of *IL-10* and *TNFS4* have been described in European, Hispanic American, and Asian populations,[4] and polymorphisms of *STAT4* have been correlated with early onset and more severe SLE.[4] Additionally, some SLE-predisposing genes have been found to be shared among ethnical groups, such as the *HLA-DR2* and *DR3* alleles among Europeans, and *HLA-DR4* and *DR8* among

TABLE 1 Summary of Genes Associated with SLE

Pathway	Genes
Apoptosis and disposal of cellular debris[a]	ACP5,[5] ATG5,[5] BACH2,[3] CRP,[3] DNASE1,[3,5] DNASE1L3,[3,5] FCGR2B,[3,5] IRF5,[3,5] TREX1,[3,5]
Phagocyte function and antigen presentation[a]	CD226,[3] CRP,[3] FCGR2B,[5] FCGR3A/B,[3,5] HLA-DRB1,[3] ICAM1/4/5,[3,5] IL10,[3,5] IRF8,[3,5] ITGAM[3,5]
TLRs and NFκB signaling[a]	ACP5,[5] IFIH1,[3,5] IRAK1,[3,5] IRF5,[3,5] IRF7/PHRF1,[3,5] IRF8,[3,5] PRDM1,[5] PRKCB,[3,5] SLC15A4,[3,5] STAT4,[3,5] TLR7,[5] TNFAIP3,[3,5] TNIP1,[3,5] TREX1,[5] TYK2,[3,5] UBE2L3[3,5]
Complement and clearance of immune complexes[a]	C1q,[3,5] C1R/C1S,[5] C2,[3,5] C4A/B,[5] CFH,[3] CFHR1/4,[3] FCGR2A/B,[3,5] FCGR3A/B[3,5]
T-cell function[a]	AFF1,[3,5] CD44/PDHX,[3] CD80,[3] CD226,[3] CSK,[3] ETS1,[3,5] HLA-DR2/DR3,[3] IKZF1,[3,5] IL10,[3,5] IL21,[3,5] IL12RB2,[3] LEF,[3] STAT4,[3,5] PDCD1,[3] PRDM1,[3,5] PTPN22,[3,5] TNFSF4,[3,5] TYK2[3,5]
B-cell function[a]	APOBEC4,[3] AFF1,[3,5] BANK1,[3,5] BLK,[3,5] CSK,[3] ELF1,[3] ETS1,[3,5] FCGR2B,[5] HLA-DR2/DR3,[3] IKZF1,[3,5] IKZF3,[3] IL10,[3,5] IL21,[3,5] IRF8,[3,5] LYN,[3,5] MSH5,[5] NCF2,[3] PRDM1,[5] PRKCB,[3,5] RASGRP3[3,5]
Signal transduction, cell cycle, growth, energy metabolism, epigenetic modifications, DNA repair[b]	ARMC3,[3] ARID5B,[3] CDKN1B,[3] CREBL2,[3] DRAM1,[3] DGUOK,[3] ICA1,[3] ITPR3,[3] LYST,[3] MECP2,[3] NMNAT2,[3] PDHX,[3] PPP2CA,[3] PTTG1,[3] PXK,[3] SCN10A,[3] SLC29A3,[3] TET3,[3] UHRF1BP1[3]
Others[c]	CLEC16A,[3] DDA1,[3] DDX6,[3] GPR19,[3] JAZF1,[3] LRRC18/WDFY4,[3] RTKN2,[3] SCUBE1,[3] SEZ6L2,[3] TMEM39A,[3] XKR6,[3] ZPBP2[3]

[a]Major pathways in SLE.
[b]Pathways altered in SLE and in other disorders.
[c]SLE-associated genes with unknown influences on immune responses;[3,5]references.

non-Europeans.[6] In particular, *HLA-DR3* has been linked to renal disease (and to anti-Ro/La autoantibodies),[7] while polymorphisms such as of *APOL1* have been associated with kidney failure in African-Americans.[4]

EPIGENETIC CONTRIBUTIONS

Epigenetic modifications help to explain part of the missing genetic heritability, as discussed in Chapter 30. For example, chromatin structure and DNA methylation, which are both sensitive to environmental factors, can significantly influence gene expression.

In SLE patients, hypomethylation in CD4+ T cells has been correlated with autoreactivity, with *ITGAL, CD70,* and *TNFS5* standing out as important genes affected by hypomethylation.[8] Also in CD4+ T cells from SLE patients with active disease, demethylation of the perforin gene has been observed in concomitance with acute flares,[8] as well as hypomethylation of genes of the type 1 interferon (IFN-I) pathway.[9]

Among the posttranscriptional modifications that influence gene expression and DNA methylation, microRNAs (miRNAs) appear to give an important contribution to SLE pathogenesis, as discussed in Chapter 27. miRNAs are small noncoding molecules that modulate target messenger RNA expression. In SLE, an overexpression of miR-126, miR-21, and miR-148a in CD4+ T cells has been shown to enhance hypomethlylation,[10,11] while in B cells, the overexpression of miR-30a and miR-181b appears to promote cell proliferation and antibody diversification, respectively.[11] Also,

miR-21 increases IL-10 levels in CD4+ T cells,[11,10] while miR-31 hyperactivity in T cells reduces IL-2 secretion and negatively regulates Foxp3 expression in regulatory T cells (Tregs).[11] For miR-146, a suppressive role in autoimmunity has been proposed, because a reduced expression of this miRNA associates with the activation of the Toll-like receptor (TLR)7/9 pathway in plasmacytoid dendritic cells (pDCs) (which sustain inflammation through IFN-α production; see Chapter 16).[10,11] Another miRNA, miR-155, acts on IFN-1 secretion from pDCs, as well as on T-cell-dependent antibody production, somatic hypermutation, and autoantibody class switch in B cells.[10,11]

GENDER

SLE mainly affects women in their reproductive age, with a female-to-male ratio of 9:1, suggesting a role for female hormones (likely favored by the presence of estrogen receptors on immune cells; see Chapter 11 for details). Studies in animal models of SLE have provided support to this hypothesis, showing that ovariectomy delays disease progression and improves survival in lupus mice.[12] Indeed, estrogens are believed to promote humoral responses and sustain B-cell autoreactivity.[13] Conversely, testosterone can suppress anti-DNA antibody production.[12]

Although in both female and male SLE patients there is an aberrant aromatase activity that could impair estrogen expression, the blockage of estrogens did not provide beneficial effects in SLE, and rather worsened hypertension and renal damage.[14] These data, along with the slight increase of SLE risk associated with the use of oral contraceptives, suggest that other factors can contribute to the gender bias that characterizes SLE. Those factors could include differences in gene methylation and X-linked predisposing loci such as *TLR7* and *FOXP3*.[9] In support of the role of X-chromosome dosage in the disease, XXY males affected by Klinefelter syndrome display a higher incidence of SLE than normal XY males.[15]

ENVIRONMENT

The link between selected environmental agents and SLE is not a simple task because of the numerous additional factors that can be possibly implied and because of the great interindividual variability in susceptibility to SLE among different individuals, as further elaborated in Chapter 9. Notwithstanding this central consideration, it is generally accepted that some environmental factors including biologic, physical, or chemical agents can facilitate the development and/or progression of SLE in predisposed subjects.

Among the biologic agents, Epstein–Barr virus has been proposed to associate with SLE pathogenesis (see Chapter 22), while for the physical agents, a known risk factor for SLE is exposure to ultraviolet light (which damages DNA, amplifying cell apoptosis and the presentation of self-antigens to immune cells). For the chemical agents, smokers have a greater risk for SLE and the development of anti-dsDNA antibodies, possibly because smoke increases cellular necrosis.[16] Occupational exposure to silica dust, petroleum, organic solvents, and mineral oils also increase the risk for SLE.[17] In this regard, the hydrocarbon oil pristane (2,6,10,14-tetramethylpentadecane), which has been used in the food, cosmetic, and pharmacological industries, has been documented to induce lupus-like disease in non-SLE-prone mice, [18]as discussed in Chapter 23. Finally, certain drugs have long been known to promote iatrogenic forms of SLE, although those effects are reversible upon drug withdrawal (see Chapter 54).

IMMUNE ABNORMALITIES IN SLE

SLE is characterized by pathologic processes that reinforce themselves in the establishment and maintenance of chronic inflammation. Among the underlying abnormalities, SLE presents altered apoptosis and clearance of cellular debris (see Chapter 21), altered antigen presentation (Chapter 16), aberrant frequency, phenotype and molecular signaling for multiple immune cell subsets (Chapters 13–15), and a dysfunctional production of soluble immune mediators (Chapters 17 and 19).

Schematically, in the pathogenesis of SLE, the impaired apoptosis (or reduced clearance of apoptotic cells) allows dying cells to provide self-determinants that are recognized by autoreactive immune cells which, as a result, undergo

phenotypic changes and secrete soluble mediators that contribute to the production of autoantibodies and the development and maintenance of tissue inflammation.[19–21] The abnormal clearance of apoptotic cells can be favored by multiple factors, such as a defective function of phagocytes, reduced levels of DNase I,[22] or complement deficiency associated with decreased levels of pentraxins and/or C3b/C4b receptors.[23,1] The sustained availability of apoptotic remnants in the germinal centers (GCs) facilitates the presentation by follicular dendritic cells (fDCs) that can activate autoreactive B cells, whose B-cell receptor (BCR) had undergone somatic hypermutation.[23] This elicits the production of autoantibodies that bind nucleic acid-containing material and promote FcγR-mediated phagocytosis, together with the secretion of pro-inflammatory cytokines such as IL-6, IL-8, IL-1β, IL-10, IL-12, and TNF-α.[23] Incidentally, an abnormal production of multiple cytokines that are derived from both innate immune cells (e.g., IFN-α) and adaptive immune cells (e.g., IL-2, IL-10) drives and sustains multiple pro-pathogenic events in SLE, ranging from the production of autoantibodies to tissue injury (see Chapters 17 and 19 for details).

Increased availability of apoptotic cell material facilitates concomitant immune abnormalities that further increase autoantibody production. For example, lupus T cells may increase their surface expression of the costimulatory molecules CD40L[24,25] or ICOS (inducible T-cell costimulator, a costimulatory molecule that plays a crucial role in the activity of follicular helper T [Tfh] cells that favor the formation of GCs).[26,27] Once autoantibodies are formed, they can bind self-antigens to form ICs (see Chapter 26), favoring tissue injury, which promotes further cell death and, together with local inflammatory mediators, the perpetration of the autoimmune process[23] (Figure 1).

Multiple players contribute to that effect. Expanded in the GCs of SLE patients, Tfh cells produce IL-21, inhibit Tregs, and promote the production of autoantibodies by providing costimulatory signals for GCs, B cells and the induction of plasmablast differentiation and class switch to IgG2a—a process that is favored by IFN-α production by pDCs.[24,28–30] The expanded pDCs in SLE (see Chapter 16) can become activated by ICs and neutrophil extracellular traps (NETs—a source of nuclear self-antigen recognized by TLR7/9) to produce IFN-α.[29,31] The pleiotropic effects of IFN-α include the induction of myeloid dendritic cells (mDCs) responses (which in turn activate T cells), monocyte differentiation, neutrophil hyperactivity, Th1 responses and, together with IL-6, the maturation of B cells into plasmacells.[22,29,31] In mDCs, the high-mobility group box protein-1 (HMGB-1)-containing nucleosomes further elicit autoantibody production via TLR-2, promoting activation of T cells.[21]

Through IL-6 and TNF-α, mDCs also favor the contraction of the pool of suppressive Tregs, promoting an expansion of pro-inflammatory Th17 cells, along with an

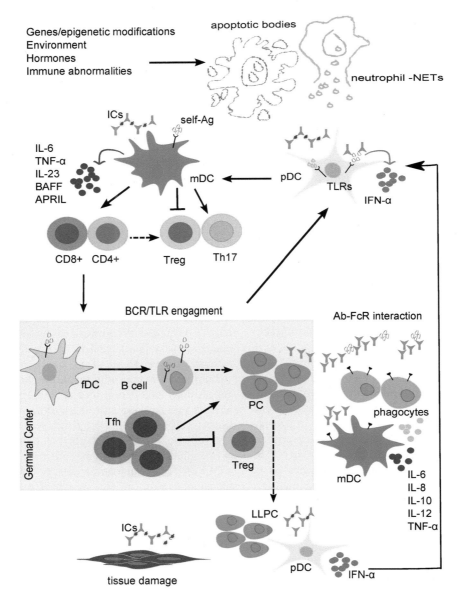

FIGURE 1   Schematic representation of the pathogenesis of SLE. Impaired apoptosis can be caused by a plethora of events and ultimately provokes the release of nuclear antigens that in turn elicit immune responses. Activated through TLR-2, mDCs can secrete pro-inflammatory cytokines (IL-6, TNF-α, IL-23), present nuclear self-antigens to T cells, induce differentiation/activation of pathogenic T cells, and limit Tregs activities. This contributes to the activation of B cells in the GCs. The process is also sustained by BAFF and APRIL produced by mDCs. In the GCs, fDCs can present self-Ag derived from apoptotic remnants, favoring B cell maturation and differentiation to PCs. This process involves the engagement of the extracellular BCR and intracellular TLR9, along with the stimulatory action of Tfh (which inhibit Tregs). Autoantibodies produced by mature PCs form complexes with circulating nucleic-acid containing apoptotic bodies and activate, via FcγR, phagocytes and mDCs, with consequent secretion of pro-inflammatory cytokines (IL-6, IL-8, IL-10, IL-12, TNF-α). PCs can migrate to inflamed tissue where they become LLPCs that make antibodies and contribute to ICs formation. pDCs also migrate to inflamed tissue-internalize antigen and sustain production of IFN-α. pDCs can also be activated by ICs and NETs (via intracellular TLR9) and B cells through BCR/TLR cross-talk. The result in an increased mDC activity and the secretion of cytokines, such as BAFF and APRIL, that support B-cell proliferation and hence ICs formation, with subsequent tissue damage due to chronic inflammation.

increase of Th17-related cytokines IL-17 and IL-23.[22] In this sense, IL-17 appears to play an important role in the pro-inflammatory events that characterize SLE, as indicated by the finding that mice genetically deficient in IL-17 were protected from the development of pristane-induced lupus manifestations, including glomerulonephritis and the production of autoantibodies,[32] The increased production of IL-17 observed in SLE patients and in lupus-prone mice[33,34] could be ascribed to the production of this cytokine by both CD4+ T cells and CD4−CD8− double negative (DN) T cells (which are expanded in the blood and kidney of SLE patients and in lupus mice[35,36]), and appeared regulated by epigenetic mechanisms, multiple transcription factors, and cytokines such as IL-23 (induced by IL-21 and required for the maintenance of IL-17). Interestingly, the genetic deficiency of the IL-23 receptor in B6/*lpr* (lupus-prone) mice associated with an amelioration of lupus nephritis and a reduced production of IL-17, together with a reduced frequency of DN T cells.[37]

Concomitant with an increase in the frequency of cells and augmented production of cytokines with pro-inflammatory activities, SLE presents with a compromised frequency and/or function of peripheral Tregs, particularly in patients with active disease.[38] A central contributor to the reduced activity of Tregs in SLE could be the decreased production of IL-2, which characterizes T cells from SLE patients and lupus-prone mice.[39] This reduced transcription of IL-2 in lupus T cells would be influenced by the transcription factors CREB and CREMα (notably, CREMα activity is indirectly modulated by hormones such as estrogens[40]) and associated with an increased activity of calcium calmodulin kinase IV (CAMKIV). Conversely, the inhibition of CaMKIV could suppress organ damage in MRL/*lpr* mice, induce Foxp3 expression, and decrease the frequency of Th17 cells.[41–44] Another factor that could negatively impact the activity of Tregs could be the activation of the mammalian target of rapamycin (mTOR).[20,1] Notwithstanding these considerations, an expansion of FoxP3+Helios+cells has been reported in subjects with active SLE,[36] together with an impairment in CD8+ Tregs,[36,45,46] suggesting that different types of Tregs could modulate SLE disease activity.

As for T cells in general, lupus T cells have an aberrant persistent mitochondrial hyperpolarization, increased production of reactive oxygen intermediates (or reduced glutathione levels) and ATP depletion,[47] as detailed in Chapter 28. At the molecular level, lupus T cells display a lowered signaling threshold associated with a reduction in the expression of the CD3 ζ chain.[48,49] Finally, lupus T cells display an aggregation of the lipid rafts that contain the TCR/CD3 complex with associated signaling molecules, differently from healthy subjects in which the lipid rafts on T cells are uniformly distributed across the cell surface membrane.[50] The dissolution ex vivo of lipid rafts on lupus T cells corrects TCR/CD3 signaling and delays disease onset in MRL/*lpr* mice.[51,52]

Other T cell abnormalities in SLE include high calcium influx, along with the activation of transcription factors (NFAT, AP1, and NF-κB) and altered differentiation.[53] Also, high levels of CD44 expression associate with increased help to B cells and T cell migration to tissue.[20,1] Additional T cell defects are discussed in Chapter 13.

For lupus B cells, an aberrant activation and subsequent production of autoantibodies are sustained by BCR and TLR co-engagement (B cells, like pDCs, express TLR7 and TLR9).[54] The BCR shuttles bound antigens to TLR7/9, inducing class switch and driving pDCs to produce IFN-α.[20,29] This promotes the expression of B-cell activating factor (BAFF) and the proliferation-inducing ligand (APRIL) in mDCs,[20] and can in part explains why sera from SLE patients have elevated levels of BAFF and why lupus B cells hyperexpress BAFF-receptor. About BAFF and APRIL, these molecules provide—in a T cell-independent manner—survival signals from the late transitional stage through memory and antibody-secreting B cells, in a process that can rescue autoreactive B cells from anergy.[20] Finally, lupus B cells display a delayed recruitment of the tyrosine kinase Lyn, with the retention of antigen by the BCR.[55]

Counteracting the activity of effector cells in SLE, in addition to the aforementioned Tregs, there are other immunoregulatory cells that attempt to keep autoimmunity under control. Those include B cells (Bregs), DCs, and invariant NK (iNK) cells. In humans, B cells expressing CD19+CD24highCD38high are considered to display suppressive properties on Th1 cells due to their elevated production of IL-10[20]. DCs appear instead to favor tolerance through the production of immunomodulatory molecules such as prostaglandin E2 (PGE2),[56] while a contraction of iNK numbers seems to associate with increased IgG levels and SLE disease activity.[57] Finally, mesenchymal stem cells in SLE patients display an increased senescence that could partly explain the delayed repair capacity in tissue injuries observed in SLE.[58]

TISSUE DAMAGE

Tissue inflammation associates with the production of chemoattractant molecules and the creation of survival niches for tissue-recruited cells. In SLE, plasmablasts can migrate to inflamed tissue where they proliferate as long-lived plasma cells (LLPCs). LLPCs can be found in the kidneys of both human and mouse, and these are believed to promote autoantibody production.[20]

More than 100 different autoantibodies have been described in SLE.[59] However, the most commonly associated with disease are anti-DNA (discussed in Chapter 24), anti-chromatin and anti-nucleosomes in lupus nephritis,[60] anti-*N*-methyl-D-aspartate receptors (a type of anti-DNA) in neuropsychiatric manifestation,[61] and anti-phospholipids and β2-glycoprotein 1 in thrombotic events.[62,63] Together with their cognate antigen, autoantibodies form ICs that can be internalized by local pDCs, with subsequent IFN-α production and plasmablast differentiation via T-dependent and T-independent mechanisms, in an autoimmune loop that sustains systemic and local inflammation (Figure 1). However, autoantibody production and disease activity in SLE are not necessarily interrelated, and the clearance of ICs (which involves complement and phagocytes) can play a key role in determining disease severity. For example, after deposition in tissue of ICs containing autoantibodies, the ability to fix complement—a key step in the initiation of tissue damage—can vary among SLE patients, and so can the local recruitment of pro-inflammatory cells and the disposal of apoptotic bodies.[63]

After tissue damage has ensued, chronic inflammation and/or tissue remodeling processes recruit the oxidative stress pathways (see Chapter 28), release metalloproteases, and activate endothelial cells in the kidney and circulation, favoring the development of complications such as renal failure or atherosclerosis, respectively.[63,1]

The infiltrating immune cells found in lupus kidney include pDCs, monocytes, macrophages, T cells (Th17, DN T cells), and B cells, together with platelet aggregates.[64] The aggregated platelets could bind CD40 on pDCs and monocytes, further promoting IFN secretion and vascular damage,[65] whereas NETs could contribute to autoantibody production, release of free radicals, and platelet activation via FCγRIIa.[64] Further details on the events involved in the generation and maintenance of renal tissue damage in SLE are provided in Chapters 33, 40, and 41.

CONCLUSIONS

There are still significant gaps in understanding the complex etiopathogenesis of SLE. As a consequence, current therapies typically employ immunosuppressive drugs with a broad spectrum of action that not only are not uniformly efficacious but also can lead to frequent side effects.

Given the multiple abnormalities in SLE—both at the level of the innate and adaptive immune response—there are significant challenges in the design of therapies that might impact key pathways involved in the pathogenesis of the disease while preserving protective immune responses. Another layer of complexity is represented by the multifaceted manifestations of the disease among SLE patients, implying the need of individual considerations for therapeutic purposes.

Yet, the progressively increased knowledge of the cellular and molecular mechanisms involved in the pathogenesis of SLE can provide hope that new targets for effective therapies with limited side effects will be identified in a near future.

REFERENCES

1. Gualtierotti R, Biggioggero M, Penatti AE, Meroni PL. Updating on the pathogenesis of systemic lupus erythematosus. *Autoimmun Rev* 2010;**10**:3–7.
2. Vaughn SE, Kottyan LC, Munroe ME, Harley JB. Genetic susceptibility to lupus: the biological basis of genetic risk found in B cell signaling pathways. *J Leukoc Biol* 2012;**92**:577–91.
3. Ramos PS, Shaftman SR, Ward RC, Langefeld CD. Genes associated with SLE are targets of recent positive selection. *Autoimmun Dis* 2014;**2014**:203435.
4. Deng Y, Tsao BP. Genetic susceptibility to systemic lupus erythematosus in the genomic era. *Nat Rev Rheumatol* 2010;**6**:683–92.
5. Rullo OJ, Tsao BP. Recent insights into the genetic basis of systemic lupus erythematosus. *Ann Rheum Dis* 2013;**72**(Suppl. 2):56–61.
6. Harley IT, Kaufman KM, Langefeld CD, Harley JB, Kelly JA. Genetic susceptibility to SLE: new insights from fine mapping and genome-wide association studies. *Nat Rev Genet* 2009;**10**:285–90.
7. Taylor KE, Chung SA, Graham RR, Ortmann WA, Lee AT, Langefeld CD, et al. Risk alleles for systemic lupus erythematosus in a large case-control collection and associations with clinical subphenotypes. *PLoS Genet* 2011;**7**:e1001311.
8. Zhang Y, Zhao M, Sawalha AH, Richardson B, Lu Q. Impaired DNA methylation and its mechanisms in CD4+ T cells of systemic lupus erythematosus. *J Autoimmun* 2013;**41**:92–9.
9. Absher DM, Li X, Waite LL, Gibson A, Roberts K, Edberg J, et al. Genome-wide DNA methylation analysis of systemic lupus erythematosus reveals persistent hypomethylation of interferon genes and compositional changes to CD4+ T-cell populations. *PLoS Genet* 2013;**9**:e1003678.
10. Shen N, Liang D, Tang Y, de Vries N, Tak PP. MicroRNAs-novel regulators of systemic lupus erythematosus pathogenesis. *Nat Rev Rheumatol* 2012;**8**:701–9.
11. Amarilyo G, La Cava A. miRNA in systemic lupus erythematosus. *Clin Immunol* 2012;**144**:26–31.
12. Verthelyi D, Ahmed SA. 17β-estradiol, but not 5 α-dihydrotestosterone, augments antibodies to double-stranded deoxyribonucleic acid in non-autoimmune C57BL/6J mice. *Endocrinology* 1994;**135**:2615–22.
13. Grimaldi CM, Cleary J, Dagtas AS, Moussai D, Diamond B. Estrogen alters thresholds for B cell apoptosis and activation. *J Clin Invest* 2002;**109**:1625–33.
14. Gilbert EL, Mathis KW, Ryan MJ. 17β-estradiol protects against the progression of hypertension during adulthood in a mouse model of systemic lupus erythematosus. *Hypertension* 2014;**63**:616–23.
15. Scofield RH, Bruner GR, Namjou B, Kimberly RP, Ramsey-Goldman R, Petri M, et al. Klinefelter's syndrome in male systemic lupus erythematosus patients: support for the notion of a gene-dose effect from the X chromosome. *Arthritis Rheum* 2008;**58**:2511–7.
16. Arnson Y, Shoenfeld Y, Amital H. Effects of tobacco on immunity, inflammation, and autoimmunity. *J Autoimmun* 2010;**34**:258–65.
17. Kuroda Y, Akaogi J, Nacionales DC, Wasdo SC, Szabo NJ, Reeves WH, et al. Distinctive patterns of autoimmune response induced by different types of mineral oil. *Toxicol Sci* 2004;**78**:222–8.
18. Reeves WH, Lee PY, Weinstein JS, Satoh M, Lu L. Induction of autoimmunity by pristane and other naturally occurring hydrocarbons. *Trends Immunol* 2009;**30**:455–64.
19. Manea ME, Mueller RB, Dejica D, Sheriff A, Schett G, Herrmann M, et al. Increased expression of CD154 and FAS in SLE patients' lymphocytes. *Rheumatol Int* 2009;**30**:181–5.
20. Gatto M, Zen M, Ghirardello A, Bettio S, Bassi N, Iaccarino L, et al. Emerging and critical issues in the pathogenesis of lupus. *Autoimmun Rev* 2013;**12**:523–36.
21. Kruse K, Janko C, Urbonaviciute V, Mierke CT, Winkler TH, Voll RE, et al. Inefficient clearance of dying cells in patients with SLE: anti-dsDNA autoantibodies, MFG-E8, HMGB-1 and other players. *Apoptosis* 2010;**15**:1098–113.
22. Chan VS, Nie YJ, Shen N, Yan S, Mok MY, Lau CS. Distinct roles of myeloid and plasmacytoid dendritic cells in systemic lupus erythematosus. *Autoimmun Rev* 2012;**11**:890–7.

23. Muñoz LE, Lauber K, Schiller M, Manfredi AA, Herrmann M. The role of defective clearance of apoptotic cells in systemic autoimmunity. *Nat Rev Rheumatol* 2010;**6**:280–9.

24. Koshy M, Berger D, Crow MK. Increased expression of CD40 ligand on systemic lupus erythematosus lymphocytes. *J Clin Invest* 1996;**98**:826–37.

25. Desai-Mehta A, Lu L, Ramsey-Goldman R, Datta SK. Hyperexpression of CD40 ligand by B and T cells in human lupus and its role in pathogenic autoantibody production. *J Clin Invest* 1996;**97**:2063–73.

26. Simpson N, Gatenby PA, Wilson A, Malik S, Fulcher DA, Tangye SG, et al. Expansion of circulating T cells resembling follicular helper T cells is a fixed phenotype that identifies a subset of severe systemic lupus erythematosus. *Arthritis Rheum* 2010;**62**:234–44.

27. Hutloff A, Büchner K, Reiter K, Baelde HJ, Odendahl M, Jacobi A, et al. Involvement of inducible costimulator in the exaggerated memory B cell and plasma cell generation in systemic lupus erythematosus. *Arthritis Rheum* 2004;**50**:3211–20.

28. Walsh ER, Pisitkun P, Voynova E, Deane JA, Scott BL, Caspi RR, et al. Dual signaling by innate and adaptive immune receptors is required for TLR7-induced B-cell-mediated autoimmunity. *Proc Natl Acad Sci USA* 2012;**109**:16276–81.

29. Pascual V, Farkas L, Banchereau J. Systemic lupus erythematosus: all roads lead to type I interferons. *Curr Opin Immunol* 2006;**18**:676–82.

30. Marshak-Rothstein A. Toll-like receptors in systemic autoimmune disease. *Nat Rev Immunol* 2006;**6**:823–5.

31. Choi J, Kim ST, Craft J. The pathogenesis of systemic lupus erythematosus - an update. *Curr Opin Immunol* 2012;**24**:651–7.

32. Amarilyo G, Lourenço EV, Shi FD, La Cava A. IL-17 promotes murine lupus. *J Immunol* 2014;**193**:540–3.

33. Wong CK, Lit LC, Tam LS, Li EK, Wong PT, Lam CW. Hyperproduction of IL-23 and IL-17 in patients with systemic lupus erythematosus: implications for Th17-mediated inflammation in autoimmunity. *Clin Immunol* 2008;**127**:385–93.

34. Apostolidis SA, Crispín JC, Tsokos GC. IL-17-producing T cells in lupus nephritis. *Lupus* 2011;**20**:120–4.

35. Crispín JC, Oukka M, Bayliss G, Cohen RA, Van Beek CA, Stillman IE, et al. Expanded double negative T cells in patients with systemic lupus erythematosus produce IL-17 and infiltrate the kidneys. *J Immunol* 2008;**181**:8761–6.

36. Mak A, Kow NY. The pathology of T cells in systemic lupus erythematosus. *J Immunol Res* 2014;**2014**:419029.

37. Kyttaris VC, Zhang Z, Kuchroo VK, Oukka M, Tsokos GC. Cutting edge: IL-23 receptor deficiency prevents the development of lupus nephritis in C57BL/6$^{lpr/lpr}$ mice. *J Immunol* 2010;**184**:4605–9.

38. La Cava A. T-regulatory cells in systemic lupus erythematosus. *Lupus* 2008;**17**:421–5.

39. Katsiari CG, Tsokos GC. Transcriptional repression of interleukin-2 in human systemic lupus erythematosus. *Autoimmun Rev* 2006; **5**:118–21.

40. Moulton VR, Holcomb DR, Zajdel MC, Tsokos GC. Estrogen upregulates cyclic AMP response element modulator a expression and downregulates interleukin-2 production by human T lymphocytes. *Mol Med* 2012;**18**:370–8.

41. Ichinose K, Juang YT, Crispín JC, Kis-Toth K, Tsokos GC. Suppression of autoimmunity and organ pathology in lupus-prone mice upon inhibition of calcium/calmodulin-dependent protein kinase type IV. *Arthritis Rheum* 2011;**63**:523–9.

42. Juang YT, Wang Y, Solomou EE, Li Y, Mawrin C, Tenbrock K, et al. Systemic lupus erythematosus serum IgG increases CREM binding to the IL-2 promoter and suppresses IL-2 production through CaMKIV. *J Clin Invest* 2005;**115**:996–1005.

43. Koga T, Ichinose K, Mizui M, Crispin JC, Tsokos GC. Calcium/calmodulindependent protein kinase IV suppresses IL-2 production and regulatory T cell activity in lupus. *J Immunol* 2012;**189**: 3490–6.

44. Koga T, Hedrich CM, Mizui M, Yoshida N, Otomo K, Lieberman LA, et al. CaMKIV-dependent activation of AKT/mTOR and CREM-α underlies autoimmunity-associated Th17 imbalance. *J Clin Invest* 2014;**124**:2234–45.

45. Gerli R, Nocentini G, Alunno A, Bocci EB, Bianchini R, Bistoni O, et al. Identification of regulatory T cells in systemic lupus erythematosus. *Autoimmun Rev* 2009;**8**:426–30.

46. Alvarado-Sanchez B, Hernandez-Castro B, Portales-Perez D, et al. Regulatory T cells in patients with systemic lupus erythematosus. *J Autoimmun* 2006;**27**:110–8.

47. Fernandez D, Perl A. Metabolic control of T cell activation and death in SLE. *Autoimmun Rev* 2009;**8**:184–9.

48. Nambiar MP, Juang YT, Krishnan S, Tsokos GC. Dissecting the molecular mechanisms of TCR z chain downregulation and T cell signaling abnormalities in human systemic lupus erythematosus. *Int Rev Immunol* 2004;**23**:245–63.

49. Krishnan S, Juang YT, Chowdhury B, Magilavy A, Fisher CU, Nguyen H, et al. Differential expression and molecular associations of Syk in systemic lupus erythematosus T cells. *J Immunol* 2008;**181**:8145–52.

50. Krishnan S, Nambiar MP, Warke VG, Fisher CU, Mitchell J, Delaney N, et al. Alterations in lipid raft composition and dynamics contribute to abnormal T cell responses in systemic lupus erythematosus. *J Immunol* 2004;**172**:7821–31.

51. Deng GM, Tsokos GC. Cholera toxin B accelerates disease progression in lupus-prone mice by promoting lipid raft aggregation. *J Immunol* 2008;**181**:4019–26.

52. Jury EC, Isenberg DA, Mauri C, Ehrenstein MR. Atorvastatin restores Lck expression and lipid raft-associated signaling in T cells from patients with systemic lupus erythematosus. *J Immunol* 2006;**177**:7416–22.

53. Moulton VR, Tsokos GC. Abnormalities of T cell signaling in systemic lupus erythematosus. *Arthritis Res Ther* 2011;**13**:207.

54. Hennessy EJ, Parker AE, O'Neill LA. Targeting Toll-like receptors: emerging therapeutics? *Nat Rev Drug Discov* 2010;**9**:293–307.

55. Flores-Borja F, Kabouridis PS, Jury EC, Isenberg DA, Mageed RA. Altered lipid raft-associated proximal signaling and translocation of CD45 tyrosine phosphatase in B lymphocytes from patients with systemic lupus erythematosus. *Arthritis Rheum* 2007;**56**:291–302.

56. Zhang Y, Liu S, Yu Y, Zhang T, Liu J, Shen Q, et al. Immune complex enhances tolerogenecity of immature dendritic cells via FcγRIIb and promotes FcγRIIb- overexpressing dendritic cells to attenuate lupus. *Eur J Immunol* 2011;**41**:1154–64.

57. Chuang YP, Wang CH, Wang NC, Chang DM, Sytwu HK. Modulatory function of invariant natural killer T cells in systemic lupus erythematosus. *Clin Dev Immunol* 2012;**2012**:478429.

58. Li X, Liu L, Meng D, Wang D, Zhang J, Shi D, et al. Enhanced apoptosis and senescence of bone-marrow-derived mesenchymal stem cells in patients with systemic lupus erythematosus. *Stem Cells Dev* 2012;**21**:2387–94.

59. Sherer Y, Gorstein A, Fritzler MJ, Shoenfeld Y. Autoantibody explosion in systemic lupus erythematosus: more than 100 different antibodies found in SLE patients. *Semin Arthritis Rheum* 2004;**34**:501–37.

60. Manson JJ, Ma A, Rogers P, Manson LJ, Berden JH, van der Vlag J, et al. Relationship between anti-dsDNA, anti-nucleosome and anti-alpha-actinin anti-bodies and markers of renal disease in patients with lupus nephritis: a prospective longitudinal study. *Arthritis Res Ther* 2009;**11**:R154.

61. Kowal C, Degiorgio LA, Lee JY, Edgar MA, Huerta PT, Volpe BT, et al. Human lupus autoantibodies against NMDA receptors mediate cognitive impairment. *Proc Natl Acad Sci USA* 2006;**103**:19854–9.

62. Ruiz-Irastorza G, Crowther M, Branch W, Khamashta MA. Antiphospholipid syndrome. *Lancet* 2010;**376**:1498–509.

63. Tsokos G. Systemic lupus erythematosus. *N Engl J Med* 2012;**366**:573–4.

64. Craft JE. Dissecting the immune cell mayhem that drives lupus pathogenesis. *Sci Transl Med* 2011;**3**:73ps9.

65. Joseph JE, Harrison P, Mackie IJ, Isenberg DA, Machin SJ. Increased circulating platelet-leucocyte complexes and platelet activation in patients with antiphospholipid syndrome, systemic lupus erythematosus and rheumatoid arthritis. *Br J Haematol* 2001;**115**:451–9.

Chapter 9

Systemic Lupus Erythematosus and the Environment

Nancy Agmon-Levin[1], Yehuda Shoenfeld[1,2]

[1]The Zabludowicz Center for Autoimmune Diseases Sheba Medical Center, Sackler Faculty of Medicine, Tel-Aviv University, Tel Aviv, Israel;

[2]Incumbent of the Laura Schwarz-Kipp Chair for Research of Autoimmune Diseases, Sackler Faculty of Medicine, Tel-Aviv University, Tel Aviv, Israel

INTRODUCTION

Systemic lupus erythematosus (SLE) is an autoimmune disease characterized by a heterogeneity of clinical manifestations, degrees of severity, and alternating phases of remission and flares, which together formed the concept that this is a syndrome encompassing a myriad of phenotypes rather than a single disease.[1–3] The etiopathogenesis of SLE, similarly to other autoimmune diseases, is defined by the *mosaic of autoimmunity*—a combination of genetic, immune-mediated, hormonal, and environmental factors that trigger and perpetuate the autoimmune process.[4] Notably, the inheritance of genes alone has not been sufficient to explain the development of most autoimmune disease and SLE in particular, even if multiple genetic and epigenetic alterations are taken into consideration. Hence, additional triggers have been suggested to contribute not only to the presentation of SLE but also to its various phenotypes.[5]

The role of environmental agents in SLE has been established and mechanisms by which these agents enable tolerance breakdown have been delineated. Both innate and adaptive pathways may be affected by the environment, such as activation of Toll-like receptor (TLR) by xenobiotics or adjuvants, modifications of self-antigens following infection, activation of T-17 cells, downregulation of T regulatory cells, activation of B cells, and the production of autoantibodies.[6] The latter are the hallmark of SLE and typically appear prior to clinical manifestations of diseases.[7] Various environmental factors, such as infectious agents, vaccines, and drugs, were found to trigger SLE-related autoantibodies production (e.g., anti-dsDNA).[8] In this chapter, we review data regarding the subtle interaction between environmental factors and the host immunity, which eventually lead to the evolution of overt disease. Notably, exposure to some of these factors may be avoided and provide primary and/or secondary prevention of SLE for those who developed this syndrome as well as for those at risk.

INFECTIOUS AGENTS, THE MICROBIOME, AND SLE

Infectious agents play a pivotal role in driving the autoimmune process. This can come about via several mechanisms, of which the principal one is molecular mimicry between infectious epitopes and self-antigens.[8] Other mechanisms have been suggested for the loss tolerance and induction of autoimmunity, such as epitope spreading, in which one epitope evolve into cryptic or neo-epitopes; bystander activation, in which infectious agents causes increases cytokine production; and T-cell activation, viral persistence, B-cell polyclonal activation, or presentation of super antigens.[9] Moreover, specific infectious agents were linked with a particular autoimmune disease and/or specific manifestations. For instance, subsets of lytic or latent viral proteins, such as Epstein–Barr virus (EBV), cytomegalovirus (CMV), and other members of the herpes viruses, parvovirus B19, rubella, mumps, retroviruses, and transfusion-transmitted viruses were associated with the triggering of SLE.[9–11] Bacteria such as mycobacteria and *Klebsiella pneumoniae* were allied with induction of anti-dsDNA antibodies, both in animal models and in humans.[8]

Among viral infections, EBV (a member of the Herpes virus family) is one of the most notorious agents with a dual association to SLE.[9,12,13] On the one hand, prior EBV infection is more prevalent among SLE patients compared to healthy controls; however, other SLE patients' immune response to this virus seems to be less efficient.[14] Notably, EBV-specific antigens are associated with production of SLE-related autoantibodies and clinical manifestations. Injection of EBV nuclear antigen-1 (EBNA-1) was found to induce the production of SLE-specific antibodies directed at Sm, Ro, and ds-DNA in animal models.[15] Moreover, in a meta-analysis of 25 case–control studies, a correlation between SLE and different EBV-specific antigens was documented, such as the anti-EBV-viral capsid antigen (VCA) IgG (OR 2.08; 95% CI; 1.15–3.76, p=0.007), anti-EBV early antigen IgG,

Systemic Lupus Erythematosus. http://dx.doi.org/10.1016/B978-0-12-801917-7.00009-7

63

and anti-VCA IgA (OR 4.5, 95% CI 3.00–11.06, p<0.00001 and OR 5.05, 95% CI 1.95–13.13, p=0.0009, respectively).[12] Furthermore, exposure to EBV is also commonly accompanied by high titers of anti-SSA/Ro antibodies and a particularly mild phenotype of SLE involving mainly the skin and joints.[9] This concept of infectious agents determining the clinical presentation of disease has been advocated for other agents, such as rubella infections and SLE central nervous system manifestations.[16] Alternatively, some infectious agents might exert opposite or "protective" effects.[10] This notion was first proposed in the *hygiene hypothesis*, which aimed to explain the inverse association between some endemic infections and allergic or autoimmune diseases. In this line of thought, infections with plasmodium or parasites correlate with a lower prevalence of SLE.[10]

In recent years, the microbiome effects on the immune system have taken center stage in the pathogenesis of autoimmune and allergic diseases.[3,17] In other words, exposure to infectious agents may be a source of immune education, and most of these interactions occur between the immune system and microbes colonizing the human gut, skin, and other cavities. Predominantly, the gut is the largest lymphoid organ with the largest interface between the outside environment and inner body core. The gut mucosal immune system is constantly bombarded with nonself antigens, food, organisms, and pathogens, and therefore must constantly distinguish between antigens that should be regulated with tolerance compare to those that should be attacked. The role of microbial community influences and SLE remains to be elucidated, although preliminary reports support a connection between intestinal dysbiosis and this autoimmune disease. Hence, one may speculate that modulation of the microbiome may affect SLE and other autoimmune diseases.

CIGARETTE SMOKING AND SLE

Cigarette smoking has an established role in the development of cancer, cardiovascular, pulmonary, and autoimmune diseases such as rheumatoid arthritis, Graves' disease, multiple sclerosis, Crohn's disease, primary biliary cirrhosis, and SLE. An elevated risk for developing SLE was reported among current smokers compared to past or nonsmokers (OR 1.50; CI 1.09–2.08) and a link between smoking and specific SLE manifestations such as cutaneous, serositis, neuropsychiatric manifestations and renal failure was observed.[18,19] This may be further illustrated by the strong association between smoking and forms of cutaneous lupus, namely discoid and subcutaneous lupus erythematosus (SCLE).[19–21]

Atherosclerosis and cardiovascular diseases are leading causes of morbidity and mortality among SLE patients.[13,22] Although the increased prevalence of atherosclerosis in SLE patients is not attributed solemnly to "traditional" risk factors (e.g., smoking, high blood pressure), the interplay

between those factors and immune-mediated ones such as chronic inflammation, endothelial cell activation, and the use of immunosuppressive drugs has been established.[20–22] Several mechanisms explaining causal relationships between smoking and SLE have been put forward. Cigarettes contain toxic chemicals including tars, nicotine, carbon monoxide, and polycyclic aromatic hydrocarbons. Free radicals either contained in cigarette smoke or endogenously produced by smoking can interact with DNA, induce tissue hypoxia and cellular necrosis that may lead to the exposure of intracellular antigens, and result in the production of autoantibodies such as anti-dsDNA antibodies. Smoking is related to chronic inflammation, documented by an increase in inflammatory markers such as C-reactive protein, adhesion molecules and selectines, production of pro-inflammatory cytokines, and stimulation of autoreactive B- and T-lymphocytes.[23] Hence, for SLE patients in particular, as for all of us, cigarette smoking avoidance and/or cessation of smoking are highly recommended.

EXPOSURE TO CHEMICALS AND RISK OF SLE

Organic and inorganic chemicals—namely xenobiotics, organic solvents, silica dusts uranium, phthalate, and pesticides—have all been related to SLE.[24] Silica dusts such as quartz and crystalline silica are minerals that can be inhaled. In lupus-prone mice, exposure to silica accelerated the development of SLE, predominantly of lupus kidney disease, and increased the production of SLE-related autoantibodies. In humans, inhalation of silica is common to certain occupations (e.g., construction, mining, powder manufacturing, farming, dental technicians). The risk of developing SLE seems to correlate with the amount of exposure, determined either by doses or length of exposure. For instance, in a cohort of 28,000 uranium miners that were heavily exposed to inhaled silica, a 10-fold increase in SLE prevalence was reported.[25] In a nested case–control study, among individuals who had resided near a uranium plant in Ohio, the presence of SLE was associated with higher levels of uranium exposure (OR 3.92, 95% CI 1.13–13.59; p<0.031).[26] Silicone implants for augmentation mammoplasty were reported in some lupus-related cases, although a causal association was difficult to ascertain. A stronger link was documented between silicone implants and scleroderma-like disease, as well as a set of clinical manifestations termed ASIA, the autoimmune/autoinflammatory syndrome induced by adjuvants.[27] Silicon has an adjuvant effects and therefore may increase production of pro-inflammatory cytokines, induce apoptosis, and affect T cells mainly by decreasing T regulatory cells. Other potential explanations include the "estrogenic" effects of uranium and silica dusts, as well as somatic and epigenetic changes observed among exposed subjects.[27]

Phthalate is commonly used in foods and biomedical devices, polyvinyl chloride polymers that are being used in children's toys, and cosmetic products including nail polish, lipsticks, and fragrances. In October 2000, the Centers for Disease Control and Prevention and the National Toxicology Program in the United States published data on increased exposure to phthalate, among women aged 20–40 years. Immunization of naïve and SLE-genetically prone animals with phthalate was shown to induce the production of anti-dsDNA antibodies and SLE-like manifestations.[28] Pesticides are a group of chemicals aimed at pest extermination, and those used against insects consist of organ chlorine compounds (e.g., DDT) and organophosphates. Occupational exposure to pesticides was associated with the risk for development of SLE in some studies.[29] Similarly to other chemicals discussed herein, exposure to pesticides was found to induce autoantibodies and aggravate SLE-like disease in animal models.[30]

ULTRAVIOLET RADIATION, VITAMIN D, AND SLE

Photosensitivity is a criterion of SLE, documented in 30–50% of patients. Increased risk of photosensitivity is observed mainly among patients who are seropositive to anti-SSA/Ro and/or anti-SSB/La antibodies. Ultraviolet (UV) radiation—both ultraviolet-A2 (UVA) and ultraviolet B (UVB)—can exacerbate skin and systemic manifestations of SLE. Markedly, this may occur following exposure to artificial lights, particularly halogen and fluorescent lamps. UV-ionized molecules can provoke DNA damage, as well as chemical- and immune-mediated reactions in the skin; in particular, UVB light induces cytotoxicity and keratinocyte apoptosis. Clearing of such apoptototic cells is somewhat defected in SLE, leading to overexpression of self-antigens and the release of pro-inflammatory cytokines. Additionally, UV light may be responsible for the redistribution of intracellular antigens such as SSA/Ro, SSB/La, and snRNP to the apoptotic cell surface, thereby enhancing their exposure to the immune system and specific antibody production.[31] UVB light, mainly in the range of 290–320 nm, is further linked with CD4+ T cells DNA hypomethylation, commonly observed in SLE. In a study of 35 SLE patients and 15 healthy controls exposed to different dosages of UVB, global DNA methylation was significantly lower among SLE patients in a dosage-dependent manner, compared to the control group.[32] In two mouse models, accelerated SLE-like systemic disease was exhibited following UV exposure. In these models, enhanced TLR-7 signaling and defected clearance of apoptotic cells were observed in the BXSB mice and NOD mice, respectively.[20]

Consequently, all of the above support the recommendation to avoid exposure to UV light for patients with SLE or those at high risk of developing the disease. However, this abstention lead to deficient levels of vitamin D, which has been linked with impaired immune functions, enhanced loss of tolerance, and severity of SLE.[20,33,34] In cross-sectional studies, significantly lower levels of vitamin D were observed among SLE patients compared with matched healthy controls. In addition, low levels of vitamin D have been related to SLE activity, severity, and the presence of anti-phospholipids-related thrombosis.[35,36] A temporal relationship between vitamin D levels and the onset of SLE flare was documented in non-African American patients, whereas relatively higher levels were suggested to protect against flares.[34,37] Last but not least, vitamin D is crucial to calcium–phosphorus homeostasis, so vitamin D deficiency may contribute to osteopenia, osteoporosis, and renal disease in SLE patients, similarly to healthy subjects.

Taken together, although further interventional studies are required, it seems prudent to recommend both avoidance of UV exposure as well as monitoring and appropriate supplementation of vitamin D.

DRUGS, VACCINES, AND SLE

Drug-induced lupus erythematosus (DILE) accounts for up to 10% of newly diagnosed SLE cases. More than 80 drugs have been associated with this adverse event, of which some (i.e., procainamide and hydralazine) confer a high risk while others (i.e., quinidine, anti-TNF) are associated with a relatively lower one.[38] DILE can present either as a systemic disease (DISLE) or as a skin disease (DICLE); the former is more common and has been frequently related to the use of hydralazine, procainamide, and minocyclin.[39] DISLE is usually comparable with typical mild SLE, along with unique features such as equal distribution between genders, a relatively older age, normal complement levels, and the presence of anti-histone antibodies in up to 95% of patients, anti-single–stranded DNA, and anti-chromatin antibodies.[40] Biological drugs (e.g., anti-TNFs and interferon [IFN] α) have been linked with DISLE, which may be irreversible. Up to 50% of patients treated with anti-TNFs (i.e., infliximab, adalimumab, or etanercept) will develop ANA reactivity, but only very few will actually develop SLE within 2–30 months following therapy.[41] Interferon-alfa (IFNα) contributes to SLE pathogenesis, and the "IFN signature" is one of the genetic hallmarks of this disease. Similarly to anti-TNF, IFN therapy may induce lupus-like disease. This biologic-related DISLE may manifest with renal and dermatologic symptoms, hypocomplementemia, high titers of anti-dsDNA antibodies, and low titers of anti-histone antibodies.[40,42]

DICLE is very similar to idiopathic SCLE, presenting with symmetric, nonscarring annular polycyclic or papulosquamous lesions. It has been reported following use of calcium channel blockers, angiotensin-converting enzyme inhibitors, thiazide diuretics, and TNF-α inhibitors.[40] The mechanisms by which drugs may induce SLE can be attributed both to the patient and to the specific drug. From the patient perspective, high-risk genes (e.g., HLA-DR4, DR2 or DR3; single C4 allele) or slow acetylation of drugs are considered pivotal. Drug-related factors such as production of reactive oxygen species, DNA methylation, and haptenization of the drug that induce an immune response against the complex drug-protein have been underscored. Noteworthy, biologic drugs may also affect control of B cell hyperactivity and induction of T cells apoptosis.[39,40]

Vaccines, similarly to drugs, are rarely linked to autoimmune phenomena via mechanisms that depend on different ingredients of the vaccine.[43,44] The infectious antigen within a vaccine may persuade autoimmunity by the same mechanisms utilized by infectious agents. Other components such as adjuvants (e.g., aluminum) may activate both the innate and adaptive immune responses, as was outlined in animal models and human studies of the ASIA syndrome induced by adjuvants.[27] In the context of SLE, injection of pristane, a hydrocarbon oil, to the peritoneum of BALB/c mice induced a lupus-like disease characterized by autoantibodies against nuclear components and clinical manifestations of SLE.[45,46] Immunization with the hepatitis B vaccine of NZBWF1 mice, which are genetically prone to develop SLE-like disease, caused exacerbation of SLE-like renal disease and neurological symptoms. Remarkably, in the latter study, aggravation of lupus nephritis was related to the infectious antigen (hepatitis B surface antigen), while neurological manifestations were associated with exposure to the adjuvant (aluminum).[47] In humans, a temporal association between SLE and immunization, particularly with hepatitis B and human papilloma vaccines, has been reported.[43,44,48,49] Nevertheless, prevention of certain infections (e.g., influenza and *Streptococcus pneumoniae*) demand particular attention in SLE patients, especially elderly ones and those receiving high dose immunosuppressive treatments. The use of nonadjuvated vaccine should be considered in such scenarios.[50]

CONCLUSION

Strong ties exist between environmental factors and SLE development, course, and outcome as well as with disease phenotypes. Moreover, it has been suggested that more exposure may aggregate the course of disease. These linkages were documented in humans by epidemiological studies and in animal models. Notably for most triggers, mechanistic explanations were either proven or suggested. This knowledge enables us to consider various measurements for primary and secondary prevention, such as avoidance of cigarette smoking, exposure to UV light, and supplementation of vitamin D (especially if low levels are documented). Refraining from occupational hazards, certain drugs, and adjuvated vaccines should be taken into consideration among SLE patients and subjects at high risk of developing this disease.

REFERENCES

1. Agmon-Levin N, Mosca M, Petri M, Shoenfeld Y. Systemic lupus erythematosus one disease or many? *Autoimmun Rev* June 2012; **11**(8):593–5.
2. Tsokos GC. Systemic lupus erythematosus. *N Engl J Med* December 1, 2011;**365**(22):2110–21.
3. Sparks JA, Costenbader KH. Genetics, environment, and gene-environment interactions in the development of systemic rheumatic diseases. *Rheum Dis Clin N Am* November 2014;**40**(4):637–57.
4. Perricone C, Toubi E, Valesini G, Shoenfeld Y. Autoinflammation and autoimmunity: pathogenic, clinical, diagnostic and therapeutic aspects. *IMAJ* October 2014;**16**(10):601–4.
5. Kamen DL. Environmental influences on systemic lupus erythematosus expression. *Rheum Dis Clin N Am* August 2014;**40**(3):401–12. vii.
6. Parks CG, Miller FW, Pollard KM, Selmi C, Germolec D, Joyce K, et al. Expert panel workshop consensus statement on the role of the environment in the development of autoimmune disease. *Int J Mol Sci* 2014;**15**(8):14269–97.
7. Yaniv G, Twig G, Shor DB, Furer A, Sherer Y, Mozes O, et al. A volcanic explosion of autoantibodies in systemic lupus erythematosus: a diversity of 180 different antibodies found in SLE patients. *Autoimmun Rev* October 16, 2014;**14**(1):75–9.
8. Agmon-Levin N, Blank M, Paz Z, Shoenfeld Y. Molecular mimicry in systemic lupus erythematosus. *Lupus* November 2009;**18**(13):1181–5.
9. Kivity S, Agmon-Levin N, Blank M, Shoenfeld Y. Infections and autoimmunity–friends or foes? *Trends Immunol* August 2009;**30**(8):409–14.
10. Rigante D, Mazzoni MB, Esposito S. The cryptic interplay between systemic lupus erythematosus and infections. *Autoimmun Rev* February 2014;**13**(2):96–102.
11. Nelson P, Rylance P, Roden D, Trela M, Tugnet N. Viruses as potential pathogenic agents in systemic lupus erythematosus. *Lupus* May 2014;**23**(6):596–605.
12. Hanlon P, Avenell A, Aucott L, Vickers MA. Systematic review and meta-analysis of the sero-epidemiological association between Epstein-Barr virus and systemic lupus erythematosus. *Arthritis Res Ther* 2014;**16**(1):R3.
13. Zimlichman E, Rothschild J, Shoenfeld Y, Zandman-Goddard G. Good prognosis for hospitalized SLE patients with non-related disease. *Autoimmun Rev* November 2014;**13**(11):1090–3.
14. Draborg AH, Jacobsen S, Westergaard M, Mortensen S, Larsen JL, Houen G, et al. Reduced response to Epstein-Barr virus antigens by T-cells in systemic lupus erythematosus patients. *Lupus Sci Med* 2014;**1**(1):e000015.
15. Poole BD, Gross T, Maier S, Harley JB, James JA. Lupus-like autoantibody development in rabbits and mice after immunization with EBNA-1 fragments. *J Autoimmun* December 2008;**31**(4):362–71.
16. Zandman-Goddard G, Berkun Y, Barzilai O, Boaz M, Ram M, Anaya JM, et al. Neuropsychiatric lupus and infectious triggers. *Lupus* May 2008;**17**(5):380–4.
17. Ma HD, Wang YH, Chang C, Gershwin ME, Lian ZX. The intestinal microbiota and microenvironment in liver. *Autoimmun Rev* October 12, 2014.
18. Boeckler P, Cosnes A, Frances C, Hedelin G, Lipsker D. Association of cigarette smoking but not alcohol consumption with cutaneous lupus erythematosus. *Arch Dermatol* September 2009;**145**(9):1012–6.
19. Takvorian SU, Merola JF, Costenbader KH. Cigarette smoking, alcohol consumption and risk of systemic lupus erythematosus. *Lupus* May 2014;**23**(6):537–44.

20. Zandman-Goddard G, Solomon M, Rosman Z, Peeva E, Shoenfeld Y. Environment and lupus-related diseases. *Lupus* March 2012; **21**(3):241–50.
21. Bockle BC, Sepp NT. Smoking is highly associated with discoid lupus erythematosus and lupus erythematosus tumidus: analysis of 405 patients. *Lupus* November 19, 2014.
22. Hollan I, Meroni PL, Ahearn JM, Cohen Tervaert JW, Curran S, Goodyear CS, et al. Cardiovascular disease in autoimmune rheumatic diseases. *Autoimmun Rev* August 2013;**12**(10):1004–15.
23. Arnson Y, Shoenfeld Y, Amital H. Effects of tobacco smoke on immunity, inflammation and autoimmunity. *J Autoimmun* May 2010; **34**(3):J258–65.
24. Parks CG, De Roos AJ. Pesticides, chemical and industrial exposures in relation to systemic lupus erythematosus. *Lupus* May 2014;**23**(6):527–36.
25. Parks CG, Cooper GS. Occupational exposures and risk of systemic lupus erythematosus: a review of the evidence and exposure assessment methods in population- and clinic-based studies. *Lupus* 2006;**15**(11):728–36.
26. Lu-Fritts PY, Kottyan LC, James JA, Xie C, Buckholz JM, Pinney SM, et al. Association of systemic lupus erythematosus with uranium exposure in a community living near a uranium-processing plant: a nested case-control study. *Arthritis Rheumatol* November 2014;**66**(11):3105–12.
27. Shoenfeld Y, Agmon-Levin N. 'ASIA' - autoimmune/inflammatory syndrome induced by adjuvants. *J Autoimmun* February 2011; **36**(1):4–8.
28. Lim SY, Ghosh SK. Autoreactive responses to environmental factors: 3. Mouse strain-specific differences in induction and regulation of anti-DNA antibody responses due to phthalate-isomers. *J Autoimmun* August 2005;**25**(1):33–45.
29. Cooper GS, Parks CG, Treadwell EL, St Clair EW, Gilkeson GS, Dooley MA. Occupational risk factors for the development of systemic lupus erythematosus. *J Rheumatol* October 2004;**31**(10):1928–33.
30. Sobel ES, Wang F, Butfiloski E, Croker B, Roberts SM. Comparison of chlordecone effects on autoimmunity in (NZBxNZW) F(1) and BALB/c mice. *Toxicology* February 1, 2006;**218**(2–3):81–9.
31. Kuhn A, Ruland V, Bonsmann G. Photosensitivity, phototesting, and photoprotection in cutaneous lupus erythematosus. *Lupus* August 2010;**19**(9):1036–46.
32. Wu Z, Li X, Qin H, Zhu X, Xu J, Shi W. Ultraviolet B enhances DNA hypomethylation of CD4+ T cells in systemic lupus erythematosus via inhibiting DNMT1 catalytic activity. *J Dermatol Sci* September 2013;**71**(3):167–73.
33. Agmon-Levin N, Theodor E, Segal RM, Shoenfeld Y. Vitamin D in systemic and organ-specific autoimmune diseases. *Clin Rev Allergy Immunol* October 2013;**45**(2):256–66.
34. Schneider L, Dos Santos AS, Santos M, da Silva Chakr RM, Monticielo OA. Vitamin D and systemic lupus erythematosus: state of the art. *Clin Rheumatol* August 2014;**33**(8):1033–8.
35. Amital H, Szekanecz Z, Szucs G, Danko K, Nagy E, Csepany T, et al. Serum concentrations of 25-OH vitamin D in patients with systemic lupus erythematosus (SLE) are inversely related to disease activity: is it time to routinely supplement patients with SLE with vitamin D? *Ann Rheum Dis* June 2010;**69**(6):1155–7.
36. Agmon-Levin N, Blank M, Zandman-Goddard G, Orbach H, Meroni PL, Tincani A, et al. Vitamin D: an instrumental factor in the antiphospholipid syndrome by inhibition of tissue factor expression. *Ann Rheum Dis* January 2011;**70**(1):145–50.
37. Birmingham DJ, Hebert LA, Song H, Noonan WT, Rovin BH, Nagaraja HN, et al. Evidence that abnormally large seasonal declines in vitamin D status may trigger SLE flare in non-African Americans. *Lupus* July 2012;**21**(8):855–64.
38. Chang C, Gershwin ME. Drugs and autoimmunity–a contemporary review and mechanistic approach. *J Autoimmun* May 2010; **34**(3):J266–75.
39. Marzano AV, Vezzoli P, Crosti C. Drug-induced lupus: an update on its dermatologic aspects. *Lupus* October 2009;**18**(11):935–40.
40. Katz U, Zandman-Goddard G. Drug-induced lupus: an update. *Autoimmun Rev* November 2010;**10**(1):46–50.
41. Takase K, Horton SC, Ganesha A, Das S, McHugh A, Emery P, et al. What is the utility of routine ANA testing in predicting development of biological DMARD-induced lupus and vasculitis in patients with rheumatoid arthritis? Data from a single-centre cohort. *Ann Rheum Dis* September 2014;**73**(9):1695–9.
42. Obermoser G, Pascual V. The interferon-alpha signature of systemic lupus erythematosus. *Lupus* August 2010;**19**(9):1012–9.
43. Agmon-Levin N, Paz Z, Israeli E, Shoenfeld Y. Vaccines and autoimmunity. *Nat Rev Rheumatol* November 2009;**5**(11):648–52.
44. Tomijenovic L, Arango MT, Agmon-Levin N. Vaccination in autoimmune animal models. *IMAJ* October 2014;**16**(10):657–8.
45. Reeves WH, Lee PY, Weinstein JS, Satoh M, Lu L. Induction of autoimmunity by pristane and other naturally occurring hydrocarbons. *Trends Immunol* September 2009;**30**(9):455–64.
46. Xu Y, Zeumer L, Reeves WH, Morel L. Induced murine models of systemic lupus erythematosus. *Methods Mol Biol* 2014;**1134**:103–30.
47. Agmon-Levin N, Arango MT, Kivity S, Katzav A, Gilburd B, Blank M, et al. Immunization with hepatitis B vaccine accelerates SLE-like disease in a murine model. *J Autoimmun* November 2014;**54**:21–32.
48. Agmon-Levin N, Zafrir Y, Kivity S, Balofsky A, Amital H, Shoenfeld Y. Chronic fatigue syndrome and fibromyalgia following immunization with the hepatitis B vaccine: another angle of the 'autoimmune (auto-inflammatory) syndrome induced by adjuvants' (ASIA). *Immunol Res* December 2014;**60**(2–3):376–83.
49. Gatto M, Agmon-Levin N, Soriano A, Manna R, Maoz-Segal R, Kivity S, et al. Human papillomavirus vaccine and systemic lupus erythematosus. *Clin Rheumatol* September 2013;**32**(9):1301–7.
50. Murdaca G, Orsi A, Spano F, Puppo F, Durando P, Icardi G, et al. Influenza and pneumococcal vaccinations of patients with systemic lupus erythematosus: current views upon safety and immunogenicity. *Autoimmun Rev* February 2014;**13**(2):75–84.

Chapter 10

Genes and Genetics in Human Systemic Lupus Erythematosus

Yun Deng, Betty P. Tsao

Division of Rheumatology, Department of Medicine, David Geffen School of Medicine, University of California, Los Angeles, Los Angeles, CA, USA

INTRODUCTION

Studies on the genetic basis of systemic lupus erythematosus (SLE) have evolved in recent decades. From candidate gene studies and linkage scans to the genome-wide association study (GWAS) and subsequent meta-analyses/large-scale replication studies, researchers have mapped more than 50 robust loci associated with SLE susceptibility predominantly in multiple ancestries.[1] Follow-up fine mapping and functional characterization of these genetic signals help to localize candidate causative variants, identify target gene(s) directly influenced by the associated variants, and elucidate pathogenic mechanisms to explain how SLE susceptibility genes affect disease risk and/or manifestations.

Most disease-associated variants lie in the noncoding regions regulating gene expression through transcriptional/posttranscriptional mechanisms or epigenetic modifications. Although fewer risk variants mapped at gene coding sequences, many have been shown to exhibit altered functions of the encoded proteins. The majority of established SLE susceptibility genes encode products involved in innate and adaptive immune responses, particularly the three key immunological pathways relevant to the pathogenesis of SLE: (1) activation of Toll-like receptor (TLR), type I interferon (IFN), and nuclear factor κB (NF-κB) signaling; (2) clearance of apoptotic cells and immune complexes (ICs); and (3) dysfunctions in lymphocyte signaling (Figure 1). In this chapter, we discuss the genes grouped by pathways that show an association with SLE risk exceeding the GWAS significance level ($p < 5 \times 10^{-8}$), with an emphasis on those that have causative variants implicated and functional consequences investigated (Table 1).

SLE-RISK GENES IN IMMUNOLOGICAL PATHWAYS

Type I IFN Pathway

Dysregulation of type I IFN has been recognized as a central driver of SLE pathogenesis.[2] The mechanisms by which elevated type I IFN affecting SLE development include promoting monocyte and plasmacytoid dendritic cell differentiation, autoreactive T/B cell activation, autoantibody production, and proinflammatory cyto/chemokine expression. Over half of the identified SLE susceptibility genes encode proteins with functions that can be directly or indirectly linked to this pathway.

Binding of ICs containing self-antigens and nucleic acids by Toll-like receptors (e.g., TLR7) or other cytosolic sensors (e.g., IFIH1) is a major trigger of type I IFN production in SLE. Studies in lupus-prone mouse models propose that TLR7-dependent MyD88 signaling is essential for activation of autoreactive lymphocytes, proliferation of dendritic cells, development of spontaneous germinal centers and autoantibody production, contributing to lupus pathogenesis.[3,4] The SLE-associated SNP of *TLR7* located within a binding site for miRNA-3148 shows allelic effect on regulating *TLR7* expression. The risk allele confers decreased degradation of *TLR7* transcripts, resulting in elevated *TLR7* levels and heightened downstream IFN response.[5,6] Genetic association of *IFIH1* with SLE could be explained by the three independent variants: one intronic and two missense SNPs.[7] Both missense variants produce phenotypic changes in apoptosis and inflammation-related gene expression. The intronic risk allele leads to decreased *IFIH1* transcript levels by disruption of binding to protein complex including nucleolin and autoantigen Ku70/80, which would be expected to promote autoantibody generation. In addition, rarely gain-of-function mutations in *IFIH1* have also been implicated in Aicardi-Goutières syndrome (AGS), an inflammatory disease characterized by type I IFN activation.[8] Similarly, rare variants of *RNASEH2*, another AGS-causal gene that encodes three subunits of the genome surveillance enzyme ribonuclease H2, increase risk for SLE and contribute to multistep initiation of autoimmunity by enhancing type I IFN responses to endogenous and external factors.[9]

Transcription factors downstream of endosomal TLRs, including IRF5, IRF7, and IRF8, are required for activating transcription of type I IFN genes. Genetic variants in or near these three genes have been implicated in SLE

Systemic Lupus Erythematosus. http://dx.doi.org/10.1016/B978-0-12-801917-7.00010-3

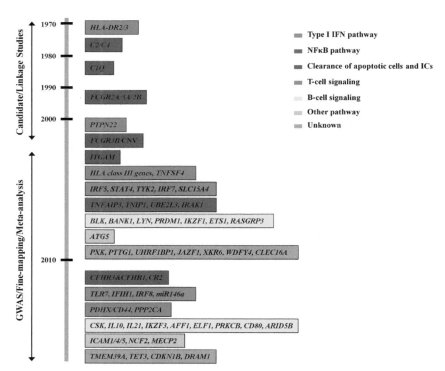

FIGURE 1 Identification of SLE-risk genes in each pathway. Abbreviations: *AFF1*, AF4/FMR2 family member 1; *ARID5B*, AT-rich interactive domain 5B; *ATG5*, autophagy-related 5; *BANK1*, B-cell scaffold protein with ankyrin repeats one; *BLK*, B lymphoid tyrosine kinase; *C1Q*, complement component 1, q subcomponent; *C2*, complement component 2; *C4*, complement component 4; *CD44*, CD44 molecule; *CD80*, CD80 molecule; *CDKN1B*, cyclin-dependent kinase inhibitor 1B; *CFHR1*, complement factor H-related 1; *CFHR3*, complement factor H-related 3; *CLEC16A*, C-type lectin domain family 16 member A; *CSK*, c-src tyrosine kinase; *CR2*, complement receptor 2; *DRAM1*, DNA-damage regulated autophagy modulator 1; *ELF1*, E74-like factor 1; *ETS1*, v-ets avian erythroblastosis virus E26 oncogene homolog 1; *FCGR2A*, Fc fragment of IgG low affinity IIa receptor; *FCGR3A*, Fc fragment of IgG low affinity IIIa receptor; *FCGR2B*, Fc fragment of IgG low affinity IIb receptor; *FCGR3B*, Fc fragment of IgG low affinity IIIb receptor; HLA, human leukocyte antigen; *ICAM1*, intercellular adhesion molecule 1; *ICAM4*, intercellular adhesion molecule 4; *ICAM5*, intercellular adhesion molecule 5; *IFIH1*, interferon induced with helicase C domain 1; *IKZF1*, IKAROS family zinc finger 1; *IKZF3*, IKAROS family zinc finger 3; *IL10*, interleukin 10; *IL21*, interleukin 21; *IRF5*, interferon regulatory factor 5; *IRF7*, interferon regulatory factor 7; *IRF8*, interferon regulatory factor 8; *IRAK1*, interleukin-1 receptor-associated kinase 1; *ITGAM*, integrin alpha M; *JAZF1*, JAZF zinc finger 1; *LYN*, v-yes-1 Yamaguchi sarcoma viral-related oncogene homolog; *MECP2*, methyl CpG binding protein 2; *miR146a*, microRNA146a; *NCF2*, neutrophil cytosolic factor 2; *PDHX*, pyruvate dehydrogenase complex component X; *PRDM1*, PR domain containing 1 with ZNF domain; *PPP2CA*, protein phosphatase 2, catalytic subunit, alpha isozyme; *PRKCB*, protein kinase C beta; *PTPN22*, protein tyrosine phosphatase non-receptor type 22; *PTTG1*, pituitary tumor-transforming 1; *PXK*, PX domain containing serine/threonine kinase; *RASGRP3*, RAS guanyl releasing protein 3; *SLC15A4*, solute carrier family 15 (oligopeptide transporter) member 4; *STAT4*, signal transducer and activator of transcription 4; *TET3*, tet methylcytosine dioxygenase 3; *TLR7*, Toll-like receptor 7; *TMEM39A*, transmembrane protein 39A; *TNFAIP3*, tumor necrosis factor alpha-induced protein 3; *TNIP1*, TNFAIP3 interacting protein 1; *TNFSF4*, tumor necrosis factor superfamily member 4; *TYK2*, tyrosine kinase 2; *UBE2L3*, ubiquitin-conjugating enzyme E2L3; *UHRF1BP1*, UHRF1 binding protein 1; *WDFY4*, WDFY family member 4; *XKR6*, XK Kell blood group complex subunit-related family member 6.

susceptibility across multiple ancestries.[10] In particular, variants at *IRF5* and *IRF7* loci have functional impact on increased serum IFN-α activity in the presence of specific autoantibodies.[11,12] Using computational approaches to model the *IRF5* locus association, a study has identified two independent genetic effects responsible for *IRF5* with SLE: one in the *IRF5* promoter present in all ancestries and one in an 85.5-kb haplotype containing genes *IRF5* and transportin 3 (*TNPO3*) present only in Europeans.[13] The risk allele of a variant tagging the promoter effect was correlated with increased binding of transcription factor ZBTB3 and elevated *IRF5* expression, supporting it as a likely causal variant in addition to the known functional

IRF5 polymorphisms.[13] Integration of genetic data with expression quantitative-trait loci (eQTL) studies leads to identification of an SNP located within the SLE-associated *IRF7* haplotype, conferring not only *cis*-eQTL effect on *IRF7* expression but also *trans*-eQTL effect on regulating type I IFN responses in activated dendritic cells.[14] This parallel progress in *IRF5* and *IRF7* suggests that advanced analytical strategy may help future studies aimed at localizing causal variants and dissecting etiological genetic effects.

Other genes related to this pathway that are associated with increased risk for SLE include *STAT4*,[15–18] *TYK2*,[19] *SLC15A4*[16,20,21] and *miR-146a*.[22] MiR-146a can inhibit key signaling proteins in the type I IFN pathway and is

TABLE 1 SLE Susceptibility Genes Grouped by Pathways That Have Causative Variants Implicated

Function	Position	Gene	OR	Population	Likely Causative Variant	References
Immunological Pathways						
Type I IFN Pathway						
	2q24	IFIH1	1.1–1.4	EA, AA	rs13023380 (A allele) results in decreased IFIH1 transcript levels; rs1990760 (A946T; A allele) and rs10930046 (H460R; A allele) confer increased apoptosis and elevated inflammation-related gene expression.	7
	5q34	miR146a	1.3	AS	rs57095329 (G allele) conferring decreased Ets-1 binding is associated with reduced miR146a levels.	22
	7q32	IRF5	1.3–1.9	EU, EA, AA, AS, HS	Four SNPs define risk haplotypes associated with increased expression of IRF5 and IFN-α. rs4728142 (A allele) tagging the promoter effect confers increased ZBTB3 binding and elevated IRF5 expression.	11,13
	11p15	IRF7	1.3–2.0	EU, EA, AA, AS	rs12805435 confers cis-eQTL effect on IRF7 expression and trans-eQTL effect on regulating type I IFN responses in activated dendritic cells.	14
	Xp22	TLR7	1.2–2.3	AS, EA, AA, HS	rs3853839 (G allele) confers increased TLR7 expression and IFN response.	5,6
NFκB Pathway						
	6q23	TNFAIP3	1.7–2.3	EU, EA, AS	TT>A polymorphic dinucleotide (deletion T followed by A transversion) with decreased NFκB binding to the promoter attenuates TNFAIP3 expression.	26,29
	Xq28	IRAK1	1.1–1.6	EA, AS, AA, HS	rs1059702 (S196F; A allele) tagging a risk haplotype confers increased NFκB activity.	27
Clearance of Apoptotic Cells and ICs						
	1q23	FCGR2A	1.3–1.4	EU, EA, AA, AS	rs1801274 (H166R; T allele) alters binding affinity of FcγRIIa and affects IC clearance.	31
		FCGR3A	1.2–1.5	EU, AA	rs396991 (F176V; T allele) alters binding affinity of FcγRIIIa and affects IC clearance.	31
		FCGR2B	1.3–2.5	AS	rs1050501 (I232T; C allele) alters binding affinity of FcγRIIb and affects IC clearance.	31
		FCGR3B	1.7–2.3	EU, AA	Decreased copy number correlates with FcγRIIIb expression and IC clearance	31
	16p11.2	ITGAM	1.3–2.1	EA, EU, AA, AS, HS	rs1143679 (R77H; A allele) impairs leukocyte phagocytosis	33
T and B Cell Signaling						
	1p13.2	PTPN22	1.4–2.4	EU, HS	rs2476601 (R620W; T allele) alters TCR and BCR signaling with enhanced B cell autoreactivity, and is associated with diminished type I IFN production in myeloid cells but enhanced functions in neutrophils.	39–42

Continued

TABLE 1 SLE Susceptibility Genes Grouped by Pathways That Have Causative Variants Implicated—cont'd

Function	Position	Gene	OR	Population	Likely Causative Variant	References
Immunological Pathways						
	1q31-q32	IL10	1.2–1.3	EU, EA	rs3122605 (G allele) tags a risk haplotype associated with increased *IL10* expression by preferentially binding to Elk-1.	53
	4q24	BANK1	1.2–1.4	EU, EA, AS, AA	rs10516487 (R61H; G allele) and rs3733197 (A383T; G allele) encode mutant BANK1; rs17266594 (T allele) alters splicing efficiency of *BANK1* transcript isoforms.	49
	7p12.2	IKZF1	1.2–1.4	EU, AS	rs4917014 (T allele) alters *IKZF1* levels in cis and regulates expression of *C1QB* and five type I IFN response genes in trans.	16,51
	8p23	BLK	1.2–1.6	EU, EA, AS, AA	rs922483 (T allele) and tri-allelic SNP rs1382568 (A, C alleles) reduce *BLK* promoter activity.	50
	15q24.1	CSK	1.3	EU	rs34933034 (A allele) is associated with increased *CSK* expression, Lyn phosphorylation, BCR-mediated activation of mature B cells and expansion of transitional B cells.	48
Others						
DNA methylation	Xq28	MECP2	1.1–1.6	EA, AS, AA, HS	rs1059702 (S196F; A allele) tagging a risk haplotype is associated with decreased *MECP2* expression.	27,55
ROS generation	1q25	NCF2	1.2–2.8	EA, AA, HS	rs17849502 (H389Q; A allele) confers decreased NADPH oxidase activity and ROS production.	57

Abbreviations: AA, African-American; AS, Asian; EA, European-American; EU, European; HS, Hispanic. OR, odds ratio.

considered as a negative regulator of immune activation.[23] The SLE-associated variant at *miR146a* promoter confers lower levels of its transcript due to decreased binding of transcription factor Ets-1 (encoded by *ETS1*, which has also been identified as a risk gene for SLE).[16,22,24]

NFκB Pathway

SLE risk genes with functions in the NFκB pathway downstream of TLR engagement include *TNFAIP3*,[16,25,26] *TNIP1*,[16,20] *UBE2L3*,[15,16,20] and *IRAK1*.[27] *TNFAIP3* encodes a deubiquitinating enzyme (A20) participating in the termination of NFκB signaling. Decreased A20 expression predisposing to autoimmunity has been demonstrated by development of lupus-like phenotypes in mice with full or conditional A20 deficiency.[28] A pair of tandem polymorphic dinucleotides (TT>A) downstream of *TNFAIP3* promoter explains genetic association of *TNFAIP3* with human SLE.[26] The risk alleles with inefficient delivery of nuclear protein complex to the *TNFAIP3* promoter attenuates A20 expression, leading to enhanced NFκB signaling activity that contributes to SLE.[29] The X-linked gene *IRAK1* encodes a kinase acting with MyD88 to regulate NFκB activation. The missense variant of *IRAK1* (S196F), which confers increased NFκB activity, captures a risk haplotype associated with SLE shared by multiple ancestries.[27]

Clearance of Apoptotic Cells and ICs

Accumulation of self-antigens resulting from inefficient clearance of apoptotic cells and ICs may initiate autoimmune response and promote chronic inflammation in SLE.[30] Deficiencies or polymorphisms in multiple members of this pathway contribute to both monogenic and polygenic forms of SLE, such as a complete deficiency in one of the classical complement pathway genes (e.g., *C1Q* and *C4*), deletion of *CFHR3/CFHR1*, decreased copy number variations of *FCGR3B*, and missense mutations of *FCGR2A/FCGR3A*.[31] CD11b (encoded by *ITGAM*) together with CD18 form the complement receptor 3 functioning in phagocytosis of complement-coated particles and ICs as well as regulation of leukocyte apoptosis, adhesion, and migration via interaction with ligands, such as ICAM1, which has also been associated with SLE.[32] The mutant CD11b encoded by the SLE-risk *ITGAM* allele with an amino acid change from Arg to His (R77H) has impaired phagocytosis of complement-opsonised targets by monocytes, neutrophils, and macrophages, which might alter IC clearance and deposition, resulting in tissue damage.[33] This is supported by the finding of increased risk in developing lupus nephritis (LN) among patients carrying the *ITGAM* risk allele.[34,35]

T-Cell Signaling

Genes implicated in T-cell regulation have been associated with SLE. The highly conserved and extended haplotypes bearing the class II *HLA-DR2* and *HLA-DR3* alleles with SLE have been well recognized in predominantly European populations.[31] HLA class II molecules mediate host defense responses through antigen presentation and immune tolerance by self/nonself recognition. Given their roles in T-cell-dependent antibody responses, cumulative studies have reported the association of class II alleles with autoantibody production, especially *HLA-DR3* with anti-Ro/La antibodies.[36] In addition, the importance of *HLA* class III genes in SLE susceptibility has been highlighted by GWAS and fine-mapping studies, including mutS homolog 5 (*MSH5*) with function in DNA repair,[15,37] RD RNA binding protein (*RDBP*), superkiller viralicidic activity 2-like (*SKIV2L*), dom-3 homolog Z (*DOM3Z*), and serine–threonine kinase 19 (*STK19*) involved in RNA processing.[38] The causal variants remain elusive due to tight linkage disequilibrium across SLE-associated *HLA* haplotypes, and intense efforts are underway to refine association signals within this complex region.

PTPN22 encodes a tyrosine phosphatase regulating immune signaling. Humans carrying the SLE-risk 620W allele and knock-in mice expressing the syntenic 619W mutation show altered T-cell receptor (TCR) and BCR signaling with enhanced B cell autoreactivity.[39] In naive and effector T-cells, PTPN22 can limit TCR signaling by weak agonists and self-antigens while not impeding responses to strong agonist antigens, which may explain the population expansion of effector and memory T-cells observed in humans and mice with either *PTPN22* variants or *Ptpn22*[−/−] alleles.[40] In nonlymphocytes, the risk 620W allele is associated with diminished TLR-induced type I IFN production in myeloid cells,[41] but with enhanced functions in neutrophils including increased transendothelial migration, Ca^{2+} release, and reactive oxygen species (ROS) production.[42] This line of investigation highlights the importance of exploring the functional consequences of disease-associated variants in diverse immune cell types.

The serine/threonine protein phosphatase 2A (PP2A) plays a key role in cellular processes including cell division, motility, and cytoskeletal dynamics. Dysregulation of its catalytic subunit PP2Ac (encoded by *PPP2CA*) associated with altered transcription factor activation, including CREB, ELF1 and SP1, has been found in T-cells from SLE patients, and such changes may affect T-cell function by reducing IL-2 production and TCR-associated signaling molecule expression.[43] Decreased CpG-DNA methylation at the *PPP2CA* promoter and compromised binding of transcription factor IKZF1 together with reduced recruitment of histone deacetylase HDAC1 to an SLE-associated variant site in the first intron of *PPP2CA* may partially explain the increased PP2Ac levels in SLE T-cells.[44–46]

The family of signaling lymphocytic activation molecules (SLAMF) comprises nine type I transmembrane glycoprotein receptors that provide co-stimulatory signals for the TCR-CD3 complex and mediate regulatory signals between immune cells. SLAMF3 and SLAMF6 molecules are expressed at higher levels on SLE T-cells, and SLAMF3/SLAMF6-mediated co-stimulation results in increased generation of T_H17 cells, enhanced shuttling of transcription factor RORγt to the nucleus, and transactivation of *IL17A*, contributing to the proinflammatory phenotype of SLE T-cells.[43] Evidence in support of the SLAMF genes associated with SLE risk comes from both human and mouse studies. Linkage studies in families with SLE have identified a susceptibility locus on chromosome 1q23 harboring the genes encoding SLAMF molecules.[47] In mice, the genomic region syntenic to human 1q23 has also been implicated in three different models of spontaneous SLE: (NZB × NZW) F1, NZM2410 and BXSB mice, and the *Sle1b* locus containing SLAMF variants (especially *Slamf6*) embedded in the C57BL/6 background may be the major candidate to be causally correlated with the *B6.Sle1b* phenotype.[47]

B-Cell Signaling

B-cells play critical roles in SLE pathogenesis through both antibody-dependent and -independent functions. Multiple genes encoding kinases, adaptor molecules, and cytokines associated with B-cell functions have been implicated in SLE susceptibility. c-Src tyrosine kinase (encoded by *CSK*) via interaction with tyrosine phosphatases regulates Src kinases (e.g., Lyn) activation in lymphocytes. The SLE-risk *CSK* variant is associated with high *CSK* expression, increased Lyn phosphorylation, enhanced BCR-mediated mature B-cells, activation, and transitional B-cells, expansion, supporting *CSK* involved in multiple developmental stages of B-cells.[48] *BANK1*, encoding an adaptor/scaffold protein, facilitates intracellular calcium release and alters B-cell activation threshold. Three functional variants that explain genetic associations of *BANK1* with SLE contribute to the sustained BCR signaling and B-cell hyperactivity characteristics of SLE.[49] *BLK*, encoding a member of the Src family kinases, functions in intracellular signaling and regulation of B-cell proliferation, differentiation, and tolerance. The SLE-risk *BLK* promoter variants confer reduced promoter activity in B-cell lines representing different B-cell developmental stages, suggesting that decreased *BLK* expression may affect development and functional responses in B-cells.[50] *IKZF1*, which encodes a transcription factor regulating lymphocyte differentiation, proliferation, and BCR signaling, has been identified as an SLE-risk gene.[16] The SLE-risk *IKZF1* variant not only alters the *IKZF1* levels in *cis* but also regulates expression of *C1QB* and five type I IFN response genes in *trans*, illustrating that *trans*-eQTL mapping can help yield insights into downstream effects of the disease-associated variants.[51]

IL-10, a pivotal cytokine with immunosuppressive and immunostimulatory properties, has been found elevated in sera from SLE patients correlating with disease activity.[52] Immune cells ubiquitously express IL10 with T-/B-cells and monocytes/macrophages as major sources. The molecular mechanism regulating *IL10* expression involves both genetic and epigenetic factors. The *IL10* risk allele confers increased *IL10* expression by preferentially binding to the activated transcription factor Elk-1 associated with disease activity in B-cells of SLE patients.[53] In addition to genetic variants, epigenetic remodeling by reduced DNA methylation and *trans*-activation of *IL10* transcription by increased Stat3/Stat5 recruitment to the *IL10* regulatory regions could promote IL-10 expression in SLE T-cells, contributing to the disease pathogenesis.[54]

Other SLE-associated genes with roles in T/B cell functions (Figure 1) await delineation of functional mechanisms to explain how they influence disease risk and/or manifestations.

SLE-RISK GENES WITH OTHER FUNCTIONS

In addition to immune signaling, other pathways containing multiple SLE susceptibility genes have potential relevance to the disease pathogenesis. For example, the role of DNA hypomethylation in SLE has been well recognized, and *MECP2* (located 2 kb upstream of *IRAK1*) encodes a transcriptional regulator modulating expression of methylation-sensitive genes. Humans carrying the SLE-risk *IRAK1-MECP2* haplotype with increased levels of a specific *MECP2* transcript isoform in stimulated T-cells showed DNA hypomethylation of IFN-regulated genes.[55] *NCF2* encodes a subunit of NADPH (nicotinamide adenine dinucleotide phosphate) oxidase complex involved in the ROS generation. Overproduction of ROS may lead to oxidative stress stimulating autoimmune responses.[56] The SLE-risk *NCF2* variant is associated with low NADPH oxidase activity and reduced ROS production, providing new insight of an anti-inflammatory role for ROS in autoimmune diseases.[57] The remaining SLE-associated loci with

unknown immune function require further fine-mapping and characterization of new pathways contributing to the development of SLE.

GENES CONNECTED TO PHENOTYPES IN SLE

Genetic effects on clinical subphenotypes have been evaluated by genotype–phenotype association studies. Multiple established SLE-risk genes are associated with anti-dsDNA autoantibody (e.g., *HLA-DR2/DR3*, *STAT4*, *IRF5/IRF7*, *IFIH1*, *ITGAM*, and *UBE2L3*)[58] and/or renal disorders (e.g., *ITGAM*, *STAT4*, *TNFSF4*, *TNFAIP3*, and *TNIP1*).[59,60] An analysis of specific manifestations with 22 validated SLE-susceptibility loci has showed cumulative genetic associations with age at diagnosis, anti-dsDNA autoantibody, oral ulcers, immunological and hematologic disorders, single marker association with renal disorders and arthritis, and no genetic association with malar/discord rash, photosensitivity, serositis, and neurological disorder.[61] Given that the gene nonmuscle myosin heavy chain 9 (*MYH9*) has been implicated in focal segmental glomerulosclerosis, hypertensive, and diabetic end-stage renal disease (ESRD), its role in LN was investigated together with the closely linked gene apolipoprotein L1 (*APOL1*). A significant association between LN and *MYH9* was found in European-Americans but not in African-Americans, Asians, Amerindians, or Hispanics.[62] The *APOL1* G1/G2 alleles strongly impact the risk and the time of progression to LN-ESRD in African-Americans, suggesting *APOL1* is associated with renal susceptibility to end organ damage in SLE.[63] This is supported by the clinical observation that kidneys from diseased donors with two *APOL1* nephropathy alleles fail more rapidly after renal transplantation than those with zero or one risk allele.[64] As more novel SLE-risk loci are emerging, our understanding of links between genotypes and disease phenotypes will be enhanced.

CONCLUSION AND FUTURE DIRECTIONS

GWAS and follow-up studies have rapidly advanced our understanding of SLE genetics. Future challenges include identification of new associations responsible for the missing heritability of SLE, localization of causal variants with functional characterization at each locus, and implication of novel pathogenic pathways contributing to the disease. Based on whole-exome/genome investigation, next-generation sequencing may accelerate the identification of novel, particularly rare variants, which may be not only functionally important but also harbor large effect sizes for SLE risk. Integration between genetic and epigenomic datasets, together with pathway- and network-based analyses, will help to narrow the search for the most likely causal variants and target genes in SLE. New technologies, like CRISPR/Cas-based methods to generate isogenic cell lines or heterozygous allele modifications in animal models, will expand our ability to validate the functional mechanisms. We expect that these approaches will enable rapid progress from genetic studies to biological knowledge, provide a better understanding of SLE molecular pathogenesis, and indicate promising new therapeutic targets for patient management.

REFERENCES

1. Deng Y, Tsao BP. Advances in lupus genetics and epigenetics. *Curr Opin Rheumatol* 2014;**26**:482–92.
2. Bronson PG, Chaivorapol C, Ortmann W, Behrens TW, Graham RR. The genetics of type I interferon in systemic lupus erythematosus. *Curr Opin Immunol* 2012;**24**:530–7.
3. Deane JA, Pisitkun P, Barrett RS, Feigenbaum L, Town T, Ward JM, et al. Control of toll-like receptor 7 expression is essential to restrict autoimmunity and dendritic cell proliferation. *Immunity* 2007;**27**:801–10.
4. Soni C, Wong EB, Domeier PP, Khan TN, Satoh T, Akira S, et al. B cell-intrinsic TLR7 signaling is essential for the development of spontaneous germinal centers. *J Immunol* 2014;**193**:4400–14.
5. Shen N, Fu Q, Deng Y, Qian X, Zhao J, Kaufman KM, et al. Sex-specific association of X-linked Toll-like receptor 7 (TLR7) with male systemic lupus erythematosus. *Proc Natl Acad Sci USA* 2010;**107**:15838–43.
6. Deng Y, Zhao J, Sakurai D, Kaufman KM, Edberg JC, Kimberly RP, et al. MicroRNA-3148 modulates allelic expression of toll-like receptor 7 variant associated with systemic lupus erythematosus. *PLoS Genet* 2013;**9**:e1003336.
7. Molineros JE, Maiti AK, Sun C, Looger LL, Han S, Kim-Howard X, et al. Admixture mapping in lupus identifies multiple functional variants within IFIH1 associated with apoptosis, inflammation, and autoantibody production. *PLoS Genet* 2013;**9**:e1003222.
8. Rice GI, del Toro Duany Y, Jenkinson EM, Forte GM, Anderson BH, Ariaudo G, et al. Gain-of-function mutations in IFIH1 cause a spectrum of human disease phenotypes associated with upregulated type I interferon signaling. *Nat Genet* 2014;**46**:503–9.
9. Gunther C, Kind B, Reijns MA, Berndt N, Martinez-Bueno M, Wolf C, et al. Defective removal of ribonucleotides from DNA promotes systemic autoimmunity. *J Clin Invest* 2015;**125**:413–24. [Epub ahead of print].
10. Jensen MA, Niewold TB. Interferon regulatory factors: critical mediators of human lupus. *Transl Res* 2015;**165**:283–95. [Epub ahead of print].
11. Niewold TB, Kelly JA, Kariuki SN, Franek BS, Kumar AA, Kaufman KM, et al. IRF5 haplotypes demonstrate diverse serological associations which predict serum interferon alpha activity and explain the majority of the genetic association with systemic lupus erythematosus. *Ann Rheum Dis* 2012;**71**:463–8.
12. Salloum R, Franek BS, Kariuki SN, Rhee L, Mikolaitis RA, Jolly M, et al. Genetic variation at the IRF7/PHRF1 locus is associated with autoantibody profile and serum interferon-alpha activity in lupus patients. *Arthritis Rheum* 2010;**62**:553–61.
13. Kottyan LC, Zoller EE, Bene J, Lu X, Kelly JA, Rupert AM, et al. The IRF5-TNPO3 association with systemic lupus erythematosus has two components that other autoimmune disorders variably share. *Hum Mol Genet* 2015;**24**:582–96.
14. Lee MN, Ye C, Villani AC, Raj T, Li W, Eisenhaure TM, et al. Common genetic variants modulate pathogen-sensing responses in human dendritic cells. *Science* 2014;**343**:1246980.
15. Harley JB, Alarcon-Riquelme ME, Criswell LA, Jacob CO, Kimberly RP, Moser KL, et al. Genome-wide association scan in women with systemic lupus erythematosus identifies susceptibility variants in ITGAM, PXK, KIAA1542 and other loci. *Nat Genet* 2008;**40**:204–10.
16. Han JW, Zheng HF, Cui Y, Sun LD, Ye DQ, Hu Z, et al. Genome-wide association study in a Chinese Han population identifies nine new susceptibility loci for systemic lupus erythematosus. *Nat Genet* 2009;**41**:1234–7.
17. Namjou B, Sestak AL, Armstrong DL, Zidovetzki R, Kelly JA, Jacob N, et al. High-density genotyping of STAT4 reveals multiple haplotypic associations with systemic lupus erythematosus in different racial groups. *Arthritis Rheum* 2009;**60**:1085–95.
18. Sanchez E, Comeau ME, Freedman BI, Kelly JA, Kaufman KM, Langefeld CD, et al. Identification of novel genetic susceptibility loci in African American lupus patients in a candidate gene association study. *Arthritis Rheum* 2011;**63**:3493–501.
19. Cunninghame Graham DS, Morris DL, Bhangale TR, Criswell LA, Syvanen AC, Ronnblom L, et al. Association of NCF2, IKZF1, IRF8, IFIH1, and TYK2 with systemic lupus erythematosus. *PLoS Genet* 2011;**7**:e1002341.
20. Gateva V, Sandling JK, Hom G, Taylor KE, Chung SA, Sun X, et al. A large-scale replication study identifies TNIP1, PRDM1, JAZF1, UHRF1BP1 and IL10 as risk loci for systemic lupus erythematosus. *Nat Genet* 2009;**41**:1228–33.
21. Baccala R, Gonzalez-Quintial R, Blasius AL, Rimann I, Ozato K, Kono DH, et al. Essential requirement for IRF8 and SLC15A4 implicates plasmacytoid dendritic cells in the pathogenesis of lupus. *Proc Natl Acad Sci USA* 2013;**110**:2940–5.
22. Luo X, Yang W, Ye DQ, Cui H, Zhang Y, Hirankarn N, et al. A functional variant in microRNA-146a promoter modulates its expression and confers disease risk for systemic lupus erythematosus. *PLoS Genet* 2011;**7**:e1002128.
23. Shen N, Liang D, Tang Y, de Vries N, Tak PP. MicroRNAs–novel regulators of systemic lupus erythematosus pathogenesis. *Nat Rev Rheumatol* 2012;**8**:701–9.
24. Yang W, Shen N, Ye DQ, Liu Q, Zhang Y, Qian XX, et al. Genome-wide association study in asian populations identifies variants in ETS1 and WDFY4 associated with systemic lupus erythematosus. *PLoS Genet* 2010;**6**:e1000841.
25. Graham RR, Cotsapas C, Davies L, Hackett R, Lessard CJ, Leon JM, et al. Genetic variants near TNFAIP3 on 6q23 are associated with systemic lupus erythematosus. *Nat Genet* 2008;**40**:1059–61.
26. Adrianto I, Wen F, Templeton A, Wiley G, King JB, Lessard CJ, et al. Association of a functional variant downstream of TNFAIP3 with systemic lupus erythematosus. *Nat Genet* 2011;**43**:253–8.
27. Kaufman KM, Zhao J, Kelly JA, Hughes T, Adler A, Sanchez E, et al. Fine mapping of Xq28: both MECP2 and IRAK1 contribute to risk for systemic lupus erythematosus in multiple ancestral groups. *Ann Rheum Dis* 2013;**72**:437–44.
28. Vereecke L, Beyaert R, van Loo G. Genetic relationships between A20/TNFAIP3, chronic inflammation and autoimmune disease. *Biochem Soc Trans* 2011;**39**:1086–91.
29. Wang S, Wen F, Wiley GB, Kinter MT, Gaffney PM. An enhancer element harboring variants associated with systemic lupus erythematosus engages the TNFAIP3 promoter to influence A20 expression. *PLoS Genet* 2013;**9**:e1003750.
30. Herrmann M, Voll RE, Kalden JR. Etiopathogenesis of systemic lupus erythematosus. *Immunol Today* 2000;**21**:424–6.
31. Deng Y, Tsao BP. Genetics of human SLE. In: Wallace DJ, Hahn BH, editors. *Dubois' lupus erythematosus and related syndromes.* Philadephia: Elsevier Inc; 2012. p. 35–45.

32. Kim K, Brown EE, Choi CB, Alarcon-Riquelme ME, Kelly JA, Glenn SB, et al. Variation in the ICAM1-ICAM4-ICAM5 locus is associated with systemic lupus erythematosus susceptibility in multiple ancestries. *Ann Rheum Dis* 2012;**71**:1809–14.

33. Fossati-Jimack L, Ling GS, Cortini A, Szajna M, Malik TH, McDonald JU, et al. Phagocytosis is the main CR3-mediated function affected by the lupus-associated variant of CD11b in human myeloid cells. *PLoS One* 2013;**8**:e57082.

34. Yang W, Zhao M, Hirankarn N, Lau CS, Mok CC, Chan TM, et al. ITGAM is associated with disease susceptibility and renal nephritis of systemic lupus erythematosus in Hong Kong Chinese and Thai. *Hum Mol Genet* 2009;**18**:2063–70.

35. Kim-Howard X, Maiti AK, Anaya JM, Bruner GR, Brown E, Merrill JT, et al. ITGAM coding variant (rs1143679) influences the risk of renal disease, discoid rash and immunological manifestations in patients with systemic lupus erythematosus with European ancestry. *Ann Rheum Dis* 2010;**69**:1329–32.

36. Morris DL, Fernando MM, Taylor KE, Chung SA, Nititham J, Alarcon-Riquelme ME, et al. MHC associations with clinical and autoantibody manifestations in European SLE. *Genes Immun* 2014;**15**:210–7.

37. Fernando MM, Freudenberg J, Lee A, Morris DL, Boteva L, Rhodes B, et al. Transancestral mapping of the MHC region in systemic lupus erythematosus identifies new independent and interacting loci at MSH5, HLA-DPB1 and HLA-G. *Ann Rheum Dis* 2012;**71**:777–84.

38. Fernando MM, Stevens CR, Sabeti PC, Walsh EC, McWhinnie AJ, Shah A, et al. Identification of two independent risk factors for lupus within the MHC in United Kingdom families. *PLoS Genet* 2007;**3**:e192.

39. Bottini N, Peterson EJ. Tyrosine phosphatase PTPN22: multifunctional regulator of immune signaling, development, and disease. *Annu Rev Immunol* 2014;**32**:83–119.

40. Salmond RJ, Brownlie RJ, Morrison VL, Zamoyska R. The tyrosine phosphatase PTPN22 discriminates weak self peptides from strong agonist TCR signals. *Nat Immunol* 2014;**15**:875–83.

41. Wang Y, Shaked I, Stanford SM, Zhou W, Curtsinger JM, Mikulski Z, et al. The autoimmunity-associated gene PTPN22 potentiates toll-like receptor-driven, type 1 interferon-dependent immunity. *Immunity* 2013;**39**:111–22.

42. Bayley R, Kite KA, McGettrick HM, Smith JP, Kitas GD, Buckley CD, et al. The autoimmune-associated genetic variant PTPN22 R620W enhances neutrophil activation and function in patients with rheumatoid arthritis and healthy individuals. *Ann Rheum Dis* 2015;**74**:1588–95. [Epub ahead of print].

43. Crispin JC, Hedrich CM, Tsokos GC. Gene-function studies in systemic lupus erythematosus. *Nat Rev Rheumatol* 2013;**9**:476–84.

44. Sunahori K, Juang YT, Kyttaris VC, Tsokos GC. Promoter hypomethylation results in increased expression of protein phosphatase 2A in T cells from patients with systemic lupus erythematosus. *J Immunol* 2011;**186**:4508–17.

45. Tan W, Sunahori K, Zhao J, Deng Y, Kaufman KM, Kelly JA, et al. Association of PPP2CA polymorphisms with systemic lupus erythematosus susceptibility in multiple ethnic groups. *Arthritis Rheum* 2011;**63**:2755–63.

46. Nagpal K, Watanabe KS, Tsao BP, Tsokos GC. Transcription factor Ikaros represses protein phosphatase 2A (PP2A) expression through an intronic binding site. *J Biol Chem* 2014;**289**:13751–7.

47. Detre C, Keszei M, Romero X, Tsokos GC, Terhorst C. SLAM family receptors and the SLAM-associated protein (SAP) modulate T cell functions. *Semin Immunopathol* 2010;**32**:157–71.

48. Manjarrez-Orduno N, Marasco E, Chung SA, Katz MS, Kiridly JF, Simpfendorfer KR, et al. CSK regulatory polymorphism is associated with systemic lupus erythematosus and influences B-cell signaling and activation. *Nat Genet* 2012;**44**:1227–30.

49. Kozyrev SV, Abelson AK, Wojcik J, Zaghlool A, Linga Reddy MV, Sanchez E, et al. Functional variants in the B-cell gene BANK1 are associated with systemic lupus erythematosus. *Nat Genet* 2008;**40**:211–6.

50. Guthridge JM, Lu R, Sun H, Sun C, Wiley GB, Dominguez N, et al. Two functional lupus-associated BLK promoter variants control cell-type- and developmental-stage-specific transcription. *Am J Hum Genet* 2014;**94**:586–98.

51. Westra HJ, Peters MJ, Esko T, Yaghootkar H, Schurmann C, Kettunen J, et al. Systematic identification of trans eQTLs as putative drivers of known disease associations. *Nat Genet* 2013;**45**:1238–43.

52. Peng H, Wang W, Zhou M, Li R, Pan HF, Ye DQ. Role of interleukin-10 and interleukin-10 receptor in systemic lupus erythematosus. *Clin Rheumatol* 2013;**32**:1255–66.

53. Sakurai D, Zhao J, Deng Y, Kelly JA, Brown EE, Harley JB, et al. Preferential binding to Elk-1 by SLE-associated IL10 risk allele upregulates IL10 expression. *PLoS Genet* 2013;**9**:e1003870.

54. Hedrich CM, Rauen T, Apostolidis SA, Grammatikos AP, Rodriguez Rodriguez N, Ioannidis C, et al. Stat3 promotes IL-10 expression in lupus T cells through trans-activation and chromatin remodeling. *Proc Natl Acad Sci USA* 2014;**111**:13457–62.

55. Koelsch KA, Webb R, Jeffries M, Dozmorov MG, Frank MB, Guthridge JM, et al. Functional characterization of the MECP2/IRAK1 lupus risk haplotype in human T cells and a human MECP2 transgenic mouse. *J Autoimmun* 2013;**41**:168–74.

56. Shah D, Mahajan N, Sah S, Nath SK, Paudyal B. Oxidative stress and its biomarkers in systemic lupus erythematosus. *J Biomed Sci* 2014;**21**:23.

57. Jacob CO, Eisenstein M, Dinauer MC, Ming W, Liu Q, John S, et al. Lupus-associated causal mutation in neutrophil cytosolic factor 2 (NCF2) brings unique insights to the structure and function of NADPH oxidase. *Proc Natl Acad Sci USA* 2012;**109**:E59–67.

58. Chung SA, Taylor KE, Graham RR, Nititham J, Lee AT, Ortmann WA, et al. Differential genetic associations for systemic lupus erythematosus based on anti-dsDNA autoantibody production. *PLoS Genet* 2011;**7**:e1001323.

59. Sanchez E, Nadig A, Richardson BC, Freedman BI, Kaufman KM, Kelly JA, et al. Phenotypic associations of genetic susceptibility loci in systemic lupus erythematosus. *Ann Rheum Dis* 2011;**70**:1752–7.

60. Caster DJ, Korte EA, Nanda SK, McLeish KR, Oliver RK, G'Sell RT, et al. ABIN1 dysfunction as a genetic basis for lupus nephritis. *J Am Soc Nephrol* 2013;**24**:1743–54.

61. Taylor KE, Chung SA, Graham RR, Ortmann WA, Lee AT, Langefeld CD, et al. Risk alleles for systemic lupus erythematosus in a large case-control collection and associations with clinical subphenotypes. *PLoS Genet* 2011;**7**:e1001311.

62. Lin CP, Adrianto I, Lessard CJ, Kelly JA, Kaufman KM, Guthridge JM, et al. Role of MYH9 and APOL1 in African and non-African populations with lupus nephritis. *Genes Immun* 2012;**13**:232–8.

63. Freedman BI, Langefeld CD, Andringa KK, Croker JA, Williams AH, Garner NE, et al. End-stage renal disease in African Americans with lupus nephritis is associated with APOL1. *Arthritis Rheumatol* 2014;**66**:390–6.

64. Reeves-Daniel AM, DePalma JA, Bleyer AJ, Rocco MV, Murea M, Adams PL, et al. The APOL1 gene and allograft survival after kidney transplantation. *Am J Transpl* 2011;**11**:1025–30.

Chapter 11

Hormones

Vaishali R. Moulton

Division of Rheumatology, Department of Medicine, Beth Israel Deaconess Medical Center, Harvard Medical School, Boston, MA USA

SEX HORMONES

Nine out of ten patients afflicted with systemic lupus erythematosus (SLE) are women, indicating that the female gender is an important factor in disease development. The gender bias in SLE reflects not only the role of sex chromosomes but also that of sex hormones. A skewed X chromosome-inactivation pattern, sex hormone defects, and reproductive history are factors that contribute to the breakdown of tolerance leading to autoimmunity.[1] Several X chromosome defects have been reported in patients with SLE. These include gene translocation causing triplication of genes, X duplication with an increased incidence of SLE in males with Klinefelter's (XXY) syndrome, and demethylation of genes such as CD40L on the X chromosome, resulting in overexpression of CD40L. The importance of the X chromosome was shown in a pristane-induced model of lupus, wherein the XX sex chromosome complement conferred increased susceptibility to disease over the XY⁻ mice.[1]

The role of sex hormones in SLE pathogenesis is supported by the fact that the disease manifests predominantly in the reproductive phase of life. Before puberty, the female-to-male prevalence is 3:1, which increases to 9:1 after the onset of puberty. In addition, there is evidence of an increased estrogenic environment in both men and women with SLE. Animal studies using both the New Zealand Black/New Zealand White (NZB/NZW) and the MRL/lpr mouse models of lupus have shown that lupus-prone female mice succumb to disease sooner than male mice. Early studies demonstrated improvement or worsening of disease with gonad removal of ovaries or testicles, respectively, suggesting a critical role of hormones in pathogenesis. Female mice survived longer after ovariectomy than castrated male mice. Administration of estrogen worsened disease while androgen supplements improved disease in both female and male castrated mice.[2,3] Accordingly, treatment with the estrogen receptor (ER) antagonist tamoxifen reduced anti-DNA antibodies, reduced immune complex deposition in the kidney and improved survival.[4] Although serum estrogen levels are not significantly altered in patients with SLE, androgen levels are found to be significantly lower. There appears to be an increase in estrogen metabolism in SLE. Increased levels of the feminizing 16-hydroxyestrone and estriol metabolites occur in the serum of patients, resulting from an increased oxidation of the androgen precursor dehydroepiandrosterone (DHEA). On the other hand, androgen levels, specifically DHEA, are low in lupus patients. Besides estrogen, the female hormone prolactin is associated with worse renal disease in lupus-prone mice while the prolactin inhibitor bromocriptine improved disease and prolonged survival in these mice.[2]

HORMONES AND THE IMMUNE RESPONSE

While hormones, especially estrogens, are considered to be important contributors in the aberrations of the immune response and expression of disease, their exact molecular role and mechanisms of action are still poorly understood. Studies have shown the effect of hormones on cytokine production by various immune cells, gene regulation in T cells, immunoglobulin production by B lymphocytes and function of granulocytes and NK cells.[5,6] Some of the first direct molecular evidence into the role of estrogen in autoimmunity came from studies performed in non-autoimmune mice transgenic for the heavy chain of a pathogenic anti-dsDNA antibody. Estrogen upregulates expression of the antiapoptotic molecule Bcl-2 and promotes survival of autoreactive B cells, allowing their escape from tolerance induction.[7] An important aspect of B-cell activation is the antibody affinity maturation, which involves somatic hypermutation and class-switch recombination, both of which require the activation-induced deaminase (AID) enzyme.[8] Estrogen was shown to directly activate transcription of AID through binding elements within the AID promoter.[9] Furthermore, estrogen enables the survival and persistence of autoreactive T cells by downregulating FasL and suppressing activation-induced cell death of human SLE T cells.[10]

Studies performed in human peripheral blood T cells have shown that estrogen increases the expression of calcineurin mRNA and the encoded protein phosphatase (PP) 2B activity in an ER-dependent manner. PP2B induces dephosphorylation of the nuclear factor of activated T cells transcription factor and subsequent nuclear

Systemic Lupus Erythematosus. http://dx.doi.org/10.1016/B978-0-12-801917-7.00011-5

translocation and binding to target genes such as CD40L. Estrogen may contribute to the increased T cell cognate help to autoreactive B cells, as estradiol administration was shown to upregulate the expression of CD40L in T cells from lupus patients but not healthy individuals.[11] Exposure of normal human peripheral blood T cells to estradiol led to increased expression of the transcriptional repressor cyclic AMP response element modulator (CREM) alpha and suppression of interleukin (IL-2) cytokine production.[12,13]

Cytokine abnormalities are an important component of the aberrant immune response in patients with SLE. The immune response in SLE is characterized by a Th2 type of cytokine environment, such that cytokines IL-4, IL-6, and IL-10 are increased in serum from patients. In addition, increased serum levels of the proinflammatory cytokine IL-17 and increased proportion of Th17 differentiated cells are observed in SLE patients and thought to contribute to autoimmune disease pathogenesis.[14] Estrogen is known to regulate the immune system by modulating cytokine production. High doses of estrogen are known to promote Th2 cytokine (IL-4, IL-10, TGFβ) production. High serum estrogen levels correlated with low IL-2 levels in the lupus-prone NZB/NZW mice. Furthermore, estrogen treatment increased tumor necrosis factor (TNF) and IL-6 levels after challenge with lipopolysaccharide (LPS) in both normal and lupus-prone MRL/lpr mice; these effects were reversed by the selective ER modulator tamoxifen. Animal studies have shown that mice treated with synthetic estrogen were susceptible to *Listeria monocytogenes* bacterial infection and their splenocytes produced less IL-2, while increased IL-17 production was seen in splenocytes from estrogen-treated mice.[15,16] Estrogen is also known to regulate the proinflammatory cytokine IFNγ and was shown to enhance CD4 responses and IFNγ producing cells from lymph nodes,[17] and the Th1 differentiation transcription factor T-bet was upregulated by estrogen in murine splenocytes.[18]

Dendritic cells (DCs) are initiators of the innate as well as adaptive immune responses and abundantly express the pattern recognition Toll-like receptors (TLRs). TLR7- and TLR9-deficient lupus-prone mice exhibit reduced disease, indicating that TLRs are important in lupus pathogenesis. DCs are defective in SLE in both humans and mice exhibiting an overstimulated phenotype and function, with increased expression of major histocompatibility complexes (MHCs) as well as costimulatory molecules CD80/86.[19] Estrogen can modulate DC differentiation and function in several ways: alter the expression of MHC proteins, costimulatory molecules, or TLR; regulate cytokine production by DCs directly or indirectly via other cell types; and modulate migratory function through changes in cytokine or chemokine production. Furthermore, estrogen is required for the activation and differentiation of DCs, specifically those bearing features of a Langerhan cell like DC.[20]

Besides the direct role of estrogen on the immune system, another notion is that the regulatory mechanisms that normally control the estrogen-induced excitation of the immune response may be abnormal in SLE patients. To this end, DNA microarray analysis of genes expressed in the peripheral blood mononuclear cells during the menstrual cycle of healthy women were compared to those from women with SLE and showed interesting differences. Specifically, tumor necrosis factor receptor superfamily member 14 (TNFRSF14; synonym: herpes virus entry mediator, HVEM) was increased in correlation with increasing serum estrogen levels in healthy women but not in SLE patients. TNFRSF14 is a ligand for B and T lymphocyte attenuator, an inhibitory receptor which dampens lymphocyte activation and is important in maintaining immune homeostasis. These results suggest that the mechanisms that regulate the immune activating effects of estrogen may be defective in SLE patients.[21]

HORMONE RECEPTORS

SLE patients experience increased disease activity and flares during pregnancy. However, in some studies, hormone levels were found to be lower in pregnant women with SLE as compared to healthy pregnant women. Thus, it is unclear if hormones alone determine disease activity.[22] Rather, the sensitivity of immune cells to hormones may be equally or more important. In this regard, the role of ERs and their contribution to disease are emerging. ER alpha (α) and beta (β) belong to the steroid hormone receptor superfamily and are intracellular receptors expressed in most immune cells, including T cells, B cells, monocytes, and DCs (Figure 1). Estradiol diffuses through the cell membrane and binds to the ER, which leads to the homo- or hetero-dimerization of the ER, which then bind with high affinity to consensus estrogen response element sites within target genes, thus functioning as transcription factors to regulate gene expression. Besides the direct binding to target genes, ER-mediated regulation of gene transcription can occur indirectly via other proteins, and they can be ligand dependent or independent. The ER can act as a transcriptional co-activator and bind to other transcription factors, such as specific protein 1 (Sp1), activator protein (AP)-1, or nuclear factor kappa-light-chain enhancer of activated B cells (NFκB). Besides the conventional intracellular ER, membrane-bound G protein-coupled receptors (GPR30) and cytoplasmic receptors have been identified, which upon estrogen ligation can induce rapid intracellular calcium fluxing and intracellular signaling in various cell types. Interestingly, the ER can function in gene regulation in a ligand-independent manner; for example, extracellular stimuli such as insulin, IGF1, EGF, and TGFβ can lead to ER phosphorylation by MAP kinases and result in gene transactivation.[23]

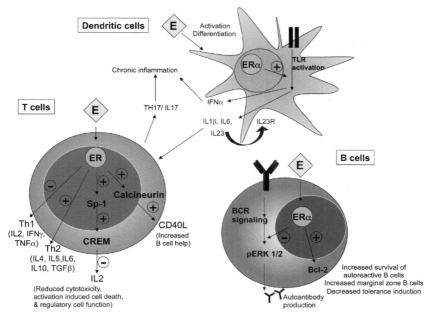

FIGURE 1   Select roles of estrogen and estrogen receptors in T cells, B cells, and dendritic cells in SLE.

ERα is required for hematopoietic and stromal development of a full-sized thymus in both male and female mice, and estrogen regulates CD4+CD8+ double-positive T cell development, which requires both ERα and ERβ. Estrogen can stimulate the production of regulatory T cells as it induced the expression of FoxP3 and IL-10 genes and promoted conversion of CD4 CD25- T cells to CD4CD25+. T regulatory cells and the ER antagonist ICI 182780 blocked this conversion. Several studies have highlighted the role of the ERs in lupus.[24] In murine lupus studies, ERα appears to be critical in disease pathogenesis; deficiency of ERα alone led to reduced renal disease and prolonged survival in lupus-prone MRL/lpr mice, although unexpectedly ERα deficiency in NZM female mice resulted in higher serum anti-dsDNA antibodies but reduced renal disease and prolonged survival.[25] In contrast, ERα-deficient NZBxNZW F1 female mice led to reduced anti-dsDNA antibodies. Studies using ERα- and β-deficient animals have shown that while both receptors regulate B-cell maturation, ERα engagement is responsible for the estrogen-induced dampening of the BCR signaling and B-cell selection and thus is an important trigger for autoimmunity.[7,26] Besides the ER-dependent functions of estrogen, a ligand-independent role of the ER in the innate immune response in SLE has recently been proposed. Reduced TLR9-mediated inflammatory cytokine (IL-6, MCP-1, IL-1β, and IL-23) production was observed from DCs of both wild-type and lupus-prone ERα-deficient mice. Furthermore, ERα-deficient DCs failed to upregulate IL-23R compared with wild-type DCs, suggesting that ERα may modulate the TLR induction of the IL-23/IL-17 pathway. These studies suggest a cross talk between the ER and

the TLR signaling that may occur in the absence of estrogen.[12] These studies implicate a role for hormones, specifically estrogen in SLE and autoimmune disease.

HORMONE THERAPY

While estrogen and ERs are potential culprits in SLE, estrogen has significant health benefits, especially in bone metabolism, and is crucial in osteoporosis treatment in postmenopausal women. Clinical trials have administered hormone replacement therapy in postmenopausal women and shown benefits in osteoporosis. The Safety of Estrogens in Lupus Erythematosus National Assessment (SELENA) studies are large multicenter randomized placebo-controlled clinical trials comprised of two separate arms—one of hormone replacement therapy and the other of combined oral contraceptive therapy in women with SLE. The results of these trials showed that hormone replacement therapy in postmenopausal women with SLE was associated with a small risk of mild-to-moderate flares. Historically, women with SLE were prohibited from using oral contraceptives for fear of exacerbating disease. However, the SELENA trials found that the use of combined estrogen-progesterone oral contraceptives in premenopausal women did not significantly increase the risk of flares in women with stable disease.

However, caution must be exercised when considering hormone therapy in patients with SLE. For example, exogenous estrogen therapy should be avoided in patients with antiphospholipid antibodies due to the increased risk of thrombosis. Clinical trials have shown some utility of prescribing DHEA to patients in terms of tapered prednisone doses, improved disease activity, and fewer flares. These studies indicate that the use of oral contraceptives and hormone therapy may be beneficial and warranted at least in some patients with SLE.[27,28]

While the role of hormones and their receptors in autoimmunity and lupus disease pathogenesis are beginning to be uncovered, further molecular mechanistic studies are needed to understand and modulate these important contributors of disease.

REFERENCES

1. Selmi C, Brunetta E, Raimondo MG, Meroni PL. The X chromosome and the sex ratio of autoimmunity. *Autoimmun Rev* May 2012;**11**(6–7): A531–7. PubMed PMID: 22155196. Epub 2011/12/14. eng.

2. Lahita RG. The role of sex hormones in systemic lupus erythematosus. *Curr Opin Rheumatol* September 1999;**11**(5):352–6. PubMed PMID: 10503654. eng.

3. Lahita RG. Gender and age in lupus. In: Lahita RG, editor. *Systemic lupus erythematosus*. 5th ed. Elsevier; 2011. p. 405–23.

4. Wu WM, Lin BF, Su YC, Suen JL, Chiang BL. Tamoxifen decreases renal inflammation and alleviates disease severity in autoimmune NZB/W F1 mice. *Scand J Immunol* October 2000;**52**(4):393–400. PubMed PMID: 11013011.

5. Karpuzoglu E, Zouali M. The multi-faceted influences of estrogen on lymphocytes: toward novel immuno-interventions strategies for autoimmunity management. *Clin Rev Allergy Immunol* February 2011;**40**(1):16–26. PubMed PMID: 19943123.

6. Oertelt-Prigione S. The influence of sex and gender on the immune response. *Autoimmun Rev* May 2012;**11**(6–7):A479–85. PubMed PMID: 22155201.

7. Cohen-Solal JF, Jeganathan V, Hill L, Kawabata D, Rodriguez-Pinto D, Grimaldi C, et al. Hormonal regulation of B-cell function and systemic lupus erythematosus. *Lupus* June 2008;**17**(6):528–32. PubMed PMID: 18539705. Epub 2008/06/10. eng.

8. Muramatsu M, Kinoshita K, Fagarasan S, Yamada S, Shinkai Y, Honjo T. Class switch recombination and hypermutation require activation-induced cytidine deaminase (AID), a potential RNA editing enzyme. *Cell* September 1, 2000;**102**(5):553–63. PubMed PMID: 11007474.

9. Pauklin S, Sernandez IV, Bachmann G, Ramiro AR, Petersen-Mahrt SK. Estrogen directly activates AID transcription and function. *J Exp Med* January 16, 2009;**206**(1):99–111. PubMed PMID: 19139166. Pubmed Central PMCID: 2626679.

10. Lang TJ. Estrogen as an immunomodulator. *Clin Immunol (Orlando, Fla)* December 2004;**113**(3):224–30. PubMed PMID: 15507385. Epub 2004/10/28. eng.

11. Rider V, Abdou NI. Gender differences in autoimmunity: molecular basis for estrogen effects in systemic lupus erythematosus. *Int Immunopharmacol* June 2001;**1**(6):1009–24. PubMed PMID: 11407298. Epub 2001/06/16. eng.

12. Moulton VR, Tsokos GC. Why do women get lupus?. *Clin Immunol (Orlando, Fla)* July 2012;**144**(1):53–6. PubMed PMID: 22659035. Epub 2012/06/05. eng.

13. Moulton VR, Holcomb DR, Zajdel MC, Tsokos GC. Estrogen upregulates cyclic AMP response element modulator alpha expression and downregulates interleukin-2 production by human T lymphocytes. *Mol Med* 2012;**18**:370–8. PubMed PMID: 22281835. Pubmed Central PMCID: 3356426. Epub 2012/01/28. eng.

14. Korn T, Bettelli E, Oukka M, Kuchroo VK. IL-17 and Th17 cells. *Annu Rev Immunol* 2009;**27**:485–517. PubMed PMID: 19132915. Epub 2009/01/10. eng.

15. Salem ML. Estrogen, a double-edged sword: modulation of TH1- and TH2-mediated inflammations by differential regulation of TH1/TH2 cytokine production. *Curr Drug Targets Inflamm Allergy* March 2004;**3**(1):97–104. PubMed PMID: 15032646. Epub 2004/03/23. eng.

16. Kassi E, Moutsatsou P. Estrogen receptor signaling and its relationship to cytokines in systemic lupus erythematosus. *J Biomed Biotechnol* 2010;**2010**:317452. PubMed PMID: 20617147. Pubmed Central PMCID: PMC2896666. Epub 2010/07/10. eng.

17. Maret A, Coudert JD, Garidou L, Foucras G, Gourdy P, Krust A, et al. Estradiol enhances primary antigen-specific CD4 T cell responses and Th1 development in vivo. Essential role of estrogen receptor alpha expression in hematopoietic cells. *Eur J Immunol* February 2003;**33**(2):512–21. PubMed PMID: 12645950.

18. Karpuzoglu E, Phillips RA, Gogal Jr RM, Ansar Ahmed S. IFN-gamma-inducing transcription factor, T-bet is upregulated by estrogen in murine splenocytes: role of IL-27 but not IL-12. *Mol Immunol* March 2007;**44**(7):1808–14. PubMed PMID: 17046061. Pubmed Central PMCID: 3097111.

19. Kis-Toth K, Tsokos GC. Dendritic cell function in lupus: independent contributors or victims of aberrant immune regulation. *Autoimmunity* March 2010;**43**(2):121–30. PubMed PMID: 20102311. Epub 2010/01/28. eng.

20. Nalbandian G, Kovats S. Understanding sex biases in immunity: effects of estrogen on the differentiation and function of antigen-presenting cells. *Immunol Res* 2005;**31**(2):91–106. PubMed PMID: 15778508. Epub 2005/03/22. eng.

21. Sekigawa I, Fujishiro M, Yamaguchi A, Kawasaki M, Inui A, Nozawa K, et al. A new hypothesis of the possible mechanisms of gender differences in systemic lupus erythematosus. *Clin Exp Rheumatol* May–Jun 2010;**28**(3):419–23. PubMed PMID: 20460035. Epub 2010/05/13. eng.

22. Walker SE. Estrogen and autoimmune disease. *Clin Rev Allergy Immunol* February 2011;**40**(1):60–5. PubMed PMID: 20182819. Epub 2010/02/26. eng.

23. Nilsson S, Makela S, Treuter E, Tujague M, Thomsen J, Andersson G, et al. Mechanisms of estrogen action. *Physiol Rev* October 2001;**81**(4): 1535–65. PubMed PMID: 11581496. Epub 2001/10/03. eng.

24. Cunningham M, Gilkeson G. Estrogen receptors in immunity and autoimmunity. *Clin Rev Allergy Immunol* February 2011;**40**(1):66–73. PubMed PMID: 20352526. Epub 2010/03/31. eng.

25. Svenson JL, EuDaly J, Ruiz P, Korach KS, Gilkeson GS. Impact of estrogen receptor deficiency on disease expression in the NZM2410 lupus prone mouse. *Clin Immunol (Orlando, Fla)* August 2008;**128**(2): 259–68. PubMed PMID: 18514033. Epub 2008/06/03. eng.

26. Cutolo M, Brizzolara R, Atzeni F, Capellino S, Straub RH, Puttini PC. The immunomodulatory effects of estrogens: clinical relevance in immune-mediated rheumatic diseases. *Ann N Y Acad Sci* April 2010;**1193**:36–42. PubMed PMID: 20398006. Epub 2010/04/20. eng.

27. Schwarz EB, Lohr PA. Oral contraceptives in women with systemic lupus erythematosus. *N Engl J Med* March 16, 2006;**354**(11):1203–4. author reply -4. PubMed PMID: 16540625. Epub 2006/03/17. eng.

28. Lateef A, Petri M. Hormone replacement and contraceptive therapy in autoimmune diseases. *J Autoimmun* May 2012;**38**(2–3):J170–6. PubMed PMID: 22261500. Epub 2012/01/21. eng.

Chapter 12

The Complement System in Systemic Lupus Erythematosus

John P. Atkinson[1], C. Yung Yu[2]

[1]Division of Rheumatology, Department of Medicine, Washington University School of Medicine, Saint Louis, MO, USA; [2]Center for Molecular and Human Genetics, The Research Institute at Nationwide Children's Hospital and Department of Pediatrics, The Ohio State University, Columbus, OH, USA

INTRODUCTION

General Comments

The complement system is a double-edged sword in lupus (Figure 1).[1,2] On the one hand, in its absence, a systemic autoimmune disease develops.[3] Thus, a *complete* deficiency of C1q, C1r, C1s, C4, or C2—early components of the classical pathway (CP)—represents a single protein deficiency state that causes lupus. More than 80% of patients with a total C1q or C4 deficiency develop SLE or a lupus-like disease. This pivotal observation, now more than four decades old, obviously has important implications relative to the etiology of this enigmatic disease.[4–13]

On the other hand, complement activation as a result of the abundant immune complexes (ICs) characteristic of SLE contributes to tissue damage. The latter is reflected by the fact that reduced serum complement levels facilitate establishing a diagnosis of SLE and then can become valuable biomarkers of disease activity. Complement fragment deposition, especially in the kidney, and reduced serum concentrations of C4 and C3 are associated with active disease and tissue damage. A return to normal levels with treatment is characteristic of a beneficial response to therapy and a much improved short- and long-term clinical outcome. Thus, "too little or too much" of this immune system underlie both the etiology and pathogenesis of SLE—a paradox still to be solved.

At this stage in our understanding of SLE, 122 patients have been reported to have a complete deficiency of C1q (74), C1r (12), C1s (8), or C4 (28) (Figure 2). Larger numbers have been noted with C2 deficiency and SLE, and most patients with these deficiencies are no longer reported. More common are genetic variants that result in a functional or partial *insufficiency*, which increases disease predisposition. Moreover, an acquired process is operating in most, if not all, patients with end-organ damage in which complement components are chronically consumed by activation of the CP secondary to immunoglobulin (Ig) G autoantibodies binding to their predominantly nuclear target autoantigens.

In this chapter, we first discuss this pathologic activation process before turning our attention to the genetic associations. The goal is to authoritatively summarize the current state of the art and to outline what are likely to become the future topics of interest relative to this paradigm of a systemic disease process featuring complement activation.

Historical Notes

The complement system was discovered in the 1880s. The Nobel Prize was awarded to Jules Bordet in 1919.[14] Complement was initially thought to be a single, labile substance in serum that rather astoundingly could lyse bacteria in seconds. To carry out this lysis, complement was one "factor" in blood, but this reaction required a second heat-stable partner, an *acquired* substance (eventually named "antibody" (Ab)) to become engaged— therefore, the term *complement*. Thus, the host in this rendition had to have had prior exposure to the bacteria before the lytic factor could be activated. This was the identification of the CP. Over 50 years later, the alternative pathway (AP) was discovered.[15,16] Initially, for almost two decades following identification of the AP in 1950s, it was thought to be an artifact. The AP was then "rediscovered" in 1970s.[17,18] Today, we know that AP is the ancient complement cascade and a key player in innate immunity. The AP is found in sponges and insects and other earlier evolutionary species, including those that lack a "pumped" circulatory system.[19,20] The lectin pathway was then a third major pathway identified in the 1980s.[21–23] In evolution, it also preceded the CP. The LP and CP, however, are similar. The differences are that an Ab in the CP versus a lectin in the LP triggers the system. Also, the initial set of proteases engaged are distinct but closely related (arose by gene duplication). Following the assembly and activation of the initiation complex, the LP and CP are identical (Figure 1, Table 1).

Systemic Lupus Erythematosus. http://dx.doi.org/10.1016/B978-0-12-801917-7.00012-7

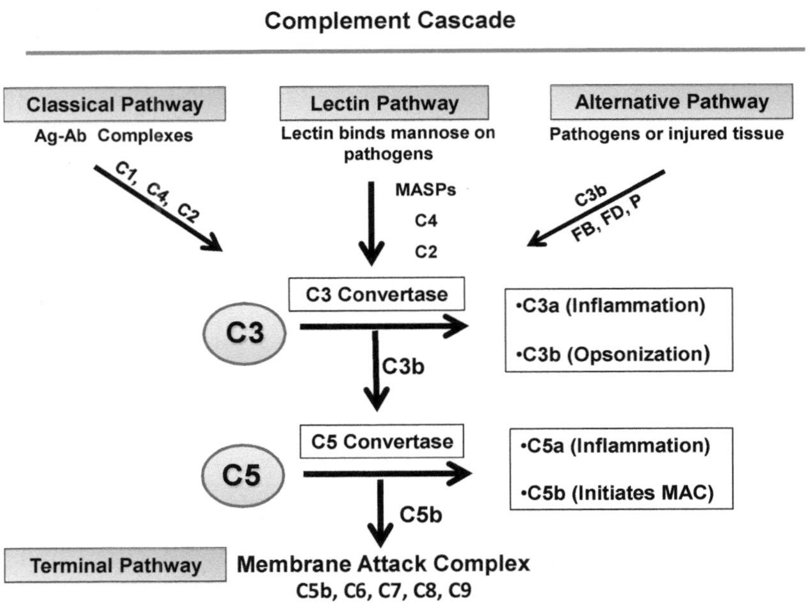

Complement Cascade

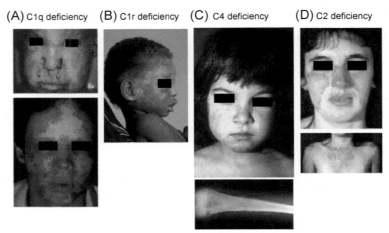

FIGURE 1 The complement cascade. The three pathways of complement activation are shown. Although each is independently triggered, they all merge at the step of C3 activation. The classical pathway is initiated by the binding of antibody to antigen and the lectin pathway by the binding of lectin to a sugar molecule. The alternative pathway turns over continuously and is further amplified in the presence of pathogens or injured tissue. Activation of the complement system leads to inflammation (release of anaphylatoxins C3a and C5a), opsonization (the coating of targets with C3b or C4b), and formation of the membrane attack complex (MAC). *Abbreviations*: MASP, MBL (mannose binding lectin)-associated serine protease; FB, factor B; FD, factor D; P, properdin. *Modified with permission from Ref. 242. For more information visit www.uptodate.com/contents/complement-pathways.*

(A) C1q deficiency **(B)** C1r deficiency **(C)** C4 deficiency **(D)** C2 deficiency

FIGURE 2 SLE patients with a homozygous deficiency of early complement components for the classical pathway (CP). Severe cutaneous lesions are common clinical presentations in SLE patients with a complete deficiency for a CP component protein. (A) A homozygous C1q-deficient male child with lupus erythematosus symptoms and cutaneous infection (*upper* panel), and with discoid LE and scarring lesions on face when he was 22 years old (*lower* panel). (B) A homozygous C1r-deficient male child with discoid lupus at 16 months old. This patient experienced generalized seizure, developed scissoring gait with toe walking, spasticity, and weakness of the legs. At 18 years old, he was diagnosed with class IV lupus nephritis and progressed to end-stage renal disease. (C) A complete C4-deficient girl at 3 years old with butterfly rash and cheilitis (*upper* panel), and osteomyelitis of the femur at 10 years old (*lower* panel). This patient died at age 12 years old because of pulmonary infection and cardiovascular failure. (D) A homozygous C2-deficient young woman with acute cutaneous LE. The *upper* panel shows the butterfly rash, the *lower* panel shows photosensitive lesions on sun exposed area. *Source of photographs: Yu CY et al. A Companion to Rheumatology-Systemic Lupus Erythematosus, 1st edition, Mosby Elsevier, Philadelphia, p185, 2007; Refs 90, 146.*

TABLE 1 Features of the Complement System

1. It works within seconds. The speed with which it can activate and amplify is amazing. In less than 100s, it can lyse cells and deposit several million C3b on a single bacterium in blood. After albumin and Ig, complement and clotting proteins are the most abundant.
2. There is a lot of complement in blood. One can dilute human serum to 1/200 and still lyse antibody-sensitized sheep red blood cells in a CH_{50} assay.
3. Both AP and CP are spontaneously turning over at ~1%/hr and thus they serve as a surveillance system for pathogens and injured tissue. This is particularly so for the AP because it has no specific activation trigger like Ab or MBL.
4. C4b and C3b bind covalently via an ester or amide to a target. This is a bond that almost is impossible to break in a physiologic system. Complement system is designed to function on a membrane—it is relatively inefficient in the fluid phase or on isolated proteins.
5. It is the guardian of the intravascular space. With the advent of pumped circulations, a quick recognition coupled to destructive, powerful force was necessary to prevent bacteria from entering and growing in nutrient-rich blood and lymphatics. Moreover, the blood flowed to locations such as the brain where bacterial infections were routinely lethal (at least until antibiotics were invented).
6. If you don't have it, you get bacterial infections or autoimmunity (primarily SLE). If you have too much, you get undesirable tissue damage—witness atypical hemolytic uremic syndrome (aHUS) and age-related macular degeneration (AMD). These diseases feature excessive AP activities for a given degree of injury secondary to a haploinsufficiency of regulators of this pathway.
7. Complement system and other innate immunity players, likely as their most important role in clinical medicine will be the processing of debris, especially as we live longer and longer—crystals (gout), misfolded proteins (AD), lipoproteinaceous debris (AMD and atherosclerosis) are some examples to consider.
8. We still have a lot to learn about how the system functions intracellularly, on cell membranes and in the extravascular/interstitial space. The role of innate immunity in special tissues is just beginning to be investigated (retina, blood vessel wall, cartilage, etc.).

Currently, the complement system is undergoing a renaissance.[3,24–26] A major contributor to this has been genetic analyses defining variants in human disease. A second contributor is the U.S. Food and Drug Administration (FDA)'s approval of a monoclonal antibody (mAb) to C5 to treat paroxysmal nocturnal hemoglobinuria (PNH) in 2009 and subsequently atypical hemolytic uremic syndrome (aHUS) in 2013. A third point is the recognition that the innate immune system directs and educates the adaptive immune system. A fourth is the resolution of crystal structures for the native proteins and large, multimolecular complexes involving C3, C4, and C5 and their associated proteins.

COMPLEMENT TESTING AND ITS INTERPRETATIONS

Complement Tests

Serum Levels and Hemolytic Activities for C4 and C3

The advantages in the clinical setting of nephelometric methodology to obtain *antigenic* measurements of C4 and C3 include simplicity, rapid turnaround, and accuracy.[27] They are time-honored and helpful tests. The CH_{50} or AP_{50} measures the lysis of red blood cells (RBCs) by the respective pathway and thus are functional tests. For example, the CH_{50} (also known as total hemolytic complement [THC]) tests the CP as all nine of its components (C1–C9) must be present to efficiently lyse the sensitized (Ab-coated) RBCs in the test mixture. A CH_{50} of 200 means that at a dilution of 1:200, a serum lysed 50% of the RBCs in the test mixture.

Both CH_{50} and AP_{50} are technically demanding functional assays that are primarily of value in the initial screening for a complete deficiency of a component.

Measuring C1q and C2

Measurements of C2 parallel those for C4 and C3 in the setting of CP activation in lupus. Because of its relatively low serum concentration, C2 is not as readily measured and usually provides little more than C4 and C3. Also, C1q has been proposed to be measured antigenically. However, even if C4, C2, and C3 are low, C1q may be normal or low. Also, Abs to C1q make interpretation of the results problematic. Therefore, C2 and C1q testing is not recommended for routine use in monitoring SLE.

Utility

In the 2012 Systemic Lupus International Collaborating Clinics (SLICC) classification criteria for SLE,[28] low complement (meaning a low C4 and low C3) had a sensitivity of 59% and a specificity of 93%. The combination of positive anti-DNA Ab test and a low complement have over 90% specificity and sensitivity for the diagnosis of SLE. Likewise, an antinuclear antibodies (ANA) titer of ≥1/640 by immunofluorescence (IF) microscopy and a low C3 also indicate that the disease process is likely SLE.

In one-third to one-half of SLE patients, as part of the initial workup and commonly upon discovery of a positive ANA, the C4 and C3 will be low (Table 2). The usual reason is that ICs via CP activation are consuming these components faster than they can be synthesized by the liver (often despite increased synthesis as part of the

TABLE 2 Complement Profiles in SLE

CH$_{50}$	C4	C3	Comments
N	N	N	Usually means mild disease (skin and joints); rarely have GN; still may be turning over excessively but compensating[a] (acute phase response)
↓	↓	↓	CP activation: anti-dsDNA Ab positive; GN common; the lower the values, the more severe the disease process tends to be; typical pattern of bad SLE
↓	N	↓	AP activation; uncommon pattern in SLE (1–5%) of patients
↓	↓	N	CP activation; milder disease; check for cryos; consider C4 CNV[b] (lack of C4A or C4B) which will require a genetic analysis; cold activation

[a]If C4 or C3 turnover studies are performed, most of these patients will have evidence of accelerated turnover which is sufficiently matched by increased synthesis to maintain the levels in the normal range; they are not necessarily normal for the patient as the predisease values are rarely available.
[b]CNV, copy-number variation; GN, glomerulonephritis; N, normal range.

acute-phase response). An example of this remarkable degree of complement turnover is the "old" lupus band test in which IgG and C3 are detected by IF on a biopsy of uninvolved skin at the dermal–epidermal junction in over 50% of lupus patients. Likewise, deposition of C1q, C4, and C3 are commonly observed in involved organs, such as the kidney, synovium, skin, pleura, and pericardium as well as on the surface of peripheral blood cells (RBCs, platelets, and lymphocytes).[29] These long-standing observations reflect substantial and continuous systemic turnover of complement in this disease. Why there is not inflammation at "uninvolved" sites (e.g., in the skin) is not clear. One explanation is that complement regulatory proteins are sufficient to prevent generation of a clinical condition. In summary, low complement levels facilitate making the diagnosis of SLE. They correlate with high titer ANAs and, especially, anti-dsDNA Abs. The pattern of low C4 and C3 represents CP activation by ICs and is strongly associated with end-organ damage, especially glomerulonephritis (GN).

Obviously, a normal complement (C4 and C3) does not rule out lupus as ~50% of patients will have serum values within the normal range. THC is usually only particularly informative if it is unmeasurably low (<10 hemolytic units). In this situation, it could be a sign of C1q, C4, or, more likely, C2 deficiency (1 in 100–200 lupus patients will have such a deficiency of C2).[25] Rarely are the C4 and C3 so consumed by ICs in lupus that the THC is < 10 hemolytic units, but this unlikely possibility is recognizable because both are proportionally very low. If on repeat measurement the CH$_{50}$ is undetectable, then antigenic assay for C2 should be obtained. If it is normal, antigenic levels of C1q should be assessed. Because of disease implications, family concerns, and increased frequency of serious bacterial infections in these deficient patients (commonly *Streptococcus pneumoniae* in C1-, C4-, or C2-deficient patients), a repeat test is recommended, including this time a functional assessment of the deficient component in question.

Interpretation of C4 and C3 Complement Tests in SLE

Consumption Versus Biosynthesis

While the large majority of low C4 and low C3 in SLE reflects accelerated consumption, C3 turnover studies in the 1980s in active lupus patients demonstrate a subset (<10%) in which the synthetic rate was decreased.[30] An explanation for this observation is still wanting. Also, in patients with "normal" complement levels, a common finding was accelerated C4 and C3 turnover, which was partially compensated by an increased synthetic rate. Furthermore, just because the C4 is 18 mg/dl (normal, 16–48 mg/dl) and the C3 is 100 mg/dl (normal, 80–160 mg/dl) does not mean that complement turnover is not accelerated. The predisease values are rarely known. For example, in the above scenario, the "normal" C4 for this patient may be 30 mg/dl and the normal C3 may be 140 mg/dl. In a lupus patient followed for several years, the highest C4 and C3 values observed during the course of disease are likely to be the closest to the patient's predisease (i.e., normal) value.

Chronically Low C4 and C3: How to Interpret?

Low C4 and C3 correlate with active disease. Institution or modification of therapy needs to be considered. Also, more than one low component almost indicates consumption of complement by immune complexes. If the patient is in a clinical remission, the excessive classical pathway turnover is causing no detectable end-organ damage. Additional therapeutic intervention(s) may or may not be indicated, but careful observation is indicated.

When C4 and C3 Are Discrepant?

The usual pattern in active lupus is that both C4 and C3 are low—that is, they commonly go "hand in hand." There are exceptions, though. A low C4 but a normal C3 has several possible explanations and is a common cause for questions to our laboratories from rheumatologists and nephrologists. Since C3 levels are normally three- to sixfold higher than C4, consumption of 20 mg/dl of each could reduce C4 below but leave C3 in the normal range. With a positive response to treatment, both will rise. The C3 may rise, for example, from 100 to 120 mg/dl and thus at least a level of 120 mg/dl was the patient's predisease C3 value. Likewise, if the C4 rose from 10 to 30 mg/dl, the predisease level was at least 30. However, there are also other issues for a clinician to consider with this scenario of a low C4 but a C3 in the normal range.

Cryoglobulins: A low C4 but a normal C3 is a commonly observed pattern in mixed cryoglobulinemia.[31–34] The reason being is that, in the case of soluble ICs (as opposed to an Ab binding to an antigen on a cell), the formation of CP C3 convertases by ICs is relatively inefficient, so less C3 is consumed.

Cold activation: This phenomenon occurs in lupus and in several other diseases featuring IC (chronic viral hepatitis). It was described by several groups in the 1970s and 1980s and seems to have been largely forgotten.[35,36] The CH_{50} is often low or undetectable but the C4 and C3 values may be normal. The ICs form during collection, freezing, and thawing of the serum sample and can activate the CP to exhaustion. The antigenic levels may be even in the normal range but they may lack any functional activity. To identify this phenomenon, the sample must either be kept at 37 °C or blood should be drawn into ethylene diamine tetraacetic acid (EDTA) to prevent complement activation. This phenomenon is often missed by clinicians. The CH_{50} is then performed on the diluted plasma. Some have argued that all complement functional tests should have their blood collected into EDTA.[35–37]

Copy-number variation: Copy-number variation (CNV) denotes how many copies of a specific gene are present in a diploid genome among different individuals. About 60% of individuals have four copies of the C4 gene, while 40% have 3 (or less) or 5 (or more).[38–40] In most Caucasian populations, 1–3% of individuals lack *both* C4A genes.[41,42] In lupus, the number of patients lacking C4A genes may increase to ~10%. Until very recently, testing for CNV has been available only in a few research laboratories.[43–46] However, commercial kits are now becoming available so that hospital or other laboratories will be able to determine C4 gene copy-number, including assessing for complete C4A deficiency. If one is C4A null, the baseline (predisease) C4 antigenic level may be 12 to 18 (~6–8 mg/dl per C4 gene). In this situation, it does not take much activation to lower the C4 out of the normal range. In an Australian study, three of 11 SLE patients with a chronically low C4 were explained by a low gene copy-number—two copies versus the ~55% of population who have four copies.[47] In Caucasians, it is usually C4A that is deficient.

Alternative pathway activation: A normal C4 but a low C3 indicates AP activation, which may be observed in 3–10% of lupus patients. Human IgM and IgG subclasses 1 and 3 activate the CP. IgE, IgD, and IgG subclasses 2 and 4 do not activate the CP. However, IgA and the nonactivating IgG subclasses may engage the AP by binding to an antigen and, if in sufficient amounts, create a milieu whereby deposited C3b is relatively protected from complement regulators like factor H, membrane cofactor protein (MCP, CD46), and decay accelerating factor (DAF, CD55). A second pathophysiologic explanation relates to the distribution of the autoantigen. For example, two IgG of subclasses that activate complement must be in close proximity (side-by-side) or possibly even a hexamer of IgGs attached to an antigen before the Fc portion of IgG can cross-link the C1q subunit of the C1 complex to initiate CP activation. Known as Ab-dependent activation of the AP, the antigenic distribution does not provide a platform for CP activation but does allow for AP activation because it provides a site that is relatively protected from the regulators.[48]

New Developments

Two other types of complement testing are available, but neither at this time has caught on in routine clinical practice. The first test is of fluid phase fragments or so-called split products, in which complement activation fragments in blood are assessed (e.g., C3a, C5a, C4d, iC3b, C3d, sC5b-9, Bb, Ba and others).[49–51] The problems are several-fold: (a) the tests are not widely available and therefore must be sent out with the confounding potential problems of a delay in getting the results and issues often arise related to cost and handling of the sample; (b) a standardized collection methodology may not be utilized (serum, EDTA-plasma, etc.) such that these fragments are generated during sample collection and preparation (serum vs plasma), and (c) even if standardization of these procurement parameters is accomplished, the interpretation of the results is problematic because of lack of clinical experience with these tests.

The second is a test of membrane fragments, where C4d and C3d fragments deposited on peripheral blood cells (RBCs, B cells, T cells, platelets) are assessed by flow cytometry.[50,52–54] Kits are now available to monitor, for example, cell-bound C4d on RBCs and B lymphocytes by flow cytometry. It is not clear, however, how much these additional and more expensive tests add to measurements of the standard C3 and C4. Also, there are several issues yet to be resolved relative to performance and interpretation of such tests, as well as the confounding issues of anti-platelet, anti-RBC, and anti-lymphocyte Abs in lupus patient populations.

Commercial Specialty Laboratories

Antigenic and functional assays for almost every complement component, regulator, or receptor are now commercially available. Examples of one of these activating proteins being produced in normal amounts but whose function is altered is very rare. In contrast, we have learned that regulators may be produced in normal amounts but may be dysfunctional, as in atypical hemolytic uremic syndrome aHUS, age-related macular degeneration and hereditary angioedema (HAE). For example, about 50% of the genetic variants in FH, MCP, and factor I (FI) in aHUS lead to an expressed protein, which has reduced or absent functional activity.[55,56] About 15% of HAE patients synthesize normal levels of a dysfunctional protein (C1-Inh deficiency type 2) such that the C1-Inh antigenic levels are normal. In lupus, however, there is almost always an agreement between antigenic levels and functional activity of a component, such as C4 and C3.

Assessing a Therapeutic Response

Interpretation

C3 and C4 antigenic tests have been utilized for over 50 years to assist in monitoring a response to therapy. A standard approach in a patient whose values are low at the time of diagnosis is to repeat the tests several weeks after the initiation of steroid and/or cytotoxic therapy. The measurements are then repeated approximately every month till they normalize and every 2–3 months thereafter. A return to normal levels at 1–3 months has repeatedly been demonstrated to indicate a good response to the treatment program and to portend better short- and long-term outcomes. As the medication intensity is reduced, a stable C3 and C4 in the normal range correlates with a remission while a reduction in C3 and/or C4 alerts the clinician to the possibility of a relapse. In our experience, each patient must be individualized. Obviously, end-organ damage is the major arbitrator of disease activity and treatment efficacy but complement measurements are of value in many patients.

Renal Biopsy

Complement C3 fragments and IgG deposition are characteristic immunofluorescent findings in renal biopsies of patients with lupus nephritis (often called a "full house biopsy").[57,58] C1q and C4 fragments will be present as well but are not commonly assessed. In addition, anti-C1q Abs in the serum are commonly detected in patients with GN.[59] Clinical renal syndromes that can occasionally mimic SLE and thus are in the differential diagnosis are C1q and C3 glomerulonephropathies.[60–62] However, neither syndrome is associated with prominent Ig deposition as is observed in lupus nephropathy, and these patients do not have the systemic features present in most lupus patients.

IMMUNOLOGY AND GENETICS OF EARLY COMPLEMENT COMPONENTS OF THE CLASSICAL PATHWAY

C1q

Biology and Genetics of C1q

The A, B, and C chains of human C1q are encoded by three different genes in a genomic region spanning 25,013 bp on chromosome 1p36.11–12. The three genes are configured in the order of C1qA-C1qC-C1qB. Each C1q gene consists of three exons, with coding sequences present in 3′ region of exon 2′ and 5′-region of exon 3.

The precursor proteins for the A, B, and C chains consist of 245, 253, and 245 amino acid residues, respectively, including a signal peptide between 22 and 28 amino acid residues. In each chain, the N-terminal region consists of a pentapeptide with a cysteine residue that is engaged in the formation of an interchain disulfide linkage. It is followed by a collagen-like region (CLR) with 27 or 28 copies of triple-helix repeats Gly-X-Y sequences, and then a globular region of 131–137 residues at the carboxyl end. In the biosynthesis of C1q, one A-chain and one B-chain form a heterodimer, and two C-chains form a homodimer, both through disulfide linkages. Two A–B heterodimers associate with one C–C homodimer to form a hexameric structure in the configuration of ABCCBA. Three of these hexamers, with a total of 18 polypeptide chains together, form the tulip-like structure of C1q with a collagenous tail and six globular regions, each which with globular heads ghA, ghB, and ghC (Figure 3(A)).

C1q is a charge pattern recognition molecule. The globular heads of C1q bind through ionic interactions to Cγ2-domains of aggregated IgG or Cμ3 domains of IgM in immune complexes.[63–65] A tetrameric structure of C1r$_2$ and C1s$_2$ associates with activated C1q to form the C1 complex that initiates the classical complement pathway.

C1q is an important opsonin to promote phagocytosis of apoptotic cells or debris. This can be achieved directly without complement activation through binding at the collagenous region of C1q to calreticulin (CRT) in apoptotic cell blebs and to CD91 on phagocytes, or indirectly with activation of the classical pathway as C1q binds to CRP ligated to phosphorylcholine/phosphatidylserine or to SAP ligated to fragmented chromatin from apoptotic cells, generating processed products C4b, C3b, iC3b, C3dg, and C3d that are ligands for CR3 and CR4 on myeloid cells to initiate phagocytosis. In cultured cells, C1q suppressed in dose-dependent manner the production of proinflammatory cytokines, such as interferon-α, IL-6, IL-8, and TNF-α by monocytes and macrophages and plasmacytoid dendritic cells (pDCs).[66] In the absence of C1q, immune complexes tended to bind to and be phagocytosed by pDCs instead of monocytes and macrophages, leading to secretion of

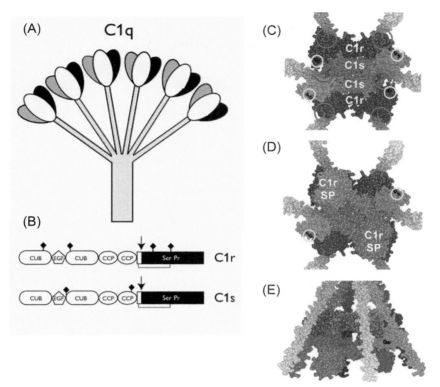

FIGURE 3 Organization and structures of the C1 complex. (A) A cartoon of the C1q with six globular heads and a collagenous tail. (B) Domain structures of C1r and C1s. *Arrows* represent proteolytic cleavage sites when the proteins are activated. Ser-Pr, serine proteinase domain; *square brackets* symbolize locations of interchain disulphide bonds; *diamonds* denote glycosylation sites. (C, D, and E) Different views of a refined, space-filled model for the assembly of the C1 complex. (C) A bottom view of the assembly between CUB1-EGF-CUB2 interaction domains of C1r/C1s and the C1q collagen stems (in *grassy green*). *Red circles*, the approximate positioning of the six C1q-binding sites contributed by C1r and C1s; *yellow circles*, the C-terminal ends of the C1r and C1s CUB2 modules. (D) A bottom view of the assembly featuring the CCP1-CCP2-SP catalytic domains of C1r, shown in *red* and *pink*. The C1s catalytic domains, emerging from the C-terminal end of both C1s CUB2 modules (*yellow circles*), are not shown for clarity. SP, serine protease domain. CCP1 and CCP2, CUB1 and CUB2 in C1r or C1s are named according to their relative positions from the N-terminus of each native protein. (E) Side view of the assembly as shown in (D). *Reproduced with permission from Refs 243, 244.*

IFN-α.[67] In mixed lymphocyte reactions, macrophages and dendritic cells that bound (or phagocytosed) C1q-opsonized apoptotic cells suppressed proliferation of inflammatory T-cell subsets Th17 and Th1.[68] In other words, C1q facilitates clearance of apoptotic cells and immune complexes under physiologic conditions, without triggering a robust inflammatory reaction, by suppressing the production of inflammatory cytokines including IFN-α and the proliferation of proinflammatory T cells.

Recently, it has been shown that C1q or its CLR is a ligand for leukocyte-associated Ig-like receptor 1 (LAIR-1 or CD305) and LAIR-2 (CD306).[69] LAIR-2 is a soluble inhibitor of LAIR-1. An association of C1q with LAIR-1 on monocyte triggered phosphorylation of its ITIM domain, leading to inhibition of monocyte differentiation. Similarly, C1q-mediated inhibition of IFN-α production by pDCs and such inhibition could be reversed by the soluble LAIR-2 or silencing RNA against LAIR-1. Thus, it was suggested that C1q limits dendritic cell differentiation and activation by engaging LAIR-1.[69] It is further shown that in

CpG-stimulated monocytes, C1q or anti-LAIR-1 antibody inhibited nuclear translocation of interferon regulatory factors IRF-3 and IRF-5 and IκBα, and thus suppressed the expression of interferon-stimulated genes. It was proposed that LAIR-1 engagement by C1q helps maintain monocyte tolerance through suppressing the TLR-9-mediated monocyte activation.[70]

Other ligands present in host cells binding to globular domain of C1q that may or may not trigger full complement activation, include adiponectin; pentraxins such as CRP, SAP, and pentraxin-3 (PTX3); and extracellular matrix proteins such as fibronectin, osteoadherin, and chondroadherin. Ligands that bind to the collagen-like region of C1q include heparin and small leucine-rich glycoproteins including decorin, biglycan, lumican, lamin, and fibronectin.

Cellular receptors using C1q as a ligand include calreticulin (cC1qR) for the C1q collagenous region and gC1qR for the C1q globular domain, with other membranous molecules including CD91, CD93, and $\alpha_2\beta_1$ integrin providing co-receptor functions.[71,72] C1q also binds

---

TABLE 3 Clinical Characteristics Complete Complement Deficiency (C1, C4, or C2)

- Early age onset, cutaneous disease often prominent (particularly subacute cutaneous lupus), commonly though looks like "bad" SLE (~50% with renal involvement).
- ANA positive in ~2/3rds. Anti-Ro more common than in general lupus population, especially in C2 deficiency.
- Complement testing in C2 deficiency:

CH_{50}	C4	C3
0	N	N

Interpretation: C2 deficiency is most likely (~1/200 SLE patients).
Repeat CH_{50}. If still zero, obtain C2 antigen test. If normal, check C1q.
Consider genetic analysis to confirm the C2 genetic variant causing the deficiency.

- Treatment. Therapy initially is similar to that for standard SLE. There are a few case reports of patients with refractory disease being treated successfully with infusion of the missing component.

---

to complement receptor CR1 but its physiologic consequence is not clear.[73,74]

Genetic Deficiency of C1q

In 2011, Schejbel and colleagues reviewed a total of 64 cases of C1q genetic deficiency, inclusive of the 42 cases summarized by Pickering and colleagues in 2001.[7,42] Many patients described were of European or Middle-East/Arabian ancestries. The clinical presentations among C1q-deficient patients varied considerably, even within families with multiple C1q-deficient subjects.[7] However, two common conditions were found to be overwhelmingly associated with a genetic deficiency of C1q: SLE or lupus-like disease in 88% of patients and recurrent bacterial infections in 41% of patients. As for SLE and lupus-like disorders, many patients had disease onset in early childhood (Table 3). The range was 6 months to 42 years.[6] The female-to-male sex ratio was close to 1:1. Many C1q-deficient patients died at a young age secondary to septicemia or renal failure. Among the C1q-deficient patients with SLE or lupus-like disease, cutaneous disorders, especially photosensitivity, were prominent with a frequency of 84%. GN and neurologic disease affected about 30% and 19% of patients, respectively. Oral ulceration occurred in 22% and arthritis/arthralgia in 16%. Immunologically, most C1q-deficient patients had normal plasma/serum levels of complement C4 and C3, high frequency of antinuclear antibodies (particularly anti-Ro), but low frequency of anti-dsDNA antibodies. As of February 2015, the number of cases of genetic deficiency of C1q has increased to about 74, including Japanese and African-American patients. High frequencies of SLE/lupus-like syndrome and recurrent bacterial infections including sepsis continue to be prominent clinical manifestations.[75–78]

Four distinct mechanisms with a total of 17 causative mutations have been identified (Table 4). The first comprises a variety of deleterious mutations resulting in the absence of biosynthesis for one of the three C1q chains. There are three types of such deleterious mutations:

1. A single point mutation that converts a codon for an amino acid to a premature stop-codon; five such distinct nonsense point mutations in C1q have been identified.
2. A deletion of a single nucleotide in the coding sequence that causes a shift in the reading frames to generate a stop-codon; three different frame-shift mutations in C1q have been discovered.
3. A point mutation at an exon-intron splice junction that disables the proper production of a mature mRNA; two such mutations identified are a 3'-splice site AG to CG of intron 1[77] and a 5'-splice site GT to TT in intron 2.[79]

The second mechanism is a missense mutation in the coding sequence that leads to the absence of the C1q plasma protein. Such defects have been noted in two families. The first was an African-American family in which the initiation codon Met of C1qA was mutated to an Arg (M1R). This abrogated the signal peptide (of 22 amino acids) required for secretion, as the next available Met codon in C1qA is at position 20. The second was an Inuit family from Greenland with no detectable C1q in serum. The defect was a G244R mutation in the globular domain of C1qB. The Gly244 (or Gly217 in the mature protein) residue is strictly conserved among all C1q-related proteins.[80] It is not clear why this C1qB with mutation did not allow assembly with C1qA and C1qC to form a high-order structure and be secreted.

The third mechanism, missense mutations, disrupts the structure and assembly of the intact C1q protein. It leads to low-molecular weight (LMW) C1q proteins being detectable in plasma. For these cases, there was often a change of the Gly-residue in the Gly-X-Y repeats to a charged Arg or Asp residue in any one of the C1q A, B, or C chain. Such mutations incapacitate the proper folding, interactions, and assembly of the CLR to form the 11S macromolecular

TABLE 4 Features of C1qA, B, C Genes, mRNA and Proteins and Causative Genetic Mutations for C1q Protein or Functional Deficiency

	C1qA	C1qB	C1qC
Gene (bp)	3058	8449	4486
Accession no.	NG_007282.1	NC_000001.11	NG_007565.1
Exons	3	3	3
mRNA (nt)	1098	1044	1205
Accession no.	NM_015991.2	NM_000491.3	NM_00114101.1
5′ UT	1–78	1–115	1–126
3′ UT	824–1098	895–1044	865–1205
Precursor protein (aa)	245	253	245
Accession no.	NP_057075.1	NP_000482.3	NP_758957.2
Signal peptide (aa)	22	27	28
Gly-X-Y repeats (copies)	27	28	27
Globular region (aa)	136	137	131
Causative mutations (17)			
	M1R	G42D	G34R
	E53fs	R177X	G55fsX83
	Q64X	G244R (globular head)	R69X
	Q208X	Intron 1, 3′ splice site: AG->CG	G61R
	W216X	Intron 2, 5′ splice site: GT->TT	Q71fsX137
		G63S (C1r binding site; no C-function)	G76R

Single-letter abbreviations are used for amino acids; fs, frame-shift; X, stop codon. Numberings are based using *initiation codon* Met as 1. Earlier numbering system was based on the N-terminus of mature proteins, which can be deduced by subtracting the numbers of the new system with number of amino acids present in signal peptide for the corresponding protein.

structure of C1q. It was observed that some patients with LMW C1q had relatively milder SLE disease.[78]

The fourth mechanism is a missense mutation leading to a functional deficiency of CP. This was found in a Middle-East Arabian patient with SLE who had central nervous system (CNS) involvement and recurrent infections. The patient died secondary to bacteria-induced septic shock leading to multiple organ failure.[75] The molecular defect was a missense mutation in the B-chain of C1q, G63S, which is a part of the C1r-binding site. Although normal quantity of plasma C1q was detectable and the binding to immunoglobulins, pentraxins, LPS and apoptotic cells were intact, there was an inability of this mutant C1q to associate with C1r and C1s to form the C1-complex, and thus a failure to activate C4 and C3. This case further underscores the importance of an intact CP to maintain immune tolerance and to fight infections.

Of the 17 causative mutations with homozygous C1q genetic deficiency, most were the results of a consanguineous marriage. Otherwise they were likely close decedents of ancestors carrying the specific deleterious mutation. Surprisingly, multiple screenings of large SLE populations in these countries to determine the prevalence of the C1q deleterious mutations all yielded negative results. This suggests that those mutations were "private" and rare with very large effect size, as documented in many complex diseases.[81,82]

Therapy and Potential Cure of C1q-deficiency

Fresh frozen plasma (FFP) is able to restore C1q activity in C1q-deficient patients temporarily, but such activity drops off rapidly within 1 to 2 weeks. Thus, weekly infusions of FFP become necessary,[77] which confers its own risk of infections and thrombotic complications from catheters.

Unlike most other component proteins of complement in blood, the primary site of biosynthesis for C1q is *not* in the liver but myeloid cells including macrophages, monocytes, and dendritic cells, which originate from the bone marrow. The effect of restoring the C1q to reconstitute complement function has been tested in mouse models. Bone marrow transplantation (BMT) of hematopoietic stem cells from wild-type animals has been shown to be effective in treating C1q-deficient animals.[83,84] Thus, BMT for hematopoietic stem cell therapy (HSCT) has been performed in a single case of a Pakistani C1q-deficient patient.[85] In this particular case of a consanguineous family, the father and five of his six sons had C1q-deficiency. The father died of chronic GN at age 38 and one of his sons died at age 17 months old secondary to *S. pneumonia* meningitis. Another son was incapacitated by a CNS vasculopathy at age 17 years old. The index patient is the third son who survived *S. pneumonia*-induced meningitis at age 3 but developed acute CNS vasculopathy at age 10. At age 16, his disease was under control through treatment with intravenous cyclophosphamide (pulse therapy) and B-cell depletion with rituximab, but he had a persistent lupus rash and increased levels of anti-Ro (SSA-60) and anticardiolipin autoantibodies (ACLAs). In view of his poor prognosis, HSCT was performed using bone marrow from his HLA-matched healthy brother, with graft-versus-host disease prophylaxis. Restoration of hematopoiesis, myelopoiesis, platelet production, and complement function with normal levels of C1q and CH50 were observed 2–4 weeks after transplantation, and he has remained stable for 5 months. Such a result gives hope to SLE patients with a C1q deficiency and a severe clinical course.

C1r and C1s

Biology and Genetics of C1r and C1s

The genes for human *C1s* and *C1r* are located on chromosome 12p11.31,[86] a region in which the Human Genome Reference sequence is still incomplete as it consists of gaps (Annotation release 106, 1/2015). Based on bioinformatic studies and past publications,[87] C1r and C1s are configured in a tail-to-tail orientation with their 3' ends separated by about 9177 bp. The human *C1s* gene spans 10.5 kb with 12 exons coding for a precursor protein of 688 amino acids, which includes a signal peptide of 15 amino acids. The human *C1r* gene probably also consists of 12 exons, but its first exon and the 5'-end of the second exon are still to be mapped.[88] The precursor protein of C1r has 705 amino acids with a signal peptide of 17 amino acids.

C1r and C1s are paralogous proteins that share 38% identity and 55% similarity. Each mature protein is a proenzyme consisting of six distinct modules: two CUB modules separated by an EGF module with a binding site for Ca^{2+}, followed by two complement controlling protein repeats CCP1 and CCP2, a linker segment and then a chymotrypsin-like serine protease domain SP at the carboxyl-terminus region (Figure 3(B)). In circulation, C1r and C1s exist as a tetramer C1s-C1r-C1r-C1s bound to C1q.

Upon activation of C1q (e.g., through binding of its globular heads to the Fc-regions of IgG or IgM in an immune complex) (Figure 3(C–E)). Autoactivation of the two C1r by proteolytic cleavages between Arg-463 and Ile-464 is followed by activation of C1s by proteolysis between Arg438 and Ile-439, which trigger the nascent C1 complex. The C1s in this C1 complex then activates C4 and then C2 to form the classical pathway C3 convertase.

Genetic Deficiency of C1r or C1s

Deficiencies in subcomponents of C1r and C1s were among the earliest reports linking complement deficiency with human glomerulonephritis or a lupus-like disease.[5,13,89] A total of 20 cases of C1r and/or C1s deficiencies have been reported, which include 12 cases of C1r deficiency from eight families and eight cases of C1s deficiency from five families. Among the C1r-deficient patients (Figure 4), there was consistent reduction in the serum protein levels of C1s to ~30% of its normal level, but highly elevated serum protein levels of C4, C2, and C1 inhibitor (200–400% of their corresponding normal ranges). C3 was also elevated by ~50%, but C1q was normal. A similar phenomenon was observable among C1s-deficient patients. C1s-deficient patients had greatly reduced serum levels of C1r; markedly elevated levels of C4, C2, C1, inhibitor and C3; and steady levels of C1q (see below).

Among the C1r/C1s-deficient subjects, all but three had recurrent bacterial, viral, or fungal infections (85%). Many patients died at a young age because of severe infections. Thirteen subjects developed SLE or a lupus-like disease (65%). The female-to-male ratio among C1r/C1s-deficient subjects with SLE was from 1.5 to 1. Mortality at young age due to fulminant infections likely explains slightly lower frequency of lupus disease association. Most patients had severe cutaneous lesions. Eight patients had renal disease due to lupus nephritis (40%). The prevalence of ANA among the SLE was about 60%. Such presentations underscore the interdependence of C1r and C1s in sustaining a stable tetrameric structure that would otherwise be susceptible to a high turnover rate. A deficiency of C1r or C1s incapacitates the formation of the C1 complex and diminishes the need for engagement of C1-inhibitor in its regulation. The classical pathway is not activated and thus consumption of C4, C2, and C3 is greatly reduced, resulting in high levels of these proteins in the circulation.[90] This and other results strongly indicate a chronic turnover of the classical pathway.[91]

The molecular defects leading to C1r or C1s deficiency were determined in one case with C1r deficiency and seven cases with C1s deficiency. For the case with C1r deficiency, the defect was a homozygous C to T substitution in exon 10 resulting in the R380X nonsense mutation in the second

(A) Genes of immunologic interest at Chromosome 12p13

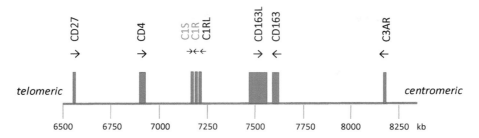

(B) Genomic structure of human C1r gene and PCR strategy

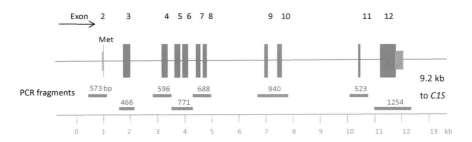

(C) Molecular basis of C1r deficiency

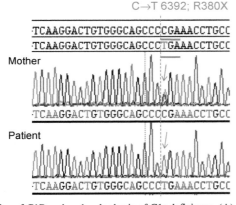

(D) High protein levels of C4 in a C1r-def patient

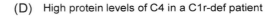
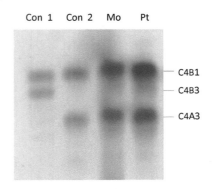

FIGURE 4 Genetics of C1R and molecular basis of C1r deficiency. (A) Genes of immunologic interest proximal to human *C1S* and *C1R* at chromosome 12p13. An arrow represents the transcriptional orientation for each gene. Numbers in kb are the sequence coordinates in the NCBI Human Genome Reference sequence, which has an undefined gap in the *C1R* gene. (B) Exon-intron structure of the human C1R gene. Data for *C1R* exon-intron structure and numbers are after GenBank entries BC035220 (for cDNA), AB083037, NT_009759.16 and NT_009714.17 (NCBI human reference sequence, version 37.1). (C) Detection of the C to T mutation at nucleotide position 6392 of the C1R gene from the C1r-deficiency patient (Pt) and his mother (Mo). This mutation changes Arg380 to a stop-codon in the CCP2 domain. An arrow shows the location of the mutation. The patient is homozygous and his mother is heterozygous. (D) Immunofixation of EDTA-plasma from the C1r-deficient patient, his mother and two controls (Con1 and Con2). Very high levels of C4A and C4B proteins (~4-5 folds higher than normal range) were detected in the patient and his mother. *Ref. 90.*

CCP domain.[90] For C1s deficiency, the deleterious mutations are (1) a C→G mutation in exon 6 leading to Y204X[92]; (2) a 4-bp deletion (TTTG) in exon 10 leading to a frameshift and a nonsense mutation[93,94]; (3) a G→T mutation in exon 12 leading to E597X[95,96]; (4) a C→T mutation in exon 12 leading to R534X[97,98]; and (5) a G→A mutation at exon 12 leading to G630E substitution.

C4A and C4B

Genetics and Biology of C4A and C4B

Together with the genes for C2 and factor B, the human C4A and C4B genes are located in the class III region of the major histocompatibility complex (MHC) on chromosome 6p21.1.[99] Human C4A and C4B genetics has been through an interesting and rather lengthy history. The initial concept was that of a single genetic locus with codominant alleles for C4A and C4B; next a two-locus model for C4A-C4B with low degree of deletions and duplications caused by unequal crossovers during meiosis; followed by continuous, multi-allelic CNV scheme from one to four copies of C4 genes on a haplotype (which equals two to eight copies of C4 genes in a diploid genome among different individuals of a population).[25] Such common CNVs are a surprising phenomenon in mammalian genetics as they deviate from the conventional one-to-one concept for a gene and a polypeptide. *Here, one-to-multiple copies of almost identical genes coexist on a chromosome and code for the same protein with limited polymorphic variation, thereby creating a gene dosage-effect for a quantitative phenotype.*

A human C4 gene consists of 41 exons coding for a transcript of 5.4 kb, which is translated to a pro-precursor protein of 1744 amino acids, including a signal peptide of 19 residues.[100–102] The primary site for C4 biosynthesis is hepatocytes, but multiple tissues also synthesize C4 for local consumption, particularly after stimulation by interferon-γ. Before secretion, the C4 protein is processed by proteolytic cleavages at two basic regions with RKKR between 676 and 679, and with RRRR between 1450 and 1453, leading to the formation of a three-chained structure, β−α−γ, linked by interchain disulfide bonds (Figure 5). Other important posttranslational modifications include (1) formation of an internal thioester bond; (2) tyrosine sulfation close to the C-terminal region of the α-chain[103]; (3) following secretion into plasma, removal of a 22-amino acid peptide from the C-terminus of the α-chain that exposes the sulfated

(A) Processing of C4 proteins

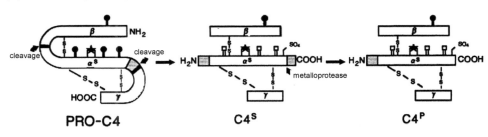

- ● - High mannose type oligosaccharide
- ⬚ - Biantennary complex type oligosaccharide
- ★ - Thioester bond
- **SO₄** - Sulfotyrosine

(B) A comparison of C4A and C4B

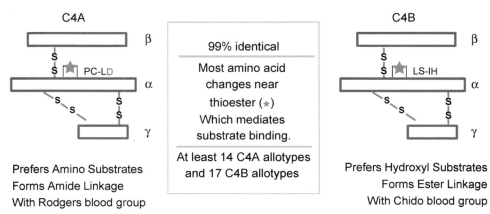

FIGURE 5   Schematic diagrams for structural features of human C4. (A) Processing of human C4. Pro-C4 is the intracellular, single chained precursor of C4. Following a series of post-translational modifications that include sulfation, glycosylation, and two proteolytic cleavages, a three-chained protein is secreted (C4ˢ). The major form of C4 in plasma, however, is C4ᵖ. This form of C4 differs from C4ˢ by removal of a 22-amino acid peptide from the caroboxyl terminal of the α-chain. The shaded are at the N-terminal region of the α-chain represents the C4a fragment. *(Modified from Chan A, Atkinson JP. J Immunol 1985;134:1790–1798, with permission.)* (B) A comparison of human C4A and C4B. Although highly homologous in sequences, the acidic C4A and basic C4B differ in binding specificities to substrates and association with blood group antigens. *Modified from Ref. 245.*

tyrosines[104]; (4) N-linked glycosylations with three complex biantennary type and one simple high mannose type[105]; and (5) one O-linked glycosylation at Thr-1244.[106–108]

A thioester bond is present in complement C4 and C3 and their related protein, α_2-macroglobulin.[109,110] In C4, the thioester bond is formed between the sulfydryl group of Cys-1010 and the carbonyl group of Gln-1013. A proteolytic cleavage by activated C1s or MASP2 at the N-terminus of the α-chain removes the 74 amino acid C4a peptide and leads to a remarkable change of conformation. The hidden thioester bond becomes exposed to the exterior. In activated C4B, one of the four isotypic residues His-1125 (as it does in activated C3) serves as a catalyst for the formation of an acyl-imidazole intermediate between Gln-1013 and His-1125. This transient facilitates a rapid nucleophilic attack by a hydroxyl group of a target on Gln-1013 to form a covalent ester linkage between activated C4B and the target surface. For activated C4A, such catalytic reaction does not exist from Asp-1125, and the Gln-1013 carbonyl *effectively* reacts with an amino group on an immune complex or a protein molecule to form a covalent amide bond.[111–114] Such a difference in chemical reactivity appears to diversify the functional roles of C4A and C4B in the clearance of immune complexes and the propagation of the activation pathways.

The covalent linkage between C4 and its activation initiator has many important outcomes. First, it localizes the complement activation and the ensuing opsonic fragments and MAC to target surfaces. Second, it tags the immune complexes or altered self materials such as apoptotic or necrotic cells for clearance through binding to complement receptors CR1 on red blood cells (immune adherence phenomenon). Some antigens or immune complexes tagged with C4b or C4d, and C3b or iC3b and C3d in circulation may be also retained in follicular regions by myeloid or dendritic cells of secondary lymphoid organs such as spleen and lymph nodes, and engaged in germinal center responses, which promote secondary immune response by reducing the threshold of B-cell activation. Meanwhile, autoreactive B cells binding to C4d-tagged autoantigens would be subjected to anergy or negative selection in peripheral tolerance. The detailed molecular mechanism behind this specific process to enhance secondary immune response and achieve long-term memory against foreign antigen and immune tolerance against self antigens through an intact CP remains enigmatic.

Downstream activation of C3 leads to the deposition of C3b on targets or cell surfaces. On microbial surfaces, the activation process proceeds to form C3 and C5 convertases. The latter activates C5 to initiate the formation of the membrane attack complex, often resulting in the cytolysis of target cells. Powerful anaphylatoxins C5a and C3a are produced during the process to facilitate the defense system. The deposition of C3b-related processed products opsonizes the tagged materials for phagocytosis by myeloid cells through binding to complement receptors

CR3 or CR4. On autologous or self surfaces, the presence of complement regulators such as membrane cofactor protein (MCP or CD46) or CR1 promotes the factor I-mediated proteolytic degradation of C4b to C4d, and C3b to iC3b, C3dg and C3d. Thus, the end-point of the activation process on most self surfaces becomes primarily C4d and, to a lesser extent, C3d. If the process were allowed to continue to the formation of MAC on self-membrane, it would cause tissue injuries and become pathogenic. It is worthy to note that the deposition of C4d on RBC in SLE may lead to calcium-dependent cytoskeleton changes and decreased membrane deformability of RBC, which could impair blood flow through capillaries and negatively affect the delivery of oxygen to tissues.[115]

In SLE, high levels of circulating autoantibodies lead to the formation of immune complexes between autoantigens and autoantibodies. C1q, r, and s are activated. The C1 complex activates C4, leading to the deposition of C4b on any nearby cell surfaces. As part of the protective mechanism against self-destruction, on healthy cells most if not all activated C4b and C3b are degraded. Increased cell-bound C4d and C3d are remarkably common features in SLE,[50,54] as these protective surfaces are overwhelmed in the setting of abundant autoantibodies and membrane/tissue damage.

Crystal Structure of C4 Proteins

Protein crystal structures are important as they offer insights to mechanisms of biologic activities, and facilitate drug development to manipulate or inhibit protein function. In 2012, the crystal structures of human C4, and a complex between C4 and CCP1-CCP2-SP domains of MASP2 (with its serine protease catalytic residue Ser-633 mutated to Ala-633) were solved with a resolution of 3.6 Å and 3.75 Å, respectively (Figure 6).[116] In 2015, the crystal and solution structure of C4b was reported.[107] Together with earlier crystal structures for the thioester domain for a mutagenized human C4A[117] and for related proteins C3, C3c, C3b, C3b-factor B-factor D complex, C3b-CRIg complex and C3b-FH complex,[118–124] a wealth of information related to structure and function became available.

The native C4 protein consists of 13 domains, with eight domains being characteristic of fibronectin type III repeats in α_2-macroglobulin-related protein family and therefore named MG1 to MG8. Each of these repeats consists of about 100 amino acids that fold into at least seven β-strands on two independent β-sheets with a three-dimensional structure like an American football. MG1-MG6 form a stable β-ring with 1.5 helical turns. Intriguingly, MG6 is interrupted by a linker region, the β–α chain junction, the anaphylatoxin domain, the C1s/MASP2 cleavage site and the N-terminal region of the α′-chain. Between MG7 and MG8 is a CUB domain that is again split into two halves by an insertion of the thioester domain (Thr 957-Arg 1336). The thioester (TE) domain folds into an α_6–α_6 barrel-like structure. The thioester bond is

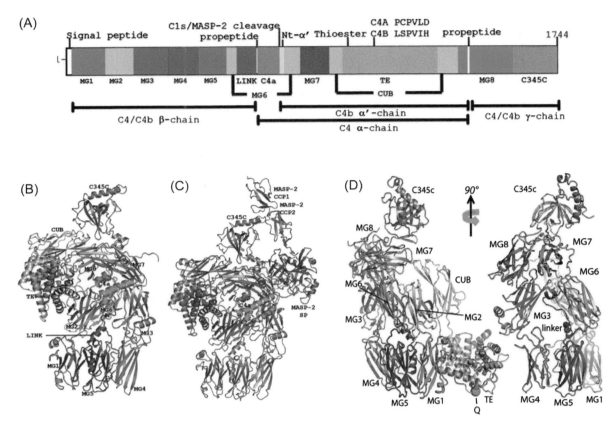

FIGURE 6 Protein structures of human C4. (A) Domain structure of the human C4. The primary structure for the precursor C4 protein consists of 1744 amino acids with a signal peptide of 19 amino acids that is removed upon secretion. The Pro-C4 protein is made up of 13 domains that include eight α_2-macroglobulin-like domains (MG1 to MG8), the anaphylatoxin domain C4a, a linker domain (LNK), a small N-terminal region (loop) of the α-chain (NT-α'), a CUB domain that is split into two halves by the insertion of the thioester (TE) domain, and a C-terminal domain that is common for complement C3, C4, and C5 (C345c). (B) Crystal structure of the native C4 protein showing the organization of the 13 domains. (C) Crystal structure of the C4 MASP-2 complex. The catalytic serine residue of MASP-2, Ser-633 was mutated to Ala-633 so that the bimolecular complex could be crystalized. Except for C4a (red) and the C345C domain (brown), C4 is shown in blue. The MASP2 CCP domains (magenta) interact with the C4 C345C domain, whereas the catalytic serine protease (SP) domain of MASP-2 (gray) recognizes C4 at the scissile bond region. (D) The crystal structure of C4b in two orientations. Notice that the C4a domain is removed after MASP-2 digestion. The TE domain translocates from the middle of the molecule to a new location next to MG1 that would be in contact with the activator surface. The position of the thioester domain (TE) glutamine residue is indicated by the red sphere marked "Q." The highly reactive carbonyl side chain of Gln-1010 would form a covalent ester bond (for C4B) or a covalent amide bond (for C4A) with the complement activator or substrate. Also note that the structures for the native C4 protein in panel B and bound structure in panel C are shown as a rotation of 180° to the structure presented in panel D. *Adapted from Refs 107, 116.*

buried in a pocket formed by hydrophobic or aromatic residues from the TE domain and the MG8 domain close to the protein surface. The α–γ-chain junction is present in MG8 and the N-terminus of the γ-chain starts at Glu-1454. Following MG8 is an anchor region and the carboxyl domain characteristic of complement C3, C4, and C5 and therefore termed C345C, which assumes a netrin-like structure.

The scissile bond in C4 for serine protease (SP) cleavage by activated C1s or MASP2 is present between Arg-756 and Ala-757 in the R-loop formed between Asp-748 and Ile-760. Besides the binding of the R-loop to the SP domain, there are additional interaction sites to enable the specific binding and cleavage. The carboxyl-terminus of plasma C4 α-chain, which consists of 11 negatively charged residues

including three sulfotyrosines, interacts electrostatically in long range with positively charged residues present in the SP domain of MASP2 and the C4a domain. Moreover, the two CCP domains of MASP2 provide an exosite with negatively charged binding patch to four positively charged Arg-residues located between 1716 and 1724 of the C345C domain in C4. Similar electrostatic interactions seem to be present between CCP1-CCP2 domains of C1s and C345C of C4, and the SP domain of C1s plus C4a with sulfotyrosine region at the carboxyl-end of the C4 α-chain.

The removal of C4a by C1s or MASP2 triggers dramatic changes in the conformation. In native C4, the thioester bond is buried at the interface between the MG8 and the thioester domain. In C4b, there is substantial movement of the thioester domain from neighboring to MG7 and MG8 (or the shoulder) to the target surface next to MG1, MG4, and MG5. The thioester bond between Cys-1010 and Gln-1013 becomes completely exposed to solvent, and the catalytic residue His-1125 from C4B (or Asp-1125 from C4A) is in close proximity with the acyl group of Gln-1013. This enables the formation of an acyl-imidazole intermediate that is highly reactive (but short-lived) toward hydroxyl nucleophiles from a target or activator. Moreover, the α'-NT on C4b consists of two electronegative motifs, EED 763–765 and DEDD 768–771, interacts with C2 to form the classical/lectin pathway C3 convertase.[107,116]

Complete Genetic Deficiencies of C4A and C4B and SLE

A total of 28 individuals have been documented with a complete genetic deficiency of both C4A and C4B. These C4-deficient subjects come from 19 families, characterized by 16 different HLA haplotypes and with European, African, and Asian ancestries. Among these C4-deficient subjects, 22 (78.6%) were diagnosed with SLE or a lupus-like disease, and four others had a renal disease including glomerulonephritis. The female-to-male ratio was 1:1. Early disease onset, a severe photosensitive skin rash, presence of anti-Ro/SSA, and high titers of ANA were common clinical presentations and immunologic findings. Many C4-deficient patients had renal disease (43%) including severe proliferative glomerulonephritis. The frequency of sepsis or severe recurrent infections was 29%. Almost all complete C4 deficiency patients were homozygous with identical HLA class I and class II markers for both copies of chromosome 6, usually because of consanguineous marriages. The molecular basis of complete C4 deficiency has been determined in 15 cases (Figure 7) and can be stratified into three groups:

1. Monomodular-long RCCX haplotypes (mono-L) with a single defective C4A gene characterized by a mini-deletion, a mini-insertion or a point mutation at exons 13, 20, or 29, leading to a nonsense mutation.[125–127]
2. Bimodular RCCX haplotypes (LS) with one long C4A gene and one short C4B gene that contained a nonsense mutation at exons 13, 29, or 36. In two haplotypes, the C4A and C4B genes had the identical mutation[126,128] and, in the third haplotype (HLA A2 B12 DR6), two different nonsense mutations were present in the two C4 genes.[129]
3. Bimodular haplotype (SS) with two short C4B genes that had identical mutations at the donor splice site of intron 28.[125]

Again, all nonsense mutations except one in these C4-deficient patients were private or restrictive mutations that were only observed in the patient's family or local community. The exception is the 2-bp insertion in exon 29

(codon 1232) of C4A gene that has an allelic frequency of about 1–4% among Europeans.[130–132]

Low Copy Number of C4 Genes and Deficiency of C4A

A comprehensive study was performed in the United States to rigorously investigate the complement C4 genetic diversities in SLE of European descent and race-matched controls, using regular genomic Southern blot analyses of *Taq*I or *Psh*AI-*Pvu*II digested DNA resolved by regular gel electrophoresis, long-range mapping by *Pme*I digested genomic DNA fragments resolved by pulsed field gel electrophoresis, and C4A and C4B protein phenotyping by immunofixation.[44,132] The primary study population included 1241 European-Americans with 233 SLE patients and 356 first-degree relatives, plus 517 unrelated healthy controls (Figure 8). In this particular study population, the gene copy-numbers of total C4 varied from 2 to 6, C4A from 0 to 5, and C4B from 0 to 4. Their corresponding median copy-numbers were 4, 2, and 2, respectively. In comparison to healthy controls, SLE patients had their total C4 and C4A, but not C4B, gene copy-number groups shifted to the lower copy-number side. Among the female SLE patients, 9.3% had only two copies of C4 genes, and 6.5% had a homozygous deficiency of C4A, compared to 1.5% and 1.3%, respectively, in healthy controls. The odds for SLE disease risk (or odds ratio, OR) for a subject with only two copies of C4 genes in a diploid genome is 6.5 times greater than those with three or more copies of C4 genes. Among the subjects with no C4A genes, the odds for SLE disease risk are 5.7 times greater than those with one or more copies of C4A genes (i.e., OR=5.7). Thus, the gene copy-number of 2 for total C4 or a homozygous deficiency of C4A are large effect size risk factors for human SLE.[82]

Parallel increases in the frequency of heterozygous C4A deficiency (GCN=1) and moderately low copy-number of total C4 (GCN=3) were also observed in the SLE population. However, their effect size (impacts on disease risk) is substantially lower. Specifically, the frequency of subjects with a single copy of C4A was 26.4% in SLE and 18.2% in controls (OR=1.6); the frequency of subjects with moderately low copy-number of total C4 was 32.9% in patients and 27.0% in controls (OR=1.3). By contrast, human subjects with high copy-numbers of total C4 or C4A genes were protected against SLE disease risk. The frequency of subjects with ≥5 copies total C4 was 6.0% in SLE patients but 12.0% in controls (OR=0.47). The frequency for subjects with ≥3 copies C4A was 15.3% in SLE patients but 23.8% in controls (OR=0.57). Thus, it was concluded that low gene copy-number of total C4 or C4A was a risk factor for, and high copy-number of total C4 or C4A was a protective factor against SLE disease susceptibility in European-Americans.[132] In the same study, family-based association tests further revealed that monomodular-short

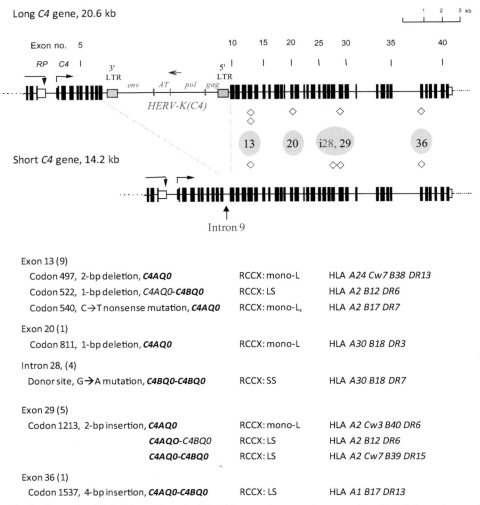

FIGURE 7   Molecular basis of complete C4 deficiency. A total of 28 subjects are known to have complete C4 deficiency. Among them, the molecular bases for the nonexpression of C4 proteins in 15 subjects have been determined. These subjects were from eight different HLA haplotypes. Molecular defects in the mutant *C4* genes include nonsense mutations caused by point mutations, mini-deletions, and mini-insertions in the coding regions, and point mutations at intron/exon splice junctions. *Filled black boxes* are the 41 exons in each *C4* gene. HERV-K(C4) is an endogenous retrovirus inserted into the intron 9 of long *C4* genes. *Modified from Ref. 126.*

RCCX haplotypes with single C4B gene and C4A deficiency was a risk factor for SLE, while haplotypes with C4A6 protein was a protective factor. C4A6 is known to have very low hemolytic activity because its R477W polymorphism leads to a defective C5 convertase and therefore dissociates the activation of the classical or lecin activation pathways from the terminal pathway.[133,134]

In two independent studies of Asian SLE in Han-Chinese and South Koreans, C4A and C4B gene copy-number was interrogated by TaqMan based real-time qualitative polymerase chain reaction (qPCR) methods.[43,135,136] Significantly lower gene copy-number of C4A and total C4 was observed in the SLE cases than race-matched controls. One common feature in those two East-Asian populations was the very low frequency of homozygous C4A deficiency in both SLE ($\leq 1\%$) and healthy controls.

In a third series of experiments for European SLE patients and controls from the United Kingdom and Spain, total C4 gene copy-numbers were determined by paralog ratio tests, followed by *Nla*IV restriction digested DNA of PCR amplified DNA to differentiate C4A and C4B.[137] Higher frequency for low gene copy-number of total C4 and C4A was apparent in both UK and Spanish SLE populations than matched controls. For the Spanish population, lower copy-number of C4B was also observed in SLE patients than controls. In comparison to the distribution of various gene copy-number groups for total C4, C4A, and C4B between the UK-European populations[137] and the US-European populations,[132] there were considerable differences in frequency, particularly, for the high copy-number groups. Thus, further replications and confirmation of C4-CNVs in European SLE and controls would be desirable.

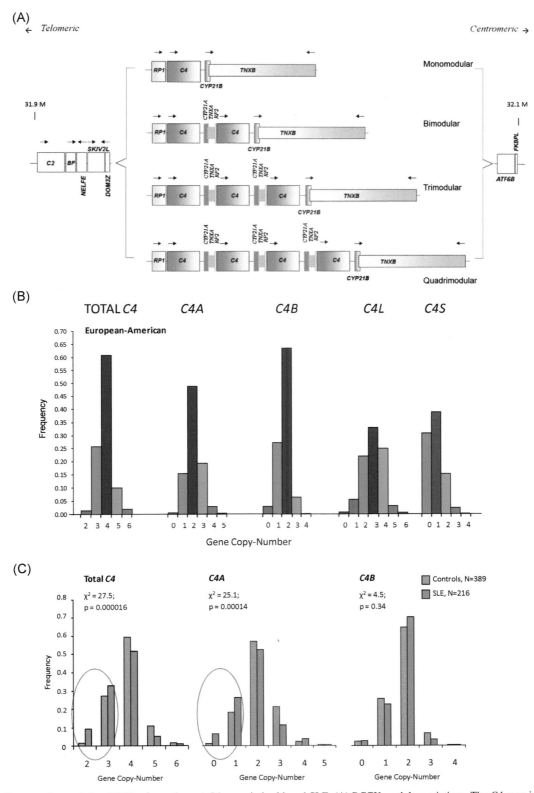

FIGURE 8 Copy-number variation (CNV) of complement *C4* genes in health and SLE. (A) RCCX modular variations. The *C4* gene is located in the class III region of the HLA on chromosome 6p21.3. On each chromosome 6, there can be one to four copies of *C4* gene. The duplication of a *C4* gene is concurrent with its three neighboring genes *RP* (*STK19*), *CYP21*, and *TNX* and thus described as RCCX modular duplication. Each *C4* gene codes either for an acidic C4A protein or a basic C4B protein. (B) Distributions of different diploid gene copy-number groups for total C4, C4A, C4B, long genes (C4L), and short genes (C4S) among healthy American subjects of European ancestry. (C) Comparisons of frequencies for total *C4*, *C4A*, and *C4B* gene copy-number groups in SLE (red) and controls (blue). SLE patients show significantly higher frequencies for low copy-numbers of total C4 and C4A but not C4B. *Modified from Ref. 132.*

As common and multiallelic CNVs are gaining attention because of their associations with many human diseases, it becomes even more important to ensure accuracy in data acquisition and interpretation. For accurate results on the pattern of variations for continuous CNVs and their associated polymorphisms, specific study designs accompanied by intra-individual (or intra-sample) data validation are critically important. It cannot be overemphasized that amplification or PCR-based technologies for quantitative CNVs are subjected to errors associated with varying qualities of the DNA samples. Therefore, independent data calls and cross-validation are essential. In the case of determining the GCNs of C4A and C4B, we suggest a minimum of three amplicons in duplicates for real-time qPCR to be performed. As such, in each sample the GCNs of total C4 = C4A + C4B. Discordance duplicates of each amplicon and unequal sums of the data sets should lead to repeats of experiments, using a new preparation of DNA samples. In addition, it is important to recognize that heteroduplexes are formed among allelic variants during the denaturation and annealing steps of PCR, and they would cause artifacts or allelic bias if the analysis is followed by restriction enzyme digest of PCR products. The issue of heteroduplexes in allelic determination of CNV can be resolved by "hotstop" PCR.[138,139]

Low Serum C4 Concentration in SLE

Several parameters affect the serum or plasma C4 protein concentration. The C4 gene copy-number, the copy-number of short C4 genes, and the body mass index are positively associated with increased C4 protein concentration.[39,140] Many SLE patients experience low or very low serum or plasma protein levels of complement C4 and C3, persistently or intermittently.[141,142] In some but not all such patients, these complement levels are biomarkers for lupus disease activity—low serum levels of C3 and/or C4 correlate with a flare and normal C3/C4 levels tend to correspond to a disease remission.[143]

It has been observed that lupus patients are characterized by high levels of degradation product C4d attached to red blood cells, reticulocytes, and platelets.[50,52–54] This phenomenon is monitored by flow cytometry using antibodies to C4. It is suggested that levels of RBC-C4d reflect complement activation in the past 60 days; the levels of reticulocyte-C4d reflect during the past 2–3 days, and platelet-C4d levels reflect complement activation during the past 5–10 days.

Longitudinal studies of serum complement protein levels in SLE patients reveal different expression profiles (Figure 9).[144] In one group of patients, there were persistently low C4 and C3 protein levels and many of these patients had a low copy-number of C4 genes. The second group of patients was marked by frequent fluctuations of C4 and C3 protein levels and SLE disease activity. The third group of patients were characterized by occasionally low C4 and C3 levels, particularly at the time of disease

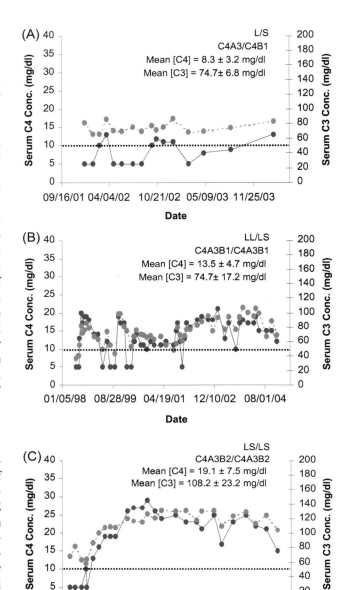

FIGURE 9 Typical complement C4 and C3 serial protein profiles in human SLE patients. Serum C4 and C3 protein levels tend to go up and down together in many SLE patients. In the first group of patients (*panel* A), levels of C4 and C3 were chronically low. In some patients, even if C3 levels rose to normal range, C4 levels remained low. This group of patients is characterized by low copy-number of C4 genes. The second group of patients had frequent and parallel fluctuations of serum protein levels for C3 and C4 (*panel* B). This group of patients has active disease, and low C3 and low C4 roughly correlate with disease activity. In the third group of patients (*panel* C), C4 and C3 protein levels stay in the normal range most of the time, except at the time of diagnosis and during a disease relapse. These patients tend to have relatively inactive disease. The second and third groups of patients have normal gene copy-number of total C4 but may have a heterozygous deficiency of C4A. The normal range for serum C4 was 16-48 mg/dL. The normal range for serum C3 was 80-160 mg/dL. C4 levels are shown as dark blue dots; C3 levels are shown as purple dots. *Modified from Ref. 144.*

diagnosis, but their levels often returned to normal. Most patients in the second and third groups had the median or higher copy-numbers of total *C4* or *C4A*, and the C4 and C3 protein concentrations roughly parallel the SLE disease activities.

Deficiency of Complement C2 or C3 in SLE

C2 Deficiency

Among individuals of European descent, C2 deficiency occurs with an estimated prevalence of 1/20,000, which probably accounts for less than 1% of SLE patients. There are two types of C2 deficiency.[145–147] Type 1C2 deficiency is caused by nonsense mutations leading to the absence of protein biosynthesis. The predominant form of such type 1 deficiency is a 28-bp deletion that removes 9-bp from the 3′ end of exon 6 and 19-bp from the 5′ end of intron 6 in the C2 gene, leading to a skipping of exon 6 in the C2 mRNA and generation of a premature stop-codon.[148] Such 28-bp deletion is present in the HLA haplotype with A10 (A25) and B18 in the class I region, BF-S, C2Q0, C4A4 and C4B2 in the class III region, and DRB1*15 (DR2) in the class II region. The second form of type 1 deficiency is present in HLA A3, B35, DR4, BF-F, C2Q0, C4A3, and C4A2.[149] The cause is a 2-bp deletion in exon two of C2 gene that leads to a nonsense mutation.

About 10% of C2 deficiency belongs to the type 2 deficiency in which the C2 protein is synthesized but not secreted. The molecular defects were found to be missense mutations C111Y, S189F, and G444R.[150,151] It is not clear how these mutations block the secretion of the C2 protein.

Unlike a deficiency of proteins for the C1 complex or C4 described earlier, the penetrance of C2 deficiency on SLE is only about 10%. Similar to other risk factors for SLE, there is a female predominance. C2-deficient SLE patients tend to have early childhood onset but a milder disease process with prominent photosensitive dermatologic manifestations, speckled ANAs (the autoantibody specificity is commonly for the Ro [SSA] antigen), and a family history of SLE. Anti-DNA antibody tests are usually negative and severe kidney disease is rare (Table 3).

In a large St. Louis kindred followed by one of the authors (JPA) for over four decades, three members were C2 deficient: a deceased male who lived into his 80s without developing SLE, a deceased female who had SLE and died at an elderly age of an unrelated disease, and a living 50-year-old female who developed life-threatening SLE in her early 20s but whose disease has now been in remission for over two decades.

Complement C3 Deficiency and SLE

C3-deficient patients are generally associated with severe infections.[152,153] Despite its prominent roles relative to the complement functions of opsonization, phagocytosis, and clearance of immune complexes, C3 deficiency is not involved in SLE predisposition in most human races except Japanese, in which five out of six C3-deficient subjects have been diagnosed with SLE.[152,154] Moreover, animals deficient in C3 including C3 knockout mice do not exhibit lupus-like phenotypes.[155,156] It is also noteworthy that development of SLE in most animals requires a permissive genetic background. Most mice and guinea pigs with C1q, C4, or C2 deficiency do not develop SLE.

COMPLEMENT RECEPTORS AND REGULATORS IN SLE

Genetic Polymorphisms and Shedding of E-CR1

Immune adherence receptor—a receptor of many names (CR1, CD35, C3b/C4b receptor)—was shown over three decades ago to be reduced in copy number on red blood cells (RBCs) in active SLE.[157] While initially thought possibly to be an inherited predisposition,[158] further analysis demonstrated that it was secondary to an acquired defect associated with IC processing.[159,160] The CR1 levels on RBC returned to normal upon remission. One mechanism of loss was that of an interaction of IC bearing RBCs with phagocytes. The fixed phagocytes in the liver and spleen induced a shedding of the receptor. Evidence for proteolytic cleavage of CR1 in the membrane was also reported. In the case of B cells or PMNs, shedding, internalization, and protease cleavage of CR1 would all be possible.[161–163]

Human CR2 and Mouse Cr2/Cr1

CR2 (CD21), CD19, and CD81 (and CD23) together form a co-receptor for B-cell receptors on B cells.[164,165] CR2's natural ligands are C3d and iC3b. Intriguingly, Epstein-Barr virus (EBV) uses CR2 as an entry to B cells.[166,167] Furthermore, IFN-α and DNA have also been shown to be ligands for CR2.[168–170]

In the mouse, Cr2/Cr1 are mainly expressed on transitional to mature B cells and follicular-dendritic cells, although in humans, CR1 and CR2 are also present on a small subset (~10%) of T cells.[171] CR2 plays a critical role on the T-dependent activation of B cells during the germinal center response in peripheral lymphoid organs[172] where immunoglobulin class switching, affinity maturation, negative selection against autoreactive B-cells and anergy occur.[173,174] In the mouse, it has been shown that immune complexes coated with C3 or C4 fragments are transferred to lymphoid tissues through binding to Cr2/Cr1 on B-cells.[175] These immune complexes are acquired by follicular-dendritic cells (FDCs), internalized and retained intact within a nondegenerative cycling compartment for long period of time. They are displayed on the cell surface of FDCs periodically and become accessible to antigen-specific B cells. Such a phenomenon offers an explanation for immunologic memory.

Mouse Cr1 and Cr2 are encoded by the same gene that produces two related transcripts through alternative splicing.[176] The Cr1/Cr2 knockout mouse exhibited reduced number of CD5+ peritoneal B-1 cells and impaired humoral immune response to T-dependent protein antigens with reduced number and size of germinal centers in splenic follicles.[177] Mice with combined deficiencies of Cr2 or C4 and CD95 (Fas) resulted in high titers of antinuclear antibodies and anti-dsDNA antibodies.[178] In transgenic mouse model system expressing soluble hen egg lysozyme (HEL, as an autoantigen) and (autoreactive) B cells with HEL-specific immunoglobulin were created to study factors contributing to autoimmunity. When crossed to Cr2/Cr1-deficient or C4-deficient mice, the percentage of HEL-specific autoreactive B cells in lymph nodes or spleens was significantly increased.[178]

Recently, it was shown that murine B cells predominantly expresses Cr2 protein, while FDC almost exclusively expresses the Cr1 protein isoform.[179] Cr1-specific knockout mice were generated through internal deletion of exons encoding domains specific to Cr1, with the Cr2 remaining intact. Cr1-deficient mice after immunization were shown to have defective antibody responses to T-dependent antigens, and the germinal centers in immunized mice were deficient of activated B cells.[179] Thus, it was concluded that murine Cr1 is required for germinal center B cell maintenance but not initiation.[180]

The murine Sle1c locus of the lupus nephritis mouse model NZM2410 is associated with the production of histone-specific autoreactive CD4+ T cells and a reduction of CD4+, CD25+, FoxP3+ regulatory T cells.[181] The murine Sle1 is present at the telomeric region of chromosome one. This is syntenic to human chromosome 1q21-42, by which the genes for human CR1 and CR2 are present. Intriguingly, DNA sequencing of Cr2 from NZM2410 and NZW revealed a nonsynonymous polymorphism, H72N, is located at the C3d-binding domain. The Asn-72 residue forms a novel N-linked glycosylation site that increases the molecular weight of Cr2 (and Cr1) and interferes with receptor dimerization, ligand binding and receptor-mediated cell signaling. Thus, it was suggested that the H72N allele of Cr2 in NZM2410 was a lupus susceptibility allele.[182]

With the background of Cr2 allele in NZM2410 as a risk factor for murine lupus, large searches of genetic variants in *human* CR2 as a risk factor have been performed. In an early study, selected single nucleotide polymorphisms (SNPs) in the regulatory, coding, and noncoding regions of CR2 gene from 400 simplex families with SLE were typed and analyzed by transmission disequilibrium test.[183] A common haplotype with three SNPs (one from the 5′-untranslated region and two from exon 10) was found to associate with SLE development with an odds ratio of 1.54. Reporter gene assays of the 5′ UT SNP (nucleotide +21 T/C, *rs3813946*) revealed differential expression between the minor and major alleles. In a more recent study that engaged 15,750 case/control subjects with genotyped and imputed genetic variants of CR2, a new SNP in the intron 1 of CR2, *rs1876453*, was found significantly associated with the presence of dsDNA antibodies in SLE patients with an odds ratio of 0.71.[184] Notably, the minor allele of this SNP correlated with increased levels mRNA and protein levels for CR1 instead of CR2, associated with reduced risk of dsDNA autoantibodies.

Human Complement Receptor CR3

Through genome-wide association studies, rs1143679, a nonsynonymous SNP for R77H in CR3 (ITGAM, CD11b/CD18, Mac-1), was identified as risk factor of SLE by multiple teams.[185–187] A meta-analysis of published results from multiple independent data sets revealed that the H77 variant of ITGAM was one of the most robust risk factors (OR = 1.76) associated with SLE from subjects of different racial backgrounds including Caucasian, Black, and Asian but not Japanese and Korean.[188,189] This missense mutation is located at the β-propeller domain and close to the ligand binding of the integrin. Human monocytes or monocyte-derived macrophages from subjects with H77 variant had a 31% reduction in phagocytosis for iC3b-opsonized sheep red blood cells.[190] Cultured cells expressing the risk variant H77 were shown to have compromised activities of adhesion to a variety of ligands including to ICAM-1 under shear flow conditions, and reduced adhesion and iC3b-dependent phagocytosis.[188,190,191]

Regulators of Complement Activation

Complement regulators have *not* been convincingly demonstrated to be involved in SLE pathogenesis. A few reports though suggest that Factor H[192] and MCP genetic variants led to slightly increased risk, or a reduction in the expression of these two regulators in SLE. A logical possibility here would be that, for example, a heterozygous deficiency of FH, FI, or MCP could predispose an individual to more severe end-organ damage mediated by complement-fixing ICs. These individuals would have a reduced capacity to control complement activation in the blood or at a tissue site and therefore be inclined to develop more severe end-organ damage.

AUTOANTIBODIES TO COMPLEMENT AND ACQUIRED DEFICIENCY OF COMPLEMENT IN SLE

There are many autoantibodies against complement proteins in SLE.[193] Most autoantibodies to complement are not directed against native proteins but neo-epitopes exposed in active or inactivated proteins, or multimolecular complexes formed during the activation process. The binding of autoantibodies to complement could lead to a state of acquired deficiency and contribute to disease pathogenesis.

Autoantibodies to C1q

About 30% of SLE patients synthesize autoantibodies to C1q. The presence of C1q autoantibodies correlates with anti-dsDNA Abs, nephritis, and low complement, and these three serologic factors are being observed in about 75% of such patients.[194–196] The development of these autoantibodies may be a secondary phenomenon that occurs when ICs bind C1q and activate the CP. Following CP activation, the C1-Inh strips the C1r and C1s proteases from the C1 complex, which is bound to Ab. C1q remains attached to the IC and therefore at the site of inflammation. Proteases at this site will next degrade the IgG and C1q and the autoantigen. Multiple proteolytic fragments of IgG and C1q are generated. Thus, it may not be surprising that anti-C1q Abs and anti-IgG or anti-IgM (rheumatoid factors) are generated in SLE patients to these potential neoantigens. Indeed, most C1q autoantibodies bind to neoepitopes of the collagen-like regions, which enabled the design for one of the detection methods to differentiate between the binding of the C1q globular heads to the Fc-regions of IgG present in immune complexes, and the binding of CLR of C1q to its autoantibodies.

On this background, a large study was recently reported in which one goal was to assess the specificity of anti-C1q Abs and its association with SLE manifestations and diagnostic tests.[59] These authors confirmed an association of anti-C1q Abs, low complement (C4 and C3), and anti-dsDNA Abs. This combination had the strongest serological association with the clinical development of renal disease. Anti-C1q Abs were seen in 28% of all SLE patients but were observed in 68% of patients with renal disease. In related rheumatic diseases, they were observed in ~5–10%. Thus, anti-C1q Abs are of limited efficacy from a diagnostic point of view but may have merit in classifying a lupus patient, particularly relative to the presence of lupus nephritis. It was suggested that the absence of anti-C1q antibodies makes a nephritis flare rare.[195]

Autoantibodies to C3 and C4

Immunoconglutinins

Immunoconglutinins are autoantibodies against solid-bound, processed fragments of C3 (and C4) such as C3b, iC3b, C3c, and C3dg but not C3d. Immunoconglutinins were among the earliest complement autoantibodies discovered,[197] which have been shown in SLE, RA, and Crohn's disease. The IgG isotype of immunoconglutinins were found to be strongly correlated with SLE disease exacerbation,[198] and IgG levels of anti-C1q in SLE.[199]

C3 and C4 Nephritic Factors

C3 and C4 nephritic factors bind to the neoepitopes present in the alternative pathway C3 convertase (C3bBb or C3bBbP) and the CP C3 convertase (C4b2a), respectively. They prolong the half-life of the convertases from minutes to hours and therefore enhance the consumption or depletion of serum C3 and variably C5 as well. Both C3 and C4 nephritic factors are associated with membranoproliferative glomerulonephritis.[200,201] In addition, C3 nephritic factors are associated with acquired partial lipodystrophy, and C4 nephritic factor with SLE and postinfectious acute glomerulonephritis.[202,203] The prevalence of C3 and/or C4 nephritic factors in SLE has not been thoroughly investigated.[201]

Autoantibodies to Other Complement Components

Autoantibodies to MBL

Autoantibodies to mannose binding lectin (MBL) have been determined in SLE patients from multiple racial backgrounds, including European, Chinese, and Asian Indians.[193,204–207] While MBL autoantibodies correlated with reduced serum levels of MBL, no association with SLE disease activities was observed.

Autoantibodies to C1s

In a study of plasma samples from 15 SLE patients, autoantibodies to C1s were found in seven SLE patients (47%).[208] The binding of autoantibodies to C1s enhanced its esterase activity for C4 that contributed to low C4 serum levels in SLE patients.

Autoantibodies to Complement Receptors

Autoantibodies to CR1

Autoantibodies against CR1 were first discovered in an SLE patient with a transiently acquired deficiency of CR1 on erythrocytes and B cells, and partial deficiency on neutrophils.[209] Such phenomenon was examined in 78 SLE patients and 90 healthy controls using recombinant CR1 bound to ELISA plates as antigens. CR1 autoantibodies were found in 3.5% of controls and 46% of SLE patients. However, it was also found that CR1 autoantibodies probably bound to neoepitopes (e.g., on CR1 with ligand, or denatured CR1 proteins) and did not recognize native CR1 protein on erythrocytes. Thus, CR1 autoantibodies probably do not play a direct role on the acquired loss of CR1 on erythrocytes in SLE.[210]

Autoantibodies to CR3

Autoantibodies against type 3 complement receptor (CR3, Mac-1 or CD11b/CD18) had been detected in patients with autoimmune neutropenia. In an early study of 50 patients with antineutrophil IgG antibodies, seven patients were detected positive for anti-CD11b/CD18 and such autoantibodies could interfere with the adhesion and opsonin functions of CR3 on neutrophils, thereby increasing the risk of infections.[211] Autoantibodies to CR3 have not been comprehensively evaluated in SLE patients.

Antibodies to Complement Regulatory Proteins

Antibodies to C1-Inhibitor

Antibodies to C1-Inh are well described and cause an acquired form of angioedema that clinically mimics hereditary angioneurotic edema (HAE). In one population study with 202 SLE patients and 134 controls, C1-Inh autoantibodies were found in 17% of SLE patients and 4% of controls. Patients with C1-Inh autoantibodies had higher SLE disease activity indices and longer duration of disease. However, the presence of C1-Inh autoantibodies did not correlate with SLE laboratory parameters, including serum levels of C4 and C3.[212]

Antibodies to Factor H

Autoantibodies to factor H account for 5–15% of cases of aHUS, which is a disease characterized by anemia because of red blood cell destruction, thrombocytopenia because of profound consumption of platelets, and acute renal failure because of platelet microaggregates in glomerular capillaries. The autoantibodies to factor H tamper with the regulatory and protective functions of factor H against complement-mediated tissue damage. Besides aHUS, factor H autoantibodies are also associated with membranoproliferative glomerulonephritis.[56,213,214]

Anticardiolipin Syndrome or Antiphospholipid Syndrome

Autoantibodies to phospholipids, cardiolipins, and beta-2-glycoprotein-1 are observed in ~30% of SLE patients. Analagous to autoantibodies to nuclear antigens, they form immune-complexes and fix complement.[215] While there is some variability in studies relative to the frequency of hypocomplementemia in patients with a moderate-to-high titer ACLA, the frequency of low complements

is similar to that in SLE. There does not appear to be an increased frequency of the anticardiolipin syndrome (ACLS) in C1q-, C4-, or C2-deficient patients. The contribution of complement to ACLS in man requires further study, but mouse studies are consistent with it having definitive pathological consequences as it does in SLE. The complement profile in antiphospholipid syndrome (APLS) in general parallels that observed in lupus with CP activation being predominant.[215–218] Complement levels though could reflect pregnancy outcomes of APLS patients. Hypocomplementemia was associated with fetal loss, preterm delivery, and lower neonatal birth weight,[219] It is not clear if low complement in APLS was secondary to a genetic deficiency, an effect of complement activation and consumption, or both.

NEW CONNECTIONS FOR LUPUS AND COMPLEMENT

Local Synthesis

Several reports have proposed a role for local synthesis of complement components on disease pathogenesis, especially in the skin and kidney. In these studies, blood and blood-derived interstitial C3 were not sufficient to trigger an optimal normal response to injury or an infectious process but local synthesis was necessary. While the large majority of attempts to show a role for local synthesis have been negative (i.e., the C3 or C4 derived from blood could mediate the event such as synovitis), there are several examples whereby a requirement for local synthesis is shown.[220–222]

Activation by Local Proteases

Multiple proteases, in cells, on cell membranes, and in the interstitial spaces, can cleave C4, C3, and C5 to liberate C4a, C3a, and C5a. These anaphylatoxins are potent activators of multiple cell types. One does not therefore necessarily need to form a C3 convertase or a C5 convertase to generate these proinflammatory fragments. A particularly informative example is that of a model system in which immune complexes were injected into the lung and thrombin was shown to be capable of cleaving C5 to C5a and C5b and mediating aspects of the inflammatory response (even in the absence of C3).[223]

Intracellular Complement Activation

In another series of reports involving primarily human T cells, intracellular C3 activation by cathepsin L of C3 stores to generate C3b and C3a was demonstrated.[224,225] In addition, in the case of C3a, its receptor was also present intracellularly. In some cases, transfer of the activated C3 products to cell membrane and extracellular space was also shown. C3 stores appear to be widespread as are proteases that can cleave C3 to C3b and C3a. These could therefore provide an assist, especially early on, to initiate a local activation process to generate an inflammatory response. One could also envision a similar system to activate C4 and C5 intracellularly, on the plasma membrane or in the extracellular milieu.

Exogenous Coating with Opsonic Fragments Lead to Endogenous Consequences

In a recent report, virus and bacteria coated with C3b, upon being internalized by immune cells, triggered an inflammasome pathway that was dependent on the microbe being coated with complement fragments.[226] This interesting work indicates that C3b coating of target not only leads to immune adherence and ingestion but, once inside the cell, the opsonic materials can engage proinflammatory pathways.

A Primitive Complement System

The hypothesis here is that the primitive complement system, particularly prior to the origin of lymphatic and vascular (pumped) circulations, could have operated intracellularly. This process is likely still important in selected sites to facilitate an early response to infection and injury.[19,224,227]

CONCLUSIONS

Why Does Lupus Develop Among Complement-Deficient Subjects?

Why do patients with genetic or acquired deficiency of complement develop SLE? For nearly four decades, a complete deficiency of an early component of the CP was the only deficiency in humans in which a single gene defect caused SLE almost 100% of the time. Over the past decade, a total efficiency of either extracellular DNaseI or extracellular DNaseIII has been shown to also regularly cause SLE. In Saudi families, the case of DNaseI deficiency was consanguineous and SLE penetrance was 100%.[228,229] Also, they developed SLE at a young age (<12 years). In addition, all were anti-dsDNA positive and had renal diseases and low C4 and C3.

While DNaseI is the major extracellular enzyme, DNaseIII (or TREX1) is the major intracellular enzyme. A deficiency of it is also strongly associated with the development of lupus as well as familial chilblains lupus.[230–235] However, a complete deficiency of this enzyme causes Aicardi-Goutieres syndrome, in retrospect it is a childhood form of lupus with primarily brain involvement.

Considering these two sets of observations, a logical explanation is that the handling of debris (garbage) containing RNA and DNA is the crux of the problem. The role of complement in this process is predicted to facilitate the identification, opsonization and proper disposal of this self debris containing DNA and RNA (Figure 10). C1q binds to necrotic and apoptotic cells and to other types of cellular

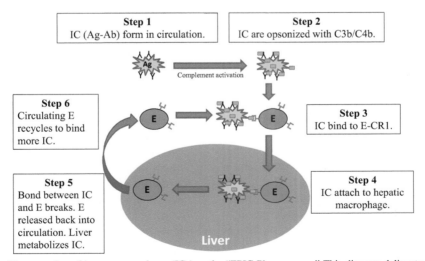

FIGURE 10 Erythrocyte (E) processing of immune complexes (ICs) or the "EPIC Phenomenon." This diagram delineates a pathway for processing (IC). Complement-coated ICs adhere to the erythrocyte (E) C3b/C4b receptor, also known as complement receptor type 1 (CR1 or CD35). This binding of IC through C3b and its receptor to E in primates and to platelets in non-primates is known as the *immune adherence phenomenon*. The erythrocyte transports, like a taxi, shuttle or ferry, the IC to the liver and spleen. In the liver, the ICs are transferred to macrophages (Kupffer cells) and destroyed. In the spleen, the ICs are transferred to B-lymphocytes, macrophages, and follicular-dendritic cells for antigen processing and presentation. The E returns to circulation, often stripped of some of its receptors, but available to again bind complement-coated IC. This model was initially defined in baboons by Hebert and colleagues; the essential elements of the scheme have now been described in humans, other primates, guinea pigs, and rabbits. Several different antigen–antibody systems, including tetanus–anti-tetanus, DNA–anti-DNA and BSA–anti-BSA, have been analyzed. *Adapted from Ref. 246.*

debris. It can both interact with C1q receptors as well as, more importantly relative to SLE, trigger the CP to deposit C4b and C3b on the DNA/RNA "trash." Likewise, natural Abs recognize modified proteins, lipids, and nucleotides. Also, lectins bind to sugars that that are modified in debris. While there are multiple pathways to assist the host with clearance of these types of materials that accumulate continuously in normal humans, at least to prevent SLE from developing, you need the CP of complement to activate through at least C4, and the presence of intracellular and extracellular DNases. The fact that 80% of C1q- or C4-deficient patients develop SLE indicates that the specific complement deficiency that leads to SLE is an inability to activate the CP.

These data raise the interesting consideration that any defect in debris handling, intracellularly or extracellularly, could be involved in lupus predisposition. Also, any condition in which the system is temporarily overloaded such as EBV infection could be a trigger.

To Treat or Not to Treat SLE with a Complement Inhibitor

Cons

1. *Clinical experience*: SLE patients feature chronic complement activation, consumption, and complement-mediated tissue injuries. Would you therefore want to inhibit these early components? It seems counterintuitive. Patients lacking a component of CP such as C1q, C1r, C1s, C4, or C2 develop SLE. Moreover, in several case reports, infusions of C1q, C4, or C2 into such patients led to the amelioration of refractory disease.
2. *Pathophysiological consequences*: Processing of immune-complexes is facilitated by CP activation; that is, deposition of C4b and C3b on the IC promotes their adherence to CR1 bearing cells and thereby safe removal by phagocytic cells in the liver and spleen. Thus, the CR1-C3b/C4b–immune complex travels via an RBC (serves the role of a ferry or taxi) and then transfers the cargo to resident monocytes-macrophages for destruction and/or antigen presentation (Figure 10). Therefore, blocking any step up to and including C3 would inhibit IC processing and possibly exacerbate SLE.
3. *Predisposition to infection*: Patients with SLE already have an increased frequency of infections (even without immunosuppression) and inhibiting the complement system could enhance this susceptibility especially to *S. pneumonia* and meningococcal infection in the case of C1q, C4, C2, or C3 blockage.

Pros

1. *Clinical experience*: Tissue damage in lupus is partly mediated by C4b/C3b, C5a/C3a, and the MAC. These activation fragments modulate membranes and produce inflammation, especially the kidney. The goal would be to curtail this cellular injury and facilitate repair.
2. *Pathophysiological consequences*: These patients have SLE. Presumably, greater than 90% do not have a major deficiency in the complement to account for the etiology of their disease. Since complement activation is responsible for some of the tissue damage, particularly in the kidney, that is mediated by C5a and C5b–C9 for which an effective inhibitor to prevent their production is FDA approved, therapeutic trials with a mAb to C5 are indicated. In aHUS, endothelial damage is mediated by the AP and inhibition of C5 cleavage is a very effective therapy.[236] While C3b and C3a themselves seem not to be the key figures in causing the damage, C3 activation is required to form a C5 convertase.
3. *Mouse models*: In mouse models, a lack of an early component of the CP led to more severe disease,[156,178,237,238] while inhibition of MAC tended to reduce disease severity.[239–241] This represents additional evidence to suggest that blocking the terminal pathway at the C5 step may be indicated in SLE.

Future Considerations

1. Complement component tests, namely C4 and C3, will continue to be of assistance in establishing the diagnosis of SLE and to have utility as a biomarker of disease activity.
2. Measurement of complement split products in plasma such as C3a, C3d, iC3b, C3d, C5a, Bb, soluble C5b–9, and others are likely to become more standardized and reliable tests for monitoring complement activation. They, however, require further study as their usefulness as biomarkers of disease activity remains to be determined. At this time, they are not ready to replace the standard antigenic levels of C4 and C3.
3. Advances in our understanding of the role of the complement system in processing debris and in instructing adaptive immunity may lead us to define the etiology and pathogenesis of lupus. In humans, the complement system and the DNases are two established pathways in which an individual lacking a protein will almost certainly develop lupus.
4. Inhibition of complement activation needs to be explored in SLE.
   a. An FDA-approved therapeutic agent is in the marketplace, which blocks C5 cleavage to C5a and C5b by the C5 convertases. Clinical trials of this mAb are indicated.
   b. Many novel agents are now in the drug pipeline to block earlier steps than C5 activation in both the CP and the AP. An attractive possibility might be to treat an acutely ill patient with, for example, an aggressive glomerulonephritis with a complement inhibitor(s) (along with cytotoxics and steroids) for several weeks to control tissue damage.

c. Because of the recognized effects of the C3a, C5a, and membrane attack complex (C5b–9) on vasculature, inhibitors of these complement fragments as well as, in the case of C3a and C5a, their specific receptors on the vasculature and on inflammatory/immune cells are attractive therapeutic targets.

5. In view of the great advances in sequencing in the era of *genomics* (the lupus patient's whole exome and whole genome sequence will soon become routine at the time of initial diagnosis), the selection of therapeutic modalities will likely in part be based on these genetic data. Rheumatologists will need to become familiar with interpreting these results, analogous to our ability to interpret serologic laboratory tests such as the ANA, RF, and antineutrophil cytoplasmic antibodies.

REFERENCES

1. Walport MJ. Complement- part I. *N Engl J Med* 2001;**344**:1058–66.
2. Walport MJ. Complement- part II. *N Engl J Med* 2001;**344**:1140–4.
3. Sturfelt G, Truedsson L. Complement in the immunopathogenesis of rheumatic disease. *Nat Rev Rheumatol* 2012;**8**:458–68.
4. Pondman KW, Cormane RH, Hannema AJ. Abnormal C'1 in a patient with systemic lupus erythematosus. *J Immunol* 1968;**101**:811.
5. Pickering RJ, Naff GB, Stroud RM, Good RA, Gewurz H. Deficiency of C1r in human serum. Effects on the structure and function of macromolecular C1. *J Exp Med* 1970;**131**:803–15.
6. Lipsker D, Hauptmann G. Cutaneous manifestations of complement deficiencies. *Lupus* 2010;**19**:1096–106.
7. Schejbel L, Skattum L, Hagelberg S, Ahlin A, Schiller B, Berg S, et al. Molecular basis of hereditary C1q deficiency–revisited: identification of several novel disease-causing mutations. *Genes Immun* 2011;**12**:626–34.
8. Gibson DJ, Glass D, Carpenter CB, Schur PH. Hereditary C2 deficiency: diagnosis and HLA gene complex associations. *J Immunol* 1976;**116**:1065–70.
9. McAdam RA, Goundis D, Reid KB. A homozygous point mutation results in a stop codon in the C1q B-chain of a C1q-deficient individual. *Immunogenetics* 1988;**27**:259–64.
10. Awdeh ZL, Ochs HD, Alper CA. Genetic analysis of C4 deficiency. *J Clin Invest* 1981;**67**:260–3.
11. Schaller JG, Gilliland BG, Ochs HD, Leddy JP, Agodoa LCY, Rosenfeld SI. Severe systemic lupus erythematosus with nephritis in a boy with deficiency of the fourth component of component. *Arthritis Rheum* 1977;**20**:1519–25.
12. Tappeiner G, Scholz S, Linert J, Albert ED, Wolff K. Hereditary deficiency of the fourth component (C4): study of a family. *Colloq Inserm/Cutan Immunopathol* 1978;**80**:399–404.
13. Moncada B, Day NK, Good RA, Windhorst DB. Lupus-erythematosus-like syndrome with a familial defect of complement. *N Engl J Med* 1972;**286**:689–93.
14. Petterson A. The Nobel lectures in immunology. The Nobel prize for physiology or medicine, 1919, awarded to Jules Bordet "for his discoveries relating to immunity". *Scand J Immunol* 1990;**32**:425–8.
15. Pillemer L, Blum L, Lepow IH, Ross OA, Todd EW, Wardlaw AC. The properdin system and immunity. I. Demonstration and isolation of a new serum protein, properdin, and its role in immune phenomena. *Science* 1954;**120**:279–85.
16. Pillemer L, Schoenberg MD, Blum L, Wurz L. Properdin system and immunity. II. Interaction of the properdin system with polysaccharides. *Science* 1955;**122**:545–9.
17. Fearon DT, Austen KF. Properdin: initiation of alternative complement pathway. *Proc Natl Acad Sci USA* 1975;**72**:3220–4.
18. Fearon DT, Austen KF. Initiation of C3 cleavage in the alternative complement pathway. *J Immunol* 1975;**115**:1357–61.
19. Sekiguchi R, Nonaka M. Evolution of the complement system in protostomes revealed by de novo transcriptome analysis of six species of Arthropoda. *Dev Comp Immunol* 2015;**50**:58–67.
20. Riesgo A, Farrar N, Windsor PJ, Giribet G, Leys SP. The analysis of eight transcriptomes from all poriferan classes reveals surprising genetic complexity in sponges. *Mol Biol Evol* 2014;**31**:1102–20.
21. Lu J, Teh C, Kishore U, Reid KB. Collectins and ficolins: sugar pattern recognition molecules of the mammalian innate immune system. *Biochim Biophys Acta* 2002;**1572**:387–400.
22. Epstein J, Eichbaum Q, Sheriff S, Ezekowitz RA. The collectins in innate immunity. *Curr Opin Immunol* 1996;**8**:29–35.
23. Endo Y, Matsushita M, Fujita T. The role of ficolins in the lectin pathway of innate immunity. *Int J Biochem Cell Biol* 2011;**43**:705–12.
24. Ricklin D, Hajishengallis G, Yang K, Lambris JD. Complement: a key system for immune surveillance and homeostasis. *Nat Immunol* 2010;**11**:785–97.
25. Atkinson JP, Yu CY. Genetic susceptibility and class III complement genes. In: Lahita RG, Tsokos G, Buyon J, Koike T, editors. *Systemic lupus erythematosus*. 5th ed. Amsterdam: Academic Press at Elsevier; 2011. p. 21–45.
26. Leffler J, Bengtsson AA, Blom AM. The complement system in systemic lupus erythematosus: an update. *Ann Rheum Dis* 2014;**73**:1601–6.
27. White RM, Buffone GJ, Savory J, Killingsworth LM. A kinetic nephelometric method for the assay of serum C3 and C4. *Ann Clin Lab Sci* 1976;**6**:525–8.
28. Petri M, Orbai AM, Alarcon GS, Gordon C, Merrill JT, Fortin PR, et al. Derivation and validation of the systemic lupus international collaborating clinics classification criteria for systemic lupus erythematosus. *Arthritis Rheum* 2012;**64**:2677–86.
29. Gaboriaud C, Ling WL, Thielens NM, Bally I, Rossi V. Deciphering the fine details of c1 assembly and activation mechanisms: "mission impossible"? *Front Immunol* 2014;**5**:565.
30. Charlesworth JA, Peake PW, Golding J, Mackie JD, Pussell BA, Timmermans V, et al. Hypercatabolism of C3 and C4 in active and inactive systemic lupus erythematosus. *Ann Rheum Dis* 1989;**48**:153–9.
31. Ng YC, Schifferli JA. Clearance of cryoglobulins in man. *Springer Semin Immunopathol* 1988;**10**:75–89.
32. Jaffe CJ, Atkinson JP, Frank MM. The role of complement in the clearance of cold agglutinin-sensitized erythrocytes in man. *J Clin Invest* 1976;**58**:942–9.
33. Monti G, Saccardo F, Castelnovo L, Novati P, Sollima S, Riva A, et al. Prevalence of mixed cryoglobulinaemia syndrome and circulating cryoglobulins in a population-based survey: the Origgio study. *Autoimmun Rev* 2014;**13**:609–14.
34. Monti G, Saccardo F, Pioltelli P, Rinaldi G. The natural history of cryoglobulinemia: symptoms at onset and during follow-up. A report by the Italian Group for the Study of Cryoglobulinemias (GISC). *Clin Exp Rheumatol* 1995;**13**(Suppl 13):S129–33.
35. Atkinson JP, Gorman JC, Curd J, Hyla JF, Deegan MJ, Keren DF, et al. Cold dependent activation of complement in systemic lupus erythematosus. A unique cause for a discrepancy between clinical and laboratory parameters. *Arthritis Rheum* 1981;**24**:592–601.

36. Newell S, Gorman JC, Bell E, Atkinson JP. Hemolytic and antigenic measurements of complement. A comparison of serum and plasma samples in normal individuals and patients. *J Lab Clin Med* 1982;**100**:437–44.

37. Wei G, Yano S, Kuroiwa T, Hiromura K, Maezawa A. Hepatitis C virus (HCV)-induced IgG-IgM rheumatoid factor (RF) complex may be the main causal factor for cold-dependent activation of complement in patients with rheumatic disease. *Clin Exp Immunol* 1997;**107**:83–8.

38. Blanchong CA, Zhou B, Rupert KL, Chung EK, Jones KN, Sotos JF, et al. Deficiencies of human complement component C4A and C4B and heterozygosity in length variants of RP-C4-CYP21-TNX (RCCX) modules in Caucasians: the load of RCCX genetic diversity on MHC-associated disease. *J Exp Med* 2000;**191**:2183–96.

39. Yang Y, Chung EK, Zhou B, Blanchong CA, Yu CY, Füst G, et al. Diversity in intrinsic strengths of the human complement system: serum C4 protein concentrations correlate with *C4* gene size and polygenic variations, hemolytic activities and body mass index. *J Immunol* 2003;**171**:2734–45.

40. Chung EK, Yang Y, Rennebohm RM, Lokki ML, Higgins GC, Jones KN, et al. Genetic sophistication of human complement *C4A* and *C4B* and *RP-C4-CYP21-TNX* (RCCX) modules in the major histocompatibility complex (MHC). *Am J Hum Genet* 2002;**71**:823–37.

41. Yang Y, Chung EK, Zhou B, Lhotta K, Hebert LA, Birmingham DJ, et al. The intricate role of complement component C4 in human systemic lupus erythematosus. *Curr Dir Autoimmun* 2004;**7**:98–132.

42. Pickering MC, Botto M, Taylor PR, Lachmann PJ, Walport MJ. Systemic lupus erythematosus, complement deficiency and apoptosis. *Adv Immunol* 2001;**76**:227–324.

43. Wu YL, Savelli SL, Yang Y, Zhou B, Rovin BH, Birmingham DJ, et al. Sensitive and specific real-time PCR assays to accurately determine copy-number variations (CNVs) of human complement *C4A*, *C4B*, *C4-Long*, *C4-Short* and RCCX modules: elucidation of *C4* CNVs in 50 consanguineous subjects with defined HLA genotypes. *J Immunol* 2007;**179**:3012–25.

44. Chung EK, Wu YL, Yang Y, Zhou B, Yu CY. Human complement components C4A and C4B genetic diversities: complex genotypes and phenotypes. In: Coligan JE, Bierer BE, Margulis DH, Shevach EM, Strober W, editors. *Current protocols in immunology*. Edison, NJ: John Wiley & Sons, Inc.; 2005. p. 13.8.1–36.

45. Paakkanen R, Vauhkonen H, Eronen KT, Jarvinen A, Seppanen M, Lokki ML. Copy number analysis of complement C4A, C4B and C4A silencing mutation by real-time quantitative polymerase chain reaction. *PLoS ONE* 2012;**7**:e38813.

46. Szilagyi A, Blasko B, Szilassy D, Fust G, Sasvari-Szekely M, Ronai Z. Real-time PCR quantification of human complement C4A and C4B genes. *BMC Genet* 2006;**7**:1.

47. Margery-Muir AA, Wetherall JD, Castley AS, Hew M, Whidborne RS, Mallon DF, et al. Establishment of gene copy number-specific normal ranges for serum C4 and its utility for interpretation in patients with chronically low serum C4 concentrations. *Arthritis Rheum* 2014;**66**:2512–20.

48. Ratnoff WD, Fearon DT, Austen KF. The role of antibody in the activation of the alternative complement pathway. *Springer Semin Immunopathol* 1983;**6**:361–71.

49. Manzi S, Rairie JE, Carpenter AB, Kelly RH, Jagarlapudi SP, Sereika SM, et al. Sensitivity and specificity of plasma and urine complement split products as indicators of lupus disease activity. *Arthritis Rheum* 1996;**39**:1178–88.

50. Manzi S, Navratil JS, Ruffing MJ, Liu CC, Danchenko N, Nilson SE, et al. Measurement of erythrocyte C4d and complement receptor 1 in systemic lupus erythematosus. *Arthritis Rheum* 2004;**50**:3596–604.

51. Buyon JP, Tamerius J, Belmont HM, Abramson SB. Assessment of disease activity and impending flare in patients with systemic lupus erythematosus. Comparison of the use of complement split products and conventional measurements of complement. *Arthritis Rheum* 1992;**35**:1028–37.

52. Liu CC, Manzi S, Kao AH, Navratil JS, Ruffing MJ, Ahearn JM. Reticulocytes bearing C4d as biomarkers of disease activity for systemic lupus erythematosus. *Arthritis Rheum* 2005;**52**:3087–99.

53. Navratil JS, Manzi S, Kao AH, Krishnaswami S, Liu CC, Ruffing MJ, et al. Platelet C4d is highly specific for systemic lupus erythematosus. *Arthritis Rheum* 2006;**54**:670–4.

54. Putterman C, Furie R, Ramsey-Goldman R, Askanase A, Buyon J, Kalunian K, et al. Cell-bound complement activation products in systemic lupus erythematosus: comparison with anti-double-stranded DNA and standard complement measurements. *Lupus Sci Med* 2014;**1**:e000056.

55. Noris M, Remuzzi G. Atypical hemolytic-uremic syndrome. *N Engl J Med* 2009;**361**:1676–87.

56. Nester CM, Barbour T, de Cordoba SR, Dragon-Durey MA, Fremeaux-Bacchi V, Goodship TH, et al. Atypical aHUS: state of the art. *Mol Immunol* 2015;**67**:31–42.

57. Popat RJ, Robson MG. Complement and glomerular diseases. *Nephron Clin Pract* 2014;**128**:238–42.

58. Mathern DR, Heeger PS. Molecules great and small: the complement system. *Clin J Am Soc Nephrol* 2015.

59. Orbai AM, Truedsson L, Sturfelt G, Nived O, Fang H, Alarcon GS, et al. Anti-C1q antibodies in systemic lupus erythematosus. *Lupus* 2015;**24**:42–9.

60. Sethi S, Fervenza FC. Membranoproliferative glomerulonephritis–a new look at an old entity. *N Engl J Med* 2012;**366**:1119–31.

61. Tortajada A, Yebenes H, Abarrategui-Garrido C, Anter J, Garcia-Fernandez JM, Martinez-Barricarte R, et al. C3 glomerulopathy-associated CFHR1 mutation alters FHR oligomerization and complement regulation. *J Clin Invest* 2013;**123**:2434–46.

62. Holers VM. Human C3 glomerulopathy provides unique insights into complement factor H-related protein function. *J Clin Invest* 2013;**123**:2357–60.

63. Duncan AR, Winter G. The binding site for C1q on IgG. *Nature* 1988;**332**:738–40.

64. Gadjeva MG, Rouseva MM, Zlatarova AS, Reid KB, Kishore U, Kojouharova MS. Interaction of human C1q with IgG and IgM: revisited. *Biochemistry* 2008;**47**:13093–102.

65. Zlatarova AS, Rouseva M, Roumenina LT, Gadjeva M, Kolev M, Dobrev I, et al. Existence of different but overlapping IgG- and IgM-binding sites on the globular domain of human C1q. *Biochemistry* 2006;**45**:9979–88.

66. Lood C, Gullstrand B, Truedsson L, Olin AI, Alm GV, Ronnblom L, et al. C1q inhibits immune complex-induced interferon-alpha production in plasmacytoid dendritic cells: a novel link between C1q deficiency and systemic lupus erythematosus pathogenesis. *Arthritis Rheum* 2009;**60**:3081–90.

67. Elkon KB, Santer DM. Complement, interferon and lupus. *Curr Opin Immunol* 2012;**24**:665–70.

68. Clarke EV, Weist BM, Walsh CM, Tenner AJ. Complement protein C1q bound to apoptotic cells suppresses human macrophage and dendritic cell-mediated Th17 and Th1 T cell subset proliferation. *J Leukoc Biol* 2015;**97**:147–60.

69. Son M, Santiago-Schwarz F, Al-Abed Y, Diamond B. C1q limits dendritic cell differentiation and activation by engaging LAIR-1. *Proc Natl Acad Sci USA* 2012;**109**:E3160–7.

70. Son M, Diamond B. C1q-mediated repression of human monocytes is regulated by leukocyte-associated Ig-like receptor 1 (LAIR-1). *Mol Med* 2014;**20**:559–68.

71. Lu JH, Teh BK, Wang L, Wang YN, Tan YS, Lai MC, et al. The classical and regulatory functions of C1q in immunity and autoimmunity. *Cell Mol Immunol* 2008;**5**:9–21.

72. Nayak A, Pednekar L, Reid KB, Kishore U. Complement and non-complement activating functions of C1q: a prototypical innate immune molecule. *Innate Immun* 2012;**18**:350–63.

73. Klickstein LB, Barbashov SF, Liu T, Jack RM, Nicholson-Weller A. Complement receptor type 1 (CR1, CD35) is a receptor for C1q. *Immunity* 1997;**7**:345–55.

74. Tas SW, Klickstein LB, Barbashov SF, Nicholson-Weller A. C1q and C4b bind simultaneously to CR1 and additively support erythrocyte adhesion. *J Immunol* 1999;**163**:5056–63.

75. Roumenina LT, Sene D, Radanova M, Blouin J, Halbwachs-Mecarelli L, Dragon-Durey MA, et al. Functional complement C1q abnormality leads to impaired immune complexes and apoptotic cell clearance. *J Immunol* 2011;**187**:4369–73.

76. Namjou B, Keddache M, Fletcher D, Dillon S, Kottyan L, Wiley G, et al. Identification of novel coding mutation in C1qA gene in an African–American pedigree with lupus and C1q deficiency. *Lupus* 2012;**21**:1113–8.

77. Higuchi Y, Shimizu J, Hatanaka M, Kitano E, Kitamura H, Takada H, et al. The identification of a novel splicing mutation in C1qB in a Japanese family with C1q deficiency: a case report. *Pediatr Rheumatol Online J* 2013;**11**:41.

78. Jlajla H, Sellami MK, Sfar I, Laadhar L, Zerzeri Y, Abdelmoula MS, et al. New C1q mutation in a Tunisian family. *Immunobiology* 2014;**219**:241–6.

79. van Schaarenburg RA, Daha NA, Schonkeren JJ, Nivine Levarht EW, van Gijlswijk-Janssen DJ, Kurreeman FA, et al. Identification of a novel non-coding mutation in C1qB in a Dutch child with C1q deficiency associated with recurrent infections. *Immunobiology* 2014.

80. Marquart HV, Schejbel L, Sjoholm A, Martensson U, Nielsen S, Koch A, et al. C1q deficiency in an Inuit family: identification of a new class of C1q disease-causing mutations. *Clin Immunol* 2007;**124**:33–40.

81. McClellan J, King MC. Genetic heterogeneity in human disease. *Cell* 2010;**141**:210–7.

82. Manolio TA, Collins FS, Cox NJ, Goldstein DB, Hindorff LA, Hunter DJ, et al. Finding the missing heritability of complex diseases. *Nature* 2009;**461**:747–53.

83. Petry F, Botto M, Holtappels R, Walport MJ, Loos M. Reconstitution of the complement function in C1q-deficient (C1qa-/-) mice with wild-type bone marrow cells. *J Immunol* 2001;**167**:4033–7.

84. Cortes-Hernandez J, Fossati-Jimack L, Petry F, Loos M, Izui S, Walport MJ, et al. Restoration of C1q levels by bone marrow transplantation attenuates autoimmune disease associated with C1q deficiency in mice. *Eur J Immunol* 2004;**34**:3713–22.

85. Arkwright PD, Riley P, Hughes SM, Alachkar H, Wynn RF. Successful cure of C1q deficiency in human subjects treated with hematopoietic stem cell transplantation. *J Allergy Clin Immunol* 2014;**133**:265–7.

86. Nguyen VC, Tosi M, Gross MS, Cohen-Haguenauer O, Jegou-Foubert C, de Tand MF, et al. Assignment of the complement serine protease genes C1r and C1s to chromosome 12 region 12p13. *Hum Genet* 1988;**78**:363–8.

87. Kusumoto H, Hirosawa S, Salier JP, Hagen FS, Kurachi K. Human genes for complement components C1r and C1s in a close tail-to-tail arrangement. *Proc Natl Acad Sci USA* 1988;**85**:7307–11.

88. Nakagawa M, Yuasa I, Irizawa Y, Umetsu K. The human complement component C1R gene: the exon-intron structure and the molecular basis of allelic diversity. *Ann Hum Genet* 2003;**67**:207–15.

89. Day NK, Geiger H, Stroud R, DeBracco M, Mancaido B, Windhorst D, et al. C1r deficiency: an inborn error associated with cutaneous and renal disease. *J Clin Invest* 1972;**51**:1102–8.

90. Wu YL, Brookshire BP, Verani RR, Arnett FC, Yu CY. Clinical presentations and molecular basis of complement C1r deficiency in a male African–American patient with systemic lupus erythematosus. *Lupus* 2011;**20**:1126–34.

91. Manderson AP, Pickering MC, Botto M, Walport MJ, Parish CR. Continual low-level activation of the classical complement pathway. *J Exp Med* 2001;**194**:747–56.

92. Amano MT, Ferriani VP, Florido MP, Reis ES, Delcolli MI, Azzolini AE, et al. Genetic analysis of complement C1s deficiency associated with systemic lupus erythematosus highlights alternative splicing of normal C1s gene. *Mol Immunol* 2008;**45**:1693–702.

93. Suzuki Y, Ogura Y, Otsubo O, Akagi K, Fujita T. Selective deficiency of C1s associated with a systemic lupus erythematosus-like syndrome. Report of a case. *Arthritis Rheum* 1992;**35**:576–9.

94. Inoue N, Saito T, Masuda R, Suzuki Y, Ohtomi M, Sakiyama H. Selective complement C1s deficiency caused by homozygous four-base deletion in the C1s gene. *Hum Genet* 1998;**103**:415–8.

95. Endo Y, Kanno K, Takahashi M, Yamaguchi K, Kohno Y, Fujita T. Molecular basis of human complement C1s deficiency. *J Immunol* 1999;**162**:2180–3.

96. Abe K, Endo Y, Nakazawa N, Kanno K, Okubo M, Hoshino T, et al. Unique phenotypes of C1s deficiency and abnormality caused by two compound heterozygosities in a Japanese family. *J Immunol* 2009;**182**:1681–8.

97. Dragon-Durey MA, Quartier P, Fremeaux-Bacchi V, Blouin J, de Barace C, Prieur AM, et al. Molecular basis of a selective C1s deficiency associated with early onset multiple autoimmune diseases. *J Immunol* 2001;**166**:7612–6.

98. Bienaime F, Quartier P, Dragon-Durey MA, Fremeaux-Bacchi V, Bader-Meunier B, Patey N, et al. Lupus nephritis associated with complete C1S deficiency efficiently treated with rituximab: a case report. *Arthritis Care Res* 2010.

99. Carroll MC, Campbell RD, Bentley DR, Porter RR. A molecular map of the human major histocompatibility complex class III region linking complement genes C4, C2 and factor B. *Nature* 1984;**307**:237–41.

100. Yu CY. The complete exon-intron structure of a human complement component C4A gene: DNA sequences, polymorphism, and linkage to the 21-hydroxylase gene. *J Immunol* 1991;**146**:1057–66.

101. Belt KT, Caroll MC, Porter RR. The structural basis of the multiple forms of human complement component C4. *Cell* 1984;**36**:907–14.

102. Belt KT, Yu CY, Carroll MC, Porter RR. Polymorphism of human complement component C4. *Immunogenetics* 1985;**21**:173–80.

103. Hortin GL, Farries TC, Graham JP, Atkinson JP. Sulfation of tyrosinbe residues increase activity of the fourth component of complement. *Proc Natl Acad Sci USA* 1989;**86**:1338–42.

104. Law SK, Gagnon J. The primary structure of the fourth component of human complement (C4)-C-terminal peptides. *Biosci Rep* 1985;**5**:913–21.

105. Yu CY, Chung EK, Yang Y, Blanchong CA, Jacobsen N, Saxena K, et al. Dancing with complement C4 and the RP-C4-CYP21-TNX (RCCX) modules of the major histocompatibility complex. *Progr Nucl Acid Res Mol Biol* 2003;**75**:217–92.

106. Halim A, Ruetschi U, Larson G, Nilsson J. LC-MS/MS characterization of O-glycosylation sites and glycan structures of human cerebrospinal fluid glycoproteins. *J Proteome Res* 2013;**12**:573–84.

107. Mortensen S, Kidmose RT, Petersen SV, Szilagyi A, Prohaszka Z, Andersen GR. Structural basis for the function of complement component C4 within the classical and lectin pathways of complement. *J Immunol* 2015;**194**:5488–96.

108. Chan AC, Karp DR, Shreffler DC, Atkinson JP. The 20 faces of the fourth component of complement. *Immunol Today* 1984;**5**:200–3.

109. Law SK, Lichtenberg NA, Levine RP. Covalent binding and hemolytic activity of complement proteins. *Proc Natl Acad Sci USA* 1980;**77**:7194–8.

110. Law SK, Dodds AW. C3, C4 and C5: the thioester site. *Biochem Soc Trans* 1990;**18**:1155–9.

111. Law SK, Dodds AW, Porter RR. A comparison of the properties of two classes, C4A and C4B, of the human complement component C4. *EMBO J* 1984;**3**:1819–23.

112. Isenman DE, Young JR. The molecular basis for the difference in immune hemolysis activity of the Chido and Rodgers isotypes of human complement component C4. *J Immunol* 1984;**132**:3019–27.

113. Yu CY, Belt KT, Giles CM, Campbell RD, Porter RR. Structural basis of the polymorphism of human complement component C4A and C4B: gene size, reactivity and antigenicity. *EMBO J* 1986;**5**:2873–81.

114. Dodds AW, Ren X-D, Willis AC, Law SKA. The reaction mechanism of the internal thioester in the human complement component C4. *Nature* 1996;**379**:177–9.

115. Ghiran IC, Zeidel ML, Shevkoplyas SS, Burns JM, Tsokos GC, Kyttaris VC. Systemic lupus erythematosus serum deposits C4d on red blood cells, decreases red blood cell membrane deformability, and promotes nitric oxide production. *Arthritis Rheum* 2011;**63**:503–12.

116. Kidmose RT, Laursen NS, Dobo J, Kjaer TR, Sirotkina S, Yatime L, et al. Structural basis for activation of the complement system by component C4 cleavage. *Proc Natl Acad Sci USA* 2012;**109**:15425–30.

117. van den Elsen JMH, Martin A, Wong V, Clemenza L, Rose DR, Isenman DE. X-ray crystal structure of the C4d fragment of human complement component C4. *J Mol Biol* 2002;**322**:1103–15.

118. Janssen BJ, Huizinga EG, Raaijmakers HC, Roos A, Daha MR, Nilsson-Ekdahl K, et al. Structures of complement component C3 provide insights into the function and evolution of immunity. *Nature* 2005;**437**:505–11.

119. Janssen BJ, Christodoulidou A, McCarthy A, Lambris JD, Gros P. Structure of C3b reveals conformational changes that underlie complement activity. *Nature* 2006.

120. Forneris F, Ricklin D, Wu J, Tzekou A, Wallace RS, Lambris JD, et al. Structures of C3b in complex with factors B and D give insight into complement convertase formation. *Science* 2010;**330**:1816–20.

121. Wiesmann C, Katschke KJ, Yin J, Helmy KY, Steffek M, Fairbrother WJ, et al. Structure of C3b in complex with CRIg gives insights into regulation of complement activation. *Nature* 2006.

122. Wu J, Wu YQ, Ricklin D, Janssen BJ, Lambris JD, Gros P. Structure of complement fragment C3b-factor H and implications for host protection by complement regulators. *Nat Immunol* 2009;**10**:728–33.

123. Abdul AA, Gunasekaran K, Volanakis JE, Narayana SV, Kotwal GJ, Murthy HM. The structure of complement C3b provides insights into complement activation and regulation. *Nature* 2006;**444**:221–5.

124. Wiesmann C, Katschke KJ, Yin J, Helmy KY, Steffek M, Fairbrother WJ, et al. Structure of C3b in complex with CRIg gives insights into regulation of complement activation. *Nature* 2006;**444**:217–20.

125. Yang Y, Lhotta K, Chung EK, Eder P, Neumair F, Yu CY. Complete complement components C4A and C4B deficiencies in human kidney diseases and systemic lupus erythematosus. *J Immunol* 2004;**173**:2803–14.

126. Wu YL, Hauptmann G, Viguier M, Yu CY. Molecular basis of complete complement C4 deficiency in two North-African families with systemic lupus erythematosus. *Genes Immun* 2009;**10**:433–45.

127. Fredrikson GN, Gullstrand B, Schneider PM, Witzel-Schlomp K, Sjoholm AG, Alper CA, et al. Characterization of non-expressed C4 genes in a case of complete C4 deficiency: identification of a novel point mutation leading to a premature stop codon. *Hum Immunol* 1998;**59**:713–9.

128. Lokki M-L, Circolo A, Ahokas P, Rupert KL, Yu CY, Colten HR. Deficiency of human complement protein C4 due to identical frameshift mutations in the C4A and C4B genes. *J Immunol* 1999;**162**:3687–93.

129. Rupert KL, Moulds JM, Yang Y, Arnett FC, Warren RW, Reveille JD, et al. The molecular basis of complete C4A and C4B deficiencies in a systemic lupus erythematosus (SLE) patient with homozygous C4A and C4B mutant genes. *J Immunol* 2002;**169**:1570–8.

130. Barba G, Rittner C, Schneider PM. Genetic basis of human complement C4A deficiency. Detection of a point mutation leading to non-expression. *J Clin Invest* 1993;**91**:1681–6.

131. Sullivan KE, Kim NA, Goldman D, Petri MA. C4A deficiency due to a 2 bp insertion is increased in patients with systemic lupus erythematosus. *J Rheumatol* 1999;**26**:2144–7.

132. Yang Y, Chung EK, Wu YL, Savelli SL, Nagaraja HN, Zhou B, et al. Gene copy number variation and associated polymorphisms of complement component C4 in human systemic erythematosus (SLE): low copy number is a risk factor for and high copy number is a protective factor against European American SLE disease susceptibility. *Am J Hum Genet* 2007;**80**:1037–54.

133. Dodds AW, Law SK, Porter RR. The origin of the very variable haemolytic activities of the common human complement component C4 allotypes including C4-A6. *EMBO J* 1985;**4**:2239–44.

134. Anderson MJ, Milner CM, Cotton RG, Campbell RD. The coding sequence of the hemolytically inactive C4A6 allotype of human complement component C4 reveals that a single arginine to tryptophan substitution at beta-chain residue 458 is the likely cause of the defect. *J Immunol* 1992;**148**:2795–802.

135. Lv Y, He S, Zhang Z, Li Y, Hu D, Zhu K, et al. Confirmation of C4 gene copy number variation and the association with systemic lupus erythematosus in Chinese Han population. *Rheumatol Int* 2012;**32**:3047–53.

136. Kim JH, Jung SH, Bae JS, Lee HS, Yim SH, Park SY, et al. Deletion variants of RABGAP1L, 10q21.3, and C4 are associated with the risk of systemic lupus erythematosus in Korean women. *Arthritis Rheum* 2013;**65**:1055–63.

137. Boteva L, Morris DL, Cortes-Hernandez J, Martin J, Vyse TJ, Fernando MM. Genetically determined partial complement C4 deficiency states are not independent risk factors for SLE in UK and Spanish populations. *Am J Hum Genet* 2012;**90**:445–56.

138. Uejima H, Lee MP, Cui H, Feinberg AP. Hot-stop PCR: a simple and general assay for linear quantitation of allele ratios. *Nat Genet* 2000;**25**:375–6.

139. Chung EK, Yang Y, Rupert KL, Jones KN, Rennebohm RM, Blanchong CA, et al. Determining the one, two, three or four long and short loci of human complement *C4* in a major histocompatibility complex haplotype encoding for C4A or C4B proteins. *Am J Hum Genet* 2002;**71**:810–22.

140. Saxena K, Kitzmiller KJ, Wu YL, Zhou B, Esack N, Hiremath L, et al. Great genotypic and phenotypic diversities associated with copy-number variations of complement C4 and RP-C4-CYP21-TNX (RCCX) modules: a comparison of Asian–Indian and European American populations. *Mol Immunol* 2009;**46**:1289–303.

141. Elliot JA, Mathieson DR. Complement in disseminated (systemic) lupus erythematosus. *A M A Arch Dermatol Syphilol* 1953;**68**:119–28.

142. Lewis EJ, Carpenter CB, Schur PH. Serum complement component levels in human glomerulonephritis. *Ann Intern Med* 1971;**75**:555–60.

143. Birmingham DJ, Irshaid F, Nagaraja HN, Zou X, Tsao BP, Wu H, et al. The complex nature of serum C3 and C4 as biomarkers of lupus renal flare. *Lupus* 2010;**19**:1272–80.

144. Wu YL, Higgins GC, Rennebohm RM, Chung EK, Yang Y, Zhou B, et al. Three distinct profiles of serum complement C4 proteins in pediatric systemic lupus erythematosus (SLE) patients: tight associations of complement C4 and C3 protein levels in SLE but not in healthy subjects. *Adv Exp Med Biol* 2006;**586**:227–47.

145. Johnson CA, Densen P, Wetsel R, Cole FS, Goeken NE, Colten HR. Molecular heterogeneity of C2 deficiency. *N Engl J Med* 1992;**326**:874.

146. Yu CY, Hauptmann G, Yang Y, Wu YL, Birmingham DJ, Rovin BH, et al. Complement deficiencies in human systemic lupus erythematosus (SLE) and SLE nephritis: epidemiology and pathogenesis. In: Tsokos GC, Gordon C, Smolen JS, editors. *Systemic lupus erythematosus: a companion to rheumatology*. Philadelphia: Elsevier; 2007. p. 183–93.

147. Agnello V. Lupus diseases associated with hereditary and acquired deficiencies of complement. *Springer Semin Immunopathol* 1986;**9**:161–78.

148. Johnson CA, Densen P, Hurford Jr RK, Colten HR, Wetsel RA. Type I human complement C2 deficiency. A 28-base pair gene deletion causes skipping of exon 6 during RNA splicing. *J Biol Chem* 1992;**267**:9347–53.

149. Wang X, Circolo A, Lokki ML, Shackelford PG, Wetsel RA, Colten HR. Molecular heterogeneity in deficiency of complement protein C2 type I. *Immunology* 1998;**93**:184–91.

150. Wetsel RA, Kulics J, Lokki ML, Kiepiela P, Akama H, Johnson CA, et al. Type II human complement C2 deficiency. Allele-specific amino acid substitutions (Ser189 --> Phe; Gly444 --> Arg) cause impaired C2 secretion. *J Biol Chem* 1996;**271**:5824–31.

151. Zhu ZB, Atkinson TP, Volanakis JE. A novel type II complement C2 deficiency allele in an African–American family. *J Immunol* 1998;**161**:578–84.

152. Reis ES, Falcao DA, Isaac L. Clinical aspects and molecular basis of primary deficiencies of complement component C3 and its regulatory proteins factor I and factor H. *Scand J Immunol* 2006;**63**:155–68.

153. Botto M, Fong KY, So AK, Rudge A, Walport MJ. Molecular basis of hereditary C3 deficiency. *J Clin Invest* 1990;**86**:1158–63.

154. Tsukamoto H, Horiuchi T, Kokuba H, Nagae S, Nishizaka H, Sawabe T, et al. Molecular analysis of a novel hereditary C3 deficiency with systemic lupus erythematosus. *Biochem Biophys Res Commun* 2005;**330**:298–304.

155. Singer L, Colten HR, Wetsel RA. Complement C3 deficiency: human, animal, and experimental models. *Pathobiology* 1994;**62**:14–28.

156. Einav S, Pozdnyakova OO, Ma H, Carroll MC. Complement C4 is protective for lupus disease independent of C3. *J Immunol* 2002;**168**:1036–41.

157. Iida K, Mornaghi R, Nussenzweig V. Complement receptor (CR1) deficiency in erythrocytes from patients with systemic lupus erythematosus. *J Exp Med* 1982;**155**:1427–38.

158. Wilson JG, Wong WW, Schur PH, Fearon DT. Mode of inheritance of decreased C3b receptors on erythrocytes of patients with systemic lupus erythematosus. *N Engl J Med* 1982;**307**:981–6.

159. Walport MJ, Ross GD, Mackworth YC, Watson JV, Hogg N, Lachmann PJ. Family studies of erythrocyte complement receptor type 1 levels: reduced levels in patients with SLE are acquired, not inherited. *Clin Exp Immunol* 1985;**59**:547–54.

160. Uko G, Dawkins RL, Kay P, Christiansen FT, Hollingsworth PN. CR1 deficiency in SLE: acquired or genetic? *Clin Exp Immunol* 1985;**62**:329–36.

161. Pascual M, Danielsson C, Steiger G, Schifferli JA. Proteolytic cleavage of CR1 on human erythrocytes in vivo: evidence for enhanced cleavage in AIDS. *Eur J Immunol* 1994;**24**:702–8.

162. Danielsson C, Pascual M, French L, Steiger G, Schifferli JA. Soluble complement receptor type 1 (CD35) is released from leukocytes by surface cleavage. *Eur J Immunol* 1994;**24**:2725–31.

163. Berger M, Wetzler E, August JT, Tartakoff AM. Internalization of type 1 complement receptors and de novo multivesicular body formation during chemoattractant-induced endocytosis in human neutrophils. *J Clin Invest* 1994;**94**:1113–25.

164. Carroll MC. The role of complement and complement receptors in induction and regulation of immunity. *Annu Rev Immunol* 1998;**16**:545–68.

165. Fearon DT, Carroll M. Regulation of B Lymphocyte responses to foreign and self-antigens by the CD19/CD21 complex. *Annu Rev Immunol* 2000;**18**:393–422.

166. Ahearn JM, Hayward SD, Hickey JC, Fearon DT. Epstein-Barr virus (EBV) infection of murine L cells expressing recombinant human EBV/C3d receptor. *Proc Natl Acad Sci USA* 1988;**85**:9307–11.

167. Lowell CA, Klickstein LB, Carter RH, Mitchell JA, Fearon DT, Ahearn JM. Mapping of the Epstein-Barr virus and C3dg binding sites to a common domain on complement receptor type 2. *J Exp Med* 1989;**170**:1931–46.

168. Delcayre AX, Salas F, Mathur S, Kovats K, Lotz M, Lernhardt W. Epstein Barr virus/complement C3d receptor is an interferon alpha receptor. *EMBO J* 1991;**10**:919–26.

169. Asokan R, Banda NK, Szakonyi G, Chen XS, Holers VM. Human complement receptor 2 (CR2/CD21) as a receptor for DNA: implications for its roles in the immune response and the pathogenesis of systemic lupus erythematosus (SLE). *Mol Immunol* 2013;**53**:99–110.

170. Asokan R, Hua J, Young KA, Gould HJ, Hannan JP, Kraus DM, et al. Characterization of human complement receptor type 2 (CR2/CD21) as a receptor for IFN-alpha: a potential role in systemic lupus erythematosus. *J Immunol* 2006;**177**:383–94.

171. Ahearn JM, Fearon DT. Structure and function of the complement receptors, CR1 (CD35) and CR2 (CD21). *Adv Immunol* 1989;**46**:183–219.

172. Croix DA, Ahearn JM, Rosengard AM, Han S, Kelsoe G, Minghe M, et al. Antibody response to a T-dependent antigen requires B cell expression of complement receptors. *J Exp Med* 1996;**183**:1857–64.

173. Victora GD, Nussenzweig MC. Germinal centers. *Annu Rev Immunol* 2012;**30**:429–57.

174. Vinuesa CG, Sanz I, Cook MC. Dysregulation of germinal centres in autoimmune disease. *Nat Rev Immunol* 2009;**9**:845–57.

175. Heesters BA, Chatterjee P, Kim YA, Gonzalez SF, Kuligowski MP, Kirchhausen T, et al. Endocytosis and recycling of immune complexes by follicular dendritic cells enhances B cell antigen binding and activation. *Immunity* 2013;**38**:1164–75.

176. Erdei A, Isaak A, Torok K, Sandor N, Kremlitzka M, Prechl J, et al. Expression and role of CR1 and CR2 on B and T lymphocytes under physiological and autoimmune conditions. *Mol Immunol* 2009;**46**:2767–73.

177. Ahearn JM, Fischer MB, Croix D, Goerg S, Ma M, Xia J, et al. Disruption of the Cr2 locus results in a reduction in B-1a cells and in an impaired B cell response to T-dependent antigen. *Immunity* 1996;**4**:251–62.

178. Prodeus AP, Goerg S, Shen LM, Pozdnyakova OO, Chu L, Alicot EM, et al. A critical role for complement in maintenance of self-tolerance. *Immunity* 1998;**9**:721–31.

179. Donius LR, Handy JM, Weis JJ, Weis JH. Optimal germinal center B cell activation and T-dependent antibody responses require expression of the mouse complement receptor Cr1. *J Immunol* 2013;**191**:434–47.

180. Donius LR, Weis JJ, Weis JH. Murine complement receptor 1 is required for germinal center B cell maintenance but not initiation. *Immunobiology* 2014;**219**:440–9.

181. Chen Y, Perry D, Boackle SA, Sobel ES, Molina H, Croker BP, et al. Several genes contribute to the production of autoreactive B and T cells in the murine lupus susceptibility locus Sle1c. *J Immunol* 2005;**175**:1080–9.

182. Boackle SA, Holers VM, Chen X, Szakonyi G, Karp DR, Wakeland EK, et al. Cr2, a candidate gene in the murine Sle1c lupus susceptibility locus, encodes a dysfunctional protein. *Immunity* 2001;**15**:775–85.

183. Wu H, Boackle SA, Hanvivadhanakul P, Ulgiati D, Grossman JM, Lee Y, et al. Association of a common complement receptor 2 haplotype with increased risk of systemic lupus erythematosus. *Proc Natl Acad Sci USA* 2007;**104**(10):3961–6.

184. Zhao J, Giles BM, Taylor RL, Yette GA, Lough KM, Ng HL, et al. Preferential association of a functional variant in complement receptor 2 with antibodies to double-stranded DNA. *Ann Rheum Dis* 2014.

185. Nath SK, Han S, Kim-Howard X, Kelly JA, Viswanathan P, Gilkeson GS, et al. A nonsynonymous functional variant in integrin-alpha(M) (encoded by ITGAM) is associated with systemic lupus erythematosus. *Nat Genet* 2008;**40**:152–4.

186. Harley JB, arcon-Riquelme ME, Criswell LA, Jacob CO, Kimberly RP, Moser KL, et al. Genome-wide association scan in women with systemic lupus erythematosus identifies susceptibility variants in ITGAM, PXK, KIAA1542 and other loci. *Nat Genet* 2008;**40**:204–10.

187. Hom G, Graham RR, Modrek B, Taylor KE, Ortmann W, Garnier S, et al. Association of systemic lupus erythematosus with C8orf13-BLK and ITGAM-ITGAX. *N Engl J Med* 2008;**358**:900–9.

188. Maiti AK, Kim-Howard X, Motghare P, Pradhan V, Chua KH, Sun C, et al. Combined protein- and nucleic acid-level effects of rs1143679 (R77H), a lupus-predisposing variant within ITGAM. *Hum Mol Genet* 2014;**23**:4161–76.

189. Han S, Kim-Howard X, Deshmukh H, Kamatani Y, Viswanathan P, Guthridge JM, et al. Evaluation of imputation-based association in and around the integrin-alpha-M (ITGAM) gene and replication of robust association between a non-synonymous functional variant within ITGAM and systemic lupus erythematosus (SLE). *Hum Mol Genet* 2009;**18**:1171–80.

190. Rhodes B, Furnrohr BG, Roberts AL, Tzircotis G, Schett G, Spector TD, et al. The rs1143679 (R77H) lupus associated variant of ITGAM (CD11b) impairs complement receptor 3 mediated functions in human monocytes. *Ann Rheum Dis* 2012;**71**:2028–34.

191. MacPherson M, Lek HS, Prescott A, Fagerholm SC. A systemic lupus erythematosus-associated R77H substitution in the CD11b chain of the Mac-1 integrin compromises leukocyte adhesion and phagocytosis. *J Biol Chem* 2011;**286**:17303–10.

192. Zhao J, Wu H, Khosravi M, Cui H, Qian X, Kelly JA, et al. Association of genetic variants in complement factor H and factor H-related genes with systemic lupus erythematosus susceptibility. *PLoS Genet* 2011;**7**:e1002079.

193. Dragon-Durey MA, Blanc C, Marinozzi MC, van Schaarenburg RA, Trouw LA. Autoantibodies against complement components and functional consequences. *Mol Immunol* 2013;**56**:213–21.

194. Walport MJ. Complement and systemic lupus erythematosus. *Arthritis Res* 2002;**4**(Suppl 3):S279–93.

195. Mahler M, van Schaarenburg RA, Trouw LA. Anti-C1q autoantibodies, novel tests, and clinical consequences. *Front Immunol* 2013;**4**:117.

196. Fremeaux-Bacchi V, Weiss L, Demouchy C, Blouin J, Kazatchkine MD. Autoantibodies to the collagen-like region of C1q are strongly associated with classical pathway-mediated hypocomplementemia in systemic lupus erythematosus. *Lupus* 1996;**5**:216–20.

197. Lachmann PJ. Conglutinin and immunoconglutinins. *Adv Immunol* 1967;**6**:479–527.

198. Nilsson B, Ekdahl KN, Sjoholm A, Nilsson UR, Sturfelt G. Detection and characterization of immunoconglutinins in patients with systemic lupus erythematosus (SLE): serial analysis in relation to disease course. *Clin Exp Immunol* 1992;**90**:251–5.

199. Ronnelid J, Gunnarsson I, Nilsson-Ekdahl K, Nilsson B. Correlation between anti-C1q and immune conglutinin levels, but not between levels of antibodies to the structurally related autoantigens C1q and type II collagen in SLE or RA. *J Autoimmun* 1997;**10**:415–23.

200. Ito S, Tamura N, Fujita T. Effect of decay-accelerating factor on the assembly of the classical and alternative pathway C3 convertases in the presence of C4 or C3 nephritic factor. *Immunology* 1989;**68**:449–52.

201. Jozsi M, Reuter S, Nozal P, Lopez-Trascasa M, Sanchez-Corral P, Prohaszka Z, et al. Autoantibodies to complement components in C3 glomerulopathy and atypical hemolytic uremic syndrome. *Immunol Lett* 2014;**160**:163–71.

202. Daha MR, van Es LA. Relative resistance of the F-42-stabilized classical pathway C3 convertase to inactivation by C4-binding protein. *J Immunol* 1980;**125**:2051–4.

203. Miller EC, Chase NM, Densen P, Hintermeyer MK, Casper JT, Atkinson JP. Autoantibody stabilization of the classical pathway C3 convertase leading to C3 deficiency and Neisserial sepsis: C4 nephritic factor revisited. *Clin Immunol* 2012;**145**:241–50.

204. Seelen MA, Trouw LA, van der Hoorn JW, Fallaux-van den Houten FC, Huizinga TW, Daha MR, et al. Autoantibodies against mannose-binding lectin in systemic lupus erythematosus. *Clin Exp Immunol* 2003;**134**:335–43.

205. Mok MY, Jack DL, Lau CS, Fong DY, Turner MW, Isenberg DA, et al. Antibodies to mannose binding lectin in patients with systemic lupus erythematosus. *Lupus* 2004;**13**:522–8.

206. Takahashi R, Tsutsumi A, Ohtani K, Goto D, Matsumoto I, Ito S, et al. Anti-mannose binding lectin antibodies in sera of Japanese patients with systemic lupus erythematosus. *Clin Exp Immunol* 2004;**136**:585–90.

207. Pradhan V, Mahant G, Rajadhyaksha A, Surve P, Rajendran V, Patwardhan M, et al. A study on anti-mannose binding lectin (anti-MBL) antibodies and serum MBL levels in Indian systemic lupus erythematosus patients. *Rheumatol Int* 2013;**33**:1533–9.

208. He S, Lin YL. In vitro stimulation of C1s proteolytic activities by C1s-presenting autoantibodies from patients with systemic lupus erythematosus. *J Immunol* 1998;**160**:4641–7.

209. Wilson JG, Jack RM, Wong WW, Schur PH, Fearon DT. Autoantibody to the C3b/C4b receptor and absence of this receptor from erythrocytes of a patient with systemic lupus erythematosus. *J Clin Invest* 1985;**76**:182–90.

210. Sadallah S, Hess C, Trendelenburg M, Vedeler C, Lopez-Trascasa M, Schifferli JA. Autoantibodies against complement receptor 1 (CD35) in SLE, liver cirrhosis and HIV-infected patients. *Clin Exp Immunol* 2003;**131**:174–81.

211. Hartman KR, Wright DG. Identification of autoantibodies specific for the neutrophil adhesion glycoproteins CD11b/CD18 in patients with autoimmune neutropenia. *Blood* 1991;**78**:1096–104.

212. Meszaros T, Fust G, Farkas H, Jakab L, Temesszentandrasi G, Nagy G, et al. C1-inhibitor autoantibodies in SLE. *Lupus* 2010;**19**:634–8.

213. Dragon-Durey MA, Loirat C, Cloarec S, Macher MA, Blouin J, Nivet H, et al. Anti-Factor H autoantibodies associated with atypical hemolytic uremic syndrome. *J Am Soc Nephrol* 2005;**16**:555–63.

214. Blanc C, Togarsimalemath SK, Chauvet S, Le QM, Moulin B, Buchler M, et al. Anti-factor H autoantibodies in c3 glomerulopathies and in atypical hemolytic uremic syndrome: one target, two diseases. *J Immunol* 2015;**194**:5129–38.

215. Shamonki JM, Salmon JE, Hyjek E, Baergen RN. Excessive complement activation is associated with placental injury in patients with antiphospholipid antibodies. *Am J Obstet Gynecol* 2007;**196**:167–75.

216. Breen KA, Seed P, Parmar K, Moore GW, Stuart-Smith SE, Hunt BJ. Complement activation in patients with isolated antiphospholipid antibodies or primary antiphospholipid syndrome. *Thromb Haemost* 2012;**107**:423–9.

217. Oku K, Atsumi T, Bohgaki M, Amengual O, Kataoka H, Horita T, et al. Complement activation in patients with primary antiphospholipid syndrome. *Ann Rheum Dis* 2009;**68**:1030–5.

218. Avalos I, Tsokos GC. The role of complement in the antiphospholipid syndrome-associated pathology. *Clin Rev Allergy Immunol* 2009;**36**:141–4.

219. De CS, Botta A, Santucci S, Salvi S, Moresi S, di PE, et al. Complementemia and obstetric outcome in pregnancy with antiphospholipid syndrome. *Lupus* 2012;**21**:776–8.

220. Hamer R, Molostvov G, Lowe D, Satchell S, Mathieson P, Ilyas R, et al. Human leukocyte antigen-specific antibodies and gamma-interferon stimulate human microvascular and glomerular endothelial cells to produce complement factor C4. *Transplantation* 2012;**93**:867–73.

221. Sheerin NS, Risley P, Abe K, Tang Z, Wong W, Lin T, et al. Synthesis of complement protein C3 in the kidney is an important mediator of local tissue injury. *FASEB J* 2008;**22**:1065–72.

222. Pratt JR, Basheer SA, Sacks SH. Local synthesis of complement component C3 regulates acute renal transplant rejection. *Nat Med* 2002;**8**:582–7.

223. Huber-Lang M, Sarma JV, Zetoune FS, Rittirsch D, Neff TA, McGuire SR, et al. Generation of C5a in the absence of C3: a new complement activation pathway. *Nat Med* 2006;**12**:682–7.

224. Liszewski MK, Kolev M, Le FG, Leung M, Bertram PG, Fara AF, et al. Intracellular complement activation sustains T cell homeostasis and mediates effector differentiation. *Immunity* 2013;**39**:1143–57.

225. Lajoie S, Wills-Karp M. New twist on an ancient innate immune pathway. *Immunity* 2013;**39**:1000–2.

226. Tam JC, Bidgood SR, McEwan WA, James LC. Intracellular sensing of complement C3 activates cell autonomous immunity. *Science* 2014;**345**:1256070.

227. Nonaka M. Evolution of the complement system. *Subcell Biochem* 2014;**80**:31–43.

228. Al-Mayouf SM, Sunker A, Abdwani R, Abrawi SA, Almurshedi F, Alhashmi N, et al. Loss-of-function variant in DNASE1L3 causes a familial form of systemic lupus erythematosus. *Nat Genet* 2011;**43**:1186–8.

229. Rice GI, Rodero MP, Crow YJ. Human disease phenotypes associated with mutations in TREX1. *J Clin Immunol* 2015;**35**:235–43.

230. Tsukumo S, Yasutomo K. DNaseI in pathogenesis of systemic lupus erythematosus. *Clin Immunol* 2004;**113**:14–8.

231. Kavanagh D, Spitzer D, Kothari PH, Shaikh A, Liszewski MK, Richards A, et al. New roles for the major human 3′– 5′ exonuclease TREX1 in human disease. *Cell Cycle* 2008;**7**.

232. Yasutomo K, Horiuchi T, Kagami S, Tsukamoto H, Hashimura C, Urushihara M, et al. Mutation of DNASE1 in people with systemic lupus erythematosus. *Nat Genet* 2001;**28**:313–4.

233. Grieves JL, Fye JM, Harvey S, Grayson JM, Hollis T, Perrino FW. Exonuclease TREX1 degrades double-stranded DNA to prevent spontaneous lupus-like inflammatory disease. *Proc Natl Acad Sci USA* 2015;**112**:5117–22.

234. Yang YG, Lindahl T, Barnes DE. Trex1 exonuclease degrades ssDNA to prevent chronic checkpoint activation and autoimmune disease. *Cell* 2007;**131**:873–86.

235. Walport MJ. Lupus, DNase and defective disposal of cellular debris. *Nat Genet* 2000;**25**:135–6.

236. Heinen S, Pluthero FG, van Eimeren VF, Quaggin SE, Licht C. Monitoring and modeling treatment of atypical hemolytic uremic syndrome. *Mol Immunol* 2013;**54**:84–8.

237. Botto M, Dell'Agnola C, Bygrave AE, Thompson EM, Cook HT, Petry F, et al. Homozygous C1q deficiency causes glomerulonephritis associated with multiple apoptotic bodies. *Nat Genet* 1998;**19**:56–9.

238. Paul E, Pozdnyakova OO, Mitchell E, Carroll MC. Anti-DNA autoreactivity in c4-deficient mice. *Eur J Immunol* 2002;**32**:2672–9.

239. Wang Y, Hu Q, Madri JA, Rollins SA, Chodera A, Matis LA. Amelioration of lupus-like autoimmune disease in NZB/WF1 mice after treatment with a blocking monoclonal antibody specific for complement component C5. *Proc Natl Acad Sci USA* 1996;**93**:8563–8.

240. Romay-Penabad Z, Carrera Marin AL, Willis R, Weston-Davies W, Machin S, Cohen H, et al. Complement C5-inhibitor rEV576 (coversin) ameliorates in-vivo effects of antiphospholipid antibodies. *Lupus* 2014;**23**:1324–6.

241. Carrera-Marin A, Romay-Penabad Z, Papalardo E, Reyes-Maldonado E, Garcia-Latorre E, Vargas G, et al. C6 knock-out mice are protected from thrombophilia mediated by antiphospholipid antibodies. *Lupus* 2012;**21**:1497–505.

242. Liszewski MK, Atkinson JP. In: Stiehm ER, Schur PH, Feldweg AM, editors. *Complement pathways*. Wolters Kluwer; 2015. www.uptodate.com/contents/complement-pathways.

243. Arlaud GJ, Gaboriaud C, Thielens NM, Rossi V, Bersch B, Hernandez JF, et al. Structural biology of C1: dissection of a complex molecular machinery. *Immunol Rev* 2001;**180**:136–45.

244. Bally I, Rossi V, Lunardi T, Thielens NM, Gaboriaud C, Arlaud GJ. Identification of the C1q-binding sites of human C1r and C1s: a refined three-dimensional model of the C1 complex of complement. *J Biol Chem* 2009;**284**:19340–8.

245. Liszewski MK, Atkinson JP, Bigazzi P. The role of complement in autoimmunity. In: Reichlin MR, editor. *Systemic autoimmunity*. New York: Marcel Dekker, Inc.; 1991. p. 13–37.

246. Hebert LA, Cosio G. The erythrocyte-immune complex-glomerulonephritis connection in man. *Kidney Int* 1987;**31**:877–85.

Chapter 13

T Cells

Noé Rodríguez-Rodríguez[1,2], Florencia Rosetti[3], José C. Crispín[3]

[1]Department of Medicine, Division of Rheumatology, Beth Israel Deaconess Medical Center, Harvard Medical School, Boston, MA, USA; [2]Department of Immunology, Universidad Complutense de Madrid, Madrid, Spain; [3]Department of Immunology and Rheumatology, Instituto Nacional de Ciencias Médicas y Nutrición Salvador Zubirán, Mexico City, Mexico

Patients with systemic lupus erythematosus (SLE) develop a chronic autoimmune response against ubiquitous, mostly intranuclear, self-antigens. This response, manifested by the presence of autoantibodies, represents the source of immune complexes and activated T cells that eventually enter target organs causing inflammation and damage.[1] T cells are key players in this process. They promote the autoimmune response by providing help to B cells and activating antigen-presenting cells through cytokine release and direct cellular contact.[2] Additionally, they infiltrate target organs where they cause inflammation. The aim of this chapter is to discuss the mechanisms through which T cells contribute to SLE and to describe how signaling abnormalities confer T cells from patients with SLE a distorted gene expression pattern that promotes their pathogenic behavior.

MECHANISMS THROUGH WHICH T CELLS PROMOTE SLE

B Cell Help

T cells develop in the thymus, where they undergo a strict selection process, central tolerance. Only cells able to interact with molecules from the major histocompatibility complex (MHC), lacking high affinity for self-antigens, are allowed to exit the thymus. This ensures that self-reactive T cells are very scarce in the repertoire. This process is not affected in lupus; accordingly, the frequency of self-reactive T cells in peripheral blood is not higher in humans and mice with lupus than in their healthy counterparts.[3]

Self-reactive B cells are eliminated from the repertoire through deletion, anergy induction, or receptor editing, at two checkpoints during a process that is less stringent than T-cell negative selection.[4] The first checkpoint occurs in the bone marrow and the second one in the periphery, before the cell becomes an immunocompetent mature naïve B cell. It has been estimated that in healthy humans this decreases the frequency of self-reactive B cells from 50–75% to 5–20%. In lupus patients, the second checkpoint is abnormally porous, and therefore the frequency of self-reactive mature B cells is significantly higher than in controls.[4] The fact that in healthy individuals the loss of tolerance toward self-antigens is rather rare, even in the presence of a relatively high abundance of self-reactive B cells (~5–20%), indicates that CD4+ T cells play an essential role in safeguarding self-tolerance and suggests that defects in T-cell regulation may allow the autoimmune response to occur in patients with SLE. The characteristics of the autoantibodies found in patients with SLE further support the notion that CD4 help is involved in their generation[2]: antibodies are mostly of high affinity, class switched, carrying somatic mutations in the V_H regions.[5]

Only a fraction of autoreactive CD4 T cells cloned from mice with lupus has the ability to promote the production of pathogenic anti-DNA antibodies and accelerate nephritis when transferred into lupus-prone mice. These CD4 T cells respond to nucleosomal antigens, in particular to peptides derived from histones.[6] Thus, self-reactive B cells able to recognize DNA may endocytose complexes of nucleic acid and associated proteins and receive help from CD4 T cells that recognize peptides derived from the protein part of the complex (e.g., histone) (Figure 1).

Follicular helper T cells (T_{FH}; CD4+ CXCR5hi PD-1hi) represent the CD4+ helper subset specialized in providing help to B cells within germinal centers (GC).[7] Naïve CD4+ T cells differentiate to T_{FH} when their priming occurs in the presence of IL-6, IL-21, and co-stimulation through inducible T cell costimulator (ICOS). This process is regulated by the balance of two transcription factors: Bcl-6 (B-cell lymphoma 6) promotes their generation, while Blimp-1 (B lymphocyte-induced maturation protein 1) inhibits it. CXCR5 surface expression allows them to migrate into the B-cell follicles in response to CXCL13, where they promote B-cell growth, differentiation, class switching, and somatic hypermutation through IL-4, IL-10, IL-21, and CD40L.[7]

Experiments in animal models have demonstrated that the expansion of T_{FH} is associated with the development of lupus-like autoimmunity, suggesting that the dysregulation

Systemic Lupus Erythematosus. http://dx.doi.org/10.1016/B978-0-12-801917-7.00013-9

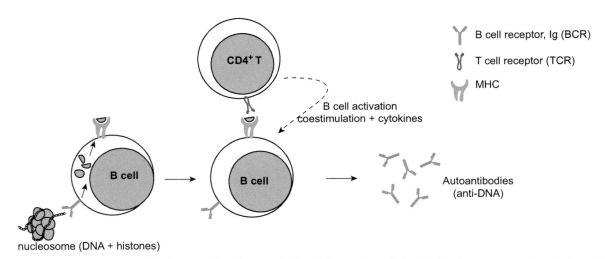

FIGURE 1   CD4 T cells provide help for the generation of autoantibodies. Self-reactive B cells bearing B-cell receptors are able to bind nucleic acids (e.g., DNA), endocytose complexes of nucleic acids and associated proteins, and present the peptides derived from the proteins to CD4 T cells.

of the germinal center can lead to tolerance failure.[8,9] In agreement with these results, deficiency of ICOS, required for the development of T_{FH}, has a protective role in MRL/*lpr* lupus-prone mice.[10] Moreover, it has been reported that a CD4[+] cell subset that resembles T_{FH} is expanded in the peripheral blood of patients with SLE, in particular during active disease,[11] suggesting an association between T_{FH} numbers and lupus activity. Intriguingly, T_{FH} cells have also been found in kidneys of patients with SLE in close association to B cells, suggesting that their pathogenic capacity extends to nonlymphoid organs.[12] Hence, T_{FH} cells are increasingly recognized as key contributors to SLE by promoting the generation of autoantibodies and assisting in the formation and/or maintenance of ectopic follicles.[13]

PRO-INFLAMMATORY ACTIVITIES

T cells from patients with SLE exhibit a number of phenotypic and functional defects that include the production of large amounts of pro-inflammatory cytokines and the expression of high levels of adhesion molecules. They infiltrate target organs, where they release mediators that promote local inflammation. Accordingly, the presence of tubulointerstitial mononuclear infiltrates in kidneys affected by lupus nephritis is a marker of bad prognosis[14] and mice lacking CXCR3, a chemokine receptor that mediates T cell migration to the kidney, develop milder lupus-like nephritis.[15]

CD4 T cells contribute to inflammation in patients with SLE by producing cytokines such as IL-17 and IFN-γ. T_H17 cells are a cell subset that arises when CD4 T cells are activated in the presence of TGF-β and certain pro-inflammatory cytokines including IL-1β, IL-6, and IL-21. T_H17 cells produce IL-17A, IL-17F, and IL-22, which promote inflammation by acting on epithelial, endothelial, and hematopoietic cells. In addition, IL-17 may protect autoreactive T cells from

apoptosis, favoring the accumulation of pathogenic T cells.[16] Patients with SLE have abnormally high levels of IL-17 in the serum and increased numbers of IL-17-producing T cells.[17,18] Furthermore, heightened generation of IL-17 in patients with SLE correlates with disease activity,[19] and IL-17-producing T cells have been found within kidney cell infiltrates of patients with lupus nephritis.[17]

IL-17 production is also increased in murine models of lupus.[20] Indeed, disease amelioration in several animal models of lupus occurred side by side with a reduction in IL-17 production.[20,21] However, the precise role of IL-17 and the extent to which it drives disease is still not clear. A report showed that, in contrast to the well-documented effects of IFN-γ blockade in murine lupus,[22] neutralization or complete absence of IL-17A had no effects on nephritis in MRL/*lpr* and NZB/WF1 mice.[23] On the other hand, IL-17 was necessary for pristane-induce lupus[24] and for glomerulonephritis driven by immune complex deposition.[25] Also, as in patients with SLE, IL17[+] T cells are abundant within kidney infiltrates of mice with lupus-like nephritis.[20]

Although it is not completely defined why IL-17 is increased in SLE, several factors common to lupus may contribute to it. From abnormalities in T-cell receptor (TCR) signaling and the metabolic profile of T cells, to imbalance in the cytokine environment. Indeed, abundance of the T_H17-promoting cytokines IL-6, IL-21, and IL-23,[26] along with reduced levels of IL-2,[27] which promotes regulatory T cell differentiation and inhibits T_H17 cell generation, could skew the CD4 T-cell priming. Thus, underlying inflammation, as well as lupus-specific factors (such as low IL-2 production), probably skew the effector differentiation of T cells toward pro-inflammatory subsets that release cytokines that amplify the autoimmune response (Figure 2).

IFN-γ is a pro-inflammatory cytokine produced by T_H1 cells, CD8 T cells, and some innate lymphoid cells.

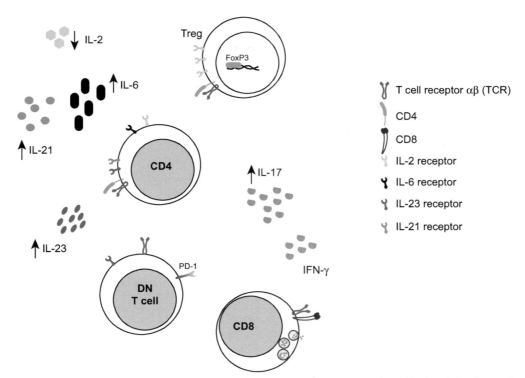

FIGURE 2 The cytokine milieu affects T-cell differentiation and function in SLE. Low production of IL-2 and abundance of pro-inflammatory cytokines probably contribute to the decreased numbers and function of regulatory T cells (Treg) while promoting the differentiation of CD4 and CD8 effector subsets that amplify inflammation.

Although some reports argue that IFN-γ production is decreased in patients with SLE,[28] this has not been uniformly found.[29] Importantly, IFN-γ-positive cells and IFN-γ RNA transcripts have been found in glomeruli from kidneys affected by lupus nephritis.[30] In murine models of lupus (e.g., NZBWF1 and MRL/lpr), IFN-γ plays a demonstrated pathogenic role.[22,31]

Chemokines and adhesion molecules lead T cells into peripheral tissues. The T-cell activation marker CD44 is an adhesion molecule that binds to hyaluronic acid and other components of the extracellular matrix. SLE T cells express increased levels of CD44, which displays heightened binding affinity, promoting migration into inflamed organs.[32] Migration is fostered as well by upregulation of CXCR4 on T cells and its ligand CXCL12 in target organs.[33] The CD44 gene can yield variant isoforms by alternative splicing. The expression of two variants, CD44v3 and v6, is increased on T cells from lupus patients and correlates with disease activity, renal disease, and anti-double-stranded DNA antibody production.[34]

The cytotoxic capacity of CD8 T cells has been reported to be hampered in SLE.[35] However, the fact that activated memory-like and self-reactive CD8 T cells are expanded in SLE patients[36,37] and that CD8 T cells produce increased amounts of perforin and granzyme B[38] argues against the idea that these cells are hyporesponsive. They may promote

disease activity by production of IFN-γ but also by directly instigating tissue damage, since they are found in cellular infiltrates in perivascular and interstitial areas in kidneys from active disease patients[39] (Figure 3).

Although not frequent in healthy humans and mice, TCR-αβ T cells lacking CD4 and CD8 (hence called double negative, DN) comprise a significant proportion of T cells in patients with SLE[17] and other autoimmune diseases.[40] They may behave as helper T cells by promoting B-cell autoantibody production,[41] they secrete pro-inflammatory cytokines, and are found among infiltrating cells in kidneys from SLE patients.[17] They are an important source of IL-17 in SLE patients.

A fraction of CD8 T cells downregulate the expression of CD8 and become DN in response to TCR-mediated activation.[42] A report has suggested that in wild-type mice, the CD8 T cells that undergo this conversion represent self-reactive T cells that lose CD8 and upregulate a set of molecules, including PD-1, that curb their activation.[43] Why DN T cells expand, infiltrate tissues, and produce cytokines in patients and mice with SLE is intriguing in view of these findings. Because a genetic variant in the gene that encodes PD-1 (*PDCD1*) has been linked to human lupus,[44] it is tempting to speculate that the consequent impaired PD-1 upregulation and function[45] may allow DN T cells to adopt a pathogenic role in SLE.

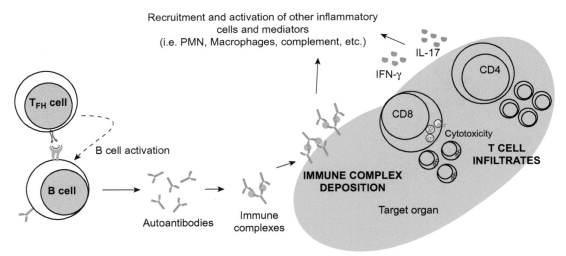

FIGURE 3 **T cells promote the autoimmune response and instigate direct organ damage.** CD4 T cells promote the production of autoantibodies that form immune complexes and deposits causing inflammation. They also infiltrate target organs, where they release cytokines that amplify and perpetuate the response.

Defective Regulation

Regulatory T cells (Treg) are T cells whose main function is the negative modulation of the immune response. Some Treg are selected during T-cell ontogeny and acquire constitutive suppressive properties (e.g., CD4$^+$ FoxP3$^+$ cells), whereas others represent conventional T cells that have undergone a functional differentiation process to gain immunosuppressive capacity, mainly by means of cytokine secretion. A wealth of evidence indicates that autoimmune diseases, including SLE, are linked to quantitative and/or qualitative deficiencies in Treg, but whether these defects represent a causal defect is still unclear.[46]

CD4$^+$ FoxP3$^+$ Treg are selected in the thymus and exert suppressive properties in a constitutive manner. They have been reported to be decreased and functionally impaired in patients with SLE, suggesting that failed immune regulation might be pathologically relevant in lupus.[47] Support for this hypothesis has been found in NZB/WF1 mice, a lupus-prone strain, where restoration of depressed Treg numbers diminished autoantibody production and ameliorated disease.[48] Nonetheless, whether low Treg numbers and defective suppressive properties actually contribute to SLE and through which mechanisms remain open questions.

Treg dysfunction might promote lupus pathology by failing to curb inflammation that causes direct organ damage and also by allowing unchecked germinal center reactions that fuel the autoimmune response by producing autoantibodies. The fact that absolute deficiency of Treg causes a phenotype very different from SLE (IPEX, immunodysregulation polyendocrinopathy enteropathy X-linked syndrome), indicates that Treg dysfunction is not a main pathogenic element in SLE but rather represents a factor that may contribute to the amplification or perpetuation of specific pathogenic processes.

Animal models have shown that failure to regulate the GC reaction can cause lupus-like tolerance failure.[9] At least two types of Treg are thought to regulate this process. Follicular regulatory T cells (T$_{FR}$), a specialized subset of CD4$^+$ FoxP3$^+$ Treg that expresses high levels of CXCR5 and PD-1,[49] and Qa-1-restricted CD8$^+$ Treg.[9] Mice that carry a mutation that inhibits the binding of Qa-1 to the T cell receptor (TCR)/ CD8 complex develop lupus-like systemic autoimmune disease driven by enhanced GC formation and antibody production.[9] Interestingly, lupus development in B6.*Yaa* mice is associated with decreased CD8 Treg suppressive capacity. Whether defects in the number or function of T$_{FR}$ or CD8$^+$ Treg cells are associated with human lupus is still unknown.

SIGNALING AND GENE EXPRESSION IN SLE T CELLS

The response to activation through the TCR is abnormal in T cells from patients with SLE. This is caused by changes in the expression of key molecules involved in signaling downstream of the TCR and is manifested by altered gene expression and cytokine production upon T-cell stimulation.

Calcium influx induced by TCR engagement is abnormally augmented in T cells from patients with SLE. This phenomenon occurs because in SLE T cells, the CD3ζ chain is deficiently expressed and TCR signaling occurs through the common γ chain of the immunoglobulin receptors (FcRγ). FcRγ binds to spleen tyrosine kinase (Syk) instead of to the canonical molecule ZAP-70 (ζ-associated protein). The result of this "rewiring" is disproportionately high signal transduction.[50] These molecular changes have not been linked to SLE-associated genetic variants and are therefore considered a consequence of acquired factors, such as chronic T cell activation. Accordingly, lipid rafts

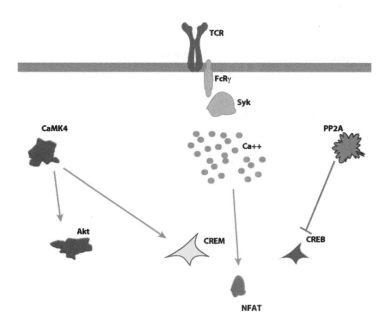

Pro-inflammatory behavior

FIGURE 4   **Signaling and gene expression defects give SLE T cells pathogenic capacities.** Distorted TCR signaling causes abnormally high calcium influx upon TCR engagement. This phenomenon, along with increased activity of CaMK4 and PP2A, alter the activity of key transcription factors and, therefore, skew gene expression toward the transcription of pro-inflammatory products.

are found preaggregated in SLE T cells. Normally, in quiescent T cells, lipid rafts are distributed throughout the cell surface and coalesce only after activation, facilitating signal transduction. In T cells from patients and mice with lupus, lipid rafts are clustered in freshly isolated T cells, indicating ongoing activation.[32]

The distorted signal transduction observed upon TCR engagement in SLE T cells leads to altered expression and activation of several transcription factors and, consequently, to an abnormal gene expression profile. Nuclear factor of activated T cells (NFAT) is a transcription factor activated by calcium influx through calcineurin. SLE T cells have increased NFAT activity as consequence of their altered calcium response.[51] Thus, the expression of certain genes regulated by NFAT is altered. For example, expression of CD40L, an important costimulatory molecule used by T cells to stimulate antibody production and dendritic cell activation, is increased.[51]

Expression and activation of transcription factors that bind to cyclic AMP response elements (CRE), the CRE-binding protein (CREB) and CRE-modulator (CREM) are also abnormal in SLE T cells.[52] The altered CREB–CREM ratio hinders the transcription of several genes, including *IL2*, *CD247* (CD3ζ), *FOS*, and *CD86*.

Calcium/calmodulin-dependent kinase IV (CaMK4) is a serine/threonine kinase that is abnormally active in SLE T cells due, at least in part, to chronic T-cell activation.[53]

Increased CaMK4 activity gives SLE T cells enhanced pro-inflammatory capacity because it phosphorylates (and thus activates CREM) and promotes the action of Akt.[21,53] Levels and activity of protein phosphatase 2A (PP2A), a serine/threonine phosphatase, are also abnormal in SLE T cells.[54] PP2A dephosphorylates CREB, contributing to the altered CREB–CREM ratio. Importantly, transgenic overexpression of the catalytic subunit of PP2A (PP2Ac) causes, in otherwise healthy mice, increased susceptibility to immune-mediated glomerulonephritis.[25] This effect is caused by abnormal levels of acetylation of histone H3, which allows the T cell to acquire a pro-inflammatory gene expression profile that includes unchecked transcription of IL-17[55] (Figure 4).

Several other epigenetic changes have been associated with altered gene expression in T cells from SLE patients. The high frequency of these, compared to the relatively few T cell-expressed genes linked to SLE in genome-wide association studies (GWAS),[56] suggest that most genetic abnormalities in SLE T cells are acquired as a consequence of the interplay between the immune system and the environment. DNA methylation acts as a suppressive epigenetic mark and DNA hypomethylation has been linked to overexpression of a large number of genes in SLE T cells.[57] In fact, DNA hypomethylation has been proposed as the triggering mechanism in drug-induced lupus because some of the drugs that cause it can inhibit DNA methylation (e.g., procainamide and hydralazine).[58]

Apoptosis Defects

Apoptosis is the main process that regulates the death of activated T cells at the end of immune responses. The importance of this clonal contraction is exemplified by the lymphoproliferative and autoimmune disorders that are caused by defects in apoptosis. In patients with SLE, T-cell apoptosis is faulty. A number of cellular changes, including abnormal elevation of the mitochondrial transmembrane potential ($\Delta\psi_m$), increased levels of reactive oxygen intermediates, and decreased amounts of ATP,[59] facilitate spontaneous apoptosis and decrease activation-induced apoptosis. Moreover, they sensitize T cells to undergo necrosis instead of apoptosis.[59] As a consequence, the rate of spontaneous apoptosis of resting CD4 T cells is increased and deletion of activated T cells is defective.[59,60] Together, these defects could contribute to lymphopenia and, paradoxically, increased survival of activated T-cell clones.

REFERENCES

1. Crispin JC, et al. Pathogenesis of human systemic lupus erythematosus: recent advances. *Trends Mol Med* 2010;**16**(2):47–57.
2. Shlomchik MJ, Craft JE, Mamula MJ. From T to B and back again: positive feedback in systemic autoimmune disease. *Nat Rev Immunol* 2001;**1**(2):147–53.
3. Andreassen K, et al. T cell autoimmunity to histones and nucleosomes is a latent property of the normal immune system. *Arthritis Rheum* 2002;**46**(5):1270–81.
4. Yurasov S, et al. B-cell tolerance checkpoints in healthy humans and patients with systemic lupus erythematosus. *Ann NY Acad Sci* 2005;**1062**:165–74.
5. van Es JH, et al. Somatic mutations in the variable regions of a human IgG anti-double-stranded DNA autoantibody suggest a role for antigen in the induction of systemic lupus erythematosus. *J Exp Med* 1991;**173**(2):461–70.
6. Mohan C, et al. Nucleosome: a major immunogen for pathogenic autoantibody-inducing T cells of lupus. *J Exp Med* 1993;**177**(5):1367–81.
7. Crotty S. T follicular helper cell differentiation, function, and roles in disease. *Immunity* 2014;**41**(4):529–42.
8. Vinuesa CG, et al. A RING-type ubiquitin ligase family member required to repress follicular helper T cells and autoimmunity. *Nature* 2005;**435**(7041):452–8.
9. Kim HJ, Cantor H. Regulation of self-tolerance by Qa-1-restricted CD8(+) regulatory T cells. *Semin Immunol* 2011;**23**(6):446–52.
10. Odegard JM, et al. ICOS-dependent extrafollicular helper T cells elicit IgG production via IL-21 in systemic autoimmunity. *J Exp Med* 2008;**205**(12):2873–86.
11. Simpson N, et al. Expansion of circulating T cells resembling follicular helper T cells is a fixed phenotype that identifies a subset of severe systemic lupus erythematosus. *Arthritis Rheum* 2010;**62**(1):234–44.
12. Liarski VM, et al. Cell distance mapping identifies functional T follicular helper cells in inflamed human renal tissue. *Sci Transl Med* 2014;**6**(230):230–46.
13. Craft JE. Follicular helper T cells in immunity and systemic autoimmunity. *Nat Rev Rheumatol* 2012;**8**(6):337–47.
14. Hsieh C, et al. Predicting outcomes of lupus nephritis with tubulointerstitial inflammation and scarring. *Arthritis Care Res Hob* 2011;**63**(6):865–74.
15. Steinmetz OM, et al. CXCR3 mediates renal Th1 and Th17 immune response in murine lupus nephritis. *J Immunol* 2009;**183**(7):4693–704.
16. Boggio E, et al. IL-17 protects T cells from apoptosis and contributes to development of ALPS-like phenotypes. *Blood* 2014;**123**(8):1178–86.
17. Crispin JC, et al. Expanded double negative T cells in patients with systemic lupus erythematosus produce IL-17 and infiltrate the kidneys. *J Immunol* 2008;**181**(12):8761–6.
18. Shah K, et al. Dysregulated balance of Th17 and Th1 cells in systemic lupus erythematosus. *Arthritis Res Ther* 2010;**12**(2):R53.
19. Talaat RM, et al. Th1/Th2/Th17/Treg cytokine imbalance in systemic lupus erythematosus (SLE) patients: correlation with disease activity. *Cytokine* 2015;**72**(2):146–53.
20. Kang HK, Liu M, Datta SK. Low-dose peptide tolerance therapy of lupus generates plasmacytoid dendritic cells that cause expansion of autoantigen-specific regulatory T cells and contraction of inflammatory Th17 cells. *J Immunol* 2007;**178**(12):7849–58.
21. Koga T, et al. CaMK4-dependent activation of AKT/mTOR and CREM-alpha underlies autoimmunity-associated Th17 imbalance. *J Clin Invest* 2014;**124**(5):2234–45.
22. Balomenos D, Rumold R, Theofilopoulos AN. Interferon-gamma is required for lupus-like disease and lymphoaccumulation in MRL-lpr mice. *J Clin Invest* 1998;**101**(2):364–71.
23. Schmidt T, et al. Function of the Th17/interleukin-17A immune response in murine lupus nephritis. *Arthritis Rheumatol* 2015;**67**(2):475–87.
24. Amarilyo G, et al. IL-17 promotes murine lupus. *J Immunol* 2014;**193**(2):540–3.
25. Crispin JC, et al. Cutting edge: protein phosphatase 2A confers susceptibility to autoimmune disease through an IL-17-dependent mechanism. *J Immunol* 2012;**188**(8):3567–71.
26. Linker-Israeli M, et al. Elevated levels of endogenous IL-6 in systemic lupus erythematosus. A putative role in pathogenesis. *J Immunol* 1991;**147**(1):117–23.
27. Alcocer-Varela J, Alarcon-Segovia D. Decreased production of and response to interleukin-2 by cultured lymphocytes from patients with systemic lupus erythematosus. *J Clin Invest* 1982;**69**(6):1388–92.
28. Tsokos GC, et al. Deficient gamma-interferon production in patients with systemic lupus erythematosus. *Arthritis Rheum* 1986;**29**(10):1210–5.
29. Basu D, et al. Stimulatory and inhibitory killer Ig-like receptor molecules are expressed and functional on lupus T cells. *J Immunol* 2009;**183**(5):3481–7.
30. Uhm WS, et al. Cytokine balance in kidney tissue from lupus nephritis patients. *Rheumatol Oxf* 2003;**42**(8):935–8.
31. Lawson BR, et al. Treatment of murine lupus with cDNA encoding IFN-gammaR/Fc. *J Clin Invest* 2000;**106**(2):207–15.
32. Li Y, et al. Phosphorylated ERM is responsible for increased T cell polarization, adhesion, and migration in patients with systemic lupus erythematosus. *J Immunol* 2007;**178**(3):1938–47.
33. Wang A, et al. Dysregulated expression of CXCR4/CXCL12 in subsets of patients with systemic lupus erythematosus. *Arthritis Rheum* 2010;**62**(11):3436–46.
34. Crispin JC, et al. Expression of CD44 variant isoforms CD44v3 and CD44v6 is increased on T cells from patients with systemic lupus erythematosus and is correlated with disease activity. *Arthritis Rheum* 2010;**62**(5):1431–7.

35. Stohl W. Impaired polyclonal T cell cytolytic activity. A possible risk factor for systemic lupus erythematosus. *Arthritis Rheum* 1995;**38**(4):506–16.

36. Contin-Bordes C, et al. Expansion of myelin autoreactive CD8⁺ T lymphocytes in patients with neuropsychiatric systemic lupus erythematosus. *Ann Rheum Dis* 2011;**70**(5):868–71.

37. Kim JS, et al. IL-7Ralphalow memory CD8⁺ T cells are significantly elevated in patients with systemic lupus erythematosus. *Rheumatol Oxf* 2012;**51**(9):1587–94.

38. Blanco P, et al. Increase in activated CD8⁺ T lymphocytes expressing perforin and granzyme B correlates with disease activity in patients with systemic lupus erythematosus. *Arthritis Rheum* 2005;**52**(1):201–11.

39. Winchester R, et al. Immunologic characteristics of intrarenal T cells: trafficking of expanded CD8⁺ T cell beta-chain clonotypes in progressive lupus nephritis. *Arthritis Rheum* 2012;**64**(5):1589–600.

40. Alunno A, et al. CD4(−)CD8(−) T-cells in primary Sjogren's syndrome: association with the extent of glandular involvement. *J Autoimmun* 2014;**51**:38–43.

41. Shivakumar S, Tsokos GC, Datta SK. T cell receptor alpha/beta expressing double-negative (CD4⁻/CD8⁻) and CD4⁺ T helper cells in humans augment the production of pathogenic anti-DNA autoantibodies associated with lupus nephritis. *J Immunol* 1989;**143**(1):103–12.

42. Crispin JC, Tsokos GC. Human TCR-alpha beta+ CD4⁻ CD8⁻ T cells can derive from CD8⁺ T cells and display an inflammatory effector phenotype. *J Immunol* 2009;**183**(7):4675–81.

43. Rodriguez-Rodriguez N, et al. Programmed cell death 1 and Helios distinguish TCR-alphabeta+ double-negative (CD4⁻CD8⁻) T cells that derive from self-reactive CD8 T Cells. *J Immunol* 2015;**161**(3):427–8.

44. Prokunina L, et al. A regulatory polymorphism in PDCD1 is associated with susceptibility to systemic lupus erythematosus in humans. *Nat Genet* 2002;**32**(4):666–9.

45. Kristjansdottir H, et al. Lower expression levels of the programmed death 1 receptor on CD4⁺CD25⁺ T cells and correlation with the PD-1.3A genotype in patients with systemic lupus erythematosus. *Arthritis Rheum* 2010;**62**(6):1702–11.

46. Fujio K, et al. Regulatory cell subsets in the control of autoantibody production related to systemic autoimmunity. *Ann Rheum Dis* 2013;**72**(Suppl 2):ii85–89.

47. Bonelli M, et al. Quantitative and qualitative deficiencies of regulatory T cells in patients with systemic lupus erythematosus (SLE). *Int Immunol* 2008;**20**(7):861–8.

48. La Cava A, Ebling FM, Hahn BH. Ig-reactive CD4⁺CD25⁺ T cells from tolerized (New Zealand Black x New Zealand White)F1 mice suppress in vitro production of antibodies to DNA. *J Immunol* 2004;**173**(5):3542–8.

49. Chung Y, et al. Follicular regulatory T cells expressing Foxp3 and Bcl-6 suppress germinal center reactions. *Nat Med* 2011;**17**(8):983–8.

50. Tsokos GC, et al. Rewiring the T-cell: signaling defects and novel prospects for the treatment of SLE. *Trends Immunol* 2003;**24**(5):259–63.

51. Kyttaris VC, et al. Increased levels of NF-ATc2 differentially regulate CD154 and IL-2 genes in T cells from patients with systemic lupus erythematosus. *J Immunol* 2007;**178**(3):1960–6.

52. Tenbrock K, Tsokos GC. Transcriptional regulation of interleukin 2 in SLE T cells. *Int Rev Immunol* 2004;**23**(3–4):333–45.

53. Juang YT, et al. Systemic lupus erythematosus serum IgG increases CREM binding to the IL-2 promoter and suppresses IL-2 production through CaMKIV. *J Clin Invest* 2005;**115**(4):996–1005.

54. Katsiari CG, et al. Protein phosphatase 2A is a negative regulator of IL-2 production in patients with systemic lupus erythematosus. *J Clin Invest* 2005;**115**(11):3193–204.

55. Apostolidis SA, et al. Protein phosphatase 2A enables expression of interleukin 17 (IL-17) through chromatin remodeling. *J Biol Chem* 2013;**288**(37):26775–84.

56. Harley IT, et al. Genetic susceptibility to SLE: new insights from fine mapping and genome-wide association studies. *Nat Rev Genet* 2009;**10**(5):285–90.

57. Jeffries MA, et al. Genome-wide DNA methylation patterns in CD4⁺ T cells from patients with systemic lupus erythematosus. *Epigenetics* 2011;**6**(5):593–601.

58. Richardson B, et al. Evidence for impaired T cell DNA methylation in systemic lupus erythematosus and rheumatoid arthritis. *Arthritis Rheum* 1990;**33**(11):1665–73.

59. Gergely Jr P, et al. Mitochondrial hyperpolarization and ATP depletion in patients with systemic lupus erythematosus. *Arthritis Rheum* 2002;**46**(1):175–90.

60. Crispin JC, et al. Induction of PP2A Bbeta, a regulator of IL-2 deprivation-induced T-cell apoptosis, is deficient in systemic lupus erythematosus. *Proc Natl Acad Sci USA* 2011;**108**(30):12443–8.

Chapter 14

Integrating Current Thinking on Peripheral B-Cell Tolerance in Lupus

Jefte M. Drijvers, Shiv Pillai

Ragon Institute of MGH, MIT and Harvard, Cambridge, MA, USA

One of the greatest intellectual challenges in biology and medicine is obtaining an understanding of the pathogenesis of complex diseases. Because autoimmune diseases involve the dysfunction of immune cells and immune cells are relatively easily accessed through the blood, it is likely that we may obtain a complete understanding of autoimmune diseases, such as type I diabetes and systemic lupus erythematosus (SLE, lupus), more easily than we will dissect the mechanisms underlying, say, autism or the metabolic syndrome.

Some perspectives on the underlying mechanisms of autoimmunity have been reviewed elsewhere.[1] The general consensus is that although these are multigene disorders and genomewide association studies and exome sequencing for rare genetic variants have yielded important information, inherited germline changes alone cannot readily explain the underlying basis of autoimmune diseases. It is assumed that both underlying genetic variation and environmentally facilitated epigenetic alterations in gene expression in immune cells contribute to disease pathogenesis. Perhaps the most tractable source of environmental alterations are changes in the intestinal microbiome. However, although the microbiome can influence immune cell function[2–4] and there is a report of alterations in the microbiome in rheumatoid arthritis,[5] there is no clear smoking gun linking changes in the human microbiome to autoimmunity in general or to lupus in particular.

Although there is marked activation of the innate immune system in lupus subjects, development of the disease requires that there be a break in central or peripheral B-cell tolerance, and that a class-switched somatically mutated humoral immune response against chromatin components must be generated. The mechanisms that contribute to the generation of antichromatin circulating immune complexes must represent a defining feature of lupus pathogenesis.

In this chapter, we address disparate mechanisms that may contribute to the processes that lead to the eventual generation of anti-self humoral immune responses in lupus subjects. We explore whether various phenomena linked to B-cell tolerance in lupus subjects are potentially causal or if they possibly occur as a consequence of the disease.

B-CELL DEPLETION THERAPY, REGULATORY B CELLS, AND LUPUS

While an important role for both T and B cells in lupus pathogenesis has long been recognized and this is consistent with the accepted pathogenic role of somatically mutated and class-switched autoantibodies in this disease, therapies targeting the adaptive immune system in lupus have generally proved disappointing.[6–8] In particular, B-cell depletion has only resulted in modest attenuation in disease severity.[9–12] It may well be that the central importance of nucleic acid dependent endosomal Toll-like receptor (TLR) activation in lupus results in the induction of long-lived plasma cells that are not susceptible to anti-CD20 mediated depletion. Another explanation for the lack of efficacy of anti-CD20 mediated depletion is that this therapy depletes regulatory B cells as well as other B-cell populations. It is postulated that regulatory B cells exhibit decreased suppressive activity in lupus patients.[13] This observation might have consequences for therapeutic strategies in lupus.

THE TYPE I INTERFERON PATHWAY IN LUPUS AND A POTENTIAL LINK TO IMMUNE TOLERANCE

The type I interferon (IFN-I) pathway may play a major role in SLE pathogenesis and potentially contribute to the break in B-cell tolerance that is presumed to be a central pathogenic event in this disorder. IFN-Is are a family of cytokines with an established role in the innate immune response to viral infections. Two of the most important IFN-Is are IFN-α (which includes the products of 13 different genes), produced primarily by plasmacytoid dendritic cells (pDCs), and IFN-β, which is synthesized by various cell types. In the context of viral infection, the expression of IFN-I is induced by members of the IFN-regulatory factor (IRF) family of

Systemic Lupus Erythematosus. http://dx.doi.org/10.1016/B978-0-12-801917-7.00014-0

transcription factors, which are induced downstream of pattern recognition receptors (PRRs), including endosomal TLRs that recognize nucleic acids.[14–16] The consequences of IFN-I signaling through the type I interferon receptor include the induction of an antiviral state, increased cytotoxic activity of NK cells, and CD8+ T cells and enhanced antigen presentation by class I MHC molecules—all of which are helpful in combating viral infection.[15,16]

The first indications of a role of IFN-I in lupus were derived both from animal models and the observation, made in the late 1970s, that IFN-I levels are elevated in the blood of human SLE patients.[17–19] More recently, an IFN-I-induced gene expression profile was described in peripheral blood mononuclear cells of lupus patients and found to correlate with disease activity.[19–22] Mechanistically, the induction of IFN-I in lupus patients likely results from the triggering of endosomal TLRs in plasmacytoid dendritic cells (pDCs) by the nucleic acid components of immune complexes consisting of nucleic acids, autoantibodies, and complement.[19,22] In this pathway, TLRs that usually initiate a signaling pathway in response to endosomal viral DNA or RNA now do the same in response to self-nucleic acids that end up in the same endosomal compartment. The result is a chronically persistent increased expression of IFN-I.[19,22]

The observation of increased IFN-I levels in lupus patients might reflect a primary role of IFN-I in lupus pathogenesis, but it could also be a consequence of the disease rather than a cause. The enhanced production of IFN-I in pDCs of lupus subjects is generally thought to be induced by nucleic acid containing immune complexes.[19,22] It may well be that although small amounts of nucleic acid containing immune complexes are generated on a daily basis by healthy individuals as well as lupus subjects, the latter may be genetically predisposed to more readily and vigorously activate endosomal TLR signaling (and possibly signaling by other nucleic acid sensors, including those in the cytosol) than control subjects. The enrichment of genetic variants that can enhance IFN-I synthesis and activate the IFN-I signaling pathway in lupus patients speaks to a possible causal role of IFN-I in disease initiation and/or progression. Genome wide association studies have identified various lupus-associated genes that are involved in endosomal TLR signaling and IFN-I production. Examples are variants in *TLR7*, a gene that encodes an endosomal TLR that recognizes single-stranded RNA; *TNFAIP3*, which limits NF-κB signaling downstream of TLRs; *IRF5* and *7*, encoding transcription factors that can induce IFN-I expression; and *IRAK1*, which encodes a kinase that contributes to IRF5 and IRF7 activation.[19,22] These gene variants linked to SLE are all potentially associated with increased IFN-I signaling. Polymorphisms leading to an increased response to IFN-I are also associated with lupus, such as *STAT4* variants.[19,22] Further evidence for a causal role of IFN-I in SLE is provided by two observations. Firstly, subjects being treated with recombinant IFN-I for

malignancy or infection develop SLE.[22–24] Secondly, Rag 2-deficient-Trex1-deficient mice (TREX1 or Three Prime Repair Exonuclease 1, a DNA-degrading enzyme), in which a lupus-like disease is induced by the Trex-deficiency, have an IFN-induced gene expression profile even though these mice lack VDJ recombination.[22,25,26] This indicates that increased IFN-I expression may occur before the appearance of autoantibodies in lupus pathogenesis.

If the IFN-I signaling pathway does indeed play a causal role in the initiation of lupus pathogenesis, two important questions remain to be answered. Firstly, how is IFN-I signaling initially induced, and can it be induced before the emergence of immune complexes? Secondly, what are the mechanisms by which IFN-I contributes to lupus pathogenesis?

With regard to the first question, one hypothesis suggests that the defective function of enzymes that degrade intracellular nucleic acids may result in cytosolic RNA or DNA in nonhematopoietic cells, which triggers cytosolic PRRs, such as cGAS, RIG-I, and MDA5. Their signaling would lead to the expression of small amounts of IFN-I, which in turn would prime other cells, including pDCs and neutrophils, to more readily induce high levels of IFN-I upon subsequent activation of PRRs.[19,22] It seems plausible that such a series of events would occur more easily in subjects with polymorphisms that make the IFN-I signaling pathway more prone to being activated. The relevance of such a mechanism is supported by the association of gene variants of *TREX1*, mentioned above, which encodes a DNase, as well as of other genes encoding proteins involved in the breakdown of nucleic acids with SLE and lupus-like syndromes.[19,22]

As for the mechanisms by which IFN-I contributes to lupus pathogenesis, it should be noted that most disease manifestations in SLE are directly caused by deposition of immune complexes made up of autoantibodies, complement, and nucleic acids and ensuing inflammation. However, there is evidence for the contribution of IFN-I as well, whether it is directly or indirectly, as IFN-induced gene expression profiles are seen in the skin and synovial tissue of lupus patients in whom the respective organs are affected.[19,27,28] A local increase in pDCs and the presence of IFN-α transcripts are observed in SLE-related kidney disease.[19,29] Furthermore, IFN-α has been shown to be able to stimulate the generation of foam cells and the activation of neurotoxic lymphocytes, underscoring potential mechanisms by which this cytokine could contribute to cardiovascular and central nervous system manifestations of SLE as well.[19,30,31]

In addition, important contributions of IFN-I to lupus pathogenesis are likely to be mediated by effects of this cytokine on immune cells.[14,19] For example, the ability of serum from lupus patients to induce dendritic cell differentiation and enhance antigen presentation, thereby potentially contributing to the presentation of self-antigens to autoreactive T cells, may reflect the activity of IFN-α in the serum.[14,19,32] Additionally, IFN-I and IL-6 secreted by pDCs have been shown to induce plasma cell differentiation.[14,33] The expression of B-cell activating factor (BAFF) was shown to be induced by IFN-α in the context of primary Sjögren's syndrome.[19,34] A similar phenomenon might be relevant to SLE as well and could be of pathogenic relevance because of the potential roles of BAFF in SLE pathogenesis (see below). Through these mechanisms, IFN-I may contribute to the activation and function of self-reactive lymphocytes in SLE, leading to a break in tolerance and the production of autoantibodies that can contribute to the formation of pathogenic immune complexes (Figure 1).

Both IFN-α as well as immune complexes can cause the activation of neutrophils to release decondensed chromatin and to form neutrophil extracellular traps (NETs). NETs can contribute to the progression of lupus by being a source of chromatin that can activate chromatin-specific B and T cells and also provide the substrate for the more abundant formation of nucleic acid containing immune complexes.[19,35]

In the previously described mechanisms, the predisposing role of gain-of-function gene variants in the PRR/IRF/IFN-I pathway was explained mostly by the increased tendency of cells like pDCs to produce IFN-I. However, an additional explanation of the association between autoantibody production and polymorphisms in IRFs, most notably IRF5 and IRF7, is that the latter may affect TLR-signaling in B cells as well. The gene variants may thereby make B cells more likely

to initiate autoantibody production.[22,36] IRF polymorphisms could thus contribute to autoantibody production directly, in addition to the described pathways involving IFN-I.

Considering the proposed role of IFN-I in lupus pathogenesis, it is not surprising that various therapeutic attempts have been undertaken to block IFN-I signaling pathways as well as to prevent the increase in IFN-I production by preventing TLR activation by nucleic acids. A possible successful example of the latter is treatment of SLE patients with hydroxychloroquine, an agent that contributes to alkalinization of lysosomes, which was shown to have a beneficial effect on lupus flares.[37]

In summary, genetic variants in the IFN-I signaling pathway may predispose patients to synthesize more IFN-I. This in turn may prime other cells to induce IFN-I more readily and may contribute to a break in tolerance and the production of autoantibodies. The resulting immune complexes stimulate IFN-I expression further via TLR-dependent mechanisms, giving rise to a positive feedback loop that likely plays a central role in lupus pathogenesis.

COMPLEMENT FUNCTION, APOPTOTIC CELL CLEARANCE, AND LUPUS

As was briefly mentioned before, most of the disease manifestations in SLE are a direct consequence of the deposition of pathogenic, pro-inflammatory immune complexes. Immune complexes containing IgG autoantibodies can initiate inflammation via activation of immune cells through

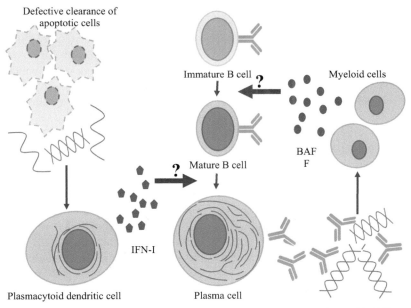

FIGURE 1 The mechanism of the break in B-cell tolerance in lupus subjects is poorly understood. Patients with SLE may have inherited or epigenetically acquired defects that contribute to defective clearance of apoptotic cells and chromatin, enhanced secretion of type I interferons by plasmacytoid dendritic cells, and increased secretion of BAFF because of an unexplained B lymphopenia or increased activation of myeloid cells by IFN-I and immune complexes. Type I interferons might contribute to a break of peripheral B cell tolerance by acting upon T cells or by driving plasma cell differentiation. BAFF may contribute to a break in tolerance at the immature or transitional B cell stages.

Fc-gamma receptors as well as complement activation. Yet, perhaps counterintuitively, defects in complement proteins, especially those involved in classical complement activation, such as C1q, C2, and C4, are strongly associated with lupus.[35] Illustratively, the vast majority of C1q-deficient subjects develop lupus-like disease,[35,38,39] and even though absolute genetic C1q deficiencies are rare, many lupus patients exhibit decreased C1q activity during active disease due to other mechanisms, including consumption, inability to upregulate production, and anti-C1q antibodies.[40–42]

An important explanation of the link between SLE and defects in the aforementioned early complement proteins is their crucial role in the clearance of apoptotic cells. Although apoptotic cell debris is cleared in a noninflammatory manner via mechanisms depending on early complement proteins, the defective function of these complement factors and inefficient clearance of apoptotic cell debris may facilitate inflammation and exposure of autoantigens, resulting in the activation of self-reactive lymphocytes.[35,43]

Another way in which defects in C1q may contribute to SLE pathogenesis is explained by the hypothesis that C1q binds and clears immune complexes. C1q binds to immune complexes and directs them to monocytes and macrophages rather than to pDCs and thus attenuates IFN-I release[35,44] as well as IFN-induced gene expression.[45] When C1q is mutated or its function is decreased, immune complexes are more likely to persist and activate pDCs, leading to IFN-I production and the ensuing sequence of pathogenic events described above. This is supported by the observation of increased serum IFN-α levels in patients with C1q defects.[35,44]

C1q not only opsonizes apoptotic bodies directly and helps clear immune complexes and diverts them away from pDCs, but it also induces signaling in macrophages that contributes to the release of anti-inflammatory cytokines such as IL-10, as well as of opsonins such as Gas6 and protein S, which can also coat apoptotic bodies.[35,46] These opsonins are recognized by a receptor that contributes to the clearance of apoptotic cells, the Mer tyrosine kinase on the surface of macrophages. The expression of Mer is also induced on these cells by C1q signaling.[35,46]

INCREASED BAFF IN LUPUS: A CONTRIBUTOR TO A BREAK IN TOLERANCE OR CONSEQUENCE OF INFLAMMATION?

Yet another pathway that has been suggested to be involved in lupus pathogenesis involves the BAFF, also known as B lymphocyte stimulator (BLyS), family of cytokines and receptors.[47] BAFF is one of the two ligands of the BAFF family, the other being APRIL. There are three receptors in the BAFF family: BAFF-R, TACI, and BCMA. BAFF-BAFF-R interactions contribute to the survival of all follicular B cells from the transitional B cell stage onward. BAFF and APRIL can interact with TACI and induce T-independent activation of B cells, inducing activation induced cytidine deaminase (AID) and consequent class-switching. The BAFF family receptor BCMA contributes to the survival of plasma cells in the bone marrow.[47]

Elevated BAFF levels have been observed in a subgroup of patients with SLE[47,48] and have been linked to disease activity.[49,50] In physiologic conditions, anergic B cells are excluded from follicles, primarily because they cannot effectively compete for the limited amount of BAFF generated within the follicle by follicular dendritic cells. The high BAFF levels seen in lupus subjects could theoretically facilitate the survival of anergic self-reactive B cells.[47] In line with this hypothesis is the observation of a strong correlation between BAFF levels and an increase in the relative numbers of B cells in the late transitional stage in SLE patients.[47,51] This could reflect the break in tolerance that may be consistent with the observation of increased proportions of mature naïve B cells expressing autoreactive antibodies in lupus patients.[47,52] Other members of the BAFF family may also be involved in lupus pathogenesis through their aforementioned roles in the later stages of B cell responses.[47] This might be exemplified by malfunction of germinal center reactions in SLE, with defective elimination of autoreactive B cells at this stage as well.[47,53]

What causes the elevation of BAFF levels in lupus subjects? One possibility is that it represents a feedback response to an underlying B cell lymphopenia commonly seen in lupus subjects.[54] While this may be the case, there is neither an understanding of the cause of the B lymphopenia in this disease nor an appreciation of the apparent B cell "counting" mechanism that regulates BAFF levels. Another possibility is that immune complex mediated activation of Fc receptors stimulates myeloid cells to secrete BAFF. Indeed, as mentioned previously, even the increased levels of IFN-I in lupus subjects might induce BAFF expression.[34] In any case, it seems likely that the increased BAFF levels seen in some lupus patients reflect a secondary rather than a primary causal process.

Two major types of therapeutics have been generated that target the BAFF-pathway in lupus. Belimumab, a monoclonal antibody blocking BAFF, was approved by the U.S. Food and Drug Administration for the treatment of SLE and was shown to decrease lupus disease activity.[47,55] However, the therapeutic benefit is modest.[56] TACI-Ig, also known as atacicept, is a receptor fusion protein that should theoretically be able to block all BAFF family receptor activation by its ability to sequester both BAFF and APRIL.[47,57] In theory, it should not only facilitate tolerance induction at the transitional B cell stage but also compromise the survival of long-lived plasma cells that secrete antinuclear antibodies. So far, TACI-Ig has also not proven to be particularly efficacious. In a phase II/III trial, a lower atacicept dose showed no benefit; a higher dose arm, which was showing some promise of benefit, had to be discontinued because of two concurrent fatal infections in this study group.[57]

REFERENCES

1. Pillai S. Rethinking mechanisms of autoimmune pathogenesis. *J Autoimmun* 2013;**45**:97–103.
2. Ivanov II , Atarashi K, Manel N, Brodie EL, Shima T, Karaoz U, et al. Induction of intestinal Th17 cells by segmented filamentous bacteria. *Cell* 2009;**139**:485–98.
3. Wu HJ, Ivanov II , Darce J, Hattori K, Shima T, Umesaki Y, et al. Gut-residing segmented filamentous bacteria drive autoimmune arthritis via T helper 17 cells. *Immunity* 2010;**32**:815–27.
4. Wen L, Ley RE, Volchkov PY, Stranges PB, Avanesyan L, Stonebraker AC, et al. Innate immunity and intestinal microbiota in the development of Type 1 diabetes. *Nature* 2008;**455**:1109–13.
5. Scher JU, Sczesnak A, Longman RS, Segata N, Ubeda C, Bielski C, et al. Expansion of intestinal Prevotella copri correlates with enhanced susceptibility to arthritis. *Elife* 2013;**2**:e01202.
6. Austin HA, Illei GG, Braun MJ, Balow JE. Randomized, controlled trial of prednisone, cyclophosphamide, and cyclosporine in lupus membranous nephropathy. *J Am Soc Nephrol* 2009;**20**:901–11.
7. ACCESS Trial Group. Treatment of lupus nephritis with abatacept: the Abatacept and Cyclophosphamide Combination Efficacy and Safety Study. *Arthritis Rheumatol* 2014;**66**:3096–104.
8. Wofsy D, Hillson JL, Diamond B. Abatacept for lupus nephritis: alternative definitions of complete response support conflicting conclusions. *Arthritis Rheum* 2012;**64**:3660–5.
9. Merrill JT, Neuwelt CM, Wallace DJ, Shanahan JC, Latinis KM, Oates JC, et al. Efficacy and safety of rituximab in moderately-to-severely active systemic lupus erythematosus: the randomized, double-blind, phase II/III systemic lupus erythematosus evaluation of rituximab trial. *Arthritis Rheum* 2010;**62**:222–33.
10. Rovin BH, Furie R, Latinis K, Looney RJ, Fervenza FC, Sanchez-Guerrero J, et al. Efficacy and safety of rituximab in patients with active proliferative lupus nephritis: the Lupus Nephritis Assessment with Rituximab study. *Arthritis Rheum* 2012;**64**:1215–26.
11. Terrier B, Amoura Z, Ravaud P, Hachulla E, Jouenne R, Combe B, et al. Safety and efficacy of rituximab in systemic lupus erythematosus: results from 136 patients from the French autoimmunity and rituximab registry. *Arthritis Rheum* 2010;**62**:2458–66.
12. Ramos-Casals M, Soto MJ, Cuadrado MJ, Khamashta MA. Rituximab in systemic lupus erythematosus: a systematic review of off-label use in 188 cases. *Lupus* 2009;**18**:767–76.
13. Blair PA, Noreña LY, Flores-Borja F, Rawlings DJ, Isenberg DA, Ehrenstein MR, et al. CD19+CD24hiCD38hi B cells exhibit regulatory capacity in healthy individuals but are functionally impaired in systemic lupus erythematosus patients. *Immunity* 2010;**32**:129–40.
14. González-Navajas JM, Lee J, David M, Raz E. Immunomodulatory functions of type I interferons. *Nat Rev Immunol* 2012;**12**:125–35.
15. Baum A, García-Sastre A. Induction of type I interferon by RNA viruses: cellular receptors and their substrates. *Amino Acids* 2010;**38**:1283–99.
16. Gessani S, Conti L, Del Corno M, Belardelli F. Type I interferons as regulators of human antigen presenting cell functions. *Toxins (Basel)* 2014;**6**:1696–723.
17. Steinberg AD, Baron S, Talal N. The pathogenesis of autoimmunity in New Zealand mice, I. Induction of antinucleic acid antibodies by polyinosinic-polycytidylic acid. *Proc Natl Acad Sci USA* 1969;**63**:1102–7.
18. Hooks JJ, Moutsopoulos HM, Geis SA, Stahl NI, Decker JL, Notkins AL. Immune interferon in the circulation of patients with autoimmune disease. *N Engl J Med* 1979;**301**:5–8.
19. Crow MK. Type I interferon in the pathogenesis of lupus. *J Immunol* 2014;**192**:5459–68.
20. Bennett L, Palucka AK, Arce E, Cantrell V, Borvak J, Banchereau J, et al. Interferon and granulopoiesis signatures in systemic lupus erythematosus blood. *J Exp Med* 2003;**197**:711–23.
21. Feng X, Wu H, Grossman JM, Hanvivadhanakul P, FitzGerald JD, Park GS, et al. Association of increased interferon-inducible gene expression with disease activity and lupus nephritis in patients with systemic lupus erythematosus. *Arthritis Rheum* 2006;**54**:2951–62.
22. Jensen MA, Niewold TB. Interferon regulatory factors: critical mediators of human lupus. *Transl Res* 2015;**165**:283–95.
23. Niewold TB, Swedler WI. Systemic lupus erythematosus arising during interferon-alpha therapy for cryoglobulinemic vasculitis associated with hepatitis C. *Clin Rheumatol* 2005;**24**:178–81.
24. Rönnblom LE, Alm GV, Oberg KE. Possible induction of systemic lupus erythematosus by interferon-alpha treatment in a patient with a malignant carcinoid tumour. *J Intern Med* 1990;**227**:207–10.
25. Stetson DB, Ko JS, Heidmann T, Medzhitov R. Trex1 prevents cell-intrinsic initiation of autoimmunity. *Cell* 2008;**134**:587–98.
26. Gall A, Treuting P, Elkon KB, Loo YM, Gale M, Barber GN, et al. Autoimmunity initiates in nonhematopoietic cells and progresses via lymphocytes in an interferon-dependent autoimmune disease. *Immunity* 2012;**36**:120–31.
27. Farkas L, Beiske K, Lund-Johansen F, Brandtzaeg P, Jahnsen FL. Plasmacytoid dendritic cells (natural interferon- alpha/beta-producing cells) accumulate in cutaneous lupus erythematosus lesions. *Am J Pathol* 2001;**159**:237–43.
28. Nzeusseu Toukap A, Galant C, Theate I, Maudoux AL, Lories RJU, Houssiau FA, et al. Identification of distinct gene expression profiles in the synovium of patients with systemic lupus erythematosus. *Arthritis Rheum* 2007;**56**:1579–88.
29. Tucci M, Quatraro C, Lombardi L, Pellegrino C, Dammacco F, Silvestris F. Glomerular accumulation of plasmacytoid dendritic cells in active lupus nephritis: role of interleukin-18. *Arthritis Rheum* 2008;**58**:251–62.
30. Li J, Fu Q, Cui H, Qu B, Pan W, Shen N, et al. Interferon-alpha priming promotes lipid uptake and macrophage-derived foam cell formation: a novel link between interferon-alpha and atherosclerosis in lupus. *Arthritis Rheum* 2011;**63**:492–502.
31. Pulliero A, Marengo B, Longobardi M, Fazzi E, Orcesi S, Olivieri I, et al. Inhibition of the de-myelinating properties of Aicardi-Goutières syndrome lymphocytes by cathepsin D silencing. *Biochem Biophys Res Commun* 2013;**430**:957–62.
32. Blanco P, Palucka AK, Gill M, Pascual V, Banchereau J. Induction of dendritic cell differentiation by IFN-alpha in systemic lupus erythematosus. *Science* 2001;**294**:1540–3.
33. Jego G, Palucka AK, Blanck J-P, Chalouni C, Pascual V, Banchereau J. Plasmacytoid dendritic cells induce plasma cell differentiation through type I interferon and interleukin 6. *Immunity* 2003;**19**:225–34.
34. Ittah M, Miceli-Richard C, Gottenberg J-E, Lavie F, Lazure T, Ba N, et al. B cell-activating factor of the tumor necrosis factor family (BAFF) is expressed under stimulation by interferon in salivary gland epithelial cells in primary Sjögren's syndrome. *Arthritis Res Ther* 2006;**8**:R51.
35. Elkon KB, Santer DM. Complement, interferon and lupus. *Curr Opin Immunol* 2012;**24**:665–70.
36. Cherian TS, Kariuki SN, Franek BS, Buyon JP, Clancy RM, Niewold TB. IRF5 systemic lupus erythematosus risk haplotype is associated with asymptomatic serologic autoimmunity and progression to clinical autoimmunity in mothers of children with neonatal lupus. *Arthritis Rheum* 2012;**64**:3383–7.

37. Crow MK, Olferiev M, Kirou KA. Targeting of type I interferon in systemic autoimmune diseases. *Transl Res* 2015;**165**:296–305.

38. Manderson AP, Botto M, Walport MJ. The role of complement in the development of systemic lupus erythematosus. *Annu Rev Immunol* 2004;**22**:431–56.

39. Pickering MC, Botto M, Taylor PR, Lachmann PJ, Walport MJ. Systemic lupus erythematosus, complement deficiency, and apoptosis. *Adv Immunol* 2000;**76**:227–324.

40. Moosig F, Damm F, Knorr-Spahr A, Ritgen M, Zeuner RA, Kneba M, et al. Reduced expression of C1q-mRNA in monocytes from patients with systemic lupus erythematosus. *Clin Exp Immunol* 2006;**146**:409–16.

41. Frémeaux-Bacchi V, Weiss L, Demouchy C, Blouin J, Kazatchkine MD. Autoantibodies to the collagen-like region of C1q are strongly associated with classical pathway-mediated hypocomplementemia in systemic lupus erythematosus. *Lupus* 1996;**5**:216–20.

42. Walport MJ, Davies KA, Botto M. C1q and systemic lupus erythematosus. *Immunobiology* 1998;**199**:265–85.

43. Benoit ME, Clarke EV, Morgado P, Fraser DA, Tenner AJ. Complement protein C1q directs macrophage polarization and limits inflammasome activity during the uptake of apoptotic cells. *J Immunol* 2012;**188**:5682–93.

44. Santer DM, Hall BE, George TC, Tangsombatvisit S, Liu CL, Arkwright PD, et al. C1q deficiency leads to the defective suppression of IFN-alpha in response to nucleoprotein containing immune complexes. *J Immunol* 2010;**185**:4738–49.

45. Santer DM, Wiedeman AE, Teal TH, Ghosh P, Elkon KB. Plasmacytoid dendritic cells and C1q differentially regulate inflammatory gene induction by lupus immune complexes. *J Immunol* 2012;**188**:902–15.

46. Galvan MD, Foreman DB, Zeng E, Tan JC, Bohlson SS. Complement component C1q regulates macrophage expression of Mer tyrosine kinase to promote clearance of apoptotic cells. *J Immunol* 2012;**188**:3716–23.

47. Scholz JL, Oropallo MA, Sindhava V, Goenka R, Cancro MP. The role of B lymphocyte stimulator in B cell biology: implications for the treatment of lupus. *Lupus* 2013;**22**:350–60.

48. Cheema GS, Roschke V, Hilbert DM, Stohl W. Elevated serum B lymphocyte stimulator levels in patients with systemic immune-based rheumatic diseases. *Arthritis Rheum* 2001;**44**:1313–9.

49. Zhao LD, Li Y, Smith MF, Wang JS, Zhang W, Tang FL, et al. Expressions of BAFF/BAFF receptors and their correlation with disease activity in Chinese SLE patients. *Lupus* 2010;**19**:1534–49.

50. Petri M, Stohl W, Chatham W, McCune WJ, Chevrier M, Ryel J, et al. Association of plasma B lymphocyte stimulator levels and disease activity in systemic lupus erythematosus. *Arthritis Rheum* 2008;**58**:2453–9.

51. Landolt-Marticorena C, Wither R, Reich H, Herzenberg A, Scholey J, Gladman DD, et al. Increased expression of B cell activation factor supports the abnormal expansion of transitional B cells in systemic lupus erythematosus. *J Rheumatol* 2011;**38**:642–51.

52. Yurasov S, Wardemann H, Hammersen J, Tsuiji M, Meffre E, Pascual V, et al. Defective B cell tolerance checkpoints in systemic lupus erythematosus. *J Exp Med* 2005;**201**:703–11.

53. Cappione A, Anolik JH, Pugh-Bernard A, Barnard J, Dutcher P, Silverman G, et al. Germinal center exclusion of autoreactive B cells is defective in human systemic lupus erythematosus. *J Clin Invest* 2005;**115**:3205–16.

54. Hepburn AL, Narat S, Mason JC. The management of peripheral blood cytopenias in systemic lupus erythematosus. *Rheumatology* 2010;**49**:2243–54.

55. Jordan N, D'Cruz DP. Belimumab for the treatment of systemic lupus erythematosus. *Expert Rev Clin Immunol* 2015;**11**:195–204.

56. Manzi S, Sanchez-Guerrero J, Merrill JT, Furie R, Gladman D, Navarra SV, et al. Effects of belimumab, a B lymphocyte stimulator-specific inhibitor, on disease activity across multiple organ domains in patients with systemic lupus erythematosus: combined results from two phase III trials. *Ann Rheum Dis* 2012;**71**:1833–8.

57. Isenberg D, Gordon C, Licu D, Copt S, Rossi CP, Wofsy D. Efficacy and safety of atacicept for prevention of flares in patients with moderate-to-severe systemic lupus erythematosus (SLE): 52-week data (APRIL-SLE randomised trial). *Ann Rheum Dis* 2014. http://dx.doi.org/10.1136/annrheumdis-2013-205067.

Chapter 15

Neutrophils in Systemic Lupus Erythematosus

Amr H. Sawalha[1,2]

[1]*Division of Rheumatology, Department of Internal Medicine, University of Michigan, Ann Arbor, MI, USA;* [2]*Center for Computational Medicine and Bioinformatics, University of Michigan, Ann Arbor, MI, USA*

INTRODUCTION

Neutrophils are the most abundant immune-competent cells in the peripheral blood, representing up to ~70% of total white blood cells. They play an important role in innate immune responses and are often at the first line of defense against infections. Neutrophils are capable of phagocytosis and produce reactive oxygen species to kill invading microorganisms. They are short-lived (half-life of ~7h in the circulation, although longer half-lives of up to 5 days have been recently reported), granulated, and characterized by the presence of multilobulated nuclei. Upon degranulation, neutrophils release immune-active peptides, such as alpha defensins, cathelicidin peptides (such as LL-37), and lactoferin, which can either directly participate in microorganism killing or trigger other components of the innate or adaptive immune response. Neutrophils express most of the toll-like receptor (TLR) family members, MHC class II, CD80, and CD86, and present antigens to T cells and can prime antigen-specific Th1 and Th17 differentiation.[1,2] Indeed, neutrophils have been demonstrated to migrate toward inflammation sites, and then "reverse migrate" away from the inflammation site to the circulation, presumably to participate in eliciting a more generalized immune response.[1] Neutrophils also produce a variety of cytokines, such as BLyS (or BAFF) and APRIL, and can therefore induce B-cell stimulation.[3,4] Neutrophils in the spleen can also produce IL-21 and have been shown to induce B-cell activation, immunoglobulin production, and immunoglobulin somatic hypermutation and class switching.[5]

A peculiar mechanism that neutrophils possess within their defensive arsenal to hinder and kill invading microorganisms is forming neutrophil extracellular traps (NETs) (Figure 1). This process, called NETosis, allows for a rapid and robust externalization of the neutrophil micobicidal content, and it is a unique cell death mechanism initially described in neutrophils in 2004.[6] During this process, chromatin and neutrophil granular proteins are released,

forming extracellular fiber-like structures that bind and "trap" invading bacterial pathogens.[6] Importantly, NETosis appears to be dependent upon the presence of reactive oxygen species and requires NADPH oxidase activity. Neutrophils stimulated in the presence of an NADPH oxidase inhibitor do not generate reactive oxygen species and do not form NETs.[7] NETosis also requires histone hypercitrulination, primarily mediated by peptidylarginine deiminase 4 (PAD4) in neutrophils. Histone hypercitrulination deconvolutes and unfolds chromatin to allow externalization and NET formation. Neutrophils from PAD4-deficient mice demonstrate an inability to form NETs upon stimulation.[8]

A role for innate immune dysfunction in the pathogenesis of lupus has been increasingly appreciated. While the lupus erythematosus (LE) cell phenomenon (neutrophil phagocytosis of a nucleus or apoptotic body) has been recognized for decades and previously used as a diagnostic tool in lupus, a pathogenic role for neutrophils in lupus has only been recently included in the paradigm of lupus pathogenesis (Table 1).

NEUTROPHIL DYSFUNCTION IN SLE

Lupus patients can develop a number of hematological abnormalities. Neutropenia, which is usually mild in lupus, has been reported in up to 50% of patients. Similar to other "cytopenias" in lupus, the pathogenesis of neutropenia is likely to be immune-mediated destruction of neutrophils. This is supported by the detection of neutrophil-recognizing antibodies in lupus patients. Further, neutropenia in lupus patients is associated with the anti-Ro antibody, which can bind and fix complement on the neutrophil surface.[9]

The percentage of apoptotic neutrophils in lupus patients is increased compared to healthy controls, and the clearance of apoptotic neutrophils in lupus seems to be impaired.[10,11] Phagocytic ability of lupus neutrophils is also defective, and purified anticardiolipin antibodies from lupus patients have been shown to inhibit phagocytosis in neutrophils.[12] Furthermore, the lupus risk genetic variant in

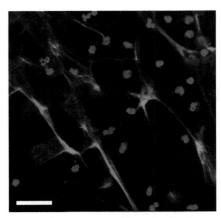

FIGURE 1   Immunofluorescence staining showing human neutrophils forming neutrophil extracellular traps (NETs) during NETosis. Cell nuclei are depicted in blue (Hoechst 33,342), and NETs are visualized in green using fluorescein isothiocyanate-conjugated antibody against neutrophil elastase. Scale bar = 25 μm. *This photograph is courtesy of Dr Jason S. Knight.*

TABLE 1 Major Aberrancies in Lupus Neutrophils That Might Play a Role in Disease Pathogenesis

Lupus Neutrophil Aberrancy	Consequences
Neutropenia	Usually mild, but if severe can predispose to infections
Increased apoptosis	Provides enhanced exposure to autoantigens
Decreased phagocytic capacity	Impairs phagocytic clearance of apoptopic debris
Increased NETosis and reduced NETs' clearance	Provides enhanced exposure to autoantigens Activates pDCs through TLR-9 Tissue damage and vascular complications
Increased IFN-α production	Activates innate and adaptive immune responses Alters B-cell development in the bone marrow Tissue damage
Increased number of LDGs	Increased IFN-α production Increased NETosis Endothelial vascular damage
Hypomethylated DNA and demethylation of IFN-regulated genes	Enhanced pDC stimulation through TLR-9? Increased hypersensitivity to IFN-α?

NETs, neutrophil extracellular traps; pDC, plasmacytoid dendritic cells; TLR-9, toll-like receptor-9; IFN, interferon; LDGs, low-density granulocytes.

ITGAM (encoding for CD11b, a subunit of Mac-1) contributes to Mac-1 dysfunction in neutrophils and is associated with impaired phagocytosis.[13] Together, these data suggest that increased neutrophil apoptosis and defective apoptotic clearance and phagocytosis might play a role in the pathogenesis of lupus by increasing autoantigen exposure and the subsequent enhanced autoimmune response. Recent evidence suggests that lupus neutrophils produce higher levels of type 1 interferon, and that neutrophil-mediated type 1 interferon production in the bone marrow can drive abnormal B-cell differentiation in lupus.[14,15]

NETosis IN THE PATHOGENESIS OF SLE

Neutrophils in lupus patients are characterized by an increased capacity to undergo NETosis, which is enhanced by exposure to antiribonucleoprotein antibodies.[16,17] In addition, the clearance of NETs in lupus is also impaired.[18] This leads to prolonged and abnormal exposure of chromatin and other intracellular immunogenic proteins included within the NETs to the immune system, which might play a role in immune-activation in lupus patients. Indeed, NETs contain a number of autoantigens, including chromatin, dsDNA, and granular proteins. NETs have been shown to directly stimulate plasmacytoid dendritic cells (pDC) in lupus through TLR-9 stimulation, and result in pDC activation and enhanced type 1 interferon production.[16,17] Type 1 interferons (especially interferon-alpha) induce NETosis, resulting in increased autoantigen exposure and pDC activation. Interferon-alpha is also produced by neutrophils in lupus.[15,19]

It has been suggested that reduced clearance of NETs in lupus patients is a result of impaired function of the serum endonuclease DNase-1, which is critical in NETs degradation.[18] The presence of antinuclear or other anti-NET antibodies that shield and therefore physically hinder DNase-1 access to NETs has been proposed. In addition, a subset of lupus patients expresses inactivating autoantibodies directed against DNase-1.[18]

A role for NETosis in organ damage in lupus has been suggested by the detection of NETs in affected skin and kidney tissues in lupus patients.[20] NETosis can also induce vascular endothelial damage and clotting, suggesting that neutrophils might play a role in accelerated atherosclerosis and vascular complications in lupus patients.[20–22] Inhibiting peptidylarginine deiminase (PAD4 is essential for NET formation) protects lupus-prone mice from kidney, skin, and vascular damage.[23,24]

LOW-DENSITY GRANULOCYTES IN SLE

A subset of "immature" or "abnormal" neutrophils has been described in lupus.[19] These cells are called low-density granulocytes (LDGs) and have a similar density to peripheral blood mononuclear cells (PBMCs). Therefore, LDGs purify with PBMCs during density gradient centrifugation of peripheral blood. Indeed, LDGs are thought to explain the granulopoeisis signature detected in gene expression profiling studies in lupus PBMCs.[25] LDGs segregate close to monocytes in flow cytometry analysis and are characterized by high expression of the neutrophil marker CD15 and low expression of the monocyte marker CD14.[19] Importantly, these cells are rare or absent in healthy individuals. They are thought to be pathogenic in lupus as they produce large amounts of type 1 interferon, interferon-gamma, and TNF-alpha, and they are more prone to NETosis than neutrophils.[19,20] LDGs have been shown to induce endothelial cell toxicity, suggesting that this granulocyte subset might be playing an important role in premature cardiovascular disease in lupus.[26]

DNA METHYLATION CHANGES IN SLE NEUTROPHILS AND LDGs

DNA methylation is an epigenetic mechanism that regulates gene expression. Abnormal DNA methylation is thought to play an important role in the pathogenesis of lupus.[27] Recent genome-wide DNA methylation studies in lupus neutrophils and LDGs identified a number of differentially methylated genetic loci compared to control neutrophils, with about two-thirds of the loci hypomethylated in lupus.[28] These data suggest that DNA in lupus neutrophils is qualitatively different, and this hypomethylation might enhance the ability of NETs to stimulate pDCs through TLR-9. This is also consistent with the described hypomethylation of LINE-1 repeats in lupus neutrophils.[29] Importantly, lupus neutrophils and LDGs show a robust DNA demethylation signature in type 1 interferon-regulated genes compared to neutrophils from healthy controls. The DNA methylome of lupus neutrophils and autologous LDGs is almost identical, suggesting that these two distinct granulocyte cell subsets are similar at the epigenomic level.

CONCLUSION

Neutrophils have been increasingly recognized to play an important role in the pathogenesis of lupus (Table 1). Neutrophils in lupus patients are characterized by impaired phagocytic ability, increased production of interferon alpha, and increased apoptosis. In addition, lupus neutrophils are more prone to NETosis, a neutrophil cell death mechanism that results in enhanced immune activation and might be involved in organ damage in lupus. A better understanding of lupus neutrophil pathophysiology can result in novel treatment options for lupus.

REFERENCES

1. Shelef MA, Tauzin S, Huttenlocher A. Neutrophil migration: moving from zebrafish models to human autoimmunity. *Immunol Rev* November 2013;**256**(1):269–81. PubMed PMID: 24117827. Pubmed Central PMCID: 4117680.

2. Abi Abdallah DS, Egan CE, Butcher BA, Denkers EY. Mouse neutrophils are professional antigen-presenting cells programmed to instruct Th1 and Th17 T-cell differentiation. *Int Immunol* May 2011;**23**(5):317–26. PubMed PMID: 21422151. Pubmed Central PMCID: 3082529.

3. Scapini P, Nardelli B, Nadali G, Calzetti F, Pizzolo G, Montecucco C, et al. G-CSF-stimulated neutrophils are a prominent source of functional BLyS. *J Exp Med* February 3, 2003;**197**(3):297–302. PubMed PMID: 12566413. Pubmed Central PMCID: 2193843.

4. Huard B, McKee T, Bosshard C, Durual S, Matthes T, Myit S, et al. APRIL secreted by neutrophils binds to heparan sulfate proteoglycans to create plasma cell niches in human mucosa. *J Clin Invest* August 2008;**118**(8):2887–95. PubMed PMID: 18618015. Pubmed Central PMCID: 2447926.

5. Puga I, Cols M, Barra CM, He B, Cassis L, Gentile M, et al. B cell-helper neutrophils stimulate the diversification and production of immunoglobulin in the marginal zone of the spleen. *Nat Immunol* February 2012;**13**(2):170–80. PubMed PMID: 22197976. Pubmed Central PMCID: 3262910.

6. Brinkmann V, Reichard U, Goosmann C, Fauler B, Uhlemann Y, Weiss DS, et al. Neutrophil extracellular traps kill bacteria. *Science* March 5, 2004;**303**(5663):1532–5. PubMed PMID: 15001782.

7. Fuchs TA, Abed U, Goosmann C, Hurwitz R, Schulze I, Wahn V, et al. Novel cell death program leads to neutrophil extracellular traps. *J Cell Biol* January 15, 2007;**176**(2):231–41. PubMed PMID: 17210947. Pubmed Central PMCID: 2063942.

8. Li P, Li M, Lindberg MR, Kennett MJ, Xiong N, Wang Y. PAD4 is essential for antibacterial innate immunity mediated by neutrophil extracellular traps. *J Exp Med* August 30, 2010;**207**(9):1853–62. PubMed PMID: 20733033. Pubmed Central PMCID: 2931169.

9. Kurien BT, Newland J, Paczkowski C, Moore KL, Scofield RH. Association of neutropenia in systemic lupus erythematosus (SLE) with anti-Ro and binding of an immunologically cross-reactive neutrophil membrane antigen. *Clin Exp Immunol* April 2000;**120**(1):209–17. PubMed PMID: 10759785. Pubmed Central PMCID: 1905619.

10. Ren Y, Tang J, Mok MY, Chan AW, Wu A, Lau CS. Increased apoptotic neutrophils and macrophages and impaired macrophage phagocytic clearance of apoptotic neutrophils in systemic lupus erythematosus. *Arthritis Rheum* October 2003;**48**(10):2888–97. PubMed PMID: 14558095.

11. Mikolajczyk TP, Skiba D, Batko B, Krezelok M, Wilk G, Osmenda G, et al. Characterization of the impairment of the uptake of apoptotic polymorphonuclear cells by monocyte subpopulations in systemic lupus erythematosus. *Lupus* November 2014;**23**(13):1358–69. PubMed PMID: 24969081.

12. Yu CL, Sun KH, Tsai CY, Wang SR. Inhibitory effects of anticardiolipin antibodies on lymphocyte proliferation and neutrophil phagocytosis. *Ann Rheum Dis* December 1991;**50**(12):903–8. PubMed PMID: 1768156. Pubmed Central PMCID: 1004578.

13. Zhou Y, Wu J, Kucik DF, White NB, Redden DT, Szalai AJ, et al. Multiple lupus-associated ITGAM variants alter Mac-1 functions on neutrophils. *Arthritis Rheum* November 2013;**65**(11):2907–16. PubMed PMID: 23918739. Pubmed Central PMCID: 3969028.

14. Knight JS, Kaplan MJ. Lupus neutrophils: 'NET' gain in understanding lupus pathogenesis. *Curr Opin Rheumatol* September 2012;**24**(5):441–50. PubMed PMID: 22617827.

15. Palanichamy A, Bauer JW, Yalavarthi S, Meednu N, Barnard J, Owen T, et al. Neutrophil-mediated IFN activation in the bone marrow alters B cell development in human and murine systemic lupus erythematosus. *J Immunol* February 1, 2014;**192**(3):906–18. PubMed PMID: 24379124. Pubmed Central PMCID: 3907774.

16. Garcia-Romo GS, Caielli S, Vega B, Connolly J, Allantaz F, Xu Z, et al. Netting neutrophils are major inducers of type I IFN production in pediatric systemic lupus erythematosus. *Sci Transl Med* March 9, 2011;**3**(73):73ra20. PubMed PMID: 21389264. Pubmed Central PMCID: 3143837.

17. Lande R, Ganguly D, Facchinetti V, Frasca L, Conrad C, Gregorio J, et al. Neutrophils activate plasmacytoid dendritic cells by releasing self-DNA-peptide complexes in systemic lupus erythematosus. *Sci Transl Med* March 9, 2011;**3**(73):73ra19. PubMed PMID: 21389263. Pubmed Central PMCID: 3399524.

18. Hakkim A, Furnrohr BG, Amann K, Laube B, Abed UA, Brinkmann V, et al. Impairment of neutrophil extracellular trap degradation is associated with lupus nephritis. *Proc Natl Acad Sci USA* May 25, 2010;**107**(21):9813–8. PubMed PMID: 20439745. Pubmed Central PMCID: 2906830.

19. Denny MF, Yalavarthi S, Zhao W, Thacker SG, Anderson M, Sandy AR, et al. A distinct subset of proinflammatory neutrophils isolated from patients with systemic lupus erythematosus induces vascular damage and synthesizes type I IFNs. *J Immunol* March 15, 2010;**184**(6):3284–97. PubMed PMID: 20164424. Pubmed Central PMCID: 2929645.

20. Villanueva E, Yalavarthi S, Berthier CC, Hodgin JB, Khandpur R, Lin AM, et al. Netting neutrophils induce endothelial damage, infiltrate tissues, and expose immunostimulatory molecules in systemic lupus erythematosus. *J Immunol* July 1, 2011;**187**(1):538–52. PubMed PMID: 21613614. Pubmed Central PMCID: 3119769.

21. Carmona-Rivera C, Zhao W, Yalavarthi S, Kaplan MJ. Neutrophil extracellular traps induce endothelial dysfunction in systemic lupus erythematosus through the activation of matrix metalloproteinase-2. *Ann Rheum Dis* February 25, 2014;**74**(7):1417–24. PubMed PMID: 24570026. Pubmed Central PMCID: 4143484.

22. Martinod K, Wagner DD. Thrombosis: tangled up in NETs. *Blood* May 1, 2014;**123**(18):2768–76. PubMed PMID: 24366358. Pubmed Central PMCID: 4007606.

23. Knight JS, Zhao W, Luo W, Subramanian V, O'Dell AA, Yalavarthi S, et al. Peptidylarginine deiminase inhibition is immunomodulatory and vasculoprotective in murine lupus. *J Clin Invest* July 1, 2013;**123**(7):2981–93. PubMed PMID: 23722903. Pubmed Central PMCID: 3696545.

24. Knight JS, Subramanian V, O'Dell A A, Yalavarthi S, Zhao W, Smith CK, et al. Peptidylarginine deiminase inhibition disrupts NET formation and protects against kidney, skin and vascular disease in lupus-prone MRL/lpr mice. *Ann Rheum Dis* August 7, 2014. pii: annrheumdis-2014-205365. http://dx.doi.org/10.1136/annrheumdis-2014-205365. PubMed PMID: 25104775.

25. Bennett L, Palucka AK, Arce E, Cantrell V, Borvak J, Banchereau J, et al. Interferon and granulopoiesis signatures in systemic lupus erythematosus blood. *J Exp Med* March 17, 2003;**197**(6):711–23. PubMed PMID: 12642603. Pubmed Central PMCID: 2193846.

26. Kaplan MJ. Neutrophils in the pathogenesis and manifestations of SLE. *Nat Rev Rheumatol* December 2011;**7**(12):691–9. PubMed PMID: 21947176. Pubmed Central PMCID: 3243068.

27. Coit P, Jeffries M, Altorok N, Dozmorov MG, Koelsch KA, Wren JD, et al. Genome-wide DNA methylation study suggests epigenetic accessibility and transcriptional poising of interferon-regulated genes in naive CD4+ T cells from lupus patients. *J Autoimmun* June 2013;**43**:78–84. PubMed PMID: 23623029. Pubmed Central PMCID: 3790645.

28. Coit P, Yalavarthi S, Ognenovski M, Zhao W, Hasni S, Wren JD, et al. Epigenome profiling reveals significant DNA demethylation of interferon signature genes in lupus neutrophils. *J Autoimmun* April 2015;**58**:59–66.

29. Sukapan P, Promnarate P, Avihingsanon Y, Mutirangura A, Hirankarn N. Types of DNA methylation status of the interspersed repetitive sequences for LINE-1, Alu, HERV-E and HERV-K in the neutrophils from systemic lupus erythematosus patients and healthy controls. *J Hum Genet* April 2014;**59**(4):178–88. PubMed PMID: 24430577.

Chapter 16

The Role of Dendritic Cells in Systemic Lupus Erythematosus

Clément Jacquemin, Patrick Blanco

University of Bordeaux, CIRID, UMR/CNRS, Bordeaux, France; CHU de Bordeaux, Bordeaux, France

Dendritic cells (DCs) were discovered in the 1970s by Ralph Steinman, primarily in mice and later in humans.[1] The early 1990s saw the description of different culture conditions, allowing the generation of large numbers of DC, and energized the study of DCs in both health and disease including autoimmune diseases. DCs represent the primary line of immune cell defense against pathogens that invade the body and form a critical interface between innate and adaptive immunity. Under steady-state conditions, DCs play important roles in the establishment of central and peripheral tolerance. Their critical role in the control of immunity and tolerance led to the hypothesis that their uncontrolled activation might drive autoimmune diseases including systemic lupus erythematosus (SLE).[2]

DENDRITIC CELL ORIGINS, SUBSETS, AND FUNCTIONS

Origins

DCs generally have a short half-life of 3–6 days and are constantly replenished from a bone marrow precursor cell, which undergoes a series of restricted differentiation programs. There is evidence that colony-stimulating factor 1 (CSF-1), Fms-like tyrosine kinase 3 ligand, and granulocyte–macrophage colony-stimulating factor (GM-CSF) are required for DC differentiation.[3] Although common lymphoid precursors can give rise to DCs, the vast majority of DCs in steady state originate from the common myeloid progenitor (MDP) cell that can differentiate into macrophages and dendritic cell progenitors.[4] The MDP gives rise to monocytes or commits toward plasmacytoid DCs (pDCs) or classical DCs. The only DC that does not originate in the bone marrow is the Langerhans cell. The Langerhans cell compartment is established before birth from fetal liver-derived monocytes, and Langerhans cells self-renew without replacement by blood-borne precursors.[5]

Subsets/Functions

Human and mouse DCs can be divided into two main subsets: plasmacytoid DCs (pDCs) and conventional/myeloid DCs (mDCs). In addition, current nomenclature describes two myeloid subsets characterized by the expression of CD1c/BDCA1 and CD141/BDCA-3 in human peripheral blood (Table 1).

Plasmacytoid DCs

pDCs represent around 1% of blood mononuclear cells in peripheral blood. In lymph nodes, they are found in the T-cell area and represent around 20% of MHC-II[+] cells. pDCs can be distinguished from mDCs and other cells by the surface markers CD123 (IL3-R), CD303 (BDCA2), and CD304 (neuropilin: BDCA4). pDCs are rare in peripheral tissues but they are rapidly recruited in inflammatory sites.[6] pDCs were initially identified in humans as natural interferon-producing cells or NIPC[7] and thus were claimed to be important in the defense against viral infections. Accordingly, within 6 h of viral activation, most of the transcriptome of human pDCs is composed of type I interferon (IFN) transcripts, and within 24 h they secrete up to 1000-fold more IFN-α than any other blood cell type, a direct consequence of their constitutive IRF7 expression. pDCs preferentially express intracellular Toll-like receptors, including TLR7 and TLR9, that can recognize ssRNA and ssDNA, respectively, and transduce signals on sensing viral and self-nucleic acids.[8] They can polarize Th1 or Th2 CD4[+] responses in a context-dependent manner.[9] pDCs have also been reported to promote peripheral tolerance through their ability to induce antigen-specific CD4[+] Foxp3[+] regulatory

TABLE 1 Phenotype for Human Dendritic Cell Subsets

		Dentritics Cells Type		
Antigen	pDCs	mDCs CD1c+	mDCs CD141+	MoDCs
CD11c	–	+	+	+
CD123	+	–	–	–
BDCA-2	+	–	–	–
BDCA-4	+	–	–	–
HLA-DR	+	+	+	+
IFNAR	+	+	+	+
CD14	–	–	–	–
CD80	+	+	+	+
CD86	+	+	+	+
CD40	+	+	+	+
CD32	+	+	+	+

+, defined positive expression of the Antigen; –, defined negative expression of the Antigen.

T cells and IL-10-producing T cells, which dampen the differentiation of antigen-specific CD4+ effector T cells induced by other DCs under both steady-state and inflammatory conditions in vivo. This tolerogenic function is abrogated, however, on activation with TLR ligands.[10]

Conventional/Myeloid DCs

Conventional DCs are a highly specialized DC subset that is efficient in antigen processing and presentation; they are present in the circulation and in lymphoid and nonlymphoid tissues. They can be divided into three main subsets based on surface marker expression and some of their functions: BDCA1/CD1c, BDCA3/CD141, and monocyte-derived dendritic cells (inflammatory DCs).[11] BDCA1 DCs secrete higher amounts of IL12 than BDCA3 DCs, whereas BDCA3 DCs secrete higher amounts of type I interferon than BDCA1.[12] Inflammatory DCs have been described recently in humans to be BDCA1/CD16+/−, and express a gene pattern similar to that of DCs and macrophages, suggesting that they derive from monocytes.[13] Under inflammatory conditions, after taking up and processing antigens from resident tissues, mDCs migrate to the peripheral draining lymph node via afferent lymph vessels to present antigen to naïve T cells, and to induce an immune response.

DCs and Tolerance

DCs in Central Tolerance

Thymic DCs contribute to CD4 and CD8 T-cell deletion as well as to natural regulatory T-cell (nTreg) generation in vivo. Medullary thymic epithelial cells are primarily responsible for the negative selection of autoreactive T cells, owing to the expression of the transcription factor autoimmune regulator (AIRE) driving the expression of tissue-specific self-antigen.[14] Thymic DCs, which are located in close interaction with medullary thymic epithelial cells (mTEC), can uptake self-antigens expressed by mTEC and cross-present them either to induce deletion or to promote the generation of nTregs.[15] Peripheral DCs can also migrate to the thymus and present peripheral self-antigens to induce clonal deletion of T cells or to induce Treg generation.[16]

DCs in Peripheral Tolerance

DCs are involved in guarding immune homeostasis in the periphery. mDCs capture apoptotic cells and migrate, without maturing, to the draining lymph node. There, they present self-peptide–MHC complexes in the absence of costimulation signals to circulating naive autoreactive T cells, resulting in anergy or deletion.[17] Immature DCs may also control peripheral tolerance through the induction and maintenance of Treg cells.[18] DCs can induce Treg cells in the presence of TGF-β and retinoic acid. Such tolerance mechanisms prevent or reduce the development of autoimmunity when dying cells are generated and processed at the time of infection.[19] Yet, constitutive ablation of DCs in autoimmunity-prone mice ameliorated rather than exacerbated the resulting disease. Thus DCs can promote or curtail an inflammatory or autoimmune response.

DCs AND SLE

pDCs

Number/Activation Status

Blood pDCs numbers are reduced in SLE patients due to an accelerated migration to inflammatory sites.[20] Although a prominent role for type I interferon in SLE pathogenesis has been known since the 1970s when high levels of type I interferon were detected in SLE patients,[21] a crucial connection between pDCs and SLE pathogenesis came with the finding that ICs can activate these cells to secrete type I IFN through the triggering of TLR7/9.[22] As an example, pDCs are enriched in kidneys of patients with glomerulonephritis, and IFN-α transcripts are present in biopsy specimens from those patients.[23] In skin biopsies, from patients with cutaneous lupus, pDCs are enriched, and Mx1 protein, a classic protein induced by type I interferon, can be detected.

In vitro systems have been used to demonstrate induction of type I Interferon-induced transcripts and/or IFN-α in PBMC or purified pDCs by serum or immune complexes from patients, and by reconstituted immune complexes that contain autoantibodies and RNA, apoptotic, or necrotic material.[24] This effect can be inhibited by blockade of the FcgammaRIIa, or degradation of RNA or DNA, and blocking the acidification of the endosomal compartment by chloroquine.[24]

In vivo, genetic ablation of type I IFN signaling ameliorates SLE development in NZB/NZW-derived lupus mouse strains.[25] Furthermore, changing the level of TLR expression by increasing *Tlr7* gene dosage, as an example, has been implicated in the development of autoimmune disease. For example BXSB/MpJ mice, which carry the Yaa (Y-linked autoimmune acceleration) translocation of the locus encoding *Tlr7* from the X chromosome onto the Y chromosome, have one extra copy of *Tlr7* and develop an SLE-like disease.[26] Specific depletion of pDCs in different murine models reduced disease manifestations including autoantibody production, glomerulonephritis, and expression of IFN-inducible genes.[27]

Chronic signaling in pDCs through TLRs during the course of SLE renders pDCs resistant to low-dose glucocorticoid-mediated NFκB inhibition. Therefore, pDCs in SLE may generate resistance to treatment and may enforce the use of higher doses of steroids, which are known to suppress the IFN signature.[28]

Implication for T-Cell Activation

When activated, pDCs produce IL-6, TNF-α, and chemokines, for example, CXCL9 (MIG), CXCL10 (IP-10), CCL3 (MIP-1α), CCL4 (MIP-1β), and CCL5 (RANTES), which are able to attract activated CD4 and CD8 T cells to the sites of inflammation and upregulate the chemokine receptor CCR7, directing them through its ligand CCL21 and CCL19 to secondary lymph organs to prime naive T cells.[29] Yet, a direct role of pDCs in autoimmune T-cell activation and/or priming remains to be established in humans.

Implication for B-Cell Activation

pDCs also activate B cells in a type I IFN-dependent manner. Indeed, virus-activated pDCs induce the maturation of TLR9-activated memory B cells into plasma cells. First, pDC-derived type I IFN promotes their differentiation into plasmablasts and then IL-6, which is also released by pDCs, induces the full differentiation into antibody-secreting plasma cells.[30] Although, not directly demonstrated in human SLE, this type I IFN/IL-6 synergistic activation of B cells could play a major role in SLE.

Myeloid DCs

Number/Activation Status

Several groups have noted that the number of cDCs is decreased in SLE, whereas there is evidence that mDCs are chronically activated. cDCs from patients spontaneously overexpress costimulatory molecules such as CD86 and CD80 and secrete proinflammatory cytokines including IL-6 and TNF-α.[31] The high-mobility group protein B1, which is attached to apoptotic chromatin, leads to the activation of mDCs via TLR2.[32] Moreover, monocytes, which represent a major source of precursors that differentiate into DCs under inflammatory conditions,[33] behave like mDCs in SLE patients. Conversely, exposure of normal monocytes to SLE serum results in the generation of DCs.[20] Thus, SLE blood represents a DC-inducing and -activating environment. Whether the BDCA1 and the BDCA3 populations are playing different role in SLE remains unclear.[2] Increased immunogenicity of cDCs has also been observed in susceptible mouse strains where autologous cDCs loaded with antigens from dying cells break self-tolerance and trigger an immune response against nuclear antigens.[34] Conversely, DC-specific deletion of several negative regulators, responsible for spontaneous DCs maturation, is sufficient to induce an SLE-like disease in vivo.[35]

Implication in T-Cell Activation

Unabated DCs activation could lead to the activation and expansion of autoreactive T cells, thus explaining many of the features of the disease. DCs generated in the presence of SLE sera (SLE-DCs) also drive the differentiation of CD8+ T cells toward fully active cytotoxic effector T lymphocytes able to generate nucleosomes and granzyme B-dependent autoantigens.[36] These autoantigens could be captured and presented by mDCs, therefore further broadening the autoimmune process.

Implication in B-Cell Activation

In lupus-prone mice, activated DCs induce B-cell proliferation and enhance antibody production. In humans, IFN-activated mDCs boost their ability to induce B-cell growth and differentiation through IL-12, IL-6, and B-cell-activating factor (BAFF).[37] Conversely, overexpression of BAFF in mice leads to the development of an SLE-like disease that is independent of T cells, and BAFF is elevated in the serum of SLE patients and correlates with disease activity.[38] Type I IFN increases the responsiveness of B cells to a proliferation-inducing ligand (APRIL), another TNF family member[38] that shares a common receptor with BAFF and is also involved in B-cell survival and T-cell-independent B-cell responses. cDCs from SLE patients can also efficiently stimulate in vitro naive and memory B cells to differentiate into IgG and IgA plasmablasts resembling those found in the blood of SLE patients. SLE-DC-mediated IgG plasmablast differentiation is dependent on BAFF and IL-10, whereas IgA plasmablast differentiation is dependent on APRIL. Importantly, SLE-DCs express CD138 and trans-present CD138-bound APRIL to B cells, leading to the induction of IgA switching and PB differentiation in an IFN-α-independent manner. Noteworthy, CD138-bound APRIL is expressed on blood monocytes from active SLE patients.[39]

OVERALL PICTURE OF DC IMPLICATION IN SLE PATHOGENESIS

IFN-α, produced by pDC, acts on monocyte and induces an mDC-like phenotype and function. mDCs migrate to the inflammatory sites and interact with effector lymphocyte cells. This interaction promotes the activation of autoreactive CD8+ cytotoxic lymphocyte T cells and CD4+ helper lymphocyte T cells, while regulatory CD4+ Foxp3+ T-cell functions are blocked. Activated

autoreactive CD4+ T cells can be differentiated into effector Th cells able to help B cells to produce autoantibodies in secondary lymphoid organs. Autoantibodies form IC with autoantigens. ICs act directly or indirectly on pDCs to induce the production of type I interferon (Figure 1).

AMPLIFYING MECHANISMS PROMOTING IFN-α SECRETION IN SLE AND ACTIVATION OF DCs

Pioneering work from Ronnblom's group showed that sera from SLE patients contained an endogenous type I interferon inducer, characterized as being immune complexes. Such ICs are internalized via the FcgammaR expressed on pDCs, reach the endosome, and stimulate the relevant TLR with subsequent production of type I interferon.[40] Interestingly, several other cells harboring FcgammaR can be activated by immune complexes and contribute to pDCs activation and type I interferon secretion.

NK Cell Help

In vitro experiments reveal that NK cells can interact with pDCs to potently enhance IFN-α production on stimulation with viruses, synthetic oligonucleotides, or RNA-containing ICs. In SLE, NK activated via the FCgammaRIIa or by cytokines including IL-12 or IL-18 release MIP-1β and

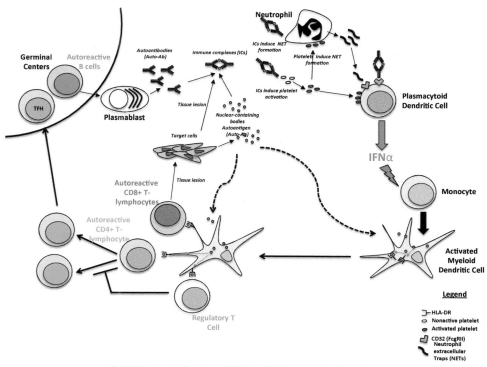

FIGURE 1   Implication of DCs in SLE immune dysfunctions.

mediate LFA-1-dependent cell–cell contact to stimulate type I interferon production by pDCs.[41]

Platelet Help

Platelet activation during SLE has been reported. Increased levels of phosphatidylserine thromboxane biosynthesis, soluble P-selectin, and platelet/monocyte aggregates can be found in SLE patients.[42] The transcriptional profile of SLE platelets disclosed a type I interferon and an activation signature.[43] Although the underlying mechanism of platelet activation in SLE relies probably on different mechanisms, immune complexes from SLE patients can directly induce platelet activation. Once activated platelets release active CD154 and modulate the adaptive immunity through their ability to activate antigen-presenting cells including dendritic cells.[44] Interestingly, platelets can interact with pDCs in SLE patients. As a consequence, activated platelets significantly increase the secretion of type I interferon on the triggering of TLR9 and TLR7 by pDCs.[45] Moreover, platelets could have a broader impact on type I interferon secretion through their ability to interact with neutrophils. Indeed, activated platelets can bind to neutrophils and promote the release of neutrophil extracellular traps (NETs), thus amplifying again the mechanism.

Neutrophil Help

On activation with certain stimuli, such as PMA, neutrophils undergo *NETosis*, a form of death characterized by the release of fibrous structures (NETs) made of decondensed chromatin as well as granular and cytoplasmic neutrophil proteins that participate in microbial killing.[46] NET formation is an active process that depends on the activation of the Raf–MEK–ERK pathway and ROS production.[47] It requires the translocation of neutrophil elastase and myeloperoxidase from cytoplasmic granules to the nucleus, which results in histone degradation and chromatin decondensation. Histone citrullination may also play a role in NETs formation, as inhibition of the major histone-citrullinating enzyme, peptidylarginine deiminase 4, interferes with NETs release.[48] Interestingly, autoanti-bodies from SLE patients that recognize either NAs or antimicrobial peptides such as LL37 (cathelicidin/CAMP) induce the release of DNA complexed with proteins by SLE but not healthy neutrophils.[49] These complexes are highly immunostimulatory as they activate pDCs to secrete type I IFN.[49,50]

REFERENCES

1. Steinman RM, Cohn ZA. Identification of a novel cell type in peripheral lymphoid organs of mice. I. Morphology, quantitation, tissue distribution. *J Exp Med* May 1, 1973;**137**(5):1142–62.
2. Blanco P, Palucka AK, Pascual V, Banchereau J. Dendritic cells and cytokines in human inflammatory and autoimmune diseases. *Cytokine Growth Factor Rev* February 5, 2008;**19**(1):41–52.
3. Maraskovsky E, Daro E, Roux E, Teepe M, Maliszewski CR, Hoek J, et al. In vivo generation of human dendritic cell subsets by Flt3 ligand. *Blood* August 1, 2000;**96**(3):878–84.
4. Doulatov S, Notta F, Eppert K, Nguyen LT, Ohashi PS, Dick JE. Revised map of the human progenitor hierarchy shows the origin of macrophages and dendritic cells in early lymphoid development. *Nat Immunol* July 2010;**11**(7):585–93.
5. Hoeffel G, Wang Y, Greter M, See P, Teo P, Malleret B, et al. Adult Langerhans cells derive predominantly from embryonic fetal liver monocytes with a minor contribution of yolk sac-derived macrophages. *J Exp Med* June 4, 2012;**209**(6):1167–81.
6. Zaba LC, Krueger JG, Lowes MA. Resident and "inflammatory" dendritic cells in human skin. *J Invest Dermatol* February 2009;**129**(2):302–8.
7. Siegal FP, Kadowaki N, Shodell M, Fitzgerald-Bocarsly PA, Shah K, Ho S, et al. The nature of the principal type 1 interferon-producing cells in human blood. *Science* June 11, 1999;**284**(5421):1835–7.
8. Gilliet M, Cao W, Liu YJ. Plasmacytoid dendritic cells: sensing nucleic acids in viral infection and autoimmune diseases. *Nat Rev Immunol* August 2008;**8**(8):594–606.
9. Grouard G, Rissoan MC, Filgueira L, Durand I, Banchereau J, Liu YJ. The enigmatic plasmacytoid T cells develop into dendritic cells with interleukin (IL)-3 and CD40-ligand. *J Exp Med* March 17, 1997;**185**(6):1101–11.
10. Ito T, Yang M, Wang YH, Lande R, Gregorio J, Perng OA, et al. Plasmacytoid dendritic cells prime IL-10-producing T regulatory cells by inducible costimulator ligand. *J Exp Med* January 22, 2007;**204**(1):105–15.
11. Haniffa M, Collin M, Ginhoux F. Ontogeny and functional specialization of dendritic cells in human and mouse. *Adv Immunol* 2013;**120**:1–49.
12. Meixlsperger S, Leung CS, Ramer PC, Pack M, Vanoaica LD, Breton G, et al. CD141+ dendritic cells produce prominent amounts of IFN-alpha after dsRNA recognition and can be targeted via DEC-205 in humanized mice. *Blood* June 20, 2013;**121**(25):5034–44.
13. Segura E, Touzot M, Bohineust A, Cappuccio A, Chiocchia G, Hosmalin A, et al. Human inflammatory dendritic cells induce Th17 cell differentiation. *Immunity* February 21, 2013;**38**(2):336–48.
14. Anderson MS, Venanzi ES, Klein L, Chen Z, Berzins SP, Turley SJ, et al. Projection of an immunological self shadow within the thymus by the aire protein. *Science* November 15, 2002;**298**(5597):1395–401.
15. Perry JS, Lio CW, Kau AL, Nutsch K, Yang Z, Gordon JI, et al. Distinct contributions of Aire and antigen-presenting-cell subsets to the generation of self-tolerance in the thymus. *Immunity* September 18, 2014;**41**(3):414–26.
16. Hadeiba H, Butcher EC. Thymus-homing dendritic cells in central tolerance. *Eur J Immunol* June 2013;**43**(6):1425–9.
17. Steinman RM, Hawiger D, Nussenzweig MC. Tolerogenic dendritic cells. *Annu Rev Immunol* 2003;**21**:685–711.
18. Vitali C, Mingozzi F, Broggi A, Barresi S, Zolezzi F, Bayry J, et al. Migratory, and not lymphoid-resident, dendritic cells maintain peripheral self-tolerance and prevent autoimmunity via induction of iTreg cells. *Blood* August 9, 2012;**120**(6):1237–45.
19. Darrasse-Jeze G, Deroubaix S, Mouquet H, Victora GD, Eisenreich T, Yao KH, et al. Feedback control of regulatory T cell homeostasis by dendritic cells in vivo. *J Exp Med* August 31, 2009;**206**(9):1853–62.
20. Blanco P, Palucka AK, Gill M, Pascual V, Banchereau J. Induction of dendritic cell differentiation by IFN-alpha in systemic lupus erythematosus. *Science* November 16, 2001;**294**(5546):1540–3.

21. Hooks JJ, Moutsopoulos HM, Geis SA, Stahl NI, Decker JL, Notkins AL. Immune interferon in the circulation of patients with autoimmune disease. *N Engl J Med* July 5, 1979;**301**(1):5–8.

22. Barrat FJ, Meeker T, Gregorio J, Chan JH, Uematsu S, Akira S, et al. Nucleic acids of mammalian origin can act as endogenous ligands for Toll-like receptors and may promote systemic lupus erythematosus. *J Exp Med* October 17, 2005;**202**(8):1131–9.

23. Tucci M, Quatraro C, Lombardi L, Pellegrino C, Dammacco F, Silvestris F. Glomerular accumulation of plasmacytoid dendritic cells in active lupus nephritis: role of interleukin-18. *Arthritis Rheum* January 2008;**58**(1):251–62.

24. Bave U, Alm GV, Ronnblom L. The combination of apoptotic U937 cells and lupus IgG is a potent IFN-alpha inducer. *J Immunol* September 15, 2000;**165**(6):3519–26.

25. Santiago-Raber ML, Baccala R, Haraldsson KM, Choubey D, Stewart TA, Kono DH, et al. Type-I interferon receptor deficiency reduces lupus-like disease in NZB mice. *J Exp Med* March 17, 2003;**197**(6):777–88.

26. Pisitkun P, Deane JA, Difilippantonio MJ, Tarasenko T, Satterthwaite AB, Bolland S. Autoreactive B cell responses to RNA-related antigens due to TLR7 gene duplication. *Science* June 16, 2006;**312**(5780): 1669–72.

27. Sisirak V, Ganguly D, Lewis KL, Couillault C, Tanaka L, Bolland S, et al. Genetic evidence for the role of plasmacytoid dendritic cells in systemic lupus erythematosus. *J Exp Med* September 22, 2014;**211**(10):1969–76.

28. Guiducci C, Gong M, Xu Z, Gill M, Chaussabel D, Meeker T, et al. TLR recognition of self nucleic acids hampers glucocorticoid activity in lupus. *Nature* June 17, 2010;**465**(7300):937–41.

29. Villadangos JA, Young L. Antigen-presentation properties of plasmacytoid dendritic cells. *Immunity* September 19, 2008;**29**(3):352–61.

30. Jego G, Palucka AK, Blanck JP, Chalouni C, Pascual V, Banchereau J. Plasmacytoid dendritic cells induce plasma cell differentiation through type I interferon and interleukin 6. *Immunity* August 2003;**19**(2):225–34.

31. Kis-Toth K, Tsokos GC. Dendritic cell function in lupus: Independent contributors or victims of aberrant immune regulation. *Autoimmunity* March 2010;**43**(2):121–30.

32. Urbonaviciute V, Furnrohr BG, Meister S, Munoz L, Heyder P, De Marchis F, et al. Induction of inflammatory and immune responses by HMGB1-nucleosome complexes: implications for the pathogenesis of SLE. *J Exp Med* December 22, 2008;**205**(13):3007–18.

33. Cheong C, Matos I, Choi JH, Dandamudi DB, Shrestha E, Longhi MP, et al. Microbial stimulation fully differentiates monocytes to DC-SIGN/CD209(+) dendritic cells for immune T cell areas. *Cell* October 29, 2010;**143**(3):416–29.

34. Bondanza A, Zimmermann VS, Dell'Antonio G, Dal Cin E, Capobianco A, Sabbadini MG, et al. Cutting edge: dissociation between autoimmune response and clinical disease after vaccination with dendritic cells. *J Immunol* January 1, 2003;**170**(1):24–7.

35. Kim SJ, Gregersen PK, Diamond B. Regulation of dendritic cell activation by microRNA let-7c and BLIMP1. *J Clin Invest* February 1, 2013;**123**(2):823–33.

36. Blanco P, Pitard V, Viallard JF, Taupin JL, Pellegrin JL, Moreau JF. Increase in activated CD8+ T lymphocytes expressing perforin and granzyme B correlates with disease activity in patients with systemic lupus erythematosus. *Arthritis Rheum* January 2005;**52**(1):201–11.

37. Le Bon A, Thompson C, Kamphuis E, Durand V, Rossmann C, Kalinke U, et al. Cutting edge: enhancement of antibody responses through direct stimulation of B and T cells by type I IFN. *J Immunol* February 15, 2006;**176**(4):2074–8.

38. Vincent FB, Morand EF, Schneider P, Mackay F. The BAFF/APRIL system in SLE pathogenesis. *Nat Rev Rheumatol* June 2014;**10**(6): 365–73.

39. Joo H, Coquery C, Xue Y, Gayet I, Dillon SR, Punaro M, et al. Serum from patients with SLE instructs monocytes to promote IgG and IgA plasmablast differentiation. *J Exp Med* July 2, 2012;**209**(7):1335–48.

40. Ronnblom L, Eloranta ML, Alm GV. Role of natural interferon-alpha producing cells (plasmacytoid dendritic cells) in autoimmunity. *Autoimmunity* December 2003;**36**(8):463–72.

41. Hagberg N, Theorell J, Schlums H, Eloranta ML, Bryceson YT, Ronnblom L. Systemic lupus erythematosus immune complexes increase the expression of SLAM family members CD319 (CRACC) and CD229 (LY-9) on plasmacytoid dendritic cells and CD319 on CD56(dim) NK cells. *J Immunol* September 15, 2013;**191**(6): 2989–98.

42. Nagahama M, Nomura S, Ozaki Y, Yoshimura C, Kagawa H, Fukuhara S. Platelet activation markers and soluble adhesion molecules in patients with systemic lupus erythematosus. *Autoimmunity* 2001;**33**(2):85–94.

43. Lood C, Amisten S, Gullstrand B, Jonsen A, Allhorn M, Truedsson L, et al. Platelet transcriptional profile and protein expression in patients with systemic lupus erythematosus: up-regulation of the type I interferon system is strongly associated with vascular disease. *Blood* September 16, 2010;**116**(11):1951–7.

44. Elzey BD, Tian J, Jensen RJ, Swanson AK, Lees JR, Lentz SR, et al. Platelet-mediated modulation of adaptive immunity. A communication link between innate and adaptive immune compartments. *Immunity* July 2003;**19**(1):9–19.

45. Duffau P, Seneschal J, Nicco C, Richez C, Lazaro E, Douchet I, et al. Platelet CD154 potentiates interferon-alpha secretion by plasmacytoid dendritic cells in systemic lupus erythematosus. *Sci Transl Med* September 1, 2010;**2**(47): 47ra63.

46. Brinkmann V, Reichard U, Goosmann C, Fauler B, Uhlemann Y, Weiss DS, et al. Neutrophil extracellular traps kill bacteria. *Science* March 5, 2004;**303**(5663):1532–5.

47. Hakkim A, Fuchs TA, Martinez NE, Hess S, Prinz H, Zychlinsky A, et al. Activation of the Raf-MEK-ERK pathway is required for neutrophil extracellular trap formation. *Nat Chem Biol* February 2010;**7**(2):75–7.

48. Dwivedi N, Radic M. Citrullination of autoantigens implicates NETosis in the induction of autoimmunity. *Ann Rheum Dis* March 2014;**73**(3):483–91.

49. Lande R, Ganguly D, Facchinetti V, Frasca L, Conrad C, Gregorio J, et al. Neutrophils activate plasmacytoid dendritic cells by releasing self-DNA-peptide complexes in systemic lupus erythematosus. *Sci Transl Med* March 9, 2011;**3**(73): 73ra19.

50. Garcia-Romo GS, Caielli S, Vega B, Connolly J, Allantaz F, Xu Z, et al. Netting neutrophils are major inducers of type I IFN production in pediatric systemic lupus erythematosus. *Sci Transl Med* March 9, 2011;**3**(73): 73ra20.

Chapter 17

Cytokines

Vaishali R. Moulton
Division of Rheumatology, Department of Medicine, Beth Israel Deaconess Medical Center, Harvard Medical School, Boston, MA, USA

CYTOKINES IN SYSTEMIC LUPUS ERYTHEMATOSUS

Cytokines produced by the cells of the innate immune system important in systemic lupus erythematosus (SLE) pathogenesis include interferon alpha (IFN-α), interleukin (IL)-1, IL-6, tumor necrosis factor (TNF), IL-10, B-cell activating factor (BAFF), and a proliferation-inducing ligand (APRIL). Cytokines produced by the adaptive immune system include those produced by the CD4 T-helper (Th) cells and are IL-2, Th1 cytokines (IFN-γ), Th2 cytokines (IL-4, IL-5, IL-9, IL-13, IL-25), and Th17 (IL-17, IL-21) cytokines.[1,2] CD4 T helper (Th) cell differentiation into distinct cell lineages is driven by specific cytokines (Figure 1). IL-12 drives a Th1 differentiation important for cell-mediated immunity against intracellular pathogens, IL-4 is required for a Th2 differentiation necessary for a humoral response against extracellular pathogens, and a combination of IL-6, TGFβ, IL-23, and IL-21 drives Th17 differentiation, important for certain types of bacterial and fungal infections.[3] TGFβ in the absence of inflammation drives regulatory T-cell (Treg) generation, and IL-6 with IL-21 leads to T follicular helper (Tfh) cell differentiation (Figure 1). The differentiation into these specific cell types is controlled by lineage-specific transcription factors. T-bet and GATA-3 are important for Th1 and Th2 differentiation, respectively. RORγt and RORα are activating factors for IL-17 transcription. FoxP3 is the transcription factor important for Tregs whereas Bcl-6 is important for Tfh-cell differentiation.

The role and regulation of a few cytokines shown to be important in SLE pathophysiology are described below.

IL-2

T cells from patients with SLE produce aberrantly low amounts of the vital cytokine IL-2. IL-2 is important in autoimmune disease not only because it is necessary for the proliferation and function of Treg cells but also because it is vital for activation-induced cell death which is important for the deletion of autoreactive T cells. In addition, IL-2 is important for cell-mediated immunity, which is crucial,

as patients with autoimmune disease are susceptible to infections either due to immunosuppressive therapy or due to dysregulated immune responses. Tregs qualified by the CD4+ CD25+ or CD4+CD25+FoxP3+ phenotype are impaired in proliferation in human autoimmune disease, accounting for their reduced numbers and function.[4] Studies in IL-2 and IL-2 receptor knockout mice have shown that these mice develop severe spontaneous autoimmune disease and succumb to lymphoproliferative disease.[5] A deficiency of Tregs in these mice is thought to account for the unchecked proliferation of lymphocytes, leading to lymphadenopathy.[6]

Whereas IL-2 production is reduced and is protective for autoimmunity, it has also been ascribed a proinflammatory role in selective target tissues rendering its role in disease complicated.[7] Whereas IL-2 knockout and FoxP3-deficient scurfy mice both develop multiorgan inflammation, the IL-2 ko mice do not develop skin and lung inflammation. It was shown that IL-2 controls the migration and localization of both Th1 and Th2 CD4 T cells in an organ-specific manner. IL-2-deficient mice demonstrated a lack of trafficking receptors and Th2 cytokines (IL-4, IL-5, IL-13) important for skin and lung inflammation, revealing a target organ-specific proinflammatory role for IL-2.

IL-2 gene expression is controlled mainly at the transcriptional and posttranscriptional levels. Transcription factors NFAT, AP1, and NFκB among others are key factors, which bind to cognate sites within the *IL-2* promoter (Figure 2). On T-cell activation, TCR signaling induces intracellular signaling cascades that ultimately lead to the translocation of NFAT and NFκB into the nucleus and initiate transcription of IL-2. In SLE T cells, reduced amounts and activity of NFκB and AP1 are thought to contribute to lower IL-2 expression. Whereas NFAT is increased in SLE T cells, hence activating CD40L expression, NFAT in conjunction with AP1 is necessary for IL-2 transcriptional activation.[8] Therefore, the lack of AP1 is important in the IL-2 defect. More recently an RNA-binding protein SRSF1 was identified to play a role in IL-2 production by activating IL-2 transcription indirectly. SRSF1 expression was reduced in patients with SLE and more so in patients with active disease. Interestingly, SRSF1 force-expressed into SLE T cells rescued IL-2 production.[9] In addition to these

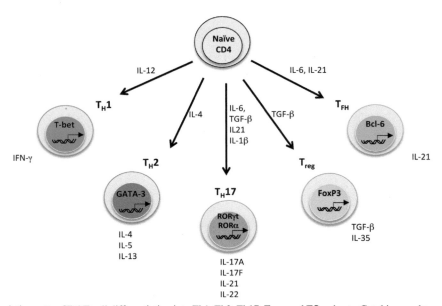

FIGURE 1 Diagram depicting naïve CD4 T-cell differentiation into Th1, Th2, Th17, Treg, and Tfh subsets. Cytokines and transcription factors involved in lineage-specific differentiation are indicated.

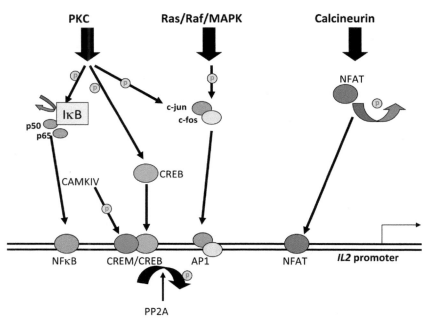

FIGURE 2 Signaling pathways and transcription factors involved in IL-2 production in T cells.

factors, a balance between the transcription factors cyclic AMP response element modulator (CREM) and CREB is important in IL-2 regulation (Figure 2). Both factors compete for binding to a CRE site at the −180 position within the *IL-2* promoter. In SLE T cells, disruption of this balance is thought to contribute to the reduced IL-2 expression. Protein kinase A (PKA) phosphorylates and PP2A dephosphorylates CREB. Reduced PKA activity and increased expression of the PP2A lead to reduced availability of pCREB.

Increased expression of CREM is attributed to the increase in transcription mediated by the SP1 transcription factor and binding to the *CREM* promoter. CREM is phosphorylated by the calcium-regulated kinase CAMKIV. CAMKIV is increased in SLE T cells and therefore increased pCREM leads to IL-2 repression. Serum from SLE patients induced the increased binding of CREM to the *IL-2* promoter through activation of CAMKIV,[10] and T cells from MRL/lpr lupus-prone mice also showed increased levels of

CAMKIV. CAMKIV inhibitor treatment was able to prevent and correct autoimmunity and disease pathology in lupus-prone mice.[11]

IL-17

IL-17 (IL-17A, IL-17F) is a proinflammatory cytokine, essential for host defense against bacteria and fungi. However its importance in autoimmune disease pathogenesis has recently been uncovered, both in patients and in animal models. IL-17 is produced by a subset of activated CD4 T cells under inflammatory conditions. Increased levels of IL-17 in the serum and increased numbers of IL-17-producing cells were demonstrated in SLE patients. Increased IL-17 was found in target organs such as skin, lungs, and kidneys, indicating a role of IL-17 in local tissue damage. Patients with lupus nephritis had increased numbers of IL-17-producing double negative T cells in the kidneys.[12] Increased expression was also noted in muscle tissue from patients with autoimmune myositis.[4] Recently, IL-17 has emerged as an important driver of pathogenic inflammation, and is considered a key underlying element in the pathogenesis of autoimmune diseases such as SLE, MS, and others.

IL-17 gene transcription is controlled by the retinoid-related orphan receptor (ROR) γ T and RORα transcription factors. RORγt drives differentiation of the Th17 cells and is exclusively expressed by Th17 cells. IL-17 is thought to be the key cytokine mediating inflammation as demonstrated in numerous autoimmune diseases including SLE and MS. Besides its role in inflammation, it also affects other cell types such as B cells. Peripheral blood mononuclear cells from patients with lupus nephritis when treated with IL-17 produced increased amounts of dsDNA autoantibodies and IL-6, suggesting its role in B-cell regulation. CD4 T cells when stimulated under proinflammatory conditions including cytokines IL-6, IL-23, IL-21, and TGFβ will differentiate into the Th17 phenotype and produce IL-17. IL-23 is necessary to initiate the IL-17 production while IL-21 is required for maintenance of IL-17. In lupus-prone mice it was shown that an IL-23 receptor deficiency lowered IL-17 production, and more importantly these mice were protected from development of disease.[13] IL-6, IL-21, and IL-23 bind to their respective receptors and through the JAK–STAT signaling pathway activate the same transcription factor STAT3, which can directly bind to the IL-17 and IL-21 genes. T cells from SLE patients were found to have increased STAT3 activity. This was also associated with their enhanced chemokine-mediated migration capacity.[1]

IL-6

IL-6 is a pleiotropic cytokine secreted by a large variety of cells and mediates its effects through activation and differentiation of immune cells including T and B lymphocytes.[14]

IL-6 exerts its effects on target cells via the IL-6 receptor, which has two components: the 80kDa IL-6R α chain, which is the IL-6-binding chain, and the IL-6R β chain (gp 130), which is the signal-transducing chain. The pathogenic role of IL-6 has been demonstrated both in human SLE and in murine lupus disease. IL-6-deficient MRL/lpr mice show delayed disease development and reduced renal pathology including IgG and C3 complement deposition.[15] In pristane-induced lupus, IL-6-deficient mice showed less severe kidney disease and reduced levels of autoantibodies.[16] In other mice models such as the BWF mice, administration of IL-6 increases, whereas blocking IL-6 reduces anti-DNA autoantibody production. Additionally, an acceleration of renal pathology, increased expression of MHC class II on mesangial cells, and increased glomerular ICAM-1 expression were observed in female BWF mice administered the human IL-6 cytokine. As in mice, elevated levels of IL-6 have been observed in patients with SLE and have been shown to correlate variably with disease severity or anti-dsDNA autoantibodies. Increased numbers of IL-6-producing cells in the PBMCs of SLE patients correlate with disease severity and autoreactive T-cell clones from patients produce high amounts of IL-6, which in turn mediates effects on B cells. IL-6 is known to promote B-cell activation and autoantibody production in SLE as evidenced by exogenous administration of IL-6 as well as by neutralizing antibodies.[17]

TNF

TNF is secreted by activated macrophages and other immune cells including monocytes and T cells. TNF mediates its effects through two distinct receptors, TNFR1 (p55) and TNFR2 (p75), and can induce either proinflammatory or anti-inflammatory pathways depending on receptor engagement.[18] Through the TNFR1, apoptosis and anti-inflammatory pathways are triggered via the Fas-associated death domain (FADD) and caspase cascade.[14] Alternatively, recruitment of TNF receptor-associated factor 2 (TRAF2) is proinflammatory via activation of NF-κB and JNK and MAP kinase pathways. These pathways are also activated when TNF engages TNFR2. The effects of these opposing functions of TNF as a proinflammatory or an immunoregulatory cytokine have been demonstrated in autoimmune disease as well. In mice, many studies have shown the pathogenic role of TNF. MRL/lpr mice were found to have increased TNF levels in serum and in kidneys, which correlated with disease,[19,20] and TNF blockade treatment proved advantageous in this mouse strain. Anti-TNF treatment also led to reduced development of autoantibodies, proteinuria, and IgG deposition in kidneys of lupus-prone mice.[21,22] On the other hand, TNF-deficient SLE mice had exacerbation of disease and recombinant TNF administration in BWF mice was beneficial.

These contradictory roles of TNF in disease reflect the dual function of this cytokine in pro- and anti-inflammatory processes. Similar to the studies in mice, data from human studies are complicated. While some studies found elevated serum TNF levels and disease correlation in patients with SLE, others did not.[23,24] Besides the circulating TNFα, tissue-specific cytokine expression may contribute locally to tissue pathology in SLE. Increased expression of TNF gene and protein expression was demonstrated in kidney biopsies from 52% of patients with lupus nephritis.[25] Reduced expression of TNF adaptor proteins TRAF2, TNF receptor 1-associated DEATH domain, FADD, and receptor interacting protein 1 in PBMCs from SLE patients may contribute to the antiapoptotic effects and increased survival of autoreactive cells,[26] whereas increased expression of these adaptor proteins was found in kidneys from lupus nephritis patients,[27] which may account for the local inflammatory effect of TNFα. Thus the systemic and local effects of TNF may be uncoupled via the distinct actions on TNF receptors and adaptor molecules such that it has a systemically immune modulatory function and a local proinflammatory effect.

IFN-α

IFN-α is a prototype member of the type I interferon family, which comprises other cytokines including IFN-β, IFN-ω, IFN-κ, and IFN ε/τ. All type I interferons bind to the IFN-α/β receptor. IFN-α is produced primarily by plasmacytoid dendritic cells and induces monocyte differentiation into myeloid DC, which are potent antigen-presenting cells. Early evidence suggested increased levels of IFN-α in the serum of SLE patients and correlated with SLE disease activity index (SLEDAI) scores, tissue damage, anti-dsDNA autoantibodies, and complement activation.[28–30] Gene expression profiling data from peripheral blood mononuclear cells and target organs of patients with SLE have shown elevated levels of genes regulated by type I interferon—the IFN signature.[31–34] Patients treated with IFN developed autoantibodies, suggesting a mechanistic role for IFN-α in SLE.[35,36] Additionally, deficiency of the IFN-α/β receptor in murine lupus ameliorated the onset and severity of disease, supporting this observation.[37,38] IFN-α can promote B-cell differentiation and autoantibody production, supporting a potential role for IFN-α in lupus pathogenesis. On the contrary, in the lupus-prone MRL/lpr mice deficient for the type I interferon receptor, a protective role for IFN-α was observed.[39]

These studies highlight an important role for cytokines in the pathogenesis of SLE. A better understanding of the regulation of cytokines and receptors can help elucidate pathogenic mechanisms underlying disease and guide effective therapies.

REFERENCES

1. Apostolidis SA, Lieberman LA, Kis-Toth K, Crispin JC, Tsokos GC. The dysregulation of cytokine networks in systemic lupus erythematosus. *J Interferon Cytokine Res* October 2011;**31**(10):769–79. PubMed PMID: 21877904. Pubmed Central PMCID: 3189553. Epub 2011/09/01. eng.

2. Davis LS, Hutcheson J, Mohan C. The role of cytokines in the pathogenesis and treatment of systemic lupus erythematosus. *J Interferon Cytokine Res* October 2011;**31**(10):781–9. PubMed PMID: 21787222. Pubmed Central PMCID: 3189549.

3. Korn T, Bettelli E, Oukka M, Kuchroo VK. IL-17 and Th17 cells. *Annu Rev Immunol* 2009;**27**:485–517. PubMed PMID: 19132915. Epub 2009/01/10. eng.

4. Wahren-Herlenius M, Dorner T. Immunopathogenic mechanisms of systemic autoimmune disease. *Lancet* August 31, 2013;**382**(9894): 819–31. PubMed PMID: 23993191. Epub 2013/09/03. eng.

5. Ma A, Koka R, Burkett P. Diverse functions of IL-2, IL-15, and IL-7 in lymphoid homeostasis. *Annu Rev Immunol* 2006;**24**:657–79. PubMed PMID: 16551262. Epub 2006/03/23. eng.

6. Setoguchi R, Hori S, Takahashi T, Sakaguchi S. Homeostatic maintenance of natural Foxp3(+) CD25(+) CD4(+) regulatory T cells by interleukin (IL)-2 and induction of autoimmune disease by IL-2 neutralization. *J Exp Med* March 7, 2005;**201**(5):723–35. PubMed PMID: 15753206. Pubmed Central PMCID: 2212841. Epub 2005/03/09. eng.

7. Ju ST, Sharma R, Gaskin F, Fu SM. IL-2 controls trafficking receptor gene expression and Th2 response for skin and lung inflammation. *Clin Immunol* October 2012;**145**(1):82–8. PubMed PMID: 22940635. Pubmed Central PMCID: PMC3444569. Epub 2012/09/04. eng.

8. Kyttaris VC, Wang Y, Juang YT, Weinstein A, Tsokos GC. Increased levels of NF-ATc2 differentially regulate CD154 and IL-2 genes in T Cells from patients with systemic lupus erythematosus. *J Immunol* February 1, 2007;**178**(3):1960–6. PubMed PMID: 17237447. eng.

9. Moulton VR, Grammatikos AP, Fitzgerald LM, Tsokos GC. Splicing factor SF2/ASF rescues IL-2 production in T cells from systemic lupus erythematosus patients by activating IL-2 transcription. *Proc Natl Acad Sci USA* January 29, 2013;**110**(5):1845–50. PubMed PMID: 23319613. Pubmed Central PMCID: PMC3562779. Epub 2013/01/16. eng.

10. Juang YT, Wang Y, Solomou EE, Li Y, Mawrin C, Tenbrock K, et al. Systemic lupus erythematosus serum IgG increases CREM binding to the IL-2 promoter and suppresses IL-2 production through CaMKIV. *J Clin Invest* April 2005;**115**(4):996–1005. PubMed PMID: 15841182. Pubmed Central PMCID: PMC1070410. Epub 2005/04/21. eng.

11. Ichinose K, Juang YT, Crispin JC, Kis-Toth K, Tsokos GC. Suppression of autoimmunity and organ pathology in lupus-prone mice upon inhibition of calcium/calmodulin-dependent protein kinase type IV. *Arthritis Rheum* February 2011;**63**(2):523–9. PubMed PMID: 20954187. Pubmed Central PMCID: 3030625. Epub 2010/10/19. eng.

12. Crispin JC, Oukka M, Bayliss G, Cohen RA, Van Beek CA, Stillman IE, et al. Expanded double negative T cells in patients with systemic lupus erythematosus produce IL-17 and infiltrate the kidneys. *J Immunol* December 15, 2008;**181**(12):8761–6. PubMed PMID: 19050297. Pubmed Central PMCID: PMC2596652. Epub 2008/12/04. eng.

13. Kyttaris VC, Zhang Z, Kuchroo VK, Oukka M, Tsokos GC. Cutting edge: IL-23 receptor deficiency prevents the development of lupus nephritis in C57BL/6-lpr/lpr mice. *J Immunol* May 1, 2010;**184**(9):4605–9. PubMed PMID: 20308633. Pubmed Central PMCID: 2926666. Epub 2010/03/24. eng.

14. Jacob N, Stohl W. Cytokine disturbances in systemic lupus erythematosus. *Arthritis Res Ther* 2011;**13**(4):228. PubMed PMID: 21745419. Pubmed Central PMCID: 3239336. Epub 2011/07/13. eng.

15. Cash H, Relle M, Menke J, Brochhausen C, Jones SA, Topley N, et al. Interleukin 6 (IL-6) deficiency delays lupus nephritis in MRL-Faslpr mice: the IL-6 pathway as a new therapeutic target in treatment of autoimmune kidney disease in systemic lupus erythematosus. *J Rheumatol* January 2010;**37**(1):60–70. PubMed PMID: 19955044. Epub 2009/12/04. eng.

16. Richards HB, Satoh M, Shaw M, Libert C, Poli V, Reeves WH. Interleukin 6 dependence of anti-DNA antibody production: evidence for two pathways of autoantibody formation in pristane-induced lupus. *J Exp Med* September 7, 1998;**188**(5):985–90. PubMed PMID: 9730900. Pubmed Central PMCID: 2213386. Epub 1998/09/09. eng.

17. Linker-Israeli M, Deans RJ, Wallace DJ, Prehn J, Ozeri-Chen T, Klinenberg JR. Elevated levels of endogenous IL-6 in systemic lupus erythematosus. A putative role in pathogenesis. *J Immunol* July 1, 1991;**147**(1):117–23. PubMed PMID: 2051017. eng.

18. Aggarwal BB. Signalling pathways of the TNF superfamily: a double-edged sword. *Nat Rev Immunol* September 2003;**3**(9):745–56. PubMed PMID: 12949498.

19. Boswell JM, Yui MA, Burt DW, Kelley VE. Increased tumor necrosis factor and IL-1 beta gene expression in the kidneys of mice with lupus nephritis. *J Immunol* November 1, 1988;**141**(9):3050–4. PubMed PMID: 3262676. Epub 1988/11/01. eng.

20. Yokoyama H, Kreft B, Kelley VR. Biphasic increase in circulating and renal TNF-alpha in MRL-lpr mice with differing regulatory mechanisms. *Kidney Int* January 1995;**47**(1):122–30. PubMed PMID: 7731137. Epub 1995/01/01. eng.

21. Edwards 3rd CK, Zhou T, Zhang J, Baker TJ, De M, Long RE, et al. Inhibition of superantigen-induced proinflammatory cytokine production and inflammatory arthritis in MRL-lpr/lpr mice by a transcriptional inhibitor of TNF-alpha. *J Immunol* August 15, 1996;**157**(4):1758–72. PubMed PMID: 8759766. Epub 1996/08/15. eng.

22. Segal R, Dayan M, Zinger H, Mozes E. Suppression of experimental systemic lupus erythematosus (SLE) in mice via TNF inhibition by an anti-TNFalpha monoclonal antibody and by pentoxiphylline. *Lupus* 2001;**10**(1):23–31. PubMed PMID: 11243506. Epub 2001/03/13. eng.

23. Gabay C, Cakir N, Moral F, Roux-Lombard P, Meyer O, Dayer JM, et al. Circulating levels of tumor necrosis factor soluble receptors in systemic lupus erythematosus are significantly higher than in other rheumatic diseases and correlate with disease activity. *J Rheumatol* February 1997;**24**(2):303–8. PubMed PMID: 9034987. Epub 1997/02/01. eng.

24. Gomez D, Correa PA, Gomez LM, Cadena J, Molina JF, Anaya JM. Th1/Th2 cytokines in patients with systemic lupus erythematosus: is tumor necrosis factor alpha protective?. *Seminars Arthritis Rheum* June 2004;**33**(6):404–13. PubMed PMID: 15190525. Epub 2004/06/11. eng.

25. Herrera-Esparza R, Barbosa-Cisneros O, Villalobos-Hurtado R, Avalos-Diaz E. Renal expression of IL-6 and TNFalpha genes in lupus nephritis. *Lupus* 1998;**7**(3):154–8. PubMed PMID: 9607638. Epub 1998/06/02. eng.

26. Zhu L, Yang X, Chen W, Li X, Ji Y, Mao H, et al. Decreased expressions of the TNF-alpha signaling adapters in peripheral blood mononuclear cells (PBMCs) are correlated with disease activity in patients with systemic lupus erythematosus. *Clin Rheumatol* September 2007;**26**(9):1481–9. PubMed PMID: 17235653. Epub 2007/01/20. eng.

27. Zhu L, Yang X, Ji Y, Chen W, Guan W, Zhou SF, et al. Up-regulated renal expression of TNF-alpha signalling adapter proteins in lupus glomerulonephritis. *Lupus* February 2009;**18**(2):116–27. PubMed PMID: 19151112. Epub 2009/01/20. eng.

28. Bengtsson AA, Sturfelt G, Truedsson L, Blomberg J, Alm G, Vallin H, et al. Activation of type I interferon system in systemic lupus erythematosus correlates with disease activity but not with antiretroviral antibodies. *Lupus* 2000;**9**(9):664–71. PubMed PMID: 11199920.

29. Lovgren T, Eloranta ML, Bave U, Alm GV, Ronnblom L. Induction of interferon-alpha production in plasmacytoid dendritic cells by immune complexes containing nucleic acid released by necrotic or late apoptotic cells and lupus IgG. *Arthritis Rheum* June 2004;**50**(6):1861–72. PubMed PMID: 15188363.

30. Kirou KA, Lee C, George S, Louca K, Peterson MG, Crow MK. Activation of the interferon-alpha pathway identifies a subgroup of systemic lupus erythematosus patients with distinct serologic features and active disease. *Arthritis Rheum* May 2005;**52**(5):1491–503. PubMed PMID: 15880830.

31. Baechler EC, Batliwalla FM, Karypis G, Gaffney PM, Ortmann WA, Espe KJ, et al. Interferon-inducible gene expression signature in peripheral blood cells of patients with severe lupus. *Proc Natl Acad Sci USA* March 4, 2003;**100**(5):2610–5. PubMed PMID: 12604793. Pubmed Central PMCID: 151388.

32. Bennett L, Palucka AK, Arce E, Cantrell V, Borvak J, Banchereau J, et al. Interferon and granulopoiesis signatures in systemic lupus erythematosus blood. *J Exp Med* March 17, 2003;**197**(6):711–23. PubMed PMID: 12642603. Pubmed Central PMCID: 2193846.

33. Crow MK. Collaboration, genetic associations, and lupus erythematosus. *N Engl J Med* February 28, 2008;**358**(9):956–61. PubMed PMID: 18204099.

34. Peterson KS, Huang JF, Zhu J, D'Agati V, Liu X, Miller N, et al. Characterization of heterogeneity in the molecular pathogenesis of lupus nephritis from transcriptional profiles of laser-captured glomeruli. *J Clin Invest* June 2004;**113**(12):1722–33. PubMed PMID: 15199407. Pubmed Central PMCID: 420500.

35. Ronnblom L, Alm GV. A pivotal role for the natural interferon alpha-producing cells (plasmacytoid dendritic cells) in the pathogenesis of lupus. *J Exp Med* December 17, 2001;**194**(12):F59–63. PubMed PMID: 11748288. Pubmed Central PMCID: 2193578.

36. Ronnblom L, Alm GV. An etiopathogenic role for the type I IFN system in SLE. *Trends Immunol* August 2001;**22**(8):427–31. PubMed PMID: 11473831.

37. Braun D, Geraldes P, Demengeot J, Type I. Interferon controls the onset and severity of autoimmune manifestations in lpr mice. *J Autoimmun* February 2003;**20**(1):15–25. PubMed PMID: 12604309.

38. Santiago-Raber ML, Baccala R, Haraldsson KM, Choubey D, Stewart TA, Kono DH, et al. Type-I interferon receptor deficiency reduces lupus-like disease in NZB mice. *J Exp Med* March 17, 2003;**197**(6):777–88. PubMed PMID: 12642605. Pubmed Central PMCID: 2193854.

39. Hron JD, Peng SL. Type I IFN protects against murine lupus. *J Immunol* August 1, 2004;**173**(3):2134–42. PubMed PMID: 15265950.

Chapter 18

Toll-Like Receptors, Systemic Lupus Erythematosus

William F. Pendergraft III[1], Terry K. Means[2]

[1]University of North Carolina Kidney Center, Chapel Hill, NC, USA; [2]Center for Immunology and Inflammatory Diseases and Division of Rheumatology, Allergy, and Immunology, Massachusetts General Hospital and Harvard Medical School, Charlestown, MA, USA

TOLL-LIKE RECEPTOR FAMILY

It has been nearly 30 years since the first Toll receptor was identified in the fruit fly *Drosophila*.[1] In 1997 the first human ortholog of the *Drosophila* Toll protein was described, a protein that was later designated Toll-like receptor 4 (TLR4).[2] In humans and mice combined, 13 TLRs have been discovered; however, their expression differs between species. Humans, but not mice, express TLR10, and only mice express TLR11, TLR12, and TLR13. TLRs are an evolutionarily conserved family of type I transmembrane receptors that have an extracellular domain compromising leucine-rich repeats and a cytoplasmic domain that shares significant homology with the mammalian type I IL-1 receptor. The TLR family can be divided into two subgroups, TLRs that are found on the cell surface and TLRs that reside in intracellular vesicles. TLR1, TLR2, TLR4, TLR5, TLR6, and TLR10 are expressed on the cell surface, with TLR2 forming heterodimers with TLR1, TLR6, or TLR10. The intracellular TLRs include TLR3, TLR7, TLR8, TLR9, TLR11, TLR12, and TLR13 and they are found localized to intracellular compartments, such as the endoplasmic reticulum, Golgi apparatus, endosomes, and lysosomes (Figure 1). TLR11, TLR12, and TLR13 are expressed in mice, but human TLR11 is a nonfunctional pseudogene and human TLR12 and TLR13 are absent from the human genome. This family of germ-line-encoded receptors recognizes a myriad of conserved pathogen-associated molecular patterns (PAMPs) found in many different microbes, such as bacteria, fungi, viruses, and parasites. TLR recognition of these PAMPs leads to the initiation of intracellular signaling pathways that elicit the expression of inflammatory genes, such as cytokines essential for host defense. In contrast, it is believed that the inappropriate activation of these receptors by endogenous self-ligands can contribute to chronic inflammatory syndromes and autoimmunity. Indeed, members of the TLR family have been implicated in the pathogenesis of several autoimmune diseases, including systemic lupus erythematosus (SLE). This chapter will describe the role of TLR7, TLR8, and TLR9 in the susceptibility, initiation, progression, and exacerbation of SLE disease. The microbial and endogenous ligands for TLRs are shown in Table 1.

TLR7

TLR7 Biology

TLR7 is expressed in intracellular compartments and mediates the recognition of guanosine- and uridine-rich ssRNA and ssRNA viruses, including influenza and vesicular stomatitis virus.[3] TLR7 also recognizes synthetic antiviral nucleoside analogs such as imiquimod (R848), gardiquimod, and loxoribine.[4] TLR7 is highly expressed in human plasmacytoid dendritic cells (pDCs), which secret high amounts of IFN-α on infection with ssRNA viruses.

TLR7 Ligands in SLE

Serologically, the hallmark of SLE is a high level of antinuclear antibodies (ANA) present in nearly all affected individuals (95–99%), with known target antigen specificities of these ANA toward DNA itself and/or nuclear proteins known to form complexes with DNA (i.e., histones) or RNA (i.e., Ro, La, Sm, RNP, others). The Smith antigen is a complex of uridine-rich small nuclear RNA (snRNA) molecules and several proteins. Several studies have demonstrated a role for snRNA-containing autoantibody complexes in the pathogenesis of SLE.[5] In addition, a correlation between the levels of RNA-containing autoantibody complexes in serum and the disease severity has been noted.[6] Furthermore, snRNA-containing immune complexes (ICs) isolated from SLE patient serum are taken up through Fc receptors and delivered to intracellular lysosomes where they stimulate TLR7[7] (Figure 2). snRNA-ICs can stimulate pDCs to produce inflammatory, immunoregulatory, and chemotatic cytokines. The specificity of TLR7 activation by snRNA-ICs

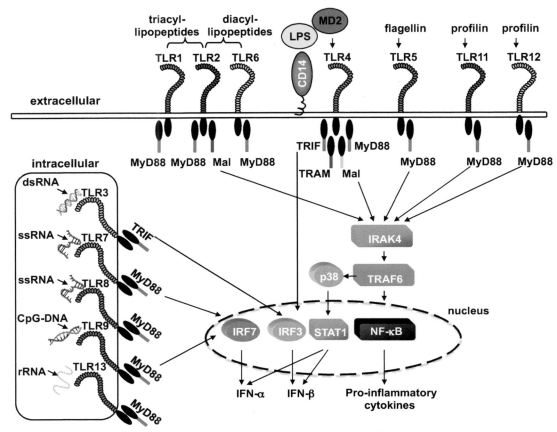

FIGURE 1 **TLR signaling pathways.** Shown is a representation of some of the known signaling intermediates in signaling pathways triggered by TLRs. TLR1, TLR2, TLR4, TLR5, TLR6, and TLR11 are expressed on the cell surface. TLR1 and TLR6 function only as a heterodimer with TLR2. TLR3, TLR7, TLR8, TLR9, TLR11, TLR12, and TLR13 are expressed in intracellular vesicular compartments. All TLRs except TLR3 signal via MyD88-dependent pathways. In addition, TLR3 and TLR4 signal via MyD88-independent pathways.

was confirmed in DCs isolated from TLR7-deficient mice and by the demonstration that oligonucleotide-based inhibitors of TLR7 blocked snRNA-IC-induced IFN-α production by pDCs.[8] Together these data suggest that snRNA molecules contained in circulating ICs found in the serum of SLE patients act as endogenous self-ligands for TLR7 and may initiate and/or exacerbate disease by inappropriately and chronically stimulating innate immune cells.

Interestingly, the recognition of ssRNA by TLR7 is selective and RNA from necrotic cells, but not apoptotic cells, induces DC activation. Furthermore, bacterial RNA is significantly more potent for inducing cell activation than mammalian DNA. One possible explanation for this is that the RNA is modified in some way. Indeed, it has been shown that RNA containing modified nucleosides is significantly less stimulatory than unmodified RNA. Most mammalian RNA is modified and less stimulatory than unmodified bacterial RNA. Thus, mammals appear to have developed a system to modify their RNA to suppress its stimulatory potential, thereby providing a mechanism for the innate immune system to distinguish between self and pathogenic sources of RNA. Still some mammalian RNAs, particularly mitochondrial RNA, have very few modifications and are

therefore a potential source for the stimulatory self-RNA contained in RNA-associated ICs that are found in SLE patients.

TLR7 Expression in SLE

PBMCs isolated from SLE patients have been reported to express significantly higher levels of TLR7 mRNA than those from healthy controls.[9] In addition the levels of TLR7 expression on SLE patient PBMCs correlated with IFN-α gene expression. TLR7 expression is equivalent in cells isolated from female versus male individuals; however, TLR7 stimulation induced significantly more IFN-α production from female than male cells.[10] While this observation was found in cells isolated from healthy subjects and needs to be repeated in cells isolated from SLE patients, it may provide an explanation for the nearly 10 times higher prevalence of SLE in females than in males.

TLR7 in Murine Lupus

In vitro experiments demonstrate that autoreactive B cells can bind self-RNA through the B-cell antigen receptor

TABLE 1 Microbial and Endogenous Host Ligands Reported to Activate Cells through Human and Murine TLRs

	Microbial Ligands	Endogenous Ligands
TLR1[a]	Triacylated lipopeptides, lipoarabinomannan *Borrelia burgdorferi* (OspA)	
TLR2	Zymosan, peptidoglycan, *M. tuberculosis* Leptospiral LPS	HSP60, HSP70, HMGB1, gp96, MSU
TLR3	dsRNA	mRNA
TLR4	LPS from Gram-negative bacteria GPI from *Trypanosoma cruz* Proteins from RSV, MMTV, and *M. tuberculosis*	HSP60, HSP70, gp96, fibrinogen hyaluron, heparin sulfate, HMGB1 MSU, β-defensin 2
TLR5	Flagellin	
TLR6[a]	Diacylated lipopeptides, lipoteichoic acid, zymosan	
TLR7	ssRNA and ssRNA viruses (VSV, NDV, parechovirus)	ssRNA/protein complexes
TLR8	ssRNA, poly(T)/imidazoquinoline complexes G-rich oligonucleotides	ssRNA/protein complexes
TLR9	CpG DNA	Chromatin, DNA/protein complexes
TLR10	Unknown	
TLR11	Profilin *Toxoplasma gondii*	
TLR12	Profilin *Toxoplasma gondii*	
TLR13	Bacterial 23S ribosomal RNA (rRNA)	

[a]*TLR1 and TLR6 function only as a heterodimer with TLR2. Murine TLR8 recognizes synthetic RNA analogue complexes (poly(T)/imidazoquinoline), but not other human TLR8 agonists. TLR10 is present only in humans and TLR11, TLR12, and TLR13 are present only in mice.*

(BCR), which delivers it to endosomes or lysosomes, where it sequentially engages TLR7[11] (Figure 2). Engagement of TLR7 then leads to B-cell activation, proliferation, and autoantibody production. In this model, self-RNA is an autoantigen that acts as an adjuvant to trigger in this case an unwanted immune response (Figure 2). Moreover, TLR7 expression on B cells can be induced by engagement of the IFN-α/β receptor on B cells[12] (Figure 2). The source of IFN-α/β can be autocrine (B cells) or paracrine (pDCs).

To test the involvement of TLR7 in the development of SLE in vivo the lupus-prone MRL[lpr/lpr] mice were crossed to TLR7-deficient mice. These mice failed to generate autoantibodies to RNA-associated antigens (Sm), but produced levels of anti-DNA autoantibodies typical for the MRL[lpr/lpr] model.[13] In addition, MRL[lpr/lpr] mice deficient in TLR7 had less activated B cells and pDCs in circulation and significantly less renal disease. In a separate study, mice engineered to express an autoreactive immunoglobulin that binds to the autoantigens ssDNA, ssRNA, and nucleosomes were created on a nonautoimmune background (C57Bl/6) called 546Igi mice.[14] The B cells in 564Igi mice escape anergy and tolerance and produce pathogenic class-switched autoantibodies that result in kidney disease. Notably, anti-RNA autoantibodies are absent in 564Igi mice deficient in

TLR7. Together these observations confirm the model that B-cell activation and regulation of autoantibody production against self-RNA-associated antigens are TLR7 dependent.

Because TLR7 serves an important role in murine lupus this receptor has been proposed as a potential therapeutic target for human SLE. Experimentally, oligonucleotide antagonists that specifically inhibit TLR7 signaling significantly decrease anti-RNA and anti-DNA autoantibody levels in the serum and reduce kidney disease when injected into lupus-prone MRL[lpr/lpr] mice. Future clinical trials using TLR7 antagonists in human SLE patients will provide answers to the specificity of the TLR7 pathway in human SLE disease.

Expression of TLR7 by B cells mediates aberrant immune cell activation, autoantibody production, and inflammation. B-cell-intrinsic TLR7 signaling promotes expansion and autoantibody production by transitional T1 B cells and the development of spontaneous germinal centers.[15] Thus, TLR7 expression by B cells permits the specific development of autoantibodies to RNA-associated protein complexes that activate TLR7 via a feedback loop, which exacerbates SLE disease.[16] Finally, the expression of TLR7 on B cells requires the expression of the cytosolic RNA sensor mitochondrial antiviral signaling protein

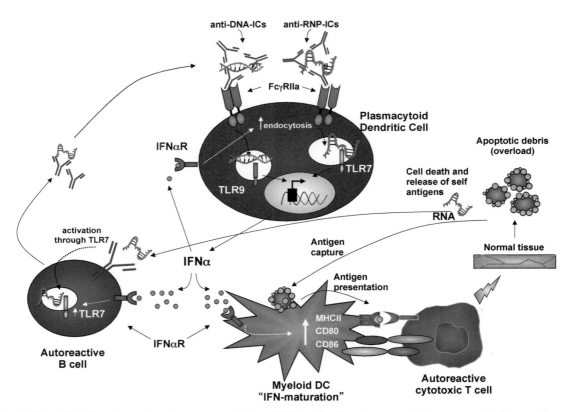

FIGURE 2 TLR7 and TLR9 activation by endogenous host RNA and DNA. This schematic represents the innate model of lupus pathogenesis. RNA and DNA released from dying or damaged cells can be recognized by the B-cell receptor on autoreactive B cells. The BCR transports RNA and DNA to intracellular lysosomes where they engage TLR7 and TLR9, respectively. Activation of TLR7 and TLR9 in B cells induces proliferation, cytokine production (IFN-β), and differentiation into plasma cells that secrete autoantibodies that can bind RNA, DNA, or RNA/DNA-associated proteins to form immune complexes. FcγRIIa (CD32), expressed by plasmacytoid dendritic cells, binds nucleic acid-containing immune complexes and transports them to intracellular lysosomes containing TLR7 and TLR9. Activation of TLR7 and TLR9 in pDCs induces proinflammatory cytokine and chemokine production, which can result in cell recruitment and a vicious cytokine storm that can lead to tissue pathogenesis. In addition, IFN-α secretion by pDCs enhances B-cell activation by nucleic acid ICs by upregulating TLR7 expression. This may provide a positive-feedback loop by further enhancing autoantibody production and B-cell proliferation leading to the exacerbation of autoimmunity.

(MAVS), also known as VISA, IPS-1, and CARDIF, suggesting that MAVS-mediated signaling may play a role in autoimmunity.[17]

TLR7 Polymorphisms and Copy Number in SLE

In 1979 the mouse strain BXSB/MP was demonstrated to develop a spontaneous lupus-like syndrome that was restricted to male mice. The susceptibility locus was mapped to the Y chromosome and called the Y-linked autoimmune accelerator (YAA) locus. Nearly 30 years later it has been shown that YAA is not a mutation but rather a duplication of X chromosomal DNA that was transposed to the Y chromosome. This duplicated 4 Mb gene segment contains TLR7 and 16 other genes.[18] The published data support a role for TLR7 as the main gene responsible for the accelerated lupus-like disease, because reduction of TLR7 copy number abrogated the YAA phenotype.[19] Furthermore, experiments

in transgenic mice demonstrated that increasing TLR7 gene dosage directly correlated with the production of autoantibodies directed against RNA autoantigens and the severity of the autoimmune disease.[19] These data suggest that strict regulation of TLR7 expression and function is critical (at least in mice) for preventing spontaneous autoimmunity. Studies examining the copy number of the TLR7 gene in human SLE patients and healthy controls have not revealed a significant association with the SLE phenotype.[20]

Several polymorphisms have been found in human TLR7, including a nonsynonymous single nucleotide polymorphism (SNP) in TLR7 that changes a glutamine to a leucine at amino acid 11 in the N-terminus. This SNP was shown not to confer a role in susceptibility or severity to SLE in a Caucasian Spanish population. In contrast, a TLR7 SNP in the 3′ untranslated region (rs3853839) and two SNPs in the intron two region (rs179019 and rs179010) of TLR7 showed significant association with susceptibility for SLE in Asian women.[21] Furthermore, the G allele of rs3853839 was associated with significantly increased TLR7 mRNA and protein levels in immune cells.[22] The increased TLR7 expression in rs3853839 cells was found to be due to the disruption of the binding site for microRNA-3138.[23] In addition, an A to G SNP at position 7926 (rs1634323) in the TLR7 gene conferred a significant risk of SLE in females.[24]

TLR8

TLR8 Biology

Similar to TLR7, TLR8 is expressed in intracellular compartments and detects guanosine- and uridine-rich ssRNA and ssRNA viruses. The TLR8 gene also lies contiguous to TLR7 on the X chromosome. While TLR7 is expressed mainly on pDCS and B cells, TLR8 is more broadly expressed on myeloid DCs, monocytes, differentiated macrophages, and regulatory T (Treg) cells.[25]

TLR8 in SLE

In mice TLR8 expression has not been extensively examined primarily because murine TLR8 was thought to be nonfunctional because it did not react to human TLR8 ligands. The natural ligands for murine TLR8 have not been described, but synthetic imidazoquinoline compounds complexed with poly(T) react specifically with murine TLR8. The role of TLR8 in human and murine lupus is less clear especially since TLR8 is not expressed on B cells or pDCs, but rather on myeloid cells. It remains plausible that immunoglobulin (Ig) G immune complexes containing unmodified forms of self-RNA may initiate or exacerbate SLE by stimulating TLR8 on myeloid DCs through the induction of IFN-α and other inflammatory cytokines.

Another interesting aspect of TLR8 is its expression and regulation of CD4+ Treg cells.[25] TLR8 signaling induced by ssRNA can reverse the suppressive function of Treg cells. This effect was shown to be independent of DCs, but dependent on TLR8 and MyD88 signaling. These data suggest that TLR8 signaling in Treg cells could play an important role in controlling immune responses. It is interesting to speculate that the reason RNA-associated ICs in serum correlate with high levels of IFN-α and renal disease in SLE is because TLR8 signaling induced by circulating RNA-associated ICs abrogates or reverses the suppressive function of Treg cells in patients with SLE.

TLR8 in Murine Lupus

In mice, deletion of TLR8 leads to spontaneous autoimmunity.[26] TLR8-deficient mice showed abnormal B-cell development, increased serum levels of autoantibodies, and development of glomerulonephritis. DCs isolated from TLR8-deficient mice overexpressed TLR7 and were hyperresponsive to TLR7 ligands. Furthermore, in lupus-prone BXSB-Yaa mice, overexpression of TLR8 correlated with podocyte injury, urinary albumin levels, and glomerulonephritis. Deletion of TLR8 in C57Bl/6 mice congenic for the Nba2 (NZB autoimmunity 2) locus and bearing the Yaa mutation, or in 564Igi knock-in mice, significantly decreased lupus disease progression.[27] Thus, in mice TLR8 deficiency exacerbates lupus disease because of an increased cellular response to TLR7 ligation that contributes to loss of B-cell tolerance, increased autoantibody production, and increased cytokine expression.[28] Together, these data suggest an important role for TLR8 in the regulation of TLR7 expression and the prevention of spontaneous autoimmunity.

TLR8 Polymorphisms in SLE

In mice and humans the TLR8 gene is located on chromosome X, 16 kb away from TLR7. The human TLR8 locus encodes two splice variants, TLR8 variant 1 (TLR8v1) and TLR8v2. TLR8v1 has an alternative translational start site that results in the addition of 15 amino acids to the N-terminus. While TLR8v2 is the predominant form of TLR8, the expression of TLR8v1 has been shown to positively regulate TLR8 signaling in certain monocyte populations.

In humans a polymorphism (rs3764880) in the start codon of TLR8 that changes ATG to GTG has been identified. The GTG allele of rs3764880 results in a variant TLR8 protein that lacks three amino acids. Several groups have noted an association between the rs3764880 polymorphism of TLR8 and the SLE in women.[22,29] The mechanism whereby the rs3764880 polymorphism of TLR8 contributes to lupus disease remains unclear, but may involve the regulation of TLR8v1 and TLR8v2 protein expression.

TLR9

TLR9 Biology

In 1984 it was demonstrated that bacterial genomic DNA was immunostimulatory and promoted antitumor responses.[30] Later, the immunostimulatory effect of bacterial DNA on B cells was shown to be mediated by the presence of unmethylated "CpG motifs."[31] In contrast to bacterial and viral DNA, CpG motifs in mammalian DNA are suppressed and mostly methylated. Thus, most mammalian DNA does not have immunostimulatory activity. TLR9 was shown to be the receptor that mediates cellular responses to CpG-DNA.[32] DCs isolated from TLR9-deficient mice did not show any response to CpG-DNA, including maturation or cytokine production. Thus TLR9 appears to have evolved to specifically recognize and differentiate microbial DNA from self-DNA. Recognition of nucleic acids by TLR9 also requires specific proteolytic processing of TLR9 within the endolysosome in a multistep process;

the ectodomain is removed by asparagine endopeptidase or cathepsin family members followed by cathepsin-mediated trimming. This appears to be required in all cell types and is needed for optimal TLR3 and TLR7 activity as well.[33] Intriguingly, it appears that the binding of DNA to TLR9 is sequence independent and enhanced by the DNA curvature-inducing proteins high mobility group protein B1 (HMGB1) and histones H2A and H2B, which enhance the DNA:TLR9 interaction.

TLR9 Expression in SLE

Anti-DNA reactivity was first discovered in the sera of patients with SLE in 1965 and it is still used clinically to aid the diagnosis of SLE because of its high specificity for SLE compared with other autoimmune diseases. Since that time several studies have demonstrated a role for DNA-specific antibodies in the pathogenesis of SLE.[5] In addition, a correlation between the levels of anti-DNA reactivity in serum and the disease severity has been noted, with DNA-specific Ig being isolated from diseased kidneys of SLE patients in some cases.[34] Notably, SLE serum containing anti-DNA antibodies activates PBMCs to secrete IFN-α.[35] Furthermore, DNA complexed with anti-DNA autoantibodies purified from SLE patient sera also stimulates PBMCs to produce IFN-α.[36] One possible explanation for this activity is that the DNA contained in DNA-anti-DNA ICs purified from SLE patient serum is stimulatory. Interestingly, DNA sequencing demonstrated that the DNA contained in some anti-DNA ICs includes CpG dinucleotides at a five times higher frequency than expected for random CpG distribution in the genome.[37] While these stimulatory dinucleotide sequences are common in bacterial and viral genomes, they are by comparison relatively suppressed in vertebrate DNA. Synthetic oligonucleotides carrying these CpG motifs are immunostimulatory and induce activation of B cells, pDCs, and monocytes exclusively through TLR9, as cells from TLR9-deficient mice lack these responses.[31,32] Furthermore, in vitro studies demonstrated that anti-DNA ICs isolated from SLE patient serum induce cell activation in a TLR9-dependent manner[38] (Figure 2). In quiescent cells TLR9 mainly resides in the endoplasmic reticulum; however, on uptake of DNA-ICs into cells, TLR9 traffics from the ER to lyosomes.[38,39] The interaction of TLR9 with DNA-ICs is rapid and specific, as other nonnucleic acid containing autoantibody complexes isolated from other rheumatic disease patients fails to activate TLR9.[6,38] In pDCs, internalization of DNA-ICs is mediated through FcγRIIa (CD32), which delivers the complexes to intracellular lysosomes containing TLR9, thereby initiating signaling and the production of inflammatory cytokines such as IFN-α[38] (Figure 2).

In addition to the two distinct mechanisms described above for DNA-IC recognition by B cells (BCR/TLR9) and pDCs (CD32/TLR9), a common third mechanism that uses HMGB1 and receptor for advanced glycation end products (RAGE) for DNA-IC recognition by B cells and pDCs has been demonstrated.[40] HMGB1 is a known ligand for RAGE. Interestingly, HMGB1 has been shown to bind to DNA with high affinity. Moreover, HMGB1 is found in DNA-ICs isolated from SLE patients. Remarkably, RAGE and HMGB1 expression were demonstrated to be required for optimal activation of pDCs and B cells by DNA-ICs.[40] Thus, TLR9 in cooperation with HMGB1/RAGE has the capacity to recognize endogenous host DNA, triggering a signaling cascade that induces inflammatory mediators that may initiate and/or exacerbate SLE disease.

TLR9 expression is higher on B cells and monocytes, but not pDCs isolated from SLE patients compared to healthy controls.[41] This increase in TLR9 expression also correlated with the presence of circulating anti-DNA antibodies in these patients and treatment of B cells isolated from healthy controls with SLE serum induced TLR9 expression.[41] In addition, inhibition of CpG-induced TLR9 stimulation with the MyD88 inhibitor ST2825 blocks autoantibody production by human B cells in vitro.[42] It was recently shown that TLR9-mediated B cell effects become exhausted or tolerant to TLR9 stimulation in patients with increasing disease activity, which requires further exploration.[43]

TLR9 in Murine Lupus

The first paper describing a role for TLR9 in autoimmunity was written by Marshak-Rothstein and colleagues.[44] They demonstrated that DNA-containing IgG complexes activated autoreactive B cells through the sequential engagement of the BCR, which delivers the complexes to intracellular vesicles containing TLR9 (Figure 2). The proliferation of autoreactive B cells induced by DNA autoantigens is TLR9 dependent, because autoreactive B cells deficient for TLR9 failed to proliferate in response to DNA-containing complexes.

Increased TLR9 expression was demonstrated in the kidneys of nephritic MRL[lpr/lpr] mice and was shown to be expressed on infiltrating macrophages. MRL[lpr/lpr] mice deficient in TLR9 made less anti-DNA antibodies, but had high levels of RNA-containing autoantibodies (anti-Sm/RNP).[45] Remarkably, despite the absence of anti-DNA antibodies, there was an increase in immune cell activation, increased renal disease, and a higher mortality rate in TLR9-deficient MRL[lpr/lpr] compared to control MRL[lpr/lpr] mice. Elegant studies involving MRLlpr/lpr mice deficient in both TLR7 and TLR9 from Nickerson and colleagues in 2010 revealed that TLR9 suppresses TLR7-dependent anti-RNA autoantibody production. Furthermore, disease exacerbation seen in TLR9-deficient mice was ameliorated in mice deficient in both TLR7 and TLR9, lending credence to the notion that TLR9 acts upstream of TLR7. This body of work also revealed that TLR7 and TLR9 are necessary and sufficient for ANA production, at least in mice.[46] Mice deficient in a subunit of the type I interferon receptor termed IFNAR1 were later shown to be protected from exacerbated autoimmune disease in TLR-deficient mice.[47] More recently, B-cell-specific TLR9 deletion resulted in decreased levels of anti-DNA antibodies; however, there was an increase in antibodies to many other lupus-related antigens as well as worse disease, suggesting the critical protective role of TLR9 on B cells.[48]

TLR9-dependent tolerance may be due to the ability of TLR9 activation to promote peritoneal B-1b-cell expansion and production of self-reactive and protective IgM.[49] In addition, using the 3H9 anti-DNA BCR transgene in the autoimmune-prone MRL/lpr mouse, it was shown that TLR9 paradoxically promotes tolerance by limiting peripheral autoreactive B-cell survival; but was also required for follicular anti-DNA B-cell activation.

TLR9 Polymorphisms and Copy Number in SLE

The TLR9 gene (chromosome 3p21.3) is located in one of the defined susceptibility regions for SLE. Several groups have investigated whether genetic variations of TLR9, which include (-1486 T$\to$C, -1237 C$\to$T, $+1174$ A$\to$G, and $+2848$ G$\to$A), are involved in susceptibility to SLE in different populations around the world. The presence of the nucleotide G at position $+1174$ in intron 1 of TLR9 was demonstrated to be significantly associated with an increased risk of SLE in a Japanese cohort.[50] Interestingly, the A$\to$G $+1174$ SNP downregulates TLR9 expression in reporter assays. These data would fit with the current model (discussed above) that TLR9 expression is protective against SLE. A significant association was also made with -1486 T$\to$C in an SLE cohort in China and $+1174$ A$\to$G in Brazil.[51,52] In contrast, other studies performed on American, British, Danish, Korean, Chinese, and Indian SLE cohorts did not detect a statistically significant association of any TLR9 gene variations with SLE susceptibility.[53] In 2012, two separate meta-analyses were performed to determine the risk of SLE with three TLR9 polymorphisms (-1486 C$\to$T, $+1174$ A$\to$G, and $+1635$ C$\to$T) in Asians, and no association was identified in either report.[54] To date, there has yet to be a proven and replicated association of TLR9 polymorphisms with SLE risk.

CONCLUSIONS

Prior to FDA approval of belimumab for SLE in 2011, there had been more than a 50 years gap since a drug had been approved by the FDA for the treatment of SLE. Furthermore, no drug has been approved for the treatment of lupus nephritis. This highlights the vital need for additional and aggressive development of novel therapies that inhibit early

steps in the pathogenesis of this refractory disease. Studies on the role of TLRs in SLE will likely lead to the development of novel therapies for SLE and other autoimmune diseases. Murine models of lupus clearly indicate that TLR7 and TLR9 are required for the generation of anti-RNA and anti-DNA autoantibodies, respectively. Thus, these receptors are potential candidates for pharmacological inhibition. Indeed, synthetic oligonucleotide-based inhibitors of TLR7 and TLR9 have already been shown to reduce SLE disease progression in mice. Hopefully, research on TLRs in SLE will continue to move forward at a rapid pace, which will help move new TLR-based therapies into the clinic.

REFERENCES

1. Anderson KV, Jurgens G, Nusslein-Volhard C. Establishment of dorsal-ventral polarity in the *Drosophila* embryo: genetic studies on the role of the Toll gene product. *Cell* 1985;**42**(3):779–89.
2. Medzhitov R, Preston-Hurlburt P, Janeway Jr CA. A human homologue of the *Drosophila* Toll protein signals activation of adaptive immunity. *Nature* 1997;**388**(6640):394–7.
3. Diebold SS, Kaisho T, Hemmi H, Akira S, Reis e Sousa C. Innate antiviral responses by means of TLR7-mediated recognition of single-stranded RNA. *Science* 2004;**303**(5663):1529–31.
4. Hemmi H, Kaisho T, Takeuchi O, Sato S, Sanjo H, Hoshino K, et al. Small anti-viral compounds activate immune cells via the TLR7 MyD88-dependent signaling pathway. *Nat Immunol* 2002;**3**(2):196–200.
5. Hahn BH. Antibodies to DNA. *N Engl J Med* 1998;**338**(19):1359–68.
6. Hua J, Kirou K, Lee C, Crow MK. Functional assay of type I interferon in systemic lupus erythematosus plasma and association with anti-RNA binding protein autoantibodies. *Arthritis Rheum* 2006;**54**(6):1906–16.
7. Vollmer J, Tluk S, Schmitz C, Hamm S, Jurk M, Forsbach A, et al. Immune stimulation mediated by autoantigen binding sites within small nuclear RNAs involves Toll-like receptors 7 and 8. *J Exp Med* 2005;**202**(11):1575–85.
8. Barrat FJ, Meeker T, Gregorio J, Chan JH, Uematsu S, Akira S, et al. Nucleic acids of mammalian origin can act as endogenous ligands for Toll-like receptors and may promote systemic lupus erythematosus. *J Exp Med* 2005;**202**(8):1131–9.
9. Komatsuda A, Wakui H, Iwamoto K, Ozawa M, Togashi M, Masai R, et al. Up-regulated expression of Toll-like receptors mRNAs in peripheral blood mononuclear cells from patients with systemic lupus erythematosus. *Clin Exp Immunol* 2008;**152**(3):482–7.
10. Berghofer B, Frommer T, Haley G, Fink L, Bein G, Hackstein H. TLR7 ligands induce higher IFN-alpha production in females. *J Immunol* 2006;**177**(4):2088–96.
11. Lau CM, Broughton C, Tabor AS, Akira S, Flavell RA, Mamula MJ, et al. RNA-associated autoantigens activate B cells by combined B cell antigen receptor/Toll-like receptor 7 engagement. *J Exp Med* 2005;**202**(9):1171–7.
12. Green NM, Laws A, Kiefer K, Busconi L, Kim YM, Brinkmann MM, et al. Murine B cell response to TLR7 ligands depends on an IFN-beta feedback loop. *J Immunol* 2009;**183**(3):1569–76.
13. Christensen SR, Shupe J, Nickerson K, Kashgarian M, Flavell RA, Shlomchik MJ. Toll-like receptor 7 and TLR9 dictate autoantibody specificity and have opposing inflammatory and regulatory roles in a murine model of lupus. *Immunity* 2006;**25**(3):417–28.

14. Berland R, Fernandez L, Kari E, Han JH, Lomakin I, Akira S, et al. Toll-like receptor 7-dependent loss of B cell tolerance in pathogenic autoantibody knockin mice. *Immunity* 2006;**25**(3):429–40.

15. Soni C, Wong EB, Domeier PP, Khan TN, Satoh T, Akira S, et al. B cell-intrinsic TLR7 signaling is essential for the development of spontaneous germinal centers. *J Immunol* 2014;**193**(9):4400–14.

16. Hwang SH, Lee H, Yamamoto M, Jones LA, Dayalan J, Hopkins R, et al. B cell TLR7 expression drives anti-RNA autoantibody production and exacerbates disease in systemic lupus erythematosus-prone mice. *J Immunol* 2012;**189**(12):5786–96.

17. Xu LG, Jin L, Zhang BC, Akerlund LJ, Shu HB, Cambier JC. VISA is required for B cell expression of TLR7. *J Immunol* 2012;**188**(1):248–58.

18. Pisitkun P, Deane JA, Difilippantonio MJ, Tarasenko T, Satterthwaite AB, Bolland S. Autoreactive B cell responses to RNA-related antigens due to TLR7 gene duplication. *Science* 2006;**312**(5780):1669–72.

19. Deane JA, Pisitkun P, Barrett RS, Feigenbaum L, Town T, Ward JM, et al. Control of toll-like receptor 7 expression is essential to restrict autoimmunity and dendritic cell proliferation. *Immunity* 2007;**27**(5):801–10.

20. Kelley J, Johnson MR, Alarcon GS, Kimberly RP, Edberg JC. Variation in the relative copy number of the TLR7 gene in patients with systemic lupus erythematosus and healthy control subjects. *Arthritis Rheum* 2007;**56**(10):3375–8.

21. Kawasaki A, Furukawa H, Kondo Y, Ito S, Hayashi T, Kusaoi M, et al. TLR7 single-nucleotide polymorphisms in the 3' untranslated region and intron 2 independently contribute to systemic lupus erythematosus in Japanese women: a case-control association study. *Arthritis Res Ther* 2011;**13**(2):R41.

22. Wang CM, Chang SW, Wu YJ, Lin JC, Ho HH, Chou TC, et al. Genetic variations in Toll-like receptors (TLRs 3/7/8) are associated with systemic lupus erythematosus in a Taiwanese population. *Sci Rep* 2014;**4**:3792.

23. Deng Y, Zhao J, Sakurai D, Kaufman KM, Edberg JC, Kimberly RP, et al. MicroRNA-3148 modulates allelic expression of toll-like receptor 7 variant associated with systemic lupus erythematosus. *PLoS Genet* 2013;**9**(2):e1003336.

24. Tian J, Ma Y, Li J, Cen H, Wang DG, Feng CC, et al. The TLR7 7926A>G polymorphism is associated with susceptibility to systemic lupus erythematosus. *Mol Med Rep* 2012;**6**(1):105–10.

25. Peng G, Guo Z, Kiniwa Y, Voo KS, Peng W, Fu T, et al. Toll-like receptor 8-mediated reversal of CD4+ regulatory T cell function. *Science* 2005;**309**(5739):1380–4.

26. Demaria O, Pagni PP, Traub S, de Gassart A, Branzk N, Murphy AJ, et al. TLR8 deficiency leads to autoimmunity in mice. *J Clin Invest* 2010;**120**(10):3651–62.

27. Tran NL, Manzin-Lorenzi C, Santiago-Raber ML. TLR8 deletion accelerates autoimmunity in a mouse model of lupus through a TLR7-dependent mechanism. *Immunology* 2015;**145**(1):60–70.

28. Desnues B, Macedo AB, Roussel-Queval A, Bonnardel J, Henri S, Demaria O, et al. TLR8 on dendritic cells and TLR9 on B cells restrain TLR7-mediated spontaneous autoimmunity in C57BL/6 mice. *Proc Natl Acad Sci USA* 2014;**111**(4):1497–502.

29. Laska MJ, Troldborg A, Hansen B, Stengaard-Pedersen K, Junker P, Nexo BA, et al. Polymorphisms within Toll-like receptors are associated with systemic lupus erythematosus in a cohort of Danish females. *Rheumatology* 2014;**53**(1):48–55.

30. Tokunaga T, Yamamoto H, Shimada S, Abe H, Fukuda T, Fujisawa Y, et al. Antitumor activity of deoxyribonucleic acid fraction from Mycobacterium bovis BCG. I. Isolation, physicochemical characterization, and antitumor activity. *J Natl Cancer Inst* 1984;**72**(4):955–62.

31. Krieg AM, Yi AK, Matson S, Waldschmidt TJ, Bishop GA, Teasdale R, et al. CpG motifs in bacterial DNA trigger direct B-cell activation. *Nature* 1995;**374**(6522):546–9.

32. Hemmi H, Takeuchi O, Kawai T, Kaisho T, Sato S, Sanjo H, et al. A Toll-like receptor recognizes bacterial DNA. *Nature* 2000;**408**(6813):740–5.

33. Ewald SE, Engel A, Lee J, Wang M, Bogyo M, Barton GM. Nucleic acid recognition by Toll-like receptors is coupled to stepwise processing by cathepsins and asparagine endopeptidase. *J Exp Med* 2011;**208**(4):643–51.

34. ter Borg EJ, Horst G, Hummel EJ, Limburg PC, Kallenberg CG. Measurement of increases in anti-double-stranded DNA antibody levels as a predictor of disease exacerbation in systemic lupus erythematosus. A long-term, prospective study. *Arthritis Rheum* 1990;**33**(5):634–43.

35. Vallin H, Blomberg S, Alm GV, Cederblad B, Ronnblom L. Patients with systemic lupus erythematosus (SLE) have a circulating inducer of interferon-alpha (IFN-alpha) production acting on leucocytes resembling immature dendritic cells. *Clin Exp Immunol* 1999;**115**(1):196–202.

36. Yasuda K, Richez C, Uccellini MB, Richards RJ, Bonegio RG, Akira S, et al. Requirement for DNA CpG content in TLR9-dependent dendritic cell activation induced by DNA-containing immune complexes. *J Immunol* 2009;**183**(5):3109–17.

37. Sato Y, Miyata M, Nishimaki T, Kochi H, Kasukawa R. CpG motif-containing DNA fragments from sera of patients with systemic lupus erythematosus proliferate mononuclear cells in vitro. *J Rheumatol* 1999;**26**(2):294–301.

38. Means TK, Latz E, Hayashi F, Murali MR, Golenbock DT, Luster AD. Human lupus autoantibody-DNA complexes activate DCs through cooperation of CD32 and TLR9. *J Clin Invest* 2005;**115**(2):407–17.

39. Latz E, Schoenemeyer A, Visintin A, Fitzgerald KA, Monks BG, Knetter CF, et al. TLR9 signals after translocating from the ER to CpG DNA in the lysosome. *Nat Immunol* 2004;**5**(2):190–8.

40. Tian J, Avalos AM, Mao SY, Chen B, Senthil K, Wu H, et al. Toll-like receptor 9-dependent activation by DNA-containing immune complexes is mediated by HMGB1 and RAGE. *Nat Immunol* 2007;**8**(5):487–96.

41. Papadimitraki ED, Choulaki C, Koutala E, Bertsias G, Tsatsanis C, Gergianaki I, et al. Expansion of toll-like receptor 9-expressing B cells in active systemic lupus erythematosus: implications for the induction and maintenance of the autoimmune process. *Arthritis Rheum* 2006;**54**(11):3601–11.

42. Capolunghi F, Rosado MM, Cascioli S, Girolami E, Bordasco S, Vivarelli M, et al. Pharmacological inhibition of TLR9 activation blocks autoantibody production in human B cells from SLE patients. *Rheumatology* 2010;**49**(12):2281–9.

43. Sieber J, Daridon C, Fleischer SJ, Fleischer V, Hiepe F, Alexander T, et al. Active systemic lupus erythematosus is associated with a reduced cytokine production by B cells in response to TLR9 stimulation. *Arthritis Res Ther* 2014;**16**(6):477.

44. Leadbetter EA, Rifkin IR, Hohlbaum AM, Beaudette BC, Shlomchik MJ, Marshak-Rothstein A. Chromatin-IgG complexes activate B cells by dual engagement of IgM and Toll-like receptors. *Nature* 2002;**416**(6881):603–7.

45. Christensen SR, Kashgarian M, Alexopoulou L, Flavell RA, Akira S, Shlomchik MJ. Toll-like receptor 9 controls anti-DNA autoantibody production in murine lupus. *J Exp Med* 2005;**202**(2):321–31.

46. Nickerson KM, Christensen SR, Shupe J, Kashgarian M, Kim D, Elkon K, et al. TLR9 regulates TLR7- and MyD88-dependent autoantibody production and disease in a murine model of lupus. *J Immunol* 2010;**184**(4):1840–8.

47. Nickerson KM, Cullen JL, Kashgarian M, Shlomchik MJ. Exacerbated autoimmunity in the absence of TLR9 in MRL.Fas(lpr) mice depends on Ifnar1. *J Immunol* 2013;**190**(8):3889–94.

48. Jackson SW, Scharping NE, Kolhatkar NS, Khim S, Schwartz MA, Li QZ, et al. Opposing impact of B cell-intrinsic TLR7 and TLR9 signals on autoantibody repertoire and systemic inflammation. *J Immunol* 2014;**192**(10):4525–32.

49. Stoehr AD, Schoen CT, Mertes MM, Eiglmeier S, Holecska V, Lorenz AK, et al. TLR9 in peritoneal B-1b cells is essential for production of protective self-reactive IgM to control Th17 cells and severe autoimmunity. *J Immunol* 2011;**187**(6):2953–65.

50. Tao K, Fujii M, Tsukumo S, Maekawa Y, Kishihara K, Kimoto Y, et al. Genetic variations of Toll-like receptor 9 predispose to systemic lupus erythematosus in Japanese population. *Ann Rheumatic Dis* 2007;**66**(7):905–9.

51. Huang CM, Huang PH, Chen CL, Lin YJ, Tsai CH, Huang WL, et al. Association of toll-like receptor 9 gene polymorphism in Chinese patients with systemic lupus erythematosus in Taiwan. *Rheumatol Int* 2012;**32**(7):2105–9.

52. dos Santos BP, Valverde JV, Rohr P, Monticielo OA, Brenol JC, Xavier RM, et al. TLR7/8/9 polymorphisms and their associations in systemic lupus erythematosus patients from southern Brazil. *Lupus* 2012;**21**(3):302–9.

53. Panda AK, Pattanaik SS, Tripathy R, Das BK. TLR-9 promoter polymorphisms (T-1237C and T-1486C) are not associated with systemic lupus erythematosus: a case control study and meta-analysis. *Hum Immunol* 2013;**74**(12):1672–8.

54. Yang Z, Liang Y, Qin B, Li C, Zhong R. TLR9 polymorphisms and systemic lupus erythematosus risk in Asians: a meta-analysis study. *Cytokine* 2012;**57**(2):282–9.

Chapter 19

The Interferon System in Lupus Erythematosus

Niklas Hagberg, Lars Rönnblom

Section of Rheumatology, Department of Medical Sciences, Uppsala University, Uppsala, Sweden

INTRODUCTION

The interferons (IFNs) are a large group of proteins defined by their capacity to interfere with viral replication in cells via induction of new mRNA and protein synthesis. They are encoded by 22 different genes, classified into three types (I–III), produced by many different cell types and act on three separate receptors. Thus, the IFNs and involved cells constitute a complex system, which is an essential part of our innate immune system. A role for IFN in the systemic lupus erythematosus (SLE) disease process was suggested already in 1979 by the observation that patients with SLE have increased serum levels of IFN.[1] Since then, a number of observations indicate a central role for the IFN system in the pathogenesis of this disease. Among them are development of SLE during type I IFN therapy, increased expression of type I IFN-regulated genes (an IFN signature) in SLE, the presence of endogenous IFN inducers in these patients, and a strong association between risk for SLE and gene variants in the IFN signaling pathway.[2] The insight that IFNs, besides the antiviral effects, also have prominent functions in the adaptive immune system can partly explain the important role of the IFN system in SLE. In this chapter the IFN system and its biology will be summarized. Our focus will be on the type I IFN system, the activation of which is one of the most prominent features in SLE.

THE INTERFERON SYSTEM

The largest group of IFNs is the type I IFNs, encompassing 17 proteins that are encoded by 13 highly homologous IFNα genes and one IFNβ, IFNω, IFNϵ, and IFNκ gene. The type II IFN, IFNγ, is encoded by one single gene, whereas the type III IFNs, IFNλ (also known as IL28 and IL29), are encoded by four separate genes (Table 1).[3,4] All type I IFN subtypes bind the ubiquitously expressed IFNα/β receptor (IFNAR), type II IFN binds the IFNγ receptor (IFNGR) expressed by most cell types, and type III IFNs bind to the IFNλ receptor (IFNLR), which is mainly expressed by epithelial cells, but also by plasmacytoid dendritic cells (pDC), B cells, and monocytes.[3,5,6] Both IFNAR and IFNLR ligation activates pathways that regulate genes containing IFN-stimulated response elements.[3,4] Due to the restricted expression of the IFNLR, type III IFNs affect less than 200 of the 2000 genes regulated by type I IFN.[7] Activation of the IFNGR results in the expression of >2000 genes containing IFNγ-activated sites.[7] This pathway can also be utilized by IFNAR and consequently, around 70% of the IFNγ-regulated genes are shared by IFNα.[8]

The majority of cell types secrete small amounts of type I IFN in response to viruses, but the most potent producer is the pDC, which after activation can synthesize up to 10^9 IFNα molecules in 24 h.[9] Type III IFNs can also be produced by many different cell types, in particular pDCs, monocytes, monocyte-derived dendritic cells (MDDC), and epithelial cells,[10] whereas type II IFNs are predominantly produced by NK cells, cytotoxic T cells, and Th1 effector cells, and in lower levels by macrophages, DCs, and B cells.[11]

In summary, the IFN system consists of a network of cells, proteins, and receptors, which has evolved to protect the body from viral infections and other pathogens.

ACTIVATION AND REGULATION OF INTERFERON PRODUCTION

Type I and type III IFNs are typically induced by viruses, bacteria, or other microbes sensed by pattern recognition receptors recognizing nucleic acids localized in either the cytosol (e.g., retinoic acid-inducible gene 1-like receptors and nucleic oligomerization domain-like receptors) or the endosomes (Toll-like receptors (TLRs) 3,7, 8, and 9).

In pDC, nucleic acids from endocytosed viruses stimulate endosomal TLR7 and TLR9 and activate the myeloid differentiation factor 88-signaling pathway, which leads to

Systemic Lupus Erythematosus. http://dx.doi.org/10.1016/B978-0-12-801917-7.00019-X

153

TABLE 1 The Type I, II, and III Interferons and Their Receptors

IFN	Genes	Sequence Homology[a]	Mainly Produced by	Receptor Usage
I	IFNA1, 2, 4, 5, 6, 7, 8, 10, 13, 14, 16, 17, 21	>75%	pDC monocytes, mDC	IFNAR
I	IFNB1	30%		IFNAR
I	IFNE1	30%		IFNAR
I	IFNK	30%		IFNAR
I	IFNW1	75%		IFNAR
II	IFNG	ns	T and NK	IFNGR
III	IFNL1, 2, 3, 4	~20%	Monocytes, MDDC, pDC, epithelial cells	IFNLR

[a]Average amino acid homology to IFNα; ns, not significant.

the phosphorylation of interferon regulatory factor (IRF) 3, IRF5, and IRF7 and the transcription of type I and III IFNs.[12,13] In addition to viral infections, type I IFN production can be triggered by self-derived type I IFN inducers found in patients with SLE and other systemic autoimmune diseases. These inducers consist of nucleic acids, released from dying cells, in complex with autoantibodies. Such immune complexes bind FcγRIIa on pDCs and are internalized to the endosomes where they trigger type I IFN production through stimulation of TLR7 and/or TLR9.[14,15]

Another class of endogenous IFN inducers is self-nucleic acids in complex with RNA- or DNA-binding proteins, such as high mobility group box chromosomal protein 1 and LL37, released in neutrophil extracellular traps (NETs) during a specific neutrophilic cell death termed NETosis.[16,17] Recent findings show that uncomplexed chromatin can induce low levels of type I IFN production in neutrophils and given their high abundance these cells have been proposed to be a source of type I IFN in lupus.[18]

The type I IFN production is strictly controlled by a network of cytokines, hormones, surface receptors, and cells, to ensure a rapid and strong, but transient response to a viral infection. An important negative regulator is complement component 1q (C1q) that attenuates type I IFN production both through interactions with the leukocyte-associated Ig-like receptor 1 on pDCs[19] and through the preferential binding of C1q-containing ICs to monocytes.[20] Activation of monocytes induces the secretion of reactive oxygen species, tumor necrosis factor α and prostaglandin E2, all potent inhibitors of the type I IFN production.[21] In contrast, natural killer cells and platelets promote the pDC-derived IFNα production through interactions with LFA-1 and CD40L, respectively.[22,23] Type I IFN itself enhances the type I IFN production, possibly through the upregulation of IRF7 and TLR7 expression.[24] This IFN effect is termed "priming" and boosts the type I IFN response once the production

is activated, which is favorable in the early phase of viral infections.

Of relevance in SLE is the observation that the female sex hormone estrogen enhances IFNα production by pDCs, whereas progesterone acts inhibitory.[25,26] These observations may thus represent cellular mechanisms contributing to the female predominance among SLE patients, as well as the suggested decreased risk for lupus in patients treated with progesterone-based contraceptives.

Type II IFN is produced in response to pathogens such as intracellular bacteria, parasites, and certain viruses and the production is mainly controlled by cytokines (e.g., IL-12 and IL-18) secreted by pathogen-sensing APCs.[27]

In conclusion, a number of different cell types have developed a multitude of sensors that can recognize invading microorganisms and elicit an IFN response. Due to the presence of endogenous IFN inducers and lack of sufficient negative control mechanisms, SLE patients have a dysregulated type I IFN production.

EFFECTS OF INTERFERONS ON THE IMMUNE SYSTEM

IFNs have numerous immune-activating functions besides the direct antiviral effects (Table 2). Type I IFNs stimulate the differentiation of DCs from monocytes and promote their maturation by inducing the expression of MCH class I and II molecules, and the costimulatory molecules CD80 and CD86.[28] Type I IFNs also enhance the cytolytic activity of cytotoxic T cells and NK cells, suppress the differentiation of T-regulatory (Treg) cells, and promote the polarization of Th1 cells.[29] In contrast, a sustained type I IFN stimulation inhibits Th1 differentiation and promotes the development of T follicular helper (Tfh) cells, which in turn supports B-cell activation.[30] In addition, type I IFNs enhance Ig class switching, promote B-cell survival

TABLE 2 Effects of Type I, II, and III Interferons on Immune Cells

Target Cell	Type I IFN	Type II IFN	Type III IFN
Dendritic cells	Maturation, enhanced antigen presentation		
Monocyte/macrophage	Upregulation of TLR, differentiation to DCs	Activation	
pDC	Enhanced type I IFN production		Enhanced type I and type III production, and pDC survival
Th cell	Th1/Tfh polarization, activation, and survival of naïve and memory T cells	Th1 polarization	–
Tc cell	Increased cytotoxicity, inhibition of apoptosis	Promotes development	–
Treg	Suppression		–
B cell	Activation and differentiation of plasmablasts to plasma cells, Ig class switch, and antibody production	Ig class switch	–
NK cells	Enhanced cytotoxicity and cytokine production		

by inducing the expression of B cell-activating factor, and together with IL-6, type I IFN induce plasma cell differentiation and antibody production.[31]

Type III IFNs have limited effects on immune cells but promote the type I IFN production and survival of pDCs,[6] whereas IFNγ promotes the cell-mediated immunity by activating monocytes/macrophages, Th1, and cytotoxic T cells and enhances humoral immunity by inducing Ig class switching in B cells.[27]

Thus, IFNs have prominent activating effects on both innate and adaptive immune cells, which are important for the immune response, but if not properly controlled these effects may lead to a disruption of the peripheral tolerance and the development of an autoimmune disease.

LUPUS AND THE INTERFERON SYSTEM

Based on the observed ongoing IFN production in SLE and the effects of IFN on the immune system, an etiopathogenic model for SLE has been proposed (Figure 1). Initially, a viral infection triggers type I IFN production and the release of nuclear material from dying cells. The proapoptotic effects of type I IFN further increase the availability of nuclear material and in individuals prone to autoimmune responses, autoantibodies to these autoantigens are formed. The defective clearance of dying cells in lupus patients facilitates the formation of ICs containing nucleic acid, which trigger pDCs to a sustained type I IFN production. This process is fueled by an IFN-mediated increase in antigen-presenting capacity of DCs, activation of Th and cytotoxic T cells, and further stimulation of B cells. Finally, a vicious circle is formed, which leads to chronic inflammation and tissue damage.

Supporting the central role of pDC-derived type I IFN in this model, data from experimental lupus models show that IFNα can drive nephritis and end-organ damage,[32,33] and that depletion of pDCs improves pathology in spontaneous murine models of lupus.[34,35]

GENES IN INTERFERON SIGNALING PATHWAY AND LUPUS

Genetic association studies have identified >70 loci that are associated with an increased risk of developing lupus;[36] see Chapter 10. A few of these are rare, highly penetrant, monogenic alterations, that is, C1q, TREX1, and TRAP1 (ACP5). Remarkably, all three genes are closely linked to the type I IFN system. C1q is a negative regulator of pDC-derived type I IFN,[19,20] and loss-of function mutations in the DNA exonuclease TREX1 or the phosphatase TRAP1 result in diseases characterized by an increased activation of the type I IFN system.[37,38]

In contrast, the majority of genetic associations are common genetic variations (SNPs) with a low effect size. Such SNPs are most often found in the noncoding region of the genome and their functional consequences have not been established yet. Nevertheless, a large proportion of these SNPs can be linked to pathways in the IFN system, including the clearance of apoptotic debris and ICs (Fc receptors, nucleases), TLR signaling (IRF5, IRF7, IRAK1), and IFNAR signaling (TYK2, STAT4). Some of these variations have been associated with phenotypical alterations in the IFN system. For instance, genetic risk variants in IRF5, IRF7, IFIH1, PTPN22, and STAT4 are all associated with an increased expression of type I IFN-induced genes and/or IFNAR sensitivity.[39,40]

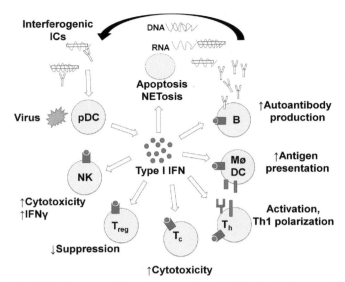

FIGURE 1 **An etiopathogenic model for SLE.** An external trigger, for example, a viral infection, induces type I IFN production and cell death resulting in the release of nucleic acid-containing material. In individuals susceptible to lupus, autoantibodies and nucleic acid-containing autoantigens form immune complexes that stimulate pDC to further type I IFN production. Type I IFN in turn promotes the production of autoantibodies leading to the formation of new interferogenic ICs. Thus a vicious circle of type I IFN production is generated. As described in the text, type I IFNs potently activate both innate and adaptive immune cells, resulting in chronic inflammation.

Several of the genetic associations linked to the IFN system are also associated with other autoimmune diseases, thus highlighting type I IFN as a central player in breaking the immune tolerance.

INTERFERONS IN THE CLINIC

Early studies demonstrated that there is an association between serum levels of IFNα and SLE disease activity and severity.[41] More recent observations derived from microarray data suggest that the activation of the IFN system in SLE is very complex and encompasses increased production of at least IFNα, IFNβ, and IFNγ.[42] In addition, type III IFN may be involved in some disease manifestations, such as skin lesions.[43] If measurements of different IFNs or IFN-regulated genes can be used as biomarkers for disease activity in SLE is at the moment unclear, but the IFN signature seems to define a disease subset with increased organ involvement, including cardiovascular and renal disease.[44,45]

High doses of both glucocorticosteroids and hydroxychloroquine downregulate the IFN signature, but during the last years several specific inhibitors of IFNα have been developed.[46] At least three monoclonal anti-IFNα antibodies have been developed, and in a recent phase IIb study of sifalimumab (MEDI-545) the drug met its primary end point (significant reduction in SLE responder index after 1 year) with an acceptable safety profile in patients with moderate to severe disease activity.[47] Another strategy to downregulate the IFN signature is to vaccinate patients with IFNα conjugated to a T-cell-dependent antigen, which induces the production of autoantibodies against IFNα.[48] A more complete inhibition of type I IFNs is to target the IFNAR, which at

least in theory could increase the risk in treated patients for viral infections. None of the type I IFN-specific therapeutic strategies will prevent the action of type II and type III IFNs, which in a subset of SLE patients may be important for the disease process or specific organ manifestations. New therapeutic concepts are to degrade the stimulatory TLR ligands in interferogenic ICs by nucleases or use inhibitory oligodeoxynucleotides to block TLR activation.[46,49] A broader therapeutic approach is to target the pDC themselves with monoclonal antibodies or proteasome inhibitors, the latter also targeting autoantibody secreting plasma cells and thus having dual beneficial effects in SLE.[50]

CONCLUSION

The importance of IFNα in the pathogenesis of lupus is supported by numerous studies. Preliminary data from clinical trials suggest that type I IFN blockade is safe and results in beneficial clinical effects in a subset of lupus patients. Given the complexity and redundant functions of the IFNs, type II and III IFNs may also be considered as therapeutic targets in future studies.

REFERENCES

1. Hooks JJ, Moutsopoulos HM, Geis SA, Stahl NI, Decker JL, Notkins AL. Immune interferon in the circulation of patients with autoimmune disease. *N Engl J Med* 1979;**301**:5–8.
2. Eloranta ML, Alm GV, Rönnblom L. Disease mechanisms in rheumatology–tools and pathways: plasmacytoid dendritic cells and their role in autoimmune rheumatic diseases. *Arthritis Rheum* 2013;**65**:853–63.

3. Baccala R, Kono DH, Theofilopoulos AN. Interferons as pathogenic effectors in autoimmunity. *Immunol Rev* 2005;**204**:9–26.

4. O'Brien TR, Prokunina-Olsson L, Donnelly RP. IFN-λ4: the paradoxical new member of the interferon lambda family. *J Interferon Cytokine Res* 2014;**34**:829–38.

5. Sommereyns C, Paul S, Staeheli P, Michiels T. IFN-lambda (IFN-λ) is expressed in a tissue-dependent fashion and primarily acts on epithelial cells in vivo. *PLoS Pathog* 2008;**4**:e1000017.

6. Yin Z, Dai J, Deng J, Sheikh F, Natalia M, Shih T, et al. Type III IFNs are produced by and stimulate human plasmacytoid dendritic cells. *J Immunol* 2012;**189**:2735–45.

7. Rusinova I, Forster S, Yu S, Kannan A, Masse M, Cumming H, et al. Interferome v2.0: an updated database of annotated interferon-regulated genes. *Nucleic Acids Res* 2013;**41**:D1040–6.

8. Hertzog P, Forster S, Samarajiwa S. Systems biology of interferon responses. *J Interferon Cytokine Res* 2011;**31**:5–11.

9. Cederblad B, Blomberg S, Vallin H, Perers A, Alm GV, Rönnblom L. Patients with systemic lupus erythematosus have reduced numbers of circulating natural interferon-α-producing cells. *J Autoimmun* 1998;**11**:465–70.

10. Coccia EM, Severa M, Giacomini E, Monneron D, Remoli ME, Julkunen I, et al. Viral infection and Toll-like receptor agonists induce a differential expression of type I and λ interferons in human plasmacytoid and monocyte-derived dendritic cells. *Eur J Immunol* 2004;**34**:796–805.

11. Frucht DM, Fukao T, Bogdan C, Schindler H, O'Shea JJ, Koyasu S. IFN-γ production by antigen-presenting cells: mechanisms emerge. *Trends Immunol* 2001;**22**:556–60.

12. Gilliet M, Cao W, Liu YJ. Plasmacytoid dendritic cells: sensing nucleic acids in viral infection and autoimmune diseases. *Nat Rev Immunol* 2008;**8**:594–606.

13. Iversen MB, Paludan SR. Mechanisms of type III interferon expression. *J Interferon Cytokine Res* 2010;**30**:573–8.

14. Båve U, Magnusson M, Eloranta ML, Perers A, Alm GV, Rönnblom L. Fc gamma RIIa is expressed on natural IFN-α-producing cells (plasmacytoid dendritic cells) and is required for the IFN-α production induced by apoptotic cells combined with lupus IgG. *J Immunol* 2003;**171**:3296–302.

15. Means TK, Latz E, Hayashi F, Murali MR, Golenbock DT, Luster AD. Human lupus autoantibody-DNA complexes activate DCs through cooperation of CD32 and TLR9. *J Clin Invest* 2005;**115**:407–17.

16. Tian J, Avalos AM, Mao SY, Chen B, Senthil K, Wu H, et al. Toll-like receptor 9-dependent activation by DNA-containing immune complexes is mediated by HMGB1 and RAGE. *Nat Immunol* 2007;**8**:487–96.

17. Garcia-Romo GS, Caielli S, Vega B, Connolly J, Allantaz F, Xu Z, et al. Netting neutrophils are major inducers of type I IFN production in pediatric systemic lupus erythematosus. *Sci Transl Med* 2011;**3**:73ra20.

18. Lindau D, Mussard J, Rabsteyn A, Ribon M, Kotter I, Igney A, et al. TLR9 independent interferon α production by neutrophils on NETosis in response to circulating chromatin, a key lupus autoantigen. *Ann Rheum Dis* 2014;**73**:2199–207.

19. Son M, Santiago-Schwarz F, Al-Abed Y, Diamond B. C1q limits dendritic cell differentiation and activation by engaging LAIR-1. *Proc Natl Acad Sci USA* 2012;**109**:E3160–7.

20. Santer DM, Hall BE, George TC, Tangsombatvisit S, Liu CL, Arkwright PD, et al. C1q deficiency leads to the defective suppression of IFN-α in response to nucleoprotein containing immune complexes. *J Immunol* 2010;**185**:4738–49.

21. Eloranta ML, Lövgren T, Finke D, Mathsson L, Rönnelid J, Kastner B, et al. Regulation of the interferon-α production induced by RNA-containing immune complexes in plasmacytoid dendritic cells. *Arthritis Rheum* 2009;**60**:2418–27.

22. Hagberg N, Berggren O, Leonard D, Weber G, Bryceson YT, Alm GV, et al. IFN-α production by plasmacytoid dendritic cells stimulated with RNA-containing immune complexes is promoted by NK cells via MIP-1β and LFA-1. *J Immunol* 2011;**186**:5085–94.

23. Duffau P, Seneschal J, Nicco C, Richez C, Lazaro E, Douchet I, et al. Platelet CD154 potentiates interferon-α secretion by plasmacytoid dendritic cells in systemic lupus erythematosus. *Sci Transl Med* 2010;**2**:47ra63.

24. Dai J, Megjugorac NJ, Amrute SB, Fitzgerald-Bocarsly P. Regulation of IFN regulatory factor-7 and IFN-α production by enveloped virus and lipopolysaccharide in human plasmacytoid dendritic cells. *J Immunol* 2004;**173**:1535–48.

25. Seillet C, Laffont S, Tremollieres F, Rouquie N, Ribot C, Arnal JF, et al. The TLR-mediated response of plasmacytoid dendritic cells is positively regulated by estradiol in vivo through cell-intrinsic estrogen receptor alpha signaling. *Blood* 2011;**119**:454–64.

26. Hughes GC, Choubey D. Modulation of autoimmune rheumatic diseases by oestrogen and progesterone. *Nat Rev Rheumatol* 2014;**10**:740–51.

27. Schoenborn JR, Wilson CB. Regulation of interferon-γ during innate and adaptive immune responses. *Adv Immunol* 2007;**96**:41–101.

28. Blanco P, Palucka AK, Gill M, Pascual V, Banchereau J. Induction of dendritic cell differentiation by IFN-α in systemic lupus erythematosus. *Science* 2001;**294**:1540–3.

29. Kadowaki N, Antonenko S, Lau JY, Liu YJ. Natural interferon α/β-producing cells link innate and adaptive immunity. *J Exp Med* 2000;**192**:219–26.

30. Osokine I, Snell LM, Cunningham CR, Yamada DH, Wilson EB, Elsaesser HJ, et al. Type I interferon suppresses de novo virus-specific CD4 Th1 immunity during an established persistent viral infection. *Proc Natl Acad Sci USA* 2014;**111**:7409–14.

31. Jego G, Palucka AK, Blanck JP, Chalouni C, Pascual V, Banchereau J. Plasmacytoid dendritic cells induce plasma cell differentiation through type I interferon and interleukin 6. *Immunity* 2003;**19**:225–34.

32. Santiago-Raber ML, Baccala R, Haraldsson KM, Choubey D, Stewart TA, Kono DH, et al. Type-I interferon receptor deficiency reduces lupus-like disease in NZB mice. *J Exp Med* 2003;**197**:777–88.

33. Fairhurst AM, Mathian A, Connolly JE, Wang A, Gray HF, George TA, et al. Systemic IFN-α drives kidney nephritis in B6.Sle123 mice. *Eur J Immunol* 2008;**38**:1948–60.

34. Rowland SL, Riggs JM, Gilfillan S, Bugatti M, Vermi W, Kolbeck R, et al. Early, transient depletion of plasmacytoid dendritic cells ameliorates autoimmunity in a lupus model. *J Exp Med* 2014;**211**:1977–91.

35. Sisirak V, Ganguly D, Lewis KL, Couillault C, Tanaka L, Bolland S, et al. Genetic evidence for the role of plasmacytoid dendritic cells in systemic lupus erythematosus. *J Exp Med* 2014;**211**:1969–76.

36. Ramos PS, Shaftman SR, Ward RC, Langefeld CD. Genes associated with SLE are targets of recent positive selection. *Autoimmune Dis* 2014;**2014**:203435.

37. Crow YJ, Hayward BE, Parmar R, Robins P, Leitch A, Ali M, et al. Mutations in the gene encoding the 3′-5′ DNA exonuclease TREX1 cause Aicardi-Goutieres syndrome at the AGS1 locus. *Nat Genet* 2006;**38**:917–20.

38. Briggs TA, Rice GI, Daly S, Urquhart J, Gornall H, Bader-Meunier B, et al. Tartrate-resistant acid phosphatase deficiency causes a bone dysplasia with autoimmunity and a type I interferon expression signature. *Nat Genet* 2011;**43**:127–31.

39. Niewold TB. Interferon alpha as a primary pathogenic factor in human lupus. *J Interferon Cytokine Res* 2011;**31**:887–92.

40. Robinson T, Kariuki SN, Franek BS, Kumabe M, Kumar AA, Badaracco M, et al. Autoimmune disease risk variant of IFIH1 is associated with increased sensitivity to IFN-α and serologic autoimmunity in lupus patients. *J Immunol* 2011;**187**:1298–303.

41. Bengtsson AA, Sturfelt G, Truedsson L, Blomberg J, Alm G, Vallin H, et al. Activation of type I interferon system in systemic lupus erythematosus correlates with disease activity but not with antiretroviral antibodies. *Lupus* 2000;**9**:664–71.

42. Chiche L, Jourde-Chiche N, Whalen E, Presnell S, Gersuk V, Dang K, et al. Modular transcriptional repertoire analyses of adults with systemic lupus erythematosus reveal distinct type I and type II interferon signatures. *Arthritis Rheumatol* 2014;**66**:1583–95.

43. Zahn S, Rehkamper C, Kummerer BM, Ferring-Schmidt S, Bieber T, Tuting T, et al. Evidence for a pathophysiological role of keratinocyte-derived type III interferon (IFNλ) in cutaneous lupus erythematosus. *J Invest Dermatol* 2011;**131**:133–40.

44. Lood C, Amisten S, Gullstrand B, Jonsen A, Allhorn M, Truedsson L, et al. Platelet transcriptional profile and protein expression in patients with systemic lupus erythematosus: up-regulation of the type I interferon system is strongly associated with vascular disease. *Blood* 2010;**116**:1951–7.

45. Baechler EC, Batliwalla FM, Karypis G, Gaffney PM, Ortmann WA, Espe KJ, et al. Interferon-inducible gene expression signature in peripheral blood cells of patients with severe lupus. *Proc Natl Acad Sci USA* 2003;**100**:2610–5.

46. Kirou KA, Gkrouzman E. Anti-interferon alpha treatment in SLE. *Clin Immunol* 2013;**148**:303–12.

47. Khamashta M, Merrill J, Werth V, Furie R, Kalunian K, Illei GG, et al. *Safety and efficacy of sifalimumab, an anti-IFN-α monoclonal antibody, in a phase 2b study of moderate to severe systemic lupus erythematosus.* Abstract presented at American College of Rheumatology. 2014.

48. Lauwerys BR, Hachulla E, Spertini F, Lazaro E, Jorgensen C, Mariette X, et al. Down-regulation of interferon signature in systemic lupus erythematosus patients by active immunization with interferon α-kinoid. *Arthritis Rheum* 2013;**65**:447–56.

49. Sun X, Wiedeman A, Agrawal N, Teal TH, Tanaka L, Hudkins KL, et al. Increased ribonuclease expression reduces inflammation and prolongs survival in TLR7 transgenic mice. *J Immunol* 2013;**190**:2536–43.

50. Ichikawa HT, Conley T, Muchamuel T, Jiang J, Lee S, Owen T, et al. Beneficial effect of novel proteasome inhibitors in murine lupus via dual inhibition of type I interferon and autoantibody-secreting cells. *Arthritis Rheum* 2012;**64**:493–503.

Chapter 20

Humoral Pathogenesis: Fcγ Receptors in Autoimmunity and End-Organ Damage

T. Ernandez[1], G. Saggu[2], T.N. Mayadas[2]

[1]Service of Nephrology, University Hospital of Geneva, Switzerland; [2]Department of Pathology, Brigham and Women's Hospital and Harvard Medical School, Boston, USA

INTRODUCTION

Antibodies are potent inducers of inflammation. A consistent feature of systemic lupus erythematosus (SLE) is the presence of autoantibodies and complement-fixing immune complexes (ICs) resulting in inflammatory lesions in multiple organ systems. Fc receptors, the receptors for immunoglobulin (Ig) G antibodies, are a group of transmembrane glycoproteins that are not only central to host defense against pathogens but, not surprisingly, can also inflict significant tissue damage when antibodies are directed against host antigens as in SLE.[1] Fc receptors are largely expressed in hematopoietic cells and mediate a wide array of immune functions such as the recruitment and activation of inflammatory cells, degranulation, antibody-dependent cell-mediated cytotoxicity (ADCC),[2] phagocytosis,[3,4] enhancement of antigen presentation, regulation of B-cell antibody production,[5] and IC clearance. Although Fc receptors exist for all the different Ig classes (IgA, IgD, IgE, IgG, IgM), our discussion will focus on the Fc receptors for IgG—the Fcγ receptors (FcγR)—because studies in mouse models suggest primary roles of FcγR in the development of SLE and functional polymorphisms in these receptors are associated with disease susceptibility in humans.

FcγRs: STRUCTURE AND FUNCTION

The extracellular region of FcγRs contains two or three extracellular Ig-like domains, which is a common feature of the Ig superfamily. In humans, three different classes of FcγRs exist—FcγRI, FcγRII, and FcγRIII—which are defined by their structural differences, signaling capacity, and variable affinity for different IgG subclasses.[6,7] Based on their role in inhibition or exacerbation of immune functions, the FcγRs are also divided into inhibitory receptors (FcγRIIB) or activating receptors (FcγRI, FcγRIIA, FcγRIIC, and FcγRIIIB). Humans also express additional FcγRs—FcRn, FcRL5, and TRIM21,[8–11] which bind IgG once internalized.

The FcγRI (CD64) and FcγRIII (CD16) are expressed as oligomeric complexes with γ (monocytes and macrophages) or ζ or β (uniquely for human FcγRIIIA in NK cells and mast cells, respectively) chain. The adaptor chains contain the cytoplasmic immunoreceptor tyrosine-based activation motif (ITAM), which links FcγRs to protein tyrosine-based intracellular signaling. Partnering with the γ chain is also required for the surface expression of both FcγRI and FcγRIII through amino acid interactions between charged residues present in the transmembrane domain of the adaptor and FcγR.[12] On the other hand, members of the FcγRII class (CD32) exist as single polypeptide transmembrane receptors containing either an activating (FcγRIIA) or inhibitory (FcγRIIB) signaling motif within their own cytoplasmic tail. A more recently recognized FcγRIIC is a crossover between FcγRIIA and IIB that contains an intracellular ITAM containing tail related to FcγRIIA and an extracellular domain homologous to FcγRIIB.[13]

Genetic deletion of FcγRs in mice has revealed primary roles for these receptors in a number of autoimmune diseases, including SLE. However, the repertoire of FcγRs between humans and mice differ in some important aspects, which should be considered when extrapolating data from mice models to human biology. Both humans and mice share a structurally common FcγRI, FcγRIIB, and FcγRIII. However, they differ in their other FcγRs. Mice express the species-specific activating FcγRIV and lack the uniquely human activating FcγRIIIB and FcγRIIA (Figure 1). The mouse FcγRIV and FcγRIII are considered orthologs of the human FcγRIIIA and FcγRIIA, respectively, based on sequence similarity in their extracellular domains.[14] The repertoire of FcγRs expressed on specific cell types can also differ between humans and mice (Figure 1). For example, human monocytes/macrophages and neutrophils express FcγRIIA, while these cell types in mice express the species-specific FcγRIV.[15] Moreover, human platelets express FcγRIIA, while mouse platelets do not express any FcγRs.[16]

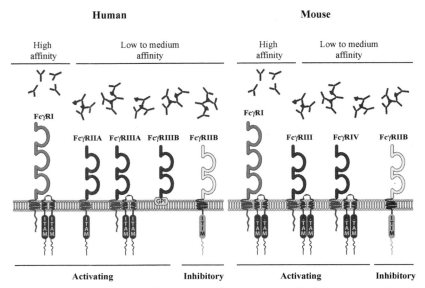

FIGURE 1   Fcγ receptor repertoire in humans and mice. Human FcγRs include the high-affinity receptor FcγRI and the low- and medium-affinity receptors FcγRIIA, FcγRIIB, FcγRIIIA, and FcγRIIIB. Mice do not express FcγRIIA and FcγRIIIB, but express a FcγRIII and a species-specific FcγRIV. The activating FcγRs are coupled to an Fcγ chain containing two immunoreceptor tyrosine-based activation motifs (ITAM) in its cytoplasmic tail. The human FcγRIIA contains an ITAM motif included in its own cytoplasmic tail. In contrast, the inhibitory FcγRIIBs of both humans and mice signal through a distinct immunoreceptor tyrosine-based inhibitory motif (ITIM) present in its cytoplasmic tail.

FcγRs are defined as high- or low-affinity receptors based on their affinity for monomeric IgG versus avidity for oligomeric ICs. Affinity values for low affinity FcγRs varies considerably between studies as the interaction with monomeric IgG has very rapid "on" and "off" rates. Nonetheless, a study conducted to assess a range of affinities of FcγRs for IgG shows that the affinity of FcγRI for IgG1-4 is in the nanomolar range compared to the micromolar range of the low-affinity receptors.[17] Notably, both high- and low-affinity receptors bind ICs with high avidity.[18]

FcγRI

The FcγRI is the only receptor able to efficiently bind monomeric IgG as well as aggregated IgG[17] and is therefore referred to as a high-affinity receptor. It differs structurally from the other FcγRs as it contains three extracellular Ig-like domains.[19] FcγRI preferentially binds IgG1 and IgG3 and to a lesser extent IgG4 and IgG2. The high-affinity IgG binding of this receptor may be due to its direct recognition of Fc glycan.[20] In contrast with the low-affinity FcγRII and FcγRIII, FcγRI is saturated with circulating monomeric IgG and triggers intracellular signals only after cross-linking with antigens, which cluster FcγRI enabling signal transduction.[14] On the other hand, cytokines induce expression of FcγRI at the cell surface and, like FcγRIIA and FcαR, rapidly increase its ability to bind ICs upon cell activation.[21] These characteristics have resulted in a hypothetical model of FcγRI activation and function: FcγRI binding of monomeric IgG and subsequent internalization

allow sampling of extracellular antigens. During inflammation, cytokines, together with subsequent IC binding, cluster FcγRI to trigger signals for cytotoxic functions, while de novo generation of FcγRI by cytokines provides additional "free" FcγRs for further IC binding.[22]

FcγRI is constitutively expressed on monocytes, macrophages, and dendritic cells and can be upregulated by interferon (IFN)-γ (and also by granulocyte-colony stimulating factor) on neutrophils, eosinophils, and glomerular mesangial cells (also IL-10).[6,23,24] Induction of FcγRI during inflammation by cytokines such as IFN-γ or interleukin (IL)-10 may trigger critical immune effector-cell functions such as phagocytosis, ADCC, and enhanced antigen presentation.[6] However, the biological role of FcγRI in autoimmunity is unclear. In humans, FcγRI deficiency does not predispose to autoimmunity[25] and no polymorphisms have been described that associate FcγRI with autoimmune disease or alter the receptor's affinity or function.[22,26] FcγRI-deficient mice or hFcγRI transgenic animals have not been reported to develop spontaneous autoimmunity. FcγRI deficiency resulted in a reduction in cartilage destruction in antigen-induced arthritis, despite an intact adaptive immune response,[27] yet it had no effect on the development of inflammatory arthritis (K/BxN) induced by the passive transfer of K/BxN mouse autoantibodies.[28,29] On the other hand, a hFcγRI transgene in mice lacking multiple endogenous murine FcγRs was sufficient to provide susceptibility to the K/BxN model.[30] The reasons for these divergent results are not clear and require further investigation.

TABLE 1 Cellular Distribution and Functions of FcγRs in Human Leukocytes

	FcγR Expression	FcγR-Mediated Functions
Neutrophils	Activating IIA, IIIB Inhibitory IIB	• Phagocytosis • Oxidative burst • Degranulation and release of proteolytic enzymes • Release of chemoattractants • ADCC
Mast cells, basophils	Activating IIA, IIIA Inhibitory IIB	• Release of vasoactive amines • Release of chemoattractants • Release of cytokines (TNFα) and prostaglandins
Macrophages	Activating I, IIA, IIIA Inhibitory IIB	• Phagocytosis • Oxidative burst • ADCC • Release of cytokines (TNFα, IL-1, IL-6)
NK cells	Activating IIIA No inhibitory FcγRs	• ADCC • Release of cytokines (TNFα, INFγ)
Dendritic cells	Activating I, IIA No inhibitory FcγRs	• Phagocytosis • Enhancement of antigen presentation • Maturation • Release of cytokines (IL-12, INFγ)
B Cells	No activating FcγRs Inhibitory IIB	• Modulation of B-cell activation • Inhibition of antibody production • Apoptosis (plasma cells)

FcγRII

The FcγRII class encompasses functionally very distinct receptors, the FcγRIIA and the FcγRIIB. It also includes the FcγRIIC, which was considered a pseudogene but then found to be expressed under certain conditions, as discussed later. FcγRIIA is an activating receptor, which signals through a noncanonical ITAM motif that may be functionally different than the common γ-chain ITAMs, perhaps through the recruitment of different signaling complexes.[31,32] Dimers of FcγRIIA bound to ICs, observed by crystallography, may play an important role in intracellular signaling.[33] FcγRIIB is an inhibitory FcγR, which signals through its immunoreceptor tyrosine-based inhibitory motif (ITIM). When co-aggregated with ITAM-containing activating receptors, FcγRIIB inhibits signals generated by the ITAM.[34,35] This inhibitory signaling extends beyond the activating FcγRs to FcεRI, FcαRI, and the B-cell receptor (BCR). Thus, FcγRIIB sets the threshold of activation and is considered an important mechanism for determining the level of cellular responses downstream of several immune receptor systems.

Both the activating FcγRIIA and the inhibitory FcγRIIB are called low-affinity receptors as they do not bind monomeric IgG, but only aggregated IgG such as ICs. Both receptors exhibit specificity for IgG1, IgG2, and IgG3 but do not bind IgG4 ICs. In general, FcγRIIB has the lowest affinity for all IgG classes compared to all other FcγRs,[26] which

may be biologically important as the ITIM-driven inhibitory signals through FcγRIIB maybe most needed only when IC concentrations increase during a normal immune response. FcγRIIA and IIB are expressed on several leukocytes (Table 1). FcγRIIA is present on neutrophils, eosinophils, basophils, platelets,[36,37] dendritic cells,[38–40] monocytes, macrophages, Langerhans cells, and transiently in immature T cells.[41,42] FcγRIIA is the most widely expressed FcγR on myeloid cells. FcγRIIA on neutrophils and macrophages promotes phagocytosis, NADPH oxidase triggered oxidative burst, leukotriene release, ADCC, cellular activation,[6] and on neutrophils supports their recruitment to IC-coated endothelium.[43,44] In dendritic cells, FcγRIIA promotes phagocytosis and facilitates the antigen-presentation required for an efficient adaptive immune response.[37,38]

In SLE, FcγRIIA may perpetuate inflammation by mediating uptake and delivery of antibody-coated chromatin to intracellular compartments containing Toll-like receptors.[45] FcγRIIA is transiently expressed in immature T cells before their T-cell receptor (TCR) rearrangement and may be important in thymocyte maturation.[41] FcγRIIA on human platelets appears to play an important role in αIIbβ3 integrin outside-in signaling and thereby, participates in platelet activation and spreading after binding of αIIbβ3 integrin to fibrinogen.[36] In platelets, this receptor may also facilitate the clearance of circulating ICs.[46] FcγRIIB is predominantly expressed on B cells but can be detected on neutrophils and monocytes at much lower levels[47–49] when associated with a specific FcγRIIB promoter haplotype, 2B.4 (see Section Fcγ Receptor Polymorphisms and Copy Number Variation in Lupus). FcγRIIB is also present on dendritic cells, but its expression is variable and may be related to the stage of cell maturation.[40,49]

The inhibitory function of FcγRIIB has been extensively studied and appears to play a critical role in maintaining peripheral tolerance (see Section Maintenance of Peripheral Tolerance)[34,35] as even a small decrease in its expression leads to a breakdown of tolerance, autoantibody production, and autoimmune disease.[50] FcγRIIB expression in other cell types also restrains the adaptive immune response, as recently demonstrated for dendritic cells. Indeed, FcγRIIB engagement in dendritic cells limits the phagocytosis of ICs as well as tumor necrosis factor (TNF)-α production, therefore impairing the antigen presentation to T cells and their subsequent activation and proliferation.[39,40,51] FcγRIIC has been detected on NK cells[52] and more recently on B cells[53] and is expressed in neutrophils and monocytes of a small number of individuals with a polymorphism that results in an open reading frame.[13].

FcγRIII

The FcγRIII class includes FcγRIIIA and FcγRIIIB, which are both low-affinity receptors. They preferentially bind IgG1 and IgG3 and exhibit virtually no binding to IgG2 and IgG4.[17] Despite a 98% identity of their extracellular domains, the two receptors are structurally distinct: the transmembrane FcγRIIIA α-chain does not contain an ITAM, and it requires interaction with the common γ-chain dimer (which contains ITAM motifs) for both expression and signaling,[6,42,54] while the FcγRIIIB attaches to the membrane through a glycosylphosphatidylinositol (GPI) anchor and lacks direct signaling capacity.[14,55,56] The FcγRIIIA is expressed on macrophages (Table 1), NK, γδ T cells, DCs[57–59] and in some reports also on a small subset of terminally differentiated αβ T cells.[60,61]

FcγRIIIA is the only FcγR expressed on NK cells and it principally mediates ADCC and proinflammatory cytokine production.[62] On γδ T cells, FcγRIIIA also mediates cytolysis via ADCC.[63] FcγRIIIA is expressed on glomerular mesangial cells after IFN-γ treatment,[6,64] where it induces the production of IL-6 and may be a key factor in the progression of glomerulonephritis.[64] In contrast to the relatively broad expression of FcγRIIIA, the GPI-linked FcγRIIIB is expressed on granulocytes (i.e., neutrophils and eosinophils)[65,66] and has recently been described on basophils.[67] It is the most abundant FcγR on neutrophils with a surface expression that is four- to fivefold greater than FcγRIIA.[68] On neutrophils, it partners with other receptors such as FcγRIIA and the complement receptor CR3 to induce neutrophil activation.[69–71]

The role of two structurally distinct activating receptors in neutrophils begs the question of whether each has evolved distinct functions. FcγRIIIB cross-linking induces calcium mobilization, triggers degranulation[72,73] and leukotriene release, oxidative burst,[70] and activation of integrins.[74] Moreover, FcγRIIIB-specific engagement triggers a robust increase in nuclear-restricted phosphorylation of ERK and the transcription factor Elk-1.[75] In vitro, human FcγRIIIB tethers neutrophils to immobilized ICs under physiological flow conditions, suggesting a role for this receptor in neutrophil recruitment.[76] Studies in transgenic mice expressing human FcγRIIIB and/or FcγRIIA on neutrophils of mice lacking their endogenous FcγRs has provided in vivo evidence that both receptors promote neutrophil recruitment that is context dependent.[44] Additionally, in mouse neutrophils, FcγRIIIB and FcγRIIA uptake soluble ICs that leads to the clearance of intravascular deposited ICs and the formation of NETs, respectively,[77] an active process of DNA extrusion from neutrophils that may be a source of autoantigen in lupus.[45] In human neutrophils, antibody blockade of FcγRIIIB but not FcγRIIA inhibits IC-induced NETosis.[77,78] In mice, the expression of FcγRIIIB alone is not sufficient for NET generation in vitro or in vivo while FcγRIIA is,[77] suggesting a complex interplay between these two receptors that requires further investigation. It is possible that FcγRIIIB plays a supportive role in FcγRIIA-induced NET formation by capturing ICs and subsequently activating FcγRIIA and/or the requirement for each FcγR in NETosis is dictated by the presence of soluble[77] versus insoluble[78] ICs.

It is noteworthy that although FcγRIIIB is a true low-affinity receptor, the FcγRIIIA in tissue macrophages is categorized as having intermediate affinity for monomeric IgG.[79] The affinity of FcγRIIIA is modulated by its glycosylation state and different glycoforms of this receptor with variable affinity pattern have been identified on monocytes/macrophages and NK cells.[80] FcγRIIIA with enhanced affinity is particularly well suited for the capture and the processing of ICs by macrophages resident in the spleen and liver, which may be critical for IC clearance from the circulation.[80] Additional complexity in the Fcγ receptor system is introduced by the presence of different allelic variants and copy number variations. These have functional consequences and may in fact dictate one aspect of the genetically predetermined susceptibility to autoimmune diseases including SLE, as detailed in the Section FcγR Polymorphisms and Copy Number Variation in Lupus.[80–83]

IgG AND FcγR INTERACTIONS

Mirroring the complex organization of FcγRs, IgG are also subdivided into four classes that exhibit different patterns of affinity for their receptors. This topic was revisited in a study where the affinity for the Fc region of the different

IgG isotypes for all four FcγRs and known allelic variants were compared in parallel in vitro.[17] The Fc fragment consists of the carboxy-terminal constant domains of the IgG heavy chains, which contain an N-glycan at Asn 297 that is essential for binding to FcγRs.[84] The differences in the degree of galactosylation, fucosylation, and sialylation can dictate selectivity in binding to particular classes of Fc receptors.[85–87] For example, α-glycosylated IgG selectively bind FcγRI, potentially bypassing inhibitory signaling by FcγRIIB.[88] On the other hand, high N-glycan galactosylation of IgG1 molecules leads to cooperative signaling between FcγRIIB and a hemi-ITAM containing receptor, Dectin-1, which in turn promotes inhibitory signaling toward chemokine receptors.[89]

Nuclear magnetic resonance studies have shown that glycan branches of an IgG are highly mobile and that this mobility allows accessibility of their glycan termini to glycan-modifying enzymes.[90] Sugars at the N-glycan termini can influence the Fc structure and in turn the FcγR binding.[91] Thus, these N-glycan modifications can give rise to a range of conformations with different affinities for the FcγRs. This may be an important regulatory mechanism in order to avoid high-affinity conformations, which may be undesirable.[92] An understanding of this also has implications in therapeutic monoclonal antibody (mAb) design. IgGs are constantly agalactosylated in serum under steady conditions. Thus, a change in their galactosylation form can lead to a change in their interactions with the receptors[93]. Notably, IgGs with altered glycosylation states (often reduced) are detected in patients with SLE[94] and rheumatoid arthritis[95] and also in mouse models of autoimmunity.[96,97] A study also showed that altered glycosylation, specifically higher exposure of fucosyl residues by immobilized IgG complexes, correlated with SLE disease activity.[98]

Mouse and human FcγRs differ in their ability to bind different subclasses of IgG. For example, FcγRI in humans can bind IgG1, IgG3, and IgG4, whereas in mice it binds only IgG2a.[22] The distinct affinity pattern of the different IgG subclasses for FcγRs may account for their variable pathogenicity both in mice and humans. For example, in mouse models of autoimmune anemia and tumor cell cytotoxicity, higher pathogenicity is attributed to IgG2a and IgG2b compared to other isotypes,[99,100] likely because of their preferential affinity for FcγRIV, which is highly proinflammatory in several models of disease in mice.[101]

Lupus-prone mice strains also predominantly express IgG2a and IgG2b: IgG2a is the dominant subclass in glomerular eluates from NZB/W mice,[102,103] whereas IgG2b is prevalent in BXSB mice.[103] IgG2a and IgG2b are equally common in MRL/lpr mice.[103] Furthermore, C57BL/6 mice genetically engineered with a deficiency in FcγRIIB develop spontaneous SLE that correlates with high serum titers and glomerular deposits of IgG (see Section Maintenance of Peripheral Tolerance).[104] Thus by extension, FcγRIV may be predicted to be the predominant FcγR responsible for tissue injury in lupus models in mice. In human SLE, IgG3 and IgG1 are the dominant isotypes involved in the anti-DNA response and preferentially engage FcγRIIA (ortholog of FcγRIV) and FcγRIIIA.[105] Anti-dsDNA IgG3 antibody appears to be more specifically involved in SLE among other connective tissue diseases,[106] and in human lupus nephritis, IgG3 and IgG1 renal deposition is the most commonly observed.[107–109] However, IgG2 deposition is also frequently observed in lupus nephritis and, interestingly, intense IgG2 deposition in the kidney was associated with FcγRIIA *R131* allele,[109] a polymorphism shown to be associated with susceptibility to SLE. The FcγRIIA R131 polymorphism exhibits a decrease in affinity for IgG2 that may result in impaired clearance of IgG2 containing IC, a subsequent increase in IC deposition, and the observed increase in lupus nephritis incidence (see Section Fcγ Receptor Polymorphisms and Copy Number Variation in Lupus).[83,110]

As discussed, the FcγRs differ in their expression pattern, their surface levels, and affinity for IgG subclasses, and the relative expression of activating versus inhibitory receptors on the cell surface.[101] All these variables are crucial in determining the immune effector response and therefore the nature of IC-mediated diseases. Thus, it is not surprising that inflammatory and/or immuno-modulatory mediators play a key role in modulating these parameters. IFN-γ and C5a upregulate the expression of FcγRI and FcγRIII and downregulate the inhibitory FcγRIIB.[23,24,111,112] On the other hand, Th-2 cytokines such as IL-4, IL-10, or TGF-β upregulate the inhibitory FcγRIIB and downregulate the activating FcγRs,[113–115] while IVIG administration, used in the treatment of inflammatory and infectious diseases, enhances FcγRIIB expression on splenic macrophages.[116]

Posttranscriptional effects of cytokines on FcγRs have also been described. For instance, inflammatory mediators promote FcγRIIIB shedding from the surface, but can also induce FcγRIIIB translocation from intracellular stores, thus increasing surface levels.[117,118] On the other hand, FcγRIIA surface levels do not change, but its activity may be regulated at the ligand-binding stage. Its binding activity for IgG-ICs was transiently increased on neutrophils following treatment with the bacterial chemotactic peptide fmlp,[71] or C5aR[119] and on eosinophils following GM-CSF, IL-3, and IL-5,[120] suggesting affinity regulation of FcγRIIA. In addition to their effects on FcγRs, cytokines regulate IgG isotype switching. The Th-1 cytokine IFN-γ preferentially induces the more pathogenic IgG2a subclass, whereas the Th-2 cytokines IL-4 induces switching to more indolent murine IgG1.[7,121]

FcγRs AND COMPLEMENT

The complement system is a major effector mechanism in innate immune responses. Complement can be activated via the classical, alternative, or mannose-binding lectin pathways, each of which converges on the activation of the central C3 component. Deficiency in components of the complement cascade and in particular the classical pathway has been strongly associated with autoimmunity and SLE.[122] Genetic variants in Factor H, a regulatory protein of the alternative pathway, have also been associated with SLE susceptibility.[123] In the classical complement pathway, the first component of the cascade, C1q, binds to and is activated by the Fc-portion of Igs in ICs.[124] C1q has protective and proinflammatory roles that have been shown to potentially contribute to the development of SLE, as discussed in detail elsewhere.[125] In particular, C1q deficiency has been linked to defects in binding and subsequent clearance of apoptotic cells, but this is likely through non-FcγR related mechanisms.[126] On the other hand, several of C1q's proinflammatory effects are manifested directly or indirectly through FcγRs. C1q may aid in the deposition of immune complexes within the vasculature,[127] which in turn triggers FcγR-mediated immune cell recruitment. Complement C1q triggers the production of C3b, which subsequently catalyzes C5 to its active form C5a[128] and these components have been shown to directly modulate FcγR functions.[48] For instance, C5a transcriptionally upregulates FcγRIII and downregulates FcγRIIB in alveolar macrophages in a murine model of acute pulmonary IC hypersensitivity.[111] Similarly, C5a induces the expression of FcγRI and FcγRIII in a model of autoimmune hemolytic anemia[129] and modulates FcγRIIA ability to bind and phagocytose IgG opsonized targets.[119] In turn, FcγRs induce the production of C5a, as shown in vitro following cross-linking on macrophages,[130,131] and in vivo in a model of autoimmune hemolytic anemia.[129]

Unexpectedly, although C5aR-deficient mice exhibit defects in FcγR-mediated inflammatory responses in the lung, peritoneum, and kidney,[132–134] C3-deficient mice are not protected. These data suggest a complex interaction between C5a and FcγR that is potentially independent of C3b production and thereby bypasses the upstream classical and alternative complement cascades.[132,135] In support of this, C5aR blockade significantly attenuated neutrophil accumulation and edema in C3-deficient mice subjected to the reverse passive Arthur's reaction.[135] It is notable that IgG can also activate the alternate pathway of complement via binding C3b,[136] which can be amplified by C5a-dependent neutrophil activation.[137] This is of interest as in mouse models of K/BxN arthritis, FcγRIII and C5aR-deficient mice are equally protected from disease development, whereas C1q-deficient mice are not. A role for the alternative pathway is also suggested by the finding that Factor B-deficient mice are protected in this model.[138] In models

that require C5aR but not complement C3, C5a may also be generated by a proteolytic pathway independent of C4b. For example, C5a can be generated by thrombin, a serine protease in the coagulation pathway.[139] Thus FcγRs and C5aRs may play codominant roles in IC-induced inflammatory responses. Clarification of the mechanisms underlying their collaboration may thereby uncover critical steps involved in autoimmune mediated end-organ damage.

The crosstalk between FcγR and C5aR has been shown to be bidirectional. A study showed that highly galactosylated IgG1-IC promotes interaction of inhibitory FcγRIIB with Dectin-1, which in turn leads to intracellular signals that suppress the C5aR-mediated effector functions in neutrophils. This inhibitory effect may serve as a feedback loop to control inflammation in autoimmunity.[89]

ACTIVATING AND INHIBITORY FcγR SIGNALING

Activating and inhibitory FcγRs are classified by their signaling properties through ITAM- and ITIM-based motifs, respectively. The activating FcγRI, FcγRIIA, FcγRIIIA, as well as the murine FcγRIII and FcγRIV, initiate signaling through ITAM motifs. FcγRI, FcγRIII, and FcγRIV need to interact with the Fcγ chain bearing two ITAM motifs, while the human FcγRIIA is a single polypeptide chain containing an ITAM motif in its own cytoplasmic domain. FcγRIIIB does not directly interact with an ITAM-bearing adaptor. It can instead transduce signals by interacting with other membrane proteins (such as CD18-integrins or FcγRIIA)[140] and accumulate in lipid rafts to trigger an activating signal through src-family tyrosine kinases, such as hck.[141,142] FcγRIIB, the only inhibitory receptor, downmodulates activating signals through an ITIM motif included in its cytoplasmic domain (Figure 2).

After the binding of ICs, FcγR clusters in lipid rafts at the cell surface, which induces the phosphorylation of the ITAM motif by an src protein kinase family member. The syk kinase is subsequently recruited by the phosphorylated ITAM through its src-homology 2 (SH2) domain leading to the formation of a signaling complex at the membrane, in which Syk phosphorylates and activates several other substrates (Figure 2).[143] As a result, the phosphatidylinositol 3-kinase (PI3K) pathway is activated and its lipid products (PIP3) mediate the membrane localization and activation of several signaling proteins including Akt and the phospholipase Cγ (PLCγ). PLCγ induces the production of inositol-3-phosphate (IP3), mediating a sustained intracellular increase in calcium (Ca^{2+}) as a result of mobilization of stores from the endoplasmic reticulum and the opening of plasma membrane Ca^{2+} channels.[144] Extracellular calcium entry is required for FcγR dependent reactive oxygen species (ROS) generation. Depletion of intracellular calcium stores is sensed by

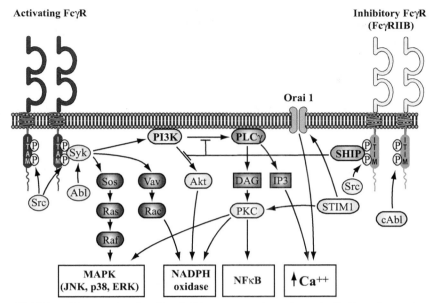

FIGURE 2   Activating and inhibitory Fcγ receptor signaling. IgG-immune complexes cluster the FcγRs at the membrane surface, which results in the phosphorylation of the ITAM motif (activating FcγRs) or the ITIM motif (inhibitory FcγRIIB) by src family kinases (Src). As depicted, this triggers opposing signaling events. ITAM signals promote proinflammatory cellular functions such as cell activation, degranulation, phagocytosis, oxidative burst, transcription, and cytokine release. ITIM signals directly counteract ITAM signals initiated by FcγR and other ITAM linked receptors such as BCR, through activation of SHIP. ITIM can also induce plasma cell apoptosis through a cAbl-dependent pathway.

stromal-interacting molecule 1 (STIM1) at the endoplasmic reticulum that then triggers the entry of external calcium.[145] Studies in phagocytes deficient in STIM1 suggest that STIM1 supports store-operated calcium entry required for ROS generation and phagocytosis following FcγR engagement.[146–148] STIM1 activation of PKCα and β phosphorylates NADPH oxidase components, and triggers two calcium binding proteins S100A8 and S100A9, that partner with NADPH oxidase cytosolic factors to support FcγR mediated ROS generation.[146,147] Moreover, FcγR dependent STIM1 activation of ORAI calcium release-activated calcium modulator 1 (Orai 1) at the plasma membrane allows extracellular Ca^{2+} influx.[146] Syk also activates the exchange factor Sos, leading to the activation of the ras-raf-MAPK pathway.[149] The Rac pathway is also activated by Syk through the Rho/Rac GTPase guanine exchange factor Vav critically involved in neutrophil and macrophage FcγR-mediated oxidative burst and cytoskeleton reorganization.[150,151] More recent data suggest that like Src kinases, the Abl family of nonreceptor tyrosine kinases, Abl and Arg may directly phosphorylate Syk to promote maximal Syk activation.[152] These signaling events can lead to cellular activation, degranulation, phagocytosis, oxidative burst, ADCC, proinflammatory genes expression, and release of cytokines.[14]

FcγRIIB, the only inhibitory FcγR, downmodulates activating signals through an ITIM motif included in its cytoplasmic domain (Figure 2). FcγRIIB triggers signaling only if co-engaged with either BCR in B cells, FcγRIII or FcεRI

in mast cells, or FcγRIII or FcγRIA in macrophages.[153] The co-aggregation of FcγRIIB induces the phosphorylation of the ITIM motif by the src-family kinase Lyn, triggering the recruitment of SH2-domain-containing phosphatases such as SHP1, SHP2, and the inositol polyphosphate 5′ phosphatase (SHIP).[154,155] As the primary substrates of SHIP are the PI3K lipid products (PIP3), FcγRIIB inhibits ITAM, activating signaling primarily by blocking the production of the second messengers IP3 and diacylglycerol (DAG) generated by PI-3k/PLCγ and therefore suppressing Ca^{2+} mobilization from intracellular stores.[34] Another ITIM- and SHIP-independent pathway engaged by FcγRIIB has also been identified in B cells. Cross-linking of FcγRIIB specifically mediates plasma cell apoptosis via an Abl-family kinase pathway. This may play an important role in eliminating autoantibody producing B cells and thereby maintaining tolerance.[156]

The importance of counterbalancing ITAM and ITIM signals in titrating effector responses emerges as a theme for other immune receptor systems as well, including TCR, BCR, and NK activating receptors.[157–160] However, it is important to recognize that ITAM-containing receptors are not always activating. For example, γ-chain associated with IgA receptor (FcαR) inhibits IgG-mediated functions in monocytes and mast cells and the ITAM-containing adaptor DAP12 limits TLR-induced cytotoxic production.[12] The switch in ITAM function may depend on the avidity of the receptor ligation, with low avidity leading to recruitment of phosphatases that cross-inhibit heterologous receptors, while high avidity receptor ligation may increase ITAM signaling and downstream activation of Syk and associated activating signals.[161] However, these are instances of heterologous receptors with distinct ligand interactions. In the case of FcγRIIB and IIA, which bind the same ligands with similar affinity, the view that ITAM is activating and ITIM is inhibitory appears to hold true with the net signaling effect depending on the ratio of activating and inhibitory signal. This ratio may be influenced by the IgG subclasses that offer differential affinity for activating and inhibitory receptors, as well as the local cytokine milieu, which directly modulates the expression of activating and inhibitory receptors at the cell surface.

ROLES OF FcγRs IN SLE

The roles of FcγRs in autoimmune disease can be divided into three distinct steps[162]:

1. Defect of FcγRIIB in controlling autoreactive B-cell activation leading to the breakdown of peripheral tolerance
2. Deficiency in clearance of circulating autoantibody IgG-containing ICs by FcγRs on macrophages in liver and spleen
3. Tissue IC deposition and activation of FcγR bearing immune effector cells (e.g., macrophages and neutrophils) that directly promote end-organ injury and clear autoantibody-opsonized circulating cells (erythrocytes, platelets), thus leading to anemia/thrombocytopenia

The available data supporting such mechanisms in SLE are detailed in this section.

Maintenance of Peripheral Tolerance

Fcγ receptors are centrally involved in the regulation and the specificity of Igs produced and are therefore an essential checkpoint in the adaptive immune response.[163] FcγRIIB plays a critical role in maintaining immune homeostasis under physiological conditions, and an increasing amount of data suggests that dysfunction of this receptor causes autoimmune disorders. The importance of FcγRIIB in tolerance maintenance has been largely elucidated following the generation of the FcγRIIB-deficient mice[164] and the discovery that a deficiency in this receptor in a C57Bl/6 background is associated with production of autoantibodies and lethal autoimmune glomerulonephritis[104] (Table 2). As FcγRIIB is the only Fcγ receptor expressed on B cells, its deficiency may be a critical determinant in development of autoreactive B cells and autoantibody production in SLE.[14,162]

However, the role of FcγRIIB deficiency in autoimmunity depends on epistatic influence of other lupus-prone genetic background. FcγRIIB deficiency was generated initially on a lupus-resistant 129Sv strain that did exhibit an enhance response to antigenic challenges, but did not develop uncontrolled production of antibodies or spontaneous inflammation.[164] When backcrossed onto C57Bl/6 background, FcγRIIB deficiency inherited from the 129Sv background triggers a spontaneous autoimmune phenotype that was however not reproduced in a BALB/c background.[104] Interestingly, FcγRIIB-deficient mice generated on a pure C57Bl/6 background produces antinuclear antibodies but do not develop lupus unless crossed to the Yaa lupus-prone strain,[165] suggesting that these antibodies are not sufficient to trigger loss of self-tolerance but are likely modifiers of autoimmune susceptibility. 129Sv mice harbor the *Sle1b* haplotype, a region of the locus *Sle1* of the chromosome 1 that is shared by all lupus-prone mouse strains and associated with lupus nephritis. The transfer of a distal region of the chromosome 1 encompassing this haplotype from the 129Sv strain onto the C57Bl/6 background is sufficient to trigger autoantibody production.[166] The initial FcγRIIB deficient 129Sv-derived mice backcrossed to C57Bl/6 mice retain this *Sle1* locus, which explains the difference of phenotype compared to the silencing of FcγRIIB in a pure C57Bl/6 strain. Altogether, FcγRIIB loss of function appears to be a critical player in autoimmunity but requires additional epistatic interactions with lupus-prone loci to manifest a loss of self-tolerance and a full-blown lupus phenotype.

The inhibitory FcγRIIB on B cells regulates the adaptive humoral immune response at two different levels: B-cell activation and plasmocyte survival.[34,167,168] First, FcγRIIB controls the magnitude and persistence of response to antigen by modulating the BCR signal. Second, this receptor excludes low-affinity or self-reactive B cells. That is, during the affinity maturation of B cells, high-affinity B cells receive a signal form both BCR and FcγRIIB when interacting with follicular dendritic cells in peripheral immune organs, while low-affinity or self-reactive lymphocytes receive a signal only through FcγRIIB and thus undergo apoptosis.[14] FcγRIIB also directly modulates plasma cell survival. In response to immunization, FcγRIIB-deficient mice have a greater number of plasma cells due to their greater production[35] and a longer lifespan.[168] With regards to the latter, cross-linking of FcγRIIB on plasma cells from wild-type mice induces apoptosis independently of BCR activation, possibly through the cAbl kinase pathway, and therefore controls their persistence in the bone marrow.[155,156,168,169] Finally, cross-linking of FcγRIIB expressed on human plasmablasts or on the human myeloma cell line (EJM) also induces apoptosis, suggesting that this mechanism is relevant in humans.[168] Thus, a dysregulation of FcγRIIB expression in B cells could enhance autoantibody production and B-cell survival, and thereby autoimmunity. This is supported by a study showing in active SLE patients a higher percentage of plasma B cells and lower levels of FcγRIIB on memory B lymphocytes (CD19+CD27+) and plasma B cells (CD19^low CD27^high) compared to normal donors.[49]

TABLE 2 FcγR Functions in Animal Models of SLE

Mouse Strain	Phenotype	FcγR Functions Involved
FcγRIIB knock out[104]		
Sv129/C57BL/6 mixed background	Normal	
BALB/c background	Normal	
C57BL/6 background	Systemic chronic inflammatory syndrome with spontaneous progressive glomerulonephritis resulting in high level of proteinuria and increased mortality. High titer of antinuclear antibodies at 4–5 months.	Impaired inhibitory signal in B cells resulting in an activated phenotype of B cells with increased number of mature IgG producing B cells. Possibilities include decreased plasma cell apoptosis[168] and/or impaired inhibitory signal in antigen presenting cells resulting in increased CD4+ lymphocytes subset.[51]
Wild-type C57BL/6 FcγRIIB restoration in BXSB background[200]	Absence of lupus syndrome. Absence of autoantibody production and glomerulonephritis. Normal lifespan.	Restoration of functional level of FcγRIIB expression in genetically impaired BXSB background (promoter polymorphism). Therefore restoration of FcγRIIB inhibitory functions in immune cells and prevention of tolerance breakdown in BXSB mice.
Fcγ chain knock out		
NZB/NZW background[198,199]	Delayed onset and reduced proteinuria in Fcγ−/− mice despite similar IC as well as C3 glomerular deposition. Prolonged survival compared to Fcγ+/− littermate.	Disruption of the FcγR-mediated response of immune effector cells.
BXSB[200]	Absence of glomerulonephritis and prolonged survival despite comparable autoantibody titers and similar IC and C3 glomerular deposition compared to BXSB Fcγ+/+.	Disruption of the FcγR-mediated response of immune effector cells. Impaired development of hyperreactive Gr-1− monocytes subset.[205]
MRL-Fas[lpr201]	Compared to Fcγ+/+ background, similar incidence of glomerulonephritis and level of proteinuria. Comparable survival. Similar levels of anti-DNA antibodies and circulating ICs.	Inflammatory syndrome and tissue damage observed in MRL-Fas[lpr] mice appear to be FcγR independent, possibly mediated by IgG3 autoantibody cryo-globulins, which do not bind FcγRs. In this mouse strain, tissue damage may be primarily mediated by complement activation.[202]

Murine models of autoimmune disorders also support the thesis that FcγRIIB regulates humoral immunity. Mouse strains susceptible to autoimmunity including SLE (NZB, MRL, BXBB, SB/Le, 129, and NOD mice) all contain a deletion in the promoter of FcγRIIB that correlates with a lower cell surface expression of this receptor on mature B cells and macrophages compared to control mouse strains (BALB/c, C57BL/6, or DBA2).[170] Furthermore, partial restoration of expression of FcγRIIB in B cells, but also in immature thymocytes and macrophages in autoimmune-prone mouse strains (NZM 2410, BXSB, B6. FcγRIIB−/−), limits autoantibody generation and greatly improves the survival of these mice.[171] The role of FcγRIIB specifically on B cells in the development of autoimmunity is also demonstrated by the finding that transgenic expression of FcγRIIB specifically in the B-cell compartment of FcγRIIB-deficient mice reduced SLE, led to early resolution of collagen-induced arthritis, and suppressed T-cell-dependent IgG immune responses. On the other hand, FcγRIIB expression in macrophages

had no effect on these parameters but decreased survival after *Streptococcus pneumoniae* infection.[172] Furthermore, Rag1- or IgH-deficient mice transplanted with bone marrow from FcγRIIB-deficient mice developed autoantibodies and glomerulonephritis in spite of FcγRIIB expression in the monocytic compartment, but not in B cells.[104] A more general immunomodulatory role for FcγRIIB is also apparent in other inflammatory mouse models. FcγRIIB-deficient mice exhibit an increase in collagen-induced arthritis[173,174] and Goodpasture-like syndrome induced by anticollagen IV antibody.[175]

Immune Complex Clearance

Effective processing of ICs diminishes their deposition in tissues and in the context of host defense may help in the delivery of antigens to specific sites where antigen presentation may occur. Defects in IC clearance are observed in many autoimmune disorders such as SLE.[176,177] However, these are complex disorders and clear evidence demonstrating a cause and effect in patients still remains elusive. Clearance of circulating ICs is accomplished by the mononuclear phagocyte system predominantly in the liver and spleen, and by erythrocytes, which bind ICs, thus preventing their interaction with the endothelium and/or extravasation into the tissues.[178,179] Then sinusoidal phagocytes remove ICs bound to erythrocytes when erythrocytes circulate through the liver and spleen.[180]

The two primary molecular mediators of IC clearance are the complement proteins and their receptors, and FcγRs. Complement prevents IC precipitation by disrupting the stability and decreasing the size of the ICs, and by coating the ICs with C4b and C3b for their safe transport within the circulation via erythrocytes bearing the C3b/C4b receptor CR1 (CD35).[181] It also mediates uptake and disposal of ICs via complement receptors present on phagocytes of the liver and spleen. Impaired processing and uptake of ICs in SLE patients is attributed to deficiencies in early complement components, decreased CR1 expression, and impaired FcγR function. A deficiency in early classical complement proteins including C1q and C4 is the strongest genetic susceptibility factor for SLE.[122] C3 deficiency and a deficiency in the complement receptor for C3, Mac-1 (Complement receptor 3, CR3), is also associated with SLE.[182–184] FcγRIIA on macrophages have been implicated in IC clearance from the circulation and patients with expression of the low IgG binding variant of FcγRIIA R131 show reduced IC endocytosis by macrophages and enhanced susceptibility to SLE.[185,186] FcγRIIB on liver sinusoidal endothelial cells, a major site of clearance of small ICs, appears to play a major role in this process. FcγRIIB-b2 isotype is highly expressed on the sinusoidal endothelial cells and FcγRIIB deficiency in mice significantly curtails the removal of passively transferred radioiodinated soluble ICs.[187]

In addition to clearance of circulating ICs, removal of tissue-deposited ICs is also required. Endothelial cells of certain vascular beds may promote endocytosis of intravascular ICs through FcγRs[188–191] and epithelial cells in close contact with the basement membrane in the glomerulus may remove trapped ICs via an active transport system involving FcRn, an IgG transport receptor.[192] Circulating phagocytes (neutrophils, monocytes) may play a role in clearing ICs deposited within the vasculature, which may be particularly important in the glomerulus, a frequent site of IC trapping.[193] Indeed, glomerular ICs can trigger transient accumulation of neutrophils that is associated with a complete clearance of the immune deposits and restoration of the structural integrity of the glomerulus within 24 h of IC deposition.[194] There is indirect evidence to suggest that FcγRIIIB plays a role in this process. FcγRIIIB promotes tethering of neutrophils to ICs under flow conditions[76] and endocytose preformed ICs both in vitro[77,195,196] and in vivo.[77] The presence of FcγRIIIB on microvilli,[197] its

predicted fast mobility in the membrane bilayer,[68] coupled with its weak signaling capacity, may suit FcγRIIIB for efficient capture and internalization of ICs deposited within the vasculature, as was shown,[77] without the potential injurious consequences of overt neutrophil activation. By extension, a potential attenuation in clearance of tissue-deposited IC as a result of impaired FcγRIIIB function may explain the observed increase in the risk of lupus nephritis in patients with a functional polymorphism in FcγRIIIB (see Section Fcγ Receptor Polymorphisms and Copy Number Variations in Lupus).

PATHOGENESIS OF LUPUS NEPHRITIS

Significant strides have been made in identifying pathogenic processes in vivo that are dependent on activating FcγRs. Using mouse models, several studies have shown that FcγRs are required for leukocyte influx and injury induced by autoimmune responses in several organs including the skin, lung, kidney, and joints. In SLE, murine activating FcγRs play an important role in the development of lupus nephritis, as disease is significantly attenuated in Fcγ chain-deficient mice bred to NZB/NZW[198] or BXSB mice[199,200] despite comparable IC deposition and complement activation (Table 2). Further confidence in these results is provided by a careful analysis of congenic strains with Fcγ chain deficiency, which has ruled out the possibility that the protective effect seen in these animals is due to the restoration of the altered inhibitory FcγRIIB function.

It is noteworthy that Fcγ chain-deficient BXSB mice had significantly less renal damage and mortality compared to wild-type BXSB mice despite comparable levels of anti-DNA autoantibodies and renal IC deposits. On the other hand, BXSB mouse strains bred to C57Bl/B6 animals to restore FcγRIIB expression levels were also protected but in this case correlated with a suppression of anti-DNA antibody production and IC deposition.[200] This set of experiments definitively showed that the protection provided by Fcγ chain deficiency in lupus models is likely related to the impaired activation of effector immune cells independently of FcγRIIB function, production of autoantibodies, and IC deposition. On the other hand, Fcγ chain deficiency in the MRL/lpr was not protective.[201] The difference may be explained by the fact that among several lupus-prone mice, including NZB/NZW and BXSB, MRL-Fas[lpr] mice produce the largest amount of IgG3 cryoglobulins (IgG that form insoluble aggregates at low temperature), which activate complement but largely fail to engage FcγRs.[202,203] This is corroborated by findings that the level of IgG3 autoantibodies correlates with lupus nephritis in the MRL-Fas[lpr] strain.[204]

A study also suggested that activating FcγRs are required for the generation of a hyperreactive Gr-1⁻ monocyte subset in BXSB mice that are characterized by high expression of activating FcγRIV and low levels of FcγRIIB. This subset, which contributes to the generation of tissue macrophages and dendritic cells, may be involved in tissue damage in this lupus-prone mouse strain. Indeed, BXSB mice lacking the Fcγ chain are protected against renal damage, as reported earlier, and do not exhibit the usual monocytosis observed in the BXSB mouse strain.[205]

With respect specifically to SLE, Fcγ chain on circulating bone marrow-derived cells has been shown to play a major role in tissue injury.[199] Genome-wide association studies in humans provide evidence that receptors highly expressed on neutrophils, FcgRIIA, FcγRIIIB and Mac-1 represent SLE susceptibility loci.[206] Further studies in mice that express human FcγRIIA selectively on neutrophils and a small percentage of monocytes, and lack endogenous murine FcγRs, have clarified the role of neutrophil FcγRs in the effector phase and end-organ injury in a model of SLE: Passive transfer of lupus patient sera containing ICs, increased glomerular neutrophil accumulation and nephritis in FcγRIIA expressing mice only when these mice additionally lack Mac-1. This suggests that FcγRIIA on neutrophils can directly contribute to end organ damage in lupus, and that Mac-1 negatively regulates FcγRIIA-mediated glomerular neutrophil accumulation.[207] FcγR may also play an important role once induced on the surface of tissue-resident cells. Mesangial cells express both FcγRIA and FcγRIIIA after stimulation with IFN-γ and engagement of FcγRIIIA on these cells triggers the production of IL-6, CCL2 (MCP-1), and CSF-1,[64,208] which can promote leukocyte recruitment in glomerulonephritis and, thereby, promote renal tissue damage.

The relative paucity of data at present examining the role of specific FcγRs directly in lupus nephritis is likely related to the complex genetic background of lupus-prone mouse strains, and the fact that a detailed and comprehensive analysis of genes of interest in lupus is both time- and labor-intensive. Lupus nephritis is common and is often a major determinant in prognosis in SLE patients. The phenotype of knockout mice subjected to anti-GBM nephritis (also referred to as nephrotoxic serum, induced by the administration of serum raised against the glomerular basement membrane) may predict the contribution of the genes of interest in lupus nephritis.[209] By this argument, FcγRI and FcγRIII shown to participate in the pathogenesis of anti-GBM nephritis may also be involved in SLE.[197,210–212] The anti-GBM model may also be useful to identify which cell type bearing the activating FcγRs may be specifically involved in the lupus nephritis pathogenesis. For instance, the specific reexpression of the γ-chain and therefore the activating FcγRs in macrophages of mice restores susceptibility to anti-GBM nephritis. However, the restoration is partial,[199] suggesting that other Fc-bearing leukocyte subsets are more important. Indeed, the specific knock-in of human FcγRIIA or FcγRIIIB in neutrophils of mice lacking their endogenous FcγRs is sufficient to restore susceptibility to nephrotoxic

nephritis, which might suggest overall a secondary role of FcγR expression in mesangial cells and macrophages in determining glomerulonephritis pathogenesis.[44] As neutrophils are consistently present in human renal biopsies from patients with membranoproliferative, crescentic and lupus glomerulonephritis,[213–215] activating FcγRs on neutrophils, may be key players in kidney injury in human SLE.

Fcγ RECEPTOR POLYMORPHISMS AND COPY NUMBER VARIATION IN LUPUS

Genetic predisposition to SLE has been known for many years. However, this heritability is a complex genetic trait, largely influenced by environmental factors and ethnic genetic backgrounds. Concordance rate among monozygotic twins is thereby lower than 50% in SLE.[216] With genome-wide linkage analysis studies, multiple genomic regions involving nearly 40 genes have been associated with increased risk of SLE.[206] Among them, the chromosomal region 1q23-24 containing the genes for the low-affinity Fcγ receptors has been repeatedly highlighted.[81] Further candidate gene analysis largely confirmed the association between polymorphisms of FcγRIIA, FcγRIIB, FcγRIIIA, FcγRIIIB, and SLE, or specifically with lupus nephritis susceptibility.[26,80]

However, the numerous influencing factors and the overall small effect of these polymorphisms in SLE susceptibility, if taken in isolation, require large cohorts or meta-analysis to achieve a sufficiently high statistical power. The observed contrasting effects of FcγR polymorphisms in different ethnic backgrounds are also suggestive of a more complex multigenic background dictating SLE susceptibility. In addition, the FcγR chromosomal region is complex, involving large gene homology and CNV that complicate genetic analysis. Careful and critical analysis of genetic data regarding technical and methodological limitations is essential to gain insights into SLE pathogenesis from such approaches. Nevertheless, although some FcγR polymorphisms such as FcγRIIIA-F/F158, FcγRIIA-R/R131, and FcγRIIIB-NA2/NA2 were not consistently associated with increased risk of SLE in different cohorts, they still appeared to influence the course of the disease and the occurrence of specific manifestations such as nephritis,[217,218] hematological manifestations,[219,220] serositis, and arthritis.[219] However, these data remain isolated and larger cohorts are required to definitively demonstrate these links.

Although such genetic information has not yet impacted clinical practice, it is still of great scientific interest to comprehend the complex pathogenesis of SLE. Indeed, a more complete genetic map of SLE susceptibility may aid in generating a network of biological pathways contributing to SLE. It may also help to better tailor treatments and predict the clinical spectrum of the disease for each patient. In this regard, early studies have reported that FcγR polymorphisms may influence clinical response to intravenous immunoglobulin (IVIG) or therapeutic mAbs (infliximab, rituximab) in Kawasaki disease, rheumatoid arthritis, idiopathic thrombocytopenic purpura (ITP), and Crohn disease.[26] To date, no such reports have been published for SLE.

In this section, we summarize the most frequently reported FcγRs polymorphisms associated with SLE or lupus nephritis (Table 3). In conjunction with functional explanations, these data may aid in the understanding of the underlying mechanisms of autoimmunity and tissue injury in SLE. Nonetheless, it is noteworthy that the FcγR encoding genes are largely present within the 1q23 locus (FcγRIIA, IIIA, IIB, IIC, IIIB) and linkage disequilibrium has been reported in some cases. Thus, association studies should include all the FcγRs rather than one particular gene.

FcγRIIA Polymorphisms

FcγRIIA R/H 131

FcγRIIA R/H 131 (rs1801274, also named FcγR2A G458A)—a polymorphism resulting in a single amino-acid substitution at position 131 (extracellular domain)—has been associated with SLE in many reports. In a meta-analysis of 17 reports, the FcγRIIA R/H 131 polymorphism is linked with SLE development. The R/R131 as well as the R/H131 genotypes were significantly associated with an increase in susceptibility to SLE in European and African descent populations, while only a minor, but still significant, association was found in Asian cohorts.[221,222] Although this risk appears to be modest (OR 1.3 for RR/RH versus HH), it may still have a significant effect at a population level as this polymorphism is codominantly expressed and the R131 is a common allele.

Mechanistically, the enhanced susceptibility may be best explained by the altered affinity for IgG2 of the low-binding R131 allele compared to the high-binding H131,[186] which may result in impaired handling of IgG2-based ICs by FcγRIIA R131. Indeed, isolated neutrophils from FcγRIIA R131 patients exhibit impaired phagocytosis of erythrocytes coated with human IgG2, while no differences were observed with erythrocytes coated with IgG1, IgG3, and IgG4.[223] The R131 allele might therefore be associated with decreased IC clearance capacity and consequently with enhanced end-organ tissue damage as a result of IC deposition. However, no

TABLE 3 FcγR Polymorphisms and Copy Number Variants Associated with SLE

Alleles	Epidemiology	Suspected Mechanism
FcγRIIA R/H 131 (rs1801274)	R131: increased SLE susceptibility in Europeans, Africans, and Asians to a lesser extent	Altered affinity for IgG2 potentially resulting in impaired IgG2-based IC clearance[106,223–225]
FcγRIIB T/I 232 (rs1050501)	T232: increase in SLE susceptibility in Asians, but not in Europeans	Exclusion of FcγRIIB from lipid rafts, resulting in altered signaling capacity and inhibitory functions[235,236]
FcγRIIB -386C-120A	Increase in SLE susceptibility in Europeans	Unclear mechanism. Possibly altered expression of FcγRIIB[51,237,238]
FcγRIIIA F/V 158 (rs39699)	F158: increased susceptibility for SLE in Europeans and in Asians, but not in Africans. Increased susceptibility for lupus nephritis in Asians, but not in Europeans or Africans	Altered affinity for IgG1 and IgG3 potentially resulting in impaired IgG1- and IgG3-based IC clearance[80,247,248]
FcγRIIIA L/R/H 66 (rs10127939)	L66: increased susceptibility to lupus nephritis in African-Americans but not European-Americans, and only in the presence of the polymorphism FcγRIIIA F158	Decreased the affinity for IgG1 and IgG3 only in the presence of FcγRIIIA F158[249]
FcγRIIIA copy number variant	Low (<2) or high (>2) copy numbers increase SLE susceptibility in a Taiwanese cohort	Decreased IC clearance in low CNV. Increased FcγRIIIA proinflammatory effects such as cytokines production by dendritic cells[250]
FcγRIIIB NA1/NA2	NA2: suspected increase in SLE susceptibility and lupus nephritis in Asians and Europeans, but not confirmed	Impaired neutrophil-mediated phagocytosis[251]
FcγRIIIB copy number variant	Low copy number: increase in susceptibility for SLE overall and possibly lupus nephritis in Europeans	Reduced surface expression of FcγRIIIB potentially resulting in impaired IC clearance[195,196] Chimeric FcγRIIB gene resulting in the ectopic expression of the FcγRIIB in NK cells, altering their function[257]

clear association between the FcγRIIA R131 allele and lupus nephritis was observed. Because IgG1 and IgG3 are predominantly involved in proliferative glomerulonephritis,[106,224,225] it was anticipated that the R131 polymorphism with altered binding to IgG2 may have mild or no effect on lupus nephritis susceptibility. Interestingly, one study links FcγRIIA R131 with SLE severity and in particular with renal involvement in IgG2 anti-C1q autoantibody-positive patients.[110] In this case, the R131 genotype may indeed lead to a specific defect in IgG2-based ICs clearance.

FcγRIIB Polymorphisms

FcγRIIB T/I 232

As the only inhibitory FcγR, FcγRIIB appears to play a critical role in immune tolerance in mouse models. Thus, any gain or loss of function of this receptor by a genetic variant may be expected to influence the susceptibility to SLE in humans. Indeed, a polymorphism of FcγRIIB, T/I 232 (rs1050501, also named T/I 187 if the signal peptide is omitted), has been associated with SLE,[226–229] although this has not been confirmed in other reports.[230,231] A meta-analysis confirms the association between the polymorphism FcγRIIB T/I 232 and an increased susceptibility for SLE in Asian-descent subjects (OR, 1.332 for the T allele) but not in Europeans.[232] However, two further studies also support an association between FcγRIIB T/I 232 polymorphism and increased SLE risk in Caucasians.[233,234] Functionally, the isoleucine (I) to threonine (T) change at amino acid position 232 located in the transmembrane domain may exclude the receptor from lipid rafts and thus prevent its association with BCR. The loss of its inhibitory function in B cells may lead to the subsequent emergence of autoreactive B cells.[235,236] However, as illustrated in mice models (see Section Maintenance of Peripheral Tolerance), this polymorphism may be interacting epistatically with a more complex susceptible genetic background and therefore is biologically significant only in certain ethnicities such as Asians. Nonetheless, these data support a regulatory role for FcγRIIB in the maintenance of tolerance with downmodulation of its function, resulting in autoimmunity in SLE.

FcγRIIB Promoter Polymorphism

The -386C-120A (2B.4) promoter polymorphism of FcγRIIB has also been associated with an increase in susceptibility to SLE in a Caucasian population (OR 1.6).[237] Although a second study confirms this association in another European cohort,[51] this link with SLE has to be cautiously interpreted because of the relatively small sample size and the absence of a convincing mechanistic explanation. Indeed, the two groups present conflicting results on the activity of this promoter haplotype. While the first group observed increased -386C-120A promoter

activity ex vivo as well as in transfected cell lines,[237,238] a finding also of another report,[239] an opposite effect was observed in the second study.[51] Therefore, further studies are required to clarify the significance of this polymorphism. The -386C-120A (2B.4) but not the more common -386G/-120T (2B.1) promoter haplotype displays increased binding to transcription factors GATA4 and Yin-Yan1, and significantly associates with FcγRIIB transcriptional activity.[237,240] Individuals with the 2B.4 haplotype (~2% frequency) exhibited stable FcγRIIB expression on neutrophils, which otherwise have low to undetectable protein levels, and higher expression on monocytes, B lymphocytes and myeloid DCs. In neutrophils, the 2B.4 associated increase in FcγRIIB expression correlates with decreased FcγRIIA mediated activation (as assessed by Mac-1 upregulation and elastase release) following stimulation with polymeric ICs.[239] The appreciation of the role of neutrophils in lupus,[45] and contribution of FcγRIIA on neutrophils in lupus-induced tissue injury,[207] predicts that a change in the balance of FcγRIIA and FcγRIIB (in individuals that do versus do not express this receptor) will dictate susceptibility to target organ injury in SLE.

FcγRIIC Polymorphisms

FcγRIIC Exon 3 Q13/Stop Polymorphism

FcγRIIC contains a polymorphism in exon 3 coding, either for a glutamine at position 13 (Q13) or for a premature stop codon. The most frequent allele (82%) is the stop codon, in which case FcγRIIC represents a pseudogene not expressed in any cell type. The minor Q13 allele codes for a functional activating FcγR expressed in NK cells, where it mediates IgG-induced cell activation.[26,52] Noteworthy, the extracellular domain of FcγRIIC is identical to FcγRIIB; no antibody (Ab) is therefore able to distinguish phenotypically this two receptors. This is certainly part of the reasons for the confusion in FcγRIIB expression pattern in NK cells, which is generally not transcriptionally expressed in this cell type.

The functional FcγRIIC Q13 is associated with increased risk of ITP. Functionally, FcγRIIC enhances the Ab-mediated cytotoxicity in NK cells, which may participate in autoimmunity.[241] However, this polymorphism has not yet been associated with SLE.

FcγRIIC Intron 7 Splicing Site Variant

Several splicing forms of FcγRIIC have been identified that may further modulate the function of this receptor. In individuals with the FcγRIIC Q13 (or ORF) variant, there is an additional polymorphism at the splicing site of the intron 7 that results in an improper splicing of exon 7 causing a frameshift with an early stop codon. This nonfunctional allele may also be protective in ITP,[13] but no data are available for SLE.

FcγRIIC Copy Number Variants

In addition to single-nucleotide polymorphisms, CNV are another type of genetic variation that can affect FcγR function. CNV are structural variations defined as DNA segments at least 1 kb in size present at variable number of copies in comparison with a reference genome. These genetic variations are being increasingly recognized as a source of gene expression modulation and thereby phenotypic variation.[242] In the 1q23-24 chromosomal region, CNV has been reported for FcγRIIIA, FcγRIIC, and FcγRIIIB, but not for FcγRIIA and FcγRIIB.[243]

FcγRIIC CNV may result in variable cell surface expression of this receptor. High CNV (>2) has been associated with an increased risk of Kawasaki disease,[13] but not with ITP,[241] and no data are available for SLE.

In addition, a large gene deletion variant involving both the FcγRIIC and FcγRIIIB genes as well as a negative regulatory element in the adjacent FcγRIIB has been reported. This results in no expression of FcγRIIC and FcγRIIIB. However, this creates a chimeric gene resulting in the expression of the inhibitory FcγRIIB in NK cells. NK cells of such individuals present with a reduced FcγRIIIA triggered antibody-mediated cytotoxicity function[13] that may influence autoimmunity (see also Section FcγRIIIB Copy Number Variants). Overall, the exact pathogenic role of FcγRIIC CNV however remains uncertain.

FcγRIIIA Polymorphisms

FcγRIIIA F/V158

Two meta-analyses have evaluated the link between the FcγRIIIA F/V158 polymorphism (rs396991, also named FCGR3A T559G and FcγRIIIA-F/V176) and SLE or lupus nephritis[244,245] finding contrasting results. These codominant alleles differ at amino acid position 158 coding for either a phenylalanine (F) or a valine (V) in the extracellular domain of the receptor. The most recent meta-analysis was the largest and the most comprehensive study.[245] Seventeen reports were analyzed, including 3493 SLE patients compared to 2426 healthy controls. A clear overall association was found between the F158 allele and SLE risk (OR 1.27) as well as lupus nephritis (OR 1.15). Furthermore, a dose–response relationship was observed for SLE with the strongest association with FF homozygosity (OR 1.68). In the ethnic subgroups analysis, the SLE association was maintained only in patients of European and Asian descent but not of African descent. The association with lupus nephritis was the strongest among patients of Asian descent, but was not significant for patients of European- or African descent.[245] A more recent study specifically analyzed a cohort of Chinese SLE patients (732 patients with SLE compared to 886 healthy controls) and found an overall increased risk of SLE in patients with the F158 allele, but no additional risk for lupus nephritis.[246] Overall, a consistent association between the FcγRIIIA F158 allele and the global risk of SLE is observed, while its influence on lupus nephritis remains uncertain and may depend on the ethnic background.

Functionally, the FcγRIIIA F158 allele has a reduced affinity for IgG1 and IgG3.[247,248] Similarly to FcγRIIA R131 polymorphism, this may influence the ability of phagocytic cells to clear ICs.[80] Although not clearly supported by genetic studies to date, this polymorphism may be particularly relevant in renal involvement as IgG1 and IgG3 ICs are predominantly implicated in the pathogenesis of proliferative glomerulonephritis.[106,224,225]

FcγRIIIA L/R/H 66

FcγRIIIA contains a second polymorphism site, FcγRIIIA L/R/H 66 (rs10127939). In the context of the low-binding FcγRIIIA F158, the FcγRIIIA L66 allele is associated with an increased risk of lupus nephritis (but not SLE per se) among African American patients, but not among European American patients.[249] In vitro, this polymorphism confer a lower ligand binding capacity that appears significant only in the context of the FcγRIIIA-176F allele.[249] Therefore, this second FcγRIIIA polymorphism further modulates the binding capacity of this receptor and may synergistically influence IC clearance by phagocytic cells.

FcγRIIIA Copy Number Variants

In a cohort of 1728 SLE patients compared with 2404 healthy controls, FcγRIIIA CNV was not associated with SLE or lupus nephritis among African American and European American patients.[249] However, low FcγRIIIA CNV (<2) was significantly associated with an increased risk of SLE as well as rheumatoid arthritis in a Taiwanese population (odd ratio 1.59). Interestingly, a high CNV (>2 compared to 2) was also associated with an increased risk of SLE.[250] As low CNV of FcγRIIIA may be associated with lower ICs clearance by phagocytic cells involved in the pathogenesis of SLE, a higher CNV may enhance the proinflammatory response triggered by the activating FcγRIIIA, such as through increased cytokine production by dentritic cells.[250]

FcγRIIIB Polymorphisms

FcγRIIIB NA1/NA2

Two main codominant allelic forms of FcγRIIIB receptor exist: NA1 and NA2. NA2 has been functionally associated with impaired phagocytosis function in neutrophils.[251] However, despite an initial report suggesting an increased risk of SLE associated with the NA2 allele,[252] two meta-analysis have shown no association between the NA2 allele and SLE or lupus nephritis in either Asian or European populations.[232,253] Interestingly, the apparent initial positive association between the NA2 allele and SLE susceptibility may have resulted from strong linkage disequilibrium with FcγRIIB, which is located in close proximity to FcγRIIIB.[228] Although the NA2 genotype is not definitively associated with SLE incidence, NA2 does appear to be associated with increased risk of lupus nephritis and hematological manifestations in some reports.[218,220]

FcγRIIIB Copy Number Variants

FcγRIIIB was the first gene CNV implicated in autoimmunity. Comparing 60 lupus nephritis patients to 109 unrelated seronegative controls, reduced number of copies of FcγRIIIB was significantly associated with lupus nephritis. Moreover, this effect was independent of the FcγRIIA R/H131 and FcγRIIIA F/V158 polymorphism in a logistic regression analysis model.[254] Further studies found contrasting results in various populations.[196,250,255] Nevertheless, a recent systematic review analyzed eight cohorts including 7460 control individuals and 5595 patients with various inflammatory diseases (rheumatoid arthritis 37.9%, SLE 32.9%, ulcerative colitis 13.4%, ANCA-associated vasculitis 10.1%, Kawasaki disease 2.8%, ITP 2.1%, and anti-GBM disease 0.8%). High FcγRIIIB CNV (>2) were not associated with autoimmunity, while low CNV (<2) was significantly associated with autoimmunity. There was a strong association between low CNV and SLE with an odds ratio of 1.59 (1.32–1.92).[256]

Functionally, a correlation between FcγRIIIB CNV and surface expression on human neutrophils has been reported.[196] Moreover, low CNV was also associated with impaired neutrophil adhesion to Ig-coated surface under flow conditions and reduced IC uptake.[196] As FcγRIIIB tethers neutrophils to immobilized ICs in vitro[197] as well as intravascular ICs in vivo[44,77] and may be able to phagocytose ICs,[77,195,196] a reduced number of copies of the FcγRIIIB gene associated with a lower expression of this receptor may impair glomerular clearance of ICs. This could potentially result in more sustained inflammation via increased production of ROS through engagement of other activating FcγR such as FcγRIIA, which in turn could result in end-organ damage and notably renal injury in SLE and possibly other autoimmune disorders.

A study found that FcγRIIIB genomic deletion might produce a chimeric juxtaposition of the 5′-regulatory sequences of the FcγRIIC with the coding sequence of FcγRIIB. This results in the ectopic expression of FcγRIIB in NK cells in patients with 0 or 1 copy of FcγRIIIB.[257] NK role in autoimmunity is not fully understood, but altered NK cell function has been observed in SLE patients.[258] Ectopic expression of the inhibitory FcγRIIB in NK cells may inhibit the function of other activating Fcγ receptor (e.g., FcγRIIIA) leading, for instance, in a reduced antibody-mediated cytotoxicity function in these cells.[257] This highlights the role of NK cells in SLE pathogenesis and constitutes an additional mechanism explaining the increased SLE risk among individuals with low FcγRIIIB CNV.

Other Polymorphisms that Potentially Influence FcγR Functions

A polymorphism of the CD18 receptor family and complement receptor Mac1 (ITGAM, CD11b/CD18, CR3) has been strongly associated with SLE (OR, 1.78) in European, African, and American populations.[182–184] This nonsynonymous polymorphism is predicted to alter the ligand binding capacity of this integrin. As Mac1 is known to interact with FcγRs at the cell surface, in particular with FcγRIIIB and FcγRIIA,[140,259] and thereby modulate their function, this polymorphism may indirectly impact FcγR-mediated functions.

FcγR TARGETED TREATMENTS

In normal homeostatic conditions, the activating and inhibiting effects of the FcγR maintain a fine balance. But in disease conditions, tipping this balance leads to inflammation and tissue damage. With several studies reporting importance of FcγRs in disease conditions and with the increased understanding of the functions and mode of action of the activating and inhibitory receptors, several potential therapeutic strategies have come to light.[18,260]

Intravenous Immunoglobulin

IVIG was the first immunosuppressive therapy targeting FcγR functions. Purification of Igs was originally developed and used to treat Ig deficiency and recurrent bacterial infections. In addition, by flooding the organism with high amount of purified normal Igs, anti-inflammatory immunomodulation occurs[261] and nowadays the primary utilization of IVIG is in inflammatory diseases. However, the immunomodulatory mechanisms involved remain poorly understood and are the topic of ongoing controversies.[262] Pooled normal polyspecific IgG obtained from healthy donors have been efficiently used for many years in the treatment of several autoimmune and systemic inflammatory diseases, such as central nervous inflammatory diseases (multiple sclerosis, Guillain–Barré syndrome, myasthenia gravis), vasculitis, ITP and antibody-mediated kidney graft rejection. Off-label prescription of IVIG also includes SLE[263,264] and antiphospholipid syndrome,[265] and shows clear benefits. However, controlled randomized clinical trials are still required to thoroughly assess a potential benefit of such treatment in lupus.

Because IVIG is an important therapeutic option in many autoimmune diseases, clarification of its anti-inflammatory function might help to elucidate key events in autoimmunity, including SLE. Furthermore, given that IVIG is available in limited supply, is a human-derived product, and is required in multiple doses to achieve efficacy, alternative approaches are needed. F(ab)2-dependent mechanisms have been speculated and specific so-called natural antibodies against molecules implicated in inflammation have been identified in IVIG preparation (for instance, anti-integrins, anti-Fas, anticytokines, or anticytokine receptors).[266–268] However, strong functional in vivo data are missing and the aforementioned effects might be anecdotal. On the other hand, the antibody Fc fragments of the pooled IVIG appear to play a dominant anti-inflammatory role. This is supported by one clinical trial with ITP that demonstrated a similar anti-inflammatory effect of both complete IVIG and isolated Fc fragments.[269] In animal models, Fc fragments have also been reported to play a significant protective role in immune thrombocytopenia, arthritis, and proliferative nephritis models.[85,116,270]

Numerous appealing explanations have been provided for these anti-inflammatory activities, such as saturation of neonatal Fc receptors (critically involved in maintaining Ig level in the serum), binding and activation of C3b and C4b leading to less complement deposition and associated tissue damage, and blockade of the activating FcγR and subsequent inhibition of proinflammatory cytokine release.[116,261] The most convincing in vivo data support the idea that IVIG works principally by upregulating the expression of the inhibitory FcγRIIB and thus counteracting the FcγR activation by IC. Indeed, the anti-inflammatory activity of IVIG is lost in FcγRIIB-deficient mice subjected to immune thrombocytopenia, arthritis, or proliferative nephritis models.[28,116,270] Another promising explanation is that IVIG is enriched in IgG glycosylated on their asparagine 297 residue, which might preferentially interact with a subtype of regulatory macrophages.[28,261] Indeed, various IgG glycovariants have been identified in humans and deglycosylated IVIG preparations have been shown to lose their anti-inflammatory effect. Moreover, enrichment of Fc fragments for terminal sialic acid residues enhanced the IVIG activity, suggesting a specific anti-inflammatory activity of this subset of salicylated antibodies.[85] Therefore, overall, IVIG may activate a specific subset of anti-inflammatory regulatory macrophages, while at the same time inhibit proinflammatory effector macrophages by engaging FcγRIIB.[261] Seemingly non-FcγR-related effects of IVIG have also been described, as reviewed in detail elsewhere.[261] Interestingly, IVIG was shown to prevent leukocyte rolling on the endothelium through effects on members of the selectin and integrin family of adhesion molecules in a model of ischemia and reperfusion.[271] Thus, IVIG, which is a complex mixture, likely engages multiple targets to reduce inflammation.

ITAM Signaling Inhibitors

Based on the structure of FcγRIIA, small molecules have been designed to inhibit FcγRIIA-IC dependent inflammation and have been effective in collagen-induced arthiritis, a FcgRIIA-dependent model.[272] A specific inhibitor of the syk kinase (R788/R406, fostamatinib) has also been developed. This inhibitor employs the alternative approach of blocking the signaling pathways of the receptor. Although the syk inhibitor blocks ITAM-activating signals downstream of FcγRs, its targets are broader because syk is downstream of many ITAM-containing receptors as well as non-ITAM receptors, such as integrins in cells of both hematopoietic and nonhematopoietic lineage.[273] Although it has been shown to efficiently reduce arthritis severity in the collagen-induced arthritis mouse model[274] and has demonstrated an encouraging effect in early clinical trials,[275–277] it has also shown limited benefits in later studies[277,278] and is associated with an unfavorable adverse effects profile, including hypertension (40%), diarrhea, neutropenia, and liver toxicity. To date, the commercial development of this drug for rheumatoid arthritis has stopped. Nevertheless, this medication has shown encouraging results in a mouse model of immune thrombocytopenia, as well as in a phase 2 clinical trial in 16 patients with chronic refractory immune thrombocytopenic purpura.[279] Fostamatinib was also efficient in reducing the severity of nephritis in NZB/NZW F1 mice[280] and MRL/lpr lupus prone-mice, as well as skin injury in BAK/BAX mice.[281] However, to date, no data are available on fostamatinib in human SLE.

Soluble FcγRs

Despite the high levels of circulating IgG and the relatively small size of FcγRs as compared to IgGs, recombinant soluble ectodomains of FcγRI, II, and III can inhibit IC-mediated inflammation in various animal models. Soluble human FcγRIA was shown to reduce inflammation in a murine model of collagen-induced arthritis.[282] A soluble humanized FcγRII substantially reduced the severity of the lupus-like disease once administered prophylactically in lupus prone NZB/NZW F1 mice.[283] Similarly, blocking activating FcγRI or FcγRIII in patients with refractory immune thrombocytopenic purpura has also produced encouraging results.[284]

Blocking Activating FcγRs

Using mAbs toward the receptors has the added advantage of specificity because recombinant soluble FcγRs does not give selective blockade of specific subtypes of the receptors. In early studies, mAbs against FcγRIII have been tested in patients with immune thrombocytopenia with some benefits.[285,286] However, overall, these antibodies have shown limited therapeutic benefit and the development of strategies using this approach has been rather slow. To develop appropriate and efficient therapies using mAbs, it needs to be first well understood which FcγRs or their combinations are involved in disease development and associated pathology. Nonetheless, anti-hFcγRII F(ab')2 fragments have shown promising results by inhibiting arthritis induction in a mouse model as well as inhibiting ROS production ex vivo in inflammatory synovial cells from rheumatoid arthritis patients.[287]

Another strategy would be to use small molecules or peptide that will specifically antagonize activating FcγRs. For instance, a synthetic peptide interfering with the IgG–FcγR interaction partially prevents kidney damage in MRL/lpr lupus-prone mice.[288] More recently, peptides designed to inhibit Fc binding to FcγRIIA prevented collagen-induced arthritis in mice.[289] Another peptide also targeting FcγRIIA limited kidney damage and improved survival of MRL/lpr mice.[290]

Activating the Inhibitory FcγRIIB

As previously discussed, loss of function of the only inhibitory receptor FcγRIIB plays a prominent role in autoantibody generation and lupus pathogenesis. It is therefore a designated therapeutic target, as any strategies aiming to enhance its function may provide anti-inflammatory effects and restore the activating-inhibitory FcRs balance in some autoimmune diseases. Several FcgRIIB-specific antibodies have been developed to induce plasma cell depletion similarly to the anti-CD20 antibody rituximab.[260] However, such antibodies provide a larger immunosuppressive effect than desired. An elegant strategy is to cross-link the FcγRIIB with the BCR on B cells to specifically trigger inhibitory signaling and lower B-cell proliferation and antibody production. This has been achieved by the production of a dual-affinity antibody, a "diabody," which targets both FcγRIIB and CD79b, a transmembrane protein part of the BCR complex. This strategy was effective in limiting arthritis in the collagen-induced arthritis mouse model.[291] Another bispecific antibody was engineered to target CD19 and FcγRIIB. This antibody potently inhibits ex vivo activation of B cells isolated from healthy or SLE donors by enhancing the FcγRIIB-mediated inhibitory signaling pathway. Furthermore, this antibody does not induce B-cell depletion in human FcγRIIB transgenic mice.[292] This molecule is in the process of starting phase 2 clinical trials in rheumatoid arthritis.

Modulating the Expression of Activating and inhibitory FcγRs

FcγRs expression profile is influenced by cytokines. For instance, TNF upregulates FcγRIIA expression while down-modulating FcγRIIB and enhancing activating Ig-mediated signaling in immune cells.[293] IL-10 also increases the expression of all ITAM-bearing FcγRs, while TGFβ, IFNγ, and macrophage stimulating factor upregulates in vitro FcγRIIIA.[293,294] Other cytokines such as IL-4 and IL-13 reduce the expression of activating FcγRs.[260,293] Altering the cytokine profile may be another effective therapeutic approach to modulate the balance between activating and inhibitory FcγRs and influence autoimmunity.[260] Similarly, in the future, targeted delivery of antisense oligonucleotides or small molecules may enable the possibility to specifically modulate FcγRs profile in specific immune cells.[260,295]

Overall, these data suggest a strong potential for the development of new anti-inflammatory drugs that target the FcγR functions, by blocking the activating receptors, modulating the expression of the inhibitory FcγRIIB, or altering the activating signaling pathway of ITAM-bearing receptors. Much progress is expected in this field in the near future.

FUTURE DIRECTIONS

Both inhibitory and activating FcγRs have been clearly identified as key regulators of the autoimmune response and end-organ damage in a wide range of autoimmune diseases, based largely on the study of genetically engineered mice in models of autoimmunity. Despite these advances, given the complexity of the FcγR family, the differences between the repertoire of murine and human receptors, and the involvement of FcγRs in several stages of autoimmune disorders from the immune response to end-stage autoimmunity-mediated inflammatory responses, it is not surprising that much more work needs to be done. Moreover, there is still a paucity of studies directly addressing the relative importance of FcγRs in mouse models of SLE and the epistatic environmental and genetic factors that dictate the FcγRIIB dependence of B-cell autoreactivity. The potential role of FcγRs in human disease is highlighted by the associations between polymorphisms in several different FcγRs and SLE disease susceptibility or disease course. The strength of these associations, however, is variable in different populations, illustrating the importance of epistatic interactions with FcγRs function. Furthermore, definitive evidence that these polymorphisms have functional consequences for development of SLE in human is needed. Advances in this area require a greater understanding of the mechanisms of FcγR function, as well as the relevant cell types bearing activating FcγRs that promote end-organ damage in SLE and other autoimmune disorders.

Another area that deserves attention is determining how the proinflammatory environment existing in SLE patients modulates FcγR expression and function. As SLE is more prevalent in women, another intriguing question is how gender can influence FcγRs function or expression. For example, gender may modulate the penetrance of certain FcγRs polymorphisms, as illustrated for instance from the significant enrichment of FcγRIIB T232 (which reduces FcγRIIB's signaling capacity) in male lupus patients compared to females.[226] These areas of study are just a small sampling of the opportunities in FcγR research that could provide insights into the mechanisms by which FcγRs promote susceptibility to autoimmunity and its manifestations.

Although our understanding of FcγR biology is increasing overall, it is also gaining complexity. Nevertheless, therapeutic targeting of FcγR function represents a formidable opportunity to improve SLE treatment and some exciting novel strategies have been proposed. In the near future, this could result in rational drug design that would restore the balance between activating and inhibitory FcγRs in autoimmunity and block the initiation of the humoral response to autoantigens, and/or targets, in a cell-specific manner. Moreover, drugs that target specific activating FcγRs that promote inflammation responsible for tissue injury may attenuate end-organ damage without profoundly affecting the adaptive immune response against pathogens.

REFERENCES

1. Nimmerjahn F. Activating and inhibitory FcgammaRs in autoimmune disorders. *Springer Semin Immunopathol* 2006;**28**:305–19.
2. Titus JA, Perez P, Kaubisch A, Garrido MA, Segal DM. Human K/natural killer cells targeted with hetero-cross-linked antibodies specifically lyse tumor cells in vitro and prevent tumor growth in vivo. *J Immunol* 1987;**139**:3153–8.
3. Young JD, Ko SS, Cohn ZA. The increase in intracellular free calcium associated with IgG gamma 2b/gamma 1 Fc receptor-ligand interactions: role in phagocytosis. *Proc Natl Acad Sci USA* 1984;**81**:5430–4.
4. Anderson CL, Shen L, Eicher DM, Wewers MD, Gill JK. Phagocytosis mediated by three distinct Fc gamma receptor classes on human leukocytes. *J Exp Med* 1990;**171**:1333–45.
5. Gergely J, Sarmay G, Rajnavolgyi E. Regulation of antibody production mediated by Fc gamma receptors, IgG binding factors, and IgG Fc-binding autoantibodies. *Crit Rev Biochem Mol Biol* 1992;**27**:191–225.
6. Gessner JE, Heiken H, Tamm A, Schmidt RE. The IgG Fc receptor family. *Ann Hematol* 1998;**76**:231–48.
7. Nimmerjahn F, Ravetch JV. Fcgamma receptors: old friends and new family members. *Immunity* 2006;**24**:19–28.
8. Franco A, Damdinsuren B, Ise T, Dement-Brown J, Li H, Nagata S, et al. Human Fc receptor-like 5 binds intact IgG via mechanisms distinct from those of Fc receptors. *J Immunol* 2013;**190**:5739–46.
9. Rath T, Baker K, Pyzik M, Blumberg RS. Regulation of immune responses by the neonatal fc receptor and its therapeutic implications. *Front Immunol* 2014;**5**:664.
10. Wilson TJ, Fuchs A, Colonna M. Cutting edge: human FcRL4 and FcRL5 are receptors for IgA and IgG. *J Immunol* 2012;**188**:4741–5.
11. Yang Y, Eversole T, Lee DJ, Sontheimer RD, Capra JD. Protein-protein interactions between native Ro52 and immunoglobulin G heavy chain. *Scand J Immunol* 1999;**49**:620–8.
12. Hamerman JA, Lanier LL. Inhibition of immune responses by ITAM-bearing receptors. *Sci STKE* 2006;**2006**:re1.
13. van der Heijden J, Breunis WB, Geissler J, de Boer M, van den Berg TK, Kuijpers TW. Phenotypic variation in IgG receptors by nonclassical FCGR2C alleles. *J Immunol* 2012;**188**:1318–24.
14. Nimmerjahn F, Ravetch JV. Fcgamma receptors as regulators of immune responses. *Nat Rev Immunol* 2008;**8**:34–47.
15. Nimmerjahn F, Bruhns P, Horiuchi K, Ravetch JV. FcgammaRIV: a novel FcR with distinct IgG subclass specificity. *Immunity* 2005;**23**:41–51.
16. McKenzie ME, Gurbel PA, Levine DJ, Serebruany VL. Clinical utility of available methods for determining platelet function. *Cardiology* 1999;**92**:240–7.
17. Bruhns P, Iannascoli B, England P, Mancardi DA, Fernandez N, Jorieux S, et al. Specificity and affinity of human Fcgamma receptors and their polymorphic variants for human IgG subclasses. *Blood* 2009;**113**:3716–25.
18. Hogarth PM, Pietersz GA. Fc receptor-targeted therapies for the treatment of inflammation, cancer and beyond. *Nat Rev Drug Discov* 2012;**11**:311–31.
19. Allen JM, Seed B. Isolation and expression of functional high-affinity Fc receptor complementary DNAs. *Science* 1989;**243**:378–81.
20. Lu J, Chu J, Zou Z, Hamacher NB, Rixon MW, Sun PD. Structure of FcgammaRI in complex with Fc reveals the importance of glycan recognition for high-affinity IgG binding. *Proc Natl Acad Sci USA* 2015;**112**:833–8.
21. van der Poel CE, Karssemeijer RA, Boross P, van der Linden JA, Blokland M, van de Winkel JG, et al. Cytokine-induced immune complex binding to the high-affinity IgG receptor, FcgammaRI, in the presence of monomeric IgG. *Blood* 2010;**116**:5327–33.
22. van der Poel CE, Spaapen RM, van de Winkel JG, Leusen JH. Functional characteristics of the high affinity IgG receptor, FcgammaRI. *J Immunol* 2011;**186**:2699–704.
23. Hoffmeyer F, Witte K, Schmidt RE. The high-affinity Fc gamma RI on PMN: regulation of expression and signal transduction. *Immunology* 1997;**92**:544–52.
24. Uciechowski P, Schwarz M, Gessner JE, Schmidt RE, Resch K, Radeke HH. IFN-gamma induces the high-affinity Fc receptor I for IgG (CD64) on human glomerular mesangial cells. *Eur J Immunol* 1998;**28**:2928–35.
25. Ceuppens JL, Baroja ML, Van Vaeck F, Anderson CL. Defect in the membrane expression of high affinity 72-kD Fc gamma receptors on phagocytic cells in four healthy subjects. *J Clin Invest* 1988;**82**:571–8.
26. Gillis C, Gouel-Cheron A, Jonsson F, Bruhns P. Contribution of human FcgammaRs to disease with evidence from human polymorphisms and transgenic animal studies. *Front Immunol* 2014;**5**:254.
27. Ioan-Facsinay A, de Kimpe SJ, Hellwig SM, van Lent PL, Hofhuis FM, van Ojik HH, et al. FcgammaRI (CD64) contributes substantially to severity of arthritis, hypersensitivity responses, and protection from bacterial infection. *Immunity* 2002;**16**:391–402.
28. Bruhns P, Samuelsson A, Pollard JW, Ravetch JV. Colony-stimulating factor-1-dependent macrophages are responsible for IVIG protection in antibody-induced autoimmune disease. *Immunity* 2003;**18**:573–81.
29. Ji H, Ohmura K, Mahmood U, Lee DM, Hofhuis FM, Boackle SA, et al. Arthritis critically dependent on innate immune system players. *Immunity* 2002;**16**:157–68.
30. Mancardi DA, Albanesi M, Jonsson F, Iannascoli B, Van Rooijen N, Kang X, et al. The high-affinity human IgG receptor FcgammaRI (CD64) promotes IgG-mediated inflammation, anaphylaxis, and antitumor immunotherapy. *Blood* 2013;**121**:1563–73.

31. Indik ZK, Park JG, Pan XQ, Schreiber AD. Induction of phagocytosis by a protein tyrosine kinase. *Blood* 1995;**85**:1175–80.

32. Van den Herik-Oudijk IE, Ter Bekke MW, Tempelman MJ, Capel PJ, Van de Winkel JG. Functional differences between two Fc receptor ITAM signaling motifs. *Blood* 1995;**86**:3302–7.

33. Ramsland PA, Farrugia W, Bradford TM, Sardjono CT, Esparon S, Trist HM, et al. Structural basis for Fc gammaRIIa recognition of human IgG and formation of inflammatory signaling complexes. *J Immunol* 2011;**187**:3208–17.

34. Bolland S, Ravetch JV. Inhibitory pathways triggered by ITIM-containing receptors. *Adv Immunol* 1999;**72**:149–77.

35. Fukuyama H, Nimmerjahn F, Ravetch JV. The inhibitory Fcgamma receptor modulates autoimmunity by limiting the accumulation of immunoglobulin G+ anti-DNA plasma cells. *Nat Immunol* 2005;**6**:99–106.

36. Boylan B, Gao C, Rathore V, Gill JC, Newman DK, Newman PJ. Identification of FcgammaRIIa as the ITAM-bearing receptor mediating alphaIIbbeta3 outside-in integrin signaling in human platelets. *Blood* 2008;**112**:2780–6.

37. Schneider DJ, Taatjes-Sommer HS. Augmentation of megakaryocyte expression of FcgammaRIIa by interferon gamma. *Arterioscler Thromb Vasc Biol* 2009;**29**:1138–43.

38. Benitez-Ribas D, Adema GJ, Winkels G, Klasen IS, Punt CJ, Figdor CG, et al. Plasmacytoid dendritic cells of melanoma patients present exogenous proteins to CD4+ T cells after Fc gamma RII-mediated uptake. *J Exp Med* 2006;**203**:1629–35.

39. Boruchov AM, Heller G, Veri MC, Bonvini E, Ravetch JV, Young JW. Activating and inhibitory IgG Fc receptors on human DCs mediate opposing functions. *J Clin Invest* 2005;**115**:2914–23.

40. Liu Y, Gao X, Masuda E, Redecha PB, Blank MC, Pricop L. Regulated expression of FcgammaR in human dendritic cells controls cross-presentation of antigen-antibody complexes. *J Immunol* 2006;**177**:8440–7.

41. Lynch RG. Rous-Whipple Award lecture. The biology and pathology of lymphocyte Fc receptors. *Am J Pathol* 1998;**152**:631–9.

42. Ravetch JV, Bolland S. IgG Fc receptors. *Annu Rev Immunol* 2001;**19**:275–90.

43. Florey OJ, Johns M, Esho OO, Mason JC, Haskard DO. Antiendothelial cell antibodies mediate enhanced leukocyte adhesion to cytokine-activated endothelial cells through a novel mechanism requiring cooperation between Fc{gamma}RIIa and CXCR1/2. *Blood* 2007;**109**:3881–9.

44. Tsuboi N, Asano K, Lauterbach M, Mayadas TN. Human neutrophil Fcgamma receptors initiate and play specialized nonredundant roles in antibody-mediated inflammatory diseases. *Immunity* 2008;**28**:833–46.

45. Kaplan MJ. Neutrophils in the pathogenesis and manifestations of SLE. *Nat Rev Rheumatol* 2011;**7**:691–9.

46. Worth RG, Chien CD, Chien P, Reilly MP, McKenzie SE, Schreiber AD. Platelet FcgammaRIIA binds and internalizes IgG-containing complexes. *Exp Hematol* 2006;**34**:1490–5.

47. Hulett MD, Hogarth PM. Molecular basis of Fc receptor function. *Adv Immunol* 1994;**57**:1–127.

48. Schmidt RE, Gessner JE. Fc receptors and their interaction with complement in autoimmunity. *Immunol Lett* 2005;**100**:56–67.

49. Su K, Yang H, Li X, Li X, Gibson AW, Cafardi JM, et al. Expression profile of FcgammaRIIb on leukocytes and its dysregulation in systemic lupus erythematosus. *J Immunol* 2007;**178**:3272–80.

50. Blank MC, Stefanescu RN, Masuda E, Marti F, King PD, Redecha PB, et al. Decreased transcription of the human FCGR2B gene mediated by the -343 G/C promoter polymorphism and association with systemic lupus erythematosus. *Hum Genet* 2005;**117**:220–7.

51. Desai DD, Harbers SO, Flores M, Colonna L, Downie MP, Bergtold A, et al. Fc gamma receptor IIB on dendritic cells enforces peripheral tolerance by inhibiting effector T cell responses. *J Immunol* 2007;**178**:6217–26.

52. Metes D, Ernst LK, Chambers WH, Sulica A, Herberman RB, Morel PA. Expression of functional CD32 molecules on human NK cells is determined by an allelic polymorphism of the FcgammaRIIC gene. *Blood* 1998;**91**:2369–80.

53. Li X, Wu J, Ptacek T, Redden DT, Brown EE, Alarcon GS, et al. Allelic-dependent expression of an activating Fc receptor on B cells enhances humoral immune responses. *Sci Transl Med* 2013;**5**:216ra175.

54. Takai T, Li M, Sylvestre D, Clynes R, Ravetch JV. FcR gamma chain deletion results in pleiotrophic effector cell defects. *Cell* 1994;**76**:519–29.

55. Simmons D, Seed B. The Fc gamma receptor of natural killer cells is a phospholipid-linked membrane protein. *Nature* 1988;**333**:568–70.

56. Ravetch JV, Perussia B. Alternative membrane forms of Fc gamma RIII(CD16) on human natural killer cells and neutrophils. Cell type-specific expression of two genes that differ in single nucleotide substitutions. *J Exp Med* 1989;**170**:481–97.

57. Groh V, Porcelli S, Fabbi M, Lanier LL, Picker LJ, Anderson T, et al. Human lymphocytes bearing T cell receptor gamma/delta are phenotypically diverse and evenly distributed throughout the lymphoid system. *J Exp Med* 1989;**169**:1277–94.

58. Angelini DF, Borsellino G, Poupot M, Diamantini A, Poupot R, Bernardi G, et al. FcgammaRIII discriminates between 2 subsets of Vgamma9Vdelta2 effector cells with different responses and activation pathways. *Blood* 2004;**104**:1801–7.

59. Lafont V, Liautard J, Liautard JP, Favero J. Production of TNF-alpha by human V gamma 9V delta 2 T cells via engagement of Fc gamma RIIIA, the low affinity type 3 receptor for the Fc portion of IgG, expressed upon TCR activation by nonpeptidic antigen. *J Immunol* 2001;**166**:7190–9.

60. Bjorkstrom NK, Gonzalez VD, Malmberg KJ, Falconer K, Alaeus A, Nowak G, et al. Elevated numbers of Fc gamma RIIIA+ (CD16+) effector CD8 T cells with NK cell-like function in chronic hepatitis C virus infection. *J Immunol* 2008;**181**:4219–28.

61. Oshimi K, Oshimi Y, Yamada O, Wada M, Hara T, Mizoguchi H. Cytotoxic T lymphocyte triggering via CD16 is regulated by CD3 and CD8 antigens. Studies with T cell receptor (TCR)-alpha beta+/CD3+16+ and TCR-gamma delta+/CD3+16+ granular lymphocytes. *J Immunol* 1990;**144**:3312–7.

62. Leibson PJ. Signal transduction during natural killer cell activation: inside the mind of a killer. *Immunity* 1997;**6**:655–61.

63. Chen Z, Freedman MS. CD16+ gammadelta T cells mediate antibody dependent cellular cytotoxicity: potential mechanism in the pathogenesis of multiple sclerosis. *Clin Immunol* 2008;**128**:219–27.

64. Radeke HH, Gessner JE, Uciechowski P, Magert HJ, Schmidt RE, Resch K. Intrinsic human glomerular mesangial cells can express receptors for IgG complexes (hFc gamma RIII-A) and the associated Fc epsilon RI gamma-chain. *J Immunol* 1994;**153**:1281–92.

65. Perussia B, Ravetch JV. Fc gamma RIII (CD16) on human macrophages is a functional product of the Fc gamma RIII-2 gene. *Eur J Immunol* 1991;**21**:425–9.

66. Li M, Wirthmueller U, Ravetch JV. Reconstitution of human Fc gamma RIII cell type specificity in transgenic mice. *J Exp Med* 1996;**183**:1259–63.

67. Meknache N, Jonsson F, Laurent J, Guinnepain MT, Daeron M. Human basophils express the glycosylphosphatidylinositol-anchored low-affinity IgG receptor FcgammaRIIIB (CD16B). *J Immunol* 2009;**182**:2542–50.

68. Selvaraj P, Rosse WF, Silber R, Springer TA. The major Fc receptor in blood has a phosphatidylinositol anchor and is deficient in paroxysmal nocturnal haemoglobinuria. *Nature* 1988;**333**:565–7.

69. Unkeless JC, Shen Z, Lin CW, DeBeus E. Function of human Fc gamma RIIA and Fc gamma RIIIB. *Semin Immunol* 1995;**7**:37–44.

70. Hundt M, Schmidt RE. The glycosylphosphatidylinositol-linked Fc gamma receptor III represents the dominant receptor structure for immune complex activation of neutrophils. *Eur J Immunol* 1992;**22**:811–6.

71. Selvaraj P, Fifadara N, Nagarajan S, Cimino A, Wang G. Functional regulation of human neutrophil Fc gamma receptors. *Immunol Res* 2004;**29**:219–30.

72. Huizinga TW, Dolman KM, van der Linden NJ, Kleijer M, Nuijens JH, von dem Borne AE, et al. Phosphatidylinositol-linked FcRIII mediates exocytosis of neutrophil granule proteins, but does not mediate initiation of the respiratory burst. *J Immunol* 1990;**144**: 1432–7.

73. Boros P, Odin JA, Muryoi T, Masur SK, Bona C, Unkeless JC. IgM anti-Fc gamma R autoantibodies trigger neutrophil degranulation. *J Exp Med* 1991;**173**:1473–82.

74. Ortiz-Stern A, Rosales C. Fc gammaRIIIB stimulation promotes beta1 integrin activation in human neutrophils. *J Leukoc Biol* 2005;**77**:787–99.

75. Garcia-Garcia E, Nieto-Castaneda G, Ruiz-Saldana M, Mora N, Rosales C. FcgammaRIIA and FcgammaRIIIB mediate nuclear factor activation through separate signaling pathways in human neutrophils. *J Immunol* 2009;**182**:4547–56.

76. Luscinskas FW, Mayadas T. FcγRs join in the cascade. *Blood* 2007;**109**:3615–6.

77. Chen K, Nishi H, Travers R, Tsuboi N, Martinod K, Wagner DD, et al. Endocytosis of soluble immune complexes leads to their clearance by FcgammaRIIIB but induces neutrophil extracellular traps via FcgammaRIIA in vivo. *Blood* 2012;**120**:4421–31.

78. Behnen M, Leschczyk C, Moller S, Batel T, Klinger M, Solbach W, et al. Immobilized immune complexes induce neutrophil extracellular trap release by human neutrophil granulocytes via FcgammaRIIIB and Mac-1. *J Immunol* 2014;**193**:1954–65.

79. Miller KL, Duchemin AM, Anderson CL. A novel role for the Fc receptor gamma subunit: enhancement of Fc gamma R ligand affinity. *J Exp Med* 1996;**183**:2227–33.

80. Li X, Ptacek TS, Brown EE, Edberg JC. Fcgamma receptors: structure, function and role as genetic risk factors in SLE. *Genes Immun* 2009;**10**:380–9.

81. Castro J, Balada E, Ordi-Ros J, Vilardell-Tarres M. The complex immunogenetic basis of systemic lupus erythematosus. *Autoimmun Rev* 2008;**7**:345–51.

82. Nath SK, Kilpatrick J, Harley JB. Genetics of human systemic lupus erythematosus: the emerging picture. *Curr Opin Immunol* 2004;**16**:794–800.

83. Tsao BP. The genetics of human systemic lupus erythematosus. *Trends Immunol* 2003;**24**:595–602.

84. Jefferis R, Lund J. Interaction sites on human IgG-Fc for FcgammaR: current models. *Immunol Lett* 2002;**82**:57–65.

85. Kaneko Y, Nimmerjahn F, Ravetch JV. Anti-inflammatory activity of immunoglobulin G resulting from Fc sialylation. *Science* 2006;**313**:670–3.

86. Matsumiya S, Yamaguchi Y, Saito J, Nagano M, Sasakawa H, Otaki S, et al. Structural comparison of fucosylated and nonfucosylated Fc fragments of human immunoglobulin G1. *J Mol Biol* 2007;**368**: 767–79.

87. Scallon BJ, Tam SH, McCarthy SG, Cai AN, Raju TS. Higher levels of sialylated Fc glycans in immunoglobulin G molecules can adversely impact functionality. *Mol Immunol* 2007;**44**:1524–34.

88. Jung ST, Reddy ST, Kang TH, Borrok MJ, Sandlie I, Tucker PW, et al. Aglycosylated IgG variants expressed in bacteria that selectively bind FcgammaRI potentiate tumor cell killing by monocyte-dendritic cells. *Proc Natl Acad Sci USA* 2010;**107**:604–9.

89. Karsten CM, Pandey MK, Figge J, Kilchenstein R, Taylor PR, Rosas M, et al. Anti-inflammatory activity of IgG1 mediated by Fc galactosylation and association of FcgammaRIIB and dectin-1. *Nat Med* 2012;**18**:1401–6.

90. Barb AW, Prestegard JH. NMR analysis demonstrates immunoglobulin G N-glycans are accessible and dynamic. *Nat Chem Biol* 2011;**7**:147–53.

91. Krapp S, Mimura Y, Jefferis R, Huber R, Sondermann P. Structural analysis of human IgG-Fc glycoforms reveals a correlation between glycosylation and structural integrity. *J Mol Biol* 2003;**325**:979–89.

92. Frank M, Walker RC, Lanzilotta WN, Prestegard JH, Barb AW. Immunoglobulin G1 Fc domain motions: implications for Fc engineering. *J Mol Biol* 2014;**426**:1799–811.

93. Arnold JN, Wormald MR, Sim RB, Rudd PM, Dwek RA. The impact of glycosylation on the biological function and structure of human immunoglobulins. *Annu Rev Immunol* 2007;**25**:21–50.

94. Tomana M, Schrohenloher RE, Koopman WJ, Alarcon GS, Paul WA. Abnormal glycosylation of serum IgG from patients with chronic inflammatory diseases. *Arthritis Rheum* 1988;**31**:333–8.

95. Parekh RB, Dwek RA, Sutton BJ, Fernandes DL, Leung A, Stanworth D, et al. Association of rheumatoid arthritis and primary osteoarthritis with changes in the glycosylation pattern of total serum IgG. *Nature* 1985;**316**:452–7.

96. Scherer HU, van der Woude D, Ioan-Facsinay A, el Bannoudi H, Trouw LA, Wang J, et al. Glycan profiling of anti-citrullinated protein antibodies isolated from human serum and synovial fluid. *Arthritis Rheum* 2010;**62**:1620–9.

97. van de Geijn FE, Wuhrer M, Selman MH, Willemsen SP, de Man YA, Deelder AM, et al. Immunoglobulin G galactosylation and sialylation are associated with pregnancy-induced improvement of rheumatoid arthritis and the postpartum flare: results from a large prospective cohort study. *Arthritis Res Ther* 2009;**11**:R193.

98. Sjowall C, Zapf J, von Lohneysen S, Magorivska I, Biermann M, Janko C, et al. Altered glycosylation of complexed native IgG molecules is associated with disease activity of systemic lupus erythematosus. *Lupus* 2014;**24**(6):569–81.

99. Fossati-Jimack L, Ioan-Facsinay A, Reininger L, Chicheportiche Y, Watanabe N, Saito T, et al. Markedly different pathogenicity of four immunoglobulin G isotype-switch variants of an antierythrocyte autoantibody is based on their capacity to interact in vivo with the low-affinity Fcgamma receptor III. *J Exp Med* 2000;**191**:1293–302.

100. Kipps TJ, Parham P, Punt J, Herzenberg LA. Importance of immunoglobulin isotype in human antibody-dependent, cell-mediated cytotoxicity directed by murine monoclonal antibodies. *J Exp Med* 1985;**161**:1–17.

101. Nimmerjahn F, Ravetch JV. Divergent immunoglobulin g subclass activity through selective Fc receptor binding. *Science* 2005;**310**:1510–2.

102. Lambert PH, Dixon FJ. Pathogenesis of the glomerulonephritis of NZB/W mice. *J Exp Med* 1968;**127**:507–22.

103. Slack JH, Hang L, Barkley J, Fulton RJ, D'Hoostelaere L, Robinson A, et al. Isotypes of spontaneous and mitogen-induced autoantibodies in SLE-prone mice. *J Immunol* 1984;**132**:1271–5.

104. Bolland S, Ravetch JV. Spontaneous autoimmune disease in Fc(gamma)RIIB-deficient mice results from strain-specific epistasis. *Immunity* 2000;**13**:277–85.

105. Maddison PJ. Autoantibodies in SLE. Disease associations. *Adv Exp Med Biol* 1999;**455**:141–5.

106. Amoura Z, Koutouzov S, Chabre H, Cacoub P, Amoura I, Musset L, et al. Presence of antinucleosome autoantibodies in a restricted set of connective tissue diseases: antinucleosome antibodies of the IgG3 subclass are markers of renal pathogenicity in systemic lupus erythematosus. *Arthritis Rheum* 2000;**43**:76–84.

107. Haas M. IgG subclass deposits in glomeruli of lupus and nonlupus membranous nephropathies. *Am J Kidney Dis* 1994;**23**:358–64.

108. Imai H, Hamai K, Komatsuda A, Ohtani H, Miura AB. IgG subclasses in patients with membranoproliferative glomerulonephritis, membranous nephropathy, and lupus nephritis. *Kidney Int* 1997;**51**:270–6.

109. Zuniga R, Markowitz GS, Arkachaisri T, Imperatore EA, D'Agati VD, Salmon JE. Identification of IgG subclasses and C-reactive protein in lupus nephritis: the relationship between the composition of immune deposits and FCgamma receptor type IIA alleles. *Arthritis Rheum* 2003;**48**:460–70.

110. Haseley LA, Wisnieski JJ, Denburg MR, Michael-Grossman AR, Ginzler EM, Gourley MF, et al. Antibodies to C1q in systemic lupus erythematosus: characteristics and relation to Fc gamma RIIA alleles. *Kidney Int* 1997;**52**:1375–80.

111. Shushakova N, Skokowa J, Schulman J, Baumann U, Zwirner J, Schmidt RE, et al. C5a anaphylatoxin is a major regulator of activating versus inhibitory FcgammaRs in immune complex-induced lung disease. *J Clin Invest* 2002;**110**:1823–30.

112. Okayama Y, Kirshenbaum AS, Metcalfe DD. Expression of a functional high-affinity IgG receptor, Fc gamma RI, on human mast cells: up-regulation by IFN-gamma. *J Immunol* 2000;**164**:4332–9.

113. Pricop L, Redecha P, Teillaud JL, Frey J, Fridman WH, Sautes-Fridman C, et al. Differential modulation of stimulatory and inhibitory Fc gamma receptors on human monocytes by Th1 and Th2 cytokines. *J Immunol* 2001;**166**:531–7.

114. Radeke HH, Janssen-Graalfs I, Sowa EN, Chouchakova N, Skokowa J, Loscher F, et al. Opposite regulation of type II and III receptors for immunoglobulin G in mouse glomerular mesangial cells and in the induction of anti-glomerular basement membrane (GBM) nephritis. *J Biol Chem* 2002;**277**:27535–44.

115. Tridandapani S, Wardrop R, Baran CP, Wang Y, Opalek JM, Caligiuri MA, et al. TGF-beta 1 suppresses [correction of supresses] myeloid Fc gamma receptor function by regulating the expression and function of the common gamma-subunit. *J Immunol* 2003;**170**:4572–7.

116. Samuelsson A, Towers TL, Ravetch JV. Anti-inflammatory activity of IVIG mediated through the inhibitory Fc receptor. *Science* 2001;**291**:484–6.

117. Huizinga TW, van der Schoot CE, Jost C, Klaassen R, Kleijer M, von dem Borne AE, et al. The PI-linked receptor FcRIII is released on stimulation of neutrophils. *Nature* 1988;**333**:667–9.

118. Middelhoven PJ, Van Buul JD, Hordijk PL, Roos D. Different proteolytic mechanisms involved in Fc gamma RIIIb shedding from human neutrophils. *Clin Exp Immunol* 2001;**125**:169–75.

119. Tsuboi N, Ernandez T, Li X, Nishi H, Cullere X, Mekala D, et al. Regulation of human neutrophil Fcgamma receptor IIa by C5a receptor promotes inflammatory arthritis in mice. *Arthritis Rheum* 2011;**63**:467–78.

120. Koenderman L, Hermans SW, Capel PJ, van de Winkel JG. Granulocyte-macrophage colony-stimulating factor induces sequential activation and deactivation of binding via a low-affinity IgG Fc receptor, hFc gamma RII, on human eosinophils. *Blood* 1993;**81**:2413–9.

121. Finkelman FD, Holmes J, Katona IM, Urban Jr JF, Beckmann MP, Park LS, et al. Lymphokine control of in vivo immunoglobulin isotype selection. *Annu Rev Immunol* 1990;**8**:303–33.

122. Karp DR. Complement and systemic lupus erythematosus. *Curr Opin Rheumatol* 2005;**17**:538–42.

123. Zhao J, Wu H, Khosravi M, Cui H, Qian X, Kelly JA, et al. Association of genetic variants in complement factor H and factor H-related genes with systemic lupus erythematosus susceptibility. *PLoS Genet* 2011;**7**:e1002079.

124. Sim RB, Reid KB. C1: molecular interactions with activating systems. *Immunol Today* 1991;**12**:307–11.

125. Lewis MJ, Botto M. Complement deficiencies in humans and animals: links to autoimmunity. *Autoimmunity* 2006;**39**:367–78.

126. Ogden CA, deCathelineau A, Hoffmann PR, Bratton D, Ghebrehiwet B, Fadok VA, et al. C1q and mannose binding lectin engagement of cell surface calreticulin and CD91 initiates macropinocytosis and uptake of apoptotic cells. *J Exp Med* 2001;**194**:781–95.

127. Stokol T, O'Donnell P, Xiao L, Knight S, Stavrakis G, Botto M, et al. C1q governs deposition of circulating immune complexes and leukocyte Fcgamma receptors mediate subsequent neutrophil recruitment. *J Exp Med* 2004;**200**:835–46.

128. Gasque P. Complement: a unique innate immune sensor for danger signals. *Mol Immunol* 2004;**41**:1089–98.

129. Kumar V, Ali SR, Konrad S, Zwirner J, Verbeek JS, Schmidt RE, et al. Cell-derived anaphylatoxins as key mediators of antibody-dependent type II autoimmunity in mice. *J Clin Invest* 2006;**116**:512–20.

130. Godau J, Heller T, Hawlisch H, Trappe M, Howells E, Best J, et al. C5a initiates the inflammatory cascade in immune complex peritonitis. *J Immunol* 2004;**173**:3437–45.

131. Skokowa J, Ali SR, Felda O, Kumar V, Konrad S, Shushakova N, et al. Macrophages induce the inflammatory response in the pulmonary Arthus reaction through G alpha i2 activation that controls C5aR and Fc receptor cooperation. *J Immunol* 2005;**174**:3041–50.

132. Baumann U, Kohl J, Tschernig T, Schwerter-Strumpf K, Verbeek JS, Schmidt RE, et al. A codominant role of Fc gamma RI/III and C5aR in the reverse Arthus reaction. *J Immunol* 2000;**164**:1065–70.

133. Welch TR, Frenzke M, Witte D, Davis AE. C5a is important in the tubulointerstitial component of experimental immune complex glomerulonephritis. *Clin Exp Immunol* 2002;**130**:43–8.

134. Bao L, Osawe I, Puri T, Lambris JD, Haas M, Quigg RJ. C5a promotes development of experimental lupus nephritis which can be blocked with a specific receptor antagonist. *Eur J Immunol* 2005;**35**:2496–506.

135. Baumann U, Chouchakova N, Gewecke B, Kohl J, Carroll MC, Schmidt RE, et al. Distinct tissue site-specific requirements of mast cells and complement components C3/C5a receptor in IgG immune complex-induced injury of skin and lung. *J Immunol* 2001;**167**:1022–7.

136. Lutz HU, Jelezarova E. Complement amplification revisited. *Mol Immunol* 2006;**43**:2–12.

137. Schwaeble WJ, Reid KB. Does properdin crosslink the cellular and the humoral immune response? *Immunol Today* 1999;**20**:17–21.

138. Karsten CM, Kohl J. The immunoglobulin, IgG Fc receptor and complement triangle in autoimmune diseases. *Immunobiology* 2012;**217**:1067–79.

139. Huber-Lang M, Sarma JV, Zetoune FS, Rittirsch D, Neff TA, McGuire SR, et al. Generation of C5a in the absence of C3: a new complement activation pathway. *Nat Med* 2006;**12**:682–7.

140. Petty HR, Worth RG, Todd 3rd RF. Interactions of integrins with their partner proteins in leukocyte membranes. *Immunol Res* 2002;**25**:75–95.

141. Stefanova I, Horejsi V, Ansotegui IJ, Knapp W, Stockinger H. GPI-anchored cell-surface molecules complexed to protein tyrosine kinases. *Science* 1991;**254**:1016–9.

142. Barabe F, Gilbert C, Liao N, Bourgoin SG, Naccache PH. Crystal-induced neutrophil activation VI. Involvment of FcgammaRIIIB (CD16) and CD11b in response to inflammatory microcrystals. *FASEB J* 1998;**12**:209–20.

143. Berton G, Mocsai A, Lowell CA. Src and Syk kinases: key regulators of phagocytic cell activation. *Trends Immunol* 2005;**26**:208–14.

144. Joshi T, Butchar JP, Tridandapani S. Fcgamma receptor signaling in phagocytes. *Int J Hematol* 2006;**84**:210–6.

145. Berna-Erro A, Woodard GE, Rosado JA. Orais and STIMs: physiological mechanisms and disease. *J Cell Mol Med* 2012;**16**:407–24.

146. Steinckwich N, Schenten V, Melchior C, Brechard S, Tschirhart EJ. An essential role of STIM1, Orai1, and S100A8-A9 proteins for Ca^{2+} signaling and FcgammaR-mediated phagosomal oxidative activity. *J Immunol* 2011;**186**:2182–91.

147. Zhang H, Clemens RA, Liu F, Hu Y, Baba Y, Theodore P, et al. STIM1 calcium sensor is required for activation of the phagocyte oxidase during inflammation and host defense. *Blood* 2014;**123**:2238–49.

148. Braun A, Gessner JE, Varga-Szabo D, Syed SN, Konrad S, Stegner D, et al. STIM1 is essential for Fcgamma receptor activation and autoimmune inflammation. *Blood* 2009;**113**:1097–104.

149. Daeron M. Fc receptor biology. *Annu Rev Immunol* 1997;**15**:203–34.

150. Utomo A, Cullere X, Glogauer M, Swat W, Mayadas TN. Vav proteins in neutrophils are required for FcgammaR-mediated signaling to Rac GTPases and nicotinamide adenine dinucleotide phosphate oxidase component p40(phox). *J Immunol* 2006;**177**:6388–97.

151. Wells CM, Bhavsar PJ, Evans IR, Vigorito E, Turner M, Tybulewicz V, et al. Vav1 and Vav2 play different roles in macrophage migration and cytoskeletal organization. *Exp Cell Res* 2005;**310**:303–10.

152. Greuber EK, Pendergast AM. Abl family kinases regulate FcgammaR-mediated phagocytosis in murine macrophages. *J Immunol* 2012;**189**:5382–92.

153. Daeron M, Latour S, Malbec O, Espinosa E, Pina P, Pasmans S, et al. The same tyrosine-based inhibition motif, in the intracytoplasmic domain of Fc gamma RIIB, regulates negatively BCR-, TCR-, and FcR-dependent cell activation. *Immunity* 1995;**3**:635–46.

154. Ono M, Bolland S, Tempst P, Ravetch JV. Role of the inositol phosphatase SHIP in negative regulation of the immune system by the receptor Fc(gamma)RIIB. *Nature* 1996;**383**:263–6.

155. Ono M, Okada H, Bolland S, Yanagi S, Kurosaki T, Ravetch JV. Deletion of SHIP or SHP-1 reveals two distinct pathways for inhibitory signaling. *Cell* 1997;**90**:293–301.

156. Tzeng SJ, Bolland S, Inabe K, Kurosaki T, Pierce SK. The B cell inhibitory Fc receptor triggers apoptosis by a novel c-Abl family kinase-dependent pathway. *J Biol Chem* 2005;**280**:35247–54.

157. Ruland J, Mak TW. From antigen to activation: specific signal transduction pathways linking antigen receptors to NF-kappaB. *Semin Immunol* 2003;**15**:177–83.

158. Dorner T, Lipsky PE. Signalling pathways in B cells: implications for autoimmunity. *Curr Top Microbiol Immunol* 2006;**305**:213–40.

159. Chung JW, Yoon SR, Choi I. The regulation of NK cell function and development. *Front Biosci* 2008;**13**:6432–42.

160. Lanier LL. Up on the tightrope: natural killer cell activation and inhibition. *Nat Immunol* 2008;**9**:495–502.

161. Ivashkiv LB. A signal-switch hypothesis for cross-regulation of cytokine and TLR signalling pathways. *Nat Rev Immunol* 2008;**8**:816–22.

162. Takai T. Roles of Fc receptors in autoimmunity. *Nat Rev Immunol* 2002;**2**:580–92.

163. Goodnow CC, Sprent J, Fazekas de St Groth B, Vinuesa CG. Cellular and genetic mechanisms of self tolerance and autoimmunity. *Nature* 2005;**435**:590–7.

164. Takai T, Ono M, Hikida M, Ohmori H, Ravetch JV. Augmented humoral and anaphylactic responses in Fc gamma RII-deficient mice. *Nature* 1996;**379**:346–9.

165. Boross P, Arandhara VL, Martin-Ramirez J, Santiago-Raber ML, Carlucci F, Flierman R, et al. The inhibiting Fc receptor for IgG, FcgammaRIIB, is a modifier of autoimmune susceptibility. *J Immunol* 2011;**187**:1304–13.

166. Bygrave AE, Rose KL, Cortes-Hernandez J, Warren J, Rigby RJ, Cook HT, et al. Spontaneous autoimmunity in 129 and C57BL/6 mice-implications for autoimmunity described in gene-targeted mice. *PLoS Biol* 2004;**2**:E243.

167. Amigorena S, Bonnerot C, Drake JR, Choquet D, Hunziker W, Guillet JG, et al. Cytoplasmic domain heterogeneity and functions of IgG Fc receptors in B lymphocytes. *Science* 1992;**256**:1808–12.

168. Xiang Z, Cutler AJ, Brownlie RJ, Fairfax K, Lawlor KE, Severinson E, et al. FcgammaRIIb controls bone marrow plasma cell persistence and apoptosis. *Nat Immunol* 2007;**8**:419–29.

169. Pearse RN, Kawabe T, Bolland S, Guinamard R, Kurosaki T, Ravetch JV. SHIP recruitment attenuates Fc gamma RIIB-induced B cell apoptosis. *Immunity* 1999;**10**:753–60.

170. Pritchard NR, Cutler AJ, Uribe S, Chadban SJ, Morley BJ, Smith KG. Autoimmune-prone mice share a promoter haplotype associated with reduced expression and function of the Fc receptor FcgammaRII. *Curr Biol* 2000;**10**:227–30.

171. McGaha TL, Sorrentino B, Ravetch JV. Restoration of tolerance in lupus by targeted inhibitory receptor expression. *Science* 2005;**307**:590–3.

172. Brownlie RJ, Lawlor KE, Niederer HA, Cutler AJ, Xiang Z, Clatworthy MR, et al. Distinct cell-specific control of autoimmunity and infection by FcgammaRIIb. *J Exp Med* 2008;**205**:883–95.

173. Kleinau S, Martinsson P, Heyman B. Induction and suppression of collagen-induced arthritis is dependent on distinct fcgamma receptors. *J Exp Med* 2000;**191**:1611–6.

174. Yuasa T, Kubo S, Yoshino T, Ujike A, Matsumura K, Ono M, et al. Deletion of fcgamma receptor IIB renders H-2(b) mice susceptible to collagen-induced arthritis. *J Exp Med* 1999;**189**:187–94.

175. Nakamura A, Yuasa T, Ujike A, Ono M, Nukiwa T, Ravetch JV, et al. Fcgamma receptor IIB-deficient mice develop Goodpasture's syndrome upon immunization with type IV collagen: a novel murine model for autoimmune glomerular basement membrane disease. *J Exp Med* 2000;**191**:899–906.

176. Herrmann M, Voll RE, Zoller OM, Hagenhofer M, Ponner BB, Kalden JR. Impaired phagocytosis of apoptotic cell material by monocyte-derived macrophages from patients with systemic lupus erythematosus. *Arthritis Rheum* 1998;**41**:1241–50.

177. Kavai M, Szegedi G. Immune complex clearance by monocytes and macrophages in systemic lupus erythematosus. *Autoimmun Rev* 2007;**6**:497–502.

178. Bogers WM, Stad RK, Van Es LA, Daha MR. Both Kupffer cells and liver endothelial cells play an important role in the clearance of IgA and IgG immune complexes. *Res Immunol* 1992;**143**:219–24.

179. Cornacoff JB, Hebert LA, Smead WL, VanAman ME, Birmingham DJ, Waxman FJ. Primate erythrocyte-immune complex-clearing mechanism. *J Clin Invest* 1983;**71**:236–47.

180. Henderson AL, Lindorfer MA, Kennedy AD, Foley PL, Taylor RP. Concerted clearance of immune complexes bound to the human erythrocyte complement receptor: development of a heterologous mouse model. *J Immunol Methods* 2002;**270**:183–97.

181. He JQ, Wiesmann C, van Lookeren Campagne M. A role of macrophage complement receptor CRIg in immune clearance and inflammation. *Mol Immunol* 2008;**45**:4041–7.

182. Harley JB, Alarcon-Riquelme ME, Criswell LA, Jacob CO, Kimberly RP, Moser KL, et al. Genome-wide association scan in women with systemic lupus erythematosus identifies susceptibility variants in ITGAM, PXK, KIAA1542 and other loci. *Nat Genet* 2008;**40**:204–10.

183. Hom G, Graham RR, Modrek B, Taylor KE, Ortmann W, Garnier S, et al. Association of systemic lupus erythematosus with C8orf13-BLK and ITGAM-ITGAX. *N Engl J Med* 2008;**358**:900–9.

184. Nath SK, Han S, Kim-Howard X, Kelly JA, Viswanathan P, Gilkeson GS, et al. A nonsynonymous functional variant in integrin-alpha(M) (encoded by ITGAM) is associated with systemic lupus erythematosus. *Nat Genet* 2008;**40**:152–4.

185. Fossati G, Bucknall RC, Edwards SW. Fcgamma receptors in autoimmune diseases. *Eur J Clin Invest* 2001;**31**:821–31.

186. Salmon JE, Millard S, Schachter LA, Arnett FC, Ginzler EM, Gourley MF, et al. Fc gamma RIIA alleles are heritable risk factors for lupus nephritis in African Americans. *J Clin Invest* 1996;**97**:1348–54.

187. Ganesan LP, Kim J, Wu Y, Mohanty S, Phillips GS, Birmingham DJ, et al. FcgammaRIIb on liver sinusoidal endothelium clears small immune complexes. *J Immunol* 2012;**189**:4981–8.

188. Groger M, Fischer GF, Wolff K, Petzelbauer P. Immune complexes from vasculitis patients bind to endothelial Fc receptors independent of the allelic polymorphism of FcgammaRIIa. *J Invest Dermatol* 1999;**113**:56–60.

189. Mousavi SA, Sporstol M, Fladeby C, Kjeken R, Barois N, Berg T. Receptor-mediated endocytosis of immune complexes in rat liver sinusoidal endothelial cells is mediated by FcgammaRIIb2. *Hepatology* 2007;**46**:871–84.

190. Sedmak DD, Davis DH, Singh U, van de Winkel JG, Anderson CL. Expression of IgG Fc receptor antigens in placenta and on endothelial cells in humans. An immunohistochemical study. *Am J Pathol* 1991;**138**:175–81.

191. Vielma S, Virella G, Gorod A, Lopes-Virella M. *Chlamydophila pneumoniae* infection of human aortic endothelial cells induces the expression of FC gamma receptor II (FcgammaRII). *Clin Immunol* 2002;**104**:265–73.

192. Akilesh S, Huber TB, Wu H, Wang G, Hartleben B, Kopp JB, et al. Podocytes use FcRn to clear IgG from the glomerular basement membrane. *Proc Natl Acad Sci USA* 2008;**105**:967–72.

193. Nangaku M, Couser WG. Mechanisms of immune-deposit formation and the mediation of immune renal injury. *Clin Exp Nephrol* 2005;**9**:183–91.

194. Fries JW, Mendrick DL, Rennke HG. Determinants of immune complex-mediated glomerulonephritis. *Kidney Int* 1988;**34**:333–45.

195. Nagarajan S, Venkiteswaran K, Anderson M, Sayed U, Zhu C, Selvaraj P. Cell-specific, activation-dependent regulation of neutrophil CD32A ligand-binding function. *Blood* 2000;**95**:1069–77.

196. Willcocks LC, Lyons PA, Clatworthy MR, Robinson JI, Yang W, Newland SA, et al. Copy number of FCGR3B, which is associated with systemic lupus erythematosus, correlates with protein expression and immune complex uptake. *J Exp Med* 2008;**205**:1573–82.

197. Coxon A, Cullere X, Knight S, Sethi S, Wakelin MW, Stavrakis G, et al. Fc gamma RIII mediates neutrophil recruitment to immune complexes: a mechanism for neutrophil accumulation in immune-mediated inflammation. *Immunity* 2001;**14**:693–704.

198. Clynes R, Dumitru C, Ravetch JV. Uncoupling of immune complex formation and kidney damage in autoimmune glomerulonephritis. *Science* 1998;**279**:1052–4.

199. Bergtold A, Gavhane A, D'Agati V, Madaio M, Clynes R. FcR-bearing myeloid cells are responsible for triggering murine lupus nephritis. *J Immunol* 2006;**177**:7287–95.

200. Lin Q, Xiu Y, Jiang Y, Tsurui H, Nakamura K, Kodera S, et al. Genetic dissection of the effects of stimulatory and inhibitory IgG Fc receptors on murine lupus. *J Immunol* 2006;**177**:1646–54.

201. Matsumoto K, Watanabe N, Akikusa B, Kurasawa K, Matsumura R, Saito Y, et al. Fc receptor-independent development of autoimmune glomerulonephritis in lupus-prone MRL/lpr mice. *Arthritis Rheum* 2003;**48**:486–94.

202. Atkinson C, Qiao F, Song H, Gilkeson GS, Tomlinson S. Low-dose targeted complement inhibition protects against renal disease and other manifestations of autoimmune disease in MRL/lpr mice. *J Immunol* 2008;**180**:1231–8.

203. Sekine H, Reilly CM, Molano ID, Garnier G, Circolo A, Ruiz P, et al. Complement component C3 is not required for full expression of immune complex glomerulonephritis in MRL/lpr mice. *J Immunol* 2001;**166**:6444–51.

204. Baudino L, Nimmerjahn F, Azeredo da Silveira S, Martinez-Soria E, Saito T, Carroll M, et al. Differential contribution of three activating IgG Fc receptors (FcgammaRI, FcgammaRIII, and FcgammaRIV) to IgG2a- and IgG2b-induced autoimmune hemolytic anemia in mice. *J Immunol* 2008;**180**:1948–53.

205. Santiago-Raber ML, Amano H, Amano E, Baudino L, Otani M, Lin Q, et al. Fcgamma receptor-dependent expansion of a hyperactive monocyte subset in lupus-prone mice. *Arthritis Rheum* 2009;**60**:2408–17.

206. Crispin JC, Hedrich CM, Tsokos GC. Gene-function studies in systemic lupus erythematosus. *Nat Rev Rheumatol* 2013;**9**:476–84.

207. Rosetti F, Tsuboi N, Chen K, Nishi H, Ernandez T, Sethi S, et al. Human lupus serum induces neutrophil-mediated organ damage in mice that is enabled by Mac-1 deficiency. *J Immunol* 2012;**189**:3714–23.

208. Hora K, Satriano JA, Santiago A, Mori T, Stanley ER, Shan Z, et al. Receptors for IgG complexes activate synthesis of monocyte chemoattractant peptide 1 and colony-stimulating factor 1. *Proc Natl Acad Sci USA* 1992;**89**:1745–9.

209. Fu Y, Du Y, Mohan C. Experimental anti-GBM disease as a tool for studying spontaneous lupus nephritis. *Clin Immunol* 2007;**124**:109–18.

210. Park SY, Ueda S, Ohno H, Hamano Y, Tanaka M, Shiratori T, et al. Resistance of Fc receptor- deficient mice to fatal glomerulonephritis. *J Clin Invest* 1998;**102**:1229–38.

211. Suzuki Y, Shirato I, Okumura K, Ravetch JV, Takai T, Tomino Y, et al. Distinct contribution of Fc receptors and angiotensin II-dependent pathways in anti-GBM glomerulonephritis. *Kidney Int* 1998;**54**:1166–74.

212. Tarzi RM, Davies KA, Claassens JW, Verbeek JS, Walport MJ, Cook HT. Both Fcgamma receptor I and Fcgamma receptor III mediate disease in accelerated nephrotoxic nephritis. *Am J Pathol* 2003;**162**:1677–83.

213. Camussi G, Cappio FC, Messina M, Coppo R, Stratta P, Vercellone A. The polymorphonuclear neutrophil (PMN) immunohistological technique: detection of immune complexes bound to the PMN membrane in acute poststreptococcal and lupus nephritis. *Clin Nephrol* 1980;**14**:280–7.

214. Hooke DH, Gee DC, Atkins RC. Leukocyte analysis using monoclonal antibodies in human glomerulonephritis. *Kidney Int* 1987;**31**:964–72.

215. Segerer S, Henger A, Schmid H, Kretzler M, Draganovici D, Brandt U, et al. Expression of the chemokine receptor CXCR1 in human glomerular diseases. *Kidney Int* 2006;**69**:1765–73.

216. Croker JA, Kimberly RP. Genetics of susceptibility and severity in systemic lupus erythematosus. *Curr Opin Rheumatol* 2005;**17**:529–37.

217. Duits AJ, Bootsma H, Derksen RH, Spronk PE, Kater L, Kallenberg CG, et al. Skewed distribution of IgG Fc receptor IIa (CD32) polymorphism is associated with renal disease in systemic lupus erythematosus patients. *Arthritis Rheum* 1995;**38**:1832–6.

218. Manger K, Repp R, Jansen M, Geisselbrecht M, Wassmuth R, Westerdaal NA, et al. Fcgamma receptor IIa, IIIa, and IIIb polymorphisms in German patients with systemic lupus erythematosus: association with clinical symptoms. *Ann Rheum Dis* 2002;**61**:786–92.

219. Dijstelbloem HM, Bijl M, Fijnheer R, Scheepers RH, Oost WW, Jansen MD, et al. Fcgamma receptor polymorphisms in systemic lupus erythematosus: association with disease and in vivo clearance of immune complexes. *Arthritis Rheum* 2000;**43**:2793–800.

220. Hong CH, Lee JS, Lee HS, Bae SC, Yoo DH. The association between fcgammaRIIIB polymorphisms and systemic lupus erythematosus in Korea. *Lupus* 2005;**14**:346–50.

221. Karassa FB, Trikalinos TA, Ioannidis JP. Role of the Fcgamma receptor IIa polymorphism in susceptibility to systemic lupus erythematosus and lupus nephritis: a meta-analysis. *Arthritis Rheum* 2002;**46**:1563–71.

222. Zhou XJ, Lv JC, Qin LX, Yang HZ, Yu F, Zhao MH, et al. Is FCGR2A a susceptibility gene to systemic lupus erythematosus in Chinese? *Lupus* 2011;**20**:1198–202.

223. Salmon JE, Edberg JC, Brogle NL, Kimberly RP. Allelic polymorphisms of human Fc gamma receptor IIA and Fc gamma receptor IIIB. Independent mechanisms for differences in human phagocyte function. *J Clin Invest* 1992;**89**:1274–81.

224. Doi T, Mayumi M, Kanatsu K, Suehiro F, Hamashima Y. Distribution of IgG subclasses in membranous nephropathy. *Clin Exp Immunol* 1984;**58**:57–62.

225. Roberts JL, Wyatt RJ, Schwartz MM, Lewis EJ. Differential characteristics of immune-bound antibodies in diffuse proliferative and membranous forms of lupus glomerulonephritis. *Clin Immunol Immunopathol* 1983;**29**:223–41.

226. Chen JY, Wang CM, Ma CC, Luo SF, Edberg JC, Kimberly RP, et al. Association of a transmembrane polymorphism of Fcgamma receptor IIb (FCGR2B) with systemic lupus erythematosus in Taiwanese patients. *Arthritis Rheum* 2006;**54**:3908–17.

227. Chu ZT, Tsuchiya N, Kyogoku C, Ohashi J, Qian YP, Xu SB, et al. Association of Fcgamma receptor IIb polymorphism with susceptibility to systemic lupus erythematosus in Chinese: a common susceptibility gene in the Asian populations. *Tissue Antigens* 2004;**63**:21–7.

228. Kyogoku C, Dijstelbloem HM, Tsuchiya N, Hatta Y, Kato H, Yamaguchi A, et al. Fcgamma receptor gene polymorphisms in Japanese patients with systemic lupus erythematosus: contribution of FCGR2B to genetic susceptibility. *Arthritis Rheum* 2002;**46**:1242–54.

229. Siriboonrit U, Tsuchiya N, Sirikong M, Kyogoku C, Bejrachandra S, Suthipinittharm P, et al. Association of Fcgamma receptor IIb and IIIb polymorphisms with susceptibility to systemic lupus erythematosus in Thais. *Tissue Antigens* 2003;**61**:374–83.

230. Li X, Wu J, Carter RH, Edberg JC, Su K, Cooper GS, et al. A novel polymorphism in the Fcgamma receptor IIB (CD32B) transmembrane region alters receptor signaling. *Arthritis Rheum* 2003;**48**:3242–52.

231. Magnusson V, Zunec R, Odeberg J, Sturfelt G, Truedsson L, Gunnarsson I, et al. Polymorphisms of the Fc gamma receptor type IIB gene are not associated with systemic lupus erythematosus in the Swedish population. *Arthritis Rheum* 2004;**50**:1348–50.

232. Lee YH, Ji JD, Song GG. Fcgamma receptor IIB and IIIB polymorphisms and susceptibility to systemic lupus erythematosus and lupus nephritis: a meta-analysis. *Lupus* 2009;**18**:727–34.

233. Niederer HA, Willcocks LC, Rayner TF, Yang W, Lau YL, Williams TN, et al. Copy number, linkage disequilibrium and disease association in the FCGR locus. *Hum Mol Genet* 2010;**19**:3282–94.

234. Willcocks LC, Carr EJ, Niederer HA, Rayner TF, Williams TN, Yang W, et al. A defunctioning polymorphism in FCGR2B is associated with protection against malaria but susceptibility to systemic lupus erythematosus. *Proc Natl Acad Sci USA* 2010;**107**:7881–5.

235. Floto RA, Clatworthy MR, Heilbronn KR, Rosner DR, MacAry PA, Rankin A, et al. Loss of function of a lupus-associated FcgammaRIIb polymorphism through exclusion from lipid rafts. *Nat Med* 2005;**11**:1056–8.

236. Kono H, Kyogoku C, Suzuki T, Tsuchiya N, Honda H, Yamamoto K, et al. FcgammaRIIB Ile232Thr transmembrane polymorphism associated with human systemic lupus erythematosus decreases affinity to lipid rafts and attenuates inhibitory effects on B cell receptor signaling. *Hum Mol Genet* 2005;**14**:2881–92.

237. Su K, Li X, Edberg JC, Wu J, Ferguson P, Kimberly RP. A promoter haplotype of the immunoreceptor tyrosine-based inhibitory motif-bearing FcgammaRIIb alters receptor expression and associates with autoimmunity. II. Differential binding of GATA4 and Yin-Yang1 transcription factors and correlated receptor expression and function. *J Immunol* 2004;**172**:7192–9.

238. Su K, Wu J, Edberg JC, Li X, Ferguson P, Cooper GS, et al. A promoter haplotype of the immunoreceptor tyrosine-based inhibitory motif-bearing FcgammaRIIb alters receptor expression and associates with autoimmunity. I. Regulatory FCGR2B polymorphisms and their association with systemic lupus erythematosus. *J Immunol* 2004;**172**:7186–91.

239. van Mirre E, Breunis WB, Geissler J, Hack CE, de Boer M, Roos D, et al. Neutrophil responsiveness to IgG, as determined by fixed ratios of mRNA levels for activating and inhibitory FcgammaRII (CD32), is stable over time and unaffected by cytokines. *Blood* 2006;**108**:584–90.

240. Smith KG, Willcocks LC, Lyons PA. Comment on "The inhibiting Fc receptor for IgG, FcgammaRIIB, is a modifier of autoimmune susceptibility". *J Immunol* 2011;**187**. 5473; author reply 5473–4.

241. Breunis WB, van Mirre E, Bruin M, Geissler J, de Boer M, Peters M, et al. Copy number variation of the activating FCGR2C gene predisposes to idiopathic thrombocytopenic purpura. *Blood* 2008;**111**:1029–38.

242. Stranger BE, Forrest MS, Dunning M, Ingle CE, Beazley C, Thorne N, et al. Relative impact of nucleotide and copy number variation on gene expression phenotypes. *Science* 2007;**315**:848–53.

243. Breunis WB, van Mirre E, Geissler J, Laddach N, Wolbink G, van der Schoot E, et al. Copy number variation at the FCGR locus includes FCGR3A, FCGR2C and FCGR3B but not FCGR2A and FCGR2B. *Hum Mutat* 2009;**30**:E640–50.

244. Karassa FB, Trikalinos TA, Ioannidis JP, Fc gamma RIIIA-SLE meta-analysis investigators. The Fc gamma RIIIA-F158 allele is a risk factor for the development of lupus nephritis: a meta-analysis. *Kidney Int* 2003;**63**:1475–82.

245. Li LH, Yuan H, Pan HF, Li WX, Li XP, Ye DQ. Role of the Fcgamma receptor IIIA-V/F158 polymorphism in susceptibility to systemic lupus erythematosus and lupus nephritis: a meta-analysis. *Scand J Rheumatol* 2010;**39**:148–54.

246. Dai M, Zhou Z, Wang X, Qian X, Huang X. Association of FcgammaRIIIa-158V/F with systemic lupus erythematosus in a Chinese population. *Int J Rheum Dis* 2013;**16**:685–91.

247. Koene HR, Kleijer M, Algra J, Roos D, von dem Borne AE, de Haas M. Fc gammaRIIIa-158V/F polymorphism influences the binding of IgG by natural killer cell Fc gammaRIIIa, independently of the Fc gammaRIIIa-48L/R/H phenotype. *Blood* 1997;**90**:1109–14.

248. Wu J, Edberg JC, Redecha PB, Bansal V, Guyre PM, Coleman K, et al. A novel polymorphism of FcgammaRIIIa (CD16) alters receptor function and predisposes to autoimmune disease. *J Clin Invest* 1997;**100**:1059–70.

249. Dong C, Ptacek TS, Redden DT, Zhang K, Brown EE, Edberg JC, et al. Fcgamma receptor IIIa single-nucleotide polymorphisms and haplotypes affect human IgG binding and are associated with lupus nephritis in African Americans. *Arthritis Rheumatol* 2014;**66**:1291–9.

250. Chen JY, Wang CM, Chang SW, Cheng CH, Wu YJ, Lin JC, et al. Association of FCGR3A and FCGR3B copy number variations with systemic lupus erythematosus and rheumatoid arthritis in Taiwanese patients. *Arthritis Rheumatol* 2014;**66**:3113–21.

251. Salmon JE, Edberg JC, Kimberly RP. Fc gamma receptor III on human neutrophils. Allelic variants have functionally distinct capacities. *J Clin Invest* 1990;**85**:1287–95.

252. Hatta Y, Tsuchiya N, Ohashi J, Matsushita M, Fujiwara K, Hagiwara K, et al. Association of Fc gamma receptor IIIB, but not of Fc gamma receptor IIA and IIIA polymorphisms with systemic lupus erythematosus in Japanese. *Genes Immun* 1999;**1**:53–60.

253. Yuan H, Ni JD, Pan HF, Li LH, Feng JB, Ye DQ. Lack of association of FcgammaRIIIb polymorphisms with systemic lupus erythematosus: a meta-analysis. *Rheumatol Int* 2011;**31**:1017–21.

254. Aitman TJ, Dong R, Vyse TJ, Norsworthy PJ, Johnson MD, Smith J, et al. Copy number polymorphism in Fcgr3 predisposes to glomerulonephritis in rats and humans. *Nature* 2006;**439**:851–5.

255. Molokhia M, Fanciulli M, Petretto E, Patrick AL, McKeigue P, Roberts AL, et al. FCGR3B copy number variation is associated with systemic lupus erythematosus risk in Afro-Caribbeans. *Rheumatol Oxf* 2011;**50**:1206–10.

256. McKinney C, Merriman TR. Meta-analysis confirms a role for deletion in FCGR3B in autoimmune phenotypes. *Hum Mol Genet* 2012;**21**:2370–6.

257. Mueller M, Barros P, Witherden AS, Roberts AL, Zhang Z, Schaschl H, et al. Genomic pathology of SLE-associated copy-number variation at the FCGR2C/FCGR3B/FCGR2B locus. *Am J Hum Genet* 2013;**92**:28–40.

258. Tsokos GC, Rook AH, Djeu JY, Balow JE. Natural killer cells and interferon responses in patients with systemic lupus erythematosus. *Clin Exp Immunol* 1982;**50**:239–45.

259. Galon J, Gauchat JF, Mazieres N, Spagnoli R, Storkus W, Lotze M, et al. Soluble Fcgamma receptor type III (FcgammaRIII, CD16) triggers cell activation through interaction with complement receptors. *J Immunol* 1996;**157**:1184–92.

260. Li X, Kimberly RP. Targeting the Fc receptor in autoimmune disease. *Expert Opin Ther Targets* 2014;**18**:335–50.

261. Nimmerjahn F, Ravetch JV. Anti-inflammatory actions of intravenous immunoglobulin. *Annu Rev Immunol* 2008;**26**:513–33.

262. Nagelkerke SQ, Kuijpers TW. Immunomodulation by IVIg and the role of Fc-gamma receptors: classic mechanisms of action after all? *Front Immunol* 2014;**5**:674.

263. Zandman-Goddard G, Blank M, Shoenfeld Y. Intravenous immunoglobulins in systemic lupus erythematosus: from the bench to the bedside. *Lupus* 2009;**18**:884–8.

264. Karim MY, Pisoni CN, Khamashta MA. Update on immunotherapy for systemic lupus erythematosus–what's hot and what's not! *Rheumatology (Oxford)* 2009;**48**:332–41.

265. Bucciarelli S, Erkan D, Espinosa G, Cervera R. Catastrophic antiphospholipid syndrome: treatment, prognosis, and the risk of relapse. *Clin Rev Allergy Immunol* 2009;**36**:80–4.

266. Basta M, Van Goor F, Luccioli S, Billings EM, Vortmeyer AO, Baranyi L, et al. F(ab)'2-mediated neutralization of C3a and C5a anaphylatoxins: a novel effector function of immunoglobulins. *Nat Med* 2003;**9**:431–8.

267. Vassilev TL, Kazatchkine MD, Duong Van Huyen JP, Mekrache M, Bonnin E, Mani JC, et al. Inhibition of cell adhesion by antibodies to Arg-Gly-Asp (RGD) in normal immunoglobulin for therapeutic use (intravenous immunoglobulin, IVIg). *Blood* 1999;**93**:3624–31.

268. Negi VS, Elluru S, Siberil S, Graff-Dubois S, Mouthon L, Kazatchkine MD, et al. Intravenous immunoglobulin: an update on the clinical use and mechanisms of action. *J Clin Immunol* 2007;**27**:233–45.

269. Debre M, Bonnet MC, Fridman WH, Carosella E, Philippe N, Reinert P, et al. Infusion of Fc gamma fragments for treatment of children with acute immune thrombocytopenic purpura. *Lancet* 1993;**342**:945–9.

270. Kaneko Y, Nimmerjahn F, Madaio MP, Ravetch JV. Pathology and protection in nephrotoxic nephritis is determined by selective engagement of specific Fc receptors. *J Exp Med* 2006;**203**:789–97.

271. Gill V, Doig C, Knight D, Love E, Kubes P. Targeting adhesion molecules as a potential mechanism of action for intravenous immunoglobulin. *Circulation* 2005;**112**:2031–9.

272. Williams RO, Feldmann M, Maini RN. Anti-tumor necrosis factor ameliorates joint disease in murine collagen-induced arthritis. *Proc Natl Acad Sci USA* 1992;**89**:9784–8.

273. Duta F, Ulanova M, Seidel D, Puttagunta L, Musat-Marcu S, Harrod KS, et al. Differential expression of spleen tyrosine kinase Syk isoforms in tissues: effects of the microbial flora. *Histochem Cell Biol* 2006;**126**:495–505.

274. Pine PR, Chang B, Schoettler N, Banquerigo ML, Wang S, Lau A, et al. Inflammation and bone erosion are suppressed in models of rheumatoid arthritis following treatment with a novel Syk inhibitor. *Clin Immunol* 2007;**124**:244–57.

275. Weinblatt ME, Kavanaugh A, Burgos-Vargas R, Dikranian AH, Medrano-Ramirez G, Morales-Torres JL, et al. Treatment of rheumatoid arthritis with a Syk kinase inhibitor: a twelve-week, randomized, placebo-controlled trial. *Arthritis Rheum* 2008;**58**:3309–18.

276. Weinblatt ME, Kavanaugh A, Genovese MC, Musser TK, Grossbard EB, Magilavy DB. An oral spleen tyrosine kinase (Syk) inhibitor for rheumatoid arthritis. *N Engl J Med* 2010;**363**:1303–12.

277. Scott IC, Scott DL. Spleen tyrosine kinase inhibitors for rheumatoid arthritis: where are we now? *Drugs* 2014;**74**:415–22.

278. Weinblatt ME, Genovese MC, Ho M, Hollis S, Rosiak-Jedrychowicz K, Kavanaugh A, et al. Effects of fostamatinib, an oral spleen tyrosine kinase inhibitor, in rheumatoid arthritis patients with an inadequate response to methotrexate: results from a phase III, multicenter, randomized, double-blind, placebo-controlled, parallel-group study. *Arthritis Rheumatol* 2014;**66**:3255–64.

279. Podolanczuk A, Lazarus AH, Crow AR, Grossbard E, Bussel JB. Of mice and men: an open-label pilot study for treatment of immune thrombocytopenic purpura by an inhibitor of Syk. *Blood* 2009;**113**:3154–60.

280. Bahjat FR, Pine PR, Reitsma A, Cassafer G, Baluom M, Grillo S, et al. An orally bioavailable spleen tyrosine kinase inhibitor delays disease progression and prolongs survival in murine lupus. *Arthritis Rheum* 2008;**58**:1433–44.

281. Deng GM, Liu L, Bahjat FR, Pine PR, Tsokos GC. Suppression of skin and kidney disease by inhibition of spleen tyrosine kinase in lupus-prone mice. *Arthritis Rheum* 2010;**62**:2086–92.

282. Ellsworth JL, Hamacher N, Harder B, Bannink K, Bukowski TR, Byrnes-Blake K, et al. Recombinant soluble human FcgammaR1A (CD64A) reduces inflammation in murine collagen-induced arthritis. *J Immunol* 2009;**182**:7272–9.

283. Werwitzke S, Trick D, Sondermann P, Kamino K, Schlegelberger B, Kniesch K, et al. Treatment of lupus-prone NZB/NZW F1 mice with recombinant soluble Fc gamma receptor II (CD32). *Ann Rheum Dis* 2008;**67**:154–61.

284. Bussel JB. Fc receptor blockade and immune thrombocytopenic purpura. *Semin Hematol* 2000;**37**:261–6.

285. Clarkson SB, Bussel JB, Kimberly RP, Valinsky JE, Nachman RL, Unkeless JC. Treatment of refractory immune thrombocytopenic purpura with an anti-Fc gamma-receptor antibody. *N Engl J Med* 1986;**314**:1236–9.

286. Psaila B, Bussel JB. Fc receptors in immune thrombocytopenias: a target for immunomodulation? *J Clin Invest* 2008;**118**:2677–81.

287. Ben Mkaddem S, Hayem G, Jonsson F, Rossato E, Boedec E, Boussetta T, et al. Shifting FcgammaRIIA-ITAM from activation to inhibitory configuration ameliorates arthritis. *J Clin Invest* 2014;**124**:3945–59.

288. Marino M, Ruvo M, De Falco S, Fassina G. Prevention of systemic lupus erythematosus in MRL/lpr mice by administration of an immunoglobulin-binding peptide. *Nat Biotechnol* 2000;**18**:735–9.

289. Pietersz GA, Mottram PL, van de Velde NC, Sardjono CT, Esparon S, Ramsland PA, et al. Inhibition of destructive autoimmune arthritis in FcgammaRIIa transgenic mice by small chemical entities. *Immunol Cell Biol* 2009;**87**:3–12.

290. Xi J, Zhang GP, Qiao SL, Guo JQ, Wang XN, Yang YY, et al. Increased survival and reduced renal injury in MRL/lpr mice treated with a human Fcgamma receptor II (CD32) peptide. *Immunology* 2012;**136**:46–53.

291. Veri MC, Burke S, Huang L, Li H, Gorlatov S, Tuaillon N, et al. Therapeutic control of B cell activation via recruitment of Fcgamma receptor IIb (CD32B) inhibitory function with a novel bispecific antibody scaffold. *Arthritis Rheum* 2010;**62**:1933–43.

292. Horton HM, Chu SY, Ortiz EC, Pong E, Cemerski S, Leung IW, et al. Antibody-mediated coengagement of FcgammaRIIb and B cell receptor complex suppresses humoral immunity in systemic lupus erythematosus. *J Immunol* 2011;**186**:4223–33.

293. Liu Y, Masuda E, Blank MC, Kirou KA, Gao X, Park MS, et al. Cytokine-mediated regulation of activating and inhibitory Fc gamma receptors in human monocytes. *J Leukoc Biol* 2005;**77**:767–76.

294. Allen JB, Wong HL, Guyre PM, Simon GL, Wahl SM. Association of circulating receptor Fc gamma RIII-positive monocytes in AIDS patients with elevated levels of transforming growth factor-beta. *J Clin Invest* 1991;**87**:1773–9.

295. Gesheva V, Szekeres Z, Mihaylova N, Dimitrova I, Nikolova M, Erdei A, et al. Generation of gene-engineered chimeric DNA molecules for specific therapy of autoimmune diseases. *Hum Gene Ther Methods* 2012;**23**:357–65.

Chapter 21

Apoptosis, Autophagy, and Necrosis

Roberto Caricchio

Department of Medicine, Section of Rheumatology and Department of Microbiology and Immunology, Temple University School of Medicine, Philadelphia, PA, USA

Two and a half millennia ago, Hippocrates used the word *apoptosis* to describe the gangrene resulting from treatment of fractures with bandages. Interestingly, he was describing a pathological form of tissue (cell) death.[1] In 1972, Kerr reused the word *apoptosis* with a different connotation, to describe a physiological form of cell demise with profound biological and pathological implications.[1] Today, this form of cell death is considered an essential mechanism in all fields of biology and has proven to be a fundamental mechanism in systemic lupus erythematous (SLE) pathogenesis.

It has become clear that cell death can occur with multiple modalities, and most forms are tightly regulated and molecularly programmed. They all play a role in SLE and are commonly defined as apoptosis and necrosis; the first is generally considered to be noninflammatory, whereas the latter is pro-inflammatory.[2]

DEFINITION

The definition of a *dead* cell is more complex than one would anticipate, and it has undergone several modifications over the last century. Currently, the Nomenclature Committee on Cell Death considers *dead* cells to be those that either exhibit irreversible plasma membrane permeabilization or have undergone complete fragmentation.[3]

Cell *death* should be divided into two main categories: accidental and regulated cell death (ACD and RCD, respectively).[3] ACD is induced by extreme physical or chemical insults, such as burns or acid exposure, and cannot be reversed or delayed; RCD, on the other hand, is extraordinarily structured and its molecular pathways are evolutionary preserved. RCD is genetically predetermined and can be modified both genetically and pharmacologically[4]; when its functions are primarily during the embryonic life or to maintain tissue homeostasis, it is described as programmed cell death. Finally, RCD is generally divided into caspase dependent and caspase independent, with the former referred to as *apoptosis* and the latter *necrosis*.[3]

APOPTOSIS

Pathways: Intrinsic versus Extrinsic

The characteristic features of an apoptotic cell are its changing morphology and the mandatory activation of genetically regulated molecular pathways. The latter can be triggered by mechanisms extrinsic and intrinsic to the cell—hence the terms *extrinsic* and *intrinsic apoptosis*.

Extrinsic factors induce death via the triggering of *trans*-membrane receptors, of which Fas is the prototype.[5] Upon trimerization of Fas by its ligand (FasL), a complex intracellular cascade is initiated by the formation of the death-inducing signaling complex (DISC). The formation and activation of DISC will lead to the activation of caspase-8, which in turn will trigger the execution phase of apoptosis where caspase-3 is activated; cellular demise is ensured by a myriad of simultaneous protein and chromatin cleavage.[5]

Intrinsic factors can induce apoptosis for example upon DNA damage or production of reactive oxygen species (ROS). However, a fundamental difference from the prior form is the involvement of mitochondrial mechanisms.[3] Given the complexity of the mitochondrial pathway, I will defer the reader to updated reviews.[3] Nevertheless, it is important to consider that the mitochondrial pathway shares the activation of the "execution" phase with caspase-3 activation.[3]

Morphology

As early as the nineteenth century, a dying cell was recognized by its dramatic morphological changes. Irrespective of the apoptotic trigger, the dying cell generally undergoes modifications of the membrane that, while preserving its integrity, exposes phospholipids, a fundamental "eat-me" signal for professional phagocytic cells[6]; there is significant shrinkage due to loss of intracellular fluids, cytoplasmic cytoskeleton, and organelles modifications and the characteristic plasma membrane blebbing. Finally, the execution phase leads to nuclear and chromatin fragmentation (karyorrhexis and formation of nucleosomes), apoptotic bodies, and microparticles, which are micronuclei surrounded by plasma membranes.[7]

Apoptosis and SLE

Defective Apoptosis

It is well established that defective molecular pathways that interfere with the homeostasis of the immune system often lead to lupus-like features. For example, the MRL/++ is a mouse strain that acquires a phenotype similar to human lupus with arthritis, glomerulonephritis, ANA, and anti-Sm autoantibodies when a loss-of-function mutation in the pro-apoptotic Fas receptor is present (MRL/*lpr*).[8] The mutation allows the survival of autoreactive T, B, and dendritic cells and the development of lupus.[9] Interestingly, genetic mutations of the intrinsic cell death pathway also lead to lupus-like manifestations, as in the case of overexpression of the pro-survival *bcl-2* or deletion of the pro-apoptotic *Bim* genes.[10]

These results clearly demonstrate how apoptosis profoundly influences the fate of autoimmunity. Nevertheless, these dramatic results in mouse models have not been replicated in human lupus disease and no profound genetic abnormalities in the apoptotic pathways have been found to date. This may be because the defects in human disease are multifactorial and implicate steps not directly involved in the apoptotic machinery per se but that nevertheless control cell death. Indeed, lupus patients have defective autoimmune B cell checkpoints, possibly due to resistance to apoptosis,[11] and have increased expression of pro-survival factor B lymphocyte stimulator (BLyS).[12] The latter discovery has lead to the first approval of a lupus-specific treatment in more than 40 years, a monoclonal antibody that specifically blocks the function of BLyS.

Excessive Apoptosis and Defective Clearance

Periods of flares and remissions characterize lupus disease, and it is quite intriguing that classic stimuli that trigger flares also induce apoptosis, such as infections and ultraviolet irradiation.[13] Initial work in mice demonstrated that repeated injections of apoptotic cells induced by ultraviolet B light or injection of antigen-presenting cells that had up-taken dead cells induced lupus-like autoimmunity in normal mice or accelerated lupus disease in genetically prone mice.[14,15] Together, these observations demonstrate that apoptotic cells are carriers of lupus autoantigens and if not properly disposed they might lead to systemic autoimmunity. Indeed the clearance of apoptotic cells by professional phagocytes is crucial to the maintenance of tolerance.[6]

Despite the numerous receptors that participate in the uptake of dead cells,[6] even the genetic disruption of a single one, such as the tyrosine kinase MER, leads to excessive circulating apoptotic cells and lupus-like autoimmunity.[16] The numerous mouse studies have been confirmed in lupus patients, in which lymph nodes have striking higher number of apoptotic cells that have not been phagocytosed compared to healthy individuals,[17] suggesting a possible impairment of the clearance mechanisms and a greater availability of autoantigens in already genetically predisposed individuals.[16]

Apoptotic Cells as Autoantigens

How does excessive apoptosis induced by external triggers or defective uptake provoke systemic autoimmunity? Seminal work in the 1980s and early 1990s demonstrated that apoptotic lymphocytes and keratinocytes redistribute lupus autoantigens such as nucleosomes, RNP, SS-A/Ro, and SS-B/La in apoptotic subcellular structures called blebs and microparticles, which then become accessible to the immune system.[18] This initial work provided the basis to demonstrate subsequently that morphological and post-translational molecular changes during apoptosis generate classic lupus autoantigens and render them available to a genetically predisposed autoimmune system.[19] Indeed, genetic or pharmacological modification of such pathways, such as the execution phase, impairs or accelerates lupus.[20]

The extraordinary changes of nuclear autoantigens during cell death due to caspase cleavage and posttranslational modifications generate the apotopes, which are self-epitopes exposed by or released from dying cells.[21] Apotopes such as nucleosomes can activate the innate immune system once recognized by autoantibodies,[22] while apotopes such as SS-A/Ro can trigger flares of subacute cutaneous lupus or damage the myocardial conductive system in neonatal lupus.[21]

Apoptotic cells, blebs, and microparticles can form immune complexes with lupus autoantibodies.[23] Once their content is uptaken by dendritic cells, it can be then presented to autoreactive T lymphocytes.[22] Interestingly, nuclear autoantigens released during excessive cell death form autoimmune complexes capable of activating the innate immune system via activation of intracellular toll-like receptors (TLRs) 7, 8, and 9, which normally recognize viral DNA and RNA.[24] This remarkable ability of autoimmune complexes is due to the engagement of pro-inflammatory Fc receptors and internalization in lysosomal compartments along with intracellular TLRs.[24] The undesirable consequences are the constant activation of type I interferon, which plays a fundamental role in the pathogenesis of lupus,[25] as well as the stimulation of dendritic cells to present autoantigens[2] and autoreactive B cells to mature into plasmablasts.[25]

NETosis: A Special Case of Cell Death

Neutrophil extracellular traps (NETs) are the manifestation of a unique type of cell death in neutrophils called NETosis;

infections and cytokines stimulate their production.[26] Their primary role is to trap bacteria and kill them by protruding filaments of fragmented chromatin coupled with antimicrobial peptides such as LL37.[26] NETosis is caspase-independent; it releases intracellular content and is regulated by nicotinamide adenine dinucleotide phosphate (NAPDH) oxidase and peptidylarginine deiminase (PAD)-4.[26] Hence, this form of cell death is often considered a regulated form of necrosis.[26]

NETosis and SLE

In the last few years, NETosis has attracted major attention as an important provider of lupus autoantigens DNA and histones.[27] Moreover, NETs also carry danger signals, such as high molecular group box (HMGB)-1 and proinflammatory cytokines such as IL-17.[28] The antimicrobial peptide LL37 contained in the NETs binds to anti-dsDNA/DNA complexes and specifically activates plasmocytoid dendritic cells to produce type I interferon, a major player in the pathogenesis of SLE.[29] Finally, lupus patients appear to have increased NETs, possibly due to delayed degradation, and the increase correlates with disease severity and activity.[30] Intriguingly, mouse models of lupus have yielded contrasting results; genetic deletion of *Nox2*, which abrogates NETosis, worsens lupus disease in the MRL/*lpr* model,[31] while PAD-4 inhibitors ameliorate disease in the New Zealand mixed (NZM) 2328 model.[32] Perhaps these results indicate that the role of NETs might be more complex than anticipated as the experiments in humans have been performed so far only and obviously in vitro.

AUTOPHAGY

Autophagy (from the Greek words *autos* meaning "self" and *phagomai* meaning "to eat") is a complex cellular function discovered more than four decades ago and initially considered just a sophisticated "rubbish-disposal" cytoplasmic mechanism.[33] Since then, autophagy instead has revealed itself to be not just a mechanism to degrade senescent, defective subcellular organelles, misfolded proteins, or infectious agents but also as a fundamental player in regulating both innate and adaptive immunity.[33] It is clear now that autophagy permeates human pathophysiology. It is implicated in multiple diseases from cancer to neurodegeneration, to the pathogenesis of lupus disease.[33]

Survival Pathway

Autophagy is primarily considered a survival mechanism. Indeed, its pathway(s) are activated during periods of cellular starvation so that intracellular nutrients can be used to maintain energy homeostasis.[33] Nevertheless, several other circumstances, such as oxidative stress, endoplasmic reticulum stress, and immune activation trigger its pathways.[33]

Autophagy is regulated by the autophagy-related genes (*Atg*)s family, which initiates the characteristic formation of the autophagosome.[34] The molecular cascade that completes the formation of the autophagosome and its fusion with lysomes and the final degradation of its content is evolutionary preserved; its key regulators are a number of ATG factors such as Beclin 1 (in the yeast ATG-6 protein), autophagy-related LC3 proteins, γ-aminobutyric acid receptor-associated proteins (in the yeast ATG-8 protein), and the serine/threonine protein kinase ULK1 (in the yeast ATG-1 protein), among others.[35]

Generally, the autophagosome is formed by a double-membrane structure due to the source of the membrane itself (i.e., a preformed intracellular membrane).[33] An exception to this rule is the membrane formed when the cell uptakes phagocytosed dead cells.[36] This form of autophagy is called LC3-associated phagocytosis (LAP) and is a mechanism to enhance the digestive capability during phagocytosis.[36] Interestingly, LAP is also triggered by particles coated with TLR agonists[37] and the Fcγ receptor-dependent uptake of immune complexes.[37]

Autophagy and SLE

Genome-wide association studies in multiple lupus cohorts have linked several single nucleotide polymorphisms (SNPs) of the *Atg5* gene to lupus susceptibility.[38] One SNP in particular has been further characterized in SLE patients, found to influence IL-10 production, and is associated with specific disease features.[39] It is well known that lupus DNA-immune complexes can stimulate the innate immunity TLR-9 to produce interferon type I, especially in dendritic cells and B cells.[24] Also, the noncanonical autophagic LAP has been shown to be necessary for the trafficking of DNA-immune complexes and TLR-9 into interferon signaling compartments and stimulate its production.[37] These results provide an explanation as to why self-DNA, once complexed with autoantibodies, is capable of activating innate immunity and perpetuate inflammation and autoimmunity itself.

Autophagy is required for the normal development of B and T cells, and data suggest that autoreactive B-cell survival depends upon increased activation of autophagy. Indeed, B cells from the NZB/W lupus mouse model, and T and B cells from lupus patients have enhanced autophagy compared to controls.[40] Moreover, the enhanced autophagy in lupus patients' peripheral T and B cells correlates with disease activity.[40] Genetic modification of the *Atg7* gene in mice confirmed these findings.[40] Interestingly, hydroxychloroquine—arguably the most prescribed medication in SLE—inhibits autophagy, especially the LAP form.[41]

NECROSIS

The pathological demise of a cell is generally called necrosis. Although this form of cell death has been known for the past two centuries, only in the last decade it has become clear it is not simply a traumatic death but occurs under very tightly controlled circumstances, regulated by molecular pathways.[26] Hence, it is now recognized as a form of caspase-independent RCD.[3] Morphologically, a necrotic cell significantly differs from apoptosis, as it quickly swells and loses cell membrane integrity, releasing pro-inflammatory danger signals[42]; chromatin undergoes condensation and then lyses due to the absence of organized fragmentation of the chromatin by caspase-activated DNase.[42] Two major pathways have been identified: *necroptosis* and *parthanatos*.

Necroptosis in SLE

Necroptosis is the prototype of necrotic cell death. It activates upon triggering of the TNF or Fas receptor and in the absence or limited activation of caspase-8.[43] The two major kinases involved are receptor interacting protein (RIP)-1 and RIP-3, which lead to oxidative stress and energy collapse.[43] Necroptosis plays an important role in sterile inflammation, such as inflammatory bowel disease and in myocardial ischemia.[4] Although it has not been thoroughly investigated in SLE, several observations make this pathway worth exploring.

Interestingly, B cells from active lupus patients express necroptosis-related genes and their rapid in vitro cell death is necroptotic.[44] T cells from SLE patients undergo necrosis, possibly due to aberrant production of ROS and mitochondrial dysfunction.[45] Some bacterial and viral infections induce macrophage necrosis as a mechanism to evade detection, and it has been previously shown that macrophage cell death accelerate autoimmunity in genetically prone mice.[46] Infections are known triggers of lupus flare; hence, the source of lupus autoantigens might not just come from apoptotic cells but also from pro-inflammatory conditions such as infection-induced necroptosis, which would promptly release nuclear autoantigens and danger signals. Moreover, necroptosis induced by bacterial infections depends on the production of type I interferon,[47] which is already increased in SLE and could further amplify the autoimmune response.[25] Finally, the TNF pathway is clearly involved in lupus nephritis and necrosis is a common histological finding; therefore, inhibition of necroptosis could be investigated as possible therapeutic target.

Parthanatos and SLE

The name of this form of necrotic cell death is derived from *Par* [poly(ADP-ribosyl)ation] and the Greek word *thanatos* ("death"). The enzyme poly(ADP)ribosyl polymerase (PARP)-1 is a DNA sentinel, which activates in response to DNA damage.[48] Its activation, once necrosis has been triggered, leads to dramatic adenosine triphosphate consumption and finally to energy collapse.[49] PARP-1 inhibition or genetic deletion protects from ischemia–reperfusion injury, septic shock, and collagen-induced arthritis.[48] These findings suggest that PARP-1 is important in tissue damage. Indeed, inhibition or absence of PARP-1 protects both spontaneous and inducible mouse models of lupus nephritis, possibly via a dual role of inhibiting necrotic cell death but also by reducing TNF alpha and VCAM-1 production.[50] Interestingly, PARP-1 appears to be beneficial only in males, possibly due to inhibition of its activity by estrogens in female.[50] Nevertheless, several inhibitors have been successfully tested in human trials, and its use could become an option during lupus nephritis in males.

Secondary Necrosis in SLE

Apoptotic cells immediately signal their imminent demise by exposing phospholipids on their membranes.[6] They are therefore rapidly cleared, as the machinery of professional phagocytic cells is very effective and redundant.[16] Nevertheless, in SLE there is a delay in their uptake and apoptosis progresses into secondary necrosis.[17] These cells behave as necrotic cells and are capable not only of releasing lupus nuclear autoantigens but also danger signals, such as HMGB-1 and interleukin 1, which will further amplify the autoimmune response.[2]

CONCLUDING REMARKS

The mechanisms by which a cell ends its existence are diverse. It has become clear that each form of cell death has a profound pathogenic relevance in systemic lupus erythematous. Apoptotic cell death provides autoantigens to fuel the aberrant immune response, and its impairment allows autoreactivity to thrive. Autophagy has implications for autoantigen presentation and survival of autoreactive B cells. Finally, necrotic cell death provides the inflammatory milieu to sustain autoimmunity. Our understanding of lupus pathogenesis has dramatically increased and has culminated in the first approval of a specific treatment after a hiatus of more than 50 years. Sophisticated manipulation of the various forms of cell death will lead to a further understanding of lupus and to innovative treatments for this still life-threatening disease.

REFERENCES

1. Diamantis A, Magiorkinis E, Sakorafas GH, Androutsos G. A brief history of apoptosis: from ancient to modern times. *Onkologie* 2008;**31**(12):702–6.
2. Gallo PM, Gallucci S. The dendritic cell response to classic, emerging, and homeostatic danger signals. Implications for autoimmunity. *Front Immunol* 2013;**4**:138.
3. Galluzzi L, Bravo-San Pedro JM, Vitale I, Aaronson SA, Abrams JM, Adam D, et al. Essential versus accessory aspects of cell death: recommendations of the NCCD 2015. *Cell Death Differ* 2015;**22**(1):58–73.

4. Linkermann A, Green DR. Necroptosis. *N Engl J Med* 2014;**370**(5): 455–65.
5. Ashkenazi A, Salvesen G. Regulated cell death: signaling and mechanisms. *Annu Rev Cell Dev Biol* 2014;**30**:337–56.
6. Poon IK, Lucas CD, Rossi AG, Ravichandran KS. Apoptotic cell clearance: basic biology and therapeutic potential. *Nat Rev Immunol* 2014;**14**(3):166–80.
7. Nagata S. DNA degradation in development and programmed cell death. *Annu Rev Immunol* 2005;**23**:853–75.
8. Kono DH, Theofilopoulos AN. Genetics of systemic autoimmunity in mouse models of lupus. *Int Rev Immunol* 2000;**19**(4–5):367–87.
9. Stranges PB, Watson J, Cooper CJ, Choisy-Rossi CM, Stonebraker AC, Beighton RA, et al. Elimination of antigen-presenting cells and autoreactive T cells by Fas contributes to prevention of autoimmunity. *Immunity* 2007;**26**(5):629–41.
10. Tischner D, Woess C, Ottina E, Villunger A. Bcl-2-regulated cell death signalling in the prevention of autoimmunity. *Cell Death Dis* 2011;**1**:e48.
11. Yurasov S, Wardemann H, Hammersen J, Tsuiji M, Meffre E, Pascual V, et al. Defective B cell tolerance checkpoints in systemic lupus erythematosus. *J Exp Med* 2005;**201**(5):703–11.
12. Stohl W. Systemic lupus erythematosus and its ABCs (APRIL/BLyS complexes). *Arthritis Res Ther* 2010;**12**(2):111.
13. Caricchio R, Reap EA, Cohen PL. Fas/Fas ligand interactions are involved in ultraviolet-B-induced human lymphocyte apoptosis. *J Immunol* 1998;**161**(1):241–51.
14. Mevorach D, Zhou JL, Song X, Elkon KB. Systemic exposure to irradiated apoptotic cells induces autoantibody production. *J Exp Med* 1998;**188**(2):387–92.
15. Bondanza A, Zimmermann VS, Dell'Antonio G, Dal Cin E, Capobianco A, Sabbadini MG, et al. Cutting edge: dissociation between autoimmune response and clinical disease after vaccination with dendritic cells. *J Immunol* 2003;**170**(1):24–7.
16. Shao WH, Cohen PL. Disturbances of apoptotic cell clearance in systemic lupus erythematosus. *Arthritis Res Ther* 2011;**13**(1):202.
17. Baumann I, Kolowos W, Voll RE, Manger B, Gaipl U, Neuhuber WL, et al. Impaired uptake of apoptotic cells into tingible body macrophages in germinal centers of patients with systemic lupus erythematosus. *Arthritis Rheum* 2002;**46**(1):191–201.
18. Casciola-Rosen LA, Anhalt G, Rosen A. Autoantigens targeted in systemic lupus erythematosus are clustered in two populations of surface structures on apoptotic keratinocytes. *J Exp Med* 1994;**179**(4):1317–30.
19. Utz PJ, Hottelet M, Schur PH, Anderson P. Proteins phosphorylated during stress-induced apoptosis are common targets for autoantibody production in patients with systemic lupus erythematosus. *J Exp Med* 1997;**185**(5):843–54.
20. Jog NR, Frisoni L, Shi Q, Monestier M, Hernandez S, Craft J, et al. Caspase-activated DNase is required for maintenance of tolerance to lupus nuclear autoantigens. *Arthritis Rheum* 2012;**64**(4):1247–56.
21. Reed JH, Jackson MW, Gordon TP. B cell apotopes of the 60-kDa Ro/SSA and La/SSB autoantigens. *J Autoimmun* 2008;**31**(3):263–7.
22. Frisoni L, McPhie L, Colonna L, Sriram U, Monestier M, Gallucci S, et al. Nuclear autoantigen translocation and autoantibody opsonization lead to increased dendritic cell phagocytosis and presentation of nuclear antigens: a novel pathogenic pathway for autoimmunity? *J Immunol* 2005;**175**(4):2692–701.
23. Dye JR, Ullal AJ, Pisetsky DS. The role of microparticles in the pathogenesis of rheumatoid arthritis and systemic lupus erythematosus. *Scand J Immunol* 2013;**78**(2):140–8.
24. Kono DH, Baccala R, Theofilopoulos AN. TLRs and interferons: a central paradigm in autoimmunity. *Curr Opin Immunol* 2013;**25**(6):720–7.
25. Crow MK. Advances in understanding the role of type I interferons in systemic lupus erythematosus. *Curr Opin Rheumatol* 2014;**26**(5): 467–74.
26. Vanden Berghe T, Linkermann A, Jouan-Lanhouet S, Walczak H, Vandenabeele P. Regulated necrosis: the expanding network of non-apoptotic cell death pathways. *Nat Rev Mol Cell Biol* 2014;**15**(2): 135–47.
27. Knight JS, Kaplan MJ. Lupus neutrophils: 'NET' gain in understanding lupus pathogenesis. *Curr Opin Rheumatol* 2012;**24**(5):441–50.
28. Radic M. Clearance of apoptotic bodies, NETs, and biofilm DNA: implications for autoimmunity. *Front Immunol* 2014;**5**:365.
29. Garcia-Romo GS, Caielli S, Vega B, Connolly J, Allantaz F, Xu Z, et al. Netting neutrophils are major inducers of type I IFN production in pediatric systemic lupus erythematosus. *Sci Transl Med* 2011;**3**(73):73ra20.
30. Leffler J, Stojanovich L, Shoenfeld Y, Bogdanovic G, Hesselstrand R, Blom AM. Degradation of neutrophil extracellular traps is decreased in patients with antiphospholipid syndrome. *Clin Exp Rheumatol* 2014;**32**(1):66–70.
31. Campbell AM, Kashgarian M, Shlomchik MJ. NADPH oxidase inhibits the pathogenesis of systemic lupus erythematosus. *Sci Transl Med* 2012;**4**(157):157ra141.
32. Knight JS, Zhao W, Luo W, Subramanian V, O'Dell AA, Yalavarthi S, et al. Peptidylarginine deiminase inhibition is immunomodulatory and vasculoprotective in murine lupus. *J Clin Invest* 2013;**123**(7):2981–93.
33. Deretic V, Kimura T, Timmins G, Moseley P, Chauhan S, Mandell M. Immunologic manifestations of autophagy. *J Clin Invest* 2015; **125**(1):75–84.
34. Noda NN, Inagaki F. Mechanisms of autophagy. *Annu Rev Biophys* 2015;**44**:101–22.
35. Kuballa P, Nolte WM, Castoreno AB, Xavier RJ. Autophagy and the immune system. *Annu Rev Immunol* 2012;**30**:611–46.
36. Martinez J, Almendinger J, Oberst A, Ness R, Dillon CP, Fitzgerald P, et al. Microtubule-associated protein 1 light chain 3 alpha (LC3)-associated phagocytosis is required for the efficient clearance of dead cells. *Proc Natl Acad Sci USA* 2011;**108**(42):17396–401.
37. Henault J, Martinez J, Riggs JM, Tian J, Mehta P, Clarke L, et al. Noncanonical autophagy is required for type I interferon secretion in response to DNA-immune complexes. *Immunity* 2012;**37**(6): 986–97.
38. Zhou XJ, Lu XL, Lv JC, Yang HZ, Qin LX, Zhao MH, et al. Genetic association of PRDM1-ATG5 intergenic region and autophagy with systemic lupus erythematosus in a Chinese population. *Ann Rheum Dis* 2011;**70**(7):1330–7.
39. Lopez P, Alonso-Perez E, Rodriguez-Carrio J, Suarez A. Influence of Atg5 mutation in SLE depends on functional IL-10 genotype. *PLoS One* 2013;**8**(10):e78756.
40. Clarke AJ, Ellinghaus U, Cortini A, Stranks A, Simon AK, Botto M, et al. Autophagy is activated in systemic lupus erythematosus and required for plasmablast development. *Ann Rheum Dis* 2015;**74**(5): 912–20.
41. Boya P, Gonzalez-Polo RA, Casares N, Perfettini JL, Dessen P, Larochette N, et al. Inhibition of macroautophagy triggers apoptosis. *Mol Cell Biol* 2005;**25**(3):1025–40.
42. Kroemer G, Galluzzi L, Vandenabeele P, Abrams J, Alnemri ES, Baehrecke EH, et al. Classification of cell death: recommendations of the Nomenclature Committee on Cell Death 2009. *Cell Death Differ* 2009;**16**(1):3–11.
43. Pasparakis M, Vandenabeele P. Necroptosis and its role in inflammation. *Nature* 2015;**517**(7534):311–20.

44. Fan H, Liu F, Dong G, Ren D, Xu Y, Dou J, et al. Activation-induced necroptosis contributes to B-cell lymphopenia in active systemic lupus erythematosus. *Cell Death Dis* 2014;**5**:e1416.

45. Lai ZW, Borsuk R, Shadakshari A, Yu J, Dawood M, Garcia R, et al. Mechanistic target of rapamycin activation triggers IL-4 production and necrotic death of double-negative T cells in patients with systemic lupus erythematosus. *J Immunol* 2013;**191**(5):2236–46.

46. Denny MF, Chandaroy P, Killen PD, Caricchio R, Lewis EE, Richardson BC, et al. Accelerated macrophage apoptosis induces autoantibody formation and organ damage in systemic lupus erythematosus. *J Immunol* 2006;**176**(4):2095–104.

47. Khan N, Lawlor KE, Murphy JM, Vince JE. More to life than death: molecular determinants of necroptotic and non-necroptotic RIP3 kinase signaling. *Curr Opin Immunol* 2014;**26**:76–89.

48. Schreiber V, Dantzer F, Ame JC, de Murcia G. Poly(ADP-ribose): novel functions for an old molecule. *Nat Rev Mol Cell Biol* 2006;**7**(7):517–28.

49. Bouchard VJ, Rouleau M, Poirier GG. PARP-1, a determinant of cell survival in response to DNA damage. *Exp Hematol* 2003;**31**(6):446–54.

50. Jog NR, Dinnall JA, Gallucci S, Madaio MP, Caricchio R. Poly(ADP-ribose) polymerase-1 regulates the progression of autoimmune nephritis in males by inducing necrotic cell death and modulating inflammation. *J Immunol* 2009;**182**(11):7297–306.

Chapter 22

Infections in Early Systemic Lupus Erythematosus Pathogenesis

Rebecka Bourn[1], Samantha Slight-Webb[1], Judith James[1,2]

[1]*Arthritis and Clinical Immunology, Oklahoma Medical Research Foundation, Oklahoma City, OK, USA;* [2]*Departments of Medicine and Pathology, Oklahoma Clinical and Translational Science Institute, University of Oklahoma Health Sciences Center, Oklahoma City, OK, USA*

INTRODUCTION

Patients with systemic lupus erythematosus (SLE) may experience malar rash, arthritis, renal damage, and a wide range of other clinical manifestations with the potential to affect any organ system. These pathologies are driven by chronic inflammation and the presence of autoantibodies, which arise through complex interactions between genetic predisposition, hormonal influences, and environmental exposures. For example, infections commonly lead to transient, low-level production of autoantibodies by stimulating the activation of cytokine pathways, differentiation and activation of immune cells, and exposure to autoantigens. In most individuals, these changes do not lead to autoimmune disease because immunoregulatory mechanisms restore tolerance to self-antigens and suppress inflammation after the infection is cleared. However, in individuals who are genetically susceptible to SLE, exposure to certain pathogens can shift the immune system toward a dysregulated state that permits the onset and progression of autoimmune disease.

PATHOGENS ASSOCIATED WITH LUPUS AUTOIMMUNITY AND CLINICAL DISEASE

Pathogens have been found to promote lupus autoimmunity and clinical SLE through mechanisms such as molecular mimicry, functional mimicry, superantigen activity, and disruption of immunoregulatory mechanisms (Figure 1).[1,2] Furthermore, an analysis identified 25 case reports of patients who initially fulfilled the American College of Rheumatology SLE classification criteria after acute viral infection (including 3 after Epstein–Barr virus (EBV) infection, 15 after parvovirus B19 infection, and 6 after cytomegalovirus (CMV) infection).[3] Human T-cell lymphotropic virus-1 (HTLV)-related endogenous sequence-1 (HRES-1), a retrovirus that is integrated into the human genome, has been linked to select clinical manifestations of SLE, including renal disease and antiphospholipid syndrome.[1] The

HRES-1/Rab4 protein can regulate the recycling of CD4 on CD4[+] T cells, which may lead to abnormal T-cell activation.[4] In addition, the HRES-1/p28 protein can elicit cross-reactive antibodies that recognize the snRNP complex, a common target of lupus autoimmunity.[1] Thus, HRES-1 can trigger autoimmunity that may lead to clinical lupus.[5]

The production of SLE-associated autoantibodies can also be stimulated by CMV and parvovirus B19.[1,6,7] Both viruses have been purported to stimulate the onset of SLE because active infections can lead to disease flares in SLE patients and may trigger SLE-like clinical manifestations in previously healthy individuals.[3,8,9] However, the mechanisms of these potential associations are unknown. Finally, pathogenic bacteria and endogenous microbial flora may stimulate autoimmunity leading to SLE. Peptides from *Vibrio cholerae* and *Streptococcus agalactiae* act as molecular mimics that elicit antibodies reactive to the lupus-associated autoantigen Sm D1.[10] In addition, bacterial superantigens can activate large numbers of T cells, including autoreactive T cells, by avidly binding to class II major histocompatibility complex molecules outside of the conventional antigen-binding clefts. Besides stimulating autoantibody production, the *Staphylococcus aureus* superantigen and cholera toxin B induce systemic, SLE-like disease in mice.[11,12] Therefore, infectious agents likely play an important role in SLE pathogenesis.

EPSTEIN–BARR VIRUS AS A MODEL INFECTION IN THE ETIOLOGY OF SLE

Epstein–Barr virus (EBV; human herpesvirus 4) is an attractive candidate in the etiology of SLE because it is nearly ubiquitous and infects B cells, which can lead to immortalization.[13] Nearly all individuals worldwide are EBV-infected by early adulthood. After an active EBV infection, EBV remains latent in memory B cells, presenting a lifelong antigenic challenge in most individuals. In addition, EBV has the potential for episodic reactivation. An association

Systemic Lupus Erythematosus. http://dx.doi.org/10.1016/B978-0-12-801917-7.00022-X

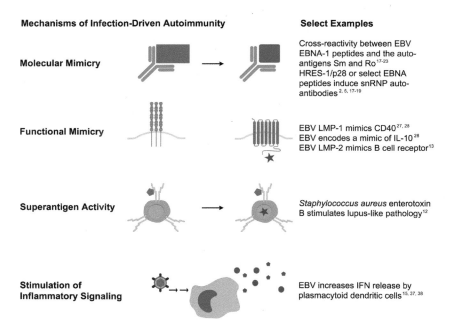

Mechanisms of Infection-Driven Autoimmunity   **Select Examples**

Molecular Mimicry   Cross-reactivity between EBV EBNA-1 peptides and the auto-antigens Sm and Ro[17-23] HRES-1/p28 or select EBNA peptides induce snRNP auto-antibodies[2, 5, 17-19]

Functional Mimicry   EBV LMP-1 mimics CD40[27, 28] EBV encodes a mimic of IL-10[26] EBV LMP-2 mimics B cell receptor[13]

Superantigen Activity   *Staphylococcus aureus* enterotoxin B stimulates lupus-like pathology[12]

Stimulation of Inflammatory Signaling   EBV increases IFN release by plasmacytoid dendritic cells[15, 37, 38]

FIGURE 1   Infections can stimulate autoimmune disease through several mechanisms. Select examples are provided for each mechanism illustrated in the figure. One example of functional mimicry is LMP-2, an EBV-encoded receptor that mimics the B-cell receptor (BCR). *(Mancao C, Hammerschmidt J. Epstein–Barr virus latent membrane protein 2A is a B-cell receptor mimic and essential for B-cell survival. Blood 2007;110:3715–21.)* Just as interactions between the BCR and Toll-like receptors (TLR) synergistically activate B cells, LMP2A also enhances TLR responses. *(Anderson LJ, Longnecker R. EBV LMP2A provides a surrogate pre-B cell receptor signal through constitutive activation of the ERK/MAPK pathway. J Gen Virol 2008;89:1563–8.)* In addition, in transgenic mice expressing LMP2A and anti-Sm, LMP2A induces hypersensitivity to TLR stimulation and activates anti-Sm B cells through the BCR/TLR pathway, thereby overcoming the regulatory checkpoint at the early pre-plasma cell stage. As a result, these mice spontaneously produce anti-Sm antibodies. *(Wang H, Nicholas MW, Conway KL, Sen P, Diz R, Tisch RM, et al. EBV latent membrane protein 2A induces autoreactive B cell activation and TLR hypersensitivity. J Immunol 2006;177:2793–802.)* Please see text and references for additional information.

between EBV seroconversion and SLE was first shown in 1969. This association was confirmed by several studies in adults and by a study showing serologic evidence of EBV infection in 99% of pediatric SLE patients, compared to only 70% of age-matched controls.[4,13,14] These serologic associations led to the hypothesis that frequent EBV reactivation might cause chronic immune stimulation, hence promoting autoimmune disease, but it was debated whether these associations were directly related to SLE etiology.[15,16] The observations that some EBV antibodies cross-react with self antigens and that cross-reactive EBV antibodies precede lupus autoimmunity support an etiological role for EBV infection in the development of SLE.[1,4,15] In addition, EBV has now been linked to SLE and other autoimmune diseases through several mechanisms, including molecular mimicry, functional mimicry, and dysregulated immune responses.[2,13]

Molecular Mimicry and Epitope Spreading

EBV infections can stimulate autoantibody production through molecular mimicry between Epstein–Barr nuclear antigen 1 (EBNA-1) and common lupus autoantigens, such as dsDNA, Ro, and Sm (Table 1).[4,14,17,18] One line of evidence for molecular mimicry is cross-reactivity between EBNA-1 sequences and early epitopes targeted by lupus autoantibodies. Antibodies targeting epitopes in Sm B′ (PPP-GMRPP) and Sm D1 ((GR)$_x$) cross-react with sequences from EBNA-1 (PPPGRRP and [GR]$_x$, respectively), and antibodies to the EBNA-1 PPPGRRP sequence can also bind Sm B′.[19–22] Finally, antibodies recognizing the carboxyl region of EBNA-1 cross-react with dsDNA, and antibodies recognizing both the carboxyl and amino regions of EBNA-1 cross-react with Sm.[15] A second line of evidence for molecular mimicry comes from immunization studies. Mice immunized with EBNA-1 protein produce antibodies that recognize dsDNA and Sm, and immunization with cross-reactive EBNA-1 peptides (outlined above) or EBNA-1 fragments leads to autoimmunity and lupus-like disease in animal models.[4,15,21,22] Another approach to EBNA-1 immunization, inoculation with EBNA-1 cDNA, results in the production of full-length EBNA-1 protein by host cells, as occurs during EBV infection. Inoculation with EBNA-1 cDNA elicits antibodies against EBNA-1, Sm, and dsDNA in BALB/c mice but not in DBA/2 mice, highlighting the importance of genetic susceptibility in the development of cross-reactive autoantibodies.[23]

Interestingly, the cross-reactive regions of EBNA-1 do not necessarily share primary sequence homology with their autoantigen counterparts. For example, by phage display library analysis, antibodies targeting the PPPGMRPP epitope

TABLE 1 Examples of Molecular Mimicry between Pathogen-Derived Antigens and Autoantigens Targeted by Lupus-Associated Antibodies

Pathogen-Derived Antigen	Autoantigen	Evidence of Molecular Mimicry
CMV		
gB	nRNP70	Anti-nRNP70 in mice inoculated with gB cDNA[7]
pp65	dsDNA	Anti-dsDNA and anti-nuclear antibodies in mice immunized with pp65.[6]
EBV		
EBNA-1	dsDNA	Antibodies against dsDNA and Sm in mice immunized with EBNA-1 peptide or EBNA-1 cDNA.[4,15,21–23] binding of dsDNA and Sm by antibodies against EBNA-1.[15] cross-reactivity of antibodies recognizing Sm B′ with the EBNA-1 PPPGRRP epitope, and of antibodies recognizing Sm D1 with the EBNA-1 (GR)$_x$ epitope.[19–22] Recognition of the EBNA-1 GGSGSGPRHRDGVRR peptide by anti-Ro.[24] antibodies against Ro169-180 and other lupus-associated epitopes in mice immunized with EBNA-1 GGSGSGPRHRDGVRR.[18,25]
	Ro	
	Sm B/B′	
	Sm D1	
Major DNA binding protein	Sm B′	Binding of the SPPEWLK peptide of EBV major DNA binding protein by anti-Sm B′ in phage display.[19]
HRES-1		
HRES-1/p28	nRNP70	Increased prevalence of serum reactivity to HRES-1/p28 in SLE patients. Peptide similarity between HRES-1 peptides and snRNP.[1,4]
S. agalactiae		
TcmP methyltransferase peptide	Sm D1	Anti-Sm D in mice immunized with peptide.[10]
V. cholerae		
Galactoside ABC transporter peptide	Sm D1	Anti-Sm D in mice immunized with peptide.[10]

in Sm B′ can also bind the SPPEWLK peptide that is found in the EBV major DNA binding protein.[19] In addition, antibodies recognizing 60kD Ro are among the earliest autoantibodies observed in SLE pathogenesis.[24] The early anti-Ro antibodies that target Ro169-180 (TKYKQRNGWSHKD) specifically recognize EBNA-1 via the EBNA-1 sequence GGSGSGPRHRDGVRR, which bears little sequence homology to Ro169-180.[24] Rabbits immunized with Ro169-180 or the EBNA-1 sequence produce antibodies against these cross-reactive epitopes as well as other lupus-associated epitopes, suggesting that epitope spreading can enhance infection-driven early autoimmunity.[18,25] In addition to producing autoantibodies, rabbits immunized with the Ro169-180 or the EBNA-1 sequence also develop lupus-like clinical features, including leukopenia, thrombocytopenia, and renal dysfunction.[25] Therefore, exposure to EBNA-1 can initiate a cross-reactive antibody response that targets autoantigens and increases the risk of developing clinical SLE.

Functional Mimicry

Functional mimicry occurs when a pathogen-derived molecule mimics the effects of a host protein.[15] For example, EBV produces viral proteins that prevent apoptosis (including a Bcl-2 homolog) and exhibit interleukin-10–like activity.[26] An EBV protein expressed during infection and reactivation, latent membrane protein-1 (LMP-1), acts as an oncogenic mimic of the host transmembrane receptor CD40.[27] Both CD40 and LMP-1 stimulate signaling pathways that lead to the activation and proliferation of B cells and other antigen presenting cells. However, CD40-stimulated signaling is tightly regulated, whereas LMP-1 is largely impervious to regulation. LMP-1 constitutively self-activates and initiates TNFR-associated factor 3 (TRAF3)- and TRAF6-dependent signaling.[27] Thus, LMP-1 expression can lead to aberrant B cell activation, contributing to the development of autoimmunity. Further linking LMP-1 to autoimmune disease, LMP-1 is expressed in peripheral blood mononuclear cells from SLE patients with baseline disease activity and during times of disease flares, and LMP-1 is expressed at higher levels in SLE patients than in healthy individuals.[15,27] Moreover, expressing a chimeric molecule with the murine CD40 extracellular domain and the LMP-1 intracellular signaling domains leads to autoantibody production and immune dysregulation in normal mice.[28] Lupus-prone mice (B6.Sle1, but not B6.Sle3) expressing the CD40-LMP-1 chimeric receptor develop enlarged lymphoid organs; greater numbers of germinal centers, B cells, CD86+ B cells, and activated and memory T cells; elevated levels of antihistone antibodies; and enhanced kidney pathology.[15] Together, these observations suggest that LMP-1 expression in genetically pre-disposed individuals may enhance autoimmunity and SLE pathogenesis. Similar immune dysregulation has been associated with LMP-2. As a constitutively active B-cell receptor mimic, LMP-2 enhances B-cell survival, alters B-cell signaling and antigen presentation, and promotes autoantibody responses (see Figure 1).[13]

Dysregulation of Immune Responses

EBV interacts with inherent susceptibility to immune dysregulation in some individuals, resulting in altered immune responses to EBV that could influence the development or progression of autoimmune disease. Approximately 90% of healthy, EBV-infected adults make antibodies directed against EBNA-1, a response dominated by antibodies binding the central region of EBNA-1.[29,30] In contrast, the humoral response against EBNA-1 in lupus patients is dominated by antibodies binding the amino and carboxyl regions of EBNA-1.[30]

The cellular response to EBV is also altered in SLE patients. Compared to healthy individuals, SLE patients have decreased EBV-specific cytotoxic T-cell responses and an increased frequency of EBV-specific CD69$^+$ CD4$^+$ T cells producing interferon-γ (IFN-γ) after EBV stimulation.[15,31,32] EBV viral loads in SLE patients are positively correlated with EBV-specific CD69$^+$ CD8$^+$ T cells, suggesting that the CD69$^+$ CD8$^+$ response in SLE patients fails to control viral replication.[15] Indeed, EBV-specific CD8$^+$ T cells from SLE patients have a reduced ability to express IFN-γ after EBV stimulation, and EBV viral loads are remarkably higher in SLE patients than in healthy individuals.[15,31,33,34] Similarly, antibodies against early antigen-D (EA/D), an indicator of EBV reactivation, are more prevalent in SLE patients (54%) than in healthy controls (17%).[33,35] Thus, a fundamentally altered response to EBV appears to make SLE patients more susceptible to viral reactivation, leading to active EBV infection.[16]

In turn, EBV infection may enhance the clinical manifestations of lupus.[36] For example, increased interferon expression, interferon-inducible gene expression profiles, and proinflammatory cytokines are now considered central to SLE pathogenesis and ongoing pathology.[15] Studies demonstrated that EBV stimulates increased IFN-α expression and increased production of proinflammatory cytokines by plasmacytoid dendritic cells.[15,37,38] Additional studies are needed to compare the plasmacytoid dendritic cell responses to EBV in SLE patients and healthy individuals. Finally, latent EBV infection of B cells can cause transactivation of the human endogenous retrovirus (HERV)-K18 superantigen, leading to the stimulation of large numbers of cells and differentiation of EBV-infected B cells to memory cells.[1,4]

Therefore, EBV can act through multiple channels to stimulate lupus autoimmunity and clinical disease in genetically predisposed individuals.

THE MICROBIOME IN AUTOIMMUNE DISEASE

In addition to pathogenic microorganisms, emerging evidence suggests that commensal microbiota may also influence the development, persistence, and presentation of autoimmune diseases. In particular, early data suggest gut microbiota may help shape immune regulation and systemic health. Specific gut microbes have been associated with multiple sclerosis, rheumatoid arthritis, and type I diabetes,[39] and early evidence supports a role for the gut microbiome in SLE pathogenesis. For example, T-cell mimicry between 60-kD Ro and peptides derived from commensal bacteria suggests that microbiota may contribute to the initiation of lupus autoimmunity.[40] Furthermore, in humans and in murine models, lupus is associated with changes in the diversity and composition of the gut microbiome.[41,42] In the mouse model, some of these differences are sex-specific, raising the possibility that microbiota could contribute to the female bias in SLE. Conversely, these changes in the gut microbiota may be driven by the immunological factors that lead to autoimmune disease. Indeed, although there is evidence of extensive cross talk between the immune system and the microbiome, it is not clear how the gut microbiota influence systemic diseases. One possibility is that gut microbiota may modulate populations of T helper 17 or other immune cell types.[39] Additional work is needed to clarify the roles of the microbiome in autoimmunity.

PATHOGEN EXPOSURES THAT MAY PROTECT AGAINST LUPUS AUTOIMMUNITY

Although considerable evidence supports infections as an important trigger of SLE, it is also possible that certain viral, bacterial, or parasitic infections might protect against the development of SLE or alleviate disease activity. It has been suggested that pathogen exposures may reduce the onset of autoimmunity through activation of regulatory mechanisms that suppress the host immune response or through bystander suppression.[2] Several infections in animal models of lupus support this hypothesis. NZB and NZBWxF1 lupus-prone mice with chronic *Toxoplamsa gondii* infection live longer and have a reduced incidence of proteinuria and immune complex deposition in the kidney compared to uninfected controls.[4] The *hygiene hypothesis* suggests that early exposure to certain pathogens may prevent autoimmune disease development by altering the lifetime level of inflammation in an individual.[4,43] For example, infection with gamma herpes virus 68 (γHV68) prior to the onset of SLE significantly decreases autoantibody production and ameliorates kidney disease in lupus-prone B6.Sle123 and MRL/MpJ-Fas*lpr* mice.[44] These changes correlate with a persistent decrease in activation of both lymphocytes and dendritic cells caused by γHV68 infection.[44] These results suggest that the timing of pathogen exposure may be critical in determining whether an infection has protective or detrimental effects in the induction of SLE, with early pathogen exposures potentially reducing the risk of SLE.

After SLE classification, infections are a leading cause of mortality, and SLE patients are twice as likely to acquire an infection compared to healthy individuals.[45] However, in clinical trials, treatment with parasites has produced positive effects for autoimmune diseases such as inflammatory bowel disease, multiple sclerosis, and autoimmune liver disease, perhaps due to skewing of the immune response to a Th2 phenotype and/or an increase in T regulatory cells.[46] Furthermore, animal models of lupus infected with *Mycobacteria, Salmonella typhimurium, Plasmodium chabaudi,* or certain viruses have increased longevity and a reversal in clinical manifestations such as kidney disease and splenomegaly.[47–50] These results raise the possibility that the increased susceptibility to infection in SLE may be driven by immunomodulatory and immunosuppressive treatments in addition to inherent immune dysfunction. Consistent with this possibility, lupus-prone MRL/MpJ-Fas*lpr* mice infected with influenza A PR/8/34 virus mount an antigen-specific T-cell response that effectively clears the virus, but develop severe pulmonary inflammation after viral clearance.[51] In contrast, lupus-prone B6.*lpr* and BXSB mice develop defective IFN-γ T-cell responses during acute *T. gondii* infection, leading to increased mortality.[52] Thus, the effects of pathogens in autoimmunity may vary, and further investigation into common infections is needed to understand the interplay between infections, inherent immune dysfunction, and immunosuppressive treatments in lupus patients. An improved understanding of the role of infections in lupus will shed light on the immune mechanisms driving development of SLE and the potential clinical benefit of targeting these pathways.

CONCLUSIONS

SLE is a complex, multifactorial disease, and we are just beginning to uncover the various combinations of risk factors that lead to the development of benign autoimmunity and the onset of clinical disease. Infections have emerged as a likely candidate in the etiology of SLE. Based on serological, molecular, and epidemiological evidence, viruses such as EBV, HRES-1, parvovirus B19, and CMV, among others, have been proposed to enhance the risk of developing SLE or to increase disease activity in SLE patients. Exposure to EBV, HRES-1, parvovirus B19, CMV, and bacterial antigens can lead to the production of lupus-associated autoantibodies through molecular mimicry, epitope spreading, and superantigen activity. These and other microorganisms can also precipitate immune dysregulation, setting genetically susceptible individuals on the path to autoimmune disease. In contrast, some microbes may reduce the risk of autoimmunity or decrease the severity of clinical manifestations, perhaps by initiating long-term changes in the background inflammatory milieu. Because current and emerging medical technologies make it possible to manipulate the timing and extent of many infections, the interplay between pathogens and immunity may be a crucial point of intervention in the development of autoimmune disease. However, the course of events leading from genetic predisposition and pathogen exposure to autoimmune disease has not been well defined. We anticipate that new research on the mechanisms of infection-mediated autoimmunity will open the door for new ways to prevent and treat SLE.

ACKNOWLEDGMENT

We thank Melissa E. Munroe, MD, PhD, for critically reading the manuscript. This work was made possible by funding from the National Institute of General Medical Sciences (U54GM104938, P30GM103510), the National Institute of Arthritis and Musculoskeletal and Skin Diseases (P30AR053483), and the National Institute of Allergy and Infectious Diseases (U19AI082714, U01AI101934) of the National Institutes of Health (NIH). The content is solely the responsibility of the authors and does not necessarily represent the official views of the NIH.

REFERENCES

1. Nelson P, Rylance P, Roden D, Trela M, Tugnet N. Viruses as potential pathogenic agents in systemic lupus erythematosus. *Lupus* 2014;**23**:596–605.

2. Rigante D, Mazzoni MB, Esposito S. The cryptic interplay between systemic lupus erythematosus and infections. *Autoimmun Rev* 2014;**13**:96–102.

3. Ramos-Casals M, Cuadrado MJ, Alba P, et al. Acute viral infections in patients with systemic lupus erythematosus: description of 23 cases and review of the literature. *Medicine* 2008;**87**:311–8.

4. Francis L, Perl A. Infection in systemic lupus erythematosus: friend or foe? *Int J Clin Rheumtol* 2010;**5**:59–74.

5. Caza TN, Fernandez DR, Talaber G, et al. HRES-1/Rab4-mediated depletion of Drp1 impairs mitochondrial homeostasis and represents a target for treatment in SLE. *Ann Rheum Dis* 2014;**73**:1888–97.

6. Hsieh AH, Jhou YJ, Liang CT, Chang M, Wang SL. Fragment of tegument protein pp65 of human cytomegalovirus induces autoantibodies in BALB/c mice. *Arthritis Res Ther* 2011;**13**:R162.

7. Halenius A, Hengel H. Human cytomegalovirus and autoimmune disease. *Biomed Res Int* 2014. http://dx.doi.org/10.1155/2014/472978. Article ID 472978.

8. Hession MT, Au SC, Gottlieb AB. Parvovirus B19-associated systemic lupus erythematosus: clinical mimicry or autoimmune induction? *J Rheumatol* 2010;**37**:2430–2.

9. Zhang J, Dou Y, Zhong Z, et al. Clinical characteristics and therapy exploration of active human cytomegalovirus infection in 105 lupus patients. *Lupus* 2014;**23**:889–97.

10. Deshmukh US, Sim DL, Dai C, et al. HLA-DR3 restricted T cell epitope mimicry in induction of autoimmune response to lupus-associated antigen SmD. *J Autoimmun* 2011;**37**:254–62.

11. Deng GM, Tsokos GC. Cholera toxin B accelerates disease progression in lupus-prone mice by promoting lipid raft aggregation. *J Immunol* 2008;**181**:4019–26.

12. Chowdhary VR, Tilahun AY, Clark CR, Grande JP, Rajagopalan G. Chronic exposure to staphylococcal superantigen elicits a systemic inflammatory disease mimicking lupus. *J Immunol* 2012;**189**:2054–62.

13. Lossius A, Johansen JN, Torkildsen O, Vartdal F, Holmoy T. Epstein-Barr virus in systemic lupus erythematosus, rheumatoid arthritis and multiple sclerosis-association and causation. *Viruses* 2012;**4**:3701–30.

14. McClain MT, Harley JB, James JA. The role of Epstein-Barr virus in systemic lupus erythematosus. *Front Biosci* 2001;**6**:E137–47.

15. James JA, Robertson JM. Lupus and Epstein-Barr. *Curr Opin Rheumatol* 2012;**24**:383–8.

16. Gross AJ, Hochberg D, Rand WM, Thorley-Lawson DA. EBV and systemic lupus erythematosus: a new perspective. *J Immunol* 2005;**174**:6599–607.

17. Poole BD, Scofield RH, Harley JB, James JA. Epstein-Barr virus and molecular mimicry in systemic lupus erythematosus. *Autoimmunity* 2006;**39**:63–70.

18. James JA, Harley JB. B-cell epitope spreading in autoimmunity. *Immunol Rev* 1998;**164**:185–200.

19. Kaufman KM, Kirby MY, Harley JB, James JA. Peptide mimics of a major lupus epitope of SmB/B'. *Ann N. Y Acad Sci* 2003;**987**:215–29.

20. James JA, Harley JB. Linear epitope mapping of an Sm B/B' polypeptide. *J Immunol* 1992;**148**:2074–9.

21. Poole BD, Gross T, Maier S, Harley JB, James JA. Lupus-like autoantibody development in rabbits and mice after immunization with EBNA-1 fragments. *J Autoimmun* 2008;**31**:362–71.

22. James JA, Mamula MJ, Harley JB. Sequential autoantigenic determinants of the small nuclear ribonucleoprotein Sm D shared by human lupus autoantibodies and MRL lpr/lpr antibodies. *Clin Exp Immunol* 1994;**98**:419–26.

23. Sundar K, Jacques S, Gottlieb P, et al. Expression of the Epstein-Barr virus nuclear antigen-1 (EBNA-1) in the mouse can elicit the production of anti-dsDNA and anti-Sm antibodies. *J Autoimmun* 2004;**23**:127–40.

24. Arbuckle MR, McClain MT, Rubertone MV, et al. Development of autoantibodies before the clinical onset of systemic lupus erythematosus. *N Engl J Med* 2003;**349**:1526–33.

25. McClain MT, Heinlen LD, Dennis GJ, Roebuck J, Harley JB, James JA. Early events in lupus humoral autoimmunity suggest initiation through molecular mimicry. *Nat Med* 2005;**11**:85–9.

26. Lindquester GJ, Greer KA, Stewart JP, Sample JT. Epstein-Barr virus IL-10 gene expression by a recombinant murine gammaherpesvirus in vivo enhances acute pathogenicity but does not affect latency or reactivation. *Herpesviridae* 2014;**5**:1.

27. Graham JP, Arcipowski KM, Bishop GA. Differential B-lymphocyte regulation by CD40 and its viral mimic, latent membrane protein 1. *Immunol Rev* 2010;**237**:226–48.

28. Stunz LL, Busch LK, Munroe ME, et al. Expression of the cytoplasmic tail of LMP1 in mice induces hyperactivation of B lymphocytes and disordered lymphoid architecture. *Immunity* 2004;**21**:255–66.

29. McClain MT, Rapp EC, Harley JB, James JA. Infectious mononucleosis patients temporarily recognize a unique, cross-reactive epitope of Epstein-Barr virus nuclear antigen-1. *J Med Virol* 2003;**70**:253–7.

30. McClain MT, Poole BD, Bruner BF, Kaufman KM, Harley JB, James JA. An altered immune response to Epstein-Barr nuclear antigen 1 in pediatric systemic lupus erythematosus. *Arthritis Rheum* 2006;**54**:360–8.

31. Tsokos GC, Magrath IT, Balow JE. Epstein-Barr virus induces normal B cell responses but defective suppressor T cell responses in patients with systemic lupus erythematosus. *J Immunol* 1983;**131**:1797–801.

32. Draborg AH, Jacobsen S, Westergaard M, et al. Reduced response to Epstein-Barr virus antigens by T-cells in systemic lupus erythematosus patients. *Lupus Sci Med* 2014;**1**:e000015.

33. Berner BR, Tary-Lehmann M, Yonkers NL, Askari AD, Lehmann PV, Anthony DD. Phenotypic and functional analysis of EBV-specific memory CD8 cells in SLE. *Cell Immunol* 2005;**235**:29–38.

34. Larsen M, Sauce D, Deback C, et al. Exhausted cytotoxic control of Epstein-Barr virus in human lupus. *PLoS Pathog* 2011;**7**:e1002328.

35. Esen BA, Yilmaz G, Uzun S, et al. Serologic response to Epstein-Barr virus antigens in patients with systemic lupus erythematosus: a controlled study. *Rheumatol Int* 2012;**32**:79–83.

36. Yu XX, Yao CW, Tao JL, et al. The expression of renal Epstein-Barr virus markers in patients with lupus nephritis. *Exp Ther Med* 2014;**7**:1135–40.

37. Severa M, Giacomini E, Gafa V, et al. EBV stimulates TLR- and autophagy-dependent pathways and impairs maturation in plasmacytoid dendritic cells: implications for viral immune escape. *Eur J Immunol* 2013;**43**:147–58.

38. Ariza ME, Rivailler P, Glaser R, Chen M, Williams MV. Epstein-Barr virus encoded dUTPase containing exosomes modulate innate and adaptive immune responses in human dendritic cells and peripheral blood mononuclear cells. *PLoS One* 2013;**8**:e69827.

39. Vieira SM, Pagovich OE, Kriegel MA. Diet, microbiota and autoimmune diseases. *Lupus* 2014;**23**:518–26.

40. Szymula A, Rosenthal J, Szczerba BM, Bagavant H, Fu SM, Deshmukh US. T cell epitope mimicry between Sjogren's syndrome Antigen A (SSA)/Ro60 and oral, gut, skin and vaginal bacteria. *Clin Immunol* 2014;**152**:1–9.

41. Hevia A, Milani C, Lopez P, et al. Intestinal dysbiosis associated with systemic lupus erythematosus. *MBio* 2014;**5**:e01548–614.

42. Zhang H, Liao X, Sparks JB, Luo XM. Dynamics of gut microbiota in autoimmune lupus. *Appl Environ Microbiol* 2014;**80**:7551–60.

43. Yazdanbakhsh M, Kremsner PG, van Ree R. Allergy, parasites, and the hygiene hypothesis. *Science* 2002;**296**:490–4.

44. Larson JD, Thurman JM, Rubtsov AV, et al. Murine gammaherpesvirus 68 infection protects lupus-prone mice from the development of autoimmunity. *Proc Natl Acad Sci USA* 2012;**109**:e1092–100.

45. Cervera R, Khamashta MA, Font J, et al. Morbidity and mortality in systemic lupus erythematosus during a 10-year period: a comparison of early and late manifestations in a cohort of 1000 patients. *Medicine* 2003;**82**:299–308.

46. Shor DB, Harel M, Eliakim R, Shoenfeld Y. The hygiene theory harnessing helminths and their ova to treat autoimmunity. *Clin Rev Allergy Immunol* 2013;**45**:211–6.

47. Castro AP, Esaguy N, Aguas AP. Effect of mycobacterial infection in the lupus-prone MRL/lpr mice: enhancement of life span of autoimmune mice, amelioration of kidney disease and transient decrease in host resistance. *Autoimmunity* 1993;**16**:159–66.

48. Matsiota-Bernard P, Hentati B, Pie S, Legakis N, Nauciel C, Avrameas S. Beneficial effect of *Salmonella typhimurium* infection and of immunoglobulins from S. typhimurium-infected mice on the autoimmune disease of (NZB x NZW) F1 mice. *Clin Exp Immunol* 1996;**104**:228–35.

49. Sato MN, Minoprio P, Avrameas S, Ternynck T. Changes in the cytokine profile of lupus-prone mice (NZB/NZW)F1 induced by *Plasmodium chabaudi* and their implications in the reversal of clinical symptoms. *Clin Exp Immunol* 2000;**119**:333–9.

50. Hayashi T, Hasegawa K, Ohta A, Maeda K. Reduction of serum interferon (IFN)-gamma concentration and lupus development in NZBxNZWF(1)mice by lactic dehydrogenase virus infection. *J Comp Pathol* 2001;**125**:285–91.

51. Slight-Webb SR, Bagavant H, Crowe SR, James JA. Influenza A (H1N1) virus infection triggers severe pulmonary inflammation in lupus-prone mice following viral clearance. *J Autoimmun* 2015;**57**:66–76. http://dx.doi.org/10.1016/j.jaut.2014.12.003.

52. Lieberman LA, Tsokos GC. Lupus-prone mice fail to raise antigen-specific T cell responses to intracellular infection. *PLoS One* 2014;**9**:e111382.

Chapter 23

Origin of Autoantibodies

Westley H. Reeves[1], Shuhong Han[1], Haoyang Zhuang[1], Yuan Xu[1], Stepan Shumyak[1], Samantha Fisher[2], Lijun Yang[3]

[1]*Division of Rheumatology & Clinical Immunology, University of Florida, Gainesville, FL, USA;* [2]*Department of Dermatology, University of Florida, Gainesville, FL, USA;* [3]*Department of Pathology, Immunology, & Laboratory Medicine, University of Florida, Gainesville, FL, USA*

SUMMARY

Systemic lupus erythematosus is associated with a characteristic serological signature, including most notably anti-dsDNA and anti-Sm/RNP autoantibodies. In humans, these autoantibodies may be regulated differently, as anti-dsDNA antibodies fluctuate with disease activity, whereas anti-Sm/RNP autoantibodies tend to remain at high levels for extended periods. Disorders of B-cell activation/survival, endosomal toll-like receptor/type I interferon signaling, and clearance of apoptotic cells are associated with partial lupus-like syndromes characterized by limited disease manifestations and autoantibodies. Clinically, these syndromes are most frequently associated with evidence of glomerulonephritis, such as renal immune complex deposition and histological changes. Interestingly, the requirements for generating anti-dsDNA autoantibodies appear less stringent than those for anti-Sm/RNP, suggesting that abnormal B-cell activation, interferon production, and phagocytosis of apoptotic cells may act synergistically to produce a more diverse autoantibody profile and more widespread disease.

Production of antinuclear antibodies (ANAs) is the most consistent manifestation of systemic lupus erythematosus (SLE; frequency ~100%) and often the earliest.[1] This is not due to a global loss of tolerance, however, as the commonly recognized antigenic targets are highly restricted. Indeed, autoantibodies against chromatin/DNA, U1 small nuclear ribonucleoproteins (snRNPs, recognized by anti-Sm and RNP antibodies), small cytoplasmic "Y" RNAs associated with Ro60, and other antigens (La, ribosomal P, RNA helicase A, and phospholipid-binding proteins) comprise the so-called serological signature of SLE. Anti-double-stranded (ds) DNA, anti-Sm, and anti-phospholipid are used diagnostically.

This chapter considers the origins of this serological signature focusing on the induction of autoantibodies and maintenance of their levels (i.e., serological memory). There are differences in the pathogenesis of polyreactive, low-affinity "natural" IgM autoantibodies and high-affinity, IgG anti-dsDNA/chromatin and anti-Sm/RNP autoantibodies. Lupus autoantibodies generally recognize the components of nucleic acid–protein complexes, the nucleic acid components of which are endogenous adjuvants.

B-CELL TOLERANCE IN SLE

B-cell activation depends on positive and negative signals transmitted through the B-cell receptor (BCR) and co-receptors as well as competition for survival factors such as B-cell activating factor (BAFF).[2,3] The balance of these positive and negative signals is influenced by regulatory T cells and determines whether a B cell becomes activated or is tolerized. Genetic polymorphisms and mutations affecting these signaling pathways are associated with increased numbers of autoreactive B cells (Table 1).

The immature BCR repertoire contains many that bind DNA or other self-antigens. Additional autoreactive B cells are generated peripherally by somatic hypermutation (SHM) in secondary lymphoid organs. Self-tolerance is mediated at both central bone marrow (BM) and peripheral checkpoints. BCRs exhibiting high affinity for ubiquitous self-antigens generally are either deleted centrally or undergo receptor editing. In contrast, autoreactive B cells that do not encounter antigen in the BM or bind with low affinity to self-antigens are censored peripherally through deletion (at the transitional B cell stage), anergy (at the follicular (FO) B-cell stage), or antigen-induced cell death. Regardless of their origin, resting B cells do not secrete immunoglobulin until they differentiate into plasma cells. Thus, autoreactive B cells can circulate without producing autoantibodies.

ALTERED BCR SIGNALING IN LUPUS

Altered BCR signaling is associated with increased autoreactive B cells (Table 1). Polymorphism of the protein tyrosine phosphatase *PTPN22* decreases B-cell responsiveness causing defective central censoring of autoreactive B cells and autoimmunity.[2] Similarly, overexpression of the Bruton's tyrosine kinase (*Btk*) gene causes spontaneous

TABLE 1 Some Genetic Abnormalities Causing Increased Numbers of Autoreactive B Cells

Gene	Defect	Checkpoint(s)	Mechanism
PTPN22	C1858T	Central and peripheral	Reduced deletion/editing in BM; regulation of memory B cells[a]
MyD88, IRAK4, or UNC93B1	Mutation	Central	Abnormal regulation of TLR signaling resulting in increased numbers of polyreactive immature B cells without autoantibody production[b]
Btk	Transgene expression in mice	Central and peripheral	Alters threshold for B cell activation and negative selection of autoreactive B cells[c]
Lyn	B-cell deficiency	Peripheral	Abnormal GC formation, increased BAFF, activation of transitional and follicular B cells with autoantibodies[d]
Fcgr2b	Deficiency in mice (knockout)	Peripheral	Increased numbers of autoreactive GC B cells[e]
Tnfsf13b (BAFF)	Transgene expression in mice	Peripheral	Hyperactive NFκB2 signaling, expanded MZ B cells, increased GC formation[f]
AICDA (aid)	Deficiency (mutation)	Central	Abnormal Ig repertoire and increased serum autoantibodies (due to decreased SHM away from autoreactivity?)[g]

[a]Rhee I, et al. Nat Immunol 2012;13:439–47; Arechiga AF, et al. J Immunol 2009;182:3343–47.
[b]Fukui R, et al. Immunity 2011;35:69–81.
[c]Kil LP, et al. Blood 2012;119:3744–56.
[d]Lamagna C, et al. J Immunol 2014;192:919–28.
[e]Tiler T. J Exp Med 2010;207:2767–78.
[f]Liu Z, et al. Trends Immunol 2011;32:388–94; Thien M. Immunity 2004;20:785–98.
[g]Meyers G, et al. Proc Natl Acad Sci USA 2011;108:11554–9.

germinal center (GC) formation, hyperresponsiveness to BCR stimulation, altered peripheral censoring of autoreactive B cells, ANAs, and lupus-like disease.[4] Deletion of the tyrosine kinase Lyn in B cells enhances signaling in transitional and FO B cells, leading to anti-Sm and anti-dsDNA autoantibodies, glomerulonephritis, poor GC formation, and increased B1a cells.[5] The autoimmune phenotype is reversed by deleting MyD88, consistent with a role of toll-like receptors (TLRs). Decreased LYN expression also is reported in human SLE.

PROPERTIES OF LUPUS AUTOANTIBODIES

DNA sequencing of the V_H and V_L regions expressed by autoantibody-producing hybridoma cells from lupus mice reveals SHM. A single somatic mutation can transform an antibody against nonself to an autoantibody.[6] Moreover, most lupus autoantibodies are derived from B cells that have undergone class switch recombination (CSR) to IgG, suggesting that they are products of T cell driven responses generated within GCs. This is further supported by evidence that autoantibody levels are maintained by long-lived plasma cells, usually derived from post-GC B cells. However, other studies show that T-cell-independent, class-switched, somatically mutated autoantibodies also can be generated extrafollicularly. There is debate over the relative importance of each pathway.

GC VERSUS EXTRAFOLLICULAR ORIGIN OF AUTOANTIBODIES

Mature B cells consist of three subsets: FO, marginal zone (MZ), and B-1, a self-renewing population located near serosal surfaces.[7] All three subsets are implicated in autoantibody formation.[8] FO B cells are involved in T-cell-dependent (TD) formation of GCs in response to protein antigens. In contrast, MZ B cells respond to particulate antigens in a T-cell-independent (TI) manner. They respond to TI-1 antigens (e.g., lipopolysaccharide, which engages TLR4) and TI-2 antigens (e.g., pneumococcal polysaccharide, which consists of highly repetitive epitopes), although they also can become GC B cells in response to TD antigens.[7] B-1 cells are the primary source of polyreactive "natural" IgM antibodies, which opsonize bacteria and like MZ B cells respond to TI-1 and TI-2 antigens. In general, FO B cells are more highly subject to SHM and CSR than MZ or B-1 cells. However, SHM and CSR can occur in all three subsets. Likewise, although memory B cell responses are considered a property of FO B cell responses to TD antigens, memory also can develop to TI-1 and TI-2 antigens.[7]

Role of GC

Tolerance of anti-Sm B cells is critically dependent on censoring at the FO B cell and pre-plasma cell stages.[9] There is considerable evidence in mice that anti-Sm and anti-dsDNA responses are mediated by post-GC B cells. Key features of the GC reaction include a requirement for T follicular helper (T_{FH}) cells and production of antibodies that have undergone SHM and CSR. Evidence for the role of GCs comes from the near-simultaneous development of anti-dsDNA autoantibodies and lupus-like disease in sanroque mice.[10] Homozygosity for a mutation of the ubiquitin ligase *Roquin* in sanroque mice causes accumulation of T_{FH}, spontaneous GC formation, autoantibodies, and glomerulonephritis.[8] B cell activation in GCs reflects competition for limited numbers of T_{FH} cells, which provide positive and negative selection signals via CD40L-CD40 and Fas-FasL signaling, respectively.[8] *Fas* mutation increases GC and memory B cells following immunization with TD antigens and causes autoantibody production in B6/*lpr* mice and lupus in MRL/*lpr* mice. Fas deficiency promotes abnormal localization of autoreactive B cells to the T cell zone, where censoring may be ineffective.[11] Whereas Fas regulates negative selection of autoreactive GC B cells,[12] Roquin affects positive selection by increasing T_{FH} cells in GCs.

Role of Extrafollicular Responses

The appearance of long-lived plasma cells and memory B cells is primarily due to FO B cells entering GCs. B-1 cells generate mainly short-lived extrafollicular plasma cells, but they also generate long-lived plasma cells in response to TI-2 antigens.[7] Likewise, MZ B cells can enter GCs following immunization with TD antigens[13] and a population of switched human MZ-derived memory B cells can be driven to plasma cell differentiation by IL-21 plus BAFF.[14]

Mouse models provide strong evidence that some autoantibodies are generated extrafollicularly. Fas deficiency causes extrafollicular localization of autoreactive anti-DNA B cells[11] and development of autoantibodies in BAFF-transgenic mice does not require T cell help.[15] BAFF, an important survival factor for FO and MZ B cells, also is over-produced in SLE patients.[15]

GC versus Extrafollicular Origin of Human Autoantibodies

Despite evidence for both GC-derived and extrafollicular B cells in murine lupus, there is only indirect evidence in humans. One line of evidence is the stability of anti-Sm/RNP and Ro60/La autoantibody levels in SLE patients, which is consistent with long-term B-cell memory and/or long-lived plasma cells. Anti-dsDNA antibodies are produced transiently with increased disease activity, suggesting that they might be produced by short-lived (extrafollicular) plasma cells. Treatment with rituximab (anti-CD20) reduces autoantibody levels, especially anti-dsDNA, but the inability to eliminate autoantibodies in most patients is consistent with long-lived plasma cells. Additional evidence comes from the defective censoring of autoreactive 9G4 idiotype+ B cells in GCs from SLE tonsils.[16] Finally, reduction of autoantibodies by anti-CD40L therapy[17] provides evidence that some autoantibody responses are derived from post-GC B cells.

ROLE OF TLR SIGNALING

Signaling through TLRs, especially endosomal TLR7, TLR8, and TLR9, may drive autoreactive B cells to undergo plasma cell differentiation.[2] TLR7 and TLR8 bind AU-rich single-stranded RNA ligands and TLR9 recognizes DNA with unmethylated CpG motifs.[18] Their primary role is sensing microbial nucleic acids, but they also recognize endogenous nucleic acids.[18] Although endogenous nucleic acids usually are degraded before reaching TLR7/8/9-containing endosomes, binding of the antimicrobial peptide LL37 or autoantibodies can allow self-nucleic acids to reach endosomal TLRs.[19] BCR binding of nucleic acid–protein complexes, such as snRNPs, delivers associated nucleic acids to endosomes where they engage TLR7/8/9, promoting autoantibody production.[20] U1 RNA, an RNA component of the Sm/RNP autoantigens, is recognized by TLR7. TLR7/8/9 signaling involves the adapter protein MyD88 and promotes type I interferon (IFN-I) production via IRF7.[21]

TLR7/8/9 are associated with the endoplasmic reticulum (ER) in resting cells, but re-localize to the Golgi and subsequently to endosomes.[18] Several ER proteins regulate TLR trafficking from the ER to endosomes, including UNC93B1, gp96, and PRAT4A.[22,23] UNC93B1 is of particular importance as it regulates levels of endosomal TLR9 (protective) and TLR7 (proinflammatory).

Endosomal TLRs and Autoantibody Production

Autoantibody production is abolished in TLR7-deficient mice. In MRL/*lpr* mice, anti-Sm autoantibodies are TLR7-dependent, whereas anti-dsDNA autoantibodies are TLR9-dependent.[24] Similarly, in pristane-induced lupus, anti-Sm/RNP autoantibodies are abolished in TLR7-deficient mice.[25] However, anti-dsDNA autoantibodies in this model also are TLR7-dependent.

Overexpression of TLR7 in BXSB male (*Yaa*) mice results in increased numbers of T_{FH} cells, increased IL-21, high anti-dsDNA levels, and glomerulonephritis.[26] B6 mice make higher levels of anti-RNA autoantibodies with increasing *TLR7* copy number.[27] In *Yaa* mice, IL-21 is overproduced both by T_{FH} cells and extrafollicular T cells, suggesting that autoantibodies may originate from both sites.[28]

Role of TLRs in Serological Memory

Most RNA-protein autoantibodies are IgG. Serum levels are high (titers ≥ 1:10^6) and often maintained for life regardless of disease activity, consistent with serological memory. In contrast, anti-dsDNA autoantibody levels are lower and they tend to be produced in mainly patients with active disease. Thus, the origins (GC vs extrafollicular) of these autoantibodies may differ. Although controversial, TLR signaling may help maintain serological memory by driving terminal differentiation of memory B cells.[29]

Autoantibodies in SLE recognize only a small subset of the thousands of cellular antigens. Most are nucleic acid–protein complexes containing immunostimulatory RNA (e.g., U1 snRNPs) or DNA (e.g., chromatin). These complexes may become immunogenic because they contain immunostimulatory nucleic acids. Thus, snRNPs bind the BCR of autoreactive B cells and then engage TLR7 following endosomal uptake.[20]

ASSOCIATION OF AUTOANTIBODIES WITH ACCUMULATION OF INTRACELLULAR NUCLEIC ACIDS

Autologous nucleic acids interact with both endosomal (TLR) and cytoplasmic (non-TLR) sensors, stimulating IFN-I production.[30,31] The role of these molecules in the pathogenesis of autoinflammatory/autoimmune diseases ("interferonopathies") is an area of recent interest. Under normal circumstances, IFN-I production is prevented by subcellular sequestration of the sensors and degradation of endogenous nucleic acids before they can engage the sensors.[32,33] Intracellular DNA activates a pathway dependent on stimulator of IFN genes (STING), an ER-associated protein that complexes with cytoplasmic DNA and bacterial cyclic di-GMP or cyclic di-AMP, activating TBK1 and IRF3 and triggering IFN-I production.[34] Gain of function mutations of the *TREM173* gene (encoding STING) cause a systemic autoinflammatory syndrome mediated by IFN-I and associated with cutaneous vasculopathy and pulmonary inflammation, but only transient low levels of ANA, c-ANCA, and antiphospholipid autoantibodies.[34]

The 3′ repair exonuclease Trex1 is a negative regulator of the STING pathway.[35] Trex-1 deficient mice develop lethal autoinflammatory disease caused by the accumulation of intracellular DNA and dysregulated IFN-I production.[36] *Trex1−/−* mice develop myocarditis with anti-cardiac myosin and junctophilin-2 autoantibodies, but not anti-DNA/chromatin or Sm/RNP. STING

deficiency rescues *Trex1−/−* mice from DNA-mediated inflammatory disease.[35] Human loss-of-function mutations affecting the exonuclease domain of *TREX1* cause familial chilblain lupus and Aicardi-Goutieres syndrome (AGS) (encephalopathy, calcification of the basal ganglia and white matter, and high levels of IFN–I in the cerebrospinal fluid).[37] *TREX1* polymorphisms outside the exonuclease domain are associated with sporadic SLE.[38] Interestingly, patients with gain-of-function mutations affecting the RNA sensor MDA5 also develop an IFN-I-mediated syndrome similar to AGS.[39]

Chilblain lupus is an erythematous/violaceous rash affecting the toes, fingers, and other sites, worsened by cold exposure but distinct from Raynaud's phenomenon and other lupus rashes (Figure 1). Familial chilblain lupus with mutation of the exonuclease domain of *TREX1* is sometimes associated with ANAs, but not anti-Sm/RNP or dsDNA.[37] In contrast, sporadic chilblain lupus can be seen in SLE and Sjogren's syndrome, often with anti-Ro antibodies, but *TREX1* mutations generally are absent.

Lysosomal nucleases, such as DNase II, normally degrade autologous nucleic acids released after phagocytosis of apoptotic cells.[33] DNase II-deficient mice die in utero from IFN-I overproduction and conditional knockout mice develop rheumatoid arthritis-like disease, with erosive polyarthritis, anti-CCP antibodies, and rheumatoid factor, but only low levels of anti-DNA (less than one-tenth that in MRL/*lpr* mice).[33] Arthritis and IFN-I production is independent of TLRs but reversed by STING deficiency.[40] Thus, despite high levels of IFN-I production, there is only limited evidence to date that *TREX1, TREM173, MDA5,* or *DNaseII* mutations lead to an autoantibody profile typical of SLE. Abnormal accumulation of cytoplasmic RNA

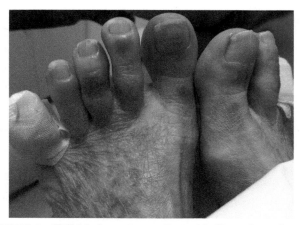

FIGURE 1 Chilblain lupus in a patient with Sjogren's syndrome. Patient is a 62-year-old white woman with sicca syndrome, high-titer anti-Ro and La autoantibodies, rheumatoid factor, interferon signature positive, and low C4 whose disease course was complicated by diffuse large B-cell lymphoma treated with rituximab. Her toes show classic findings of chilblain lupus (red-purple patches with uncomfortable fissuring).

is associated with a more robust pattern of autoantibody production. Mice deficient in Ro60, a chaperone for misfolded cytoplasmic RNA, develop glomerulonephritis and autoantibodies to ribosomal P, dsDNA, histones, and nucleosomes.[41]

RELATIONSHIP OF IFN-I TO AUTOANTIBODY PRODUCTION

Endosomal or cytoplasmic sensing of DNA/RNA results in IFN-I production, which is strongly implicated in autoimmunity. IFN-I includes multiple IFNα species, IFNβ, and other isoforms.[42] Although downstream effects vary, all IFN-I isoforms bind the type I interferon receptor (IFNAR), initiating a STAT1-regulated signaling cascade and increasing transcription of ~100 IFN-stimulated genes. This gene expression program, seen in peripheral blood mononuclear cells from most SLE patients and in mice with pristane-induced lupus, is termed the "interferon signature," and is associated with anti-dsDNA and Sm/RNP autoantibodies and nephritis.[25,43]

ANAs and anti-dsDNA antibodies develop in many patients treated with IFNα and individuals with three copies of the type I interferon gene cluster overexpress IFN-I and develop autoimmune manifestations, including anti-RNP and anti-Ro60 autoantibodies.[44] Moreover, lupus is accelerated by IFNα in NZB/W mice, whereas autoantibody production and nephritis are abolished in pristane-treated BALB/c IFNAR−/− mice.[25,45] The effect of IFN-I is likely due in part to increased TLR7 expression.[20] IFN-I production is downregulated by TNFα.[46] Up to 60% of patients treated with TNFα inhibitors develop ANAs and 20% anti-dsDNA autoantibodies. TNFα-deficient mice do not produce autoantibodies spontaneously, but they produce substantially more IFN-I and anti-RNP/Sm following pristane treatment, probably due to increased circulating PDCs.

ASSOCIATION OF AUTOANTIBODIES WITH ABNORMAL CLEARANCE OF APOPTOTIC CELLS

There is considerable evidence that the ligands driving TLR7-mediated IFN-I production are derived from dead cells. Inefficient clearance of apoptotic cells is associated with lupus-like autoimmunity in animal models.[33]

Phosphatidylserine (PtdSer) Receptors

PtdSer expressed on the surface of apoptotic cells is recognized by diverse macrophage receptors.[33] The secreted protein MFG-E8 (produced by macrophages and dendritic cells) and two serum proteins, Gas6 and protein S, bind PtdSer. MFG-E8 associates with the integrins $\alpha_v\beta_3$ and $\alpha_v\beta_5$, whereas Gas6 and protein S bind to the TAM receptors Tyro3, Axl, and Mertk, facilitating phagocytosis.[33] TAM receptors mediate the IFNAR-dependent, noninflammatory, clearance of apoptotic cells by broadly suppressing TLR signaling. In the absence of Mertk, the phagocytic capacity of macrophages for apoptotic cells is nearly eliminated, whereas absence of Axl or Tyro3 reduces it by half.[47] Mice deficient in Mertk or other TAM receptors develop lupus-like disease, with production of anti-dsDNA and anti-phospholipid (but not anti-Sm/RNP or Ro/La) autoantibodies, renal disease, and arthritis. *Mfge8−/−* mice also develop anti-dsDNA, but not anti-Sm/RNP or Ro/La autoantibodies.[33] Although Tim4 is another PtdSer receptor expressed by resident macrophages, Tim4-deficient mice do not develop lupus.[48]

MFG-E8 expression by tingible body macrophages and follicular dendritic cells may aid the clearance of B cells undergoing deletion in GCs and *Mfge8−/−* mice accumulate dead cells within GCs.[33] Human SLE also is associated with abnormal accumulation of apoptotic cells in GCs (tingible body macrophages).[49]

Role of Complement Proteins

Deficiency of the early classical complement pathway components C1q, C4, and C2 is strongly associated with lupus-like disease.[38] The risk in C1q-deficient patients is 93%, but lupus is uncommon in C3 deficient patients (3 of 23 cases, none ANA positive). C1q deficient mice develop autoantibodies, glomerular accumulation of apoptotic cells, nephritis, and anti-Sm (but not anti-DNA) autoantibodies. C1q binds PtdSer on apoptotic cells, followed by recognition of C1q by the scavenger receptor SCARF1.[50] Clearance of apoptotic cells is decreased in C1q-deficient mice and SCARF1 deficient mice develop lupus-like disease with dermatitis, nephritis, and antinucleosome antibodies, but not anti-dsDNA or anti-Sm/RNP.

AUTOANTIBODY PRODUCTION INDUCED BY PRISTANE

Treatment of non-autoimmune-prone mice with the inflammatory hydrocarbon pristane induces a lupus-like syndrome manifested by glomerulonephritis, arthritis, diffuse alveolar hemorrhage, and hematological abnormalities and associated with a broad spectrum of lupus autoantibodies (anti-dsDNA/chromatin, anti-Sm/RNP, and others).[25] Pristane causes TLR7-mediated IFN-I production, abnormal apoptotic cell clearance, and B cell hyperresponsiveness, suggesting that defects which by themselves produce a limited lupus-like syndrome (Table 2) may act together to cause more severe disease.

TABLE 2 Autoantibody Production in Selected Lupus-like Disorders

Disorder	Clinical Features	Autoantibodies		
		Anti-dsDNA	Anti-Sm/RNP	Other
Increased B Cell Activation or Survival				
Lyn deficiency[m]	GN, myeloproliferation	Yes	Yes	N/A
BAFF overexpression[m]	GN	Yes	N/A	RF, histone
Increased IFN-I Production				
TLR7 overexpression (Yaa)[m]	GN, myeloproliferation	Yes	No	RNA
Trex1 deficiency[m]	Myocarditis	No	No	Cardiac myosin,
STING gain of function[m]	Cutaneous vasculopathy, pulmonary inflammation	No	No	c-ANCA, phospholipid (low levels)
Pristane-lupus[m]	GN, alveolar hemorrhage, arthritis, hematologic	Yes	Yes	Su, ribosomal P, chromatin
IFNα therapy[m,h]	Arthritis, fever	Yes	Rare	c-ANCA, Ro
TNFα inhibitor therapy[h]	Arthritis, serositis	Yes	Rare	c-ANCA
Decreased Clearance of Apoptotic Cells				
Mertk deficiency[m]	GN, arthritis	Yes	No	Phospholipid
MFG-E8 deficiency[m]	GN, splenomegaly	Yes	No	N/A
Tim4 deficiency[m]	None	No	No	None
C1q deficiency[m]	GN	No	Yes	N/A
SCARF1 deficiency[m]	GN, dermatitis	No	No	Nucleosomes

[m]Mouse.
[h]Human.

REFERENCES

1. Arbuckle MR, McClain MT, Rubertone MV, Scofield RH, Dennis GJ, James JA, et al. Development of autoantibodies before the clinical onset of systemic lupus erythematosus. *N Engl J Med* 2003;**349**(16): 1526–33.

2. Giltiay NV, Chappell CP, Clark EA. B-cell selection and the development of autoantibodies. *Arthritis Res Ther* 2012;**14**(Suppl. 4):S1. Epub 2013/01/11.

3. Mackay F, Schneider P. Cracking the BAFF code. *Nat Rev Immunol* 2009;**9**(7):491–502.

4. Kil LP, de Bruijn MJ, van Nimwegen M, Corneth OB, van Hamburg JP, Dingjan GM, et al. Btk levels set the threshold for B-cell activation and negative selection of autoreactive B cells in mice. *Blood* 2012;**119**(16):3744–56. Epub 2012/03/03.

5. Lamagna C, Hu Y, DeFranco AL, Lowell CA. B cell-specific loss of Lyn kinase leads to autoimmunity. *J Immunol* 2014;**192**(3):919–28. Epub 2014/01/01.

6. Diamond B, Scharff MD. Somatic mutation of the T15 heavy chain gives rise to antibody with autoantibody specificity. *Proc Natl Acad Sci USA* 1984;**81**:5841–4.

7. Vinuesa CG, Chang PP. Innate B cell helpers reveal novel types of antibody responses. *Nat Immunol* 2013;**14**(2):119–26. Epub 2013/01/22.

8. Vinuesa CG, Sanz I, Cook MC. Dysregulation of germinal centres in autoimmune disease. *Nat Rev Immunol* 2009;**9**(12):845–57.

9. Clarke SH. Anti-Sm B cell tolerance and tolerance loss in systemic lupus erythematosus. *Immunol Res* 2008;**41**(3):203–16.

10. Linterman MA, Rigby RJ, Wong RK, Yu D, Brink R, Cannons JL, et al. Follicular helper T cells are required for systemic autoimmunity. *J Exp Med* 2009;**206**(3):561–76.

11. William J, Euler C, Christensen S, Shlomchik MJ. Evolution of autoantibody responses via somatic hypermutation outside of germinal centers. *Science* 2002;**297**(5589):2066–70.

12. Hao Z, Duncan GS, Seagal J, Su YW, Hong C, Haight J, et al. Fas receptor expression in germinal-center B cells is essential for T and B lymphocyte homeostasis. *Immunity* 2008;**29**(4):615–27.

13. Song H, Cerny J. Functional heterogeneity of marginal zone B cells revealed by their ability to generate both early antibody-forming cells and germinal centers with hypermutation and memory in response to a T-dependent antigen. *J Exp Med* 2003;**198**(12):1923–35.

14. Ettinger R, Sims GP, Robbins R, Withers D, Fischer RT, Grammer AC, et al. IL-21 and BAFF/BLyS synergize in stimulating plasma cell differentiation from a unique population of human splenic memory B cells. *J Immunol* 2007;**178**(5):2872–82.

15. Groom JR, Fletcher CA, Walters SN, Grey ST, Watt SV, Sweet MJ, et al. BAFF and MyD88 signals promote a lupuslike disease independent of T cells. *J Exp Med* 2007;**204**(8):1959–71.

16. Cappione A, Anolik JH, Pugh-Bernard A, Barnard J, Dutcher P, Silverman G, et al. Germinal center exclusion of autoreactive B cells is defective in human systemic lupus erythematosus. *J Clin Invest* 2005;**115**(11):3205–16.

17. Grammer AC, Slota R, Fischer R, Gur H, Girschick H, Yarboro C, et al. Abnormal germinal center reactions in systemic lupus erythematosus demonstrated by blockade of CD154-CD40 interactions. *J Clin Invest* 2003;**112**(10):1506–20.

18. Ewald SE, Barton GM. Nucleic acid sensing Toll-like receptors in autoimmunity. *Curr Opin Immunol* 2011;**23**(1):3–9. Epub 2010/12/15.

19. Lande R, Gregorio J, Facchinetti V, Chatterjee B, Wang YH, Homey B, et al. Plasmacytoid dendritic cells sense self-DNA coupled with antimicrobial peptide. *Nature* 2007;**449**(7162):564–9.

20. Lau CM, Broughton C, Tabor AS, Akira S, Flavell RA, Mamula MJ, et al. RNA-associated autoantigens activate B cells by combined B cell antigen receptor/Toll-like receptor 7 engagement. *J Exp Med* 2005;**202**(9):1171–7.

21. Kawai T, Akira S. TLR signaling. *Semin Immunol* 2007;**19**(1):24–32. Epub 2007/02/06.

22. Saitoh S, Miyake K. Regulatory molecules required for nucleotide-sensing Toll-like receptors. *Immunol Rev* 2009;**227**(1):32–43.

23. Fukui R, Saitoh S, Kanno A, Onji M, Shibata T, Ito A, et al. Unc93B1 restricts systemic lethal inflammation by orchestrating Toll-like receptor 7 and 9 trafficking. *Immunity* 2011;**35**(1):69–81. Epub 2011/06/21.

24. Christensen SR, Shupe J, Nickerson K, Kashgarian M, Flavell RA, Shlomchik MJ. Toll-like receptor 7 and TLR9 dictate autoantibody specificity and have opposing inflammatory and regulatory roles in a murine model of lupus. *Immunity* 2006;**25**(3):417–28.

25. Reeves WH, Lee PY, Weinstein JS, Satoh M, Lu L. Induction of autoimmunity by pristane and other naturally occurring hydrocarbons. *Trends Immunol* 2009;**30**(9):455–64.

26. Subramanian S, Tus K, Li QZ, Wang A, Tian XH, Zhou J, et al. A Tlr7 translocation accelerates systemic autoimmunity in murine lupus. *Proc Natl Acad Sci USA* 2006;**103**(26):9970–5.

27. Deane JA, Pisitkun P, Barrett RS, Feigenbaum L, Town T, Ward JM, et al. Control of toll-like receptor 7 expression is essential to restrict autoimmunity and dendritic cell proliferation. *Immunity* 2007;**27**(5):801–10.

28. Bubier JA, Sproule TJ, Foreman O, Spolski R, Shaffer DJ, Morse III HC, et al. A critical role for IL-21 receptor signaling in the pathogenesis of systemic lupus erythematosus in BXSB-Yaa mice. *Proc Natl Acad Sci USA* 2009;**106**(5):1518–23.

29. Bernasconi NL, Traggiai E, Lanzavecchia A. Maintenance of serological memory by polyclonal activation of human memory B cells. *Science* 2002;**298**(5601):2199–202.

30. Desmet CJ, Ishii KJ. Nucleic acid sensing at the interface between innate and adaptive immunity in vaccination. *Nat Rev Immunol* 2012;**12**(7):479–91. Epub 2012/06/26.

31. Rice GI, Forte GM, Szynkiewicz M, Chase DS, Aeby A, Abdel-Hamid MS, et al. Assessment of interferon-related biomarkers in Aicardi-Goutieres syndrome associated with mutations in TREX1, RNASEH2A, RNASEH2B, RNASEH2C, SAMHD1, and ADAR: a case-control study. *Lancet Neurol* 2013;**12**(12):1159–69. Epub 2013/11/05.

32. Barton GM, Kagan JC. A cell biological view of Toll-like receptor function: regulation through compartmentalization. *Nat Rev Immunol* 2009;**9**(8):535–42.

33. Nagata S, Hanayama R, Kawane K. Autoimmunity and the clearance of dead cells. *Cell* 2010;**140**(5):619–30. Epub 2010/03/10.

34. Liu Y, Jesus AA, Marrero B, Yang D, Ramsey SE, Montealegre Sanchez GA, et al. Activated STING in a vascular and pulmonary syndrome. *N Engl J Med* 2014;**371**(6):507–18. Epub 2014/07/17.

35. Gall A, Treuting P, Elkon KB, Loo YM, Gale Jr M, Barber GN, et al. Autoimmunity initiates in nonhematopoietic cells and progresses via lymphocytes in an interferon-dependent autoimmune disease. *Immunity* 2012;**36**(1):120–31. Epub 2012/01/31.

36. Stetson DB, Ko JS, Heidmann T, Medzhitov R. Trex1 prevents cell-intrinsic initiation of autoimmunity. *Cell* 2008;**134**(4):587–98. Epub 2008/08/30.

37. Rice G, Newman WG, Dean J, Patrick T, Parmar R, Flintoff K, et al. Heterozygous mutations in TREX1 cause familial chilblain lupus and dominant Aicardi-Goutieres syndrome. *Am J Hum Genet* 2007;**80**(4):811–5. Epub 2007/03/16.

38. Crispin JC, Hedrich CM, Tsokos GC. Gene-function studies in systemic lupus erythematosus. *Nat Rev Rheumatol* 2013;**9**(8):476–84. Epub 2013/06/05.

39. Rice GI, del Toro Duany Y, Jenkinson EM, Forte GM, Anderson BH, Ariaudo G, et al. Gain-of-function mutations in IFIH1 cause a spectrum of human disease phenotypes associated with upregulated type I interferon signaling. *Nat Genet* 2014;**46**(5):503–9. Epub 2014/04/02.

40. Ahn J, Gutman D, Saijo S, Barber GN. STING manifests self DNA-dependent inflammatory disease. *Proc Natl Acad Sci USA* 2012;**109**(47):19386–91. Epub 2012/11/08.

41. Xue D, Shi H, Smith JD, Chen X, Noe DA, Cedervall T, et al. A lupus-like syndrome develops in mice lacking the Ro 60-kDa protein, a major lupus autoantigen. *Proc Natl Acad Sci USA* 2003;**100**(13):7503–8.

42. Crow MK. Advances in understanding the role of type I interferons in systemic lupus erythematosus. *Curr Opin Rheumatol* 2014;**26**(5):467–74. Epub 2014/07/11.

43. Baechler EC, Batliwalla FM, Karypis G, Gaffney PM, Ortmann WA, Espe KJ, et al. Interferon-inducible gene expression signature in peripheral blood cells of patients with severe lupus. *Proc Natl Acad Sci USA* 2003;**100**(5):2610–5.

44. Zhuang H, Kosboth M, Lee P, Rice A, Driscoll DJ, Zori R, et al. Lupus-like disease and high interferon levels with trisomy of the Type I interferon cluster on chromosome 9p. *Arthritis Rheum* 2006;**54**(5):1573–9.

45. Mathian A, Weinberg A, Gallegos M, Banchereau J, Koutouzov S. IFN-alpha induces early lethal lupus in preautoimmune (New Zealand Black x New Zealand White) F1 but not in BALB/c mice. *J Immunol* 2005;**174**(5):2499–506.

46. Palucka AK, Blanck JP, Bennett L, Pascual V, Banchereau J. Cross-regulation of TNF and IFN-alpha in autoimmune diseases. *Proc Natl Acad Sci USA* 2005;**102**(9):3372–7.

47. Seitz HM, Camenisch TD, Lemke G, Earp HS, Matsushima GK. Macrophages and dendritic cells use different Axl/Mertk/Tyro3 receptors in clearance of apoptotic cells. *J Immunol* 2007;**178**(9):5635–42. Epub 2007/04/20.

48. Wong K, Valdez PA, Tan C, Yeh S, Hongo JA, Ouyang W. Phosphatidylserine receptor Tim-4 is essential for the maintenance of the homeostatic state of resident peritoneal macrophages. *Proc Natl Acad Sci USA* 2010;**107**(19):8712–7. Epub 2010/04/28.

49. Baumann I, Kolowos W, Voll RE, Manger B, Gaipl U, Neuhuber WL, et al. Impaired uptake of apoptotic cells into tingible body macrophages in germinal centers of patients with systemic lupus erythematosus. *Arthritis Rheum* 2002;**46**(1):191–201. Epub 2002/01/31.

50. Ramirez-Ortiz ZG, Pendergraft 3rd WF, Prasad A, Byrne MH, Iram T, Blanchette CJ, et al. The scavenger receptor SCARF1 mediates the clearance of apoptotic cells and prevents autoimmunity. *Nat Immunol* 2013;**14**(9):917–26. Epub 2013/07/31.

Chapter 24

Anti-DNA Antibodies

Susan Malkiel, Betty Diamond
Autoimmune & Musculoskeletal Disease Center, Feinstein Institute for Medical Research, North Shore LIJ Health System, Manhasset, NY, USA

INTRODUCTION

Elevated anti-double-stranded (ds) DNA antibody titers are diagnostic and prognostic markers of systemic lupus erythematosus (SLE), and their presence is well documented to correlate with lupus nephritis. These antibodies are often deposited in the glomeruli and can be eluted from the kidneys of SLE patients and lupus mice. Moreover, passively transferring anti-dsDNA antibodies into mice can induce proteinuria. The observation that a subset of anti-dsDNA antibodies cross-reacts to the N-methyl-D-aspartate receptor (NMDAR) on neurons has led to the discovery of another pathogenic role for these antibodies in neuropsychiatric lupus. Finally, these antibodies form immune complexes, and, in so doing, facilitate the entry of DNA, a toll-like receptor (TLR)-9 ligand, into the cell to activate downstream inflammatory pathways.

CELLULAR SOURCE OF ANTI-DNA ANTIBODIES

There are two B-cell lineages in mice; one gives rise to B1 cells and one to marginal zone and follicular B cells. Presumably, these same two lineages are present in humans. B1 cells originate in the fetal liver, self-renew, have a limited repertoire of immunoglobulin genes, and respond to antigen without cognate T-cell help. Marginal zone and follicular B cells arise in the bone marrow, and they continue to arise from hematopoietic stem cells throughout adult life. Marginal zone B cells, like B1 cells, have a relatively limited repertoire and respond to antigen without a requirement for cognate T-cell help. Many autoreactive B cells that are present in healthy individuals and produce the antibodies that help clear apoptotic debris have a marginal zone phenotype.[1] Follicular B cells express a diverse repertoire and require both antigen and cognate T-cell help to differentiate into short-lived plasma cells or to form a germinal center and become memory cells or long-lived plasma cells. In mice, it is clear that B1 cells, marginal zone, or follicular B cells can each be the source for pathogenic anti-DNA antibodies.[2,3] In patients, most data suggest that follicular B cells are the source, as the antibodies are formed from a diverse set of immunoglobulin genes. The presence of high interferon (IFN) in many SLE patients may skew activated B cells to a short-lived plasma cell phenotype, and so lead to relatively rapid alterations in anti-dsDNA antibody titers.[4]

CONTRIBUTION OF ANTIGEN SELECTION

One persistent question is whether anti-DNA antibodies arise as a consequence of nonspecific polyclonal activation or develop in an antigen-driven fashion, undergoing class-switch recombination, somatic mutation, and affinity maturation in a germinal center. Analysis of anti-ds DNA antibodies on a molecular level, both in murine models of lupus and in SLE patients, has provided much evidence for antigen-driven selection.[5] In early studies, this was established by finding high frequencies of replacement mutations in the complementarity determining regions (CDRs) of both the heavy- and light-chain variable region genes (V_H and V_L) encoding anti-dsDNA antibodies. Comparisons of monoclonal anti-DNA antibodies from the autoimmune MRL/*lpr* strain to sequences of germline variable region genes, and to other anti-DNA antibodies, demonstrated oligoclonal expansion, and nonrandom somatic hypermutation, leading to specificity for dsDNA.[6,7] Anti-DNA antibodies in lupus-prone NZB/W mice similarly exhibited clonal relatedness between anti-DNA immunoglobulin (Ig) M and IgG antibodies and antigen-driven selection.[8] Rigorous analysis of the somatic mutations in mouse and human anti-dsDNA IgG antibodies found high frequencies of replacements to the charged amino acids arginine, asparagine, and lysine in the CDRs.[9,10] Site-directed mutagenesis was used to revert somatic mutations found in these antibodies to their germline configuration, and stepwise maturation from a non-dsDNA reactive antibody into a high-affinity anti-DNA antibody was observed.[11] Backmutation analysis of IgM anti-dsDNA antibodies derived from peripheral blood B cells of SLE patients similarly showed a loss of reactivity to dsDNA, and emphasized that anti-dsDNA antibodies can develop from non-DNA reactive B cells in the periphery.[12,13] In contrast, other observations

Systemic Lupus Erythematosus. http://dx.doi.org/10.1016/B978-0-12-801917-7.00024-3

have suggested that some human anti-DNA antibodies derive from autoreactive B cells that mature to immunocompetence in the autoimmune host, which may become activated in an inflammatory milieu.[12,14]

TRIGGERS: CHROMATIN AND ENVIRONMENTAL EXPOSURES

Whether the antigen (or antigens) that triggers the production of anti-dsDNA antibodies in lupus is chromatin itself or a cross-reactive foreign antigen is still debated. Although different forms of DNA are immunogenic (synthetic single-stranded or ds polynucleotides, or Z-DNA), "pure" native B-helical dsDNA is not immunogenic unless complexed with polypeptides or proteins as in chromatin.[15] The release of chromatin from damaged or dead cells has been shown to be proinflammatory and capable of activating an immune response. The demonstration that lupus-prone mice develop autoantibodies to nucleosomes, which are comprised of DNA and histones, prior to developing reactivity to naked dsDNA supports chromatin as an initiating antigen.[16,17] Additionally, autoreactive T-helper cells specific for histones were shown to have the capacity to activate an anti-dsDNA antibody response in both mouse and humans.[18–20] Some studies have shown that lupus patients have increased levels of nucleosomes in their blood.[21] The increased chromatin in SLE is thought to arise from a variety of associated deficiencies in the clearance of apoptotic cells and nuclear debris.[22,23] Deficits encompass molecules ranging from opsonins that coat dying cells (C1q,[24] mannose-binding lectin,[25] C-reactive protein[26]) to receptors on phagocytes that recognize them (class A scavenger receptors,[27,28] the tyrosine kinase c-mer,[29] or CD44[30]), and include early complement components C2 and C4,[24] and bridging molecules (milk fat globule epidermal growth factor 8[31,32]). Impaired DNase I activity,[23] degradation of neutrophil extracellular traps in SLE,[33] and microparticles[34] provide other sources of DNA to promote autoantibody production.

Environmental triggers may also elicit the production of anti-dsDNA antibodies. An early discovery that an antimicrobial antibody could become an autoreactive anti-dsDNA antibody by a single amino acid substitution suggested that these autoantibodies could be generated in the course of a protective immune response to infection.[35] Subsequent studies demonstrated that immunization with phosphorylcholine, a dominant epitope on the polysaccharide of various infectious microbes, including *Streptococcus pneumoniae*, induces the generation of cross-reactive anti-dsDNA B cells. These B cells do not enter the memory compartment, suggesting a tolerance checkpoint within the germinal center.[36,37] Cross-reactive anti-dsDNA antibodies can also be elicited after immunization with EBNA-1, a major nuclear antigen of the Epstein–Barr virus, commonly linked to SLE.[38] Alternatively, immunogenic microbial or

viral DNA-binding proteins may complex with chromatin fragments from the host to induce the production of anti-dsDNA antibodies. This paradigm was demonstrated in non-autoimmune mice immunized with Fus1, a DNA-binding peptide from a *Trypanosoma cruzi* protein,[39] and in normal Balb/c mice expressing the polyomaviral T antigen[40] or immunized with the BK polyomavirus.[41] SLE patients are susceptible to high-titer polyomaviral infection, yet a causal relationship between dsDNA reactivity and polyomavirus in SLE patients is controversial.[42] Although anti-dsDNA responses elicited in the context of an infectious agent in a nonautoimmune host have been shown to be transient, SLE susceptibility genes may convert transient to persistent autoreactivity.

MECHANISMS OF INJURY IN THE KIDNEY AND BRAIN

Lupus nephritis is initiated by the deposition of anti-dsDNA antibodies in the kidney parenchyma, either by directly binding cross-reactive glomerular antigens or indirectly binding to nucleosomes or DNA trapped in the glomerular basement membrane. Factors that influence their pathogenicity in the kidney include fine specificity and isotype.[43,44] The detection of highly cationic anti-dsDNA antibodies in the serum of patients with active lupus nephritis, but not in patients without renal disease, and the demonstration that these antibodies bind heparan sulfate, a highly acidic polysaccharide expressed ubiquitously in the glomeruli basement membrane, supports the former mechanism.[45,46] Other cross-reactive antigens shown to mediate binding of anti-dsDNA antibodies to glomeruli include collagen IV, fibronectin, and laminin in the basement membrane, and α-actinin on mesangial cells.[47] However, other data suggest that anti-dsDNA antibodies deposit in the kidney by the indirect binding of immune complexes to renal tissue.[48] By vigorously removing nucleosomal material from anti-dsDNA antibodies using stringent purification methods, reactivity to heparin sulfate was also removed and binding to glomerular basement membrane was prevented.[49] In addition, cross-reactive anti-DNA antibodies have been observed exclusively within chromatin-rich electron dense structures in nephritic kidneys.[50] Thus, both the direct and indirect binding of immunoglobulin in the glomeruli are mechanisms through which pathogenic antibodies deposit in the kidneys of SLE patients. It is of interest that a study suggests that the kidney-infiltrating B cells are not the source of anti-DNA antibodies in patients; rather, they may be produced in lymphoid organs.[51]

Damage to kidney cells may occur through the internalization of anti-dsDNA antibodies, as a small number of mouse and human anti-DNA antibodies have been shown to penetrate the cell, and even the nucleus, bind to DNA, and alter cellular functions.[47] However, the majority of renal injury most likely occurs following immune complex deposition in the glomeruli and FcR-mediated cellular activation, the activation of complement, and the recruitment of infiltrating immune cells.

Neuropsychiatric manifestations in lupus are a major complication affecting over 50% of patients and frequently involve cognitive dysfunction and memory loss.[52] The discovery that the sequence of a peptide mimetope of dsDNA (DWEYS) is present in the extracellular domain of the NMDAR on neurons led to the identification of a subset of cross-reactive antibodies that can induce neuronal death in vitro and in vivo.[53] The NMDAR is an ionotropic glutamate receptor important for controlling synaptic plasticity and memory. Interestingly, anti-DNA, anti-NMDAR antibodies have been found in the cerebrospinal fluid of SLE patients and titers correlate with nonfocal neuropsychiatric symptoms.[54] Further studies demonstrated that upon breach of the blood–brain barrier in mice, the transfer of human serum from SLE patients with reactivity to DNA and NMDAR induced hippocampal-dependent memory impairment.[55] Ex vivo examination of synaptic signaling in hippocampal sections revealed that low concentrations of a cross-reactive mouse (R4A) or human (G11) anti-NMDAR monoclonal antibody amplify NMDAR-mediated signaling, preferentially binding to the NMDAR pore of an activated synapse, and presumably increasing the duration of the active state and increasing calcium influx.[56] High concentrations of the same antibodies promote excitotoxicity, which was measured by mitochondrial permeability transition (or mitochondrial collapse) on hippocampal sections.[56]

Human and mouse antibodies with reactivity to dsDNA and NMDAR were found to also bind C1q.[57] One important role of C1q is to clear immune complexes and apoptotic debris from the circulation. The ex vivo binding of monoclonal cross-reactive antibodies to DNAse-treated glomeruli suggested that the targeted antigen in the glomeruli could be C1q itself, rather than DNA.[57] This was confirmed by demonstrating that an intravenously administered, cross-reactive murine monoclonal antibody showed diminished deposition in kidneys of C1q-deficient mice.[57] Aside from targeting C1q in the kidney, anti-C1q antibodies may exacerbate systemic inflammation by removing soluble C1q from the circulation, attenuating its ability to suppress monocyte and dendritic cell (DC) activation and inflammatory cytokine and IFN production.[58,59]

IMMUNE COMPLEXES AND MYELOID CELL ACTIVATION

Immune complexes containing DNA play a crucial role in sustaining systemic inflammation in lupus by participating in an autoamplification feedback loop between the innate and adaptive immune response. IFNα is a key component

of innate immunity, and it has been associated with lupus in both humans and mouse models. The fundamental demonstration that purified anti-dsDNA antibodies from SLE sera, when complexed to unmethylated plasmid DNA, induced the production of IFNα by plasmacytoid DCs spurred new insight into IFNα production in SLE.[60,61] Subsequently, SLE sera were shown to have the capacity to induce the differentiation of monocytes from healthy donors into myeloid DCs that were capable of inducing the proliferation of autologous CD4+ T cells,[62] also mediated by TLR activation. The interaction of anti-dsDNA B cells with activated cognate T-helper cells would also increase the production of autoantibodies.[63] Moreover, IFNα itself can augment T-independent stimulation of B cells through mechanisms involving TLRs and B cell activating factor.

SUMMARY

Studies of anti-DNA antibodies continue to provide insight into SLE pathogenesis. Understanding the mechanisms responsible for their production in individual patients will advance precision medicine, and may yield an improved efficacy to toxicity ratio in therapeutic regimens.

REFERENCES

1. Cerutti A, Cols M, Puga I. Marginal zone B cells: virtues of innate-like antibody-producing lymphocytes. *Nat Rev Immunol* 2013;**13**:118–32.
2. Jacobi AM, Diamond B. Balancing diversity and tolerance: lessons from patients with systemic lupus erythematosus. *J Exp Med* 2005;**202**:41–4.
3. Sang A, Zheng YY, Morel L. Contributions of B cells to lupus pathogenesis. *Mol Immunol* 2014;**62**:329–38.
4. Liu Z, Zou YR, Davidson A. Plasma cells in systemic lupus erythematosus: the long and short of it all. *Eur J Immunol* 2011;**41**:588–91.
5. Schroeder K, Herrmann M, Winkler TH. The role of somatic hypermutation in the generation of pathogenic antibodies in SLE. *Autoimmunity* 2013;**46**:121–7.
6. Shlomchik MJ, Marshak-Rothstein A, Wolfowicz CB, Rothstein TL, Weigert MG. The role of clonal selection and somatic mutation in autoimmunity. *Nature* 1987;**328**:805–11.
7. Shlomchik M, et al. Anti-DNA antibodies from autoimmune mice arise by clonal expansion and somatic mutation. *J Exp Med* 1990;**171**:265–92.
8. Tillman DM, Jou NT, Hill RJ, Marion TN. Both IgM and IgG anti-DNA antibodies are the products of clonally selective B cell stimulation in (NZB x NZW)F1 mice. *J Exp Med* 1992;**176**:761–79.
9. Radic MZ, Weigert M. Genetic and structural evidence for antigen selection of anti-DNA antibodies. *Annu Rev Immunol* 1994;**12**:487–520.
10. Rahman A, Giles I, Haley J, Isenberg D. Systematic analysis of sequences of anti-DNA antibodies–relevance to theories of origin and pathogenicity. *Lupus* 2002;**11**:807–23.
11. Wellmann U, et al. The evolution of human anti-double-stranded DNA autoantibodies. *Proc Natl Acad Sci USA* 2005;**102**:9258–63.
12. Zhang J, Jacobi AM, Wang T, Diamond B. Pathogenic autoantibodies in systemic lupus erythematosus are derived from both self-reactive and non-self-reactive B cells. *Mol Med* 2008;**14**:675–81.
13. Tsuiji M, et al. A checkpoint for autoreactivity in human IgM+ memory B cell development. *J Exp Med* 2006;**203**:393–400.

14. Zhang J, et al. Polyreactive autoantibodies in systemic lupus erythematosus have pathogenic potential. *J Autoimmun* 2009;**33**:270–4.

15. Rekvig OP. Anti-dsDNA antibodies as a classification criterion and a diagnostic marker for systemic lupus erythematosus: critical remarks. *Clin Exp Immunol* 2015;**179**:5–10.

16. Burlingame RW, Rubin RL, Balderas RS, Theofilopoulos AN. Genesis and evolution of antichromatin autoantibodies in murine lupus implicates T-dependent immunization with self antigen. *J Clin Invest* 1993;**91**:1687–96.

17. Laderach D, Koutouzov S, Bach JF, Yamamoto AM. Concomitant early appearance of anti-ribonucleoprotein and anti-nucleosome antibodies in lupus prone mice. *J Autoimmun* 2003;**20**:161–70.

18. Mohan C, Adams S, Stanik V, Datta SK. Nucleosome: a major immunogen for pathogenic autoantibody-inducing T cells of lupus. *J Exp Med* 1993;**177**:1367–81.

19. Kaliyaperumal A, Mohan C, Wu W, Datta SK. Nucleosomal peptide epitopes for nephritis-inducing T helper cells of murine lupus. *J Exp Med* 1996;**183**:2459–69.

20. Voll RE, et al. Histone-specific Th0 and Th1 clones derived from systemic lupus erythematosus patients induce double-stranded DNA antibody production. *Arthritis Rheum* 1997;**40**:2162–71.

21. Mehra S, Fritzler MJ. The spectrum of anti-chromatin/nucleosome autoantibodies: independent and interdependent biomarkers of disease. *J Immunol Res* 2014;**2014**:368274.

22. Munoz LE, Lauber K, Schiller M, Manfredi AA, Herrmann M. The role of defective clearance of apoptotic cells in systemic autoimmunity. *Nat Rev Rheumatol* 2010;**6**:280–9.

23. Shao WH, Cohen PL. Disturbances of apoptotic cell clearance in systemic lupus erythematosus. *Arthritis Res Ther* 2011;**13**:202.

24. Truedsson L, Bengtsson AA, Sturfelt G. Complement deficiencies and systemic lupus erythematosus. *Autoimmunity* 2007;**40**:560–6.

25. Cai Y, Zhang W, Xiong S. Mannose-binding lectin blunts macrophage polarization and ameliorates lupus nephritis. *PloS One* 2013;**8**:e62465.

26. Kelley JM, Edberg JC, Kimberly RP. Pathways: Strategies for susceptibility genes in SLE. *Autoimmun Rev* 2010;**9**:473–6.

27. Wermeling F, et al. Class A scavenger receptors regulate tolerance against apoptotic cells, and autoantibodies against these receptors are predictive of systemic lupus. *J Exp Med* 2007;**204**:2259–65.

28. Rogers NJ, et al. A defect in Marco expression contributes to systemic lupus erythematosus development via failure to clear apoptotic cells. *J Immunol* 2009;**182**:1982–90.

29. Cohen PL, et al. Delayed apoptotic cell clearance and lupus-like autoimmunity in mice lacking the c-mer membrane tyrosine kinase. *J Exp Med* 2002;**196**:135–40.

30. Yung S, Chan TM. The role of hyaluronan and CD44 in the pathogenesis of lupus nephritis. *Autoimmune Dis* 2012;**2012**:207190.

31. Hanayama R, et al. Autoimmune disease and impaired uptake of apoptotic cells in MFG-E8-deficient mice. *Science* 2004;**304**:1147–50.

32. Yamaguchi H, et al. Milk fat globule EGF factor 8 in the serum of human patients of systemic lupus erythematosus. *J Leukoc Biol* 2008;**83**:1300–7.

33. Yu Y, Su K. Neutrophil extracellular traps and systemic lupus erythematosus. *J Clin Cell Immunol* 2013;**4**.

34. Dye JR, Ullal AJ, Pisetsky DS. The role of microparticles in the pathogenesis of rheumatoid arthritis and systemic lupus erythematosus. *Scand J Immunol* 2013;**78**:140–8.

35. Diamond B, Scharff MD. Somatic mutation of the T15 heavy chain gives rise to an antibody with autoantibody specificity. *Proc Natl Acad Sci USA* 1984;**81**:5841–4.

36. Ray SK, Putterman C, Diamond B. Pathogenic autoantibodies are routinely generated during the response to foreign antigen: a paradigm for autoimmune disease. *Proc Natl Acad Sci USA* 1996;**93**:2019–24.

37. Kuo P, Bynoe M, Diamond B. Crossreactive B cells are present during a primary but not secondary response in BALB/c mice expressing a bcl-2 transgene. *Mol Immunol* 1999;**36**:471–9.

38. Yadav P, et al. Antibodies elicited in response to EBNA-1 may crossreact with dsDNA. *PloS One* 2011;**6**:e14488.

39. Desai DD, Krishnan MR, Swindle JT, Marion TN. Antigen-specific induction of antibodies against native mammalian DNA in nonautoimmune mice. *J Immunol* 1993;**151**:1614–26.

40. Moens U, et al. In vivo expression of a single viral DNA-binding protein generates systemic lupus erythematosus-related autoimmunity to double-stranded DNA and histones. *Proc Natl Acad Sci USA* 1995;**92**:12393–7.

41. Rekvig OP, et al. Molecular analyses of anti-DNA antibodies induced by polyomavirus BK in BALB/c mice. *Scand J Immunol* 1995;**41**:593–602.

42. Rianthavorn P, Posuwan N, Payungporn S, Theamboonlers A, Poovorawan Y. Polyomavirus reactivation in pediatric patients with systemic lupus erythematosus. *Tohoku J Exp Med* 2012;**228**:197–204.

43. Krishnan MR, Wang C, Marion TN. Anti-DNA autoantibodies initiate experimental lupus nephritis by binding directly to the glomerular basement membrane in mice. *Kidney Int* 2012;**82**:184–92.

44. Doria A, Gatto M. Nephritogenic-antinephritogenic antibody network in lupus glomerulonephritis. *Lupus* 2012;**21**:1492–6.

45. Kohro-Kawata J, Wang P, Kawata Y, Matsuzaki M, Nakamura K. Highly cationic anti-DNA antibodies in patients with lupus nephritis analyzed by two-dimensional electrophoresis and immunoblotting. *Electrophoresis* 1998;**19**:1511–5.

46. Suzuki N, Harada T, Mizushima Y, Sakane T. Possible pathogenic role of cationic anti-DNA autoantibodies in the development of nephritis in patients with systemic lupus erythematosus. *J Immunol* 1993;**151**:1128–36.

47. Yung S, Chan TM. Anti-DNA antibodies in the pathogenesis of lupus nephritis–the emerging mechanisms. *Autoimmun Rev* 2008;**7**:317–21.

48. Seredkina N, Van Der Vlag J, Berden J, Mortensen E, Rekvig OP. Lupus nephritis: enigmas, conflicting models and an emerging concept. *Mol Med* 2013;**19**:161–9.

49. van Bavel CC, van der Vlag J, Berden JH. Glomerular binding of anti-dsDNA autoantibodies: the dispute resolved? *Kidney Int* 2007;**71**:600–1.

50. Mjelle JE, Rekvig OP, Van Der Vlag J, Fenton KA. Nephritogenic antibodies bind in glomeruli through interaction with exposed chromatin fragments and not with renal cross-reactive antigens. *Autoimmunity* 2011;**44**:373–83.

51. Kinloch AJ, et al. Vimentin is a dominant target of in situ humoral immunity in human lupus tubulointerstitial nephritis. *Arthritis Rheumatol* 2014;**66**:3359–70.

52. Lauvsnes MB, Omdal R. Systemic lupus erythematosus, the brain, and anti-NR2 antibodies. *J Neurol* 2012;**259**:622–9.

53. DeGiorgio LA, et al. A subset of lupus anti-DNA antibodies crossreacts with the NR2 glutamate receptor in systemic lupus erythematosus. *Nat Med* 2001;**7**:1189–93.

54. Yoshio T, Onda K, Nara H, Minota S. Association of IgG anti-NR2 glutamate receptor antibodies in cerebrospinal fluid with neuropsychiatric systemic lupus erythematosus. *Arthritis Rheum* 2006;**54**:675–8.

55. Kowal C, et al. Human lupus autoantibodies against NMDA receptors mediate cognitive impairment. *Proc Natl Acad Sci USA* 2006;**103**: 19854–9.

56. Faust TW, et al. Neurotoxic lupus autoantibodies alter brain function through two distinct mechanisms. *Proc Natl Acad Sci USA* 2010; **107**:18569–74.

57. Franchin G, et al. Anti-DNA antibodies cross-react with C1q. *J Autoimmun* 2013;**44**:34–9.

58. Son M, Santiago-Schwarz F, Al-Abed Y, Diamond B. C1q limits dendritic cell differentiation and activation by engaging LAIR-1. *Proc Natl Acad Sci USA* 2012;**109**:E3160–7.

59. Son M, Diamond B. C1q-Mediated repression of human monocytes is regulated by leukocyte-associated Ig-like receptor 1 (LAIR-1). *Mol Med* 2015;**20**:559–68.

60. Vallin H, Perers A, Alm GV, Ronnblom L. Anti-double-stranded DNA antibodies and immunostimulatory plasmid DNA in combination mimic the endogenous IFN-alpha inducer in systemic lupus erythematosus. *J Immunol* 1999;**163**:6306–13.

61. Vallin H, Blomberg S, Alm GV, Cederblad B, Ronnblom L. Patients with systemic lupus erythematosus (SLE) have a circulating inducer of interferon-alpha (IFN-alpha) production acting on leucocytes resembling immature dendritic cells. *Clin Exp Immunol* 1999;**115**:196–202.

62. Blanco P, Palucka AK, Gill M, Pascual V, Banchereau J. Induction of dendritic cell differentiation by IFN-alpha in systemic lupus erythematosus. *Science* 2001;**294**:1540–3.

63. Liu Z, et al. Interferon-alpha accelerates murine systemic lupus erythematosus in a T cell-dependent manner. *Arthritis Rheum* 2011;**63**: 219–29.

Chapter 25

Antihistone and Antispliceosome Antibodies

Minoru Satoh[1,2,3], Marvin J. Fritzler[4], Edward K.L. Chan[5]

[1]Department of Clinical Nursing, University of Occupational and Environmental Health, Japan, Kitakyushu, Fukuoka, Japan; [2]Department of Medicine, University of Florida, Gainesville, FL, USA; [3]Department of Pathology, Immunology, and Laboratory Medicine, University of Florida, Gainesville, FL, USA; [4]Department of Biochemistry and Molecular Biology, Cumming School of Medicine, University of Calgary, Calgary, AB, Canada; [5]Department of Oral Biology, University of Florida, Gainesville, FL, USA

List of Abbreviations

ANA Antinuclear antibody
DID Double immunodiffusion
DIL Drug-induced lupus
ELISA Enzyme-linked immunosorbent assay
ENA Extractable nuclear antigens
MCTD Mixed connective tissue disease
PHA Passive hemagglutination
snRNA U-rich small nuclear RNAs
snRNP Small nuclear ribonucleoprotein
UCTD Undifferntiated connective tissue disease

Autoantibodies directed against intracellular antigens are characteristic features of systemic lupus erythematosus (SLE) and other systemic autoimmune diseases. Studies have provided strong evidence that autoantibodies are produced by antigen-driven responses and they can be reporters from the immune system, revealing the identity of antigens involved in the pathognomonic mechanism. Some of these autoantibodies serve as disease-specific markers and are directed against intracellular macromolecular complexes or particles such as nucleosomes, small nuclear ribonucleoproteins (snRNPs), and Ro and La cytoplasmic ribonucleoproteins (RNPs). This chapter discusses the finer specificity of these autoantibodies.

ANTIHISTONE ANTIBODIES

The identification of lupus erythematosus (LE) cell phenomenon by Hargraves et al.[1] led to the recognition of autoimmune reactivity as a major feature of SLE. The LE cell phenomenon—which was based on the observation that cellular components released during cell death (particularly nuclei) can be phagocytosed by neutrophils in the milieu of certain plasma factors—is a classic immunoassay that was included in the previous criterion for classification of SLE.[2]

Subsequent studies showed that antibodies to histones were a key requirement for the LE cell phenomenon and they hold a distinguished position in the recognition of the autoimmune nature of SLE, which lead to the discovery of many other antinuclear antibodies (ANA). It was concluded from these early studies that autoantibodies to deoxyribonucleoprotein recognize histone–DNA complexes, and this specificity was directly related to the LE cell factor.

Histones are Key Protein Components of Chromatin

Histones are bound to genomic DNA and organized into a macromolecular complex referred to as native chromatin. In addition to DNA and histones, which constitute 80% of its mass, chromatin contains nonhistone proteins, many of which are also autoantibody targets in rheumatic diseases—proteins such as the centromere and high-mobility group proteins.[3] Histones and DNA constitute the repeat subunit of chromatin called the nucleosome, which consists of two molecules of each of the "core" histones—H2A, H2B, H3, and H4—forming an octamer, along with a histone H1 molecule and of approximately 200 base pairs of DNA. An artificial complex of the H2A-H2B dimer and DNA can be formed in vitro at physiological conditions. This (H2A-H2B)-DNA complex is an important antigenic target in patients with SLE and drug-induced lupus (DIL).

Assays for Antihistone Antibodies

In SLE, most autoantibodies to the histone-DNA complexes can be detected as a homogeneous or diffuse indirect immunofluorescence staining pattern of the nuclei and the condensed mitotic chromatin (Figure 1(A)). A similar pattern is also seen with other autoantibodies, notably those directed

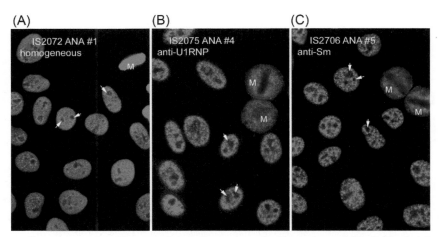

FIGURE 1 **Indirect immunofluorescence of antihistone and antispliceosome antibodies on human HEp-2 cells.** Staining patterns of standard sera from the Centers for Disease Control and Prevention (CDC) IS2072 for anti-DNA homogeneous pattern (A), IS2075 anti-U1RNP (B), and IS2076 anti-Sm (C). *HEp-2 substrate was obtained from INOVA Diagnostics, Inc., San Diego (CA, USA). M, mitotic cell; arrows, nucleoli. Original magnification 400×. Note that variations in staining patterns may depend on HEp-2 cell substrates (manufacturer and lot).*

against dsDNA. This pattern must be discriminated from the dense fine speckled pattern which also stains interphase nuclei and metaphase chromatin and is the hallmark of autoantibodies to DFS70/LEDGF antigens. Sera with antibodies to certain histone classes (e.g., H1, H3, H4) or hidden determinants (cryptotopes) on native or denatured histones may show a weak or even negative ANA; thus, more specific assays employing purified analytes are preferable.

Solid Phase Enzyme-Linked Immunosorbent Assays for Antihistone Antibodies

Enzyme-linked immunosorbent assays (ELISAs) are often used to detect specific antihistone and antichromatin antibodies, and this platform can be adapted to measure reactivity to individual histones, macromolecular histone complexes, and chromatin. Most immunoassays for the detection of antihistone antibodies in the past two decades have relied on histones purified from various cells or tissues, such as calf thymus. Subnucleosome structures have also been adapted to ELISA formats, which allow measurement of autoantibodies requiring these higher-ordered structures.

Problems and Discrepancies in Measuring Antihistone Antibodies

There are many possible explanations for discrepancies in the literature on the prevalence and fine specificity of antihistone antibodies. The quality of histones used as antigens can be highly variable, and histones from commercial sources were often degraded or contaminated with nonhistone proteins. In addition, the propensity for histones to bind nascent DNA in serum and other biological fluids can result in artifacts, such as false-positive reactions with anti-DNA antibodies. Such factitious binding to histone/DNA complexes that are formed in vitro is a phenomenon that is generally indistinguishable

from bona fide antihistone antibody reaction.[4] DNA existing in serum in the form of mono- and oligonucleosomes may also have pathologic significance in that circulating nucleohistone binding to the negatively charged residues on heparin sulfate of the glomerular basement membrane may mediate the binding of DNA and anti-DNA antibodies to the glomerulus.

Antibodies to denatured purified histones detected by most immunoassays are common in systemic rheumatic diseases and appear to have limited value as specific diagnostic marker.[4] Other assays which use histone-DNA complexes, including LE cells, chromatin, soluble (H1-stripped) chromatin, (poly) nucleosomes, and (H2A-H2B)-DNA complexes would more likely be detecting reactivity to native autoepitopes. It is possible that in some immunoassays there is overlap of available epitopes in denatured histones and native (DNA-bound) histones; however, for the most part, autoantibodies directed to histones and to nucleosome-related antigens should be considered distinct and one cannot be substituted for the other. In the context of autoimmunity, the terms chromatin, nucleosome, and polynucleosome tend to be used interchangeably.[5]

Prevalence and Disease Association of Antihistone and Antinucleosome Antibodies

Reports of antihistone antibodies in various diseases are summarized in Table 1. Although antihistone antibodies have been observed in various rheumatic diseases, most studies have focused on SLE or DIL. Reported prevalence ranged from 17% to 95% in SLE and 67–100% in DIL.[4] Antihistone antibodies have also been consistently observed in rheumatoid arthritis and juvenile idiopathic arthritis. In some cases, a remarkably high prevalence was observed in other diseases, especially in primary biliary cirrhosis, autoimmune hepatitis, and ANA-positive neoplastic diseases.

In addition to the antibodies reactive with isolated histones, patients with up to ~75% lupus-like disorders

Antihistone in SLE

Studies on the association of antihistone antibodies with disease activity or severity, or with specific clinical features or organ involvement, have been inconsistent.[4] In recent years, studies that used nucleosome antigens have shown strong correlation with symptomatic SLE and a clinical specificity in such patients that was 95–99%. Antichromatin and anti-[(H2A-H2B)-DNA] antibodies were significantly correlated with glomerulonephritis and were more specific for this feature than anti-DNA. A higher prevalence and/or amount of antichromatin antibodies in SLE patients with kidney disease, progression to renal failure, or overall disease activity score have been reported, although association with disease activity was not seen in all studies (see Ref. 6 and references therein). Other studies have shown that nucleosomes can be found in the circulation due to aberrations during apoptosis and/or an ineffective clearance in SLE and during apoptosis, histones can be modified through acetylation and possibly other modifications, thereby possibly making them more immunogenic. While more definitive comparative studies are still required, current studies indicate that native nucleosomes are substantially better analytes for monitoring SLE than assays using purified histones, and many studies have concluded that antinucleosome antibodies are a better biomarker for SLE than anti-DNA, although this concept has been challenged.[7]

Antihistone in Drug-Induced Lupus

Histone-reactive antibodies have been reported in 50–100% of patients with DIL (Table 1), depending on the drug and the assay employed. The drugs most commonly implicated in DIL include procainamide, hydralazine, quinidine, and isoniazid; however, these drugs are currently rarely used, except isoniazid, and a variety of other drugs have been implicated as well. However, most patients who are treated with procainamide and other lupus-inducing drugs eventually develop antihistone antibodies, even though symptomatic disease occurs in only 10–20% of patients. Thus, most antihistone antibodies in this clinical setting are apparently relatively benign, consistent with the seemingly innocuous occurrence of histone-reactive antibodies in many rheumatic and nonrheumatic diseases (Table 1). However, examination of their class and fine specificity has revealed that antihistone antibodies in asymptomatic patients are predominantly IgM and display broad reactivity with all the individual histones. In contrast, patients with symptomatic DIL develop predominantly IgG antihistone antibodies that display pronounced reactivity with the H2A-H2B complex, especially when bound to DNA. In fact, anti-(H2A-H2B) has been observed to precede overt clinical symptoms and therefore may have predictive as well as diagnostic value. Anti-(H2A-H2B) has a sensitivity approaching 100% and a specificity of >90% for symptomatic procainamide-induced lupus compared to asymptomatic procainamide-treated

TABLE 1 Prevalence of Antihistone/Antinucleosome Antibodies in Human Diseases

Disease/Syndrome[a]	Prevalence[b]
Rheumatic Diseases	
SLE	24–95%
Drug-induced lupus	50–100%
Drug-induced ANA	22–95%
Rheumatoid arthritis	0–80%
Vasculitis	31–75%
Felty's syndrome	79%
Juvenile chronic arthritis	42–75%
Mixed connective tissue disease	45–90%
Sjögren's syndrome	8–67%
Systemic sclerosis	23–67%
Polymyositis/dermatomyositis	17%
Other Diseases	
Primary biliary cirrhosis	50–81%
Hepatic cirrhosis/autoimmune hepatitis	35–50%
Inflammatory bowel disease/ulcerative colitis	13–15%
Neoplastic diseases	14–79%

[a]Modified from Fritzler and Rubin.[4]
[b]Prevalence of elevated IgG and/or IgM antibody to total histone or to at least one histone class.

commonly have autoantibodies to chromatin (nucleosomes). In this context, it is important to appreciate that antinucleosome and anti-dsDNA responses appear to be particularly sensitive to corticosteroid therapy. Other studies from various geographic regions reported 38–86% sensitivity of antinucleosome antibodies in SLE. Most patients with lupus induced by procainamide, penicillamine, isoniazid, acebutolol, methyldopa, timolol, and sulfasalazine also have antinucleosome antibodies, predominately reactive with the (H2A-H2B)-DNA complex. Several groups reported antinucleosome antibodies in almost half the patients with autoimmune hepatitis. Antinucleosome antibodies have also been reported in 25–50% of patients with SSc (systemic sclerosis, scleroderma), but the specificity of these antibodies may be different from bona fide antichromatin antibodies as discussed below. A high prevalence of antinucleosome antibodies have generally not been reported in other rheumatic diseases and are remarkably lower in healthy cohorts, resulting in an overall sensitivity for SLE of 63% and when compared to other rheumatic diseases, a specificity for SLE of 95%.[5]

patients and an even higher specificity when an (H2A-H2B)-DNA complex is used as the screening antigen.

A convincing argument that chromatin drives the bulk of the histone-reactive antibody response in SLE and most DIL can be made from the data that compare the antigenicity of various forms of histones. Antibodies from patients with SLE and DIL as well as antibodies from murine lupus bound prominently to a structural epitope in the (H2A-H2B)-DNA complex. Antibodies in some patients with SLE also bound native DNA and (H3-H4)$_2$-DNA, but reactivity with individual histones was much lower. In murine lupus, antibodies to (H2A-H2B)-DNA were found early in disease, before antibodies to native DNA and (H3-H4)$_2$-DNA arose. Absorption with chromatin removed most of the antibody reactivity to subnucleosome structures, indicating that regions buried in chromatin were not antigenic in SLE, DIL, or murine lupus. Thus, antihistone antibodies in SLE can be most readily explained by autoimmunization with native chromatin accompanied by sequential loss of tolerance first to the (H2A-H2B)-DNA region and then to (H3-H4)$_2$-DNA and native DNA. Loss of immune tolerance to epitopes on DNA-free histones, which can be considered "denatured histones," and to "denatured DNA" (and to other nuclear antigens) may accompany the immune dysregulation associated with lupus-related disorders; however, because of the complexity of these epitopes and the heterogeneity of this immune response, only with nucleosome-reactive antibodies can a strong case be made for the putative in vivo existence of a chromatin-like immunogen.[4] More recent evidence links the antichromatin response to the release of DNA neutrophil extracellular traps (NETs).[8]

ANTISPLICEOSOME ANTIBODIES

The major autoantigens in spliceosome are snRNP and autoantibodies to snRNPs have been a focus of research and clinical immunological studies related to autoantibodies in rheumatic diseases for over three decades. Anti-Sm antibodies, identified over 40 years ago, were one of the first described to target nonhistone proteins in systemic autoimmune rheumatic diseases. Anti-Sm antibodies are highly specific (>90%) markers for SLE, although the prevalence in SLE is 5–30%. The Sm antigen was defined as proteins bound to U-rich small nuclear RNAs (snRNAs) and these autoantibodies have served as useful probes to help investigate the molecular and cellular functions of the spliceosome, which is responsible for pre-mRNA splicing of heterogeneous nuclear RNA to mature messenger RNA (mRNA). In this section, we discuss the major classes of autoantibodies to snRNP including anti-Sm (Smith), anti-U1RNP (also known as anti-nRNP), anti-U1/U2RNP, and briefly review minor autoantibodies to other classes of UsnRNPs, such as LSm (Like Sm) proteins.

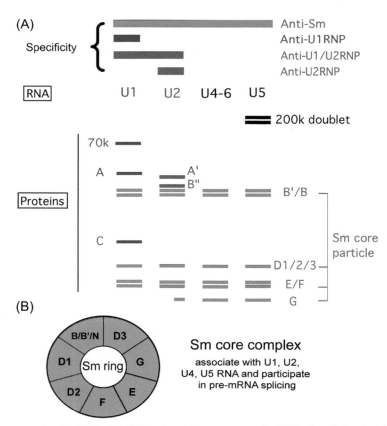

FIGURE 2   **Structure and components of snRNPs.** (A) RNA and protein components of snRNPs. Specificity of anti-Sm (red), -U1RNP (blue), -U1/U2RNP, and -U2RNP (green), and RNA and protein components of each snRNP are shown. (B) Components of Sm ring. Seven-member Sm ring has structural similarity to a doughnut. The center of the structure is involved in binding to single-stranded RNA.

Cellular Localization and Function of snRNP

Components of snRNPs. snRNPs are classified by association with specific snRNAs including the most abundant U1, U2, U4, U5, and U6 RNAs (Figure 2(A)). U6snRNP uses one of the LSm rings, which are structurally similar to the Sm ring, as its core complex (Figure 2(B)). Each snRNP is an RNA-protein macromolecule of corresponding UsnRNA complexed with several proteins. Common anti-snRNPs autoantibodies are classified into anti-U1RNP that recognize U1snRNPs and anti-Sm that recognize U1, U2, U4-6, and U5 snRNPs (Figure 2(A), see specificity). The Sm core proteins B or B' (27/28 kDa), D1/D2/D3 (14 kDa), E (12 kDa), F (11 kDa), and G (9 kDa), which are organized as seven-member ring structures (Figure 2(B), Sm ring, Sm core particle) are shared by U1, U2, U4/U6, and U5 snRNPs. Because these shared Sm core proteins are recognized by anti-Sm antibodies, U1, U2, U4/U6, and U5 snRNAs are immunoprecipitated by anti-Sm antibodies versus only U1RNA immunoprecipitated by anti-U1RNP antibodies (Figure 2(A)).

In addition to the Sm core particle, each snRNP is associated with several unique proteins. U1snRNPs (U1RNP) has U1snRNP specific proteins U1-70k (68/70kD), A (33kD), and C (22kD). U2snRNP has two unique proteins, U2-A' and B''. U4/U6snRNP and U5snRNP have several unique proteins in addition to the Sm core particle that are not included in Figure 2(A), except the U5-200kD doublet.

Reactivity of Anti-snRNPs Autoantibodies

Following immunoprecipitation (IP) using sera with anti-snRNP autoantibodies, RNA and protein components can be analyzed (Figure 3). U1RNA is seen in anti-U1RNP immunoprecipitates (lane U1RNP), while U1, U2, U4, U5, and U6 RNAs are detectable with anti-Sm serum (lane Sm, Figure 3(A)). Protein components are usually analyzed by IP using ^{35}S-methionine labeled cell extract (Figure 3(B)).

To identify which proteins are directly recognized, western blot using affinity-purified snRNPs is the standard method. Anti-U1RNP sera frequently react with U1-70k, A, B'/B, and less frequently with C, in various combination

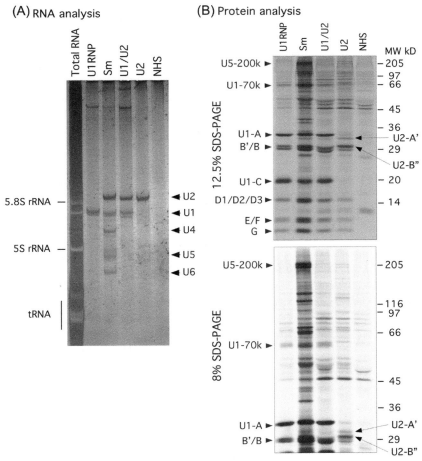

FIGURE 3 **Immunoprecipitation using anti-snRNPs antibodies.** A. RNA components immunoprecipitated from cell extract by human sera were extracted, run on urea-polyacrylamide gel, and identified by silver staining. B. snRNP associated proteins metabolically radiolabeled with ^{35}S-methionine were immunoprecipitated from cell extracts of K562 cells by human autoimmune sera and fractionated by 12.5% or 8% SDS-polyacrylamide gel electrophoresis (SDS-PAGE) and visualized by autoradiography.

of reactivity. Anti-Sm antibodies react with Sm-B′/B and D1/D2/D3 proteins. Because virtually all human anti-Sm sera also have anti-U1RNP antibodies, reactivity with U1 unique proteins are also seen in anti-Sm positive sera. In contrast to short linear epitopes for T-cells, classic characteristic of autoimmune B-cell epitopes are discontinuous conformational epitopes as shown within each polypeptide of the snRNPs.[9] In addition, autoantibodies that recognize the conformational structure of the multiprotein complexes, possibly quaternary structure, have been described, including EFG complex[10] and U1-C-Sm core particle.[11] Autoantibodies to LSm4 and LSm complex also were reported.[12]

History of Detection of Autoantibodies to snRNPs and Potential Problems

Our understanding of the difference in reactivity of anti-U1RNP versus anti-Sm is incomplete, and changes in technology further complicate the issue. Assay technologies started with Ouchterlony double immunodiffusion (DID) followed by passive hemagglutination (PHA), IP detection of UsnRNA and protein components, western blot detection of reactivity to individual protein components, eventually evolving to line immunoassays (LIA), ELISA, addressable laser bead immunoassays (ALBIA), chemiluminescence immunoassay (CIA), and other multiplexed immunoassays. The source of antigens (analytes) used in various immunoassays also has been changed; antigens have spanned the spectrum from calf or rabbit thymus extract to human cell lines and recombinant proteins.

Historically, DID was one of the first assays used to detect anti-Sm reactivity. Anti-U1RNP was originally reported as anti-Mo that recognizes soluble nuclear ribonucleoprotein (nRNP) and makes a distinctive precipitin line from anti-Sm in DID. At about the same time, the same group of specificities (anti-snRNPs) were reported as anti-ENA that was based on a classification into RNase sensitive anti-ENA (correspond to anti-U1RNP) and RNase-resistant anti-ENA (correspond to anti-Sm). After this period, the source of antigens used for immunoassays had gradually shifted from calf or rabbit thymus tissues to human culture cell lines and recombinant human proteins. This was paralleled by a switch in ANA substrates from cryopreserved animal tissue to human culture cell lines such as HEp-2 (laryngeal cancer).

Detection of Antibodies to snRNPs in Clinical Practice

Antibodies to U1RNP and anti-Sm are autoantibody specificities that show a typical nuclear speckled pattern in ANA by immunofluorescence (Figure 1(B) and (C)). There are many other autoantibody specificities that show a similar ANA pattern but, certainly, anti-U1RNP and Sm are specificities that should be considered when the nuclear speckled pattern is observed. The titer of ANA is often very high,

1:1280 or even higher, particularly in patients with overlapping features of SLE, SSc, PM/DM—referred to as mixed connective tissue diseases (MCTD)—as well as in certain SLE or undifferentiated connective tissue disease (UCTD).

To confirm anti-U1RNP, -Sm specificities, a commonly used assay in the diagnostic laboratory is ELISA using recombinant or affinity purified antigens. Although ELISA will identify the majority of true positives, it may be troubled by a significant percentage of false positives, in particular anti-Sm.[13] Improved sensitivity of the anti-U1RNP ELISA using recombinant U1-70k, A, and C proteins was accomplished by adding U1RNA, via the formation of new epitopes resulted from interaction of U1RNA with the proteins antigens.[14] Other improvements in ELISA were the use of symmetric dimethylarginine modified Sm-D derived peptide to detect anti-Sm antibodies[15] based on earlier studies indicating the importance of this posttranslational modification in anti-Sm antibody reactivity.

DID was the original method to detect and define the anti-U1RNP and Sm specificities, but it was less commonly used after the 1990s. With the recent emergence of large, high-throughput laboratories, the emphasis has shifted to assays, such as ELISA and ALBIA, which can be automated, effecting cost savings and rapid turnaround times.[16] More recently, LIA, which is similar to dot blot immunoassay but contains multiple autoantigens individually printed on membrane strips, has been adopted by some laboratories. Other new types of assays include ALBIA, in which individual antigens are covalently bound to beads of different composition. Advantages of these assays include the detection of multiple autoantibodies in a single assay and the requirement for only small amounts (typically $10\,\mu l$) of serum sample.

Clinical Significance of Antibodies to snRNPs

Distribution and Coexistence of Anti-U1RNP and Anti-Sm Antibodies. Although anti-U1RNP and Sm often coexist, there are major differences in clinical significance of these two specificities. Anti-Sm antibodies are highly specific for the diagnosis of SLE, whereas anti-U1RNP can be found in patients with various diagnoses, particularly MCTD, as well as unclassified conditions, such as UCTD, and is not specific for SLE (Figure 4). The prevalence of anti-U1RNP in UCTD is 6–22% while anti-Sm is only 1–3%.[17]

Anti-U1RNP and anti-Sm antibodies have a unique interrelationship. Virtually all anti-Sm positive patients also have anti-U1RNP, with anti-Sm alone rarely found. However, only a fraction of patients with anti-U1RNP have anti-Sm antibodies. In SLE, usually 25–40% of anti-U1RNP positive patients have anti-Sm. This ratio (anti-Sm/anti-U1RNP) becomes much lower when all anti-U1RNP positive cases are analyzed because anti-U1RNP can be seen in diseases other than SLE and unclassified conditions (Figure 4).

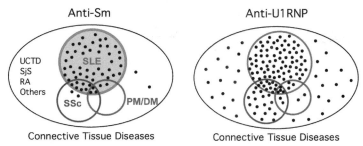

FIGURE 4   **Distribution patterns of anti-Sm versus U1RNP in patients with connective tissue diseases.** Typical distribution pattern of anti-Sm versus anti-U1RNP in SLE, SSc, PM/DM, and other connective tissue diseases is illustrated. Data are only to illustrate the trend and not based on actual numbers from two reports.[13]

Clinical Association of Anti-Sm and U1RNP Antibodies. Anti-Sm is highly specific for the diagnosis of SLE and is one of the most established and widely utilized disease marker antibodies. It is under the immunologic criteria, along with anti-dsDNA and anti-phospholipid antibodies, in the SLICC Classification system for SLE.[18] Many anti-Sm positive patients have typical SLE; however, anti-Sm is often seen in patients with SLE-overlap syndromes, which also have features of SSc and/or PM/DM (Figure 4) and some of them have more than one disease marker antibody. Because the production of specific autoantibodies usually precedes the development of typical clinical manifestation,[19] a small number of patients may not meet the classification criteria for SLE. In contrast, although anti-U1RNP antibodies are common in SLE patients, they can be found in SSc, PM/DM, Sjögren's syndrome and other conditions, and were associated with certain clinical manifestations such as Raynaud's phenomenon, swollen hand, sausage-like fingers, leukopenia, regardless of the diagnosis. Although, by definition, virtually all patients with MCTD are positive for anti-U1RNP antibodies, they are not a specific biomarker for MCTD. Why different clinical diagnosis and features are associated with anti-U1RNP versus anti-Sm, with both recognizing closely related UsnRNPs, is not known.

The clinical association and significance of anti-U1RNP and anti-Sm described above appears to be consistent regardless of ethnicity and certain other demographic variables; however, studies on detailed clinical association are more inconsistent. The reasons may be due to the differences in immunoassays used, genetic and environmental backgrounds of patients, focus and methods in clinical analysis, as well as treatment and follow-up.

The fact that most anti-Sm positive sera are also positive for anti-U1RNP makes anti-U1RNP antibodies a major confounding factor in clinical analysis. The only practical option to analyze the clinical associations of anti-Sm may be an analysis of anti-Sm+U1RNP versus anti-U1RNP cohorts. Similarly, clinical associations and immunological cross-reactivity of anti-Sm with anti-ribosomal P or with anti-dsDNA may also bias the data on clinical associations of anti-Sm. This might be part of the reason why clinical manifestations associated with anti-Sm were also associated with either anti-U1RNP or

anti-dsDNA antibodies. Some reports suggested that the titers of anti-Sm antibodies correlate with the disease activity, milder renal and central nervous involvement, or late-onset renal disease, but these findings are controversial.[20]

A clinical concept of MCTD characterized by overlapping features of SLE, SSc, and PM/DM was proposed. MCTD has a high prevalence of Raynaud's phenomenon, edema of the fingers, arthritis/arthralgia, myositis, serositis, favorable response to steroid treatment, and a relative absence of renal disease. Although early studies emphasized a good prognosis of MCTD, long-term follow-up studies reported premature death in a subset of patients. Pulmonary hypertension and interstitial lung disease are particularly known as life-threatening comorbidities associated with anti-U1RNP antibodies.[21]

When anti-U1RNP antibodies are present alone in high titer, patients often present with typical features of MCTD; however, anti-U1RNP antibodies are also detected in other systemic rheumatic diseases. Because of the clinical relevance of the titers observed in systemic rheumatic diseases, consideration of the levels of antibodies may be important because patients with high levels of anti-U1RNP antibodies tend to have more typical features of classical MCTD.

Some SLE and MCTD sera bind most of the snRNP polypeptides, whereas others bind to little, if any, U1-70k or C polypeptides. The observed high frequency of anti-U1-70k antibodies in MCTD has been supported in several studies and reported to be as high as 76–95% in MCTD, while the range of reactivity in SLE is 8–50%, although the frequency is highly variable. It has been suggested that the presence of anti-U1-70k is primarily associated with classical features of MCTD, such as Raynaud's phenomenon, esophageal dysmotility, and myositis, and it is a negative indicator for the presence of renal disease. Although antibodies to the U1-70k, A, or C protein quantitatively vary during the disease course, there is little evidence that they correlate with disease activity or that they are involved in disease pathogenesis.

An association of the presence of anti-U1RNP in cerebrospinal fluid (CSF) and increased anti-U1RNP index [(CSF anti-U1RNP/serum anti-U1RNP)/(CSF IgG/serum IgG)] with neuropsychiatric symptoms in SLE and MCTD patients has been reported.[22] Anti-U1RNP antibodies in

CSF also were correlated with increased interferon-α and MCP-1 in CSF.[23] These observations suggest intrathecal production of anti-U1RNP antibodies and the possible role of anti-U1RNP antibodies in neuropsychiatric symptoms.

Other Anti-snRNPs Antibodies

Anti-U1/U2RNP antibodies were reported in patients with overlapping feature of SLE, SSc, and/or PM/DM. Antibodies to U4/U6RNP, U5RNP, and trimethylguanosine cap structure of UsnRNA that recognize U1-U5RNAs were also reported in some cases. Antibodies to UsnRNPs were originally thought to target only protein components; however, later studies showed that patients with autoantibodies to snRNPs often (35–38%) have antibodies directed to U1RNA.

Immunologic Characteristics of Anti-U1RNP and Sm Antibodies

Anti-U1RNP and Sm antibodies have been associated with hypergammaglobulinemia, with reported levels up to 20–30%, 8.6 mg/ml, of the total IgG, in striking contrast to relatively low concentrations of anti-dsDNA antibodies, 1–3 μg/ml. It has been emphasized in early studies that the titers of anti-U1RNP do not fluctuate significantly over time. Although this is true for many patients with MCTD, the levels of anti-U1RNP antibodies may not be as stable as originally believed, particularly in SLE patients. This issue was revisited recently because of the new concept of autoantibody production by short-lived plasmablasts in lymphoid tissue versus long-lived plasma cells in bone marrow[24] and of B-cell depleting therapy using rituximab.[25] B-cell depletion dramatically reduced the levels of anti-dsDNA antibodies but did not affect the levels of anti-U1RNP, Sm, Ro, and La, or total immunoglobulin levels.[25] These data are consistent with the interpretation that anti-U1RNP and Sm antibodies are mainly produced by long-lived plasma cells and may explain their relatively stable production.

Mechanism of Production

Despite various hypothesis and observations, the mechanisms of production of autoantibodies in SLE, and in particular the mechanism of selection of the target antigens, are incompletely understood. Different mechanism may play a role in breaking tolerance, spreading epitopes, and sustaining autoantibody production. Molecular mimicry may be a trigger, while intermolecular-intrastructural help mechanisms may be responsible for the epitope spreading. Apoptosis, microbody release, and Toll-like receptor (TLR) stimulation are also likely key factors in these processes. Thus, the actual mechanism is likely multifactorial and, to a certain extent, specific to individual patients based on genotype, environment, and epigenetic factors.

Production of anti-snRNPs antibodies in murine models of SLE appears to be dependent on IFN-γ, IL-12, and type I IFN (I-IFN). Levels of I-IFN inducible genes Mx1 and others were higher in patients with autoantibodies to U1RNP/Sm versus patients without antibodies to RNA-protein complex,[26,27] suggesting the association between I-IFN production and anti-U1RNP/Sm antibodies. However, it is not known whether high I-IFN in these patients is responsible for anti-snRNPs antibody production or if this is a result of I-IFN induction by anti-snRNPs immune complex. Studies indicate that anti-U1RNP immune complexes can be internalized via Fc receptor and released U1RNA stimulate TLR-7 to induce I-IFN.[28]

REFERENCES

1. Hargraves MM, Richmond H, Morton R. Presentation of two bone marrow elements: the "Tart" cell and the "L.E." cell. *Proc Staff Mtg Mayo Clin* 1948;**23**:25–8.
2. Tan EM, Cohen AS, Fries JF, Masi AT, McShane DJ, Rothfield NF, et al. The 1982 revised criteria for the classification of systemic lupus erythematosus. *Arthritis Rheum* 1982;**25**:1271–7.
3. Fritzler MJ, Chan EKL, Lahita RG. *Antibodies to nonhistone antigens in systemic lupus erythematosus. Systemic lupus Erythematosus.* San Diego: Elsevier Academic Press; 2004. pp.348–76.
4. Fritzler MJ, Rubin RL. Antibodies to histones and nucleosome-related antigens. In: Wallace DJ, Hahn BH, editors. *Dubois' lupus erythematosus.* Philadelphia (PA): Lippincott Williams & Wilkins; 2007. pp. 464–86.
5. Burlingame RW. Recent advances in understanding the clinical utility and underlying cause of antinucleosome (antichromatin) autoantibodies. *Clin Appl Immunol Rev* 2004;**4**:351–66.
6. Stinton LM, Barr SG, Tibbles LA, Yilmaz S, Sar A, Benedikttson H, et al. Autoantibodies in lupus nephritis patients requiring renal transplantation. *Lupus* 2007;**16**:394–400.
7. Steiman AJ, Urowitz MB, Ibanez D, Li TT, Gladman DD, Wither J. Anti-dsDNA and Antichromatin Antibody Isotypes in Serologically active Clinically Quiescent Systemic Lupus Erythematosus. *J Rheumatol* March 1, 2015;**42**(5):810–6.
8. Mehra S, Fritzler MJ. The spectrum of anti-chromatin/nucleosome autoantibodies: independent and interdependent biomarkers of disease. *J Immunol Res* 2014;**2014**:368274.
9. Mahler M, Fritzler MJ. Epitope specificity and significance in systemic autoimmune diseases. *Ann NY Acad Sci* January 2010;**1183**:267–87.
10. Brahms H, Raker VA, van Venrooij WJ, Luhrmann R. A major, novel systemic lupus erythematosus autoantibody class recognizes the E, F, and G Sm snRNP proteins as an E-F-G complex but not in their denatured states. *Arthritis Rheum* April 1997;**40**:672–82.
11. Satoh M, Richards HB, Hamilton KJ, Reeves WH. Human antinuclear ribonucleoprotein antigen autoimmune sera contain a novel subset of autoantibodies that stabilizes the molecular interaction of U1RNP-C protein with the Sm core proteins. *J Immunol* 1997;**158**:5017–25.
12. Eystathioy T, Peebles CL, Hamel JC, Vaughn JH, Chan EKL. Autoantibody to hLSm4 and the heptameric LSm complex in anti-Sm sera. *Arthritis Rheum* March 2002;**46**:726–34.
13. Satoh M, Chan EKL, Sobel ES, Kimpel DL, Yamasaki Y, Narain S, et al. Clinical implication of autoantibodies in patients with systemic rheumatic diseases. *Expert Rev Clin Immunol* September 2007;**3**:721–38.

14. Murakami A, Kojima K, Ohya K, Imamura K, Takasaki Y. A new conformational epitope generated by the binding of recombinant 70-kd protein and U1 RNA to anti-U1 RNP autoantibodies in sera from patients with mixed connective tissue disease. *Arthritis Rheum* December 2002;**46**:3273–82.

15. Mahler M, Fritzler MJ, Bluthner M. Identification of a SmD3 epitope with a single symmetrical dimethylation of an arginine residue as a specific target of a subpopulation of anti-Sm antibodies. *Arthritis Res Ther* 2005;**7**:R19–29.

16. Fritzler MJ, Fritzler ML. Microbead-based technologies in diagnostic autoantibody detection. *Expert Opin Med Diagn* 2009;**3**:81–9.

17. Vaz CC, Couto M, Medeiros D, Miranda L, Costa J, Nero P, et al. Undifferentiated connective tissue disease: a seven-center cross-sectional study of 184 patients. *Clin Rheumatol* August 2009;**28**:915–21.

18. Petri M, Orbai AM, Alarcon GS, Gordon C, Merrill JT, Fortin PR, et al. Derivation and validation of the Systemic Lupus International Collaborating Clinics classification criteria for systemic lupus erythematosus. *Arthritis Rheum* August 2012;**64**:2677–86.

19. Arbuckle MR, McClain MT, Rubertone MV, Scofield RH, Dennis GJ, James JA, et al. Development of autoantibodies before the clinical onset of systemic lupus erythematosus. *N Engl J Med* October 16, 2003;**349**:1526–33.

20. Craft J. Antibodies to snRNPs in systemic lupus erythematosus. *Rheum Dis Clin North Am* 1992;**18**:311–35.

21. Lundberg IE. The prognosis of mixed connective tissue disease. *Rheum Dis Clin North Am* August 2005;**31**:535–47. vii-viii.

22. Sato T, Fujii T, Yokoyama T, Fujita Y, Imura Y, Yukawa N, et al. Anti-U1 RNP antibodies in cerebrospinal fluid are associated with central neuropsychiatric manifestations in systemic lupus erythematosus and mixed connective tissue disease. *Arthritis Rheum* December 2010;**62**:3730–40.

23. Yokoyama T, Fujii T, Kondo-Ishikawa S, Yamakawa N, Nakano M, Yukawa N, et al. Association between anti-U1 ribonucleoprotein antibodies and inflammatory mediators in cerebrospinal fluid of patients with neuropsychiatric systemic lupus erythematosus. *Lupus* February 3, 2014;**23**:635–42.

24. Manz RA, Hauser AE, Hiepe F, Radbruch A. Maintenance of serum antibody levels. *Annu Rev Immunol* 2005;**23**:367–86.

25. Cambridge G, Leandro MJ, Teodorescu M, Manson J, Rahman A, Isenberg DA, et al. B cell depletion therapy in systemic lupus erythematosus: effect on autoantibody and antimicrobial antibody profiles. *Arthritis Rheum* November 2006;**54**:3612–22.

26. Kirou KA, Lee C, George S, Louca K, Peterson MG, Crow MK. Activation of the interferon-alpha pathway identifies a subgroup of systemic lupus erythematosus patients with distinct serologic features and active disease. *Arthritis Rheum* May 2005;**52**:1491–503.

27. Zhuang H, Narain S, Sobel E, Lee PY, Nacionales DC, Kelly KM, et al. Association of anti-nucleoprotein autoantibodies with upregulation of Type I interferon-inducible gene transcripts and dendritic cell maturation in systemic lupus erythematosus. *Clin Immunol* December 2005;**117**:238–50.

28. Lee PY, Kumagai Y, Li Y, Takeuchi O, Yoshida H, Weinstein J, et al. TLR7-dependent and Fc{gamma}R-independent production of type I interferon in experimental mouse lupus. *J Exp Med* December 1, 2008;**205**:2995–3006.

Chapter 26

Immune Complexes in Systemic Lupus Erythematosus

Mark H. Wener

Departments of Laboratory Medicine & Medicine, University of Washington, Seattle, WA, USA

Antigen-antibody complexes (immune complexes (ICs)) are responsible for glomerulonephritis, vasculitis, and a variety of other systemic lupus erythematosus (SLE) manifestations. This traditional view of ICs implicates them as the cause of end-organ damage in lupus.[1] Increasingly, ICs are recognized for a regulatory role, interacting with Fc receptors (FcRs) and complement receptors on cells of the adaptive and innate immune system, and upregulating or modulating inflammatory pathways either directly (i.e., as an IC), or indirectly by enhancing cellular delivery of antigens such as RNA and DNA that then upregulate the immune response in lupus.

BASIC IMMUNOCHEMISTRY OF IMMUNE COMPLEXES: THE PRECIPITIN CURVE AND COMPLEMENT ACTIVATION

Adding increasing amounts of antigen to a constant amount of antibody demonstrates a bell-shaped *precipitin curve* with three general regions: the zone of antibody excess (pro-zone) on the left, the zone of equivalence in the middle, and the zone of antigen excess (post-zone) on the right. ICs formed in the zone of far antigen or antibody excess are relatively small and soluble. Large-lattice ICs containing immunoglobulin (Ig) G, formed at antigen–antibody ratios close to the zone of equivalence, tend to precipitate, and have multiple IgG Fc-regions available for interaction with C1q complement proteins, and therefore activate complement efficiently via the classical pathway.

C3 complement peptides may covalently bind to ICs and inhibit their lattice formation. Once immune precipitates are formed, their size can be reduced, leading to solubilization of preformed immunoprecipitates via activation of the alternative pathway of complement.[2] Activation of the classical pathway of complement can inhibit IC growth by preventing extended lattice formation. Thus, in the presence of complement, the precipitin curve can be more properly considered a precipitin surface (Figure 1). Higher concentrations of complement components or excess of antigen or antibody relative to the concentration ratio at the zone of equivalence leads to smaller ICs or reduced immune precipitation. Complement activation thus serves as a negative regulator of IC lattice extension.

IMMUNE COMPLEXES AND END-ORGAN DAMAGE

Active renal SLE is associated with high serum concentrations of anti-double-stranded DNA (antidsDNA) antibodies, and enrichment of anti-DNA within glomerular eluates of patients with SLE, supporting the role of anti-DNA in the pathogenesis of SLE. DNA-anti-DNA ICs are central in the pathogenesis of lupus nephritis.[1] Several investigators have found evidence for circulating DNA-anti-DNA ICs and other circulating ICs in SLE patients and experimental models.

Antibodies to the collagen-like region of C1q (anti-C1q) also are concentrated in the glomerular basement membranes of lupus patients.[3] Together with data demonstrating a strong association between lupus nephritis and serum levels of anti-C1q, these data strongly implicate anti-C1q in the pathogenesis of lupus nephritis. Anti-C1q tends to be present if there are multiple autoantibodies (including antidsDNA, antiSSA, antiSm, and/or others) present and enriched in glomerular basement membrane fragments from kidneys of patients with SLE, suggesting a role for anti-C1q in promoting aggregation of diverse ICs in the basement membrane.[4,5]

Immunoglobulins and complement components are detected in the walls of blood vessels with lupus vasculitis. Immunoglobulin deposits with a discontinuous, discrete, granular distribution are presumed to be caused by ICs. The granular pattern is seen in SLE, including in the microvasculature comprising the renal glomerulus, and

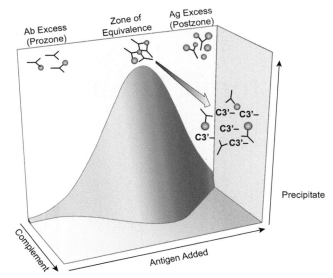

FIGURE 1 Immune complex precipitin curve or precipitin surface. Increasing amount of antigen added to a constant amount of antibody leads to increasing immune complex precipitation, until a maximum amount of precipitate is formed. At this ratio of antigen and antibody, the zone of equivalence, an extended lattice of immune complexes is formed based on optimum cross-linking of antigen epitopes and antibody binding sites. In the presence of complement, antigens and antibodies within immune complexes bind complement C3 fragments (**C3′**), preventing extension of nascent lattice formation or disrupting lattices, leading to smaller immune complexes. **Y** = antibody; ◯ = antigen.

small-vessel vasculitis contributes to glomerulonephritis and other pathologic lesions in SLE.

IMMUNE COMPLEXES AS INITIATORS AND REGULATOR OF THE AUTOIMMUNE RESPONSE

ICs are critical in causing tissue damage in SLE. ICs also initiate and enhance the immune dysregulation observed in SLE. They play a central role by harnessing the specificity of the acquired immune system (high-affinity autoantibodies) to augment the potent but less-specific inflammatory response of the innate immune response (Figure 2).

Dysfunctional overactivity of the type I interferon system is a central factor in SLE.[6] The trigger for type I interferon production by pDCs in response to infection is viral DNA and/or RNA, enhancing protection from infection. In lupus and related conditions, type I interferon enhances autoimmune responses. ICs composed of nucleic acids and IgG from SLE patients are potent inducers of type I interferon production by pDCs.[7] Both IgG and viral nucleic acids are required to achieve a maximum response, with IgG effects mediated via FcγRIIA.[8] The requirement for IgG (acting through FcR) as a costimulant for maximum interferon response is not unique to autoimmunity, since the optimum interferon response to virus

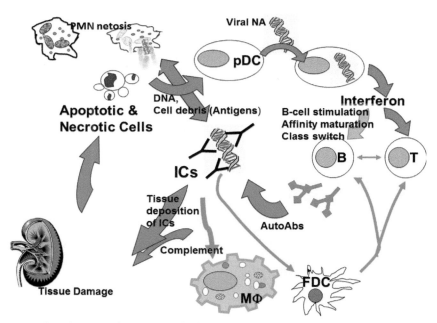

FIGURE 2 Role of immune complexes in augmenting and regulating immune response and causing tissue damage in SLE. Immune complexes deposit in target tissues and organs such as the kidney, activate complement, and lead to tissue damage including release of DNA, nuclear material, and cell debris as sources of antigens. Immune complexes are formed by nuclear protein and nucleic acid antigens (released by dysregulated cell apoptosis, necrosis, and neutrophil netosis) that combine with antibodies directed against those antigens. Antinuclear antibodies also combine with DNA and RNA from viruses and other exogenous sources of activating DNA. Facilitated by Fcγ receptor binding of immune complexes, activating DNA and RNA bind to TLRs and markedly upregulate production of type I interferon by pDCs, a central feature of the altered inflammatory and immune milieu in SLE. Type I pDCs secrete cytokines which activate B-cells and T-cells, increasing the immune response. In germinal centers, immune complexes interact with FDCs, also augmenting the response of T-cells and B-cells (green arrows). Activated B- and T-lymphocytes together lead to production of inflammatory cytokines, high levels of high-affinity autoantibodies, and generation of a mature autoimmune response. Fc and complement receptors on macrophages and other phagocytic cells remove immune complexes, and help to downregulate the immune complex-mediated inflammatory processes. pDC = plasmacytoid dendritic cell. FDC = follicular dendritic cells.

also requires IgG and Fcγ receptors.[9] Internalization of the ICs is mediated by Fcγ receptors, and the internalized nucleic acid then binds to toll-like receptors (TLRs) including TLR 9. ICs binding to germinal center follicular dendritic cells (FDC) facilitates antigen presentation by FDCs and thereby promotes the ability of FDCs to interact with B cells and cause affinity maturation and class switching. It has been proposed that IC-bearing FDCs may be required for development of high-affinity IgG antibodies, including anti-DNA.[10]

Increasingly, neutrophil netosis has been implicated in the pathogenesis of lupus. The extensive pericellular mesh of decondensed DNA with associated neutrophil granule proteins and trapped microbes could provide antigens to promote immune responses to autoantigens. ICs promote neutrophil netosis by binding to neutrophil FcRs.[11]

C1q binding and activation of complement modulates the regulatory effect of ICs. For example, complement proteins bound to ICs tend to promote immune adherence and clearance by mononuclear phagocytes, but ICs in the absence of the early complement components tend to bind to dendritic cells and promote an interferon signature.[12,13] Not only does the presence of C1q direct ICs towards mononuclear phagocytes and away from DCs, but C1q also inhibits PDC production of interferon alpha induced by RNA-containing ICs, DNA, and herpes simplex virus.[14] Furthermore, antibodies to C1q, which are associated with lupus and particularly with proliferative lupus nephritis, could impair the C1q-mediated clearance.[15] ICs also enhance development of lymph node lymphatic vessels, by stimulating production of vascular endothelial growth factor A.[16] Of interest, the inflammatory response to ICs may be modulated by cholinergic stimulation either directly or through the nervous system.[17]

ICs interact with a variety of cells via the cellular FcRs. The FcRs for IgG (FcγRs) differ in their avidity to bind monomeric IgG versus ICs, differ in their relative avidity for IgG subclasses, differ in their cellular distribution, and differ in function (Table 1). Binding of ICs to most FcRs has an activating role via the immunoreceptor tyrosine-based activation motif in the cytoplasmic domain of the multichain receptor. As shown in Table 1, these activation effects are present in many immune and inflammatory cells, including B and T cells in adaptive immunity, and dendritic cells, macrophages, natural killer (NK) cells, and neutrophils of the innate immune system. The corresponding inhibitory motif leads to inhibition mediated via FcγRIIB, which is particularly important for B cells.

Genetic studies of patients with lupus support the importance of complement and FcR function in SLE (reviewed in Chapter 20).[18] Genetically determined deficiency in complement proteins (complete deficiency of C1q, copy number variants of C2 and C4) are strongly linked to SLE. Polymorphisms in Fcγ receptors, in complement receptor CR2 and in C3 receptors (CD11b or ITGAM), associated

with relatively decreased IC clearance are linked to SLE. A common coding variant in ITGAM, which forms half of the heterodimeric complement receptor 3 (CR3), is associated with SLE and has been shown to impair CR3-mediated phagocytosis.[19] The strongest single gene genetic linkage with SLE is C1q deficiency, which leads to SLE in over 90% of patients affected, probably because of defects in clearance of apoptotic cells and ICs.

Interactions between ICs and FcRs are influenced by the glycosylation of the immunoglobulin proteins. Glycosylated Fc region of the immunoglobulin models interferes with the interaction between conventional FcRs and IgG in ICs. In contrast, lectin receptors, by binding to immunoglobulin glycoproteins via their glycosylation sites, provide another type of cellular receptor for immunoglobulins. It has been suggested that immunoglobulins binding to lectin receptors such as DC-SIGN on cells provide a downregulatory mechanism for ICs.[20]

The interaction of ICs with FcRs and with complement proteins and complement receptors plays a multifaceted role, with a variety of diverse and interacting functions. Antibodies recognizing autoantigens and a myriad of exogenous antigens provide the specificity for antigen/ligand interaction with proteins of the complement system and with cells of adaptive and innate/inflammatory immune system. Because FcRs and complement proteins and complement receptors have both activating and inhibitory functions, and because the antigen within the IC also influences the upregulation and downregulation of the immune response, the regulatory role of ICs is dynamic and dependent on multiple interactions. This complex situation, with the presence of positive as well as negative feedback regulation, may help explain why lupus can dramatically flare after relatively minor environmental triggers.

IMMUNE COMPLEX CLEARANCE AND LOCALIZATION

The mononuclear phagocyte system plays the central role in removing ICs from the circulation, with clearance mediated by families of Fc and complement receptors on mononuclear phagocytes, neutrophils, and other cells. The presence of C3 receptors on primate erythrocytes provides an IC removal and transfer mechanism.[21,22] ICs that had activated complement and bound C3 in the circulation bind to the complement receptor CR1 on the erythrocyte, which are transported to the liver and spleen while bound to the red cell, where those ICs are phagocytized by cells of the mononuclear phagocyte system via Fc and complement receptors. Although phagocytosis of an entire IC-covered cell may take place, in some situations ICs are removed with portions of the adjacent cell membrane while leaving the remainder of the cell intact—a process termed trogocytosis.[23]

In experimental models, administration of preformed ICs into the blood results in mesangial and subendothelial

TABLE 1 Fcγ Receptors

Class	FcγRI (CD64)	Canonical Fcγ Receptors					Other Potential Fcγ Receptors
		FcγRII (CD32)			FcγRIII (CD16)		C-Type Lectin (Preferential Binding to Sialylated Fc)
	FcγRI	FcγRIIa	FcγRIIb	FcγRIIc	FcγRIIIa	FcγRIIIb	DC-SIGN
Name	FcγRI	FcγRIIa	FcγRIIb	FcγRIIc	FcγRIIIa	FcγRIIIb	DC-SIGN
Gene	FCGR1A	FCGR2A	FCGR2B	FCGR2C	FCGR3A	FCGR3b	CD209
SLE genetics linkage		SNP	SNP	SNP, CNV	SNP	SNP, CNV	
Monomeric IgG avidity	High	Low	Low	Low	Intermediate	Low	Intermediate
IgG subclass avidity	1=3>4>>2	3~1>2>>4 polymorphic 1>>3>4>2	3~1>4>>2		3>1>4>2	1=3>>>2,4	Sialylated IgG
Activate/inhibit	A	A	I	A	A	A	I
DCs	+	+	+		(+)		+
Macrophages	+				+		+ (some)
PMNs	+ (induced)	+				+	
B cells			+				
Myeloid		+	+				
T cells					+ (γ/δ T cells)		
NK cells				+	+		
Monocytes	+	+			+ (some)		+
Endothelium							+
Platelets		+					

Canonical Fcγ receptors and alternative lectin IgG receptor implicated in immune complex homeostasis, clearance, and regulation of the immune response.
Genetic linkages in population studies linked to either single nucleotide polymorphisms (SNPs), some of which have established functional associations, or copy number variants (CNV).
DC-SIGN (**D**endritic **C**ell-**S**pecific **I**ntercellular adhesion molecule-3-**G**rabbing **N**on-integrin) is a lectin (i.e., a ligand for carbohydrates). It has been proposed as a cellular receptor for glycosylated immunoglobulins, which may facilitate an immunomodulatory role for immune complexes. A theory suggesting that therapeutic intravenous gamma globulin may be mediated by glycosylated IgG has been controversial (Pincetic,[20] Schoenfeld).
Adapted from Refs. 18,20,38.

localization of ICs within renal glomeruli. ICs that form in situ within the kidney tend to localize in the subepithelial region of glomeruli.[24] Formation of complexes in situ occurs because of direct binding of antigens or antibodies, initially because of interaction between the circulating molecule and structures within the kidney. Once deposited in tissues, ICs cause inflammation. Complement-mediated injury is the dominant mechanism responsible.

Deposition of antigens or antibodies could be augmented or facilitated also by antigen-specific receptors within the tissues. ICs containing DNA may be removed in part by DNA receptors.[25]

AUTOANTIBODIES TO THE COLLAGEN-LIKE REGION OF C1q

Antibodies to C1q also augment aggregation of ICs in tissues. AntiC1q antibodies are found in association with lupus nephritis, and are less commonly demonstrable in serum of patients with nonrenal lupus.[26] Rising concentrations of IgG antiC1q generally are associated with flares of lupus nephritis, and high levels of antiC1q are associated with proliferative forms of lupus glomerulonephritis and active disease.[27] Antibodies to the collagen-like region of C1q are present and enriched in the glomeruli of many patients with lupus and are associated with proliferative lupus nephritis.[3] Antibodies to C1q play a pathogenic role in the proliferative forms of lupus nephritis.

By binding to different molecules of C1q which have bound to ICs composed of different antigen–antibody systems, antibodies to C1q promote aggregation of those different types of ICs, leading to larger, more persistent, and more pathogenic immune deposits. AntiC1q tends to be found in lupus kidneys when multiple autoantibodies are identified in the kidney, supporting the idea that antiC1q could be promoting the aggregation of different antigen–antibody systems. A murine model employing monoclonal antimurine C1q has demonstrated that antiC1q contributes to the pathogenesis of experimental glomerulonephritis only if C1q-containing ICs have already deposited in the kidney.[4] Thus, antiC1q augments pathogenic complement activation in the kidney, but by itself does not appear to be sufficient to cause glomerulonephritis.

TISSUE EFFECTS OF IMMUNE COMPLEXES

Once deposited in tissues, ICs cause inflammation. Complement-mediated injury is the dominant mechanism responsible. Clinically and experimentally, activation of complement can be demonstrated in serum, on blood cells, at tissue sites, in urine, and on circulating blood cells (where cell-bound complement activation products are found).[28] The well-known pro-inflammatory chemotactic role of complement fragments is believed to lead to recruitment of inflammatory cells into the lesion. IgG Fc receptors (FcγR) have an important role in mediating IC disease.

ICs themselves have a variety of other immunomodulatory effects. For example, binding of ICs to FcRs leads to aggregation of those receptors, triggering intracellular signaling pathways. ICs augment the responsiveness of both B cells and T cells to antigen stimulation.[29,30] Nucleic acid-containing ICs can augment activation of cells by engagement of TLRs, such as TLR9.[12] ICs can attract neutrophils to sites of inflammation, and also lead to neutrophil netosis (release of intracellular DNA forming antibacterial DNA nets) via neutrophil FcRIIA.[31]

DEVELOPMENT OF THERAPIES BASED ON IMMUNE COMPLEXES

Therapeutic approaches based on removing ICs, while plausible, are largely unproven. In extreme or refractory disease, plasmapheresis and immunoadsorption (e.g., with immunoglobulin-binding molecules such as staphylococcal protein A) have been used for treatment, with suggestive evidence that these treatments may be efficacious.[32] However, a controlled clinical trial of plasmapheresis in patients with lupus nephritis demonstrated no efficacy.[33]

An intriguing approach to targeted, specific immunotherapy has been proposed based on inhibition of pathogenic antigen–antibody binding by using small molecules, such as peptides, that preferentially bind the pathogenic antibody. This approach has been used to inhibit DNA–antiDNA antibody formation.[34] The antigen–antibody complexes formed by this approach are likely to be stable, small (because there is only one epitope per small molecule) and noninflammatory. The net effect is anti-inflammatory because formation of the more pro-inflammatory ICs are inhibited.

DETECTION OF IMMUNE COMPLEXES

Analyzing tissue biopsies using direct immunofluorescence microscopy, immunoglobulins, and complement components are routinely identified within vessels affected by IC forms of vasculitis and IC nephritis. The detection of these immune deposits depends in part on technical issues. Biopsy material ideally should be obtained from new, "fresh" lesions, because immune deposits are transient and may be undetectable in older lesions. A portion of tissue biopsies should be snap-frozen to prevent degradation of immune deposits. For some biopsies, such as small punch biopsies of skin, one specimen may be obtained for routine histology and a second obtained for freezing and immunofluorescence studies. Specimens should be sent to an experienced laboratory because background staining, specificity of antibodies, and other factors can influence interpretation of results.

Circulating ICs have been measured by a multitude of techniques, few of which are available.[35] For the clinician, probably the most important IC assay is the assay for cryoglobulins. The test for cryoglobulins is frequently inaccurate because of problems with specimen handling: blood should be allowed to remain at 37°C while clotting, and should be kept warm while the clot is centrifuged. Phlebotomists and laboratory personnel should be alerted to the suspected presence of cryoglobulins and should be reminded of the special handling requirements.

Autoantibodies to C1q can be measured by variations of the C1q solid-phase binding test for ICs.[27,36] Cell-bound complement activation products are a promising biomarker for complement activation in lupus, presumably reflecting the presence of ICs on and around cells in the circulation.[37]

SUMMARY

Inflammation caused by ICs in tissues remains the single most important mechanism for clinical manifestations of SLE, particularly for lupus nephritis. While substantial progress is being made investigating genetic contributions to clearance mechanisms of ICs, questions remain about the site and mechanism of IC formation and about factors that influence localization and pathogenicity at different sites. Although the role of anti-DNA as a contributor to lupus IC disease has been studied, the role of other antibodies (e.g., those directed to nucleoprotein complexes, C1q, and phospholipids) as constituents of ICs remains another relatively unexplored area of investigation. The role of complement and FcR activation in the pathogenesis of IC disease remains uncertain, in part because of their mixed inflammatory and anti-inflammatory potential. Although ICs are one of the fundamental causes of inflammation in autoimmune rheumatic diseases, many mysteries remain concerning their pathophysiology.

REFERENCES

1. Koffler D, Agnello V, Thoburn R, Kunkel HG. Systemic lupus erythematosus: prototype of immune complex nephritis in man. *J Exp Med* 1971;**134**:169s–79s.
2. Takahashi M, Czop J, Ferreira A, Nussenzweig V. Mechanism of solubilization of immune aggregates by complement. Implications for immunopathology. *Transpl Rev* 1976;**32**:121–39.
3. Mannik M, Wener MH. Deposition of anitbodies to the collagen-like region of C1q in renal glomeruli of patients with proliferative lupus glomerulonephritis. *Arthritis Rheum* 1997;**40**:1504–11.
4. Trouw LA, Groeneveld TW, Seelen MA, Duijs JM, Bajema IM, Prins FA, et al. Anti-C1q autoantibodies deposit in glomeruli but are only pathogenic in combination with glomerular C1q-containing immune complexes. *J Clin Invest* September 2004;**114**(5):679–88.
5. Mannik M, Merrill CE, Stamps LD, Wener MH. Multiple autoantibodies form the glomerular immune deposits in patients with systemic lupus erythematosus. *J Rheumatol* July 2003;**30**(7):1495–504.
6. Baechler EC, Gregersen PK, Behrens TW. The emerging role of interferon in human systemic lupus erythematosus. *Curr Opin Immunol* December 2004;**16**(6):801–7.
7. Lovgren T, Eloranta ML, Kastner B, Wahren-Herlenius M, Alm GV, Ronnblom L. Induction of interferon-alpha by immune complexes or liposomes containing systemic lupus erythematosus autoantigen- and Sjogren's syndrome autoantigen-associated RNA. *Arthritis Rheum* June 2006;**54**(6):1917–27.
8. Bave U, Magnusson M, Eloranta ML, Perers A, Alm GV, Ronnblom L. Fc gamma RIIa is expressed on natural IFN-alpha-producing cells (plasmacytoid dendritic cells) and is required for the IFN-alpha production induced by apoptotic cells combined with lupus IgG. *J Immunol* September 15, 2003;**171**(6):3296–302.
9. Palmer P, Charley B, Rombaut B, Daeron M, Lebon P. Antibody-dependent induction of type I interferons by poliovirus in human mononuclear blood cells requires the type II fcgamma receptor (CD32). *Virology* December 5, 2000;**278**(1):86–94.
10. Aydar Y, Sukumar S, Szakal AK, Tew JG. The influence of immune complex-bearing follicular dendritic cells on the IgM response, Ig class switching, and production of high affinity IgG. *J Immunol* May 1, 2005;**174**(9):5358–66.
11. Behnen M, Leschczyk C, Moller S, Batel T, Klinger M, Solbach W, et al. Immobilized immune complexes induce neutrophil extracellular trap release by human neutrophil granulocytes via FcγRIIIB and Mac-1. *J Immunol* August 15, 2014;**193**(4):1954–65.
12. Elkon KB, Santer DM. Complement, interferon and lupus. *Curr Opin Immunol* December 2012;**24**(6):665–70.
13. Santer DM, Wiedeman AE, Teal TH, Ghosh P, Elkon KB. Plasmacytoid dendritic cells and C1q differentially regulate inflammatory gene induction by lupus immune complexes. *J Immunol* January 15, 2012;**188**(2):902–15.
14. Lood C, Gullstrand B, Truedsson L, Olin AI, Alm GV, Ronnblom L, et al. C1q inhibits immune complex-induced interferon-alpha production in plasmacytoid dendritic cells: a novel link between C1q deficiency and systemic lupus erythematosus pathogenesis. *Arthritis Rheum* October 2009;**60**(10):3081–90.
15. Pang Y, Yang XW, Song Y, Yu F, Zhao MH. Anti-C1q autoantibodies from active lupus nephritis patients could inhibit the clearance of apoptotic cells and complement classical pathway activation mediated by C1q in vitro. *Immunobiology* December 2014;**219**(12):980–9.
16. Clatworthy MR, Harford SK, Mathews RJ, Smith KG. FcγRIIb inhibits immune complex-induced VEGF-A production and intranodal lymphangiogenesis. *Proc Natl Acad Sci USA* December 16, 2014;**111**(50):17971–6.
17. Vukelic M, Qing X, Redecha P, Koo G, Salmon JE. Cholinergic receptors modulate immune complex-induced inflammation in vitro and in vivo. *J Immunol* August 15, 2013;**191**(4):1800–7.
18. Li X, Kimberly RP. Targeting the Fc receptor in autoimmune disease. *Expert Opin Ther Targets* March 2014;**18**(3):335–50.
19. Lee YH, Bae SC. Association between the functional ITGAM rs1143679 G/A polymorphism and systemic lupus erythematosus/lupus nephritis or rheumatoid arthritis: an update meta-analysis. *Rheumatol Int* May 2015;**35**(5):815–23.
20. Pincetic A, Bournazos S, DiLillo DJ, Maamary J, Wang TT, Dahan R, et al. Type I and type II Fc receptors regulate innate and adaptive immunity. *Nat Immunol* August 2014;**15**(8):707–16.
21. Kimberly RP, Edberg JC, Merriam LT, Clarkson SB, Unkeless JC, Taylor RP. In vivo handling of soluble complement fixing Ab/dsDNA immune complexes in chimpanzees. *J Clin Invest* September 1989;**84**(3):962–70.
22. Craig ML, Bankovich AJ, Taylor RP. Visualization of the transfer reaction: tracking immune complexes from erythrocyte complement receptor 1 to macrophages. *Clin Immunol* October 2002;**105**(1):36–47.

23. Taylor RP. Gnawing at Metchnikoff's paradigm. *Blood* October 24, 2013;**122**(17):2922–4.

24. Nangaku M, Couser WG. Mechanisms of immune-deposit formation and the mediation of immune renal injury. *Clin Exp Nephrol* September 2005;**9**(3):183–91.

25. Emlen W, Mannik M. Clearance of circulating DNA-anti-DNA immune complexes in mice. *J Exp Med* 1982;**155**:1210–5.

26. Trendelenburg M. Antibodies against C1q in patients with systemic lupus erythematosus. *Springer Semin Immunopathol* November 2005;**27**(3):276–85.

27. Akhter E, Burlingame RW, Seaman AL, Magder L, Petri M. Anti-C1q antibodies have higher correlation with flares of lupus nephritis than other serum markers. *Lupus* October 2011;**20**(12):1267–74.

28. Batal I, Liang K, Bastacky S, Kiss LP, McHale T, Wilson NL, et al. Prospective assessment of C4d deposits on circulating cells and renal tissues in lupus nephritis: a pilot study. *Lupus* January 2012;**21**(1): 13–26.

29. Marusic-Galesic S, Pavelic K, Pokric B. Cellular immune response to antigen administered as an immune complex. *Immunology* 1991;**72**: 526–31.

30. Chauhan AK, Moore TL. Immune complexes and late complement proteins trigger activation of Syk tyrosine kinase in human CD4(+) T cells. *Clin Exp Immunol* February 2012;**167**(2):235–45.

31. Chen K, Nishi H, Travers R, Tsuboi N, Martinod K, Wagner DD, et al. Endocytosis of soluble immune complexes leads to their clearance by FcγRIIIB but induces neutrophil extracellular traps via FcγRIIA in vivo. *Blood* November 22, 2012;**120**(22):4421–31.

32. Loo CY, Mohamed Said MS, Mohd R, Abdul Gafor AH, Saidin R, Halim NA, et al. Immunoadsorption and plasmapheresis are equally efficacious as adjunctive therapies for severe lupus nephritis. *Transfus Apher Sci* December 2010;**43**(3):335–40.

33. Lewis EJ, Hunsicker LG, Lan SP, Rohde RD, Lachin JM. A controlled trial of plasmapheresis therapy in severe lupus nephritis. The Lupus Nephritis Collaborative Study Group. *N Engl J Med* 1992;**326**:1373–9.

34. Bloom O, Cheng KF, He M, Papatheodorou A, Volpe BT, Diamond B, et al. Generation of a unique small molecule peptidomimetic that neutralizes lupus autoantibody activity. *Proc Natl Acad Sci USA* June 21, 2011;**108**(25):10255–9.

35. Lambert PH, Dixon FJ, Zubler RH, Agnello V, Cambiaso C, Casali P, et al. A WHO collaborative study for the evaluation of eighteen methods for detecting immune complexes in serum. *J Clin Lab Immunol* 1978;**1**:1–15.

36. Kohro-Kawata J, Wener MH, Mannik M. The effect of high salt concentration on detection of serum immune complexes and autoantibodies to C1q in patients with systemic lupus erythematosus. *J Rheumatol* 2002;**29**:84–9.

37. Putterman C, Furie R, Ramsey-Goldman R, Askanase A, Buyon J, Kalunian K, et al. Cell-bound complement activation products in systemic lupus erythematosus: comparison with anti-double-stranded DNA and standard complement measurements. *Lupus Sci Med* October 1, 2014;**1**(1):e000056. eCollection 2014.

38. Karsten CM, Kohl J. The immunoglobulin, IgG Fc receptor and complement triangle in autoimmune diseases. *Immunobiology* November 2012;**217**(11):1067–79.

Chapter 27

MicroRNA in Systemic Lupus Erythematosus

Bo Qu[1], Nan Shen[1,2,3]

[1]*Shanghai Institute of Rheumatology, Renji Hospital, Shanghai Jiao Tong University School of Medicine, Shanghai, China;* [2]*Institute of Health Sciences, Shanghai Institutes for Biological Sciences (SIBS) & Shanghai Jiao Tong University School of Medicine (SJTUSM), Chinese Academy of Sciences (CAS), Shanghai, China;* [3]*Division of Rheumatology, The Center for Autoimmune Genomics and Etiology (CAGE), Cincinnati Children's Hospital Medical Center, Cincinnati, OH, USA*

SUMMARY

MicroRNAs (miRNAs) are endogenous small noncoding RNAs that fine-tune cellular gene expression. There is compelling evidence showing that miRNAs can control immune cell development and regulate innate and adaptive immunity in physiological and pathological conditions. Abnormal miRNA expression occurs in many autoimmune diseases, including systemic lupus erythematosus (SLE). Many dysregulated miRNAs are involved in the immune abnormalities and major organ damage in SLE. Studies of miRNA expression in peripheral blood cells, body fluid, and target tissues of SLE patients have revealed unique miRNA signatures of SLE and its associated organ damage. These findings suggest that miRNAs could be used as specific biomarkers for diagnosing SLE and assessing disease activity. Here, we review our current knowledge about the cellular and molecular mechanisms that are possibly used by miRNAs in the pathogenesis of SLE, and the future applications of miRNAs as therapeutic targets in the management of SLE.

BIOLOGY OF miRNAs

Biogenesis of miRNAs

A large proportion of miRNA genes are located within the intronic regions of a genome, with a few located in exonic regions.[1] RNA polymerase II is responsible for the transcription of most miRNA genes.[2] After transcription, the primary transcripts of miRNA genes (pri-miRNA) undergo complex processing, the detailed steps of which are reviewed elsewhere.[3] Briefly, pri-miRNAs are cleaved by Drosha in the nucleus, and small hairpin RNAs (pre-miRNA) are released and exported to the cytoplasm by Exportin 5. In the cytoplasm, Dicer dices the pre-miRNA into a ~22-nt-long duplex RNA containing two mature miRNA strands. Finally, one of the two strands is incorporated into the RNA-induced silencing complex (RISC), which contains a member of the Argonaut (Ago) protein family as a functional core. The transcriptional regulation of the expression of miRNA confers them with cell-type-specific and spatiotemporal expression patterns. Because of their complicated maturation process, posttranscriptional regulation by accessory factors (e.g., DGCR8, DDX5, TRBP) in the miRNA processing pathway fine-tunes the exact expression level of miRNA in specific cells.

Function of miRNA

By base-pairing of their seed region to the 3′UTR of a target mRNA, in some cases the coding region of the target mRNA, mature miRNAs can direct RISC to its targets and thus destabilize or cause translational inhibition of mRNAs.[4] The nature of miRNA's targeting strategy endows each mature miRNA with the ability to target multiple different mRNAs. Furthermore, a particular mRNA can be bound by multiple miRNAs, which regulate the expression of this same gene expression in concert. Similar to miRNA biogenesis, the function of an miRNA can be affected by many protein factors[5] or the presence of regulatory circular RNAs.[6] Therefore, by fine-tuning gene expression, miRNAs function as key regulators in many physiological processes (e.g., cell proliferation and development) and pathogenic processes (e.g., tumorigenesis and cardiovascular diseases).[7–9] Many studies have also demonstrated that miRNAs play key regulatory roles in important immune pathways,[10] and abnormal expression or dysfunction of miRNAs was found to be responsible for many autoimmune diseases, including (SLE).[11,12]

Systemic Lupus Erythematosus. http://dx.doi.org/10.1016/B978-0-12-801917-7.00027-9

ROLE OF miRNAs IN SLE

The original discovery that linked the miRNA machinery to SLE was that certain autoantibodies in the sera of lupus patients can target epitopes of the key components of the miRNA pathway, such as GW182 and Ago2.[13] The miRNA expression profiles of lupus patients and mouse models revealed that miRNAs are relevant to the pathogenesis of SLE.[14,15] Investigations into the functions of abnormally expressed miRNAs have shed light on the mechanisms involved in the development of SLE (Figure 1).[16]

Genetic Risk Factors Associated with miRNAs in SLE

As a complex systemic autoimmune disease, many genetic factors that affect immune responses and end-organ damage have been found to contribute to the risk of developing SLE.[17] Several genetic susceptibility loci of SLE were reported to be functionally associated with miRNAs. For example, rs57095329, which is located in the promoter region of miR-146a, is enriched in SLE patients and contributes to the decreased expression of miR-146a, allowing overactivation of the Toll-like receptor (TLR) signaling pathway and excessive production of inflammatory cytokines.[18] Another genetic variant, rs2341697, was associated

with reduced miR-146a expression in European SLE patients, which emphasizes the importance of miR-146a in the pathogenesis of SLE.[19] MiR-3148 targets TLR7 by binding to its 3′UTR and a genetic variant in the 3′UTR of TLR7 was found to contribute to the overexpression of TLR7 in SLE.[20] Similarly, a single nucleotide polymorphism in the 3′UTR of SPI1, which affects its binding to miR-569, is associated with increased SPI1 expression and susceptibility to SLE.[21]

miRNAs in Innate Immunity of SLE

Innate immune cells are sentinels of our body. They use pattern recognition receptors (PRRs) to recognize dangerous signals from pathogens or damaged cells.[22] Ligand binding to PRRs triggers signaling cascades, activates downstream transcription factors, and leads to the secretion of inflammatory cytokines and upregulation of costimulatory molecules, amplifying inflammation and activating the adaptive immune response. Tight regulation of innate immune signaling keeps the host's immune responses under control and protects against autoimmune diseases.

Type I interferon is one of the most important proinflammatory cytokines involved in the development of SLE.[23] Because PRRs play key roles in the induction of type I interferon, their involvement in the pathogenesis

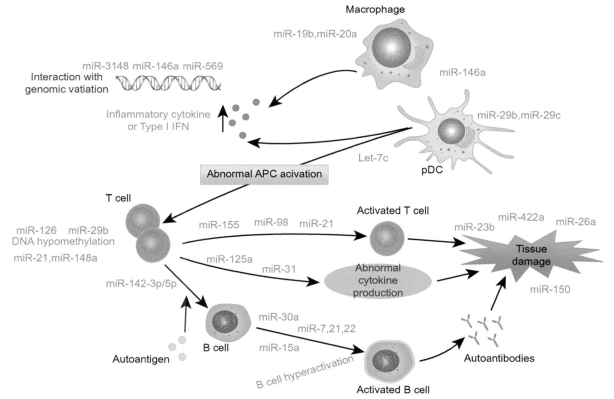

FIGURE 1   Selected miRNAs involved in SLE pathogenesis.

of SLE is well established.[24] Recent studies indicate that deficient elimination of cytosolic DNA by three prime repair exonuclease 1(TREX1) and subsequent chronic activation of the stimulator of interferon gene (STING)-dependent signaling pathway may contribute to type I interferon production in SLE.[25]

Several miRNAs were found to be essential in innate immunity and these regulatory mechanisms are involved in the abnormal activation of innate immunity in SLE.[26]

For example, MiR-146a can suppress NFκB activity and the production of proinflammatory cytokines by targeting multiple key molecules in the TLR or RIG-I signaling pathways in a negative feedback manner.[27,28] Subsequent studies have revealed that miR-146a is underexpressed in SLE,[29] and the identification of two new targets (STAT1 and IRF5) of miR-146a and the reverse correlation between its level and the expression of interferon-inducible genes and SLE disease activity indicates that miR-146a has a critical role in the pathogenesis of lupus.[29]

Numerous miRNAs contribute to different aspects of the abnormal innate immune responses in SLE. For example, elevated let-7c expression was found to be responsible for the proinflammatory phenotype (increased expression of MHCII and proinflammatory cytokines) of Blimp1-deficient DCs by inhibiting Blimp1 and SOCS1. Evidence for a similar regulatory mechanism and analogous phenotypic changes was also found in DCs obtained from lupus patients carrying the Blimp1 SLE-risk allele.[30] In addition, by targeting Mcl-1 and Bcl-2, miR-29b and miR-29c are possibly involved in TLR-inhibited glucocorticoid-induced plasmacytoid DC apoptosis in SLE.[31] Meanwhile, downregulation of miR-19b and miR-20a contributes to increased tissue factor expression and the hypercoagulable state in SLE patients.[32] Furthermore, recent studies have identified dynamic miRNA expression patterns during ALD-DNA-induced macrophage M2b polarization, indicating a crucial role of miRNA in controlling macrophage polarization in SLE.[33]

miRNAs in Adaptive Immunity of SLE

Adaptive immunity provides the host with antigen-specific protection against pathogens. Based on the fact that autoantibodies are elevated in SLE, it is recognized that overactivated T cells and B cells are important mediators of the pathogenesis of SLE.[34]

The genomic DNA of CD4+ T cells from SLE patients was demonstrated to be hypomethylated, which, from an epigenetic perspective, explains why there is excessive T-cell activation in SLE.[35,36] However, the exact mechanism underlying this hypomethylation is still unclear. Recent studies have shown that several miRNAs are involved in establishing this hypomethylated DNA status. In particular, miR-21 and miR-148a were found to be upregulated in

lupus CD4+ T cells and contributed to DNA hypomethylation of CD4+ T cells in SLE by targeting DNMT1.[37] Further studies found that, in addition to DNMT1, miR-21 can inhibit the RAS–MAPK–ERK signaling pathway upstream of DNMT1 in T cells. Two other miRNAs (miR-126 and miR-29b) were also reported to be upregulated in SLE CD4+ T cells, where they modulate DNA methylation by directly targeting DNMT1.[38,39] Taken together, these findings provide comprehensive insight into DNA hypomethylation of CD4+ T cells in SLE.

Altered expression of cytokines and chemokines in T cells has crucial roles in SLE. The expression of IL2, which has an indispensable role in peripheral maintenance of natural regulatory T cells,[40] is dramatically lower in T cells of SLE patients than those of normal people.[41] miR-31, which is underexpressed in SLE T cells, was responsible for impaired IL2 expression by targeting RhoA, a negative regulator of NFAT.[42,43] MiR-125a is significantly downregulated in PBMCs of SLE patients and is selectively expressed in T cells. It was reported that miR-125a plays an important role in the excessive secretion of CCL5 by SLE T cells by targeting KLF13, which might promote the infiltration of immune cells and lupus-associated tissue damage.[44]

miRNAs also participate in the overactivation of T cells in SLE. In addition to its role in regulating DNA methylation, miR-21 was found to target PDCD4 and enhance T-cell proliferation, IL10 production, CD40L expression, and the capacity to drive B-cell maturation in SLE.[45] MiR-142-3p and miR-142-5p were reported to be downregulated in SLE T cells, allowing enhanced translation of their target genes (i.e., SAP, CD84, and IL10), providing an alternative mechanism for the overactivated T-cell phenotype in SLE.[46]

In humans, elevated expression of miR-30a was reported to be responsible for the underexpression of Lyn and excessive production of IgG antibodies and B-cell proliferation in SLE.[47] Additionally, miR-7, miR-21, and miR-22, which can inhibit PTEN expression, were reported to be increased in SLE B cells, and may contribute to the abnormalities of SLE B cells.[48] The autoantibodies in lupus patients are high affinity, somatically mutated, and Ig-switched, indicating that there are defects in the germinal center (GC) response in SLE.[49] Transgenic mice that overexpress miRNAs within the miR-17~92 cluster developed lymphoproliferative disease and autoimmune symptoms, like SLE.[50] Additionally, miRNAs within the miR-17~92 cluster were shown to target PTEN and PHLPP2 to regulate follicular helper T-cell differentiation and its function in the GC response.[51,52] Another study demonstrated that elevated miR-15a was responsible for the defective differentiation of B10 cells, a regulatory B-cell subpopulation.[53] These findings indicate that miRNAs are extensively involved in B-cell abnormalities in SLE and more studies are needed to investigate the function of miRNAs in human SLE B cells.

miRNAs in Target Tissues of SLE

As a systemic autoimmune disease, SLE patients suffer from many types of organ damage, with lupus nephritis contributing most to SLE morbidity and mortality.[54] MiRNAs play important roles in renal physiology and pathology.[55] A comparison of renal biopsies showed marked differences in the expression of miRNAs between lupus nephritis and healthy controls.[56] In particular, miR-422a was reported to regulate kallikrein expression in renal tissues.[57] MiR-23b was reported to be underexpressed in the target tissues of patients with SLE or RA, and in corresponding mouse models.[58] MiR-23b can target TAB2, TAB3, and IKK-α to inhibit IL17, TNFα, or IL1β signaling. Thus decreased miR-23b expression enhances local inflammation and emphasizes that tissue resident cells are also important in organ damage processes. In specific cell types, let-7a, which is increased in mesangial cells of NZB/W F1 mice compared with age-matched NZW mice, was shown to promote IL6 production in these cells.[59] Additional studies suggested that let-7a might also contribute to hyperplasia and the pro-inflammatory responses in lupus nephritis.[60] In podocytes, miR-26a was reported to be decreased in lupus nephritis and that it regulates podocyte differentiation and cytoskeletal integrity.[61] Furthermore, the expression of miR-150 was found to be positively correlated with chronicity scores and the expression of profibrotic proteins. Also it was indicated that miR-150 mediated renal fibrosis in lupus nephritis by targeting SOCS1, as a downstream effector of TGFβ, in renal proximal tubular and mesangial cells.[62]

miRNAs as Biomarkers for SLE

Many reports have focused on the translational aspects of miRNAs in SLE. miRNA signatures were found to be associated with lupus nephritis.[63] Since the discovery of the differential expression of miRNAs in circulation between SLE patients and healthy controls or other autoimmune diseases,[64] miRNAs have been proposed to be an ideal biomarker for SLE. It was reported that circulating miRNAs were systematically altered and a signature of four miRNAs could be used to diagnose SLE, while another set of miRNAs was found to be associated with lupus nephritis.[65] Another study identified specific changes in urinary miRNA expression that were associated with lupus nephritis.[66] Recently, the differential miRNA expression between SLE patients with distinct autoantibodies was analyzed, which will help us to identify novel biomarkers for SLE.[67]

miRNAs as Therapeutic Targets for SLE

Another translational aspect of miRNA research in SLE is to explore the possibility of using miRNAs as therapeutic targets for SLE. Steroids and immunosuppressive drugs are the front-line treatment for SLE. They are effective but they frequently have serious side effects.[68] MiRNAs have been proposed to be potential therapeutic agents for many diseases, including SLE.[69,70] Some studies have shown that miR-98 and miR-155 are involved in the mechanisms by which glucocorticoids and methylprednisolone modulate immune responses.[71,72] MiR-155 was demonstrated to target CD62L and might promote the defects in the Treg cells in the MRL/lpr murine model of SLE.[73] As an important regulatory factor of B-cell effector functions and antibody production, miR-155 deficiency reduced autoantibody production and alleviated kidney inflammation in MRL/lpr lupus-prone mice.[74] Another study showed that application of a synthetic miR-155 antagomir to mice could ameliorate lupus-associated pulmonary hemorrhage induced by pristane.[75] Similar results are that in vivo silencing of miR-21 by seed-targeting LNA reversed splenomegaly, altered the CD4/CD8 T-cell ratio, and reduced Fas receptor-expressing lymphocyte populations.[76] Administration of miR-146a, an extensively studied miRNA, inhibited autoantibody production and enhanced resistance to hemorrhagic pulmonary capillaritis in lupus mouse models.[77,78] Although there are still issues to be addressed, particularly the identification of efficient chemical modifications and delivery approaches, we believe that miRNAs are still a promising choice as a therapeutic intervention for SLE in the future.

CONCLUSION

We are still in the early stage of exploring the essential roles of miRNAs in SLE.[79] We also need to conduct more comprehensive analyses of the miRNA expression patterns in patients and to obtain more knowledge about the function and regulation of miRNAs in SLE pathogenesis. Using such data, we will be able to develop novel biomarkers and therapeutic interventions.

REFERENCES

1. Rodriguez A, Griffiths-Jones S, Ashurst JL, Bradley A. Identification of mammalian microRNA host genes and transcription units. *Genome Res* 2004;**14**(10a):1902–10.
2. Lee Y, Kim M, Han J, Yeom KH, Lee S, Baek SH, et al. MicroRNA genes are transcribed by RNA polymerase II. *EMBO J* 2004;**23**(20):4051–60.
3. Ha M, Kim VN. Regulation of microRNA biogenesis. *Nat Rev Mol Cell Biol* 2014;**15**(8):509–24.
4. Bartel DP. MicroRNAs: target recognition and regulatory functions. *Cell* 2009;**136**(2):215–33.
5. Krol J, Loedige I, Filipowicz W. The widespread regulation of microRNA biogenesis, function and decay. *Nat Rev Genet* 2010;**11**(9):597–610.
6. Memczak S, Jens M, Elefsinioti A, Torti F, Krueger J, Rybak A, et al. Circular RNAs are a large class of animal RNAs with regulatory potency. *Nature* 2013. advance online publication.

7. Bushati N, Cohen SM. MicroRNA Functions. *Annu Rev Cell Dev Biol* 2007;**23**(1):175–205.

8. Croce CM. Causes and consequences of microRNA dysregulation in cancer. *Nat Rev Genet* 2009;**10**(10):704–14.

9. Condorelli G, Latronico MV, Cavarretta E. MicroRNAs in cardiovascular diseases: current knowledge and the road ahead. *J Am Coll Cardiol* 2014.

10. Baltimore D, Boldin MP, O'Connell RM, Rao DS, Taganov KD. MicroRNAs: new regulators of immune cell development and function. *Nat Immunol* 2008;**9**(8):839–45.

11. Hu R, O'Connell RM. MicroRNA control in the development of systemic autoimmunity. *Arthritis Res Ther* 2013;**15**(1).

12. Ceribelli A, Yao B, Dominguez-Gutierrez PR, Nahid MA, Satoh M, Chan EKL. MicroRNAs in systemic rheumatic diseases. *Arthritis Res Ther* 2011;**13**(4).

13. Pauley KM, Cha S, Chan EK. MicroRNA in autoimmunity and autoimmune diseases. *J Autoimmun* 2009;**32**(3):189–94.

14. Dai Y, Huang YS, Tang M, Lv TY, Hu CX, Tan YH, et al. Microarray analysis of microRNA expression in peripheral blood cells of systemic lupus erythematosus patients. *Lupus* 2007;**16**(12):939–46.

15. Dai R, Zhang Y, Khan D, Heid B, Caudell D, Crasta O, et al. Identification of a common lupus disease-associated microRNA expression pattern in three different murine models of lupus. *PLoS One* 2010;**5**(12):e14302.

16. Shen N, Liang D, Tang Y, de Vries N, Tak P-P. MicroRNAs-novel regulators of systemic lupus erythematosus pathogenesis. *Nat Rev Rheumatol* 2012;**8**(12):701–9.

17. Dai C, Deng Y, Quinlan A, Gaskin F, Tsao BP, Fu SM. Genetics of systemic lupus erythematosus: immune responses and end organ resistance to damage. *Curr Opin Immunol* 2014;**31**:87–96.

18. Luo X, Yang W, Ye D-Q, Cui H, Zhang Y, Hirankarn N, et al. A functional variant in microRNA-146a promoter modulates its expression and confers disease risk for systemic lupus erythematosus. *PLoS Genet* 2011;**7**(6):e1002128.

19. Lofgren SE, Frostegard J, Truedsson L, Pons-Estel BA, D'Alfonso S, Witte T, et al. Genetic association of miRNA-146a with systemic lupus erythematosus in Europeans through decreased expression of the gene. *Genes Immun* 2012;**13**(3):268–74.

20. Deng Y, Zhao J, Sakurai D, Kaufman KM, Edberg JC, Kimberly RP, et al. MicroRNA-3148 modulates allelic expression of toll-like receptor 7 variant associated with systemic lupus erythematosus. *PLoS Genet* 2013;**9**(2):e1003336.

21. Hikami K, Kawasaki A, Ito I, Koga M, Ito S, Hayashi T, et al. Association of a functional polymorphism in the 3'-untranslated region of SPI1 with systemic lupus erythematosus. *Arthritis Rheum* 2011;**63**(3):755–63.

22. Akira S, Uematsu S, Takeuchi O. Pathogen recognition and innate immunity. *Cell* 2006;**124**(4):783–801.

23. Banchereau J, Pascual V. Type I interferon in systemic lupus erythematosus and other autoimmune diseases. *Immunity* 2006;**25**:383–92.

24. Kontaki E, Boumpas DT. Innate immunity in systemic lupus erythematosus: sensing endogenous nucleic acids. *J Autoimmun* 2010;**35**(3):206–11.

25. Barber GN. STING-dependent cytosolic DNA sensing pathways. *Trends Immunol* 2014;**35**(2):88–93.

26. Luo X, Ranade K, Talker R, Jallal B, Shen N, Yao Y. MicroRNA-mediated regulation of innate immune response in rheumatic diseases. *Arthritis Res Ther* 2013;**15**(2):210.

27. Taganov KD, Boldin MP, Chang K-J, Baltimore D. NF-κB-dependent induction of microRNA miR-146, an inhibitor targeted to signaling proteins of innate immune responses. *Proc Natl Acad Sci* 2006;**103**(33):12481–6.

28. Hou J, Wang P, Lin L, Liu X, Ma F, An H, et al. MicroRNA-146a feedback inhibits RIG-I-dependent Type I IFN production in macrophages by targeting TRAF6, IRAK1, and IRAK2. *J Immunol* 2009;**183**(3):2150–8.

29. Tang Y, Luo X, Cui H, Ni X, Yuan M, Guo Y, et al. MicroRNA-146a contributes to abnormal activation of the type I interferon pathway in human lupus by targeting the key signaling proteins. *Arthritis Rheum* 2009;**60**(4):1065–75.

30. Kim SJ, Gregersen PK, Diamond B. Regulation of dendritic cell activation by microRNA let-7c and BLIMP1. *J Clin Invest* 2013;**123**(2):823–33.

31. Hong Y, Wu J, Zhao J, Wang H, Liu Y, Chen T, et al. miR-29b and miR-29c are involved in Toll-like receptor control of glucocorticoid-induced apoptosis in human plasmacytoid dendritic cells. *PLoS One* 2013;**8**(7).

32. Teruel R, Perez-Sanchez C, Corral J, Herranz MT, Perez-Andreu V, Saiz E, et al. Identification of miRNAs as potential modulators of tissue factor expression in patients with systemic lupus erythematosus and antiphospholipid syndrome. *J Thromb Haemost* 2011;**9**(10):1985–92.

33. Xiao P, Dong C, Yue Y, Xiong S. Dynamic expression of microRNAs in M2b polarized macrophages associated with systemic lupus erythematosus. *Gene* 2014;**547**(2):300–9.

34. Tsokos GC. Systemic lupus erythematosus. *N Engl J Med* 2011;**365**(22):2110–21.

35. Richardson B, Scheinbart L, Strahler J, Gross L, Hanash S, Johnson M. Evidence for impaired T cell DNA methylation in systemic lupus erythematosus and rheumatoid arthritis. *Arthritis Rheum* 1990;**33**(11):1665–73.

36. Zhao M, Liu S, Luo S, Wu H, Tang M, Cheng W, et al. DNA methylation and mRNA and microRNA expression of SLE CD4+T cells correlate with disease phenotype. *J Autoimmun* 2014;**54**:127–36.

37. Pan W, Zhu S, Yuan M, Cui H, Wang L, Luo X, et al. MicroRNA-21 and microRNA-148a contribute to DNA hypomethylation in lupus CD4+ T cells by directly and indirectly targeting DNA methyltransferase 1. *J Immunol* 2010;**184**(12):6773–81.

38. Zhao S, Wang Y, Liang Y, Zhao M, Long H, Ding S, et al. MicroRNA-126 regulates DNA methylation in CD4+ T cells and contributes to systemic lupus erythematosus by targeting DNA methyltransferase 1. *Arthritis Rheum* 2011;**63**(5):1376–86.

39. Qin H, Zhu X, Liang J, Wu J, Yang Y, Wang S, et al. MicroRNA-29b contributes to DNA hypomethylation of CD4+T cells in systemic lupus erythematosus by indirectly targeting DNA methyltransferase 1. *J Dermatol Sci* 2013;**69**(1):61–7.

40. Setoguchi R, Hori S, Takahashi T, Sakaguchi S. Homeostatic maintenance of natural Foxp3(+) CD25(+) CD4(+) regulatory T cells by interleukin (IL)-2 and induction of autoimmune disease by IL-2 neutralization. *J Exp Med* 2005;**201**(5):723–35.

41. Alcocer-Varela J, Alarcon-Segovia D. Decreased production of and response to interleukin-2 by cultured lymphocytes from patients with systemic lupus erythematosus. *J Clin Invest* 1982;**69**(6):1388.

42. Fan W, Liang D, Tang Y, Qu B, Cui H, Luo X, et al. Identification of microRNA-31 as a novel regulator contributing to impaired interleukin-2 production in T cells from patients with systemic lupus erythematosus. *Arthritis Rheum* 2012;**64**(11):3715–25.

43. Crispin JC, Tsokos GC. Transcriptional regulation of IL-2 in health and autoimmunity. *Autoimmun Rev* 2009;**8**(3):190–5.

44. Zhao X, Tang Y, Qu B, Cui H, Wang S, Wang L, et al. MicroRNA-125a contributes to elevated inflammatory chemokine RANTES levels via targeting KLF13 in systemic lupus erythematosus. *Arthritis Rheum* 2010;**62**(11):3425–35.

45. Stagakis E, Bertsias G, Verginis P, Nakou M, Hatziapostolou M, Kritikos H, et al. Identification of novel microRNA signatures linked to human lupus disease activity and pathogenesis: miR-21 regulates aberrant T cell responses through regulation of PDCD4 expression. *Ann Rheum Dis* 2011;**70**(8):1496–506.

46. Ding S, Liang Y, Zhao M, Liang G, Long H, Zhao S, et al. Decreased microRNA-142-3p/5p expression causes CD4+T cell activation and B Cell hyperstimulation in systemic lupus erythematosus. *Arthritis Rheum* 2012;**64**(9):2953–63.

47. Liu Y, Dong J, Mu R, Gao Y, Tan X, Li Y, et al. MicroRNA-30a promotes B cell hyperactivity in patients with systemic lupus erythematosus by direct interaction with Lyn. *Arthritis Rheum* 2013;**65**(6): 1603–11.

48. Wu X-N, Ye Y-X, Niu J-W, Li Y, Li X, You X, et al. Defective PTEN regulation contributes to B cell hyperresponsiveness in systemic lupus erythematosus. *Sci Transl Med* 2014;**6**(246).

49. Grammer AC, Slota R, Fischer R, Gur H, Girschick H, Yarboro C, et al. Abnormal germinal center reactions in systemic lupus erythematosus demonstrated by blockade of CD154-CD40 interactions. *J Clin Invest* 2003;**112**(10):1506–20.

50. Xiao C, Srinivasan L, Calado DP, Patterson HC, Zhang B, Wang J, et al. Lymphoproliferative disease and autoimmunity in mice with increased miR-17-92 expression in lymphocytes. *Nat Immunol* 2008;**9**(4):405–14.

51. Baumjohann D, Kageyama R, Clingan JM, Morar MM, Patel S, de Kouchkovsky D, et al. The microRNA cluster miR-17~92 promotes TFH cell differentiation and represses subset-inappropriate gene expression. *Nat Immunol* 2013;**14**(8):840–8.

52. Kang SG, Liu W-H, Lu P, Jin HY, Lim HW, Shepherd J, et al. MicroRNAs of the miR-17~92 family are critical regulators of TFH differentiation. *Nat Immunol* 2013;**14**(8):849–57.

53. Yuan Y, Kasar S, Underbayev C, Vollenweider D, Salerno E, Kotenko SV, et al. Role of microRNA-15a in autoantibody production in interferon-augmented murine model of lupus. *Mol Immunol* 2012;**52**(2):61–70.

54. Bomback AS, Appel GB. Updates on the treatment of lupus nephritis. *J Am Soc Nephrol* 2010;**21**(12):2028–35.

55. Akkina S, Becker BN. MicroRNAs in kidney function and disease. *Transl Res* 2011;**157**(4):236–40.

56. Dai Y, Sui W, Lan H, Yan Q, Huang H, Huang Y. Comprehensive analysis of microRNA expression patterns in renal biopsies of lupus nephritis patients. *Rheumatol Int* 2009;**29**(7):749–54.

57. Krasoudaki E, Stagakis E, Loupasakis K, Papagianni A, Alexopoulos E, Bertsias G, et al. MicroRNA analysis of human lupus nephritis: evidence for modulation of kallikrein 4 By MIR-422a. *Ann Rheum Dis* 2012;**71**:472–3.

58. Zhu S, Pan W, Song X, Liu Y, Shao X, Tang Y, et al. The microRNA miR-23b suppresses IL-17-associated autoimmune inflammation by targeting TAB2, TAB3 and IKK-alpha. *Nat Med* 2012;**18**(7):1077–86.

59. Chafin CB, Regna NL, Dai R, Caudell DL, Reilly CM. MicroRNA-let-7a expression is increased in the mesangial cells of NZB/W mice and increases IL-6 production in vitro. *Autoimmunity* 2013;**46**(6):351–62.

60. Chafin CB, Regna NL, Caudell DL, Reilly CM. MicroRNA-let-7a promotes E2F-mediated cell proliferation and NF kappa B activation in vitro. *Cell Mol Immunol* 2014;**11**(1):79–93.

61. Ichii O, Otsuka-Kanazawa S, Horino T, Kimura J, Nakamura T, Matsumoto M, et al. Decreased miR-26a expression correlates with the progression of podocyte injury in autoimmune glomerulonephritis. *PloS One* 2014;**9**(10).

62. Zhou H, Hasni SA, Perez P, Tandon M, Jang SI, Zheng C, et al. miR-150 promotes renal fibrosis in lupus nephritis by downregulating SOCS1. *J Am Soc Nephrol: JASN* 2013;**24**(7):1073–87.

63. Te JL, Dozmorov IM, Guthridge JM, Nguyen KL, Cavett JW, Kelly JA, et al. Identification of unique microRNA signature associated with lupus nephritis. *PloS One* 2010;**5**(5):e10344.

64. Zeng L, Cui J, Wu H, Lu Q. The emerging role of circulating microRNAs as biomarkers in autoimmune diseases. *Autoimmunity* 2014;**47**(7):419–29.

65. Carlsen AL, Schetter AJ, Nielsen CT, Lood C, Knudsen S, Voss A, et al. Circulating microRNA expression profiles associated with systemic lupus erythematosus. *Arthritis Rheum* 2013;**65**(5):1324–34.

66. Goilav B, Ben-Dov IZ, Blanco I, Loudig O, Wahezi DM, Putterman C. Next-generation sequencing of urinary microRNA in human lupus nephritis. *Arthritis Rheum* 2012;**64**(10):S135.

67. Chauhan SK, Singh VV, Rai R, Rai M, Rai G. Differential microRNA profile and post-transcriptional regulation exist in systemic lupus erythematosus patients with distinct autoantibody specificities. *J Clin Immunol* 2014;**34**(4):491–503.

68. Koutsokeras T, Healy T. Systemic lupus erythematosus and lupus nephritis. *Nat Rev Drug Discov* 2014;**13**(3):173–4.

69. Wahid F, Khan T, Kim YY. MicroRNA and diseases: therapeutic potential as new generation of drugs. *Biochimie* 2014;**104C**:12–26.

70. Rigby RJ, Vinuesa CG. SiLEncing SLE: the power and promise of small noncoding RNAs. *Curr Opin Rheumatol* 2008;**20**(5):526–31.

71. Davis TE, Kis-Toth K, Szanto A, Tsokos GC. Glucocorticoids suppress T cell function by up-regulating microRNA-98. *Arthritis Rheum* 2013;**65**(7):1882–90.

72. Davis TE, Kis-Toth K, Tsokos GC. A114: methylprednisolone-induced inhibition of miR-155 expression increases SOCS1-driven suppression of cytokine signaling. *Arthritis Rheumatol (Hoboken, NJ)* 2014;**66**(Suppl. 11):S151.

73. Divekar AA, Dubey S, Gangalum PR, Singh RR. Dicer insufficiency and microRNA-155 overexpression in lupus regulatory T cells: an apparent paradox in the setting of an inflammatory milieu. *J Immunol* 2011;**186**(2):924–30.

74. Thai TH, Patterson HC, Pham DH, Kis-Toth K, Kaminski DA, Tsokos GC. Deletion of microRNA-155 reduces autoantibody responses and alleviates lupus-like disease in the Fas(lpr) mouse. *Proc Natl Acad Sci USA* 2013;**110**(50):20194–9.

75. Zhou SY, Liang D, Huang XF, Xiao CY, Tang YJ, Jia Q, et al. In vivo therapeutic Success of microRNA-155 (miR-155) antagomir in a mouse model of lupus pulmonary hemorrhage. *Arthritis Rheum* 2013;**65**:S246–7.

76. Garchow BG, Bartulos Encinas O, Leung YT, Tsao PY, Eisenberg RA, Caricchio R, et al. Silencing of microRNA-21 in vivo ameliorates autoimmune splenomegaly in lupus mice. *EMBO Mol Med* 2011;**3**(10):605–15.

77. Pan Y, Jia T, Zhang Y, Zhang K, Zhang R, Li J, et al. MS2 VLP-based delivery of microRNA-146a inhibits autoantibody production in lupus-prone mice. *Int J Nanomed* 2012;**7**:5957–67.

78. Liang D, Zhou SY, Liu Z, Shan ZY, Brohawn P, Yao YH, et al. In vivo administration of MiR-146a protects C57BL/6 mice from pristane-induced pulmonary hemorrhage via suppressing type I interferon response. *Arthritis Rheum* 2013;**65**:S1162.

79. Liang D, Shen N. MicroRNA involvement in lupus: the beginning of a new tale. *Curr Opin Rheumatol* 2012;**24**(5):489–98.

Chapter 28

Oxidative Stress in Systemic Lupus Erythematosus: Causes, Consequences, and Treatment

Andras Perl

Division of Rheumatology, Department of Medicine, College of Medicine, Upstate Medical University, State University of New York, Syracuse, NY, USA; Department of Microbiology and Immunology, College of Medicine, Upstate Medical University, State University of New York, Syracuse, NY, USA

INTRODUCTION

The pathogenesis of systemic lupus erythematosus (SLE) is widely attributed to immune cell malfunction that results in the production of antinuclear autoantibodies (ANA).[1] Current therapies that rely on cytotoxic agents[2] and B-cell blockade have limited clinical efficacy.[3,4] Selective depletion of T cells (e.g., CD4+ cells) blocks lupus;[6] however, such therapy creates a state of severe immunodeficiency similar to that caused by HIV.[7] Although other cell types, such as macrophages, dendritic cells, and neutrophils may not be essential to disease pathogenesis, their production of (i) proinflammatory metabolites such as nitric oxide (NO),[8] (ii) cytokines, as type I interferon,[9] and phagocytosis of infecting organisms also contribute to the pathogenesis.[10,11]

Oxidative stress, i.e., the production of reactive oxygen intermediates (ROI), has long been considered only as a toxic by-product of aerobic existence. However, ROI are increasingly viewed as essential modulators of various signal-transduction pathways, including epigenetic regulation of gene transcription,[18] mRNA translation,[19] and protein folding,[20] as well as degradation and recycling of organelles via autophagy.[21] In accordance with these diverse functions, oxidative stress seems to mediate T-cell dysfunction in SLE at multiple levels.[13] Such T-cell defects result in aberrant immune responses and, in concert with oxidative autoantigenesis, elicit the inflammatory pathology and comorbidities of SLE.[13]

In turn, redox signaling is tightly controlled by intracellular antioxidant systems that mainly rely on the availability of reduced glutathione (GSH).[13] Oxidative stress in SLE was initially revealed by the increased levels of mitochondrial ROI production, which is caused by the elevation of mitochondrial transmembrane potential ($\Delta\Psi$m) or mitochondrial hyperpolarization (MHP) in T lymphocytes.[22,23] ROI production is mainly increased by complex I of the mitochondrial electron transport chain (ETC) in lupus T cells.[24]

Although increased blood levels of lipid hydroperoxides, malonaldehyde, hydroxynonenal (HNE), and other reactive aldehydes provide evidence for an overall increased oxidative stress in patients with SLE, paradoxically, further increase of oxidative stress in highly proliferative autoreactive B cells and T cells may also be beneficial. Therefore, it is important to consider that compartmentalized oxidative stress may prevent SLE. Along these lines, a loss of NADPH oxidase (NOX) activity, due to deficiency of NOX2 isozyme, is a common genetic cause of chronic granulomatous disease (CGD) that can predispose to lupus in such patients[25] as well as in MRL/lpr mice.[26] Given that antioxidants such as *N*-acetylcysteine (NAC) show overall benefit both in patients[27] and in mice,[28] and other antioxidant treatments also improved lupus disease activity, at least in mice,[29–31] a better understanding of redox signaling is relevant for overall disease pathogenesis, mechanisms of flares, and identification of biomarkers and targets for treatment. Therefore, this chapter critically evaluates the causes and consequences of oxidative stress in SLE.

ACCUMULATION OF DYSFUNCTIONAL MITOCHONDRIA IS THE SOURCE OF OXIDATIVE STRESS IN T CELLS

In most nucleated cells, mitochondria are the main source of ROI. The transfer of electrons to molecular oxygen (O_2) during ETC activity generates ROI, primarily superoxide anion, O_2^-. This is a by-product of ETC activity, which generates electrical energy, stored as $\Delta\Psi$m. In turn, this chemical energy is transformed into chemical energy in the form of ATP by the terminal ETC complex, complex V, or F_0F_1 ATPase.[32] ETC activity is increased in lupus T cells, primarily at complex I,[24] which has been proposed as a potential source of ROI production in mammalian mitochondria.[33]

ETC complex I activity is elevated in "untouched" T cells of SLE patients over twofold relative to healthy and nonlupus psoriatic and rheumatoid arthritis (RA) disease controls studied in parallel.[24] O_2 consumption and ETC activity are also increased relative to greater mitochondrial mass and MHP in lupus T cells.[24] In a state of mitochondrial hyperpolarization, H^+ ions are extruded from the mitochondrial matrix and cytochromes within the ETC become more reduced, promoting the transfer of electrons onto O_2, thus generating more O_2^- and oxidative stress.[13] Among the ROI, the most toxic moiety is the hydroxyl radical (OH^-), which cannot be eliminated without causing oxidative damage. OH^- is generated from O_2^- and H_2O_2 in the presence of metal ions through the Fenton reaction or UV light.[34] The generation of OH^- is primarily controlled by prevention via fully functional, endogenous antioxidant mechanisms, as described below, that is, converting O_2^- into relatively stable, nonradical hydrogen peroxide (H_2O_2) by superoxide dismutases and then into water by catalase.[35] Besides ROI, redox signaling also involves reactive nitrogen intermediates, such as NO and peroxynitrite ($ONOO^-$), the latter of which is generated by the reaction of NO with O_2^-.

The accumulation of mitochondria contributes to oxidative stress in lupus T cells. This is caused in part by NO-induced MHP[36] and mitochondrial biogenesis.[37] As more recently uncovered, NO also induces the expression of the lupus susceptibility gene, HRES-1/Rab4,[38] which, in turn, inhibits mitophagy.[39,40] Thus, the accumulation of mitochondria is favored by both increased biogenesis and diminished turnover in lupus T cells. These mechanisms of altered mitochondrial homeostasis are detectable in patients with SLE as well as in lupus-prone NZB/WF1, Sle1.Sle2. Sle3 triple congenic, MRL, and MRL/lpr mice.[39]

Genetic data also support mitochondrial dysfunction in SLE. Sle1c2 (a sublocus of the major lupus susceptibility locus Sle1) have been identified as estrogen-related receptor γ (ESRRG). Sle1c2 congenic mice exhibit increased mitochondrial mass, as evidenced by elevated voltage-dependent anion channel protein levels, CD4 T-cell hyperreactivity, and cGVHD susceptibility.[41] These findings are consistent with a role of ESRRG as a transcription factor involved in NO-dependent mitochondrial biogenesis.[42,43] Genetic polymorphisms in human mitochondrial DNA have also been associated with SLE.[44] The nt4917 and nt9055 mtDNA polymorphisms cause amino acid substitutions: (i) D→N in the ND2 subunit of ETC complex I and (ii) A→T in the ATP6 subunit of complex V.[44] The functional consequences of these amino acid changes are yet to be determined. Moreover, inactive alleles of mitochondrial uncoupling protein 2 (UCP2), a protein that reduces oxidative stress, are associated with susceptibility to several autoimmune diseases, including SLE, multiple sclerosis, RA, granulomatosis with polyangiitis, Crohn's disease, and ulcerative colitis.[45]

EXTRAMITOCHONDRIAL GENERATION OF OXIDATIVE STRESS

In addition to mitochondria, phagocytic cells and endothelial cells generate ROI by NOX enzymes, mainly NOX2 (Figure 1).[46,47] Macrophages and granulocytes express NOX2, which produces ROI for the killing of ingested bacteria.[46] Oxidative stress contributes to the destruction of organisms in phagocytic cells: ROI, generated by the respiratory burst with the involvement of NOX2, participate in elimination of bacteria by neutrophils. Leftover DNA-persistent bacteria are thought to chronically stimulate the innate immune system and trigger SLE.[48] Genetic mutations of NOX2 lead to CGD, which is characterized by recurrent bacterial infections due to NOX2 deficiency in phagocytic cells. Discoid lupus was significantly associated with the X chromosome-linked recessive form of CGD relative to autosomal chromosome-linked recessive CGD.[25] NOX2 deficiency exacerbated lupus disease activity in MRL/lpr mice, thus supporting a role for defective ROI generation in neutrophils. Paradoxically, the formation of neutrophil extracellular traps (NET) or NETosis was reduced in NOX2-deficient MRL/lpr mice.[26] This is in contrast to increased NETosis in patients with SLE.[49] Polymorphism in CYBB, which encodes the NOX2 subunit cytochrome b-245 heavy chain, has been associated with SLE in a Chinese population.[50] Along these lines, polymorphism of NCF2, encoding a 67-kDa activating cytosolic subunit of NOX2, has been associated with SLE in another Chinese cohort[51] and in patients in the United States.[52]

OXIDATIVE STRESS DUE TO DIMINISHED REDUCING POWER

$\Delta\Psi m$ is regulated by the equilibrium of ROI, pyridine nucleotides (NADH–NAD and NADPH–NADP), and GSH–GSSG.[53] The regeneration of GSH from GSSG requires NADPH, as the ultimate reducing equivalent. The net production of NADPH relies on the pentose phosphate pathway (PPP).[53] In addition, NADPH is required for the activity of thioredoxin reductase, catalase, and NOS.[53] As previously noted, GSH is depleted in PBL of SLE patients[22] as well as in lupus-prone NZB/W(F1)[28] and MRL/lpr mice.[29] Depletion of GSH in lupus PBL and T cells has been confirmed.[38,54–56] The extent of GSH depletion, 20–30%, in lupus PBL relative to matched healthy subjects[22,27] is comparable to that noted in erythrocytes of patients with G6PD deficiency.[57,58] Given that the nonoxidative PPP enzyme transaldolase is only expressed in nucleated cells but absent in erythrocytes,[59] its overexpression in "untouched," negatively isolated T cells indicates an involvement of this enzyme in oxidative stress of SLE patients.[38]

Beyond enzymes directly involved in the production and metabolism of NADPH and GSH, the loss of a transcription factor, nuclear factor erythroid 2-related factor 2

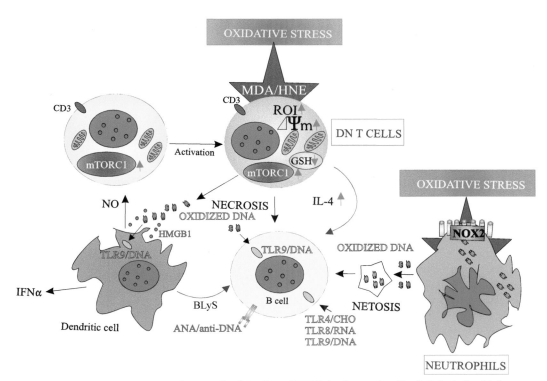

FIGURE 1 The generation of oxidative stress by mitochondria of T cells and NOX2 in phagocytic cells. Pathological oxidative stress is proposed to originate in CD4$^-$CD8$^-$ double-negative (DN) T cells, which play a central role in orchestrating dysfunction of the immune system in SLE. Accumulated mitochondria are shown in T cells that exhibit oxidative stress. Elevation of the mitochondrial transmembrane potential ($\Delta\Psi$m) or mitochondrial hyperpolarization (MHP), accumulation of mitochondria, and oxidative stress cause proinflammatory mTORC1 activation in lupus T cells, most prominently affecting DN T cells that exhibit increased production of IL-17 and IL-4, thus stimulating B cells and contracting CD4$^+$CD25$^+$FoxP3$^+$Tregs. Following activation, necrosis-prone T cells release oxidized DNA and high mobility group protein-1 (HMGB1), which stimulate B cells, macrophages, and dendritic cells (DC). In turn, macrophages and DC produce NO, which stimulate MHP of T cells and BLyS (B lymphocyte stimulator), which activates B cells. B lineage cells produce ANA. NETosis depicts the extrusion and sensing of foreign DNA containing NETS. NOX2-dependent oxidative stress facilitates destruction of infectious organisms in phagocytic cells, potentially limiting NETosis and stimulation of B cells through Toll-like receptors (TLRs) that detect foreign DNA containing NETs. TLRs 4, 8, and 9 detect bacterial carbohydrates (CHO), RNA, and DNA, respectively. While oxidative stress emanating from T cells is clearly pathogenic, NOX-2-mediated ROI production by neutrophils also protects against SLE.

(Nrf2), which orchestrates the expression of a wide array of antioxidant enzymes, predisposes to lupus-like autoimmunity. Nrf2-deficient female mice have reduced life spans and increased lipid peroxidation, with development of anti-DNA autoantibodies, splenomegaly, mesangial deposits, and massive granular deposits of IgG, IgM, and C3 along renal capillary walls, and glomerulonephritis.[60] Moreover, polymorphism of *NRF2* has been linked to the development of nephritis in 362 patients with childhood-onset SLE when compared to 379 matched controls.[61] Enhanced expression of Nrf2 has been found to mediate the therapeutic benefit of several antioxidants that have been found to improve nephritis in lupus-prone mice.[30,31]

BIOMARKERS OF OXIDATIVE STRESS REFLECT DISEASE ACTIVITY IN SLE

Increased production of ROI is directly detectable in peripheral blood T cells of SLE patients,[22,62] including the circulation of patients with lupus nephritis,[63] as well as in the nephritic

kidneys of lupus-prone mice.[30] Serum ONOO$^-$ levels positively correlate with disease activity in patients with nephritis.[8] HNE-modified albumin in the serum correlates with disease activity in patients with SLE.[64] In the urine, levels of F2 isoprostane are associated with nephritis.[65] Oxidized β2GPI is highly specific for detection of APS in the setting of thrombosis.[66] Oxidized phospholipids such as 1-palmitoyl-2-arachidonoyl-*sn*-3-glycero-phosphorylcholine accumulate in atherosclerotic lesions and are serum markers of oxidative stress in inflammatory diseases, including SLE.[67] oxHDL is a biomarker of cardiovascular disease,[68] and it is also associated with atherosclerosis in SLE.[69]

OXIDATIVE STRESS IS A TARGET FOR TREATMENT IN SLE

UV-induced oxidative stress can be prevented by wearing photo-resistant fabrics and covering the skin with cream containing sun protection factor >50.[5] As summarized in Table 1, antioxidant therapies of SLE include NAC[27,70]

TABLE 1 Antioxidant Treatment Approaches in SLE

Drug	Molecular Target	Mechanism of Action	References
N-acetylcysteine	GSH depletion, mTORC1	T-cell skewing	22,23
Rapamycin	mTORC1	T-cell skewing	67,70,71
CLA	GSH depletion, Nrf2	Anti-oxidant gene expression	24,72
Antroquinonol	Nrf2	Anti-oxidant gene expression	25
CDDO-ME	Nrf2	Anti-oxidant gene expression	26
Hydroxychloroquine	Endosome acidification	Netosis, atherosclerosis	73

and dietary antioxidant nutrients such as CLA.[29] Natural and synthetic terpenoids have been found to inhibit nephritis through activating NRF2.[30,31] These treatments may not only limit oxidative stress generated by the disease process but also reduce the toxicity of prooxidant immunosuppressive therapies, such as cyclophosphamide. In addition to targeting autoreactive T and B cells, these drugs damage myeloid cells of the bone marrow and hepatocytes, as well as intestinal and urinary tract epithelial cells.[5] Among the antioxidant treatments, NAC has shown clinical efficacy both in animal models and in clinical trials. NAC prevents the decline of GSH:GSSG ratios, reduces autoantibody production and development of nephritis, and prolongs the survival of lupus-prone mice.[28] As recently documented, a phase I–phase II double-blind placebo-controlled randomized clinical trial of NAC in 36 patients with SLE showed remarkable safety and promising clinical benefits.[27,70] Excellent tolerability of NAC has been attributed to the improvements in fatigue[27] and cognition.[70] The clinical efficacy of NAC was associated with the reversal of GSH depletion, the profound blockade of mTOR complex 1 (mTORC1) activation, moderate expansion of CD4+CD25+FoxP3+ regulatory T cells, and reduced anti-DNA antibody production.[27] NAC depletes CD4−CD8−double-negative T cells, which exhibit the most prominent mTORC1 activation before treatment.[27,71] They are held responsible for promoting anti-DNA autoantibody production by B cells.[72,73] The remarkable safety and selectivity of NAC for mTORC1 activation in T cells offer an inexpensive, alternative, and potentially synergistic approach to B-cell blockade in SLE. This 3-month pilot study warrants confirmation in larger cohorts and with longer treatment duration.

ACKNOWLEDGMENTS

This work was supported in part by Grants AI 048079, AI 061066, and AI 072648, AT 4332 from the National Institutes of Health and the Central New York Community Foundation. Due to space limitations, important discoveries of oxidative stress research in SLE may have only been referenced through reviews.

REFERENCES

1. Perl A. Systems biology of lupus: mapping the impact of genomic and environmental factors on gene expression signatures, cellular signaling, metabolic pathways, hormonal and cytokine imbalance, and selecting targets for treatment. *Autoimmunity* 2010;**43**: 32–47.
2. Ginzler EM, Dooley MA, Aranow C, Kim MY, Buyon J, Merrill JT, et al. Mycophenolate mofetil or intravenous cyclophosphamide for lupus nephritis. *N Engl J Med* 2005;**353**:2219–28.
3. Merrill JT, Neuwelt CM, Wallace DJ, Shanahan JC, Latinis KM, Oates JC, et al. Efficacy and safety of rituximab in moderately-to-severely active systemic lupus erythematosus: the randomized, double-blind, phase II/III systemic lupus erythematosus evaluation of rituximab trial. *Arth Rheum* 2010;**62**(1):222–33.
4. Navarra SV, Guzman RM, Gallacher AE, Hall S, Levy RA, Jimenez RE, et al. Efficacy and safety of belimumab in patients with active systemic lupus erythematosus: a randomised, placebo-controlled, phase 3 trial. *Lancet* 2011;**377**(9767):721–31.
5. Francis L, Perl A. Pharmacotherapy of systemic lupus erythematosus. *Expert Opin Pharmacother* 2009;**10**(9):1481–94.
6. Wofsy D, Seaman WE. Successful treatment of autoimmunity in NZB/NZW F1 mice with monoclonal antibody to L3T4. *J Exp Med* 1985;**161**(2):378–91.
7. Molina JF, Citera G, Rosler D, Cuellar ML, Molina J, Felipe O, et al. Coexistence of human immunodeficiency virus infection and systemic lupus erythematosus. *J Rheumatol* 1995;**22**(2):347–50.
8. Gilkeson G, Cannon C, Oates J, Reilly C, Goldman D, Petri M. Correlation of serum measures of nitric oxide production with lupus disease activity. *J Rheumatol* 1999;**26**(2):318–24.
9. Kirou KA, Lee C, George S, Louca K, Peterson MG, Crow MK. Activation of the interferon-alpha pathway identifies a subgroup of systemic lupus erythematosus patients with distinct serologic features and active disease. *Arth Rheum* 2005;**52**:1491–503.
10. Midgley A, Watson L, Beresford MW. New insights into the pathogenesis and management of lupus in children. *Arch Dis Child* 2014;**99**(6):563–7.
11. Carmona-Rivera C, Kaplan MJ. Low-density granulocytes: a distinct class of neutrophils in systemic autoimmunity. *Semin Immunopathol* 2013;**35**(4):455–63.
12. Tsokos GC. Systemic lupus erythematosus. *N Engl J Med* 2011; **365**(22):2110–21.
13. Perl A. Oxidative stress in the pathology and treatment of systemic lupus erythematosus. *Nat Rev Rheumatol* 2013;**9**:674–86.

14. Anolik J, Sanz I. B cells in human and murine systemic lupus erythematosus. *Curr Opin Rheumatol* 2004;**16**:505–12.

15. Jenks SA, Ia S. Altered B cell receptor signaling in human systemic lupus erythematosus. *Autoimmun Rev* 2009;**8**(3):209–13.

16. Majai G, Kiss E, Tarr T, Zahuczky G, Hartman Z, Szegedi G, et al. Decreased apopto-phagocytic gene expression in the macrophages of systemic lupus erythematosus patients. *Lupus* 2014;**23**(2):133–45.

17. Chi H. Regulation and function of mTOR signalling in T cell fate decisions. *Nat Rev Immunol* 2012;**12**(5):325–38.

18. Cyr AR, Domann FE. The redox basis of epigenetic modifications: from mechanisms to functional consequences. *Antiox Redox Signal* 2011;**15**(2):551–89.

19. Gerashchenko MV, Lobanov AV, Gladyshev VN. Genome-wide ribosome profiling reveals complex translational regulation in response to oxidative stress. *Proc Natl Acad Sci USA* 2012;**109**(43):17394–9.

20. Margittai E, Sitia R. Oxidative protein folding in the secretory pathway and redox signaling across compartments and cells. *Traffic* 2011;**12**(1):1–8.

21. Caza TN, Talaber G, Perl A. Metabolic regulation of organelle homeostasis in lupus T cells. *Clin Immunol* 2012;**144**(3):200–13.

22. Gergely PJ, Grossman C, Niland B, Puskas F, Neupane H, Allam F, et al. Mitochondrial hyperpolarization and ATP depletion in patients with systemic lupus erythematosus. *Arth Rheum* 2002;**46**:175–90.

23. Gergely PJ, Niland B, Gonchoroff N, Pullmann Jr R, Phillips PE, Perl A. Persistent mitochondrial hyperpolarization, increased reactive oxygen intermediate production, and cytoplasmic alkalinization characterize altered IL-10 signaling in patients with systemic lupus erythematosus. *J Immunol* 2002;**169**:1092–101.

24. Doherty E, Oaks Z, Perl A. Increased mitochondrial electron transport chain activity at complex I is regulated by N-acetylcysteine in lymphocytes of patients with systemic lupus erythematosus. *Antioxid Redox Signal* 2014;**21**:56–65.

25. Winkelstein JA, Marino MC, Johnston RBJ, Boyle J, Curnutte J, Gallin JI, et al. Chronic granulomatous disease: report on a national registry of 368 patients. *Medicine* 2000;**79**(3).

26. Campbell AM, Kashgarian M, Shlomchik MJ. NADPH oxidase inhibits the pathogenesis of systemic lupus erythematosus. *Sci Transl Med* 2012;**4**(157).

27. Lai Z-W, Hanczko R, Bonilla E, Caza TN, Clair B, Bartos A, et al. N-acetylcysteine reduces disease activity by blocking mTOR in T cells of lupus patients. *Arthritis Rheum* 2012;**64**(9):2937–46.

28. Suwannaroj S, Lagoo A, Keisler D, McMurray RW. Antioxidants suppress mortality in the female NZB×NZW F1 mouse model of systemic lupus erythematosus (SLE). *Lupus* 2001;**10**:258–65.

29. Bergamo P, Maurano F, Rossi M. Phase 2 enzyme induction by conjugated linoleic acid improves lupus-associated oxidative stress. *Free Rad Biol Med* 2007;**43**(1):71–9.

30. Tsai PY, Ka SM, Chang JM, Lai JH, Dai MS, Jheng HL, et al. Antroquinonol differentially modulates T cell activity and reduces interleukin-18 production, but enhances Nrf2 activation, in murine accelerated severe lupus nephritis. *Arth Rheum* 2012;**64**(1):232–42.

31. Wu T, Ye Y, Min SY, Zhu J, Khobahy E, Zhou J, et al. Targeting multiple signaling axes and oxidative stress using a synthetic triterpenoid prevents murine lupus nephritis. *Arthritis Rheum* 2014;**66**:3129–39.

32. Skulachev VP. Mitochondrial physiology and pathology; concepts of programmed death of organelles, cells and organisms. *Mol Asp Med* 1999;**20**:139–40.

33. St Pierre J, Buckingham JA, Roebuck SJ, Brand MD. Topology of superoxide production from different sites in the mitochondrial electron transport chain. *J Biol Chem* 2002;**277**(47):44784–90.

34. Halliwell B, Gutteridge JM. Role of free radicals and catalytic metal ions in human disease: an overview. *Meth Enzymol* 1990;**186**:1–85.

35. Ortona E, Maselli A, Delunardo F, Colasanti T, Giovannetti A, Pierdominici M. Relationship between redox status and cell fate immunity and autoimmunity. *Antioxid Redox Signal* 2014;**21**(1):103–22.

36. Nagy G, Koncz A, Perl A. T cell activation-induced mitochondrial hyperpolarization is mediated by Ca^{2+}- and redox-dependent production of nitric oxide. *J Immunol* 2003;**171**:5188–97.

37. Nagy G, Barcza M, Gonchoroff N, Phillips PE, Perl A. Nitric oxide-dependent mitochondrial biogenesis generates Ca^{2+} signaling profile of lupus T cells. *J Immunol* 2004;**173**(6):3676–83.

38. Fernandez DR, Telarico T, Bonilla E, Li Q, Banerjee S, Middleton FA, et al. Activation of mTOR controls the loss of TCRzeta in lupus T cells through HRES-1/Rab4-regulated lysosomal degradation. *J Immunol* 2009;**182**:2063–73.

39. Caza TN, Fernandez D, Talaber G, Oaks Z, Haas M, Madaio MP, et al. HRES-1/RAB4-Mediated depletion of DRP1 impairs mitochondrial homeostasis and represents a target for treatment in SLE. *Ann Rheum Dis* 2014;**73**:1887–97.

40. Talaber G, Miklossy G, Oaks Z, Liu Y, Tooze SA, Chudakov DM, et al. HRES-1/Rab4 promotes the formation of LC3+ autophagosomes and the accumulation of mitochondria during autophagy. *PLoS One* 2014;**9**(1):e84392.

41. Perry DJ, Yin Y, Telarico T, Baker HV, Dozmorov I, Perl A, et al. Murine lupus susceptibility locus Sle1c2 mediates CD4+ T cell activation and maps to estrogen-related receptor gamma. *J Immunol* 2012;**189**(2):793–803.

42. Poidatz D, Dos Santos E, Brule A, De Mazancourt P, Dieudonne MN. Estrogen-related receptor gamma modulates energy metabolism target genes in human trophoblast. *Placenta* 2012;**33**(9):688–95.

43. Hock MB, Kralli A. Transcriptional control of mitochondrial biogenesis and function. *Ann Rev Physiol* 2009;**71**(1):177–203.

44. Vyshkina T, Sylvester A, Sadiq S, Bonilla E, Canter JA, Perl A, et al. Association of common mitochondrial DNA variants with multiple sclerosis and systemic lupus erythematosus. *Clin Immunol* 2008;**129**:31–5.

45. Yu X, Wieczorek S, Franke A, Yin H, Pierer M, Sina C, et al. Association of UCP2 -866 G/A polymorphism with chronic inflammatory diseases. *Genes Immun* 2009;**10**(6):601–5.

46. Bedard K, Krause KH. The NOX family of ROS-generating NADPH oxidases: physiology and pathophysiology. *Physiol Rev* 2007;**87**(1):245–313.

47. Jackson SH, Devadas S, Kwon J, Pinto LA, Williams MS. T cells express a phagocyte-type NADPH oxidase that is activated after T cell receptor stimulation. *Nat Immunol* 2004;**5**(8):818–27.

48. Pisetsky DS. The origin and properties of extracellular DNA: from PAMP to DAMP. *Clin Immunol* 2012;**144**(1):32–40.

49. Villanueva E, Yalavarthi S, Berthier CC, Hodgin JB, Khandpur R, Lin AM, et al. Netting neutrophils induce endothelial damage, infiltrate tissues, and expose immunostimulatory molecules in systemic lupus erythematosus. *J Immunol* 2011;**187**(1):538–52.

50. Tang FY, Xie XW, Ling GH, Liu FY. Endothelial nitric oxide synthase and nicotinamide adenosine dinucleotide phosphate oxidase p22phox gene (C242T) polymorphisms and systemic lupus erythematosus in a Chinese Population. *Lupus* 2010;**19**(2):192–6.

51. Yu B, Chen Y, Wu Q, Li P, Shao Y, Zhang J, et al. The association between single-nucleotide polymorphisms of NCF2 and systemic lupus erythematosus in Chinese mainland population. *Clin Rheumatol* 2011;**30**(4):521–7.

52. Jacob CO, Eisenstein M, Dinauer MC, Ming W, Liu Q, John S, et al. Lupus-associated causal mutation in neutrophil cytosolic factor 2 (NCF2) brings unique insights to the structure and function of NADPH oxidase. *Proc Natl Acad Sci USA* 2012;**109**(2):E59–67.

53. Perl A, Hanczko R, Telarico T, Oaks Z, Landas S. Oxidative stress, inflammation and carcinogenesis are controlled through the pentose phosphate pathway by transaldolase. *Trends Mol Med* 2011;**7**: 395–403.

54. Shah D, Aggarwal A, Bhatnagar A, Kiran R, Wanchu A. Association between T lymphocyte sub-sets apoptosis and peripheral blood mononuclear cells oxidative stress in systemic lupus erythematosus. *Free Rad Res* 2011;**45**(5):559–67.

55. Shah D, Kiran R, Wanchu A, Bhatnagar A. Oxidative stress in systemic lupus erythematosus: relationship to Th1 cytokine and disease activity. *Immunol Lett* 2010;**129**(1):7–12.

56. Li KJ, Wu CH, Hsieh SC, Lu MC, Tsai CY, Yu CL. Deranged bioenergetics and defective redox capacity in T lymphocytes and neutrophils are related to cellular dysfunction and increased oxidative stress in patients with active systemic lupus erythematosus. *Clin Dev Immunol* 2012;**2012**. http://dx.doi.org/10.1155/2012/548516.

57. Huang CS, Sung YC, Huang MJ, Yang CS, Shei WS, Tang TK. Content of reduced glutathione and consequences in recipients of glucose-6-phosphate dehydrogenase deficient red blood cells. *Am J Hematol* 1998;**57**(3):187–92.

58. Shimo H, Nishino T, Tomita M. Predicting the kinetic properties associated with redox imbalance after oxidative crisis in G6PD-deficient erythrocytes: a simulation study. *Adv Hematol* 2011;**2011**.

59. Grossman CE, Qian Y, Banki K, Perl A. ZNF143 mediates basal and tissue-specific expression of human transaldolase. *J Biol Chem* 2004;**279**:12190–205.

60. Yoh K, Itoh K, Enomoto A, Hirayama A, Yamaguchi N, Kobayashi M, et al. Nrf2-deficient female mice develop lupus-like autoimmune nephritis. *Kidney Int* 2001;**60**(4):1343–53.

61. Cordova EJ, Velazquez-Cruz R, Centeno F, Baca V, Orozco L. The NRF2 gene variant, -653G/A, is associated with nephritis in childhood-onset systemic lupus erythematosus. *Lupus* 2010;**19**(10): 1237–42.

62. Misra R, Matera AG, Schmid CW, Rush MG. Recombination mediates production of an extrachromosomal circular DNA containing a transposon-like human element, THE-1. *Nucleic Acids Res* October 25, 1989;**17**(20):8327–41.

63. Moroni G, Novembrino C, Quaglini S, De Giuseppe R, Gallelli B, Uva V, et al. Oxidative stress and homocysteine metabolism in patients with lupus nephritis. *Lupus* 2010;**19**(1):65–72.

64. Wang G, Pierangeli SS, Papalardo E, Ansari GAS, Khan MF. Markers of oxidative and nitrosative stress in systemic lupus erythematosus: correlation with disease activity. *Arth Rheum* 2010;**62**(7):2064–72.

65. Avalos I, Chung CP, Oeser A, Milne GL, Morrow JD, Gebretsadik T, et al. Oxidative stress in systemic lupus erythematosus: relationship to disease activity and symptoms. *Lupus* 2007;**16**(3):195–200.

66. Ioannou Y, Zhang JY, Qi M, Gao L, Qi JC, Yu DM, et al. Novel assays of thrombogenic pathogenicity in the antiphospholipid syndrome based on the detection of molecular oxidative modification of the major autoantigen beta2-glycoprotein I. *Arth Rheum* 2011;**63**(9):2774–82.

67. Leitinger N. The role of phospholipid oxidation products in inflammatory and autoimmune diseases: evidence from animal models and in humans. *Sub-cellular Biochem* 2008;**49**:325–50.

68. Viigimaa M, Abina J, Zemtsovskaya G, Tikhaze A, Konovalova G, Kumskova E, et al. Malondialdehyde-modified low-density lipoproteins as biomarker for atherosclerosis. *Blood Press* 2010;**19**(3):164–8.

69. Skaggs BJ, Hahn BH, McMahon M. Accelerated atherosclerosis in patients with SLE–mechanisms and management. *Nat Rev Rheumatol* 2012;**8**(4):214–23.

70. Garcia RJ, Francis L, Dawood M, Lai Z-W, Faraone SV, Perl A. Attention deficit and hyperactivity disorder scores are elevated and respond to NAC treatment in patients with SLE. *Arthritis Rheum* 2013;**65**:1313–8.

71. Lai Z-W, Borsuk R, Shadakshari A, Yu J, Dawood M, Garcia R, et al. mTOR activation triggers IL-4 production and necrotic death of double-negative T cells in patients with systemic lupus eryhthematosus. *J Immunol* 2013;**191**:2236–46.

72. Shivakumar S, Tsokos GC, Datta SK. T cell receptor alpha/beta expressing double-negative (CD4−/CD8−) and CD4+ T helper cells in humans augment the production of pathogenic anti-DNA autoantibodies associated with lupus nephritis. *J Immunol* 1989;**143**(1):103–12.

73. Sieling PA, Porcelli SA, Duong BT, Spada F, Bloom BR, Diamond B, et al. Human double-negative T cells in systemic lupus erythematosus provide help for IgG and are restricted by CD1c. *J Immunol* 2000;**165**(9):5338–44.

Chapter 29

Reactive Nitrogen Intermediates in the Pathogenesis of Systemic Lupus Erythematosus

Gary S. Gilkeson, Jim C. Oates

Medical Research Service, Ralph H. Johnson VA Medical Center, Charleston, SC, USA; Department of Medicine, Division of Rheumatology, Medical University of South Carolina, Charleston, SC, USA

INTRODUCTION

Systemic lupus erythematosus (SLE) is a prototypic autoimmune disease characterized by the production of autoantibodies with subsequent immune complex deposition resulting in inflammatory injury to target organs. Reactive intermediates (RIs) and for the purpose of this chapter, specifically reactive nitrogen intermediates (RNI), are important mediators of the innate immune system, tissue damage, and organ/cellular function in health and in lupus. RNI are under tight physiologic control due to the potency of their biologic activities. In SLE, enhanced production of RNI and/or impaired regulation may contribute to a break in immune tolerance, increase tissue damage, and alter enzyme function. This chapter reviews the latest evidence from both animal and human studies on the role of RNI in the pathogenesis of SLE.

BIOLOGY OF REACTIVE INTERMEDIATES

RIs are short-lived molecules produced by normal cellular metabolism and are critical to a multitude of physiological and pathological processes. Nitrogen-based RIs are known as RNI (Table 1), while those that are oxygen-based are known as reactive oxygen intermediates (ROI). They were initially regarded as toxic by-products,[1] but later recognized to act as signaling molecules that are under tight physiologic control.[2] RNI are primarily produced by reactions involving the nitric oxide synthases (NOSs).[3] The biologic action of RNI is limited by a number of processes and properties including the short half-life of RIs,[4] and the negative feedback mechanisms that regulate the enzymatic production of RIs (e.g., the nitric oxide (NO) negative feedback inhibition of NOS).[5] A balance must be tightly maintained between the RNI production and the clearance; any perturbation in this balance leads to pathology and cellular injury.[6] In most cases low to moderate levels of RNI are physiologic and aid in normal cellular function including proliferation[7] and muscle relaxation.[8] High levels of RNI cause direct cellular injury by reacting with lipids, amino acids, and DNA[9–11] or indirect cellular injury by skewing the normal pathways that govern cellular processes.[6] In SLE,[12] overproduction of RNI may augment autoreactivity, disrupt normal enzyme function, and amplify tissue damage.[13]

The study of RI biology is hindered by a number of obstacles that are related to the nature of RIs as well as the lack of sensitive scientific tools that can detect and modulate these molecules in real time. For instance, RIs can interact with each other and modulate the function of one another. Thus, the outcome of reducing the level of a given reactive species (A) can be due to the primary effect of the reduced level, or the secondary effect of another species (B) that is modulated by the first species (A). For example, when NO and superoxide (SO) are produced in close proximity, peroxynitrite ($ONOO^-$) is produced, while SO and NO are consumed.[14,15] If NO levels are reduced in the system, the functional outcome could be due to reduced effects of NO, increased availability of SO, or reduced levels of $ONOO^-$.

Reactive Oxygen Intermediates

Due to the multiple interactions between RNI and ROI, it is important to consider the two together when discussing the biologic activity of one or the other. ROI encompass all oxygen-based radical (SO, hydroxyl radical (OH radical)) and nonradical (hydrogen peroxide (H_2O_2), hypochlorous

TABLE 1 Important Reactive Nitrogen Intermediates

RNI	Source	Mode of Action	Half-Life
Nitric oxide (NO)	Nitric oxide synthases	Nitrosylation of metal centers Redox signaling	3–30 s
Peroxynitrite ($ONOO^-$)	Reaction between NO and SO	Nitration Oxidation Oxidative stress	1 s
Nitrogen dioxide radical	Reaction between NO and O_2	Nitration Oxidation Oxidative stress	7×10^{-6} s
Dinitrogen trioxide	Reaction between NO and NO_2	Nitrosation Nitrosative stress	7×10^{-4} s

acid (HOCl)) reactive species. High ROI production is associated with SLE as evident by oxidative protein modifications, lipid peroxidation,[16] and lipoprotein oxidation.[17] SO stands at the center of major physiologic and pathologic processes that take place in a wide variety of biological systems.[18,19] The mitochondrion is a major source of endogenous SO production. It is estimated that 1% to 3% of electrons passing through the mitochondrial electron transport chain "leak" and bind with molecular oxygen to form the SO anion. SO is also produced by a number of enzymes including nicotine adenine dinucleotide phosphate (NAD(P)H) oxidases,[20] xanthine oxidase,[21] 5-lipoxygenase,[22] cyclooxygenase,[23] and uncoupled NOS.[24] In phagocytes, NAD(P)H oxidase produces high levels of SO that create an oxidative antimicrobial environment, the respiratory burst.[25] This burst activates redox-sensitive signaling pathways such as nuclear factor-kappa B (NF-κB) and activator protein-1 that in turn induce the transcription of proinflammatory proteins such as cytokines.[26]

SO is a reactive molecule with a very short half-life ($t_{1/2} = 10^{-9}$ s).[27] It can be converted into H_2O_2 either enzymatically (major pathway) under action of SO dismutases[28] or nonenzymatically (minor pathway).[29] H_2O_2, in turn, can be converted into water under the action of catalases and peroxidases[30] or OH radical. H_2O_2 is involved in many cellular processes such as proliferation,[31] differentiation,[32] and immune cell activation.[33] It acts on a number of key proteins and enzymes such as transcription factors, kinases, and phosphatases by oxidizing susceptible cysteine residues in these proteins.[30] An OH radical can be very detrimental to the cell because of its rapid reactivity with macromolecules. Reactions with DNA can induce mutations,[34] while reactions with lipids can initiate cycles of lipid peroxidation and membrane damage.[35] Another important oxygen-derived RI is HOCl, a potent bactericide and the active ingredient in bleach.[36] HOCl is produced by the action of myeloperoxidase (MPO),

which catalyzes the oxidation of chloride (Cl^-) by H_2O_2.[37] Stimulated phagocytes release their MPO-rich azurophilic granules into phagosomes as well as sites of inflammation to generate HOCl that chlorinates and oxidizes bacterial components killing the microorganism.[38] An important role of HOCl and the modulation of redox signaling was demonstrated in the pathogenesis of a number of diseases such as atherosclerosis.[39,40] Examples of modulation of redox signaling by HOCl are the depletion of NO by oxidizing available NO,[41] the uncoupling of endothelial NOS,[42] the chlorination of NOS arginine substrate,[43] and the reduction of endothelial NOS transcript stability by a chlorinated form of high density lipoprotein (HDL).[44]

Reactive Nitrogen Intermediates

RNI[45] encompass all nitrogen-based reactive species including NO and its nitrogen oxide derivatives (nitrogen dioxide (NO_2), nitrogen trioxide (N_2O_3), and $ONOO^-$; Table 1). NO is a membrane-permeable free radical molecule synthesized by NOSs[46] using arginine and oxygen as substrates. There are three known NOS each transcribed by a separate gene. All three NOS dimerize in the presence of cofactors to become active. Each monomer contains a reductase and an oxygenase domain. The reductase domain catalyzes the transfer of two electrons to heme iron in the oxygenase domain. Calmodulin, nicotinamide adenine dinucleotide phosphate, flavin adenine dinucleotide, and flavin mononucleotide are required cofactors for the reductase domain. Electrons from the reductase domain are transferred to the oxygenase domain of the adjacent monomer, where heme and tetrahydrobiopterin act as cofactors. Here, a reaction between O_2 and L-arginine is catalyzed, resulting in the formation of NO and citrulline.

Two NOS (endothelial or eNOS/NOS1 and neuronal or nNOS/NOS3) are considered constitutively expressed and are dependent on sufficient concentrations of calcium for activity. Each, however, can be activated by external physical factors or bioactive compounds. In the vascular system, NO produced by eNOS is a potent vasodilator and regulator of vascular tone. Sheer stress induces increased activity of eNOS. Nitroglycerin mimics the activity of eNOS by acting as a donor of NO.[47] The beneficial effects of NO, produced by the constitutively expressed NOS isoforms, are negated when NO is produced in an environment high in ROI, as discussed later.

A third NOS gene (iNOS2) produces an inducible isoform (iNOS)[46] that is primarily expressed in immune cells, most notably macrophages and macrophage-like cells. In murine cells, iNOS activity is enhanced in response to a number of inflammatory stimuli. Among these stimuli are several cytokines and toll-like receptor ligands such as lipopolysaccharide, interleukin-6 (IL6), interferon-γ (IFNγ), IL1β, and tumor necrosis factor-α (TNFα). In human cells, induction of iNOS is not as simple as in murine cells as complex mixtures of cytokines are necessary for induction. In most cells, inducing signaling pathways converge on the janus kinase/signal transducer and activator of transcription cascade and/or NF-κB-dependent pathways.[48] Nuclear hormone receptors also play a role in regulation of iNOS activity. Estrogen acts as an inducer[49] and PPARγ ligands act as inhibitors[50] of iNOS induction in response to IFNγ or IFNγ+LPS stimulation, respectively, in murine cells. iNOS is expressed during pathologic states in human endothelial cells, synovial fibroblasts, polymorphonuclear cells, lymphocytes, and natural killer cells.[51] In nonpathologic states, iNOS, expression is present as a baseline in myocytes, skeletal muscle, and Purkinje cells.[52]

iNOS produces log-fold higher amounts of NO than the constitutively expressed eNOS and nNOS. In a low arginine environment, iNOS cannot transfer nitrogen to molecular oxygen, and electrons from the reductase domain combine with oxygen to produce SO.[53] NO, when combined with SO, forms $ONOO^-$, a more reactive and toxic molecule than NO itself. $ONOO^-$, produced by immune cells, is capable of killing intracellular pathogens and tumor cells. Glutathione peroxidase, catalase, SO dismutase, heme oxygenase, and antioxidants protect host cells during inflammatory states by reducing ROI that contributes to $ONOO^-$ production.[54,55] Thus, RNI production depends on catalytic enzyme activity and substrate availability as well as the amount of and activity of detoxifying enzymes.

Despite its simple diatomic structure, NO can induce different and often opposite biologic effects.[56,57] These confusing effects are attributable to the unique chemical properties of NO, the variability of the biological milieu where NO signaling takes place, and the wide range of NO-responsive targets.[58] The interaction between NO and its targets can be direct or indirect. Direct interactions, occurring at low levels of NO (<400nM), are mediated by reactions between NO and targets such as metal centers

and organic free radicals to form nitrosyl adducts. A typical example is the nitrosylation of heme iron in soluble guanylate cyclase (sGS)[59] and the reaction with alkoxyl radicals limiting lipid peroxidation.[60] Indirect effects, dominant at higher levels of NO (>400nM), are mediated by nitrogen oxide derivatives of NO and its target.[58,61] NO can react with oxygen and SO to produce NO_2 and $ONOO^-$, respectively; both species are strong oxidants and mediators of oxidative stress.[56] NO_2 can further react with NO to give N_2O_3, a strong nitrosating agent and mediator of nitrosative stress.[56] Thus, the relative flux of NO with respect to SO in a given biological system determines the nature of indirect NO interactions. When the NO level is higher than that of SO, N_2O_3 and nitrosative stress dominate, manifested by nitrosation of thiol, lysine, and zinc fingers.[62] When SO and NO levels are equimolar, $ONOO^-$ and oxidative stress dominate, manifested by nitration and oxidation of macromolecules.[63]

The activation of NO targets is concentration dependent. A given target of NO is not activated unless the concentration of NO reaches a threshold specific to that molecule. Nitrosylation of sGS is achieved at low levels of NO (1–30nM) in endothelial cells.[61] In the 30–100nM concentration range, the Akt pathway is activated, leading to phosphorylation of BAD and caspase-6, both of which lead to cell survival.[58] At 100nM, hypoxia-induced factor 1α is stabilized, increasing proliferation and protection against cellular injury. Above 400 nM, p53 is phosphorylated and acetylated, leading to cell cycle arrest and apoptosis.

The complex effect of NO on cellular processes can appear paradoxical, as demonstrated by the effects of RNI on apoptosis. S-Nitrosation of caspases by NO in the cytoplasm has an antiapoptotic effect. Mitochrondrial NO combines with SO to form $ONOO^-$. $ONOO^-$ nitrates cytochrome c and leads to mitochondrial-mediated apoptosis.[64] In addition, synergistic effects are present in the interaction between RNI and eicosanoid synthesis. NO produced in the presence of SO, as is often seen in inflamed tissues,[65] results in the formation of $ONOO^-$ that in turn nitrates and inhibits the activity of prostacyclin synthase.[66] $ONOO^-$ also acts as a peroxide substrate to cyclooxygenase-2 (COX2) and increases its activity.[67] This may result in increased availability of prostaglandin H_2 (PGH_2) substrate for thromboxane and PGE_2 synthases in the vasculature and glomerulus. The inhibition of prostacyclin synthase and activation of COX2 can reverse the vasodilatory and antithrombotic effects of PGI_2 and increase the formation and thus inflammatory effects of TXA_2 and PGE_2.

RNI IN MURINE MODELS OF LUPUS

While iNOS activity suppresses parasitemia and tumor growth in murine models, its overexpression in the setting of lupus leads to organ damage and an altered immune response. Several studies involving murine models of lupus support this hypothesis. Both MRL/MpJ-*Fas^lpr*/J (MRL/lpr) and (New Zealand Black × New Zealand White)$_{F1}$ (NZB/W) mice develop spontaneous proliferative lupus nephritis. MRL/lpr mice develop increasing levels of urinary NO metabolites (nitrate + nitrite or NO$_x$) in parallel with the onset of glomerulonephritis.[68] This increase in NO production is associated with formation of 3-nitrotyrosine (3NTyr), a product of ONOO$^-$ or NO$_2$ and tyrosine.[69] Tyr nitration additionally reduces the activity of catalase in the MRL/lpr kidney. Because of its role in removing H$_2$O$_2$, catalase inactivation exposes cells to increased oxidative stress.[70] iNOS expression is increased in NZB/W brain tissue compared to control BALB/c brain tissue and is associated with an increase in p53 expression. The proapoptotic role of p53 in brain cells activated by iNOS may promote brain injury in patients with SLE.[71]

Autoantibody immune complex formation and tissue deposition precede increased iNOS activity in murine lupus and do not appear to require increased iNOS activity to be formed. iNOS inhibitors, while improving renal histopathology, had no effect on glomerular immune complex deposition in MRL/lpr mice.[68] The enhanced expression of iNOS in lupus nephritis thus appears a result of downstream innate immune responses to immune complex glomerular deposition. Enhanced iNOS expression/3NTyr formation is observed in passive transfer models of anti-glomerular basement membrane and MPO antibody glomerulonephritis.

MECHANISMS OF INCREASED iNOS EXPRESSION IN LUPUS

Several studies in murine models of lupus investigated mechanisms of increased iNOS expression in disease. Epigenetic regulation may effect iNOS expression as the histone deacetylase inhibitor trichostatin A, which attenuated renal disease in MRL/lpr mice, also inhibited NO production in cultured MRL/lpr mesangial cells.[72] Interferon regulatory factor 1 (IRF1) may also play a role in iNOS expression. LPS/IFNγ-induced iNOS expression in MRL/lpr mesangial cells was abrogated through inactivation of the (IRF1) gene. MRL/lpr mice lacking a functional IRF1 gene also had reduced expression of splenic cell iNOS. It is difficult to conclude whether the lack of IRF1 directly reduces iNOS expression in MRL/lpr mice, as IRF1 deficiency also reduced anti-dsDNA antibody production and glomerular immune complex deposition.[73] In NZB/W mesangial cells, IL20 and IL20 receptors are upregulated, and addition of IL20 induces expression of iNOS along with IL6, RANTES, IP10, and MCP-1.[74] Some interventions that do not directly inhibit iNOS enzyme in vitro can reduce expression of iNOS/NO production in vivo. For instance, chemical induction of heme oxygenase-1 and oral administration of mycophenolate mofetil both effectively reduced glomerulonephritis in MRL/lpr mice while concurrently reducing iNOS expression in the kidney and not impacting iNOS expression in vitro.[75–77] These data suggest that glomerular iNOS expression in murine models can be induced through several independent mechanisms. iNOS expression, however, is not required for development of glomerulonephritis in vivo, as iNOS-deficient MRL/lpr mice developed renal disease similar to that of their wild-type littermates. This unexpected result is discussed in more detail below.

iNOS INHIBITION IN MURINE LUPUS

Several studies utilizing competitive inhibitors of iNOS suggest that iNOS activity is pathogenic in murine lupus. Inhibiting iNOS activity in MRL/lpr mice, before disease onset, with the nonspecific arginine analog L-N^G-monomethyl-L-arginine (L-NMMA) reduced 3NTyr formation in the kidney, partially restored renal catalase activity, and inhibited cellular proliferation and necrosis within the glomerulus.[68,70,78] Improved renal disease and survival in the iNOS-deficient mice occurred despite no significant decrease in immunoglobulin or complement deposition in the glomerulus. These findings suggest that increased iNOS expression occurred downstream of immune complex deposition and complement activation.[68] The partially selective iNOS inhibitor L-N^6-(1-iminoethyl)lysine (L-NIL) had a similar effect when used to treat MRL/lpr mice prior to disease onset. L-NIL-treated mice exhibited significant improvement in glomerular histopathology compared to vehicle-treated littermates and similar protection against renal disease compared to L-NMMA-treated mice. However, proteinuria was only partially inhibited in the L-NIL-treated mice, whereas L-NMMA-treated mice developed no significant proteinuria.[78] L-NMMA therapy in NZB/W mice, that already had significant clinical nephritis, was also partially protective, but treatment postonset of disease was less effective as measured by proteinuria and renal histopathology than preventative therapy. L-NMMA, as monotherapy for the treatment of active disease, was less effective at renal protection in the rapidly progressive MRL/lpr disease model than in the more chronic progression model in NZB/NZW mice.[79]

In contrast to the effectiveness of pharmacologic iNOS inhibition in murine lupus, MRL/lpr mice genetically lacking iNOS, while having reduced vasculitis and IgG rheumatoid factor production, had similar proteinuria and glomerular pathology as their MRL/lpr wild-type littermates.[80] To address whether the beneficial effect of L-NMMA in lupus was unrelated to iNOS, MRL/lpr NOS2$^{-/-}$ mice were administered an iNOS-selective inhibitor prior to and throughout the progression of disease. NOS2$^{-/-}$ mice had elevated anti-dsDNA antibody levels and had, as observed in the past, no significant reductions in glomerular pathology or proteinuria. However, L-NMMA significantly reduced proteinuria and evidence of podocyte flattening and endothelial cell swelling by electron microscopy in iNOS-deficient mice.[81] These results indicate that L-NMMA therapy reduces pathologic changes in podocytes and endothelial cell pathology in an iNOS-independent (and possibly eNOS-dependent) fashion.

Studies of eNOS-deficient mice provided further insight into the role of NO in disease. In studies in MRL/lpr mice, the eNOS-deficient mice had markedly decreased survival due to development of severe vasculitis and crescentic glomerulonephritis.[82] Thus, low levels of NO produced by eNOS are anti-inflammatory and protective against vasculitis. High levels of NO production by iNOS are proinflammatory and enhance vasculitis.[83]

POTENTIAL MECHANISMS FOR PATHOGENICITY OF RNI IN MURINE MODELS OF LUPUS

As noted before, iNOS activity can lead to $ONOO^-$ production only if it occurs within or in close proximity to a cell with equimolar SO levels. One mechanism for production of SO and NO in close proximity is through the parallel production of SO by the reductase domain of iNOS itself. This process occurs in murine macrophages.[53] Support of this mechanism in lupus comes from the experiments with pharmacologic inhibition of iNOS in the MRL/lpr and NZB/W models. Mice given L-NIL or L-NMMA demonstrated significant reductions in markers of systemic oxidant stress (urine F2-isoprostanes) compared to vehicle-treated mice.[84] Thus some of the pathogenic effects of iNOS activity in SLE may arise from its ability to produce ROI in proximity to NO.

$ONOO^-$, a by-product of iNOS activity, can nitrate protein amino acids and change the catalytic activity of enzymes. One such enzyme, catalase, serves to protect host tissues from free radical attack.[70] In vascular tissue, prostacyclin synthase[85] and eNOS[86] are inactivated by $ONOO^-$, leading to vasoconstriction. These observations suggest that one mechanism through which iNOS activity is pathogenic is via deactivation of tissue protective enzymes.

Increasing attention in autoimmune diseases is being focused on whether immune tolerance can be broken by presentation of autoantigens in a novel manner. Two such processes are noteworthy: (1) presentation of nuclear antigens in the proinflammatory context of late apoptotic blebs and (2) posttranslational modification of self-antigens to form novel epitopes or neoepitopes. Because nuclear antigens are presented in late apoptotic blebs,[87] regulation of apoptosis and clearance of apoptotic cells are important areas of investigation. NO and $ONOO^-$ are both integral in regulating nonreceptor-mediated apoptosis.[88] To investigate the role of iNOS activity in apoptosis, MRL/lpr mice with active disease were treated with L-NMMA. Compared to controls, L-NMMA-treated mice exhibited reduced levels of splenocyte apoptosis. In vitro treatment of cultured splenocytes, isolated from mice with active disease, with an NO donor resulted in increased levels of apoptosis.[89] NO or other RNI appear to increase nonreceptor-mediated apoptosis despite the well-described defect in Fas receptor-mediated apoptosis in MRL/lpr mice.[90]

Another mechanism for inducing autoimmunity is via formation of neoepitopes in autoantigens. Both $ONOO$ and NO_2 can nitrate self-antigens in a manner that leads to a break in immune tolerance. For instance, normal mice immunized with nitrated IgG produced anti-nitrotyrosine antibodies that cross-reacted with single-stranded DNA (ssDNA).[91]

REACTIVE INTERMEDIATES IN HUMAN LUPUS

Due to the toxicity of iNOS inhibitors developed thus far, there have been no trials of a NOS inhibitor in human lupus. However, several studies demonstrated elevated markers of NO production in lupus patients compared to controls and a significant correlation between markers of systemic NO production and lupus disease activity.[13] One study demonstrated more prominent increases in markers of NO production among African–Americans with lupus disease activity.[92] A predisposition to produce increased NO in response to inflammatory stimuli may be inherited. Two NOS2 promoter polymorphisms were more prevalent in female African–American SLE subjects than race-matched controls. Increased markers of systemic NO production and improved malaria survival were observed in some African populations with these polymorphisms.[93] In GWAS studies done to date, however, there was not a significant association between SNPs in any of the NOS genes and lupus. The two malaria iNOS SNPs were not included on the arrays used for the GWAS studies. In a separate analysis, in African Americans, there were a higher number of SNPs in genes in the RI gene family than expected. These findings suggest that there may be a genetic link between lupus and RI genes in African Americans.[94] These combined observations engender the hypothesis that polymorphisms that are protective for specific infectious diseases may predispose to developing lupus due to their overall immune activation function.

iNOS Expression in the Lupus Skin Rash

The skin often mirrors or heralds disease activity in SLE. iNOS expression in this organ appears to be induced by a known trigger of SLE flares, UV light exposure. Immunostaining for iNOS protein and levels of NOS2 mRNA were elevated in 33% of epidermal tissue from cutaneous lupus subjects before exposure to ultraviolet B (UVB) irradiation, but expression was increased to 100% of skin tissue biopsied after UVB exposure.[95] SLE patients with photosensitivity are often Ro positive. The Ro protein Ro52 is normally expressed in the cytoplasm. In cutaneous lupus patients, Ro52 localizes to the nucleus in the presence of iNOS. In cultured primary keratinocytes in vitro, exogenous NO induces such a translocation from the cytoplasm to the nucleus, a phenomenon often seen in stressed cells.[46] These combined observations suggest that UV-induced iNOS expression in cutaneous lupus patients has a functional consequence on Ro52.

iNOS EXPRESSION IN PROLIFERATIVE NEPHRITIS

More recent longitudinal observational studies demonstrate increased systemic NO production (serum NO_x) in lupus patients with proliferative lupus nephritis when compared to those with nonproliferative renal disease or those without nephritis. In nephritis patients, those who did not achieve renal response to therapy had significantly higher serum NO_x levels in the first three months of therapy than those who achieved a renal response.[96] How sustained RNI production may mediate renal damage in LN is not completely understood, but several studies shed light on possible mechanisms.

Increased iNOS expression is consistently found in proliferative lupus nephritis.[92,97,98] In such proliferative lesions, citrulline staining increased in parallel with iNOS staining, suggesting that iNOS catalyzed the conversion of arginine to citrulline.[99] Glomerular iNOS staining also colocalized with markers of apoptosis and staining for p53, a redox-sensitive transcription factor that can signal for apoptosis in the presence of damaged DNA.[98] This is consistent with the known effect of higher levels of NO on p53 phosphorylation and activation.[58] Renal biopsies from patients with proliferative LN expressed increased glomerular, tubular, and interstitial cell iNOS levels. Tubulointerstitial iNOS levels correlated with the extent of proteinuria and reduced creatinine clearance at the time of biopsy. INOS and NF-κB colocalized with apoptotic cells in the glomerulus.[100] These data suggest two mechanisms for iNOS-mediated glomerular damage in proliferative nephritis: (1) increased signaling for apoptosis via increased p53 activity and; (2) inflammation through activation of NF-κB.

ROLE OF RNI IN VASCULAR DISEASE IN SLE

As described in the background, the ultimate effects of NOS activity are determined by the location and concentration of NO production combined with the proximity of this production to reactive oxygen. Several studies suggest that in SLE patients, NO production is increased in combination with reduced antioxidant capacity. So-called proinflammatory

HDL (piHDL) cannot prevent oxidation of LDL and aid in cholesterol reverse transport as can normal HDL. The presence of piHDL was significantly associated with carotid plaque in lupus patients. Apolipoprotein A-1 (Apo A1) is an HDL protein with both antioxidant and cholesterol efflux properties. SLE patients have increased levels of antibodies to Apo A1 that interfere with function. The presence of these antibodies was associated with elevations in markers of systemic NO production and reductions in total antioxidant capacity.[101] This interference with the antioxidant and anti-inflammatory properties of HDL resulted in a more conducive environment for atherosclerosis progression. Recently neutrophil nets were shown to have a pathogenic role in lupus as well as possibly the enhanced atherosclerotic disease in lupus. Neutrophil nets contain both ROI and RNI. HDL from patients with lupus contained higher levels of nitrotyrosine and chlorotyrosine. Lupus-derived HDL also had decreased antiatherogenic properties, further implicating RNI and ROI in the increased atherosclerosis seen in lupus patients[102]

ONOO⁻ can also modify lipids. Peroxidation of arachidonate by ONOO⁻ can lead to formation of isoprostanes,[103] known to stimulate monocyte adhesion to endothelial cells[104] and induce vasoconstriction in smooth muscles.[105] ONOO⁻ can also oxidize LDL. Oxidized, but not native LDL, complexes with β2-glycroprotein I. This antibody/antigen complex enhances influx of oxidized LDL into foamy macrophages, providing a plausible mechanism for accelerated atherosclerosis in SLE.[106] Some phospholipids within oxidized LDL have platelet-activating factor-like activity and can stimulate growth of smooth muscle cells.[69] Nitrogen dioxide derived from MPO, but not iNOS, can lead to nitration of tryptophan 166 in apo A1 within HDL. Nitration of this amino acid leads to a loss of cholesterol efflux capacity of HDL,[107] and this modification along with chlorination of this site confers a 6- to 16-fold risk for cardiovascular disease in nonlupus patients that is independent of Framingham risk factors.[108] The extent to which this phenomenon enhances atherosclerosis in SLE subjects is unknown.

Lupus patients often have reduced endothelial function that is manifested by decreased endothelium-dependent vasodilation.[109] The mechanism driving this defect is unclear, but increased levels of circulating endothelial cells, observed in lupus subjects, may be a marker of ongoing endothelial injury. This endothelial damage appears related to complement activation and is associated with iNOS activity. The level of circulating endothelial cells in lupus subjects correlated positively with disease activity and inversely with complement split product levels. Circulating endothelial cells stained positive for nitrotyrosine, a marker of iNOS or MPO activity.[110] This observation, combined with the observation that endothelial cells stain for iNOS even in nonlesional skin,[111] suggests an immune complex-mediated production of

ONOO⁻ or NO_2 by iNOS or MPO in endothelial cells.[110,111] Thus, reactive nitrogen and oxygen stress in SLE patients may lead to combined reductions in the protective effects of endothelial and HDL function.

PATHOGENIC MECHANISMS OF RNI PRODUCTION IN LUPUS PATIENTS

In SLE, one mechanism through which NO can be pathogenic is through ONOO⁻ or NO_2-mediated nitration of self-antigens. This nitration can form neoantigens and serve to break tolerance to self-antigens. This is supported by evidence that SLE serum bound more avidly to nitrated poly-L-tyrosine than native poly-L-tyrosine. Binding of SLE serum with dsDNA antibodies was inhibited by preincubation with nitrated poly-L-tyrosine, nitrated BSA, nitrated DNA, and nitrated chromatin much more effectively than native forms of these antigens. In addition, poly-L-tyrosine immunization of experimental animals induced antibodies that bound avidly to dsDNA and chromatin.[112] Similarly, peroxynitrite-treated DNA is more antigenic than native DNA when used in anti-dsDNA antibody testing of serum from lupus patients.[113,114] Thus ONOO⁻ and NO_2 modifications of self-antigens can create neoepitopes with increased binding affinity over native antigens and induce humoral autoimmunity.

NO production can also lead to T-cell dysfunction. Normal T cells express eNOS and nNOS but not iNOS following anti-CD3/CD28 costimulation. The resulting NO production induced an increase of mitochondrial hyperpolarization (MHP) in normal human T cells.[115] In contrast, T lymphocytes of SLE patients exhibited persistent MHP and mitochondrial mass, accounting for increased production of ROI. These data suggest that mitochondrial dysfunction leading to ATP depletion is ultimately responsible for diminished activation-induced apoptosis and sensitizes lupus T cells to necrosis.[116-118] NO-induced MHP in SLE T cells also leads to activation of mTOR, a sensor of mitochondrial potential and target of the drug rapamycin.[119]

CONCLUSION

Observational studies indicate a strong association between SLE and reactive oxygen and nitrogen intermediate production in animal models and humans. Moreover, expression of iNOS is increased in lupus and correlates with disease severity. Conflicting results from murine studies using pharmacologic or genetic manipulation of NOS highlight the complex biology of RIs in lupus. Future studies should investigate potential sources of RIs other than iNOS, define the key reactive species that are dominant in lupus, and address how the interplay between RNI and ROI may lead to a break in immune tolerance and enhanced lupus disease activity.

REFERENCES

1. Harman D. Aging: a theory based on free radical and radiation chemistry. *J Gerontol* 1956;**11**:298–300. PubMed PMID: 13332224.
2. Valko M, Leibfritz D, Moncol J, Cronin MTD, Mazur M, Telser J. Free radicals and antioxidants in normal physiological functions and human disease. *Int J Biochem Cell Biol* 2007;**39**:44–84. PubMed PMID: 16978905.
3. Wei C-C, Wang Z-Q, Durra D, Hemann C, Hille R, Garcin ED, et al. The three nitric-oxide synthases differ in their kinetics of tetrahydrobiopterin radical formation, heme-dioxy reduction, and arginine hydroxylation. *J Biol Chem* 2005;**280**:8929–35. PubMed PMID: 15632185.
4. Squadrito GL, Pryor WA. Oxidative chemistry of nitric oxide: the roles of superoxide, peroxynitrite, and carbon dioxide. *Free Radic Biol Med* 1998;**25**:392–403. PubMed PMID: 9741578.
5. Droge W. Free radicals in the physiological control of cell function. *Physiol Rev* 2002;**82**:47–95. PubMed PMID: 11773609.
6. D'Autreaux B, Toledano MB. ROS as signalling molecules: mechanisms that generate specificity in ROS homeostasis. *Nat Rev Mol Cell Biol* 2007;**8**(10):813–24. http://www.nature.com/nrm/journal/v8/n10/suppinfo/nrm2256_S1.html.
7. Sauer H, Wartenberg M, Hescheler J. Reactive oxygen species as intracellular messengers during cell growth and differentiation. *Cell Physiol Biochem* 2001;**11**:173–86. PubMed PMID: 11509825.
8. Ji LL, Gomez-Cabrera M-C, Vina J. Role of free radicals and antioxidant signaling in skeletal muscle health and pathology. *Infect Disord Drug Targets* 2009;**9**:428–44. PubMed PMID: 19689384.
9. Valko M, Rhodes CJ, Moncol J, Izakovic M, Mazur M. Free radicals, metals and antioxidants in oxidative stress-induced cancer. *Chem Biol Interact* 2006;**160**:1–40. PubMed PMID: 16430879.
10. Campos ACE, Molognoni F, Melo FHM, Galdieri LC, Carneiro CRW, D'Almeida V, et al. Oxidative stress modulates DNA methylation during melanocyte anchorage blockade associated with malignant transformation. *Neoplasia* 2007;**9**:1111–21. PubMed PMID: 18084618.
11. Kavak S, Ayaz L, Emre M, Inal T, Tamer L, Günay I. The effects of rosiglitazone on oxidative stress and lipid profile in left ventricular muscles of diabetic rats. *Cell Biochem Funct* 2008;**26**(4):478–85.
12. Gomez-Mejiba SE, Zhai Z, Akram H, Deterding LJ, Hensley K, Smith N, et al. Immuno-spin trapping of protein and DNA radicals: "tagging" free radicals to locate and understand the redox process. *Free Radic Biol Med* 2009;**46**(7):853–65.
13. Oates JC, Gilkeson GS. The biology of nitric oxide and other reactive intermediates in systemic lupus erythematosus. *Clin Immunol* 2006;**121**:243–50. http://dx.doi.org/10.1016/j.clim.2006.06.001. Epub 25.07.06. PII:S1521-6616(06)00767-4. PubMed PMID: 16861040; PubMed Central PMCID: PMC2765327.
14. Trostchansky A, O'Donnell VB, Goodwin DC, Landino LM, Marnett LJ, Radi R, et al. Interactions between nitric oxide and peroxynitrite during prostaglandin endoperoxide H synthase-1 catalysis: a free radical mechanism of inactivation. *Free Radic Biol Med* 2007;**42**:1029–38. PubMed PMID: 17349930.
15. Pacher P, Mukhopadhyay P, Rajesh M, Batkai S, Hasko G, Szabo C. Interplay of superoxide, nitric oxide and peroxynitrite in doxorubicin-induced cell death. *FASEB J* 2008;**22** (1_MeetingAbstracts):970.12-.
16. Kurien BT, Scofield RH. Free radical mediated peroxidative damage in systemic lupus erythematosus. *Life Sci* 2003;**73**:1655–66. PubMed PMID: 12875898.

17. Craig WY. Autoantibodies against oxidized low density lipoprotein: a review of clinical findings and assay methodology. *J Clin Lab Anal* 1995;**9**:70–4. PubMed PMID: 7722776.

18. Kopkan L, Castillo A, Navar LG, Majid DSA. Enhanced superoxide generation modulates renal function in ANG II-induced hypertensive rats. *Am J Physiol Ren Physiol* 2006;**290**(1):F80–6. http://dx.doi.org/10.1152/ajprenal.00090.2005.

19. Brand MD, Affourtit C, Esteves TC, Green K, Lambert AJ, Miwa S, et al. Mitochondrial superoxide: production, biological effects, and activation of uncoupling proteins. *Free Radic Biol Med* 2004;**37**:755–67. PubMed PMID: 15304252.

20. Vignais PV. The superoxide-generating NADPH oxidase: structural aspects and activation mechanism. *Cell Mol Life Sci* 2002;**59**:1428–59. PubMed PMID: 12440767.

21. Vorbach C, Harrison R, Capecchi MR. Xanthine oxidoreductase is central to the evolution and function of the innate immune system. *Trends Immunol* 2003;**24**:512–7. PubMed PMID: 12967676.

22. Bonizzi G, Piette J, Merville MP, Bours V. Cell type-specific role for reactive oxygen species in nuclear factor-kappaB activation by interleukin-1. *Biochem Pharmacol* 2000;**59**:7–11. PubMed PMID: 10605929.

23. Feng L, Xia Y, Garcia GE, Hwang D, Wilson CB. Involvement of reactive oxygen intermediates in cyclooxygenase-2 expression induced by interleukin-1, tumor necrosis factor-alpha, and lipopolysaccharide. *J Clin Invest* 1995;**95**:1669–75. PubMed PMID: 7706475.

24. Satoh M, Fujimoto S, Haruna Y, Arakawa S, Horike H, Komai N, et al. NAD(P)H oxidase and uncoupled nitric oxide synthase are major sources of glomerular superoxide in rats with experimental diabetic nephropathy. *Am J Physiol Ren Physiol* 2005;**288**(6):F1144–52. http://dx.doi.org/10.1152/ajprenal.00221.2004.

25. Keisari Y, Braun L, Flescher E. The oxidative burst and related phenomena in mouse macrophages elicited by different sterile inflammatory stimuli. *Immunobiology* 1983;**165**:78–89. PubMed PMID: 6309652.

26. Rahman I, Yang S-R, Biswas SK. Current concepts of redox signaling in the lungs. *Antioxid Redox Signal* 2006;**8**:681–9. PubMed PMID: 16677111.

27. Zahrt TC, Deretic V. Reactive nitrogen and oxygen intermediates and bacterial defenses: unusual adaptations in *Mycobacterium tuberculosis*. *Antioxid Redox Signal* 2002;**4**:141–59. PubMed PMID: 11970850.

28. Deby C, Goutier R. New perspectives on the biochemistry of superoxide anion and the efficiency of superoxide dismutases. *Biochem Pharmacol* 1990;**39**:399–405. PubMed PMID: 2154984.

29. Steinbeck MJ, Khan AU, Karnovsky MJ. Extracellular production of singlet oxygen by stimulated macrophages quantified using 9,10-diphenylanthracene and perylene in a polystyrene film. *J Biol Chem* 1993;**268**:15649–54. PubMed PMID: 8340389.

30. Veal EA, Day AM, Morgan BA. Hydrogen peroxide sensing and signaling. *Mol Cell* 2007;**26**:1–14. PubMed PMID: 17434122.

31. Foreman J, Demidchik V, Bothwell JHF, Mylona P, Miedema H, Torres MA, et al. Reactive oxygen species produced by NADPH oxidase regulate plant cell growth. *Nature* 2003;**422**:442–6. PubMed PMID: 12660786.

32. Li J, Stouffs M, Serrander L, Banfi B, Bettiol E, Charnay Y, et al. The NADPH oxidase NOX4 drives cardiac differentiation: role in regulating cardiac transcription factors and MAP kinase activation. *Mol Biol Cell* 2006;**17**:3978–88. PubMed PMID: 16775014.

33. Geiszt M, Leto TL. The Nox family of NAD(P)H oxidases: host defense and beyond. *J Biol Chem* 2004;**279**:51715–8. PubMed PMID: 15364933.

34. Brandon M, Baldi P, Wallace DC. Mitochondrial mutations in cancer. *Oncogene* 2006;**25**(34):4647–62.

35. Stadler K, Bonini MG, Dallas S, Jiang J, Radi R, Mason RP, et al. Involvement of inducible nitric oxide synthase in hydroxyl radical-mediated lipid peroxidation in streptozotocin-induced diabetes. *Free Radic Biol Med* 2008;**45**(6):866–74.

36. Mütze S, Hebling U, Stremmel W, Wang J, Arnhold J, Pantopoulos K, et al. Myeloperoxidase-derived hypochlorous acid antagonizes the oxidative stress-mediated activation of iron regulatory protein 1. *J Biol Chem* 2003;**278**(42):40542–9. http://dx.doi.org/10.1074/jbc.M307159200.

37. Winterbourn CC, Vissers MC, Kettle AJ. Myeloperoxidase. *Curr Opin Hematol* 2000;**7**:53–8. PubMed PMID: 10608505.

38. Hampton MB, Kettle AJ, Winterbourn CC. Inside the neutrophil phagosome: oxidants, myeloperoxidase, and bacterial killing. *Blood* 1998;**92**(9):3007–17.

39. Lau D, Baldus S. Myeloperoxidase and its contributory role in inflammatory vascular disease. *Pharmacol Ther* 2006;**111**:16–26. PubMed PMID: 16476484.

40. Nicholls SJ, Hazen SL. Myeloperoxidase and cardiovascular disease. *Arterioscler Thromb Vasc Biol* 2005;**25**(6):1102–11. http://dx.doi.org/10.1161/01.ATV.0000163262.83456.6d.

41. Eiserich JP, Baldus S, Brennan M-L, Ma W, Zhang C, Tousson A, et al. Myeloperoxidase, a leukocyte-derived vascular NO oxidase. *Science* 2002;**296**:2391–4. PubMed PMID: 12089442.

42. Xu J, Xie Z, Reece R, Pimental D, Zou M-H. Uncoupling of endothelial nitric oxidase synthase by hypochlorous acid: role of NAD(P)H oxidase-derived superoxide and peroxynitrite. *Arterioscler Thromb Vasc Biol* 2006;**26**(12):2688–95. http://dx.doi.org/10.1161/01.atv.0000249394.94588.82.

43. Zhang C, Yang J, Jacobs JD, Jennings LK. Interaction of myeloperoxidase with vascular NAD(P)H oxidase-derived reactive oxygen species in vasculature: implications for vascular diseases. *Am J Physiol Heart Circ Physiol* 2003;**285**:2563–72. PubMed PMID: 14613914.

44. Marsche G, Heller R, Fauler G, Kovacevic A, Nuszkowski A, Graier W, et al. 2-chlorohexadecanal derived from hypochlorite-modified high-density lipoprotein-associated plasmalogen is a natural inhibitor of endothelial nitric oxide biosynthesis. *Arterioscler Thromb Vasc Biol* 2004;**24**:2302–6. PubMed PMID: 15514213.

45. Migliorini P, Pratesi F, Bongiorni F, Moscato S, Scavuzzo M, Bombardieri S. The targets of nephritogenic antibodies in systemic autoimmune disorders. *Autoimmun Rev* 2002;**1**(3):168–73.

46. Espinosa A, Oke V, Elfving A, Nyberg F, Covacu R, Wahren-Herlenius M. The autoantigen Ro52 is an E3 ligase resident in the cytoplasm but enters the nucleus upon cellular exposure to nitric oxide. *Exp Cell Res* 2008;**314**(20):3605–13. http://dx.doi.org/10.1016/j.yexcr.2008.09.011. Epub 11.10.08. PII:S0014-4827(08)00360-1. PubMed PMID: 18845142.

47. Alderton WK, Cooper CE, Knowles RG. Nitric oxide synthases: structure, function and inhibition. *Biochem J* 2001;**357**:593–615. PubMed PMID: 11463332.

48. Kleinert H, Pautz A, Linker K, Schwarz PM. Regulation of the expression of inducible nitric oxide synthase. *Eur J Pharmacol* 2004;**500**(1–3):255–66. PubMed PMID: 15464038.

49. Karpuzoglu E, Ahmed SA. Estrogen regulation of nitric oxide and inducible nitric oxide synthase (iNOS) in immune cells: implications for immunity, autoimmune diseases, and apoptosis. *Nitric Oxide* 2006;**15**. PubMed PMID: 16647869.

50. Reilly CM, Oates JC, Sudian J, Crosby MB, Halushka PV, Gilkeson GS. Prostaglandin J(2) inhibition of mesangial cell iNOS expression. *Clin Immunol* 2001;**98**(3):337–45.

51. Lincoln J, Hoyle CHV, Burnstock G. In: Lucy JA, editor. *Nitric oxide in health and disease*. New York (NY): Cambridge University Press; 1997. 363 pp.

52. *NOS2A in normal tissues Uppsala: human proteome resource program*. 2005. [cited 19.05.06.]. Available from: http://www.hpr.se/tissue_profile.php?antibody_id=2014.

53. Xia Y, Zweier JL. Superoxide and peroxynitrite generation from inducible nitric oxide synthase in macrophages. *Proc Natl Acad Sci USA* 1997;**94**(13):6954–8.

54. Gaertner SA, Janssen U, Ostendorf T, Koch KM, Floege J, Gwinner W. Glomerular oxidative and antioxidative systems in experimental mesangioproliferative glomerulonephritis. *J Am Soc Nephrol* 2002;**13**(12):2930–7. PubMed PMID: 12444211.

55. Abraham NG, Kappas A. Heme oxygenase and the cardiovascular-renal system. *Free Radic Biol Med* 2005;**39**(1):1–25. PubMed PMID: 15925276.

56. Wink DA, Feelisch M, Fukuto J, Chistodoulou D, Jourd'heuil D, Grisham MB, et al. The cytotoxicity of nitroxyl: possible implications for the pathophysiological role of NO. *Arch Biochem Biophys* 1998;**351**:66–74. PubMed PMID: 9501920.

57. Wink DA, Mitchell JB. Chemical biology of nitric oxide: insights into regulatory, cytotoxic, and cytoprotective mechanisms of nitric oxide. *Free Radic Biol Med* 1998;**25**:434–56. PubMed PMID: 9741580.

58. Thomas DD, Ridnour LA, Isenberg JS, Flores-Santana W, Switzer CH, Donzelli S, et al. The chemical biology of nitric oxide: implications in cellular signaling. Epub 29.04.08. *Free Radic Biol Med* 2008; **45**(1):18–31. http://dx.doi.org/10.1016/j.freeradbiomed.2008.03.020. PII:S0891-5849(08)00175-5. PubMed PMID: 18439435.

59. Kharitonov VG, Sharma VS, Magde D, Koesling D. Kinetics of nitric oxide dissociation from five- and six-coordinate nitrosyl hemes and heme proteins, including soluble guanylate cyclase. *Biochemistry* 1997;**36**:6814–8. PubMed PMID: 9184164.

60. Padmaja S, Huie RE. The reaction of nitric oxide with organic peroxyl radicals. *Biochem Biophys Res Commun* 1993;**195**:539–44. PubMed PMID: 8373394.

61. Thomas DD, Ridnour LA, Espey MG, Donzelli S, Ambs S, Hussain SP, et al. Superoxide fluxes limit nitric oxide-induced signaling. *J Biol Chem* 2006;**281**(36):25984–93. http://dx.doi.org/10.1074/jbc.M602242200.

62. Ridnour LA, Thomas DD, Mancardi D, Espey MG, Miranda KM, Paolocci N, et al. The chemistry of nitrosative stress induced by nitric oxide and reactive nitrogen oxide species. Putting perspective on stressful biological situations. *Biol Chem* 2005;**385**(1):1–10. http://dx.doi.org/10.1515/bc.2004.001.

63. Salvemini D, Doyle TM, Cuzzocrea S. Superoxide, peroxynitrite and oxidative/nitrative stress in inflammation. *Biochem Soc Trans* 2006;**34**(Pt 5):965–70. http://dx.doi.org/10.1042/bst0340965.

64. Leon L, Jeannin JF, Bettaieb A. Post-translational modifications induced by nitric oxide (NO): implication in cancer cells apoptosis. *Nitric Oxide* 2008;**19**(2):77–83. http://dx.doi.org/10.1016/j.niox.2008.04.014. Epub 14.05.08. PII:S1089-8603(08)00067-0. PubMed PMID: 18474258.

65. Delgado Alves J, Mason LJ, Ames PR, Chen PP, Rauch J, Levine JS, et al. Antiphospholipid antibodies are associated with enhanced oxidative stress, decreased plasma nitric oxide and paraoxonase activity in an experimental mouse model. *Rheumatology (Oxford)* 2005;**44**(10):1238–44. PubMed PMID: 15987712.

66. Zou MH, Yesilkaya A, Ullrich V. Peroxynitrite inactivates prostacyclin synthase by heme-thiolate-catalyzed tyrosine nitration. *Drug Metab Rev* 1999;**31**(2):343–9.

67. Goodwin DC, Landino LM, Marnett LJ. Reactions of prostaglandin endoperoxide synthase with nitric oxide and peroxynitrite. *Drug Metab Rev* 1999;**31**(1):273–94. http://dx.doi.org/10.1081/DMR-100101918. Epub 05.03.99. PubMed PMID: 10065376.

68. Weinberg JB, Granger DL, Pisetsky DS, Seldin MF, Misukonis MA, Mason SN, et al. The role of nitric oxide in the pathogenesis of spontaneous murine autoimmune disease: increased nitric oxide production and nitric oxide synthase expression in MRL-lpr/lpr mice, and reduction of spontaneous glomerulonephritis and arthritis by orally administered NG-monomethyl-L- arginine. *J Exp Med* 1994;**179**(2):651–60. PubMed PMID:7507509.

69. Heery JM, Kozak M, Stafforini DM, Jones DA, Zimmerman GA, McIntyre TM, et al. Oxidatively modified LDL contains phospholipids with platelet-activating factor-like activity and stimulates the growth of smooth muscle cells. *J Clin Invest* 1995;**96**(5):2322–30.

70. Keng T, Privalle CT, Gilkeson GS, Weinberg JB. Peroxynitrite formation and decreased catalase activity in autoimmune MRL-lpr/lpr mice. *Mol Med* 2000;**6**(9):779–92. Epub 09.11.00. PubMed PMID: 11071272; PubMed Central PMCID: PMC1949981.

71. Wang HP, Hsu TC, Hsu GJ, Li SL, Tzang BS. Cystamine attenuates the expressions of NOS- and TLR-associated molecules in the brain of NZB/W F1 mice. *Eur J Pharmacol* 2009;**607**(1–3): 102–6. http://dx.doi.org/10.1016/j.ejphar.2009.02.039. Epub 10.03.09. PII:S0014-2999(09)00196-4. PubMed PMID: 19268457.

72. Mishra N, Reilly CM, Brown DR, Ruiz P, Gilkeson GS. Histone deacetylase inhibitors modulate renal disease in the MRL-lpr/lpr mouse. *J Clin Invest* 2003;**111**(4):539–52. http://dx.doi.org/10.1172/JCI16153. PubMed PMID: 12588892; PubMed Central PMCID: PMC151922.

73. Reilly CM, Olgun S, Goodwin D, Gogal Jr RM, Santo A, Romesburg JW, et al. Interferon regulatory factor-1 gene deletion decreases glomerulonephritis in MRL/lpr mice. *Eur J Immunol* 2006;**36**(5): 1296–308. http://dx.doi.org/10.1002/eji.200535245. Epub 17.03.06. PubMed PMID: 16541466.

74. Li HH, Cheng HH, Sun KH, Wei CC, Li CF, Chen WC, et al. Interleukin-20 targets renal mesangial cells and is associated with lupus nephritis. *Clin Immunol* 2008;**129**(2):277–85. http://dx.doi.org/10.1016/j.clim.2008.07.006. Epub 06.09.08. PII:S1521-6616(08)00713-4. PubMed PMID: 18771958.

75. Takeda Y, Takeno M, Iwasaki M, Kobayashi H, Kirino Y, Ueda A, et al. Chemical induction of HO-1 suppresses lupus nephritis by reducing local iNOS expression and synthesis of anti-dsDNA antibody. *Clin Exp Immunol* 2004;**138**(2):237–44. PubMed PMID: 15498032.

76. Lui SL, Tsang R, Wong D, Chan KW, Chan TM, Fung PC, et al. Effect of mycophenolate mofetil on severity of nephritis and nitric oxide production in lupus-prone MRL/lpr mice. *Lupus* 2002;**11**(7):411–8. PubMed PMID: 12195781.

77. Yu CC, Yang CW, Wu MS, Ko YC, Huang CT, Hong JJ, et al. Mycophenolate mofetil reduces renal cortical inducible nitric oxide synthase mRNA expression and diminishes glomerulosclerosis in MRL/lpr mice. *J Lab Clin Med* 2001;**138**(1):69–77. PubMed PMID: 11433230.

78. Reilly CM, Farrelly LW, Viti D, Redmond ST, Hutchison F, Ruiz P, et al. Modulation of renal disease in MRL/lpr mice by pharmacologic inhibition of inducible nitric oxide synthase. *Kidney Int* 2002;**61**(3): 839–46. http://dx.doi.org/10.1046/j.1523-1755.2002.00230.x. Epub 19.02.02. PubMed PMID: 11849435.

79. Oates JC, Ruiz P, Alexander A, Pippen AM, Gilkeson GS. Effect of late modulation of nitric oxide production on murine lupus. *Clin Immunol Immunopathol* 1997;**83**(1):86–92. Epub 01.04.97. PII:S0090122997943324. PubMed PMID:9073540.

80. Gilkeson GS, Mudgett JS, Seldin MF, Ruiz P, Alexander AA, Misukonis MA, et al. Clinical and serologic manifestations of autoimmune disease in MRL-lpr/lpr mice lacking nitric oxide synthase type 2. *J Exp Med* 1997;**186**(3):365–73. Epub 04.08.97. PubMed PMID:9236188; PubMed Central PMCID: PMC2199001.

81. Njoku C, Self SE, Ruiz P, Hofbauer AF, Gilkeson GS, Oates JC. Inducible nitric oxide synthase inhibitor SD-3651 reduces proteinuria in MRL/lpr mice deficient in the NOS2 gene. *J Investig Med* 2008;**56**(7):911–9. http://dx.doi.org/10.231/JIM.0b013e3181889e13. Epub 18.09.08. PubMed PMID: 18797415; PubMed Central PMCID: PMC2637653.

82. Gilkeson GS, Mashmoushi AK, Ruiz P, Caza TN, Perl A, Oates JC. Endothelial nitric oxide synthase reduces crescentic and necrotic glomerular lesions, reactive oxygen production, and MCP1 production in murine lupus nephritis. *PLoS One* 2013;**8**(5):e64650. http://dx.doi.org/10.1371/journal.pone.0064650. PubMed PMID: 23741359; PubMed Central PMCID: PMC3669382.

83. Oates JC, Mashmoushi AK, Shaftman SR, Gilkeson GS. NADPH oxidase and nitric oxide synthase-dependent superoxide production is increased in proliferative lupus nephritis. *Lupus* 2013;**22**(13): 1361–70. http://dx.doi.org/10.1177/0961203313507988. PubMed PMID: 24106214; PubMed Central PMCID: PMC3839955.

84. Njoku CJ, Patrick KS, Ruiz Jr P, Oates JC. Inducible nitric oxide synthase inhibitors reduce urinary markers of systemic oxidant stress in murine proliferative lupus nephritis. *J Investig Med* 2005;**53**(7):347–52. PubMed PMID: 16297360.

85. Zou MH, Cohen R, Ullrich V. Peroxynitrite and vascular endothelial dysfunction in diabetes mellitus. *Endothelium* 2004;**11**(2):89–97. PubMed PMID: 15370068.

86. Zou MH, Shi C, Cohen RA. Oxidation of the zinc-thiolate complex and uncoupling of endothelial nitric oxide synthase by peroxynitrite. *J Clin Invest* 2002;**109**(6):817–26. PubMed PMID: 11901190.

87. Casciola-Rosen LA, Anhalt G, Rosen A. Autoantigens targeted in systemic lupus erythematosus are clustered in two populations of surface structures on apoptotic keratinocytes. *J Exp Med* 1994;**179**(4):1317–30.

88. Boyd CS, Cadenas E. Nitric oxide and cell signaling pathways in mitochondrial-dependent apoptosis. *Biol Chem* 2002;**383**(3–4):411–23. PubMed PMID: 12033432.

89. Oates JC, Gilkeson GS. Nitric oxide induces apoptosis in spleen lymphocytes from MRL/lpr mice. *J Investig Med* 2004;**52**(1):62–71. Epub 03.03.04. PubMed PMID: 14989372.

90. Singh AK. Lupus in the fast lane? *J R Coll Physicians Lond* 1995;**29**(6):475–8.

91. Ohmori H, Oka M, Nishikawa Y, Shigemitsu H, Takeuchi M, Magari M, et al. Immunogenicity of autologous IgG bearing the inflammation-associated marker 3-nitrotyrosine. *Immunol Lett* 2005;**96**(1):47–54. PubMed PMID: 15585307.

92. Oates JC, Christensen EF, Reilly CM, Self SE, Gilkeson GS. Prospective measure of serum 3-nitrotyrosine levels in systemic lupus erythematosus: correlation with disease activity. *Proc Assoc Am Physicians* 1999;**111**(6):611–21.

93. Oates JC, Levesque MC, Hobbs MR, Smith EG, Molano ID, Page GP, et al. Nitric oxide synthase 2 promoter polymorphisms and systemic lupus erythematosus in African-Americans. *J Rheumatol* 2003;**30**(1):60–7. Epub 01.01.03. PII:0315162X-30-60. PubMed PMID: 12508391.

94. Ramos PS, Oates JC, Kamen DL, Williams AH, Gaffney PM, Kelly JA, et al. Variable association of reactive intermediate genes with systemic lupus erythematosus in populations with different African ancestry. *J Rheumatol* 2013;**40**(6):842–9. http://dx.doi.org/10.3899/jrheum.120989. PubMed PMID: 23637325; PubMed Central PMCID: PMC3735344.

95. Kuhn A, Fehsel K, Lehmann P, Krutmann J, Ruzicka T, Kolbbachofen V. Aberrant timing in epidermal expression of inducible nitric oxide synthase after UV irradiation in cutaneous lupus erythematosus. *J Invest Dermatol* 1998;**111**(1):149–53.

96. Oates JC, Shaftman SR, Self SE, Gilkeson GS. Association of serum nitrate and nitrite levels with longitudinal assessments of disease activity and damage in systemic lupus erythematosus and lupus nephritis. *Arthritis Rheum* 2008;**58**(1):263–72. http://dx.doi.org/10.1002/art.23153. Epub 01.01.08. PubMed PMID: 18163495; PubMed Central PMCID: PMC2733831.

97. Furusu A, Miyazaki M, Abe K, Tsukasaki S, Shioshita K, Sasaki O, et al. Expression of endothelial and inducible nitric oxide synthase in human glomerulonephritis. *Kidney Int* 1998;**53**(6):1760–8.

98. Wang JS, Tseng HH, Shih DF, Jou HS, Ger LP. Expression of inducible nitric oxide synthase and apoptosis in human lupus nephritis. *Nephron* 1997;**77**(4):404–11. Epub 01.01.97. PubMed PMID:9434061.

99. Bollain YGJJ, Ramirez-Sandoval R, Daza L, Esparza E, Barbosa O, Ramirez D, et al. Widespread expression of inducible NOS and citrulline in lupus nephritis tissues. *Inflamm Res* 2009;**58**(2):61–6. http://dx.doi.org/10.1007/s00011-009-7215-1. Epub 03.02.09. PubMed PMID: 19184355.

100. Zheng L, Sinniah R, IHH S. Renal cell apoptosis and proliferation may be linked to nuclear factor-kappaB activation and expression of inducible nitric oxide synthase in patients with lupus nephritis. *Hum Pathol* 2006;**37**(6):637–47. PubMed PMID: 16733202.

101. Batuca JR, Ames PR, Amaral M, Favas C, Isenberg DA, Delgado Alves J. Anti-atherogenic and anti-inflammatory properties of high-density lipoprotein are affected by specific antibodies in systemic lupus erythematosus. *Rheumatology (Oxford)* 2009;**48**(1):26–31. http://dx.doi.org/10.1093/rheumatology/ken397. Epub 13.11.08. PubMed PMID: 19000993.

102. Ahmad R, Ahsan H. Role of peroxynitrite-modified biomolecules in the etiopathogenesis of systemic lupus erythematosus. *Clin Exp Med* 2014;**14**(1):1–11. http://dx.doi.org/10.1007/s10238-012-0222-5. PubMed PMID: 23179301.

103. Moore KP, Darley-Usmar V, Morrow J, Roberts 2nd LJ. Formation of F2-isoprostanes during oxidation of human low-density lipoprotein and plasma by peroxynitrite. *Circ Res* 1995;**77**(2):335–41.

104. Huber J, Bochkov VN, Binder BR, Leitinger N. The isoprostane 8-iso-PGE2 stimulates endothelial cells to bind monocytes via cyclic AMP- and p38 MAP kinase-dependent signaling pathways. *Antioxid Redox Signal* 2003;**5**(2):163–9. PubMed PMID: 12716476.

105. Fukunaga M, Makita N, Roberts 2nd LJ, Morrow JD, Takahashi K, Badr KF. Evidence for the existence of F2-isoprostane receptors on rat vascular smooth muscle cells. *Am J Physiol* 1993;**264** (6 Pt 1):C1619–24.

106. Lopez LR, Kobayashi K, Matsunami Y, Matsuura E. Immunogenic oxidized low-density lipoprotein/beta2-glycoprotein I complexes in the diagnostic management of atherosclerosis. *Clin Rev Allergy Immunol* 2008;**37**. http://dx.doi.org/10.1007/s12016-008-8096-8. Epub 05.11.08. PubMed PMID: 18982458.

107. Peng DQ, Brubaker G, Wu Z, Zheng L, Willard B, Kinter M, et al. Apolipoprotein A-I tryptophan substitution leads to resistance to myeloperoxidase-mediated loss of function. *Arterioscler Thromb Vasc Biol* 2008;**28**(11):2063–70. http://dx.doi.org/10.1161/ATVBAHA.108.173815. Epub 09.08.08. PII:ATVBAHA.108.173815. PubMed PMID: 18688016.

108. Nicholls SJ, Hazen SL. Myeloperoxidase, modified lipoproteins, and atherogenesis. *J Lipid Res* 2009;**50**(Suppl):S346–51. http://dx.doi.org/10.1194/jlr.R800086-JLR200. Epub 19.12.08. PII:R800086-JLR200. PubMed PMID: 19091698.

109. El-Magadmi M, Bodill H, Ahmad Y, Durrington PN, Mackness M, Walker M, et al. Systemic lupus erythematosus: an independent risk factor for endothelial dysfunction in women. *Circulation* 2004;**110**(4):399–404. PubMed PMID: 15262847.

110. Clancy R, Marder G, Martin V, Belmont HM, Abramson SB, Buyon J. Circulating activated endothelial cells in systemic lupus erythematosus: further evidence for diffuse vasculopathy. *Arthritis Rheum* 2001;**44**(5):1203–8. PubMed PMID: 11352255.

111. Belmont HM, Levartovsky D, Goel A, Amin A, Giorno R, Rediske J, et al. Increased nitric oxide production accompanied by the up-regulation of inducible nitric oxide synthase in vascular endothelium from patients with systemic lupus erythematosus. *Arthritis Rheum* 1997;**40**(10):1810–6. PubMed PMID:9336415.

112. Khan F, Ali R. Antibodies against nitric oxide damaged poly L-tyrosine and 3-nitrotyrosine levels in systemic lupus erythematosus. *J Biochem Mol Biol* 2006;**39**(2):189–96. PubMed PMID: 16584635.

113. Dixit K, Ali R. Role of nitric oxide modified DNA in the etiopathogenesis of systemic lupus erythematosus. *Lupus* 2004;**13**(2):95–100. PubMed PMID: 14995001.

114. Habib S, Moinuddin, Ali R. Peroxynitrite-modified DNA: a better antigen for systemic lupus erythematosus anti-DNA autoantibodies. *Biotechnol Appl Biochem* 2006;**43**(Pt 2):65–70. PubMed PMID: 16232128.

115. Nagy G, Koncz A, Perl A. T cell activation-induced mitochondrial hyperpolarization is mediated by Ca^{2+}- and redox-dependent production of nitric oxide. *J Immunol* 2003;**171**(10):5188–97. PubMed PMID: 14607919.

116. Gergely Jr P, Niland B, Gonchoroff N, Pullmann Jr R, Phillips PE, Perl A. Persistent mitochondrial hyperpolarization, increased reactive oxygen intermediate production, and cytoplasmic alkalinization characterize altered IL-10 signaling in patients with systemic lupus erythematosus. *J Immunol* 2002;**169**(2):1092–101. PubMed PMID: 12097418.

117. Nagy G, Barcza M, Gonchoroff N, Phillips PE, Perl A. Nitric oxide-dependent mitochondrial biogenesis generates Ca^{2+} signaling profile of lupus T cells. *J Immunol* 2004;**173**(6):3676–83. PubMed PMID: 15356113.

118. Gergely Jr P, Grossman C, Niland B, Puskas F, Neupane H, Allam F, et al. Mitochondrial hyperpolarization and ATP depletion in patients with systemic lupus erythematosus. *Arthritis Rheum* 2002;**46**(1):175–90. PubMed PMID: 11817589.

119. Fernandez DR, Telarico T, Bonilla E, Li Q, Banerjee S, Middleton FA, et al. Activation of mammalian target of rapamycin controls the loss of TCRzeta in lupus T cells through HRES-1/Rab4-regulated lysosomal degradation. *J Immunol* 2009;**182**(4):2063–73. http://dx.doi.org/10.4049/jimmunol.0803600. Epub 10.02.09. PubMed PMID: 19201859.

Chapter 30

Epigenetics

Christian M. Hedrich

Children's Hospital Dresden, Pediatric Rheumatology and Immunology Section, University Medical Center Carl Gustav Carus, TU Dresden, Dresden, Germany

INTRODUCTION

The pathophysiology of the systemic autoimmune disease systemic lupus erythematosus (SLE) is only partially understood.[1] In rare cases, SLE or lupus-like disorders are conferred by disease-causing mutations in single genes, such as the complement genes *C1*, *C2*, and *C4*.[2] In "classical" SLE, a strong genetic component is evident by a 25- to 30-fold increased risk of first-degree relatives of SLE patients to also develop the disease, which is even further enhanced in genetically identical monozygotic twins. However, this "only" results in 3–5% concordance rates in dizygotic twins or "normal" siblings, and 25–40% in identical twins.[1] These numbers are significantly too low to assume monogenic causes, following Mendelian traits. Thus, additional factors have been attributed to nongenetic, namely environmental, and hormonal factors, since postpubertal girls and women are 9–10 times more frequently affected than men (Figure 1).[1–3] Some of the environmental factors cause epigenetic modifications that have been recently implicated in the pathophysiology of SLE.[3–5]

The term epigenetics summarizes a group of gene regulatory mechanisms, governing gene expression in a stable, sometimes heritable fashion. Epigenetic alterations to the DNA itself or packing proteins, so-called histones, define gene expression patterns. The most central epigenetic mechanisms are DNA methylation, posttranslational histone modifications, and micro-RNAs. Together, those mechanisms regulate gene expression in a cell- and tissue-specific manner without altering the underlying DNA sequence.[3–5] Regardless of recent efforts mapping the "epigenome" in health and disease, epigenetic patterns are only partially understood. However, more recently it became increasingly clear that epigenetic marks are tightly regulated and that they can result in gene dysregulation, potentially contributing to a large number of autoimmune-inflammatory disorders.[3–8] The systemic autoimmune disease SLE is characterized by a profound dysregulation of immune function, the expression of a wide range of autoantibodies, and altered cytokine expression, resulting in a proinflammatory phenotype and

tissue damage.[1,2] A constantly growing body of literature supports a central involvement of epigenetic disturbances in the pathophysiology of SLE. Since most data on epigenetic alterations in SLE were generated in T cells, this chapter will mainly focus on selected key epigenetic mechanisms in such.

DNA METHYLATION IN T CELLS FROM SLE PATIENTS

Addition of a methyl group to the 5' position of the cytosine pyrimidine ring is a potent mechanism, attenuating the binding of transcription factors and RNA polymerases to DNA regulatory regions. In nonembryonic tissues, DNA methylation predominantly occurs at cytosine–phosphate–guanosine (CpG) dinucleotides and is established and controlled by DNA methyltransferases (DNMT). DNMT1 is mainly responsible for remethylation of the primarily unmethylated daughter strand during cell division, using the ancestor cells' methylation status as template. Thus, impaired activity of DNMT1 can result in gradual DNA demethylation and disrupted gene expression patterns. DNMT3a and DNMT3b are so-called de novo methyltransferases, mainly conferring DNA methylation to previously unmethylated CpG sites. An involvement of DNMT1 in de novo methylation has recently been documented, suggesting a more complex situation than the historic division into "maintenance" and de novo DNMTs (Figure 2).[3,4,6–9]

B and T cells from patients with SLE exhibit altered DNA methylation patterns. The relationship between reduced DNA methylation in T lymphocytes and SLE was first discovered in the 1990s by Bruce Richardson and his group.[10] In a series of publications, the authors demonstrated that T cells from SLE patients exhibit reduced DNA methylation, which correlated with disease activity.[9–11] In agreement with these findings, Javierre et al. more recently determined globally reduced DNA methylation in PBMCs from individuals with SLE as compared to their disease-discordant, genetically identical monozygotic twins.[6,12] Differences

Systemic Lupus Erythematosus. http://dx.doi.org/10.1016/B978-0-12-801917-7.00030-9

in DNA methylation were especially pronounced in several genes that are involved in immune regulation. More recently, a number of SLE-associated genes have been demonstrated to undergo epigenetic remodeling, exhibiting distinct, gene-specific methylation patterns. Next to DNA hypomethylation in many genes, a number of genes, however, exhibit increased DNA methylation in SLE T cells, suggesting a complex epigenetic pattern determining the proinflammatory effector T-cell phenotype in SLE patients.

In the following, DNA methylation patterns of several genes that are relevant to SLE pathogenesis and mechanisms contributing to such changes will be discussed.[3,4,6,9]

Receptors and Coreceptors

A number of methylation-sensitive (co)receptor and signaling molecule genes are expressed at increased levels in T and B cells from SLE patients.

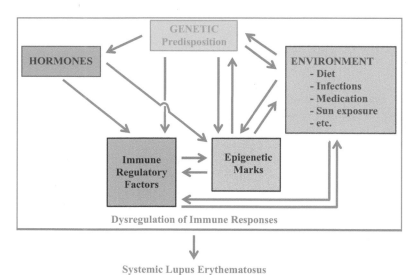

FIGURE 1 **Pathophysiology of systemic lupus erythematosus.** Genetic predisposition plays a central role in SLE pathophysiology. Some rare lupus-like disorders are caused by mutations in single genes (such as complement factor genes). In most cases, individuals have a more or less strong genetic predisposition for disease expression. However, additional factors need to be present to develop clinical SLE, including hormonal (estrogen) or environmental (infections, medication, etc.) factors, immune regulatory factors, and epigenetic marks. The sum effect of such alterations can be the disruption per se of physiological immune mechanisms and the development of autoimmune responses.

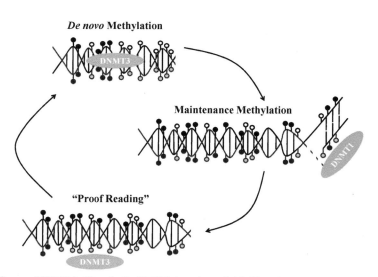

FIGURE 2 **DNA methyltransferases (DNMTs).** Historically DNMTs have been divided into de novo and maintenance enzymes. DNMT3a and b are generally responsible for the methylation of previously unmethylated genes or "proof reading" during cell division and subsequent remethylation of hemi-methylated CpGs. DNMT1 is responsible for the remethylation of the newly synthesized DNA daughter strand during cell division. Impaired function of DNMTs may therefore result in gradual demethylation of DNA and expression of previously silent genes.

CD11A, also referred to as integrin alpha L (ITGAL), along with CD18, forms the leukocyte function-associated antigen 1 that plays a central role during cellular adhesion and costimulation.[13] CD11A expression is increased in T cells from SLE patients and in response to treatment with DNA methylation inhibitors, such as procainamide or 5-azacytidine. Increased CD11A expression in SLE T cells is caused by reduced methylation of regulatory regions flanking the *ITGAL* gene.[5,10,14–16] Adoptive transfer of T cells overexpressing CD11A results in lupus-like symptoms in mice, indicating that hypomethylation of DNA in T cells mediates autoimmune responses that are at least partially due to the increased expression of CD11A.[16]

The **CD70 receptor** is encoded by the *TNFSF7* (tumor necrosis factor (TNF) super family 7) gene. CD70 is the cell-bound ligand of CD27, a TNF receptor family member. CD70 is transiently expressed on activated T cells.[17] CD27:CD70 interactions play a role during B-cell activation and IgG synthesis, as well as costimulatory signals for T-cell expansion. Interestingly, T-cell immunodeficiency has been reported to be induced by chronic costimulation through CD27:CD70 interactions.[18] This is of special interest, since T cells from SLE patients and lupus-prone mice as well as T cells treated with DNMT inhibitors express increased amounts of CD70, resulting in increased B-cell stimulation and IgG production. Those effects were reversible by CD70 inhibition.[3,9,17]

The **CD40 ligand (CD40L)**, also referred to as CD154, is a member of the TNF superfamily primarily expressed on activated T cells. CD40L binds the CD40 receptor on antigen-presenting cells (APCs). CD40:CD40L interactions mediate various events, depending on the target cell type.[19] On T cells, particularly on T follicular helper cells (T$_{FH}$ cells), CD40L acts as a costimulatory molecule. CD40:CD40L interactions between T$_{FH}$ cells and B cells promote their maturation and activation.[20] The absence of CD40L, on the other hand, abrogates the formation of germinal centers. CD40L is encoded by the *TNFSF5* gene on the X chromosome. In women, one X chromosome is inactivated through a complex epigenetic event, involving DNA methylation and histone modifications. Since women are 9- to 10-fold more frequently affected by SLE when compared to men, the question of whether reduced DNA methylation plays a role in the increased expression of CD40L in T cells from female SLE patients appears important.[3,5] Indeed, demethylation of *TNFSF5* resulted in increased CD40L expression in T cells from women. Likewise, female SLE patients exhibited reduced DNA methylation of *TNFSF5* on the second, usually methylated, X chromosome. Since increased CD40L expression results in increased B-cell costimulation and subsequent antibody production, this could be a central mechanism in the pathogenesis of SLE and may partially explain the female predominance in SLE.[21–23]

However, DNA methylation in SLE is even more complex, since gene-specific changes occur in either direction: hypo- or hypermethylation.[3] We documented the *CD8* **(cluster of differentiation 8) gene locus** undergoing epigenetic remodeling through DNA methylation in CD8+ T cells from SLE patients, contributing to the downregulation of surface CD8 coreceptors and the generation of CD3+TCR+CD4−CD8−, so-called double negative (DN) T cells.[24] DN T cells have been demonstrated to play a role in the pathophysiology of SLE through their increased expression of the proinflammatory effector cytokine IL-17A and their recruitment to inflamed tissues, including the kidneys, contributing to tissue damage.[25,26] The downregulation of CD8 has been linked to several molecular mechanisms, depending on the activating transcription factor CREM-α (cAMP response element activator-α).[27] CD4+ and CD8+ T cells from SLE patients produce increased amounts of CREM-α when compared to controls. We demonstrated that CREM-α recruits to regulatory elements within the *CD8* cluster, thus contributing to the silencing of gene expression. CREM-α *trans*-represses the *CD8B* promoter and induces epigenetic remodeling through the recruitment of DNMT3a, resulting in DNA methylation and stable silencing of *CD8* (Figure 3).[24,28]

Cytokine and Cytolysine Genes

Interleukin (IL-)2 is a pluripotent cytokine necessary for the proliferation and activation of T cells. Conversely, a lack of IL-2 or IL-2 signaling results in autoimmune

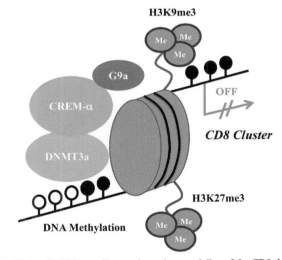

FIGURE 3 **CREM-α mediates epigenetic remodeling of the *CD8* cluster.** In eukaryotic cells, DNA is coiled around histone octamers (orange), which regulate its accessibility to transcription factors and RNA polymerases. In CD8+ T cells from SLE patients, CREM-α *trans*-represses the *CD8A* promoter. Furthermore, CREM-α instructs epigenetic remodeling of the entire *CD8* cluster through the recruitment of DNMT3a, and the histone methyltransferase G9a, resulting in DNA methylation and histone trimethylation at amino acid residues H3K9 and H3K27. The sum effect of these mechanisms is stable silencing of *CD8*, contributing to the generation of TCR+CD3+CD4−CD8− "double negative" T cells.

pathology in humans and mice.[29] Attenuated IL-2 production and IL-2 receptor signaling are hallmarks of SLE T cells. Reduced IL-2 expression has been linked to the impaired generation of regulatory T cells (T regs) and reduced activation-induced cell death, both contributing to enhanced activity and longer survival of autoreactive T cells.[29,30] The failure to produce IL-2 in T cells from SLE patients has been linked to several molecular mechanisms, all depending on CREM-α.[3,4,27] As aforementioned, SLE T cells produce increased amounts of CREM-α. We demonstrated CREM-α recruitment to regulatory elements within the *IL2* promoter centrally contributing to the silencing of gene expression. CREM-α *trans*-repressed *IL2* promoter activity and induces epigenetic remodeling through the recruitment of DNMT1 and DNMT3a.[31–33]

The proinflammatory effector cytokine **interleukin (IL-)17** consists of several isoforms: IL-17A through IL-17F. All IL-17 isoforms are key players in the host defense against bacteria and fungi. IL-17 cytokines have also been implicated in the development and course of autoimmune disorders, including SLE.[34] IL-17 is mainly produced by T cells, NK cells, mast cells, and neutrophils. Its function is, e.g., die induction of chemokines, additional cytokines, and the recruitment of neutrophils to inflamed tissues. Thus, IL-17A plays a central role in the development of tissue damage.[31,34] The expression of IL-17A is increased in T cells from SLE patients.[31] We demonstrated that, conversely

to *IL2*, the transcription factor CREM-α *trans*-activates *IL17A*.[27,32,35–37] CREM-α furthermore mediates DNA demethylation of the entire *IL17* gene locus in a yet to be determined fashion. Thus, CREM-α appears central to the generation of effector T-cell phenotypes in SLE and impaired cytokine expression.[27]

Interleukin (IL-10) is an immune-regulatory cytokine, ubiquitously expressed by immune cells and most other tissues. IL-10 modulates T-cell responses through several mechanisms, including the inhibition of MHC (major histocompatibility complex) II expression, reduced costimulation, and impaired proinflammatory cytokine expression from APCs.[38,39] Conversely, IL-10 contributes to the differentiation, proliferation, survival, and activation of B cells and induces antibody production. Thus, IL-10 has been implicated in the pathophysiology of SLE.[40] Indeed, IL-10 expression from immune cells and IL-10 serum levels are increased in SLE patients, reflecting disease activity.[41] IL-10 blockade with antibodies reduced disease activity in a subset of SLE patients.[35] We and others documented reduced DNA methylation of the *IL10* promoter and an enhancer element in the fourth intron of T cells from SLE patients, allowing for increased transcription factor binding and gene expression (Figure 4).[41–45]

Perforin, encoded by the perforin gene (*PRF1*), is a cytolytic protein produced by CD8+ T cells and NK cells. After degranulation, perforin inserts into target cells, forming a pore subsequently resulting in immune-mediated cell lysis.[46]

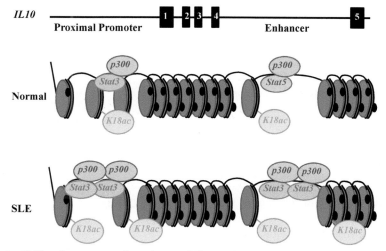

FIGURE 4 Stat3 *trans*-activates *IL10* and promotes epigenetic remodeling. *IL10* consists of five exons, a 5′ proximal promoter, which is considered to harbor the main regulatory elements, and an enhancer element in the fourth intron (upper panel). T cells from SLE patients are characterized by increased Stat3 phosphorylation, resulting in an overabundance of Stat3 in the nucleus. The middle and lower panels depict the epigenetic conformation of the *IL10* gene in health (normal) and disease (SLE). Blue cylinders symbolize histone octamers, the black lines symbolize DNA, and filled black circles DNA methylation. Histone modifications are depicted as orange circles (K18ac: histone 3 lysine 18 acetylation). Under physiological conditions (middle panel) and in SLE (lower panel), Stat3 recruits to the *IL10* proximal promoter. In healthy T cells, mainly Stat5 recruits to the enhancer. Both Stat3 and Stat5 *trans*-activate *IL10* and instruct epigenetic remodeling through the histone acetyltransferase p300, mediating histone acetylation (H3K18ac) and "opening" of the *IL10* gene. In SLE T cells, impaired DNA methylation "opens" additional Stat response elements within the proximal promoter. Reduced DNA methylation, together with increased nuclear levels of Stat3 in SLE T cells, results in increased Stat3 recruitment to the proximal promoter and replacement of Stat5 at the enhancer, allowing for *trans*-activation and epigenetic remodeling through p300.

CD4+ T cells from clinically active SLE patients abnormally produce perforin, while CD8+ T cells produce increased amounts. Perforin expression was linked to DNA demethylation of the *PRF1* promoter in both CD4+ and CD8+ T cells and a 3′ enhancer element particularly in CD4+ T cells from SLE patients.[47–49] It has been postulated that increased perforin production from CD4+ T cells in SLE results in increased macrophage/monocyte apoptosis and subsequent autoantibody production and organ damage.[9,50]

HISTONE MODIFICATIONS

Nucleosomes are the basic subunit of chromatin, consisting of 146 bp of DNA coiled around histone octamers consisting of two copies of each H2A, H2B, H3, and H4. Histones regulate gene expression and the structure of whole chromosomes. Posttranslational modifications to amino-termini of histone proteins influence their electric charge, strongly impacting nucleosome function. Modifications include histone acetylation, methylation, ubiquitination, phosphorylation, and many others. Each of these modifications and their combination facilitate specific changes to nucleosome arrangement and chromatin structure.[3,4,7,8,51] Histone modifications and DNA methylation often concur and can even be translated into one another. At present, we are only beginning to understand the molecular mechanisms mediating epigenetic patterns. Experimental data on the involvement of an altered histone code in SLE are limited. Histone modifications in SLE, however, appear to be even more complex when compared to DNA methylation. Histone acetylation in some regions is associated with disease activity whereas it is protective in other regions. Most data on disturbed histone marks in SLE are available for the surface coreceptors *CD8A* and *CD8B* and several cytokine genes.[4,24,27,31,32,37,52–54]

Receptors and Coreceptors

The *CD8* **(cluster of differentiation 8) gene locus** is regulated through DNA methylation and histone modifications.[24,55,56] During the generation of DN T cells from CD8+ T cells, CREM-α recruits to various regulatory elements within the *CD8* cluster instructing DNMT3a and histone methyltransferase G9a corecruitment to the CD8 cluster. This contributed to epigenetic silencing through DNA and histone methylation, resulting in stable silencing of *CD8A* and *CD8B* (Figure 3).[24,28]

Cytokine Genes

As aforementioned, **interleukin (IL-)2** centrally contributes to T-cell proliferation and activation, and also the generation of T regs and the termination of inflammatory responses.[1,29,30] Histone marks have been documented as centrally contributing to the control of IL-2 expression.[32,57,58] In T cells from SLE

patients, histone modifications reflect disrupted DNA methylation of the *IL2* gene. Reduced histone acetylation and increased histone methylation enhance the effects of DNA methylation. We linked these epigenetic modifications to the overexpression of CREM-α in SLE T cells.[32,33] CREM-α recruits histone deacetylase (HDAC)1 to the *IL2* promoter, mediating histone deacetylation.[31,32] Since CREM-α physically interacts with G9a mediating G9a recruitment and histone methylation at other genes (*CD8A* and *CD8B*),[24] this mechanism likely contributes to the silencing of *IL2*.[32] However, this has not experimentally been proven for the *IL2* gene yet.

Also, the proinflammatory cytokine genes *IL17A* **and** *IL17F* undergo chromatin remodeling through histone modifications.[3,31,53] In T cells from patients with SLE, increased histone acetylation and reduced histone methylation reflect reduced DNA methylation of the *IL17* gene cluster.[4,24,28,31,32,53] Interestingly, epigenetic modifications, though antithetic to the changes at the *IL2* gene, are also mediated by CREM-α.[32] The exact molecular mechanisms, however, remain to be determined.

Expression of the immune-regulatory **interleukin (IL-10)** is also governed by histone modifications.[36,39,41,43,59–61] In T cells from SLE patients, the *IL10* promoter and an intronic enhancer undergo activating histone modifications. The aforementioned preexistingly reduced DNA methylation of the *IL10* promoter and the intronic enhancer allows for increased transcription factor binding in SLE.[41,62] This, together with increased nuclear levels of Stat3 in SLE T cells, results in increased Stat3 recruitment to *IL10* regulatory regions. Subsequently, Stat3 mediates *trans*-activation and the recruitment of histone acetyltransferase (HAT) p300, resulting in enhanced histone acetylation (H3K18ac) and gene expression (Figure 4).[41]

MICRO-RNAs IN SLE

Micro-RNAs are small RNAs, spanning 21 to 23 bp. They function as posttranscriptional and/or posttranslational regulators of gene expression. Micro-RNAs derive from larger transcripts that are transcribed from intergenic DNA. Intergenic transcription contributes to chromatin remodeling, since a tight correlation between the chromatin structure and the presence of intergenic transcription permits interactions between proximal and distal regulatory regions. After transcription, intergenic transcripts are cleaved by the nuclear ribonuclease Drosha and exported into the cytoplasm. There, Dicer further processes the transcripts into mature micro-RNAs. The function of micro-RNAs can be executed by duplex formation with target genes and subsequent downregulation of gene expression, mRNA cleavage, or translational arrest. A large number of micro-RNAs are suspected to control at least one-third of human gene transcription and are involved in cell and tissue differentiation, cell cycle programming, programmed cell death, and the regulation of immune responses. Thus, micro-RNAs

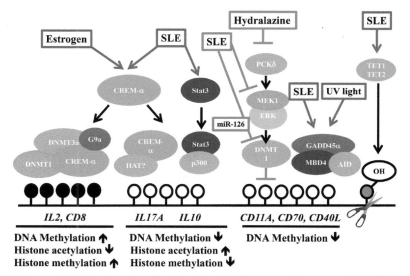

FIGURE 5   Molecular mechanisms contributing to epigenetic alterations in SLE. Epigenetic patterns in SLE T cells are complex with increased DNA and histone methylation (*IL2, CD8*) in some and reduced DNA and histone methylation (*IL17, IL10, CD11A, CD70, CD40L*) in other areas. A number of molecular mechanisms have been documented central to epigenetic disruption in T cells from SLE patients. Environmental factors and the disease itself can activate (green boxes) or inhibit (red boxes) molecular events. The transcription factor CREM-α is expressed at increased levels in T cells from SLE patients, and estrogen receptor signaling has been reported to increase CREM-α expression. CREM-α centrally contributes to disrupted epigenetic marks in SLE T cells. Through its interactions with DNMT1, DNMT3a, and the histone methyltransferase G9a, it contributes to epigenetic silencing of *IL2* and *CD8A/B*. Conversely, CREM-α instructs the epigenetic "opening" of *IL17* in a yet to be determined manner. Stat3, another transcription factor that is overactivated in SLE T cells, mediates epigenetic remodeling of *IL10* through the interaction with the histone acetyltransferase p300. Several molecular events have been linked with DNA demethylation in SLE T cells. Defective ERK pathway activation, particularly through the protein kinase PCK-δ that can be inhibited by hydralazine, mediates reduced activity of DNMT1 and gradual DNA demethylation. Furthermore, DNMT1 expression can be reduced by miR-126, which is expressed at increased levels in SLE T cells. Growth arrest and DNA damage-inducible protein alpha (GADD45α), which is overexpressed in T cells from SLE patients and inducible by UV irradiation, mechanisms contributing to SLE flares, mediates DNA demethylation in conjunction with two enzymes: activation-induced deaminase (AID), and methyl-CpG-binding domain (MBD)4-related G:T glycosylase. Another potential, most recently reported mechanism involves Ten–eleven translocation (TET) proteins (TET). TET1 and TET2 are expressed at increased levels in T cells from SLE patients and have been claimed as mediating hydroxymethylation (-OH) of DNA, an intermediate of several active demethylation pathways.

are interesting targets in the search for molecular pathomechanisms and potential biomarkers in SLE. To date, several micro-RNAs have been implicated in the pathophysiology of SLE and can be divided into three groups[4,63]: (1) micro-RNAs that are involved in the regulation of innate immune responses (miR-146a),[64] (2) micro-RNAs involved in anti-inflammatory responses (miR-125a),[65] and (3) micro-RNAs that regulate DNA methylation and histone modifications (DNA methylation, e.g., miR-126 (Figure 5),[66] miR-21, miR-148a[67]; histone modifications, miR-181a[68]). Conversely, the presence of intergenic transcripts and subsequently the expression of micro-RNAs are largely affected by other epigenetic events, namely DNA methylation and histone modifications. Thus, DNMT and HDAC inhibitors have been demonstrated, upregulating micro-RNA expression.[4,39]

MOLECULAR MECHANISMS OF PATHOLOGICAL EPIGENETIC REMODELING IN SLE

Recently, a number of molecular mechanisms have been established contributing to epigenetic disruption of various genes in immune cells from SLE patients.

Transcription Factors Mediate Epigenetic Changes in SLE T Cells

Recent work focused on disrupted transcription factor networks mediating epigenetic alterations in SLE T cells. Transcription factors contribute to the establishment and maintenance of tightly balanced gene expression programs during the differentiation of cells and tissues.[4,9,38,39,41] In addition to their *trans*-regulatory capacities, transcription factors orchestrate epigenetic remodeling of target genes. We established the involvement of the transcription factors CREM-α and Stat3, both of which are overactivated in SLE T cells, in chromatin remodeling of cytokine genes in health and disease.[27,41] CREM-α affects the expression of cytokine genes in a diametric fashion. As aforementioned, CREM-α *trans*-represses *IL2* and instructs epigenetic silencing through DNMT1, DNMT3, and G9a, while *trans*-activating *IL17A*.[31,32,37,53] Furthermore, CREM-α instructs DNA demethylation and histone acetylation of *IL17A* in a yet to be determined fashion.[31] CREM-α has been demonstrated to centrally contribute to the generation of DN T cells from CD8+ T cells in SLE.[24,28] Thus, CREM-α contributes to the determination of effector

T-cell phenotypes and T-cell subset distribution in SLE. Both Stat3 and Stat5 regulate the immune-modulatory cytokine IL-10.[38,39,41,44,45] In T cells from SLE patients, reduced levels of DNA methylation and increased nuclear concentrations of Stat3 result in increased transcription factor recruitment to regulatory elements and the replacement of Stat5 at an intronic enhancer. Both transcription factors, Stat3 and Stat5, corecruit the HAT p300, which is increased in SLE, further contributing to enhanced IL-10 expression.[41] Thus, transcription factor blockade has promising potential as future treatment options in autoimmune-inflammatory disorders, including SLE (Figure 5).

The Extracellular Signal-Regulated Kinase Pathway and Reduced DNA Methylation in SLE T Cells

Reduced DNA methylation in T cells from patients with SLE has been linked to the extracellular signal-regulated kinase (ERK) pathway. In patients with active SLE, defective activation of ERK results in reduced mitogen-activated protein kinase signaling and impaired DNMT1 activity. In concordance with these findings, the phenotype of SLE T cells can be mimicked through inhibition of the ERK pathway by MEK1 inhibitors. The contribution of impaired ERK activation in SLE is further supported by findings in mice that developed autoimmune phenotypes in response to MEK blockade or in animals with defective ERK signaling. In these systems, reduced DNMT1 activity results in gradual DNA demethylation and increased expression of CD11a, CD70, and CD40L (in female mice), the development of anti-dsDNA antibodies, and increased expression of interferon-regulated genes. Furthermore, inhibition of protein kinase C (PKC)δ with hydralazine centrally contributes to reduced ERK activation and that oxidative stress induced PCKδ phosphorylation. This observation is in agreement with PCKδ-deficient mice developing lupus-like symptoms, including glomerulonephritis and lymphocyte infiltration of several organ systems (Figure 5).[3,4,9]

GADD45α, AID, and MBD4 Mediate Reduced DNA Methylation in SLE

Three additional molecules have been implicated in DNA hypomethylation in SLE: the growth arrest and DNA damage-inducible protein alpha (GADD45α), activation-induced deaminase (AID), and methyl-CpG-binding domain (MBD)4-related G:T glycosylase. GADD45α has been documented as expressed at increased levels in SLE T cells and suspected to promote DNA demethylation in a complex mechanism through interaction with AID and MBD4. Interestingly, GADD45 has also been demonstrated to be upregulated by UV irradiation, a mechanism contributing to SLE flares (Figure 5).[3,4,9]

DNA Hydroxymethylation in SLE T Cells

Recently, the oxidation of 5-methylcytosine into 5-hydroxymethylcytosine by Ten–eleven translocation (TET) proteins has been documented as a central mechanism in the active regulation of DNA methylation. In SLE T cells, TET proteins TET1 and TET2 have been reported as increased and suspected to mediate active DNA demethylation (Figure 5).[3,5]

EPIGENETIC MODIFICATION AS PROMISING TARGETS FOR FUTURE TREATMENT

Epigenetic alterations in lymphocytes from SLE patients result in impaired gene expression and immune function, thus promising potential applications for reshaping the epigenome in future SLE treatment. In the following, epigenetic effects of existing treatment options and potential future interventions will be discussed.

Epigenetics as Targets of Already Existing Treatments

Though SLE is a highly heterogeneous disease with large interindividual variability in organ involvement and resulting damage, treatment options are not particularly target directed. Current protocols at best suggest "more or less" individualized treatment strategies with various immune-suppressing drugs, based on the severity and distribution of organ involvement. Treatment regimens include (1) antimalarial agents for almost all SLE patients, (2) corticosteroids, and (3) immunosuppressives, which are based on organ involvement. In selected cases, novel, antibody-based biological treatments can be discussed. All treatment regimens have the potential of severe side effects with an overall more or less disappointing outcome.[1]

1. **Antimalarial agents** (chloroquine, hydroxychloroquine) have beneficial effects on the course of SLE, resulting in fewer flares. Their mechanism of action, however, is not fully understood. Pharmacoepigenetic studies documented altered micro-RNA expression in response to hydroxychloroquine treatment in mice.[51,69]
2. **Corticosteroids** directly or indirectly regulate the transcription of genes.[70] Because of their rapid anti-inflammatory and immune-suppressive effects, corticosteroids are widely used in SLE treatment. Corticosteroids have been discussed as inducing RNA-binding proteins, and modulating micro-RNA expression.[71] Furthermore, corticosteroids have been reported as modifying histone acetylation through the induction of nuclear factor interleukin-3-regulated (NFIL3)/E4BP4 expression, a transcription factor, that in turn alters histone acetylation and methylation, e.g., at the *CD40L* promoter.[72] These effects may explain some of the effects of corticosteroids in SLE.[51]

3. Several **immune-suppressive drugs**, including methotrexate (MTX), have been documented as modifying epigenetic patterns in cancer. MTX inhibits DNA synthesis through targeting the enzyme dihydrofolate reductase, which is used in cancer treatment. MTX has been discussed as blocking DNMT activity by depleting the synthesis of the DNMT substrate *S*-adenosylmethionine. This may contribute to some of the beneficial effects in autoimmune disorders.[73,74] Cyclophosphamide (CPM), an alkylating agent widely used in cancer treatment, exerts cytotoxic effects through the inhibition of DNA replication. The precise mechanisms of action in SLE treatment, however, are poorly understood. Recently, CPM treatment has been suggested as mediating increased DNA methylation through the induction of DNMT1 expression.[75] These partially conflicting explanations for MTX's and CPM's mechanisms in SLE underscore the complexity of epigenetic patterns in lupus and their potentially region-, cell-, and tissue-specific contributions to the pathophysiology of this complex disease.[3,4,51]

Epigenetic Alterations as Targets for Potential Future Strategies in SLE Therapy

Modulating altered DNA methylation and/or histone modifications are promising candidates in the search for effective, individually tailored, and well-tolerated therapeutic options in SLE. Modulating disrupted DNMT function and recruitment to certain genes in SLE T cells appears logical and possible. DNA methylation patterns, however, are complex with regions of hyper- (*IL2, CD8,* etc.) or hypomethylation (*IL17, IL10, PRF, CD40L, CD70,* etc.). While some lupus-associated epigenetic alterations may be reversed by such strategies, "unwanted" hypomethylation in other genomic regions may result in "SLE phenotypes." Furthermore, HDACs, HDAC inhibitors, and HATs have been discussed as potential treatment options. Currently available therapeutic agents, however, are not target-gene directed. Histone alterations in SLE are highly complex with regions of hyper- (e.g., *IL17, IL10,* etc.) and hypoacetylation (e.g., *IL2*). Furthermore, global changes in "one direction" may activate physiologically silenced genes or silence others (e.g., tumor suppressor genes). Thus, currently available therapeutics carry the risk of severe side effects or complications, such as autoimmune-inflammatory responses, or even the development of cancer. Next to the lack of selectivity, unwanted events are the most obvious and challenging obstacle in the search for novel treatment strategies, targeting the epigenome in SLE.[3,4,51]

Disrupted transcription factor networks have been implicated in the molecular pathophysiology of SLE. They have been demonstrated as contributing to defective epigenetic patterns in SLE T cells. Thus, modulating transcription factor expression and/or activation may be promising in the search for novel therapeutic strategies. We and other demonstrated increased transcription factor expression and/or activation in T cells from SLE patients. Particularly the activated (phosphorylated) forms of CREM-α and Stat3 are increased in the nucleus of SLE T cells. Both transcription factors were documented as contributing to epigenetic dysregulation in SLE through their interactions with "epigenetic modifiers" (CREM-α: HDAC1, DNMT1, DNMT3A, G9a; Stat3: p300). Thus, transcription factor blockade with antibodies, micro-RNAs, or small molecules promise to be future, target-directed, and tolerable treatment options in SLE. Since CREM has more than 20 isoforms with sometimes high sequence homology, specific blockade of CREM-α is challenging and holds the risk of severe side effects.[3,4,27,41]

CONCLUSIONS

Epigenetic alterations in immune cells centrally contribute to the expression of SLE in genetically predisposed individuals. Epigenetic marks, however, are highly complex and we are only beginning to understand their specific patterns and contribution to disease pathology. Still, epigenetic marks promise high potential as biomarkers for disease activity and predictors of individual clinical courses and outcomes, and may be used as future individualized, effective, and target-directed therapeutic options. Currently available "epigenetic drugs" are unable to selectively target epigenetic alterations at single genes or gene clusters in specific cells or tissues. Thus, therapeutic interventions hold the risk of severe side effects and/or complications. A better understanding of the molecular events contributing to gene- and tissue-specific epigenetic alterations may be the key for developing disease biomarkers and treatment strategies, targeting epigenetic patterns in SLE.

REFERENCES

1. Tsokos GC. Systemic lupus erythematosus. *N Engl J Med* 2011;**365**(22):2110–21.
2. Crispin JC, Hedrich CM, Tsokos GC. Gene-function studies in systemic lupus erythematosus. *Nat Rev Rheumatol* 2013;**9**(8):476–84.
3. Hedrich CM, Crispin JC, Tsokos GC. Epigenetic regulation of cytokine expression in systemic lupus erythematosus with special focus on T cells. *Autoimmunity* 2014;**47**(4):234–41.
4. Hedrich CM, Tsokos GC. Epigenetic mechanisms in systemic lupus erythematosus and other autoimmune diseases. *Trends Mol Med* 2011;**17**(12):714–24.
5. Zhao M, Liu S, Luo S, Wu H, Tang M, Cheng W, et al. DNA methylation and mRNA and microRNA expression of SLE CD4+ T cells correlate with disease phenotype. *J Autoimmun* 2014;**54**:127–36.
6. Ballestar E. Epigenetics lessons from twins: prospects for autoimmune disease. *Clin Rev Allergy Immunol* 2010;**39**(1):30–41.

7. Ballestar E. An introduction to epigenetics. *Adv Exp Med Biol* 2011;**711**:1–11.

8. Ballestar E. Epigenetic alterations in autoimmune rheumatic diseases. *Nat Rev Rheumatol* 2011;**7**(5):263–71.

9. Zhang Y, Zhao M, Sawalha AH, Richardson B, Lu Q. Impaired DNA methylation and its mechanisms in CD4(+)T cells of systemic lupus erythematosus. *J Autoimmun* 2013;**41**:92–9.

10. Richardson BC, Strahler JR, Pivirotto TS, Quddus J, Bayliss GE, Gross LA, et al. Phenotypic and functional similarities between 5-azacytidine-treated T cells and a T cell subset in patients with active systemic lupus erythematosus. *Arthritis Rheum* 1992;**35**(6):647–62.

11. Oelke K, Lu Q, Richardson D, Wu A, Deng C, Hanash S, et al. Over-expression of CD70 and overstimulation of IgG synthesis by lupus T cells and T cells treated with DNA methylation inhibitors. *Arthritis Rheum* 2004;**50**(6):1850–60.

12. Javierre BM, Fernandez AF, Richter J, Al-Shahrour F, Martin-Subero JI, Rodriguez-Ubreva J, et al. Changes in the pattern of DNA methylation associate with twin discordance in systemic lupus erythematosus. *Genome Res* 2010;**20**(2):170–9.

13. Hogg N, Laschinger M, Giles K, McDowall A. T-cell integrins: more than just sticking points. *J Cell Sci* 2003;**116**(Pt 23):4695–705.

14. Quddus J, Johnson KJ, Gavalchin J, Amento EP, Chrisp CE, Yung RL, et al. Treating activated CD4+ T cells with either of two distinct DNA methyltransferase inhibitors, 5-azacytidine or procainamide, is sufficient to cause a lupus-like disease in syngeneic mice. *J Clin Invest* 1993;**92**(1):38–53.

15. Richardson B, Powers D, Hooper F, Yung RL, O'Rourke K. Lymphocyte function-associated antigen 1 overexpression and T cell autoreactivity. *Arthritis Rheum* 1994;**37**(9):1363–72.

16. Yung R, Powers D, Johnson K, Amento E, Carr D, Laing T, et al. Mechanisms of drug-induced lupus. II. T cells overexpressing lymphocyte function-associated antigen 1 become autoreactive and cause a lupus-like disease in syngeneic mice. *J Clin Invest* 1996;**97**(12):2866–71.

17. Hedrich CM, Rauen T. Epigenetic patterns in systemic sclerosis and their contribution to attenuated CD70 signaling cascades. *Clin Immunol* 2012;**143**(1):1–3.

18. Tesselaar K, Arens R, van Schijndel GM, Baars PA, van der Valk MA, Borst J, et al. Lethal T cell immunodeficiency induced by chronic costimulation via CD27–CD70 interactions. *Nat Immunol* 2003;**4**(1):49–54.

19. Zhang B, Wu T, Chen M, Zhou Y, Yi D, Guo R. The CD40/CD40L system: a new therapeutic target for disease. *Immunol Lett* 2013;**153** (1–2):58–61.

20. Vinuesa CG, Linterman MA, Goodnow CC, Randall KL. T cells and follicular dendritic cells in germinal center B-cell formation and selection. *Immunol Rev* 2010;**237**(1):72–89.

21. Sawalha AH, Wang L, Nadig A, Somers EC, McCune WJ, Michigan Lupus C, et al. Sex-specific differences in the relationship between genetic susceptibility, T cell DNA demethylation and lupus flare severity. *J Autoimmun* 2012;**38**(2–3):J216–22.

22. Zhou Y, Yuan J, Pan Y, Fei Y, Qiu X, Hu N, et al. T cell CD40LG gene expression and the production of IgG by autologous B cells in systemic lupus erythematosus. *Clin Immunol* 2009;**132**(3):362–70.

23. Lu Q, Wu A, Tesmer L, Ray D, Yousif N, Richardson B. Demethylation of CD40LG on the inactive X in T cells from women with lupus. *J Immunol* 2007;**179**(9):6352–8.

24. Hedrich CM, Crispin JC, Rauen T, Ioannidis C, Koga T, Rodriguez Rodriguez N, et al. cAMP responsive element modulator (CREM) alpha mediates chromatin remodeling of CD8 during the generation of CD3+ CD4– CD8– T cells. *J Biol Chem* 2014;**289**(4):2361–70.

25. Crispin JC, Oukka M, Bayliss G, Cohen RA, Van Beek CA, Stillman IE, et al. Expanded double negative T cells in patients with systemic lupus erythematosus produce IL-17 and infiltrate the kidneys. *J Immunol* 2008;**181**(12):8761–6.

26. Crispin JC, Tsokos GC. Human TCR-alpha beta+ CD4– CD8– T cells can derive from CD8– T cells and display an inflammatory effector phenotype. *J Immunol* 2009;**183**(7):4675–81.

27. Rauen T, Hedrich CM, Tenbrock K, Tsokos GC. cAMP responsive element modulator: a critical regulator of cytokine production. *Trends Mol Med* 2013;**19**(4):262–9.

28. Hedrich CM, Rauen T, Crispin JC, Koga T, Ioannidis C, Zajdel M, et al. cAMP-responsive element modulator alpha (CREMalpha) trans-represses the transmembrane glycoprotein CD8 and contributes to the generation of CD3+CD4–CD8– T cells in health and disease. *J Biol Chem* 2013;**288**(44):31880–7.

29. Lieberman LA, Tsokos GC. The IL-2 defect in systemic lupus erythematosus disease has an expansive effect on host immunity. *J Biomed Biotechnol* 2010;**2010**:740619.

30. Crispin JC, Liossis SN, Kis-Toth K, Lieberman LA, Kyttaris VC, Juang YT, et al. Pathogenesis of human systemic lupus erythematosus: recent advances. *Trends Mol Med* 2010;**16**(2):47–57.

31. Hedrich CM, Crispin JC, Rauen T, Ioannidis C, Apostolidis SA, Lo MS, et al. cAMP response element modulator alpha controls IL2 and IL17A expression during CD4 lineage commitment and subset distribution in lupus. *Proc Natl Acad Sci USA* 2012;**109**(41):16606–11.

32. Hedrich CM, Rauen T, Tsokos GC. cAMP-responsive element modulator (CREM)alpha protein signaling mediates epigenetic remodeling of the human interleukin-2 gene: implications in systemic lupus erythematosus. *J Biol Chem* 2011;**286**(50):43429–36.

33. Tenbrock K, Juang YT, Leukert N, Roth J, Tsokos GC. The transcriptional repressor cAMP response element modulator alpha interacts with histone deacetylase 1 to repress promoter activity. *J Immunol* 2006;**177**(9):6159–64.

34. Martin JC, Baeten DL, Josien R. Emerging role of IL-17 and Th17 cells in systemic lupus erythematosus. *Clin Immunol* 2014;**154**(1):1–12.

35. Lauwerys BR, Garot N, Renauld JC, Houssiau FA. Interleukin-10 blockade corrects impaired in vitro cellular immune responses of systemic lupus erythematosus patients. *Arthritis Rheum* 2000;**43**(9):1976–81.

36. Lee CG, Kang KH, So JS, Kwon HK, Son JS, Song MK, et al. A distal cis-regulatory element, CNS-9, controls NFAT1 and IRF4-mediated IL-10 gene activation in T helper cells. *Mol Immunol* 2009;**46**(4):613–21.

37. Rauen T, Hedrich CM, Juang YT, Tenbrock K, Tsokos GC. cAMP-responsive element modulator (CREM)alpha protein induces interleukin 17A expression and mediates epigenetic alterations at the interleukin-17A gene locus in patients with systemic lupus erythematosus. *J Biol Chem* 2011;**286**(50):43437–46.

38. Hofmann SR, Rosen-Wolff A, Tsokos GC, Hedrich CM. Biological properties and regulation of IL-10 related cytokines and their contribution to autoimmune disease and tissue injury. *Clin Immunol* 2012;**143**(2):116–27.

39. Hedrich CM, Bream JH. Cell type-specific regulation of IL-10 expression in inflammation and disease. *Immunol Res* 2010;**47**(1–3):185–206.

40. Liu Y, Zhu T, Cai G, Qin Y, Wang W, Tang G, et al. Elevated circulating CD4+ ICOS+ Foxp3+ T cells contribute to overproduction of IL-10 and are correlated with disease severity in patients with systemic lupus erythematosus. *Lupus* 2011;**20**(6):620–7.

41. Hedrich CM, Rauen T, Apostolidis SA, Grammatikos AP, Rodriguez Rodriguez N, Ioannidis C, et al. Stat3 promotes IL-10 expression in lupus T cells through trans-activation and chromatin remodeling. *Proc Natl Acad Sci USA* 2014;**111**(37):13457–62.

42. Grant LR, Yao ZJ, Hedrich CM, Wang F, Moorthy A, Wilson K, et al. Stat4-dependent, T-bet-independent regulation of IL-10 in NK cells. *Genes Immun* 2008;**9**(4):316–27.

43. Hofmann SR, Moller J, Rauen T, Paul D, Gahr M, Rosen-Wolff Z, et al. Dynamic CpG-DNA methylation of Il10 and Il19 in CD4⁺ T lymphocytes and macrophages: effects on tissue-specific gene expression. *Klin Padiatrie* 2012;**224**(2):53–60.

44. Tsuji-Takayama K, Suzuki M, Yamamoto M, Harashima A, Okochi A, Otani T, et al. IL-2 activation of STAT5 enhances production of IL-10 from human cytotoxic regulatory T cells, HOZOT. *Exp Hematol* 2008;**36**(2):181–92.

45. Tsuji-Takayama K, Suzuki M, Yamamoto M, Harashima A, Okochi A, Otani T, et al. The production of IL-10 by human regulatory T cells is enhanced by IL-2 through a STAT5-responsive intronic enhancer in the IL-10 locus. *J Immunol* 2008;**181**(6):3897–905.

46. Thiery J, Lieberman J. Perforin: a key pore-forming protein for immune control of viruses and cancer. *Sub-Cell Biochem* 2014;**80**:197–220.

47. Kaplan MJ, Lu Q, Wu A, Attwood J, Richardson B. Demethylation of promoter regulatory elements contributes to perforin overexpression in CD4⁺ lupus T cells. *J Immunol* 2004;**172**(6):3652–61.

48. Lu Q, Wu A, Ray D, Deng C, Attwood J, Hanash S, et al. DNA methylation and chromatin structure regulate T cell perforin gene expression. *J Immunol* 2003;**170**(10):5124–32.

49. Luo Y, Zhang X, Zhao M, Lu Q. DNA demethylation of the perforin promoter in CD4(+) T cells from patients with subacute cutaneous lupus erythematosus. *J Dermatol Sci* 2009;**56**(1):33–6.

50. Denny MF, Chandaroy P, Killen PD, Caricchio R, Lewis EE, Richardson BC, et al. Accelerated macrophage apoptosis induces autoantibody formation and organ damage in systemic lupus erythematosus. *J Immunol* 2006;**176**(4):2095–104.

51. Guo Y, Sawalha AH, Lu Q. Epigenetics in the treatment of systemic lupus erythematosus: potential clinical application. *Clin Immunol* 2014;**155**(1):79–90.

52. Apostolidis SA, Rauen T, Hedrich CM, Tsokos GC, Crispin JC. Protein phosphatase 2A enables expression of interleukin 17 (IL-17) through chromatin remodeling. *J Biol Chem* 2013;**288**(37):26775–84.

53. Hedrich CM, Rauen T, Kis-Toth K, Kyttaris VC, Tsokos GC. cAMP-responsive element modulator alpha (CREMalpha) suppresses IL-17F protein expression in T lymphocytes from patients with systemic lupus erythematosus (SLE). *J Biol Chem* 2012;**287**(7):4715–25.

54. Rauen T, Grammatikos AP, Hedrich CM, Floege J, Tenbrock K, Ohl K, et al. cAMP-responsive element modulator alpha (CREMalpha) contributes to decreased Notch-1 expression in T cells from patients with active systemic lupus erythematosus (SLE). *J Biol Chem* 2012;**287**(51):42525–32.

55. Kappes DJ, He X, He X. CD4–CD8 lineage commitment: an inside view. *Nat Immunol* 2005;**6**(8):761–6.

56. Kioussis D, Ellmeier W. Chromatin and CD4, CD8A and CD8B gene expression during thymic differentiation. *Nat Rev Immunol* 2002;**2**(12):909–19.

57. Adachi S, Rothenberg EV. Cell-type-specific epigenetic marking of the IL2 gene at a distal cis-regulatory region in competent, nontranscribing T-cells. *Nucleic Acids Res* 2005;**33**(10):3200–10.

58. Tao R, de Zoeten EF, Ozkaynak E, Chen C, Wang L, Porrett PM, et al. Deacetylase inhibition promotes the generation and function of regulatory T cells. *Nat Med* 2007;**13**(11):1299–307.

59. Hedrich CM, Ramakrishnan A, Dabitao D, Wang F, Ranatunga D, Bream JH. Dynamic DNA methylation patterns across the mouse and human IL10 genes during CD4⁺ T cell activation; influence of IL-27. *Mol Immunol* 2010;**48**(1–3):73–81.

60. Im SH, Hueber A, Monticelli S, Kang KH, Rao A. Chromatin-level regulation of the IL10 gene in T cells. *J Biol Chem* 2004;**279**(45):46818–25.

61. Kang KH, Im SH. Differential regulation of the IL-10 gene in Th1 and Th2 T cells. *Ann NY Acad Sci* 2005;**1050**:97–107.

62. Zhao M, Tang J, Gao F, Wu X, Liang Y, Yin H, et al. Hypomethylation of IL10 and IL13 promoters in CD4⁺ T cells of patients with systemic lupus erythematosus. *J Biomed Biotechnol* 2010;**2010**:931018.

63. Carlsen AL, Schetter AJ, Nielsen CT, Lood C, Knudsen S, Voss A, et al. Circulating microRNA expression profiles associated with systemic lupus erythematosus. *Arthritis Rheum* 2013;**65**(5):1324–34.

64. Tang Y, Luo X, Cui H, Ni X, Yuan M, Guo Y, et al. MicroRNA-146A contributes to abnormal activation of the type I interferon pathway in human lupus by targeting the key signaling proteins. *Arthritis Rheum* 2009;**60**(4):1065–75.

65. Zhao X, Tang Y, Qu B, Cui H, Wang S, Wang L, et al. MicroRNA-125a contributes to elevated inflammatory chemokine RANTES levels via targeting KLF13 in systemic lupus erythematosus. *Arthritis Rheum* 2010;**62**(11):3425–35.

66. Wang H, Peng W, Ouyang X, Li W, Dai Y. Circulating microRNAs as candidate biomarkers in patients with systemic lupus erythematosus. *Transl Res J Lab Clin Med* 2012;**160**(3):198–206.

67. Pan W, Zhu S, Yuan M, Cui H, Wang L, Luo X, et al. MicroRNA-21 and microRNA-148a contribute to DNA hypomethylation in lupus CD4⁺ T cells by directly and indirectly targeting DNA methyltransferase 1. *J Immunol* 2010;**184**(12):6773–81.

68. Lashine YA, Seoudi AM, Salah S, Abdelaziz AI. Expression signature of microRNA-181-a reveals its crucial role in the pathogenesis of paediatric systemic lupus erythematosus. *Clin Exp Rheumatol* 2011;**29**(2):351–7.

69. Chafin CB, Regna NL, Hammond SE, Reilly CM. Cellular and urinary microRNA alterations in NZB/W mice with hydroxychloroquine or prednisone treatment. *Int Immunopharmacol* 2013;**17**(3):894–906.

70. Rhen T, Cidlowski JA. Antiinflammatory action of glucocorticoids–new mechanisms for old drugs. *N. Engl J Med* 2005;**353**(16):1711–23.

71. Stellato C. Posttranscriptional gene regulation: novel pathways for glucocorticoids' anti-inflammatory action. *Transl Med UniSa* 2012;**3**:67–73.

72. Zhao M, Liu Q, Liang G, Wang L, Luo S, Tang Q, et al. E4BP4 overexpression: a protective mechanism in CD4⁺ T cells from SLE patients. *J Autoimmun* 2013;**41**:152–60.

73. Chan ES, Cronstein BN. Methotrexate–how does it really work? *Nat Rev Rheumatol* 2010;**6**(3):175–8.

74. Nihal M, Wu J, Wood GS. Methotrexate inhibits the viability of human melanoma cell lines and enhances Fas/Fas-ligand expression, apoptosis and response to interferon-alpha: rationale for its use in combination therapy. *Arch Biochem Biophysics* 2014;**563**:101–7.

75. Zhang J, Yuan B, Zhang F, Xiong L, Wu J, Pradhan S, et al. Cyclophosphamide perturbs cytosine methylation in Jurkat-T cells through LSD1-mediated stabilization of DNMT1 protein. *Chem Res Toxicol* 2011;**24**(11):2040–3.

Chapter 31

What Do Mouse Models Teach Us about Human Systemic Lupus Erythematosus?

Yong Du, Chandra Mohan

Department of Biomedical Engineering, University of Houston, Houston, TX, USA

Systemic lupus erythematosus (SLE) is a prototypic auto-immune disease characterized by extensive immunopathological aberrations and peripheral organ damage. From 1965 to 2015, murine models have provided valuable insights in elucidating the mechanisms underlying lupus pathogenesis, identifying potential therapeutic targets, and examining the efficacy of potential treatment approaches.[1]

COMMONLY USED MURINE LUPUS MODELS

The earliest murine lupus models comprised various inbred strains that developed systemic autoimmunity and lupus nephritis spontaneously. These spontaneous lupus nephritis models, including NZB/W F1, BXSB/*yaa*, and MRL/*lpr* strains, demonstrate many characteristic features of human SLE and mirror human SLE pathogenesis remarkably well. When the NZB strain of mice is bred with either the relatively normal New Zealand White (NZW) or the Swiss–Webster mice, the F1 progeny, designated as NZB/W F1 and SNF1, respectively, develop early onset immune complex-mediated glomerulonephritis (GN) and enhanced autoantibody production. Both the NZB/W F1 and the SNF1 strains exhibit a female predominance, closely resembling that of lupus patients. The BXSB/*yaa* mouse model is a recombinant inbred strain derived from the backcross of (B6×SB/Le) F1 to SB/Le, where the ensuing male-predominant disease is dependent on the duplication of Toll-like receptor 7 (*TLR7*) gene.[2]

Another mouse strain that develops lupus spontaneously is Murphy's recombinant large (MRL)/*lpr* strain, which carries the lymphoproliferation (*lpr*) mutation in the *Fas* gene on the lupus-prone MRL background. This strain also exhibits more widespread systemic involvement and some unique phenotypes rarely observed in NZB/W F1 and BXSB/*yaa*, such as sialoadenitis, inflammatory arthritis, skin damage, and neuropsychiatric symptoms, not unlike the disease seen in humans. Beside these strains, accidental brother–sister mating between NZB/W F1 and NZW led to the generation of the New Zealand

Mixed (NZM) strains. Among them, the NZM2410 and NZM2328 strains have also provided researchers additional insights on lupus pathogenesis.

A more recent category of lupus mouse models include congenic strains developed by several groups, including the B6.*Sle1*, B6.*Sle2*, and B6.*Sle3* strains.[1,3] These congenic lupus models are commonly generated by introgressing a susceptibility locus from a disease-prone strain onto a disease-free or resistant strain (e.g., B6), through a process called "selective breeding."[4] Congenic strains are unique in that each mouse harbors a particular susceptibility locus on a common immune disease-free genetic background. This characteristic renders the congenic mouse model a powerful tool for genetic dissection analysis, because one can readily compare the congenic strain bearing the disease locus with a genomically matched background strain to decipher the function of each disease locus very precisely, something that can never be done with humans.

Besides these spontaneous models, lupus can also be experimentally triggered using pristane or by inducing chronic graft versus host disease. Both models facilitate the rapid analysis of how various cells and molecules impact lupus development, and the testing of immunomodulatory agents on disease, relatively quickly. Finally, genetically engineered murine models represent a very powerful tool for studying the role of individual genes in the development of lupus. Indeed, a large number of transgenic mouse models (where a particular gene is hyperexpressed) and gene-knockout models (where the function of a gene is ablated) have taught us how various genes could potentially impact lupus development, as reviewed.[5]

MURINE LUPUS STRAINS CONSTITUTE EXCELLENT MODELS FOR DEFINING THE GENETIC ARCHITECTURE OF SLE

Since the 1980s, more than 100 genomic regions have been identified to be associated with increased susceptibility to lupus in mice. Though linkage and association studies have

Systemic Lupus Erythematosus. http://dx.doi.org/10.1016/B978-0-12-801917-7.00031-0

been carried out in murine and human lupus, murine strains have facilitated research in a very important way—murine lupus geneticists were able to establish "gene–function" relationships through the construction of congenic strains.[3] From 2005 to 2015, an increasing number of double congenic and triple congenic strains have demonstrated that not only can lupus be genetically dissected into its functional components it can also be reconstituted back to full blown disease, as illustrated by the B6.*Sle1.Sle2.Sle3* triple congenic strain.[6]

Congenic strains contribute in another important fashion. By progressively shortening the chromosomal interval of interest, scientists can reduce the pool of potential candidate genes encompassed within the genetic interval, and then eventually identify the causative disease genes. Importantly, several such murine lupus genes identified by congenic studies have been validated by genetic association studies in human SLE. For example, the *Sle1c* locus is linked to increased circulating IgG antibodies and immune alterations in T cells.[7] *Cr2*, a gene encoding complement receptor type 2 that functions as a B-cell coreceptor, has been considered as a candidate gene within this locus. A point mutation in *Cr2* leads to alterations in B-cell responses and germinal center formation. Similarly, in human SLE, a common three single-nucleotide polymorphism *Cr2* haplotype has been associated with lupus susceptibility. Several functional variants in this gene also alter gene transcription, splicing efficiency, or the formation of multiple protein–DNA complexes. Thus, besides underscoring the fact that the same gene can be causative in murine and human lupus, murine studies may also offer potential mechanisms by which *Cr2* could contribute to the development of lupus. In general, there is limited overlap between the lupus genes described in mice and those described in humans, although the functional pathways implicated may be similar in both species.

THE PRESENCE OF AUTOANTIBODIES IS NOT A PREREQUISITE FOR THE DEVELOPMENT OF END ORGAN DAMAGE

A large body of work from murine lupus models has demonstrated the importance of autoantibodies, especially anti-DNA antibodies, in the pathogenesis of lupus. Several groups have eluted these antibodies from the inflamed kidneys of experimental mouse models, while the passive transfer of human or murine anti-DNA antibodies triggers lupus-like syndromes in nonautoimmune mouse strains.[8–10]

Autoantibodies have been shown to bind to cell surface antigens or components of the glomerular matrix through direct cross-reactivity or indirectly via chromatin-containing bridges. Once autoantibodies deposit onto the glomerular matrix, FcχR and complement play essential roles in mediating end organ damage, and it has been shown that the

development of lupus nephritis is FcχR and complement dependent.[11–13] However, not all autoantibodies exhibit a similar capacity to engage Fc receptors or trigger the activation of complement. Differences in pathogenicity can be explained by the nature of somatic mutations in the complementarity determining regions (CDRs) of anti-DNA antibodies. CDRs of anti-DNA antibodies bear charged amino acid residues, such as arginine, asparagine, and lysine. Murine studies have clearly demonstrated that the presence and position of these amino acids greatly influence antibody–DNA interaction and pathogenicity.[14,15]

On the other hand, the presence of autoantibodies is not always a prerequisite for the development of end organ damage, as a couple of murine models are documented to develop lupus nephritis in the absence of anti-DNA antibodies, including the *TLR9* knockout mice,[16] NZM2328.*Lc4* congenic mice,[17] and mIgM.MRL/*lpr* transgenic mice.[18] Interestingly, antibodies eluted from the kidneys of NZM2328.*Lc4* congenic mice reacted with several renal antigens but not with dsDNA.[17] Conversely, other strains have been reported where there is discordance between the presence of IgG anti-dsDNA antibodies and the development of nephritis, including the B6.Sle1.CD19 mice, B6.*Sle1*.BAFF Tg, and B6.*Nba2*.BAFF Tg strains.

Extrapolating from these findings, it appears that although IgG anti-dsDNA antibodies may be important drivers of LN in most murine lupus strains and patients, antibodies of other antigenic specificities and renal-intrinsic factors can also profoundly impact the development of nephritis. In this context, the protective role of IgM antibodies against LN cannot be underestimated.[19,20]

THE PATHOGENIC ROLE OF LEUKOCYTES IN LUPUS

B Cells: More Than Just a Source of Autoantibodies

A growing body of evidence indicates that B cells play other roles in SLE, besides simply producing autoantibodies. In this context, murine models engineered by Shlomchik and colleagues have been particularly instructive.[18,20] The JHD-MRL/*lpr* strain bears a targeted JH deletion on the lupus-prone MRL/*lpr* background; it lacks B cells and is concomitantly free from nephritis, indicating a critical role for B cells However, in this model, reduced renal disease could have been due to the absence of autoantibodies or abnormalities of other B-cell functions. In order to distinguish between these possibilities, they generated a second mouse model, mIgM.MRL/MpJ.Faslpr (mIgM strain), an MRL/*lpr* mutant mouse line with B cells that only expressed surface Ig but not secreted autoantibodies. Hence, this strain is B-cell intact but autoantibody deficient. These mice developed nephritis associated with cellular infiltration, indicating that B cells, in the absence of autoantibodies, are sufficient to induce several aspects of nephritis. Another antibody-independent function of B cells in SLE is cytokine and chemokine release. In particular, IL-6, IL-10, TNF-α, and INF-γ are all elevated both in murine lupus and in human SLE, as discussed elsewhere. Importantly, the relative role of autoantibody production versus other functions that B cells play in LN could not have been dissected out without murine models!

B cells also exhibit protective or regulatory properties in the development of autoimmune diseases, including SLE. Regulatory B cells secrete IL-10, a cytokine with anti-inflammatory properties and the capacity to induce regulatory T cells. In general, the absence of these regulatory B cells accentuates autoimmunity (lupus or otherwise), while the adoptive transfer of these B cells dampens autoimmunity. All in all, B cells play a preponderant role in driving lupus pathogenesis, though the contribution of regulatory B cells cannot be overlooked.

T Cells: Manifold Contributions to Lupus

Murine studies were the first to show an essential role for T cells in lupus pathogenesis,[21] partly by delivering help to B cells.[22] Indeed, pathogenic autoantibody-inducing Th-cell clones or IFN-γ-expressing CD4+ T-cell clones alone were sufficient to induce and promote nephritis in recipient mice.[23] Datta and colleagues have demonstrated that lupus T cells may be specific for nucleosomes or histone,[24] whereas T cells cloned from MRL/*lpr* mice exhibited proliferation to antigens from renal TEC and mesangial cells. The intrarenal role of T cells in LN has been supported by the observations that the abrogation of nephritis by CD4 ablation or anti-CD4 mAb treatment was related to the loss of CD4+ T cells, but not the extent of immune complex deposition in glomeruli.[25]

T cells not only promote autoantibody production by B cells they also play a role in clonal selection and cationic charge evolution of anti-DNA antibodies, through T cell–MHC class II interactions. One important cytokine produced by T cells is IFN-γ. The pathogenic role of this cytokine is supported by its role in immunoglobulin class switching to pathogenic isotypes of anti-DNA autoantibodies, and the protective effects of IFN-γ deficiency in lupus mice.[26] Moreover, IFN-γ administration accelerated nephritis in NZB/W F1 mice, while blocking IFN-γ receptors with mAbs or soluble IFN-γ receptors dampened disease activity in NZB/W F1 mice, as reviewed.[27]

Two T-cell subsets, Th17 cells and Treg cells, have garnered much attention from 2005 to 2015. The pathogenic role of the IL23/IL17 axis in lupus has been demonstrated by several studies, as exemplified by those of Tsokos and colleagues.[28] Generally, IL-17 has been regarded as a proinflammatory cytokine acting as a potent neutrophil chemoattractant, and an inducer of other cytokines and chemokines. Increased IL-17-producing T cells have been reported in murine lupus, associated with disease activity. Nonautoimmune mice exhibited immune complex-mediated GN when transferred with IL-23 pretreated MRL/*lpr* lymphocytes.[28] On the other hand, administering histone-derived peptide to SNF1 mice or ROCK inhibitors to MRL/*lpr* mice ameliorated autoimmunity, accompanied by decreased IL-17-producing cells and IL-17 production. Treg cells, with documented suppressor function, are critical to the maintenance of immune cell homeostasis. Their protective role in SLE is supported by adoptively transferring Treg cells into lupus prone mice or challenging mouse models with tolerogenic peptides, where improved autoimmunity and renal function have been attributed to Treg cells.[29,30] In contrast to these murine studies, although alterations in Treg number and function have been reported in numerous human SLE studies, the precise role of Treg cells in patients can only be inferred, but not directly verified.

MACROPHAGE: THE UNDEFINED ROLE OF MACROPHAGE SUBTYPES IN SLE

The role of macrophages in lupus nephritis is quite similar to that of T cells: they constitute major infiltrating inflammatory cells within the nephritic kidneys. Renal infiltrating macrophages express high levels of CD11b, CD80, and CD86 cell surface markers and secrete high amounts of proinflammatory cytokines, and their numbers are strongly associated with the onset of proteinuria in murine lupus.[31] The pathogenic role of macrophages in lupus is supported by macrophage depletion studies and migration inhibitory factor treatment, where improved nephritis was directly associated with decreased macrophage infiltration in murine models.[32,33] Once again, although intrarenal macrophages are also prevalent in human LN, their functional role can only be inferred.

Macrophages are not monolithic, but rather heterogeneous.[34] Researchers have defined proinflammatory M1 macrophages, profibrotic M2a macrophages, anti-inflammatory M2c macrophages, and other subtypes. Interestingly, both M2a and M2c subset macrophages and their molecular hallmarks, such as MHC II and mannose receptors, are likely to be decreased, while M2b subtype macrophages and their products, including IL-10 and TNF-α, appear to be increased in SLE, as reviewed.[34] In addition, a population of regulatory macrophages, just like B10 and Treg cells, might exist, characterized by the expression of Foxp3, and the secretion of PGE2 and PDGF. Further studies are needed not only to better define different macrophage subsets and explore their biological functions in the context of lupus but also to investigate their possible therapeutic implications in SLE.

DCs: TIPPING THE BALANCE FROM IMMUNE TOLERANCE TOWARD AUTOIMMUNITY

Dendritic cells or DCs are major APCs in the body, serving primarily to activate antigen-specific T cells. The first clue indicating the pathogenic role of DCs in SLE has been generated from an early study in which DC transfers induced the breach of tolerance, leading to autoantibody production.[35] Besides their APC function, a subset of DCs called pDCs are major producers of type I interferons (IFN-I). Recently, studies of two novel genetically engineered mouse models underscore the importance of pDCs in lupus. In the first model, the monoallelic loss of the Tcf4 gene that encode E2-2, a pDC-specific transcription factor, leads to specific impairment of pDC function. The loss of pDC function in these mice abrogated both autoimmunity and GN.[36] In a second model, early, transient, selective depletion of pDCs before disease onset improved most lupus-associated phenotypes, including GN, autoantibody production, and splenomegaly, and these beneficial effects could be sustained even though pDCs recovered later.[37]

Conversely, subsets of DCS have immunoregulatory or tolerizing roles. Hence, the use of "tolerogenic DCs" (tolDCs) to reestablish immune tolerance for immunotherapy has become an attractive approach. tolDCs are characterized by the low expression of MHC II and costimulatory receptors, reduced proinflammatory cytokines production (e.g., IL-6), and enhanced anti-inflammatory cytokine release (e.g., IL-10). Datta and colleagues reported that administering nucleosomal histone-loaded tolDCs ameliorated autoimmunity and nephritis in SNF1 lupus-prone mice, accompanied by an expansion of functional Treg cells, increased TGFβ levels, and decreased IL-17 production.[38] Similarly, Sela et al. reported that the beneficial effects of hCDR1, a peptide derived from the complementarity determining region-1 of anti-DNA autoantibody, were mediated by the induction of immature, tolerogenic DCs.[39] The precise, relative roles of pDCs, toIDCs, and other DC subsets in normal immunity and autoimmunity continue to be an active area of investigation, primarily using murine models.

DCs present within nephritic kidneys can also contribute to renal injury. Increased infiltrating DCs have been documented in the kidneys of lupus-prone mice.[40] Unlike the normal kidney where DCs reside in the tubulointerstitial area, DCs in inflamed kidneys are distributed in both the glomeruli and the tubulointerstitium.[40,41] These DCs exhibit more immature, proinflammatory phenotypes, with elevated expression of the IFN signature preceding lupus onset.[42]

MULTIPLE CYTOKINES AND CHEMOKINES ALSO CONTRIBUTE TO LUPUS PATHOGENESIS

Cytokines play diverse roles in normal immunity and autoimmunity.[27] Some cytokines act predominantly in a systemic fashion with little direct effect on end organ damage. One such example is the B-cell activating factor (BAFF). This cytokine is absolutely required for B-cell development, as mice deficient in BAFF lack follicular and marginal zone B lymphocytes. In contrast, transgenic overexpression of BAFF leads to lupus-like phenotypes, including autoantibody production and immune complex-mediated GN.[43] In parallel with the murine findings, the levels of soluble BAFF are strongly correlated with the titers of anti-dsDNA autoantibodies in lupus patients. The therapeutic effects of blocking BAFF in lupus have been documented by either selective BAFF neutralization or combined BAFF and APRIL neutralization in several murine lupus models.[44] These successful preclinical studies have led to several promising clinical trials and the first drug approved by FDA for SLE treatment from 1965 to 2015, *belimumab*.

Many other cytokines exert their impact on both systemic autoimmunity and end organ damage, including IL-6, IL-17, TGF-β, and IFN-I. Like BAFF, IL-6, a proinflammatory cytokine, is also closely linked with B-cell differentiation and autoantibody production. Several studies have collectively demonstrated enhanced IL-6 expression in both SLE patients and lupus-prone mouse models both systemically (e.g., serum, urine) and within the renal tissue, as reviewed.[45] Evidence for the pathogenicity of this hyperexpressed cytokine arises from murine studies. IL-6 deficiency or blockade in lupus-prone mice ameliorates autoantibody production and nephritis, while IL-6 administration and the IL-6 transgene enhanced autoantibody production, as reviewed.[45] These findings led to an open-label phase I dosage-escalation study of *tocilizumab*, where SLE patients demonstrated an improvement of disease activity, decreased anti-dsDNA Ab levels, and circulating plasma cells.

The role of IFN-I in SLE has been extensively studied, as SLE patients exhibit an IFN signature, which refers to an increased expression of IFN-I-regulated genes both in PBMC and within the target organs. In vitro studies and murine studies revealed that IFN-I contributes to SLE through many avenues, including promoting DC maturation, enhancing costimulatory molecule expression, and triggering B-cell differentiation and autoantibody production, as reviewed.[27] The administration of IFNα results in accelerated nephritis and death in several lupus-prone mouse models, including NZB/W F1, (NZW×BXSB)F1 mice, B6.*Sle123* mice, and NZM2328 mice (199–201), associated with an expansion of short-lived plasma cells.[46] Similarly, improved nephritis has been observed in NZB/W F1 and NZM2383 lupus-prone mice following IFNα receptor ablation.[47] In contrast to the above cytokines, the role of TGF-β in autoimmunity has been quite complex. TGF-β exhibits diverse biological functions, including anti-inflammatory and immunosuppressive effects on systemic immunity and fibrogenic effects in the end organs. Murine studies have shown that TGF-β may play a protective role in systemic lupus but a pathogenic role in renal lupus.[48] Hence, it may not be a surprise that lupus patients exhibit lower serum, but higher intrarenal TGF-β levels.

Chemokines are a family of chemotactic cytokines that are able to induce the migration of different cell types. Therefore, chemokines and their receptors are important in recruiting inflammatory cells into the end organs, including the kidneys. The chemokine MCP-1 is overexpressed in the kidneys from lupus mice, and cyclophosphamide treatment reverses its expression and consequent inflammatory cell infiltration, suggesting that elevated MCP-1 might act as a signal for inflammatory cells to infiltrate the kidney in lupus nephritis. Likewise, MRL/*lpr* mice with MCP-1 deficiency exhibited reduced nephritis and lower mortality, accompanied by significantly decreased inflammatory cell infiltration.[49] Similarly, several therapies targeting MCP-1, such as anti-MCP-1 spiegemer and MCP-1 synthesis inhibitor, have exhibited beneficial effects in murine lupus.[50] Not surprisingly, a small scale SLE clinical study using *bindarit*, an MCP-1 synthesis inhibitor, has also shown positive results.

LESSONS FROM THERAPEUTIC STUDIES IN MURINE LUPUS MODELS

Based on the knowledge gained from murine lupus studies, various biologically based drugs have been advanced to clinical trials over the past from 1965 to 2015. One of them, *belimumab*, a humanized mAb that binds soluble BAFF, is the first drug approved for SLE treatment by FDA from 1965 to 2015. Other biodrugs that have progressed to clinical trials in patients following successful murine studies include *tocilizumab* (an anti-IL-6R), *ocrelizumab* (an anti-CD20 mAb), and *epratuzumab* (an anti-CD22 mAb). These success stories underscore the importance of preclinical murine studies in SLE. However, there are still some limitations in evaluating lupus therapies in murine models. First, renal involvement is a key feature of murine lupus while other phenotypes, such as skin rash, neuropsychiatric symptoms, and cardiovascular disease are rarely observed. Hence, the drug efficacy documented in preclinical mouse models may only be effective for a subset of symptoms seen in patients. Second, the short time course of the murine lupus model makes it challenging to examine the efficacy of different combination therapies or sequential treatment

regimes, or long-term treatments. Third, murine preclinical studies can be executed in one or a few genetic backgrounds at most, and whether the observed outcomes from such studies can be extrapolated to an outbred, genetically heterogeneous human population remains uncertain. These and other reasons explain the reality that multiple therapies are reported as being successful in murine models but only a small subset of these turn out to be equally promising in SLE patients.

CONCLUDING THOUGHTS

Since 1965, multiple murine models have allowed researchers to carefully study the stepwise evolution of SLE and to systemically detail the pathogenic mechanisms, cells, and molecules that mediate disease systemically as well as within the end organs such as the kidneys. Thanks to mouse models, we now know a great deal about the mechanisms and molecular cascades that lead to the emergence of anti-DNA antibodies. Thanks also to mouse models, our knowledge of the molecular cascades leading to renal inflammation has also significantly evolved.

Murine models have also allowed geneticists to advance our understanding of the disease one step further—by performing congenic dissection researchers can identify and isolate the functional pathways leading to lupus, each of which is under distinct genetic control. In addition to a long list of mouse-to-human translational studies in lupus, an increasing number of human-to-mouse translational studies are also being performed, where genes and molecules first identified in human SLE can be studied in engineered murine models. Finally, the advances we have made in lupus therapeutics would have been significantly delayed if not for the availability of murine preclinical models. The laboratory mouse continues to be the best tool in our ongoing efforts to unravel the mystery enshrouding the most complex autoimmune disease, lupus.

REFERENCES

1. Liu K, Mohan C. What do mouse models teach us about human SLE? *Clin Immunol* 2006;**119**(2):123–30.
2. Pisitkun P, Deane JA, Difilippantonio MJ, Tarasenko T, Satterthwaite AB, Bolland S. Autoreactive B cell responses to RNA-related antigens due to TLR7 gene duplication. *Science* 2006;**312**(5780):1669–72.
3. Morel L, Mohan C, Yu Y, Croker BP, Tian N, Deng A, et al. Functional dissection of systemic lupus erythematosus using congenic mouse strains. *J Immunol* 1997;**158**(12):6019–28.
4. Wakeland E, Morel L, Achey K, Yui M, Longmate J. Speed congenics: a classic technique in the fast lane (relatively speaking). *Immunol Today* 1997;**18**(10):472–7.
5. Guo Y, Orme J, Mohan C. A genopedia of lupus genes – lessons from gene knockouts. *Curr Rheumatol Rev* 2013;**9**(2):90–9.

6. Morel L, Croker BP, Blenman KR, Mohan C, Huang G, Gilkeson G, et al. Genetic reconstitution of systemic lupus erythematosus immunopathology with polycongenic murine strains. *Proc Natl Acad Sci USA* 2000;**97**(12):6670–5.

7. Boackle SA, Holers VM, Chen X, Szakonyi G, Karp DR, Wakeland EK, et al. Cr2, a candidate gene in the murine Sle1c lupus susceptibility locus, encodes a dysfunctional protein. *Immunity* 2001;**15**(5):775–85.

8. Van Bruggen MC, Kramers C, Hylkema MN, Smeenk RJ, Berden JH. Significance of anti-nuclear and anti-extracellular matrix autoantibodies for albuminuria in murine lupus nephritis; a longitudinal study on plasma and glomerular eluates in MRL/l mice. *Clin Exp Immunol* 1996;**105**(1):132–9.

9. Dang H, Harbeck RJ. The in vivo and in vitro glomerular deposition of isolated anti-double-stranded-DNA antibodies in NZB/W mice. *Clin Immunol Immunopathol* 1984;**30**(2):265–78.

10. Liang Z, Xie C, Chen C, Kreska D, Hsu K, Li L, et al. Pathogenic profiles and molecular signatures of antinuclear autoantibodies rescued from NZM2410 lupus mice. *J Exp Med* 2004;**199**(3):381–98.

11. Clynes R, Dumitru C, Ravetch JV. Uncoupling of immune complex formation and kidney damage in autoimmune glomerulonephritis. *Science* 1998;**279**(5353):1052–4.

12. Bao L, Zhou J, Holers VM, Quigg RJ. Excessive matrix accumulation in the kidneys of MRL/lpr lupus mice is dependent on complement activation. *J Am Soc Nephrol* 2003;**14**(10):2516–25.

13. Bao L, Haas M, Boackle SA, Kraus DM, Cunningham PN, Park P, et al. Transgenic expression of a soluble complement inhibitor protects against renal disease and promotes survival in MRL/lpr mice. *J Immunol* 2002;**168**(7):3601–7.

14. Katz JB, Limpanasithikul W, Diamond B. Mutational analysis of an autoantibody: differential binding and pathogenicity. *J Exp Med* 1994;**180**(3):925–32.

15. Radic MZ, Weigert M. Genetic and structural evidence for antigen selection of anti-DNA antibodies. *Annu Rev Immunol* 1994;**12**:487–520.

16. Christensen SR, Kashgarian M, Alexopoulou L, Flavell RA, Akira S, Shlomchik MJ. Toll-like receptor 9 controls anti-DNA autoantibody production in murine lupus. *J Exp Med* 2005;**202**(2):321–31.

17. Waters ST, McDuffie M, Bagavant H, Deshmukh US, Gaskin F, Jiang C, et al. Breaking tolerance to double stranded DNA, nucleosome, and other nuclear antigens is not required for the pathogenesis of lupus glomerulonephritis. *J Exp Med* 2004;**199**(2):255–64.

18. Chan OT, Hannum LG, Haberman AM, Madaio MP, Shlomchik MJ. A novel mouse with B cells but lacking serum antibody reveals an antibody-independent role for B cells in murine lupus. *J Exp Med* 1999;**189**(10):1639–48.

19. Jiang C, Zhao ML, Scearce RM, Diaz M. Activation-induced deaminase-deficient MRL/lpr mice secrete high levels of protective antibodies against lupus nephritis. *Arthritis Rheum* 2011;**63**(4):1086–96.

20. Chan O, Shlomchik MJ. A new role for B cells in systemic autoimmunity: B cells promote spontaneous T cell activation in MRL-lpr/lpr mice. *J Immunol* 1998;**160**(1):51–9.

21. Peng SL, Craft J. T cells in murine lupus: propagation and regulation of disease. *Mol Biol Rep* 1996;**23**(3–4):247–51.

22. Ando DG, Sercarz EE, Hahn BH. Mechanisms of T and B cell collaboration in the in vitro production of anti-DNA antibodies in the NZB/NZW F1 murine SLE model. *J Immunol* 1987;**138**(10):3185–90.

23. Knupp CJ, Uner AH, Tatum AH, Kakanar JR, Gavalchin J. IdLNF1-specific T cell clones accelerate the production of IdLNF1 + IgG and nephritis in SNF1 mice. *J Autoimmun* 1995;**8**(3):367–80.

24. Mohan C, Adams S, Stanik V, Datta SK. Nucleosomes: a major immunogen for pathogenic autoantibody-inducing T cells of lupus. *J Exp Med* 1993;**177**:1367–81.

25. Chesnutt MS, Finck BK, Killeen N, Connolly MK, Goodman H, Wofsy D. Enhanced lymphoproliferation and diminished autoimmunity in CD4-deficient MRL/lpr mice. *Clin Immunol Immunopathol* 1998;**87**(1):23–32.

26. Peng SL, Moslehi J, Craft J. Roles of interferon-gamma and interleukin-4 in murine lupus. *J Clin Invest* 1997;**99**(8):1936–46.

27. Davis LS, Hutcheson J, Mohan C. The role of cytokines in the pathogenesis and treatment of systemic lupus erythematosus. *J Interferon Cytokine Res* 2011;**31**(10):781–9.

28. Zhang Z, Kyttaris VC, Tsokos GC. The role of IL-23/IL-17 axis in lupus nephritis. *J Immunol* 2009;**183**(5):3160–9.

29. Scalapino KJ, Tang Q, Bluestone JA, Bonyhadi ML, Daikh DI. Suppression of disease in New Zealand Black/New Zealand White lupus-prone mice by adoptive transfer of ex vivo expanded regulatory T cells. *J Immunol* 2006;**177**(3):1451–9.

30. Weigert O, von Spee C, Undeutsch R, Kloke L, Humrich JY, Riemekasten G. CD4+Foxp3+ regulatory T cells prolong drug-induced disease remission in (NZBxNZW) F1 lupus mice. *Arthritis Res Ther* 2013;**15**(1):R35.

31. Schiffer L, Bethunaickan R, Ramanujam M, Huang W, Schiffer M, Tao H, et al. Activated renal macrophages are markers of disease onset and disease remission in lupus nephritis. *J Immunol* 2008;**180**(3):1938–47.

32. Varghese B, Haase N, Low PS. Depletion of folate-receptor-positive macrophages leads to alleviation of symptoms and prolonged survival in two murine models of systemic lupus erythematosus. *Mol Pharm* 2007;**4**(5):679–85.

33. Leng L, Chen L, Fan J, Greven D, Arjona A, Du X, et al. A small-molecule macrophage migration inhibitory factor antagonist protects against glomerulonephritis in lupus-prone NZB/NZW F1 and MRL/lpr mice. *J Immunol* 2011;**186**(1):527–38.

34. Orme J, Mohan C. Macrophage subpopulations in systemic lupus erythematosus. *Discov Med* 2012;**13**(69):151–8.

35. Georgiev M, Agle LM, Chu JL, Elkon KB, Ashany D. Mature dendritic cells readily break tolerance in normal mice but do not lead to disease expression. *Arthritis Rheum* 2005;**52**(1):225–38.

36. Sisirak V, Ganguly D, Lewis KL, Couillault C, Tanaka L, Bolland S, et al. Genetic evidence for the role of plasmacytoid dendritic cells in systemic lupus erythematosus. *J Exp Med* 2014;**211**(10):1969–76.

37. Rowland SL, Riggs JM, Gilfillan S, Bugatti M, Vermi W, Kolbeck R, et al. Early, transient depletion of plasmacytoid dendritic cells ameliorates autoimmunity in a lupus model. *J Exp Med* 2014;**211**(10):1977–91.

38. Kang HK, Liu M, Datta SK. Low-dose peptide tolerance therapy of lupus generates plasmacytoid dendritic cells that cause expansion of autoantigen-specific regulatory T cells and contraction of inflammatory Th17 cells. *J Immunol* 2007;**178**(12):7849–58.

39. Sela U, Sharabi A, Dayan M, Hershkoviz R, Mozes E. The role of dendritic cells in the mechanism of action of a peptide that ameliorates lupus in murine models. *Immunology* 2009;**128**(S1):e395–405.

40. Bagavant H, Deshmukh US, Wang H, Ly T, Fu SM. Role for nephritogenic T cells in lupus glomerulonephritis: progression to renal failure is accompanied by T cell activation and expansion in regional lymph nodes. *J Immunol* 2006;**177**(11):8258–65.

41. Krüger T, Benke D, Eitner F, Lang A, Wirtz M, Hamilton-Williams EE, et al. Identification and functional characterization of dendritic cells in the healthy murine kidney and in experimental glomerulonephritis. *J Am Soc Nephrol* 2004;**15**(3):613–21.

42. Sriram U, Varghese L, Bennett HL, Jog NR, Shivers DK, Ning Y, et al. Myeloid dendritic cells from B6.NZM Sle1/Sle2/Sle3 lupus-prone mice express an IFN signature that precedes disease onset. *J Immunol* 2012;**189**(1):80–91.

43. Mackay F, Woodcock SA, Lawton P, Ambrose C, Baetscher M, Schneider P, et al. Mice transgenic for BAFF develop lymphocytic disorders along with autoimmune manifestations. *J Exp Med* 1999;**190**(11):1697–710.

44. Ramanujam M, Bethunaickan R, Huang W, Tao H, Madaio MP, Davidson A. Selective blockade of BAFF for the prevention and treatment of systemic lupus erythematosus nephritis in NZM2410 mice. *Arthritis Rheum* 2010;**62**(5):1457–68.

45. Tackey E, Lipsky PE, Illei GG. Rationale for interleukin-6 blockade in systemic lupus erythematosus. *Lupus* 2004;**13**(5):339–43.

46. Mathian A, Weinberg A, Gallegos M, Banchereau J, Koutouzov S. IFN-α induces early lethal lupus in preautoimmune (New Zealand Black x New Zealand White) F1 but not in BALB/c mice. *J Immunol* 2005;**174**:2499–506.

47. Agrawal H, Jacob N, Carreras E, Bajana S, Putterman C, Turner S, et al. Deficiency of type I IFN receptor in lupus-prone New Zealand mixed 2328 mice decreases dendritic cell numbers and activation and protects from disease. *J Immunol* 2009;**183**(9):6021–9.

48. Saxena V, Lienesch DW, Zhou M, Bommireddy R, Azhar M, Doetschman T, et al. Dual roles of immunoregulatory cytokine TGF-beta in the pathogenesis of autoimmunity-mediated organ damage. *J Immunol* 2008;**180**(3):1903–12.

49. Tesch GH, Maifert S, Schwarting A, Rollins BJ, Kelley VR. Monocyte chemoattractant protein 1-dependent leukocytic infiltrates are responsible for autoimmune disease in MRL-Fas (lpr) mice. *J Exp Med* 1999;**190**(12):1813–24.

50. Hasegawa H, Kohno M, Sasaki M, Inoue A, Ito MR, Terada M, et al. Antagonist of monocyte chemoattractant protein 1 ameliorates the initiation and progression of lupus nephritis and renal vasculitis in MRL/lpr mice. *Arthritis Rheum* 2003;**48**(9):2555–66.

Genes and Genetics of Murine Systemic Lupus Erythematosus

Dwight H. Kono, Argyrios N. Theofilopoulos

Department of Immunology and Microbial Science, The Scripps Research Institute, La Jolla, CA, USA

INTRODUCTION

Systemic lupus erythematosus (SLE) is inherited as a multifactorial trait with genetic predisposition playing a major role. Consequently, there has been considerable interest in defining the genetics of this disease. Progress in this area has advanced tremendously over the past few years, resulting in the identification of more than 50 genes associated with lupus risk variants.[1] This effort has been greatly facilitated by studies in the mouse, which because of a seemingly natural susceptibility to lupus, a similar immune system and overall genomic composition to humans, and the ease of genetic and immune system manipulation, has made it the de facto model species of choice. Accordingly, there has been an increasing body of complementary information on the genetics of lupus in mouse models with over 120 genes associated with increased susceptibility and at least 70 other genes that when modified inhibit disease. This chapter will provide an overview of the model systems used in defining genetic predisposition to lupus and briefly describe the major mechanistic pathways that have been implicated.

MOUSE MODELS OF LUPUS USED IN GENETIC STUDIES

Models of lupus can be classified into three general types: spontaneous, modified, and induced. In the first group, lupus arises spontaneously as a polygenetic trait sometimes associated with a major risk variant, e.g., the *Fas^lpr* in MRL-*Fas^lpr* mice and the *Yaa* (TLR7 duplication on Y chromosome) in BXSB males. The "modified" group consists of genetically manipulated mice that spontaneously develop lupus because of a single known engineered variant. Their background can be either nonautoimmune or lupus predisposed with the latter used to detect less potent lupus variants. Genetic-modified lupus mice are also used to define genes and corresponding pathways and affected cell types critical for disease pathogenesis.

The spontaneous group includes strains, recombinant inbred (RI) mice, and related congenics and is genetically heterogeneous (Table 1). The most commonly studied strains or crosses are the MRL-*Fas^lpr*, female (NZBxNZW) F1 hybrid, and male BXSB, which all develop hypergammaglobulinemia, antinuclear antibodies, and glomerulonephritis (GN). The MRL-*Fas^lpr* also develops a mild arthritis and accumulates CD4⁻CD8⁻ (double negative, DN) T cells, NZB acquires autoimmune hemolytic anemia, and a marked monocytosis is found in BXSB mice.[2,3] (NZWxBXSB)F1 males produce high autoantibody titers to phospholipids and platelets and develop antiphospholipid syndrome and immune thrombocytopenia. Importantly, the distinct characteristics of individual lupus models clearly demonstrate the central role genetics can play in lupus susceptibility. Notably, each exhibits a unique lupus phenotype with consistent disease course, autoantibody profiles, and types of end-organ pathology.

Several RI lines, generated from autoimmune and normal strains, also develop spontaneous lupus. These include RI lines derived from NZB and NZW strains (NZM/Aeg2410 and NZM/Aeg2328) and the BXD2 line derived from the nonautoimmune C57BL/6 (B6) and DBA/2 strains. The latter is unique in developing severe erosive arthritis associated with rheumatoid factor and anti-CCP in addition to lupus[4] and is an example of the presence of significant lupus genetic variants in so-called normal strains. Interval-specific congenic mice containing susceptibility loci have been instrumental in defining the contribution of specific loci and in identifying candidate genes. A notable example is the B6.*Sle* set of congenics that contain individually or in combination the full length or subintervals of the three *Sle1–3* loci.[5]

The genetic-modified group, generated by transgenic, knockout, knockin, or mutagenic modification of genes in nonautoimmune and autoimmune background strains, is already the largest and continues to expand in part because many are serendipitously discovered to exhibit features of lupus. Genetic manipulation models yield not only insights

Systemic Lupus Erythematosus. http://dx.doi.org/10.1016/B978-0-12-801917-7.00032-2

TABLE 1 Mouse Models of Lupus[a]

Natural-Occurring

  New Zealand and related strains

  NZB, NZW, (NZBxNZW)F$_1$, NZM2410, NZM2328

  MRL-*Fas^{lpr}* (B6-*Fas^{lpr}*)

  BXSB (B6-*Yaa*)

  BXD2

Genetic-Modified

  B6.129-*Fcgr2$^{-/-}$*

  B6-*Lyn$^{-/-}$*

  B6-*Tlr7 Tg*

Induced

  Pristane (TMPD)-induced

  Heavy metal-induced autoimmunity

  Chronic graft-versus-host disease

[a]*Representative list of mouse models used in genetic studies.*

into the potential contribution of individual genes, alone or combined with other predisposing alleles, but also a way to directly examine human SLE risk variants.[6] Importantly, compilation of these genes provides a scaffold for constructing a model of the central pathways in lupus immunopathology.

The induced models allow more rapid testing of genetic variants and modified genes for their effects on systemic autoimmunity, although uncertainty about relevance to conventional lupus is a potential drawback in part because autoimmunity is induced in nonautoimmune strains. The most common models used for this purpose include exposure of mice to tetramethylpentadecane (pristane) or mercury and chronic graft-versus-host disease. Susceptibility in the induced models is also strain dependent and genetic studies have with few exceptions produced results concordant with the spontaneous-occurring models.

PREDISPOSING LOCI AND GENES IN NATURAL-OCCURRING LUPUS MODELS

Over 80 loci distributed over autosomal and sex chromosomes have been identified in natural-occurring models by directed and genome-wide approaches. Some loci, identified in different strains, appear to represent the same variant, whereas most are unique. Susceptibility in each model therefore appears to be most likely the consequence of a few, but different, loci rather than a large number of common ones. Many of these loci have been confirmed in interval congenic mice, including *Sle1, Cgnz1, Nba2, Bxsb1–4,*

Sle16 (chromosome (chr) 1); *Sle18* (chr 3); *Sle2, Adnz1, Lbw2,* and *Lmb1* (chr 4); *Lmb2* (chr 5); *Sle3, Sle5, Nba5, Lmb3* (chr 7); *Lmb4* (chr 10); *Ssb2* (chr 12); *Sgp3* (chr 13); and *Sles1* (chr 17) (reviewed in Ref. 7).

Sle16, a 129-derived chromosome 1 locus, will be briefly mentioned because of its implication for studies of lupus in genetic-modified mice.[8] Congenic mice containing the 129-*Sle16* interval on the B6 background despite being generated from nonautoimmune strains were found to develop autoantibodies and even GN.[9–12] As gene knockout mice are commonly generated using 129 embryonic stem cells and backcrossing to the B6 strain, the resulting 129/B6 mixed background instead of the gene modification could cause lupus to develop. Awareness of this problem has led to greater attention to reducing the possibility of lupus arising from background genes and the use of B6 embryonic stem cells.

Several lupus risk variants have been identified in natural-occurring models (Table 2). These include genes involved in apoptosis (*Fas, Fasl*), lymphocyte activation (*Ly108, Fcgr2b, Cr2*), transcription regulation (*Pbx-1d*), oxidative metabolism (*Essrg*), the cell cycle (*Cdkn2c*), actin dynamics (*Coro1a*), TLR-mediated cell activation (*TLR7, Yaa*), and antigen presentation (*H-2*).

Several general conclusions about the genetics of mouse models of lupus can be deduced. Notably, the contribution of individual lupus variants on disease manifestations is context dependent. As an example, for even highly penetrant lupus alleles, such as *Fas^{lpr}* and *Yaa*, other susceptibility genes are required to determine the type of autoimmune disease, i.e., nephritis or autoimmune hemolytic anemia, and to develop tissue pathology. Most lupus variants have small effect sizes and many require the presence of other risk alleles for autoimmunity to develop, making characterization a challenge. Additive and epistatic interactions are common and a single locus often consists of a cluster of loci. Candidate gene selection is complicated by the large number of genes that could potentially influence lupus. Defining how a risk variant promotes autoimmunity is often difficult because of expression in multiple potentially relevant immune cell types. Finally, like human SLE, risk variants are often located in noncoding regions that manifest as alterations in gene expression, splicing, or other functions. Taken together, they support the presence of a large heterogeneous pool of lupus variants.

LUPUS PREDISPOSING VARIANTS THAT PROMOTE LUPUS IN NONAUTOIMMUNE MICE

A game changer in defining the genetics of SLE has come from the application of genome manipulation in mice. No longer is the field constrained by a limited number of spontaneous lupus strains, but instead virtually any

TABLE 2 Spontaneous Lupus Susceptibility or Resistant Genes

Gene	Chr	Locus or Allele	Strain[a]	Type of Change[b]	Gene Function	Lupus
Fasl[54]	1	gld	C3H	LOF	Apoptosis	Promotes
Fcgr2b[55,56]	1		NZB, NZW	LOF	Inhibitory signal: B cells, DC	Promotes
Pbx-1d[57]	1	Sle1a1	NZW	GOF	Transcription regulation	Promotes
Ly108, Slamf6[58,59]	1	Sle1b, Sle16	NZW, 129	GOF, no Ly 108-H1 (decoy)	Costimulation	Promotes
Cr2[60]	1	Sle1c	NZW	LOF	Complement receptor	Promotes
Esrrg[61]	1	Sle1c2	NZW	LOF	Oxidative metabolism	Promotes
Cdkn2c[18,62,63]	4	Sle2c1	NZB	LOF	Cell cycle inhibition	Promotes
Coro1a[64]	7	Lmb3	B6-Fas^lpr/Scr	LOF	Actin dynamics	Inhibits
H-2	17	H2	NZW, BXSB	Variant	Antigen presentation	Modifies severity
Fas[65]	19	Lpr	MRL-Fas^lpr	LOF	Apoptosis	Promotes
Tlr7[66,67]	Y	Yaa	BXSB	GOF	ssRNA receptor	Promotes

[a]Original strain.
[b]GOF, gain-of-function; LOF, loss-of-function.

gene and noncoding allelic variation can now be directly probed using mouse models for their effects on lupus, a disease that can only be replicated in intact animals. Early on, gene-modified lupus models were often the unintentional consequence of autoimmunity serendipitously occurring in transgenic or knockout mice produced for other purposes,[13] but with advancing technologies, mice with specific variations relevant to lupus are being generated.[6]

More than 80 genes associated with the development of lupus in nonautoimmune strains have been identified in genetically modified lines (Table 3)[6,7,14–33] along with over 40 others that can enhance susceptibility in lupus-predisposed models (partial list in Table 3 legend).[34–43] Although the relevance of many of these genes to human SLE is not known, they have nevertheless been useful in defining the areas in lupus pathogenesis that can be promoted by genetic susceptibility and in identifying common mechanisms. When combined with genes identified in spontaneous models they can be loosely grouped by functions that span both the innate (self-antigen disposal, dendritic cell-related, innate cytokines) and the adaptive responses (B and T cells, antigen presentation, and costimulation) (Table 3).

A particularly interesting group comprises genes responsible for the generation and clearance of apoptotic cells and cellular debris. This category of risk variant genes is rather specific to lupus and is consistent with the current model of lupus pathogenesis discussed

later. The number and diverse functions of genes in this group suggest a lack of redundancy that involves different aspects of disposal, including clearance of apoptotic debris (*C1qa, C4*), degradation of nuclear material (*Trex1, DNase1*), and regulation of phagocytes (*Mertk/ Tyro3/Axl, Scarf1*). Within the innate immune system, another group of genes enhances DC function while other genes are related to the production and response to innate cytokines. Notably *Ifih1* is associated with type I IFN production.[17,23]

The largest group of genes affects B cells, consistent with studies showing that breach of tolerance in lupus models is often B cell intrinsic.[6,44] Included are genes involved in antigen receptor signaling (*Blk, Cd22, CD72, Fcgr2b, Lyn, Prkcd* (PKC-δ), *Ptpn6* (SHP-1), *Ptpn22, Prprc* (CD45), *Sema4d* (CD100), survival (*Tnfsf13b* (BAFF), *Tnfrsf13b* (TACI), Cd40lg), and nucleic acid TLRs (*Tlr7, Tlr8*)).

Several genes affecting primarily T cells have also been associated with the development of lupus. In slight contrast to B cells, they are less concentrated in antigen receptor signaling (*Mgat5, Lat, Def6, Usp9x*) and involve more diverse functions such as negative regulation (*Ctla4, Pdcd1* (PD-1)), costimulation (*Tnfsf14* (LIGHT), *Rc3h1* (Roquin; repressor of ICOS)), and proliferation and survival (*Cblb, Gpr132* (G2A), *E2f2, Gadd45*). Modification of several apoptosis and cell cycle genes that affect multiple immune cell types has also been shown to promote lupus (Table 3).

276 PART | II Pathogenesis

TABLE 3 Genes Associated with the Development of Lupus in Nonautoimmune Mice

Self-Antigen Production and Clearance
LOF variants: *Axl,* **C1qa, C4, DNase1,** *Mertk, Mfge8, Pparg, Rxra, Scarf1,* **Trex1,** *Trove2, Tyro3*
DC Function
LOF: *Clec4a2,* **Prdm1, Tnfaip3**
Type I IFN and Other Cytokines
LOF: **Mir146a,** *Zfp36, Zc3h12a*
GOF: **Ifih1,** *Ifng, Tnf*
B-cell Activation and Survival
LOF: **Blk,** *Cd22, Cd72,* **Ets1, Fcgr2b, Ikzf1, Ikzf3, Lyn,** *Pecam1, Prkcd, Ptpn6,* **Ptpn22,** *Ptprc, Sema4d, Shc1, Shc2, Tlr8, Tnfrsf13b,* **Tnip1,** *Traf3ip2*
GOF: *Cd19, Cd40lg, Fli1, Mirc1* (miR-17–92), *Plcg2,* **Tlr7,** *Tnfsf13b*
T-cell Activation and Differentiation
LOF: *Cblb, Ctla4, Def6, E2f2, Gadd45a, Gadd45b, Gpr132, Icmt, Il2, Il2ra, Lat, Mgat5, Pdcd1, Socs1, Tgfb1, Usp9x*
GOF: *Il4, Roquin, Tnfrsf14*
Apoptosis
LOF: *Bcl2l11, Fas, Fasl, Pten, Sh2d2a, Stra1*
GOF: *Bcl2, Ier3*
Cell Cycle Regulation
LOF: *Cdkn1a, Rassf5, Cdkn2c*
Other Mechanisms
Variant: **H2** (antigen presentation)
LOF: *Man2a1* (glycosylation), *Mark2* (cellular processes), **Mecp2** (chromatin methylation), *Nrf2* (oxidation), *Mta2* (nucleosome remodeling), *Slamf4* (costimulation)

Genes are categorized by predominant or likely mechanism, and listed by the effect of the predisposing allele on gene function. Lupus includes autoantibody production, immune-complex deposition, and glomerulo-nephritis, but not lymphoproliferation or inflammation alone. In bold are human SLE genes.[1] Additional human lupus genes implicated in genetic studies of lupus-prone mice: *Cd80, Icam1, Il10, Il21, Irak1, Irf5, Irf8, Itgam, Prkcb, Slc15a4,* and *Stat4.* LOF, loss-of-function; GOF, gain-of-function.

GENES AFFECTING SUSCEPTIBILITY TO END-ORGAN PATHOLOGY

In addition to genes associated with the early stages of lupus pathogenesis, i.e., generation of autoantibodies and immune complexes, several genes that affect the development of end-organ disease independent of the presence of autoantibodies or immune complex have been identified using genetic-modified lupus-background models. These include *Icam1, Nos2,* and *Selp* for skin disease[35,45–47] and *AT1a, Bloc1s4, C5ar1, Ccl1* (MCP-1), *Fcer1g* (FcR g-chain), *Igh-8, Mif, Selp,* and Tdt for GN.[47–53] Several different processes were implicated including cell migration (*Icam1, Selp*), inflammation (*Nos2, C5ar1, Ccl1, Fcer1g, Mif*), podocyte injury (*Bloc1s4*), and autoantibody characteristics (*Igh-8, Tdt*).

SUSCEPTIBILITY GENES AFFECT SEVERAL KEY STAGES IN LUPUS PATHOGENESIS

The cumulative data suggest several stages of lupus pathogenesis commonly targeted by genetic susceptibility (Figure 1). These span a wide range of processes extending from the elimination of autoantigens to inflammation caused by autoantibodies and immune complexes. Particularly notable are three key steps, the disposal of nuclear debris, loss-of-tolerance and autoantibody production by B cells for which many genes are intrinsic to B cells, and end-organ susceptibility to injury for which genes are usually but not required to be expressed in the target organ. Other factors such as cytokines and dendritic cells also contribute. The clustering of predisposing risk variant genes at certain common stages also provides a mechanism for the similar clinical manifestations in lupus despite diverse genetic causes.

COMPARISON WITH HUMAN SLE GENES

Currently there are about 55 genes associated with confirmed SLE risk variants that have mouse homologs.[1] Of these, 19 have been implicated in mice in nonautoimmune backgrounds and 12 others have been shown to modify disease in lupus models, thus accounting for over half of human risk variants (Table 3, indicated in bold). Most of the other genes have yet to be adequately investigated in mice. Interestingly, genes affecting B-cell activation and survival are the most prominent followed by genes affecting clearance of apoptotic material, DC function, cytokine production, or response.

CONCLUSION

As the emphasis in lupus genetics increasingly morphs from identifying susceptibility genes to defining their specific contributions to immunopathology, the mouse will remain an essential resource that will continue to yield key insights not otherwise possible to obtain.

ACKNOWLEDGMENTS

This is Publication Number 12345-IMM from the Department of Immunology & Microbial Science, The Scripps Research Institute, 10550 North Torrey Pines Road, La Jolla, CA 92037. The work of the authors reported herein was supported by National Institutes of Health Grants HL114408, AR060181, AR065919. The authors thank Dr Hua Huang for assistance with the figure and M. Kat Occhipinti for editing.

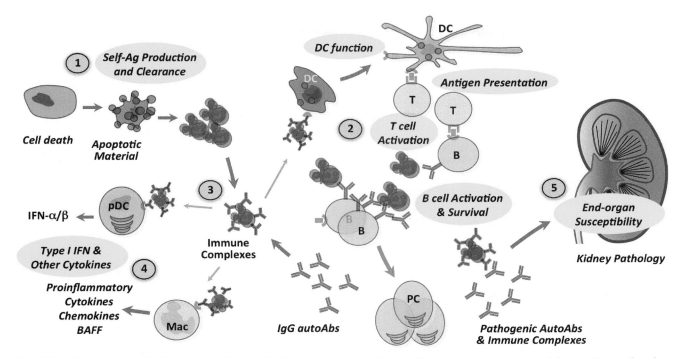

FIGURE 1 **Postulated contribution of lupus risk genes in disease pathogenesis.** Several of the stages in lupus pathogenesis impacted by predisposing mouse variants are highlighted in yellow. These contribute to: (1) impaired clearance of apoptotic material, (2) autoimmune T-cell-dependent B-cell activation and plasma-cell production of pathogenic IgG autoantibodies, (3) the formation of nucleic acid-containing immune complexes that activate pDCs, DCs, macrophages, and other cell types via endosomal TLR stimulation, (4) the overproduction or altered response to type I IFN or other cytokines, and (5) heightened susceptibility to end-organ damage.

REFERENCES

1. Dai C, Deng Y, Quinlan A, Gaskin F, Tsao BP, Fu SM. Genetics of systemic lupus erythematosus: immune responses and end organ resistance to damage. *Curr Opin Immunol* 2014;**31**:87–96.

2. Theofilopoulos AN, Dixon FJ. Murine models of systemic lupus erythematosus. *Adv Immunol* 1985;**37**:269–390.

3. Theofilopoulos AN, Kono DH. Murine lupus models: gene-specific and genome-wide studies. In: Lahita RG, editor. *Systemic lupus erythematosus*. San Diego: Academic Press; 1999. p. 145–81.

4. Mountz JD, Yang P, Wu Q, Zhou J, Tousson A, Fitzgerald A, et al. Genetic segregation of spontaneous erosive arthritis and generalized autoimmune disease in the BXD2 recombinant inbred strain of mice. *Scand J Immunol* 2005;**61**:128–38.

5. Morel L. Mapping lupus susceptibility genes in the NZM2410 mouse model. *Adv Immunol* 2012;**115**:113–39.

6. Dai X, James RG, Habib T, Singh S, Jackson S, Khim S, et al. A disease-associated PTPN22 variant promotes systemic autoimmunity in murine models. *J Clin Invest* 2013;**123**:2024–36.

7. Kono DH, Theofilopoulos AN. Genetics of lupus in mice. In: Lahita RG, editor. *Systemic lupus erythematosus*. San Diego: Academic Press; 2011. p. 63–105.

8. Bygrave AE, Rose KL, Cortes-Hernandez J, Warren J, Rigby RJ, Cook HT, et al. Spontaneous autoimmunity in 129 and C57BL/6 mice-implications for autoimmunity described in gene-targeted mice. *PLoS Biol* 2004;**2**:E243.

9. Heidari Y, Fossati-Jimack L, Carlucci F, Walport MJ, Cook HT, Botto M. A lupus-susceptibility C57BL/6 locus on chromosome 3 (Sle18) contributes to autoantibody production in 129 mice. *Genes Immun* 2009;**10**:47–55.

10. Heidari Y, Bygrave AE, Rigby RJ, Rose KL, Walport MJ, Cook HT, et al. Identification of chromosome intervals from 129 and C57BL/6 mouse strains linked to the development of systemic lupus erythematosus. *Genes Immun* 2006;**7**:592–9.

11. Fossati-Jimack L, Cortes-Hernandez J, Norsworthy PJ, Cook HT, Walport MJ, Botto M. Regulation of B cell tolerance by 129-derived chromosome 1 loci in C57BL/6 mice. *Arthritis Rheum* 2008;**58**:2131–41.

12. Carlucci F, Cortes-Hernandez J, Fossati-Jimack L, Bygrave AE, Walport MJ, Vyse TJ, et al. Genetic dissection of spontaneous autoimmunity driven by 129-derived chromosome 1 loci when expressed on C57BL/6 mice. *J Immunol* 2007;**178**:2352–60.

13. Kono DH, Theofilopoulos AN. Genetics of SLE in mice. *Springer Semin Immunopathol* 2006;**28**:83–96.

14. Katagiri K, Ueda Y, Tomiyama T, Yasuda K, Toda Y, Ikehara S, et al. Deficiency of Rap1-binding protein RAPL causes lymphoproliferative disorders through mislocalization of p27kip1. *Immunity* 2011;**34**:24–38.

15. Brown DR, Calpe S, Keszei M, Wang N, McArdel S, Terhorst C, et al. Cutting edge: an NK cell-independent role for Slamf4 in controlling humoral autoimmunity. *J Immunol* 2011;**187**:21–5.

16. Roszer T, Menendez-Gutierrez MP, Lefterova MI, Alameda D, Nunez V, Lazar MA, et al. Autoimmune kidney disease and impaired engulfment of apoptotic cells in mice with macrophage peroxisome proliferator-activated receptor gamma or retinoid X receptor alpha deficiency. *J Immunol* 2011;**186**:621–31.

17. Funabiki M, Kato H, Miyachi Y, Toki H, Motegi H, Inoue M, et al. Autoimmune disorders associated with gain of function of the intracellular sensor MDA5. *Immunity* 2014;**40**:199–212.

18. Potula HH, Xu Z, Zeumer L, Sang A, Croker BP, Morel L. Cyclin-dependent kinase inhibitor Cdkn2c deficiency promotes B1a cell expansion and autoimmunity in a mouse model of lupus. *J Immunol* 2012;**189**:2931–40.

19. Wang D, John SA, Clements JL, Percy DH, Barton KP, Garrett-Sinha LA. Ets-1 deficiency leads to altered B cell differentiation, hyperresponsiveness to TLR9 and autoimmune disease. *Int Immunol* 2005;**17**:1179–91.

20. Kool M, van Loo G, Waelput W, De Prijck S, Muskens F, Sze M, et al. The ubiquitin-editing protein A20 prevents dendritic cell activation, recognition of apoptotic cells, and systemic autoimmunity. *Immunity* 2011;**35**:82–96.

21. Kim SJ, Gregersen PK, Diamond B. Regulation of dendritic cell activation by microRNA let-7c and BLIMP1. *J Clin Invest* 2013;**123**:823–33.

22. Hodge DL, Berthet C, Coppola V, Kastenmuller W, Buschman MD, Schaughency PM, et al. IFN-gamma AU-rich element removal promotes chronic IFN-gamma expression and autoimmunity in mice. *J Autoimmun* 2014;**53**:33–45.

23. Boldin MP, Taganov KD, Rao DS, Yang L, Zhao JL, Kalwani M, et al. miR-146a is a significant brake on autoimmunity, myeloproliferation, and cancer in mice. *J Exp Med* 2011;**208**:1189–201.

24. Caster DJ, Korte EA, Nanda SK, McLeish KR, Oliver RK, G'Sell RT, et al. ABIN1 dysfunction as a genetic basis for lupus nephritis. *J Am Soc Nephrol* 2013;**24**:1743–54.

25. Nanda SK, Venigalla RK, Ordureau A, Patterson-Kane JC, Powell DW, Toth R, et al. Polyubiquitin binding to ABIN1 is required to prevent autoimmunity. *J Exp Med* 2011;**208**:1215–28.

26. Ramirez-Ortiz ZG, Pendergraft 3rd WF, Prasad A, Byrne MH, Iram T, Blanchette CJ, et al. The scavenger receptor SCARF1 mediates the clearance of apoptotic cells and prevents autoimmunity. *Nat Immunol* 2013;**14**:917–26.

27. Naik E, Webster JD, DeVoss J, Liu J, Suriben R, Dixit VM. Regulation of proximal T cell receptor signaling and tolerance induction by deubiquitinase Usp9X. *J Exp Med* 2014;**211**:1947–55.

28. Desnues B, Macedo AB, Roussel-Queval A, Bonnardel J, Henri S, Demaria O, et al. TLR8 on dendritic cells and TLR9 on B cells restrain TLR7-mediated spontaneous autoimmunity in C57BL/6 mice. *Proc Natl Acad Sci USA* 2014;**111**:1497–502.

29. Kil LP, de Bruijn MJ, van Nimwegen M, Corneth OB, van Hamburg JP, Dingjan GM, et al. Btk levels set the threshold for B-cell activation and negative selection of autoreactive B cells in mice. *Blood* 2012;**119**:3744–56.

30. Deane JA, Pisitkun P, Barrett RS, Feigenbaum L, Town T, Ward JM, et al. Control of toll-like receptor 7 expression is essential to restrict autoimmunity and dendritic cell proliferation. *Immunity* 2007;**27**:801–10.

31. Koelsch KA, Webb R, Jeffries M, Dozmorov MG, Frank MB, Guthridge JM, et al. Functional characterization of the MECP2/IRAK1 lupus risk haplotype in human T cells and a human MECP2 transgenic mouse. *J Autoimmun* 2013;**41**:168–74.

32. Wu YY, Georg I, Diaz-Barreiro A, Varela N, Lauwerys B, Kumar R, et al. Concordance of increased B1 cell subset and lupus phenotypes in mice and humans is dependent on BLK expression levels. *J Immunol* 2015;**194**(12):5692–702.

33. Wojcik H, Griffiths E, Staggs S, Hagman J, Winandy S. Expression of a non-DNA-binding Ikaros isoform exclusively in B cells leads to autoimmunity but not leukemogenesis. *Eur J Immunol* 2007;**37**:1022–32.

34. Liang B, Gee RJ, Kashgarian MJ, Sharpe AH, Mamula MJ. B7 costimulation in the development of lupus: autoimmunity arises either in the absence of B7.1/B7.2 or in the presence of anti-B7.1/B7.2 blocking antibodies. *J Immunol* 1999;**163**:2322–9.

35. Bullard DC, King PD, Hicks MJ, Dupont B, Beaudet AL, Elkon KB. Intercellular adhesion molecule-1 deficiency protects MRL/MpJ-Fas(lpr) mice from early lethality. *J Immunol* 1997;**159**:2058–67.

36. Gutierrez T, Mayeux JM, Ortega SB, Karandikar NJ, Li QZ, Rakheja D, et al. IL-21 promotes the production of anti-DNA IgG but is dispensable for kidney damage in lyn-/- mice. *Eur J Immunol* 2013;**43**:382–93.

37. Jacob CO, Zhu J, Armstrong DL, Yan M, Han J, Zhou XJ, et al. Identification of IRAK1 as a risk gene with critical role in the pathogenesis of systemic lupus erythematosus. *Proc Natl Acad Sci USA* 2009;**106**:6256–61.

38. Tada Y, Kondo S, Aoki S, Koarada S, Inoue H, Suematsu R, et al. Interferon regulatory factor 5 is critical for the development of lupus in MRL/lpr mice. *Arthritis Rheum* 2011;**63**:738–48.

39. Baccala R, Gonzalez-Quintial R, Blasius AL, Rimann I, Ozato K, Kono DH, et al. Essential requirement for IRF8 and SLC15A4 implicates plasmacytoid dendritic cells in the pathogenesis of lupus. *Proc Natl Acad Sci USA* 2013;**110**:2940–5.

40. Shi Y, Tsuboi N, Furuhashi K, Du Q, Horinouchi A, Maeda K, et al. Pristane-induced granulocyte recruitment promotes phenotypic conversion of macrophages and protects against diffuse pulmonary hemorrhage in Mac-1 deficiency. *J Immunol* 2014;**193**:5129–39.

41. Oleksyn D, Pulvino M, Zhao J, Misra R, Vosoughi A, Jenks S, et al. Protein kinase Cbeta is required for lupus development in Sle mice. *Arthritis Rheum* 2013;**65**:1022–31.

42. Kobayashi T, Shimabukuro-Demoto S, Yoshida-Sugitani R, Furuyama-Tanaka K, Karyu H, Sugiura Y, et al. The histidine transporter SLC15A4 coordinates mTOR-dependent inflammatory responses and pathogenic antibody production. *Immunity* 2014;**41**:375–88.

43. Singh RR, Saxena V, Zang S, Li L, Finkelman FD, Witte DP, et al. Differential contribution of IL-4 and STAT6 vs STAT4 to the development of lupus nephritis. *J Immunol* 2003;**170**:4818–25.

44. Kono DH, Baccala R, Theofilopoulos AN. TLRs and interferons: a central paradigm in autoimmunity. *Curr Opin Immunol* 2013;**25**:1–8.

45. Lloyd CM, Gonzalo JA, Salant DJ, Just J, Gutierrez-Ramos JC. Intercellular adhesion molecule-1 deficiency prolongs survival and protects against the development of pulmonary inflammation during murine lupus. *J Clin Invest* 1997;**100**:963–71.

46. Gilkeson GS, Mudgett JS, Seldin MF, Ruiz P, Alexander AA, Misukonis MA, et al. Clinical and serologic manifestations of autoimmune disease in MRL-lpr/lpr mice lacking nitric oxide synthase type 2. *J Exp Med* 1997;**186**:365–73.

47. He X, Schoeb TR, Panoskaltsis-Mortari A, Zinn KR, Kesterson RA, Zhang J, et al. Deficiency of P-selectin or P-selectin glycoprotein ligand-1 leads to accelerated development of glomerulonephritis and increased expression of CC chemokine ligand 2 in lupus-prone mice. *J Immunol* 2006;**177**:8748–56.

48. Clynes R, Dumitru C, Ravetch JV. Uncoupling of immune complex formation and kidney damage in autoimmune glomerulonephritis. *Science* 1998;**279**:1052–4.

49. Tesch GH, Maifert S, Schwarting A, Rollins BJ, Kelley VR. Monocyte chemoattractant protein 1-dependent leukocytic infiltrates are responsible for autoimmune disease in MRL-Fas(lpr) mice. *J Exp Med* 1999;**190**:1813–24.

50. Hoi AY, Hickey MJ, Hall P, Yamana J, O'Sullivan KM, Santos LL, et al. Macrophage migration inhibitory factor deficiency attenuates macrophage recruitment, glomerulonephritis, and lethality in MRL/lpr mice. *J Immunol* 2006;**177**:5687–96.

51. Crowley SD, Vasievich MP, Ruiz P, Gould SK, Parsons KK, Pazmino AK, et al. Glomerular type 1 angiotensin receptors augment kidney injury and inflammation in murine autoimmune nephritis. *J Clin Invest* 2009;**119**:943–53.

52. Greenspan NS, Lu MA, Shipley JW, Ding X, Li Q, Sultana D, et al. IgG3 deficiency extends lifespan and attenuates progression of glomerulonephritis in MRL/lpr mice. *Biol Direct* 2012;**7**:3.

53. Conde C, Weller S, Gilfillan S, Marcellin L, Martin T, Pasquali JL. Terminal deoxynucleotidyl transferase deficiency reduces the incidence of autoimmune nephritis in (New Zealand Black × New Zealand White)F1 mice. *J Immunol* 1998;**161**:7023–30.

54. Suda T, Takahashi T, Golstein P, Nagata S. Molecular cloning and expression of the Fas ligand, a novel member of the tumor necrosis factor family. *Cell* 1993;**75**:1169–78.

55. Rahman ZS, Manser T. Failed up-regulation of the inhibitory IgG Fc receptor Fc gamma RIIB on germinal center B cells in autoimmune-prone mice is not associated with deletion polymorphisms in the promoter region of the Fc gamma RIIB gene. *J Immunol* 2005;**175**:1440–9.

56. Jiang Y, Hirose S, Sanokawa-Akakura R, Abe M, Mi X, Li N, et al. Genetically determined aberrant down-regulation of FcgammaRIIB1 in germinal center B cells associated with hyper-IgG and IgG autoantibodies in murine systemic lupus erythematosus. *Int Immunol* 1999;**11**:1685–91.

57. Cuda CM, Li S, Liang S, Yin Y, Potula HH, Xu Z, et al. Pre-B cell leukemia homeobox 1 is associated with lupus susceptibility in mice and humans. *J Immunol* 2012;**188**:604–14.

58. Kumar KR, Li L, Yan M, Bhaskarabhatla M, Mobley AB, Nguyen C, et al. Regulation of B cell tolerance by the lupus susceptibility gene Ly108. *Science* 2006;**312**:1665–9.

59. Dutta M, Schwartzberg PL. Characterization of Ly108 in the thymus: evidence for distinct properties of a novel form of Ly108. *J Immunol* 2012;**188**:3031–41.

60. Boackle SA, Holers VM, Chen X, Szakonyi G, Karp DR, Wakeland EK, et al. Cr2, a candidate gene in the murine Sle1c lupus susceptibility locus, encodes a dysfunctional protein. *Immunity* 2001;**15**:775–85.

61. Perry DJ, Yin Y, Telarico T, Baker HV, Dozmorov I, Perl A, et al. Murine lupus susceptibility locus Sle1c2 mediates CD4+ T cell activation and maps to estrogen-related receptor gamma. *J Immunol* 2012;**189**:793–803.

62. Xu Z, Potula HH, Vallurupalli A, Perry D, Baker H, Croker BP, et al. Cyclin-dependent kinase inhibitor Cdkn2c regulates B cell homeostasis and function in the NZM2410-derived murine lupus susceptibility locus Sle2c1. *J Immunol* 2011;**186**:6673–82.

63. Potula HH, Morel L. Genetic variation at a Yin-Yang 1 response site regulates the transcription of cyclin-dependent kinase inhibitor p18INK4C transcript in lupus-prone mice. *J Immunol* 2012;**188**:4992–5002.

64. Haraldsson MK, Louis-Dit-Sully CA, Lawson BR, Sternik G, Santiago-Raber ML, Gascoigne NR, et al. The lupus-related Lmb3 locus contains a disease-suppressing Coronin-1A gene mutation. *Immunity* 2008;**28**:40–51.

65. Watanabe-Fukunaga R, Brannan CI, Copeland NG, Jenkins NA, Nagata S. Lymphoproliferative disorder in mice explained by defects in Fas antigen that mediates apoptosis. *Nature* 1992;**356**:314–7.

66. Subramanian S, Tus K, Li QZ, Wang A, Tian XH, Zhou J, et al. A Tlr7 translocation accelerates systemic autoimmunity in murine lupus. *Proc Natl Acad Sci USA* 2006;**103**:9970–5.

67. Pisitkun P, Deane JA, Difilippantonio MJ, Tarasenko T, Satterthwaite AB, Bolland S. Autoreactive B cell responses to RNA-related antigens due to TLR7 gene duplication. *Science* 2006;**312**:1669–72.

Part III

Mechanisms of Tissue Damage

Mechanisms of Renal Damage in Systemic Lupus Erythematosus

Shu Man Fu[1,2,3], Chao Dai[1,2], Hongyang Wang[1,3], Sun-Sang J. Sung[1,2], Felicia Gaskin[4]

[1]*Division of Rheumatology, Department of Medicine, University of Virginia, Charlottesville, VA, USA;* [2]*Center for Immunity, Inflammation, and Regenerative Medicine, Department of Medicine, University of Virginia, Charlottesville, VA, USA;* [3]*Department of Microbiology, Immunology, and Cancer Biology, School of Medicine, University of Virginia, Charlottesville, VA, USA;* [4]*Department of Psychiatry and Neurobehavioral Sciences, School of Medicine, University of Virginia, Charlottesville, VA, USA*

INTRODUCTION

Renal involvement of systemic lupus erythematosus (SLE) was first reported by W. Osler in 1895.[1] "Wire loop" glomeruli, the pathological lesions that are characteristic of lupus nephritis (LN) as shown in Figures 1(A) and 1(B), were described by Baehr et al. in 1935.[2] With the advent of immunofluorescence microscopy (Figure 1(C)), Ig deposits in the kidneys of LN were recognized[3,4] and complement deposition was demonstrated.[5,6] Subsequently Ig was eluted from diseased kidney.[7–9] The eluted Ig was shown to be enriched in antibodies (Abs) to DNA and other nuclear antigens (Ags). By electron microscopy (EM), electron-dense deposits in subendothelial space and subepithelial space with foot process effacement (Figure 1(D)) correlated with the presence of wire loop lesions in LN. The nature of these deposits was shown by Dixon et al.[10] to be immune complex (IC) deposition. These and other observations led Kunkel and his colleagues[11] to propose SLE as a prototype of IC nephritis in Man. Careful morphological studies on the kidneys of patients with LN by Koffler et al.[12] showed the variable patterns of Ig and complement deposition in the kidneys in patients with SLE. It appeared that linear and mesangial deposition of Ig and complement was seen first. These depositions do not correlate with clinical or histological evidence of renal disease. This was followed by granular and lumpy deposits of IG and complement with clinical evidence of renal disease. Since the early 1970s, there have been numerous studies identifying the Ags in the IC that are deposits in the glomeruli.

In order to discuss mechanisms of renal damage, it is paramount to understand that the kidney is a complex organ. Figure 2 shows the structures in the kidney and sites where renal damage may occur. In the glomeruli, the intrinsic renal cells are mesangial cells, endothelial cells, and podocytes that represent epithelial components of the glomeruli. Glomerular injury can be classified into three patterns of injury.[13] In the mesangial pattern, IC accumulation with the mesangial cells with mesangial proliferation is seen. This pattern is seen in class II LN. The endothelial pattern is characterized by leucocyte accumulation, endothelial injury, and endocapillary proliferation. These changes are accompanied by capillary wall destruction, mesangial cell proliferation, IC deposits, and crescent formation. These changes are seen in class III and class IV LN. In the epithelial pattern, the IC deposit in the linear fashion. IC deposition with complement activation leads to podocyte injury. This is seen in class V LN. With advanced sclerosis and fibrosis, class VI LN results. It is often that more than one pattern are seen in patients' renal biopsies. Thus it is obvious that the 2003 International Society of Nephrology (ISN)/Renal Pathology Society (RPS) classification of LN is mainly based on glomerular changes, although some consideration of tubular damage is made.[13]

The role of immune cells in renal damage and the mechanisms of tissue injury have been studied in many mouse models of LN (reviewed in Refs 14 and 15). Many aspects of these topics are detailed in other chapters in this book and will not be reviewed here. In this chapter, selective mechanisms of renal damage that are less emphasized or less recognized will be reviewed. The mechanisms of renal damage to be discussed are limited to class III and class IV LN.

dsDNA IS NOT THE ONLY AUTOANTIGEN IN LN

Since the identification of DNA as a target Ag of ANA by Holman and Kunkel,[16] the importance of DNA as an autoantigen in SLE in general and in LN in particular

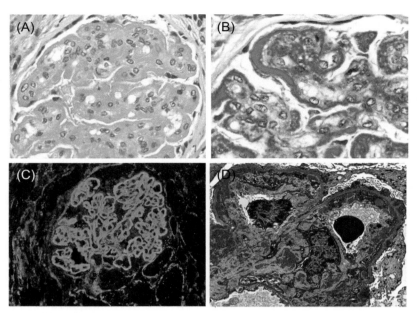

FIGURE 1 Pathology of class IV diffuse proliferative lupus glomerulonephritis. (A) H&E shows frequent round capillary luminal deposits, referred to as hyaline thrombi. In addition, numerous large confluent subendothelial deposits, known as wire-loop lesions are present. (B) Masson trichrome stain can highlight the wire-loop subendothelial deposits (bright red). (C) Immunofluorescence in proliferative lupus glomerulonephritis shows numerous glomerular capillary loop deposits, wire loops by light microscopy, and extraglomerular deposits involving tubular basement membranes and interstitium. (D) EM shows numerous subendothelial and mesangial deposits with well-developed basement membrane duplication. There are scattered subepithelial deposits with basement membrane response in the form of spikes. *Composite photographs from Atlas of Medical Renal Pathology by Dr Stephen M. Bonsib, published in 2013 by Springer New York. Permission to use these photographs has been obtained from both the publisher and Dr Bonsib.*

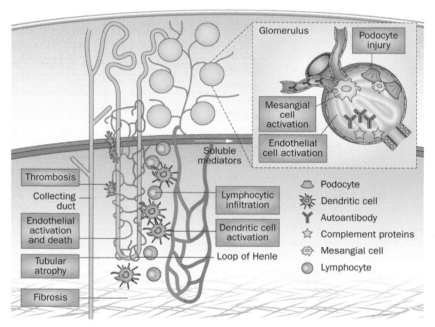

FIGURE 2 Pathogenesis of lupus nephritis. Immune complex deposition and complement activation in the glomeruli lead to the activation of endothelial cells and mesangial cells and induction of inflammatory mediators, resulting in efflux of inflammatory cells. Inflammatory cytokines interact with tubular epithelial cells, which in turn secrete cytokines. These events lead to infiltration of lymphocytes and macrophages and the activation of resident macrophages, dendritic cells, and lymphocytes. Microangiopathic changes occur in the blood vessels surrounding renal tubules with endothelial cell activation and death. These events in the interstitium cause tubular atrophy and dilatation and interstitial fibrosis, the hallmarks of chronic glomerulonephritis. (Figure 1 in Ref. 14).

has received significant recognition. This impression was reinforced by the seminal papers from the laboratory of the late Henry Kunkel that show the presence of anti-dsDNA Abs–dsDNA IC in the diseased kidney of patients with LN.[8,9] However, it was recognized that other Ag–Ab systems were involved. This was evident in the original series of patients, three of whom had no anti-dsDNA Abs despite the presence of severe LN.[9] Furthermore rheumatoid factor activity was demonstrated in some of the kidney eluates.[17] The concept that multiple Ab–Ag systems operate in LN is further supported by the finding of Mannik et al.[18] that the Abs to dsDNA, the collagen-like region of C1q, Sm, SSA, SSB, and chromatin were enriched in the glomerular extract of kidneys from patients who died of LN. In addition, the identifiable Ag specificities of the eluted Ab account for less than 10% of the Abs. Thus the bulk of Abs were reactive to yet to be identified Ags.

ANTI-dsDNA Abs MAY NOT BE THE Abs THAT INITIATE LN

From the preceding discussion, it is obvious that anti-dsDNA Abs may not be the most important or the only Abs that cause LN in patients or at least in some patients. There may be reservations regarding studies with postmortem kidneys because the kidneys were either from patients with advanced renal disease or from patients who died of severe infections. With the advances in proteomics, it is now feasible to study Abs from renal biopsy samples. In the studies by Bruschi et al.,[19,20] 20 biopsies from LN patients (one class II, three class III, nine class IV, two class IV + V, three class V, and two undetermined) were microdissected with laser capture and eluted Abs were analyzed with podocyte Ags by two-dimensional electrophoresis.[19] The identified spots were characterized by MALD–MS and LC–MS. Eleven podocyte proteins were identified to be present in one or more samples. It is of interest that Abs to α-enolase and annexin A1 were identified in 11 and 10 biopsy samples, respectively. These 11 proteins are termed Ags intrinsic to the podocytes and are targeted by auto-Abs to form IC. Bruschi et al.[20] identified Abs that were reactive with histones (H2A, H3, and H4), DNA, and C1q as planted Ags because of their charge interaction with the glomerular basement membrane. The frequencies of Abs reactive with DNA, histone, and C1q were 50%, 55%, and 70%, respectively. It is of considerable interest that circulating anti-DNA Abs were detected in the patients whose kidneys did not have Abs to DNA. The lack of anti-DNA Abs in many of the renal biopsy samples and the presence of circulating anti-DNA Abs without their renal deposits suggest that anti-DNA and antinucleosome may not be the starter of LN. In addition the divergence of anti-DNA

and anti-α-enolase/annexin A1 Abs rules out that cross-reactivity often detected with anti-DNA Abs is responsible for the observation that α-enolase and annexin A1 are the most common auto-Ag detected in LN.

BREAKING TOLERANCE TO DNA, NUCLEOSOME, AND OTHER NUCLEAR Ags IS NOT REQUIRED FOR THE PATHOGENESIS OF LN

Genetic evidence has been obtained that breaking tolerance to DNA, nucleosome, and other nuclear Ags is not required in the pathogenesis of LN.[21] NZM2328 has been established as a model for human LN.[22] Approximately 70% of the female mice of NZM2328 develop severe proteinuria, end stage renal disease, and early mortality. The renal pathology resembles that of human proliferative LN. As shown in Figure 3, three stages of the renal pathology of LN in NZM2328 can be identified readily: normal, acute GN (aGN), and chronic GN (cGN). aGN is characterized by hypercellular glomeruli with little glomerulosclerosis and without interstitial fibrosis and tubular atrophy/dilatation. At this stage, affected female mice have moderate proteinuria (1 – 2 + by dipstick measurements) with normal renal function. In contrast, cGN is characterized by extensive glomerulosclerosis, interstitial fibrosis, and tubular atrophy/dilatation. At this stage, 3+ proteinuria is present with impaired renal function. Both male and female mice produce ANA and anti-dsDNA Abs. With ANA, anti-dsDNA, aGN, and cGn as phenotypes, the analysis of a cohort of female mice of the backcross (C57L/JXNZM2328)F1XNZM2328 identified five lupus-susceptible genetic intervals.[22] A single locus Cgnz1 on chromosome 1 was significantly linked to cGN. Three genetic intervals, Agnz1 distal to Cgnz1 on chromosome 1, the H-2 complex, and Agnz2 distal to H-2 on chromosome 17 were suggestively linked to aGN. A single locus Adnz1 on chromosome 4 was identified to be linked to elevated ANA and anti-dsDNA Abs. Two congenic strains, NZM2328.C57L/Jc1 (NZM.C57Lc1) and NZM2328.C57L/Jc4 (NZM.C57Lc4) were generated. Their derivation is depicted in Figure 4. Female mice of NZM.C57Lc4 had little circulating ANA or anti-dsDNA Abs. No anti-dsDNA Abs were detected in kidney eluates from diseased kidneys. However, they developed cGN with severe proteinuria and early mortality in the same manner as that of the parental NZM2328.[21] This finding provides genetic evidence that LN pathogenesis does not require breaking tolerance to dsDNA, nucleosome, and nuclear Ags, adding support to the thesis that LN is due to multiple Abs to different auto-Ags. Thus the prevailing view that anti-dsDNA Abs are the main LN player in LN should be modified.

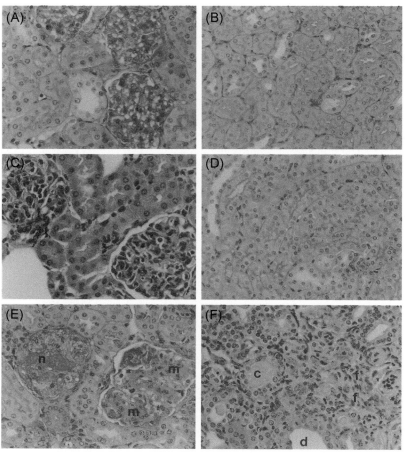

FIGURE 3   Renal histopathology of NZM2328 mice. (A and B) The kidney sections of a 12-month-old female mouse with no proteinuria. Shown are glomeruli with normal cellularity (A) and normal tubules without interstitial cellular infiltrate, fibrosis, or tubular atrophy (B). (C and D) Renal pathology of a 12-month-old female mouse with diffuse proliferative glomerulonephritis without severe proteinuria shows hypercellular glomeruli with many exudative mononuclear cells within the capillary lumen (C) and normal tubules without interstitial nephritis (D). (E and F) The kidney sections of a 6-month-old female mouse, which was morbid-bound and sacrificed, show severe and diffuse glomerulonephritis with high chronicity index. In (E), glomeruli show expansion of the mesangial space with increased matrix material, designated m, and one necrotic glomerulus designated n. In (F), dilated tubules, d, proteinaceous casts, c, and interstitial fibrosis, f, are shown (hematoxylin and periodic acid–Schiff stain with 200× magnification).[22]

IC DEPOSITION WITH COMPLEMENT ACTIVATION IS NOT SUFFICIENT FOR LN TO PROGRESS FROM aGN TO cGN AND END STAGE RENAL DISEASE

The female mice of the NZM.C57Lc1 congenic line (Figure 4) do not develop ANA, anti-dsDNA Abs, and severe proteinuria.[21] The genetic interval introgressed from C57L/J contains the loci *Agnz1* and *Cgnz1*. An informative intrachromosomal recombinant line NZM.Lc1R27 (R27) with the introgression of genetic interval containing only the allele of *Cgnz1* from C57L/J to NZM2328 was characterized.[23] As shown in Figure 5, female mice of R27 developed IC-mediated aGN without progression to cGN and end stage renal failure. The R27 mice develop anti-kidney Abs early and their kidneys have Ig deposits with complement activation. They have mild proteinuria (1–2 plus).

A cohort of these mice has been followed for more than 18 months without the development cGN and severe proteinuria. It is of interest that no significant differences have been observed in intrarenal cytokines and kidney infiltrating monocytes and macrophages between NZM2328 and R27, many of which have been shown to be important in the pathogenesis of LN and renal damage.[24,25] These observations led us to postulate that the *Cgnz1* allele confers end organ resistance to damage. This hypothesis was initially supported by data showing that R27 kidneys were resistant to damage by nephrotoxic anti-GBM Abs.[23] R27 mice were shown to be resistant to the development of cGN, which is accelerated in the parental line NZM2328 with the injection of adeno-IFNα, although treated R27 had higher titers of anti-dsDNA Abs and more intense deposits of Ig and complement.[26] Thus Ic deposition and complement activation with cellular infiltration are not sufficient in

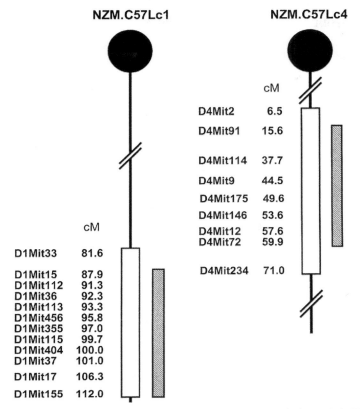

NZM.C57Lc1

cM

D1Mit33	81.6
D1Mit15	87.9
D1Mit112	91.3
D1Mit36	92.3
D1Mit113	93.3
D1Mit456	95.8
D1Mit355	97.0
D1Mit115	99.7
D1Mit404	100.0
D1Mit37	101.0
D1Mit17	106.3
D1Mit155	112.0

NZM.C57Lc4

cM

D4Mit2	6.5
D4Mit91	15.6
D4Mit114	37.7
D4Mit9	44.5
D4Mit175	49.6
D4Mit146	53.6
D4Mit12	57.6
D4Mit72	59.9
D4Mit234	71.0

FIGURE 4 NZM.C57Lc1 and NZM.C57Lc4 congenic lines were derived by replacing the genetic intervals in NZM2328 with those from C57L/J (hatched bars). The genetic intervals with SLE susceptibility genes in NZM2328 delineated by informative microsatellite markers are shown (open bars). Chromosome intervals are not drawn to scale.[21]

causing irreversible damage if the host has genetic elements that confer end organ resistance to damage. These observations suggest that intrinsic renal cells actively participate in the pathogenesis of LN. In this regard, it was documented that proliferating glomerular epithelial cells are the main cellular components in the crescents in an anti-GBM GN model.[27]

MULTIPLE CELLS AND CYTOKINES ARE INVOLVED IN THE PATHOGENESIS OF LN

Thus far the role of IC with complement activation has been discussed. It is apparent that resident immune cells, intrinsic renal cells, and infiltrating cells interact in a complex fashion to influence the outcome of LN. Some of these cell types will be briefly discussed.

The role of T cells in LN has been well recognized.[28-38] It should be recognized that both CD8 and CD4 T cells have been identified to be in LN kidneys and these T cells have cytotoxic potentials. Wofsy and his colleagues have shown that anti-CD4 mAb can prevent the development of LN in (NZBxNZW)F1 female mice[29] and can reverse established LN with reduction of anti-dsDNA Abs and prolonged survival.[30] The absence of Tαβ cells in BXSB

prevents the development of LN in males.[31] It should be stated that the absence of Tαβ cells did not have a similar effect in MLR/*lpr*.[32] It was formally shown that Tγδ cells could support the development of LN in MRL/*lpr*.[33] This strain difference is due to the fact that MRL/*lpr* is primarily an autoinflammatory disorder. We have shown that activation and expansion of nephritogenic T cells in the regional lymph nodes are associated with the progression of nephritis to renal failure in NZM2328.[34] In man, Winchester et al. showed that clonally expanded CD4+ and CD8+ T cells with memory effector cell markers are in the kidneys of LN.[35] Both T cells are found in the periglomerular region. CD8+ T cells were present in all biopsy samples and adhered to Bowman's capsule and infiltrate tubular epithelium. These findings suggest that both CD4+ and CD8+ T cells have the potential to mediate renal injury. Recently Th17 were shown to be present in the kidney and their role in autoimmunity in general and in LN in particular has been updated by Konya et al.[36] The role of Treg cells in LN remains unsettled. In one study by Bagavant and Tung,[37] the infusion of the number of Treg cells that could suppress autoimmune thyroiditis did not suppress the development of LN in NZM2328. However, Scalapino et al. showed that infusion of Treg that achieved 80-fold ex vivo expansion achieved

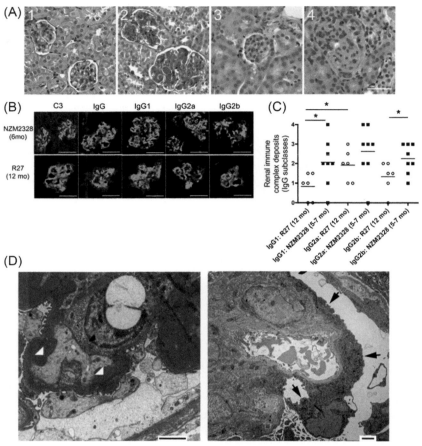

FIGURE 5 Morphological studies on NZM2328 and R27 kidneys. (A) PAS staining of R27 kidneys and H&E staining of NZM2328 kidneys. R27 females without aGN[1] and with aGN[2] are shown. PAS-positive material in the glomerular capillary lumen is shown in 2. Kidneys of NZM2328 at age of 8 weeks and NZM2328 at 36 weeks are shown in 3 and 4, respectively. Bar, 50 μm. (B) Immunofluorescent staining for detecting IgG subclasses and C3 in the glomeruli. Bars, 100 μm. (C) Semiquantitative estimates of IgG subclass staining of kidneys of NZM2328 and in R27 at different ages are shown. Horizontal bars show means. $P < 0.05$ is denoted by *. (D) Transmission electron micrographs of the kidney of a 12-month-old R27 mouse (left photo; bar, 1 μm) and that of an 8-month-old NZM2328 mouse (right photo; bar, 5 μm). In the left photo, the arrowheads show subendothelial deposits. Despite the massive deposits, the foot processes are well preserved. In the right photo, effacement of the foot processes is shown by the arrows.[23]

significant suppression of LN in (NZBxNZW)F1.[38] These different results may be simply due to the number of transfused Treg cells. In summary, there is substantial evidence to support a major role of T cells in LN. The elucidation of the antigenic specificity of the nephritogenic T cells will help us to understand further the role of T cells in LN.

The intrarenal macrophages have been considered an important player (reviewed in Ref. 14). The requirement of macrophages for the participation of LN was formally documented in an anti-GBM nephritis model.[39] The depletion of macrophages by GW2528, a selective inhibitor of CSF-1 (the colony stimulating factor 1) receptor kinase, prevented the development of proteinuria and increase in serum creatinine and BUN in mice treated with a rabbit anti-GBM antiserum, although the treated mice developed anti-rabbit Ig Abs to the same extent as those treated with control rabbit serum.

Intrarenal B cells have been demonstrated in human LN kidneys. Germinal center-like structures have been shown to be present in some LN kidneys that have marked tubular abnormalities disproportional to the glomerular destruction.[40] Microdissection of B cells with BCR amplification shows that anti-vimentin is the dominant target in human lupus tubulointerstitial nephritis.[41] The significance of this finding has been put into proper perspective by Anne Davidson in her editorial accompanying the paper.[42] The disproportional tubulointerstitial nephritis signals the progression from acute kidney injury to chronic renal disease. The role of the anti-vimentin Abs in this transition remains to be defined in view of circulating auto-Abs that may also interact with tubular cells to secrete multiple cytokines, among which TGF-β1 plays an important role in fibrosis.[43] In addition, acute renal injuries occur quite often with increase in creatinine and BUN. These episodes are often subclinical.

These injuries subject patients with SLE and LN to have tubulointerstitial abnormalities out of proportion of glomerular disease.

Many proinflammatory cytokines are identified to be involved in LN (reviewed in Ref. 14). Recently our laboratory has obtained data showing interactions among podocytes, infiltrating macrophages, and mesangial cells. As LN nephritis progresses from aGN to cGN, there is polarization of cytokine production. It appears that activated podocytes make IL-1β, infiltrating macrophages make TNFα, and mesangial cells make IL-6. Within the diseased glomeruli, a cytokine network is established to regulate intraglomerular inflammation (Sung, S-S J et al., unpublished observation and manuscript in preparation). This novel observation has significant implications in how we should approach the treatment of LN.

KIDNEY DISEASE IN LUPUS IS NOT ALWAYS "LUPUS NEPHRITIS"

It should be evident that not all kidney disease in lupus is always "lupus nephritis." Systemic inflammation, interstitial infiltration by inflammatory cells, and activation of resident immune cells often lead to renal tubular epithelial cell activation, leading to the expression of MHC class II molecules and other costimulatory molecules such as B7-1 and CD40.[44] Further interaction of the activated tubular cells with immune cells leads to release of inflammatory cytokines. Some of these events are depicted in Figure 2: dendritic cell and lymphocyte activation, endothelial activation and death and thrombosis leading to vascular dropout and tubular atrophy, and interstitial fibrosis as results of attempts to repair the acute kidney damage. Other processes contributing to kidney damage in lupus are hypertension and previous subclinical acute kidney damage. Types of kidney disease in patients with SLE are summarized: IC glomerulonephritis, IC tubulointerstitial nephritis, minimal change nephrotic syndrome, thrombotic microangiopathy, infectious ascending tubulointerstitial disease, opportunistic renal infections, renal drug-induced toxicity, renal injuries due to concomitant diseases such as diabetes mellitus and hypertension and amyloidosis.[45] From the list of the conditions that may contribute to renal failure in patients with SLE, it is apparent that many of these conditions are not related directly to IC-mediated GN seen in proliferative LN.

REGENERATION AND FIBROSIS ARE KEYS TO RECOVERY FROM LN

Much of our therapeutic approach has been centered on controlling immunological processes that result from IC deposition and complement activation. It is often neglected that regeneration and fibrosis are two important processes that control the recovery of renal function. Better understanding of podocyte progenitor biology may help us to repair podocyte loss, a characteristics of all glomerulopathies.[46] Excessive fibrosis will lead to end stage renal failure. Recently perivascular Gli1+ progenitors have been identified to be key contributors to injury-induced organ fibrosis.[47] In the kidney, pericytes that are branched mesenchymal cells surrounding endothelial cells in the capillary bed and postcapillary venules have been identified to have a key role in regeneration and fibrosis.[48] Pericytes have been linked to mesenchymal stem cells and some of them have been suggested to be mesenchymal stem cells. These cells play a significant role in kidney homeostasis, injury, and repair. They contribute to the myofibroblast pool. Their detachment from endothelial cells is a major event in acute renal injury and subsequent fibrosis that leads to end stage renal failure. Our better understanding of the function of these cells would lead us to a rational approach to balance regeneration and fibrosis that ultimately reestablish renal homeostasis.

CONCLUDING REMARKS

LN is a complex disease. The prognosis of the disease is not very good in that a significant population of the affected patients will progress to end stage renal disease. The mechanisms of renal damage are complex. Recently studies in our laboratory have led us to postulate the separation of autoimmunity from end organ damage.[49] This hypothesis of lupus pathogenesis is depicted in Figure 6. This would remind us that the end organ, i.e., kidney is not a passive participant in the pathogenesis of LN. We should consider that IC-mediated LN causes aGN and the interaction of the immune response with intrinsic renal cells ultimately leads to cGN in susceptible hosts. This scheme will enable us to identify useful markers for monitoring responses to therapies. From this brief discussion it should be obvious that to achieve good therapeutic results in our treatment of LN, multitarget (drug) approaches should be undertaken. This is illustrated by the recent report that tacrolimus plus mycophenolate mofetil is superior to intravenous cyclophosphamide in a control clinical trial.[50] Further understanding of the mechanisms of renal damage in lupus renal disease will lead us to design logical protocols for the treatment of LN. It would be appropriate to conclude by citing the first paragraph in the editorial in *Lupus* by Whittier and Reiser[51]: (In *Through the Looking Glass*, Lewis Carroll's sequel to *Alice in Wonderland*, Alice learns that things on the other side of the metaphorical mirror (looking glass) are not always what they seem. She enters a world of riddles and challenges, and learns that she cannot always expect to find logic in the situations she encounters. Over the last 60 years, as we similarly "reflect" on the history of our understanding of LN, our world has been consumed with the obvious

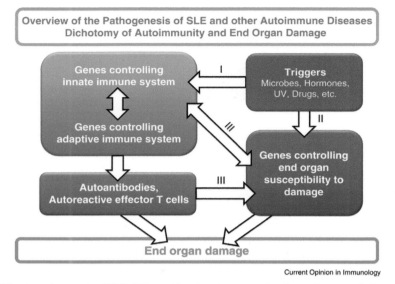

FIGURE 6 Interactive model for the pathogenesis of SLE. This model makes the assumption that environmental triggers act on susceptible hosts. The triggers act on both genes controlling immune responsiveness and genes for end organ damage. These are two independent yet interactive pathways. Pathway I leads to the generation of autoantibodies and autoreactive effector T cells. Pathway II provides autoantigens and/or soluble mediators that influence immune responsiveness. Pathways I and II interact at several levels as indicated by III. These interactions can lead to end organ damage. In the context of this chapter the end organ is the kidney and the autoimmune response is the production of autoantibodies to multiple autoantigens that forms immune complexes to be deposited in the kidney.[49]

immune aggregates seen in the glomeruli on immunofluorescence microscopy and likewise tries to explain many, if not all, of the clinical manifestations of this disease by these immune complexes. In fact, LN is commonly known as the "prototypical immune complex mediated disease." The unwillingness to look beyond the immune aggregates has made alternative views on pathophysiology of this complicated disease difficult to appreciate.) http://lup.sagepub.com/content/24/6/533.long - ref-2.

ACKNOWLEDGMENT

This work is supported in part by grants from the National Institute of Arthritis and Musculoskeletal and Skin Diseases (R01-AR047988 and R01-AR049449) and a grant (TIL187966) from the Alliance for Lupus Research, New York.

REFERENCES

1. Osler W. On the visceral complications of erythema exudativum multiforme. *Am J Med Sci* 1895;**110**:629–46.
2. Baehr G, Klemperer P, Schifren A. A diffuse disease of the peripheral circulation (usually associated with lupus erythematosus and endocarditis). *Trans Assoc Am Phys* 1935;**50**:139–55. 63–69.
3. Vazquez JJ, Dixon FJ. Immunohistochemical study of lesions in rheumatic fever, systemic lupus erythematosus, and rheumatoid arthritis. *Lab Invest* 1957;**6**:205–17.
4. Mellors RC, Ortega CG, Holman HR. Role of gamma globulins in pathogenesis of renal lesions in systemic lupus erythematosus and chronic membranous glomerulonephritis with an observation on the lupus erythematosus cell reaction. *J Exp Med* 1957;**106**:191–202.
5. Lachmann PJ, Muller-Eberhard HJ, Kunkel HG, Paronetto F. The localization of in vivo bound complement in tissue sections. *J Exp Med* 1962;**115**:63–82.
6. Freedman P, Markowitz AS. Gamma globulin and complement in the diseased kidney. *J Clin Invest* 1962;**41**:328–34.
7. Krishnan C, Kaplan MH. Immunopathologic studies of systemic lupus erythematosus. II. Antinuclear reaction of γ-globulin eluted from homogenates and isolated glomeruli of kidneys from patients with lupus nephritis. *J Clin Invest* 1967;**46**:569–79.
8. Koffler D, Schur PH, Kunkel HG. Immunological studies concerning the nephritis of systemic lupus erythematosus. *J Exp Med* 1967;**126**:607–24.
9. Kunkel HG. Mechanisms of renal injury in systemic lupus erythematosus. *Arthritis Rheum* 1966;**9**:725–6.
10. Dixon FJ, Feldman JD, Vazquez JJ. Experimental glomerulonephritis. The pathogenesis of a laboratory model resembling the spectrum of human glomerulonephritis. *J Exp Med* 1961;**113**:899–920.
11. Koffler D, Agnello V, Thoburn R, Kunkel HG. Systemic lupus erythematosus: prototype of immune complex nephritis in man. *J Exp Med* 1971;**134**:169s–79s.
12. Koffler D, Agnello V, Carr RI, Kunkel HG. Variable patterns of immunoglobulin and complement deposition in the kidneys of patients with systemic lupus erythematosus. *Am J Pathol* 1969;**56**:305–16.
13. Weening JJ, D'Agati VD, Schwartz MM, Seshan SV, Alpers CE, Appel GB, et al. The classification of glomerulonephritis in systemic lupus erythematosus revisited. *J Am Soc Nephrol* 2004;**15**:241–50.
14. Davidson A, Arano C. Lupus nephritis: lessons from murine models. *Nat Rev Rheumatol* 2010;**6**:13–20.
15. Nowling TK, Gilkeson GS. Mechanisms of tissue injury in lupus nephritis. *Arthritis Res Ther* 2011;**13**:250.
16. Holman RH, Kunkel HG. Affinity between the lupus erythematosus serum factor and cell nuclei and nucleoprotein. *Science* 1957;**126**:162–3.

17. Agnello V, Koffler D, Kunkel HG. Immune complex systems in the nephritis of systemic lupus erythematosus. *Kidney Int* 1973;**3**:90–9.

18. Mannik M, Merrill CE, Stamps LD, Wener MH. Multiple autoantibodies form the glomerular immune deposits in patients with systemic lupus erythematosus. *J Rheumatol* 2003;**30**:1495–504.

19. Bruschi M, Sinico RA, Moroni G, Pratesi F, Migliorini P, Galetti M, et al. Glomerular autoimmune multicomponents of human lupus nephritis in vivo: α-enolase and annexin AI. *J Am Soc Nephrol* 2014;**25**:2483–98.

20. Bruschi M, Galetti M, Sinica RA, Moroni G, Bonanni A, Radice A, et al. Glomerular autoimmune multicomponents of human lupus nephritis in vivo (2): planted antigens. *J Am Soc Nephrol* 2014;**25**:2483–98.

21. Waters ST, McDuffie M, Bagavant H, Deshmukh US, Gaskin F, Jiang C, et al. Breaking tolerance to double stranded DNA, nucleosome and other nuclear antigens is not required for the pathogenesis of lupus glomerulonephritis. *J Exp Med* 2004;**199**:255–64.

22. Waters ST, Fu SM, Gaskin F, Deshmukh US, Sung SS, Kannapell CC, et al. NZM2328: a new mouse model of systemic lupus erythematosus with unique genetic susceptibility loci. *Clin Immunol* 2001;**100**:372–83.

23. Ge Y, Jiang C, Sung S-SJ, Bagavant H, Dai C, Wang H, et al. *Cgnz1* allele confers kidney resistance to damage preventing progression of immune complex-mediated acute lupus glomerulonephritis. *J Exp Med* 2013;**210**:2387–401.

24. Schiffer L, Bethunaickan R, Ramanujam M, Huang W, Schiffer M, Tao H, et al. Activated renal macrophages are markers of disease onset and disease remission in lupus nephritis. *J Immunol* 2008;**180**:1938–47.

25. Bethunaickan R, Berthier CC, Ramanujam M, Sahu R, Zhang W, Sun Y, et al. A unique hybrid renal mononuclear phagocyte activation phenotype in murine systemic lupus erythematosus nephritis. *J Immunol* 2011;**186**:4994–5003.

26. Dai C, Wang H, Sung SS, Sharma R, Kannapell C, Han W, et al. Interferon alpha on NZM2328.Lc1R27: enhancing autoimmunity and immune complex-mediated glomerulonephritis without end stage renal failure. *Clin Immunol* 2014;**154**:66–71.

27. Ophascharoensuk V, Pippin JW, Gordon KL, Shankland SJ, Couser WG, Johnson RJ. Role of intrinsic renal cells versus infiltrating cells in glomerular crescent formation. *Kidney Int* 1998;**54**:416–25.

28. Tipping PG, Holdsworth SR. T cells in glomerulonephritis. *Springer Semin Immunopathol* 2003;**24**:377–93.

29. Wofsy D, Seaman WE. Successful treatment of autoimmunity in NZB/NZW F₁ mice with monoclonal antibody to L3T4. *J Exp Med* 1985;**161**:378–91.

30. Wofsy D, Seaman WE. Reversal of advanced murine lupus in NZB/NZW F₁ mice by treatment with monoclonal antibody to L3T4. *J Immunol* 1987;**138**:3247–53.

31. Lawson BR, Koundouris SI, Barnhouse M, Dummer W, Baccala R, Kono WH, et al. The role of αβ⁺ T cells and homeostatic T cell proliferation in Y-chromosome-associated murine lupus. *J Immunol* 2001;**167**:2354–60.

32. Peng SL, Madaio MP, Hughes DPM, Crispe JN, Owen MJ, Wen L, et al. Murine lupus in the absence of αβ T cells. *J Immunol* 1996;**156**:4041–9.

33. Peng SL, Madaio MP, Hayday AC, Craft J. Propagation and regulation of systemic autoimmunity by γδ T cells. *J Immunol* 1996;**157**:5689–97.

34. Bagavant H, Deshmukh US, Wang H, Ly T, Fu SM. Role for nephritogenic T cells in lupus glomerulonephritis: progression to renal failure is accompanied by T cell activation and expansion in regional lymph nodes. *J Immunol* 2006;**177**:8258–65.

35. Winchester R, Wiesendanger M, Zhang H-Z, Steshenko V, Peterson K, Geraldino-Pardilla L, et al. Immunologic characteristics of intrarenal T cells. Trafficking of expanded CD8⁺ T cell β-Chain clonotypes in progressive lupus nephritis. *Arthritis Rheum* 2012;**64**:1589–600.

36. Konya C, Paz Z, Apostolidis SA, Tsokos GC. Update on the role of Interleukin 17 in rheumatologic autoimmune diseases. *Cytokine* 2015;**75**:205–15.

37. Bagavant H, Tung KS. Failure of CD25⁺ T cells from lupus-prone mice to suppress lupus glomerulonephritis and sialoadenitis. *J Immunol* 2005;**175**(2):944–50.

38. Scalapino KJ, Tang Q, Bluestone JA, Bonyhadi ML, Daikh DI. Suppression of disease in New Zealand Black/New Zealand White lupus-prone mice by adoptive transfer of ex vivo expanded regulatory T cells. *J Immunol* 2006;**177**:1451–9.

39. Chalmers SA, Chitu V, Herlitz LC, Sahu R, Stanley ER, Putterman C. Macrophage depletion ameliorates nephritis induced by pathogenic antibodies. *J Autoimmun* 2015;**57**:42–52.

40. Hsieh C, Chang A, Brandt D, Guttikonda R, Utset TO, Clark MR. Predicting outcomes of lupus nephritis with tubulointerstitial inflammation and scarring. *Arthritis Care Res (Hoboken)* 2011;**63**:865–74.

41. Kinloch AJ, Chang A, Ko K, Dunand CJH, Henderson S, Maienschein-Cline M, et al. Vimentin is a dominant target of in situ humoral immunity in human lupus tubulointerstitial nephritis. *Arthritis Rheumatol* 2014;**66**:3359–70.

42. Davidson A. Editorial: autoimmunity to vimentin and lupus nephritis. *Arthritis Rheumatol* 2014;**66**(12):3251–4.

43. Yung S, Ng CY, Ho SK, Cheung KF, Chan KW, Zhang Q, et al. Anti-dsDNA antibody induces soluble fibronectin secretion by proximal renal tubular epithelial cells and downstream increase of TGF-β1 and collagen synthesis. *J Autoimmun* 2015;**58**:111–22.

44. Cantaluppi V, Quercia AD, Dellepiane S, Ferrario S, Camussi G, Biancone L. Interaction between systemic inflammation and renal tubular epithelial cells. *Nephrol Dial Transpl* 2014;**29**:2004–11.

45. Anders H-J, Weening JJ. Kidney disease in lupus is not always 'Lupus Nephritis'. *Arthritis Res Ther* 2013;**15**:108.

46. Shankland SJ, Pippin JW, Duffield JS. Progenitor cells and podocyte regeneration. *Semin Nephrol* 2014;**34**:418–28.

47. Kramann RK, Schneider RK, Ebert BL, Humphreys BD. Perivascular Gli1⁺ progenitors are key contributors to injury-induced organ fibrosis. *Cell Stem Cell* 2015;**16**:51–66.

48. Kramann R, Humphreys BD. Kidney pericytes: roles in regeneration and fibrosis. *Semin Nephrol* 2014;**34**:374–83.

49. Dai C, Deng Y, Quinlan A, Gaskin F, Tsao BP, Fu SM. Genetics of systemic lupus erythematosus: immune responses and end organ resistance to damage. *Curr Opin Immunol* 2014;**31**:87–96.

50. Liu Z, Zhang H, Liu Z, Xing C, Fu P, Ni Z, et al. Multitarget therapy for induction treatment of lupus nephritis; a randomized, controlled trial. *Ann Intern Med* 2015;**162**:18–26.

51. Whittier WL, Reiser J. Lupus nephritis: through the looking-glass. *Lupus* 2015;**24**:533–5.

Chapter 34

Mechanisms of Vascular Damage in Systemic Lupus Erythematosus

Sarfaraz A. Hasni, Mariana J. Kaplan

National Institute of Arthritis and Musculoskeletal and Skin Diseases, National Institutes of Health, Bethesda, MD, USA

SUMMARY

Cardiovascular (CV) disease is one of the most important causes of morbidity and mortality in systemic lupus erythematosus (SLE), occurring primarily as a result of accelerated atherosclerosis. CV risk is particularly increased in young women when compared to age- and gender-matched controls, and it cannot be explained by traditional risk factors. Indeed, immune dysregulation characteristic of SLE appears to play a prominent role in enhancing CV risk in patients affected by this disease. Among putative pathways implicated in the enhancement of CV risk, aberrant innate immune responses present in SLE may promote early damage to the vasculature, followed by inability to repair the damaged endothelium and progression of plaque formation and thrombosis. This chapter describes several of these pro-atherogenic pathways in SLE, including the role of type I Interferons, neutrophils and their production of extracellular traps, autoantibodies and modified lipoproteins, as well as the potential for modulation of vascular risk.

EPIDEMIOLOGY OF VASCULAR DAMAGE IN SYSTEMIC LUPUS ERYTHEMATOSUS

Accelerated atherosclerosis leading to cardiovascular (CV) events is a well-established cause of morbidity and mortality in patients with systemic lupus erythematosus (SLE).[1,2] A bimodal mortality pattern in SLE was recognized in the 1970s,[3] and these observations of enhanced mortality late in the course of SLE disease due primarily to CV disease (CVD) have been replicated in several other cohorts. Indeed, enhanced relative risk for vascular disease is well documented in SLE[4] and is particularly enhanced in young women with lupus, who are 50 times more likely to develop a myocardial infarction when compared to women of similar age without SLE.[1] In population-based studies, several risk factors for CV events in women with SLE have been identified, including older age at the time of lupus diagnosis, disease duration, length of corticosteroid use,

hypercholesterolemia, and postmenopausal status. However, the rate of CVD in SLE patients is much higher than what would be expected based on the Framingham risk equation alone.[5] Furthermore, there is high prevalence of noncalcified coronary plaques in SLE (54%), as assessed by multidetector computed tomography scans,[6] which may promote a higher propensity to acute coronary syndromes.

RISK OF VASCULAR DAMAGE: TRADITIONAL VERSUS NONTRADITIONAL FACTORS

While traditional risk factors for atherosclerosis cannot fully account for the increased risk of CVD in SLE, they likely contribute to vascular complications. Among the traditional risk factors, age and smoking have been associated with CV events in SLE.[7,8] While hypertension has been reported as an independent predictor of mortality in SLE, the frequent use of antihypertensive medications in patients with lupus nephritis, even in the absence of hypertension, complicates the assessment of the role of this risk factor in CVD.[9,10]

Patients with SLE are frequently found to have abnormal lipid profiles, with increased low-density lipoprotein (LDL) and triglycerides and decreased high-density lipoprotein (HDL). The prevalence of metabolic syndrome is close to 10% in SLE, a rate significantly higher than what is reported in age- and gender-matched controls,[11] and it is associated with endothelial injury and coronary atherosclerosis. Overall, it is considered that the presence of any of the Framingham CV risk factors, in association with various nontraditional SLE-specific risk factors for atherosclerosis, may promote additive or synergistic effects on vascular injury.

Several mechanisms unique to SLE have been proposed to contribute to vascular damage and premature atherosclerosis.[12] There is convincing evidence placing atherosclerosis as a chronic inflammatory condition,[13] where a sophisticated interplay of various components of the innate and adaptive arms of the immune system, including cytokines, autoantibodies, T and B lymphocytes, neutrophils, macrophages, and dendritic cells play key roles in contributing to endothelial cell injury. However, several features that characterize SLE are atypical, when considering what is known about promoters of atherogenesis in the general population: (1) young women without SLE are considered protected from plaque formation, while young women with lupus are at risk[1]; (2) the "classical" inflammatory burden associated to atherosclerosis in the general population[14,15] (i.e., elevated high-sensitivity C-reactive protein) is not traditionally observed in a high proportion of SLE patients[15]; (3) while trials have been overall small, it is unclear if statins play a prominent role in preventing CV risk in SLE.[16,17] These observations indicate that immune dysregulation

characteristic of SLE may play a key role in the promotion of vascular damage and progression to atherosclerosis in this disease (Figure 1).

ROLE OF CYTOKINES IN VASCULAR DAMAGE IN SLE

Type I Interferons: Human and murine studies indicate that type I interferons (IFNs) may play an important role in promoting pleiotropic damaging effects in the vasculature of SLE patients. An imbalance between vascular damage and endothelial repair has been reported in SLE, and this phenomenon may accelerate plaque development.[18] Levels of circulating apoptotic endothelial cells are increased in SLE in association with development of endothelial

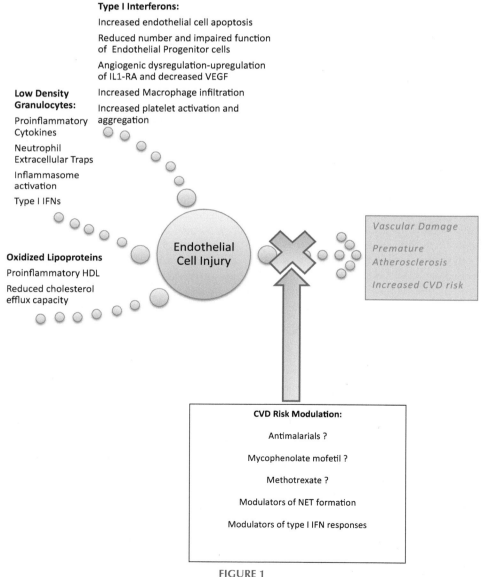

FIGURE 1

dysfunction and generation of tissue factor.[19] In addition, SLE patients have decreased levels and function of endothelial progenitor cells (EPCs),[18] previously implicated in repairing the vasculature following an insult and inversely associated with the incidence of CVD and vascular damage risk factors in the general population.[20] We have reported that enhanced apoptosis and functional impairments in EPC differentiation in SLE are mediated by type I IFNs, as neutralization of these cytokines restores a normal phenotype.[18]

The pathways by which type I IFNs promote abnormal vasculogenesis are still being characterized. One mechanism appears to be transcriptional repression of the proangiogenic molecules interleukin (IL)-1β and vascular endothelial growth factor (VEGF), as well as enhancement of inflammasome activation, with subsequent upregulation of IL-18.[21,22] Furthermore, type I IFNs promote transcriptional upregulation of the antiangiogenic IL-1 receptor antagonist (IL1-RA). Antiangiogenic pathways are operational in vivo in SLE, as demonstrated by decreased vascular density and increased vascular rarefaction in renal blood vessels in vivo, in association with upregulation of IL-1-RA and decreased VEGF-A both in the tissues and in serum.[22] Indeed, there is evidence that angiogenic dysregulation induced by type I IFNs may not only promote atherogenesis but may also be involved in the vasculopathy associated with preeclampsia or progression of renal dysfunction in SLE.[22,23]

In addition to dysregulating vascular repair, type I IFNs have other proatherogenic roles. Type I IFN-induced signaling and IFN-α- producing plasmacytoid dendritic cells (pDCs) are increased in atherosclerotic plaques in patients without SLE, while pDC depletion is protective in murine atherosclerosis models.[24-26] There is also evidence that IFN-α sensitizes and/or activates plaque-residing myeloid DCs and CD4+ T cells, leading to downstream proinflammatory effects that can promote plaque rupture.[25] Importantly, mice exposed to enhanced levels of type I IFNs display increased macrophage infiltration of vessel walls,[27,28] while in vitro priming of macrophages with IFN-α enhances their capacity to take up oxidized LDL and differentiate into foam cells.[29] Importantly, abrogation of type I IFN pathways in atherosclerosis-prone mice decreases plaque burden, macrophage, and T-cell arterial wall infiltration.[27] Finally, lupus platelets are activated in response to exposure to type I IFNs[30] and lupus-prone and/or atherosclerosis-prone mice exposed to increased levels of type I IFNs display accelerated thrombosis, enhanced platelet activation, and formation of leukocyte:platelet aggregates.[27] Overall, these observation suggest a crucial role for type I IFNs in the promotion of premature vascular damage in acute coronary syndrome in SLE and, potentially, in the general population. Further supporting this hypothesis, SLE patients with high type I IFN serum activity have lower flow mediated dilatation of the brachial artery and peripheral arterial tone (both indicators of endothelial dysfunction), higher carotid intima media thickness, and higher calcification scores of coronaries by computed tomography.[31]

Role of other cytokines: Interleukin-6 may play a prominent role in lupus pathogenesis but the effects on SLE-associated vascular risk remain to be determined, as both proatherogenic (through promotion of aberrant lipoprotein profiles) and antiatherogenic anti-inflammatory roles have been described.[32,33] Similarly, the role of other cytokines found to be elevated in subsets of lupus patients (IL-10, IL-17, etc.), with regards to atherosclerosis risk, remains to be determined.

AUTOANTIBODIES AND IMMUNE COMPLEXES

Patients with SLE generate a myriad of autoantibodies, and some of them could potentially have atherogenic effects. Besides their prothrombotic role, the significance of antiphospholipid (APL) antibodies as drivers of atherosclerosis remains a matter of debate.[34] Autoantibodies to the main protein in HDL, Apo A-1, and lipoprotein lipase are elevated in SLE and increase with disease flares, but whether they play an atherogenic role in this disease is not known.[35] Anti-Ro antibodies are associated with EPC dysfunction.[21] There is preliminary evidence that natural IgM antibodies could carry atheroprotective roles in SLE, an area that requires further investigation.[36] The role of complement activation and immune complexes in driving plaque formation in SLE remains unclear, but they are certainly implicated in endothelial damage and could be important as drivers of vascular insult. Complement consumption and a reduction in the uptake of apoptotic/necrotic debris has been hypothesized to promote atherogenesis in SLE,[37] similar to the hypothesis of aberrant efferocytosis in idiopathic atherosclerosis.[38]

CELLULAR MEDIATORS

Adaptive immune responses: The role of T and B cells in CV risk in SLE is not well characterized. Dysregulated CD4+ T cells from lupus-prone mice can accelerate plaque development in atherosclerosis-prone mice[39]; furthermore, murine models of atherosclerosis display increased vascular inflammation and CD4+ T-cell infiltration in arterial plaques following bone marrow transplantation from SLE-prone donor mice.[40] The precise role that distinct T- and B-cell subsets play in induction and prevention of vascular damage and plaque development remains unclear and how immunomodulatory therapies modulate CV risk should be explored.

Innate immune responses: Lupus monocytes and macrophages appear to have enhanced activation status, characterized by their increased capacity to synthesize proinflammatory cytokines and upregulation of various surface markers of activation[41] and with potential association to atherosclerosis burden.[42] Furthermore, macrophages pried with type I IFNs are more prone to become foam cells.[29] The cytokine macrophage migration inhibitory factor (MIF) plays a role in activation of macrophages and lymphocytes and has been shown to be increased in SLE, while murine models of atherosclerosis indicate that MIF is involved in plaque development and monocyte recruitment. The specific role of MIF in lupus-related vascular disease remains to be determined.[43]

Evidence has implicated neutrophils as putative mediators of atherothrombosis.[44] Neutrophils contribute to recruitment of classical monocytes by release of granular proteins. In addition, neutrophil extracellular traps (NETs) can promote lesional macrophage accumulation, coagulation, and type I IFN release from pDCs, further amplifying plaque formation.[44] A distinct subset of low-density granulocytes (LDGs) isolated from SLE patients displays enhanced capacity to synthesize proinflammatory cytokines and type I IFNs and induces EC cytotoxicity while impairing vascular repair.[45] These LDGs display exuberant capacity to form NETs ex vivo and this may be an additional mechanism contributing to atherothrombosis and endothelial damage through externalization of vasculopathic proteins[46,47] and oxidation of lipoproteins like HDL, thereby impairing their function.[48] Bactericidal proteins present in the NETs, including the cathelicidin LL-37, may be important in atheroma formation.[49] Inhibition of NET formation through modulation of peptidylarginine deiminase pathways, using small molecules, decreases endothelial dysfunction, limits type I IFN responses, abrogates prothrombotic phenotype and limits plaque burden in animal models of lupus and atherosclerosis.[50–52] Overall, these observations suggest a prominent interplay between type I IFNs and aberrant neutrophils that promote endothelial damage and progression to atherothrombosis, an effect that may be particularly amplified in SLE.

OXIDIZED LIPOPROTEINS

In its native form, HDL has vasoprotective properties, due in part to its capacity to remove excess cholesterol from arterial wall macrophages, as well as through pleiotropic anti-inflammatory effects, including paraoxonase-1 activity. When HDL is oxidized in specific residues, it loses vasoprotective capabilities, has impaired cholesterol efflux capacity and gains proinflammatory activity. SLE patients have increased levels of oxidized HDL and impaired cholesterol efflux capacity, in association with subclinical atherosclerosis.[48,53] Enzymes present in NETs carry all the oxidative machinery necessary for HDL oxidation, and lupus-prone mice treated in vivo with an inhibitor of NETs display reduced HDL oxidation.[48] Also in murine lupus, autoantibodies against the most abundant protein in HDL,

Apo A-I, contribute to reducing HDL levels and paraoxonase activity,[54] with potential contributions to CV risk.

MODULATION OF CV RISK IN SLE

While no drug to date has proven to effectively decrease CV risk in SLE, there is evidence that some of the drugs typically used to treat this disease may have effects on the vasculature. Antimalarial use in SLE has been associated with enhanced endothelial function and decreased prevalence of subclinical atherosclerosis, and there are indications that this drug decreases the risk of developing diabetes.[55] Mycophenolate mofetil can promote immunoregulatory effects on arterial T cells and modulate atherosclerosis in mouse models.[56,57] An antiatherogenic effect form methotrexate use has been proposed, but whether this applies to SLE patients remains to be determined.[58] Further studies are required to better understand the impact of medications used in the treatment of SLE.

REFERENCES

1. Manzi S, Meilahn EN, Rairie JE, Conte CG, Medsger Jr TA, Jansen-McWilliams L, et al. Age-specific incidence rates of myocardial infarction and angina in women with systemic lupus erythematosus: comparison with the Framingham study. *Am J Epidemiol* 1997;**145**:408–15.
2. Nikpour M, Gladman DD, Urowitz MB. Premature coronary heart disease in systemic lupus erythematosus: what risk factors do we understand? *Lupus* 2013;**22**:1243–50.
3. Urowitz MB, Bookman AA, Koehler BE, Gordon DA, Smythe HA, Ogryzlo MA. The bimodal mortality pattern of systemic lupus erythematosus. *Am J Med* 1976;**60**:221–5.
4. Hak AE, Karlson EW, Feskanich D, Stampfer MJ, Costenbader KH. Systemic lupus erythematosus and the risk of cardiovascular disease: results from the nurses' health study. *Arthritis Rheum* 2009;**61**: 1396–402.
5. Esdaile JM, Abrahamowicz M, Grodzicky T, Li Y, Panaritis C, du Berger R, et al. Traditional Framingham risk factors fail to fully account for accelerated atherosclerosis in systemic lupus erythematosus. *Arthritis Rheum* 2001;**44**:2331–7.
6. Kiani AN, Vogel-Claussen J, Magder LS, Petri M. Noncalcified coronary plaque in systemic lupus erythematosus. *J Rheumatol* 2010;**37**:579–84.
7. Gustafsson J, Gunnarsson I, Borjesson O, Pettersson S, Moller S, Fei GZ, et al. Predictors of the first cardiovascular event in patients with systemic lupus erythematosus – a prospective cohort study. *Arthritis Res Ther* 2009;**11**:R186.
8. Gustafsson JT, Simard JF, Gunnarsson I, Elvin K, Lundberg IE, Hansson LO, et al. Risk factors for cardiovascular mortality in patients with systemic lupus erythematosus, a prospective cohort study. *Arthritis Res Ther* 2012;**14**:R46.
9. Abu-Shakra M, Urowitz MB, Gladman DD, Gough J. Mortality studies in systemic lupus erythematosus. Results from a single center. II. Predictor variables for mortality. *J Rheumatol* 1995;**22**:1265–70.
10. Seleznick MJ, Fries JF. Variables associated with decreased survival in systemic lupus erythematosus. *Semin Arthritis Rheum* 1991;**21**:73–80.

11. Mok CC, Poon WL, Lai JP, Wong CK, Chiu SM, Wong CK, et al. Metabolic syndrome, endothelial injury, and subclinical atherosclerosis in patients with systemic lupus erythematosus. *Scand J Rheumatol* 2010;**39**:42–9.

12. Bruce IN, Urowitz MB, Gladman DD, Ibanez D, Steiner G. Risk factors for coronary heart disease in women with systemic lupus erythematosus: the Toronto Risk Factor Study. *Arthritis Rheum* 2003;**48**:3159–67.

13. Ross R. Atherosclerosis–an inflammatory disease. *N Engl J Med* 1999;**340**:115–26.

14. Libby P, Ridker PM. Inflammation and atherosclerosis: role of C-reactive protein in risk assessment. *Am J Med* 2004;**116**(Suppl. 6A):9S–16S.

15. Enocsson H, Sjowall C, Skogh T, Eloranta ML, Ronnblom L, Wettero J. Interferon-alpha mediates suppression of C-reactive protein: explanation for muted C-reactive protein response in lupus flares? *Arthritis Rheum* 2009;**60**:3755–60.

16. Schanberg LE, Sandborg C, Barnhart HX, Ardoin SP, Yow E, Evans GW, et al. Atherosclerosis prevention in pediatric lupus erythematosus I. Use of atorvastatin in systemic lupus erythematosus in children and adolescents. *Arthritis Rheum* 2012;**64**:285–96.

17. Petri MA, Kiani AN, Post W, Christopher-Stine L, Magder LS. Lupus atherosclerosis prevention study (laps). *Ann Rheum Dis* 2011;**70**:760–5.

18. Denny MF, Thacker S, Mehta H, Somers EC, Dodick T, Barrat FJ, et al. Interferon-alpha promotes abnormal vasculogenesis in lupus: a potential pathway for premature atherosclerosis. *Blood* 2007;**110**:2907–15.

19. Rajagopalan S, Somers EC, Brook RD, Kehrer C, Pfenninger D, Lewis E, et al. Endothelial cell apoptosis in systemic lupus erythematosus: a common pathway for abnormal vascular function and thrombosis propensity. *Blood* 2004;**103**:3677–83.

20. Werner N, Kosiol S, Schiegl T, Ahlers P, Walenta K, Link A, et al. Circulating endothelial progenitor cells and cardiovascular outcomes. *N Engl J Med* 2005;**353**:999–1007.

21. Kahlenberg JM, Thacker SG, Berthier CC, Cohen CD, Kretzler M, Kaplan MJ. Inflammasome activation of IL-18 results in endothelial progenitor cell dysfunction in systemic lupus erythematosus. *J Immunol* 2011;**187**:6143–56.

22. Thacker SG, Berthier CC, Mattinzoli D, Rastaldi MP, Kretzler M, Kaplan MJ. The detrimental effects of IFN-alpha on vasculogenesis in lupus are mediated by repression of IL-1 pathways: potential role in atherogenesis and renal vascular rarefaction. *J Immunol* 2010;**185**:4457–69.

23. Andrade D, Kim M, Blanco LP, Karumanchi SA, Koo GC, Redecha P, et al. Interferon-alpha and angiogenic dysregulation in pregnant lupus patients destined for preeclampsia. *Arthritis Rheumatol* 2014;**16**(1):A28.

24. Niessner A, Sato K, Chaikof EL, Colmegna I, Goronzy JJ, Weyand CM. Pathogen-sensing plasmacytoid dendritic cells stimulate cytotoxic T-cell function in the atherosclerotic plaque through interferon-alpha. *Circulation* 2006;**114**:2482–9.

25. Niessner A, Shin MS, Pryshchep O, Goronzy JJ, Chaikof EL, Weyand CM. Synergistic proinflammatory effects of the antiviral cytokine interferon-alpha and toll-like receptor 4 ligands in the atherosclerotic plaque. *Circulation* 2007;**116**:2043–52.

26. Macritchie N, Grassia G, Sabir SR, Maddaluno M, Welsh P, Sattar N, et al. Plasmacytoid dendritic cells play a key role in promoting atherosclerosis in apolipoprotein E-deficient mice. *Arterioscler Thromb Vasc Biol* 2012;**32**:2569–79.

27. Thacker SG, Zhao W, Smith CK, Luo W, Wang H, Vivekanandan-Giri A, et al. Type I interferons modulate vascular function, repair, thrombosis, and plaque progression in murine models of lupus and atherosclerosis. *Arthritis Rheum* 2012;**64**:2975–85.

28. Goossens P, Gijbels MJ, Zernecke A, Eijgelaar W, Vergouwe MN, van der Made I, et al. Myeloid type I interferon signaling promotes atherosclerosis by stimulating macrophage recruitment to lesions. *Cell Metab* 2010;**12**:142–53.

29. Li J, Fu Q, Cui H, Qu B, Pan W, Shen N, et al. Interferon-alpha priming promotes lipid uptake and macrophage-derived foam cell formation: a novel link between interferon-alpha and atherosclerosis in lupus. *Arthritis Rheum* 2011;**63**:492–502.

30. Lood C, Amisten S, Gullstrand B, Jonsen A, Allhorn M, Truedsson L, et al. Platelet transcriptional profile and protein expression in patients with systemic lupus erythematosus: up-regulation of the type I interferon system is strongly associated with vascular disease. *Blood* 2010;**116**:1951–7.

31. Somers EC, Zhao W, Lewis EE, Wang L, Wing JJ, Sundaram B, et al. Type I interferons are associated with subclinical markers of cardiovascular disease in a cohort of systemic lupus erythematosus patients. *PloS One* 2012;**7**:e37000.

32. Shirota Y, Yarboro C, Fischer R, Pham TH, Lipsky P, Illei GG. Impact of anti-interleukin-6 receptor blockade on circulating T and B cell subsets in patients with systemic lupus erythematosus. *Ann Rheum Dis* 2013;**72**:118–28.

33. Souto A, Salgado E, Maneiro JR, Mera A, Carmona L, Gomez-Reino JJ. Lipid profile changes in patients with chronic inflammatory arthritis treated with biologic agents and tofacitinib in randomized clinical trials: a systematic review and meta-analysis. *Arthritis Rheumatol* 2015;**67**:117–27.

34. Farzaneh-Far A, Roman MJ, Lockshin MD, Devereux RB, Paget SA, Crow MK, et al. Relationship of antiphospholipid antibodies to cardiovascular manifestations of systemic lupus erythematosus. *Arthritis Rheum* 2006;**54**:3918–25.

35. O'Neill SG, Giles I, Lambrianides A, Manson J, D'Cruz D, Schrieber L, et al. Antibodies to apolipoprotein A-I, high-density lipoprotein, and C-reactive protein are associated with disease activity in patients with systemic lupus erythematosus. *Arthritis Rheum* 2010;**62**:845–54.

36. Gronwall C, Reynolds H, Kim JK, Buyon J, Goldberg JD, Clancy RM, et al. Relation of carotid plaque with natural IgM antibodies in patients with systemic lupus erythematosus. *Clin Immunol* 2014;**153**:1–7.

37. Lewis MJ, Malik TH, Fossati-Jimack L, Carassiti D, Cook HT, Haskard DO, et al. Distinct roles for complement in glomerulonephritis and atherosclerosis revealed in mice with a combination of lupus and hyperlipidemia. *Arthritis Rheum* 2012;**64**:2707–18.

38. Thorp E, Tabas I. Mechanisms and consequences of efferocytosis in advanced atherosclerosis. *J Leukoc Biol* 2009;**86**:1089–95.

39. Wilhelm AJ, Rhoads JP, Wade NS, Major AS. Dysregulated CD4+ T cells from SLE-susceptible mice are sufficient to accelerate atherosclerosis in LDLr-/- mice. *Ann Rheum Dis* 2015;**74**:778–85.

40. Gautier EL, Huby T, Ouzilleau B, Doucet C, Saint-Charles F, Gremy G, et al. Enhanced immune system activation and arterial inflammation accelerates atherosclerosis in lupus-prone mice. *Arterioscler Thromb Vasc Biol* 2007;**27**:1625–31.

41. Burbano C, Vasquez G, Rojas M. Modulatory effects of CD14+CD16++ monocytes on CD14++CD16- monocytes: a possible explanation of monocyte alterations in systemic lupus erythematosus. *Arthritis Rheumatol* 2014;**66**:3371–81.

42. Korman BD, Huang CC, Skamra C, Wu P, Koessler R, Yao D, et al. Inflammatory expression profiles in monocyte-to-macrophage differentiation in patients with systemic lupus erythematosus and relationship with atherosclerosis. *Arthritis Res Ther* 2014;**16**:R147.

43. Ayoub S, Hickey MJ, Morand EF. Mechanisms of disease: macrophage migration inhibitory factor in SLE, RA and atherosclerosis. *Nat Clin Pract Rheumatol* 2008;**4**:98–105.

44. Doring Y, Drechsler M, Soehnlein O, Weber C. Neutrophils in atherosclerosis: from mice to man. *Arterioscler Thromb Vasc Biol* 2015;**35**:288–95.

45. Denny MF, Yalavarthi S, Zhao W, Thacker SG, Anderson M, Sandy AR, et al. A distinct subset of proinflammatory neutrophils isolated from patients with systemic lupus erythematosus induces vascular damage and synthesizes type I IFNs. *J Immunol* 2010;**184**:3284–97.

46. Carmona-Rivera C, Zhao W, Yalavarthi S, Kaplan MJ. Neutrophil extracellular traps induce endothelial dysfunction in systemic lupus erythematosus through the activation of matrix metalloproteinase-2. *Ann Rheum Dis* 2015;**74**(7):1417–24.

47. Villanueva E, Yalavarthi S, Berthier CC, Hodgin JB, Khandpur R, Lin AM, et al. Netting neutrophils induce endothelial damage, infiltrate tissues, and expose immunostimulatory molecules in systemic lupus erythematosus. *J Immunol* 2011;**187**:538–52.

48. Smith CK, Vivekanandan-Giri A, Tang C, Knight JS, Mathew A, Padilla RL, et al. Neutrophil extracellular trap-derived enzymes oxidize high-density lipoprotein: an additional proatherogenic mechanism in systemic lupus erythematosus. *Arthritis Rheumatol* 2014;**66**:2532–44.

49. Doring Y, Drechsler M, Wantha S, Kemmerich K, Lievens D, Vijayan S, et al. Lack of neutrophil-derived CRAMP reduces atherosclerosis in mice. *Circ Res* 2012;**110**:1052–6.

50. Knight JS, Luo W, O'Dell AA, Yalavarthi S, Zhao W, Subramanian V, et al. Peptidylarginine deiminase inhibition reduces vascular damage and modulates innate immune responses in murine models of atherosclerosis. *Circ Res* 2014;**114**:947–56.

51. Knight JS, Subramanian V, O'Dell AA, Yalavarthi S, Zhao W, Smith CK, et al. Peptidylarginine deiminase inhibition disrupts NET formation and protects against kidney, skin and vascular disease in lupus-prone MRL/lpr mice. *Ann Rheum Dis* 2014; http://dx.doi.org/10.1136/annrheumdis-2014-205365.

52. Knight JS, Zhao W, Luo W, Subramanian V, O'Dell AA, Yalavarthi S, et al. Peptidylarginine deiminase inhibition is immunomodulatory and vasculoprotective in murine lupus. *J Clin Invest* 2013;**123**:2981–93.

53. McMahon M, Grossman J, FitzGerald J, Dahlin-Lee E, Wallace DJ, Thong BY, et al. Proinflammatory high-density lipoprotein as a biomarker for atherosclerosis in patients with systemic lupus erythematosus and rheumatoid arthritis. *Arthritis Rheum* 2006;**54**:2541–9.

54. Srivastava R, Yu S, Parks BW, Black LL, Kabarowski JH. Autoimmune-mediated reduction of high-density lipoprotein-cholesterol and paraoxonase 1 activity in systemic lupus erythematosus-prone gld mice. *Arthritis Rheum* 2011;**63**:201–11.

55. Chen YM, Lin CH, Lan TH, Chen HH, Chang SN, Chen YH, et al. Hydroxychloroquine reduces risk of incident diabetes mellitus in lupus patients in a dose-dependent manner: a population-based cohort study. *Rheumatology* 2015.

56. van Leuven SI, Mendez-Fernandez YV, Wilhelm AJ, Wade NS, Gabriel CL, Kastelein JJ, et al. Mycophenolate mofetil but not atorvastatin attenuates atherosclerosis in lupus-prone LDLr(-/-) mice. *Ann Rheum Dis* 2012;**71**:408–14.

57. David KM, Morris JA, Steffen BJ, Chi-Burris KS, Gotz VP, Gordon RD. Mycophenolate mofetil vs. azathioprine is associated with decreased acute rejection, late acute rejection, and risk for cardiovascular death in renal transplant recipients with pre-transplant diabetes. *Clin Transplant* 2005;**19**:279–85.

58. Choi HK, Hernan MA, Seeger JD, Robins JM, Wolfe F. Methotrexate and mortality in patients with rheumatoid arthritis: a prospective study. *Lancet* 2002;**359**:1173–7.

Chapter 35

The Mechanism of Skin Damage

Xin Huang[1], Haijing Wu[1], Christopher Chang[2], Qianjin Lu[1]

[1]Department of Dermatology, Hunan Key Laboratory of Medical Epigenomics, Second Xiangya Hospital, Central South University, Changsha, Hunan, China; [2]Division of Rheumatology, Allergy and Clinical Immunology, University of California at Davis, Davis, CA, USA

INTRODUCTION

Lupus erythematosus (LE) comprises a broad spectrum of chronic inflammatory autoimmune disorders that display many diverse symptoms. Localized cutaneous LE (CLE) and severe systemic LE (SLE) represent the two ends of the spectrum of LE. The various cutaneous manifestations of LE are divided into LE-specific and LE-nonspecific skin disease based on histopathological findings.[1,2] The underlying cause of a lupus-like lesion is unknown, but it is generally believed that the pathogenesis involves a genetic predisposition triggered by environmental factors. These environmental triggers include ultraviolet radiation (UVR), infection, hormones, and exposure to drugs and chemicals.[3–5] To date, a growing body of literature indicates that the activation of intrinsic and extrinsic pathways of apoptosis by UVR and externalization of autoantigens initiate skin injury in LE.[3,6–11] UVR can stimulate the immune response through the activation and recruitment of dendritic cells (DCs), B cells, and effector T cells.[3,12] During this process, the type 1 interferon (IFN-1) pathway plays an important role in the interaction of immune cells.[3,4,9,13–15] Through the influence of various inflammatory factors (e.g., interleukins and tumor necrosis factor family) and chemokines, activated immune cells migrate into different layers of the dermis and epidermis, causing lupus-like lesions.[8,9,13,14,16–27]

In this chapter, we focus on the clinical aspects associated with skin damage and elucidate the recent advances in the pathogenesis of skin lesions of LE.

CLINICAL ASPECTS

The various cutaneous manifestations of LE can present as LE-specific or LE-nonspecific manifestations.[1,2] LE-specific skin manifestations can be further subdivided into acute CLE (ACLE), subacute CLE (SCLE), chronic CLE (CCLE), and intermittent CLE (ICLE)[28–30] (for information on the manifestations of different subsets of LE, see Chapter 39). Histological findings of skin lesions are essentially identical for SLE and CLE. Direct histological examination of skin biopsies shows the appearance of characteristic skin changes, which are always organ-specific and meaningful for distinguishing LE from other conditions in the differential diagnosis. The most common histologic findings are abnormal keratinocyte distribution, perivascular, and periappendageal lymphocytic infiltration, smudged appearance of the dermoepidermal junction, and thickened basement membrane (Figure 1).[31] Direct immunofluorescence (DIF) is able to detect the deposition of immunoglobulins and complement component C3 at the dermoepidermal junction. This test is also known as the *lupus band test* (Figure 2).[28] Although positive findings in nonlesional, sun-protected skin strongly support a diagnosis of SLE, it is not exclusive because similar deposits can also be found in normal or sun-damaged skin. Different subsets of LE may share similar histological changes and, in certain cases of LE, will undergo a consequent epidermal and dermal transformation throughout the entire disease process.

PATHOGENESIS OF SKIN DAMAGE

Ultraviolet Radiation and Skin Damage

Skin lesions in patients with LE can be induced and exacerbated by UVR exposure. The reaction to UV light varies between different subtypes of CLE. Among them, SCLE, discoid lupus erythematosus (DLE), and lupus erythematosus tumidus (LET) may be the most relevant subsets.

Photosensitivity and Photoprovocation

The term *photosensitivity* is briefly defined by the American College of Rheumatology (ACR) as a "skin rash as a result of unusual reaction to sunlight by patient history or physician observation."[32] Because this is a very broad definition, a variety of other diseases such as polymorphic light eruption (PLE), photoallergic contact dermatitis, and dermatomyositis can also fall within this description. Some researchers have tried to define photosensitivity more specifically as an induction of skin lesions following extensive

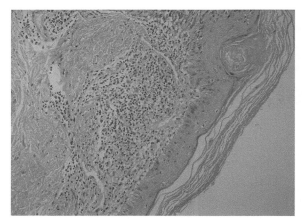

FIGURE 1 Histopathological features of DLE: Marked hyperkeratesis with follicular horny plugs, atrophy of epidermis with extensive liquefaction degeneration of basal cells, interface dermatitis of the epidermis and follicles accompanied by perivascular and periappendageal lymphocytic infiltrates in the upper and lower dermis.

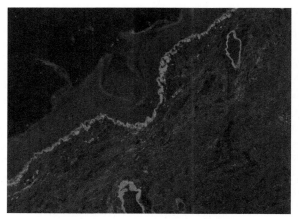

FIGURE 2 DIF shows significant deposits of IgG at the basement membrane.

sun exposure (including sunburn), or they may add spring and summer aggravation into the definition.[4,33] Photosensitivity is listed as one of the ACR criteria for the classification of SLE. However, subsequently Albreht and his colleagues remarked that "malar rash" is often not distinguishable from photosensitivity in SLE patients. Thus, the two ACR criteria are not independent of each other.[4,34]

The photoprovocation experiment (or test) is an approach to objectively define photosensitivity. To artificially test for photosensitivity of LE patients, the characterization of the action spectrum, or *morbific wavelength*, is needed. The testing regimen combining ultraviolet (UV) B and UVA received much attention because the ability to reproduce skin lesions in patients with LE by irradiation of UVB plus UVA was reported. This still represents an optimal model for clinical and experimental studies. Besides this, an optimized protocol for photoprovocation testing should also include the selected testing area, the dose of UV exposure,

and frequency of irradiation.[4] UV-induced LE-specific lesions are significantly slower to appear and persist longer than reaction of other photosensitivity-related diseases. Nonetheless, there is a latency time before the observation of related positive testing resulting from experimental photoprovocation, making the relationship of UVR and the induction of skin lesions sometimes elusive.

UV-Triggered Apoptotic Cells

Apoptosis, or programmed cell death, is the most common form of cell death in the human body. Several processes are involved, such as caspase activation, exposure of negatively charged phospholipids, generation of reactive oxygen species (ROS), and DNA cleavage.[35] The final step in the apoptotic process is the removal of apoptotic cells, which is performed in an immunologically silent fashion, without the unwanted release of intracellular danger-associated molecules (DAMPS) and potential autoantigens, such as high-mobility group protein B1 (HMGB1) and histone–DNA complexes.[7] The induction of apoptosis is mediated via extrinsic or intrinsic pathways. The extrinsic pathway is activated following ligation of the so-called death receptors, such as CD95/Fas, tumor necrosis factor receptor 1 (TNF-R1), or tumor necrosis factor related apoptosis induce ligand (TRAIL) receptors.[35,36] In the pathogenesis of LE-like lesion, both the abnormal generation and/or defective engulfment of apoptotic cells have been implicated in this disease. It has been observed by Kuhn et al. that an increased number of apoptotic cells exist in the skin of CLE and SLE patients, when compared with healthy controls.[15]

UVR can lead to exposure to autoantigens and nucleic acids, such as Ro52, ani-Ro, and anti-La antibody. The UV-oxidized DNA is resistant to degradation by cytosolic nucleases such as TREX1, potentiating subsequent activation of the apoptosis related cascade (Figure 3). An important tumor suppressor gene p53 was found to be increasingly expressed in CLE, and activation of p53 promotes apoptosis through direct effects on bax and bcl-2 and by induction of p21. Some conductors of extrinsic pathway of apoptosis such as CD95/Fas, TRAIL-R1, and caspase 8 have also been shown to be highly expressed in the skin of CLE patients.[37] UVR can also affect the oxidation process by increasing local nitric oxide production in the skin through stimulation of inducible NO synthase (iNOS) and generation of ROS. It has been reported that iNOS is expressed in the lesional skin of CLE after UVR.[9] Moreover, mice with C1q (an important complement component in clearing apoptosis debris) deficiency develop an SLE-like disease and patients with complete congenital C1q deficiency develop LE-like photosensitive eruptions, suggesting that a disrupted clearance process mediated by C1q is strongly associated with the development of CLE.[38]

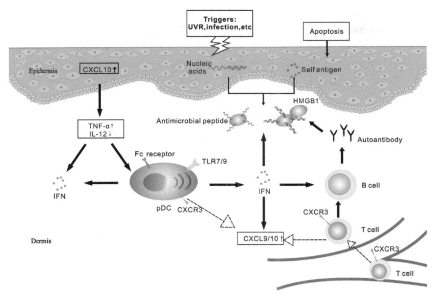

FIGURE 3   The pathogenesis of skin damage in LE.

Immune Cells, Cytokines and Chemokines

UVR-related skin damage, apoptosis of keratinocytes, and inflammatory infiltrations are mediated by the interaction of immune cells, primarily including T cells, B cells, and DCs. A group of cytokines and chemokines, such as IFN-1 and tumor necrosis factor alpha (TNF-α), are upregulated as a result of this interaction, and the interaction is also highly regulated to produce a more specific and precise immune response.[3,4,7–12,14–17,19,27,39–43]

Dendritic Cells and T-Cell Subtypes

DCs are a part of the innate immune system, and they play pivotal roles in the induction of effective cellular immune responses and in the maintenance of peripheral tolerance. Based on their surface markers and typical functions, DCs are divided into two groups: conventional DCs (cDCs) and plasmacytoid DCs (pDCs). Although decreased numbers of pDCs are found in the peripheral blood of SLE patients, their presence and accumulation in cutaneous lesions has been demonstrated.[27] pDCs have the unique capacity to rapidly produce huge amounts of IFN-α upon recognition of viral RNA and DNA through Toll-like receptors (TLRs)-7 and 9 and other pattern recognition receptors (PRR).[41] The distribution of pDCs in skin shows two distinct patterns. Most of them are observed within perivascular inflammatory nodules in the dermis (D-pDCs). The others are found along the dermal–epithelial junction (J-pDCs).[12] Exposure to UVR or other environmental factors can give rise to the release of nuclear components and endogenous autoantigens from apoptotic debris, leading to a sustained production of IFN-α.[10,41] Under the influence of IFN-α, pDCs secrete high

amounts of TNF and IL-6. In the presence of TNF, additional apoptosis takes place.[14] Meanwhile, Mendez-Reguera et al. found that pathogenic CCR6⁺cDCs resulting from in situ phenotypic changes exist in the skin lesions of DLE patients and may mediate the inflammatory response via DAMPS.[43]

Skin-infiltrating activated leukocytes are thought to play a crucial role in the induction and maintenance of UV-induced cutaneous LE lesions. The majority of inflammatory infiltrated leukocytes are memory T lymphocytes, and these cells display a CD4 phenotype. Th1 cells are thought to be the predominant driver in CLE pathogenesis—a concept that is supported by the shift toward Th1-associated chemokines, which has been reported in all types of CLE.[11,39] Imbalanced Th17 cells and regulatory T cells ratio have also been reported to contribute to the unwanted autoimmune response in CLE.[17,19] Moreover, a subset of CD8⁺ T cell may also possess inflammatory activity by transforming to TCRαβ+CD4⁻CD8 double-negative (DN) T cells, which then exert their inflammatory effects by altering the number of CD4⁺ regulatory T cells in a IL-2 dependent manner.[44–46]

Type 1 Interferon and Tumor Necrosis Factor

Type 1 IFNs (α and β) have a specific role in the immunological interface between the innate and the adaptive immune system. The most widely accepted biologic effects include activating DCs, promoting proliferation, survival, and differentiation of monocytes and B cells, stimulating the Th1 pathway, and preventing apoptosis of activated cytotoxic T cells.[39] IFN-1 can be produced by macrophages, DCs, and epithelial cells. Evidence suggests that the recruitment of inflammatory effector T cells and DCs is directly linked to the accumulation of pDCs and IFN-1 in the skin lesions of CLE patients.[27,39,42] Additionally, a new class of IFNs, type 3 or IFN-k, which is likely produced by keratinocytes expressing CXCL9, has also been shown to be involved in the pathogenesis of CLE (Table 1).[47]

Exogenous stimuli (bacterial and viral pathogens) can activate pattern recognition receptors (PRRs), such as TLR7/9 and TLR3, which then give rise to the activation of IFN-regulatory factor (IRF) 7 and IRF 3, the key regulators of IFN-1 transcription. Endogenous elements such

TABLE 1 The Role of Cytokines and Chemokines in the Pathogenesis of Skin Damage in LE

Cytokine/ Chemokine	Major Functions	Expression in Lupus Condition	Mechanism of Action
Type 1 IFN	Activates DCs and monocytes, stimulates the Th1 pathway, suppresses Treg cells	Highly expressed in the skin lesion and serum of all the subtype of CLE and SLE	Activates numerous lymphocytes, promotes the secretion of cytokines and causes an inflammatory feedback loop[27,39,42]
Type 3 IFN	Antiviral immunity	Highly expressed by keratinocytes in the skin lesion of CLE patient	Induces the production of pro-inflammatory cytokines, such as CXCL9[47]
TNF-α	Induces the production of cytokines, attracts inflammatory cells	High levels in skin and serum of SCLE patients. Contradictory findings in murine models	Upregulates Ro52, stimulates TNFRI signaling pathway and can be induced by IL-18[11,40,49,50]
IL-6	Induces the differentiation of B cell and cytotoxic T cell, promotes Ig production	Highly expressed in skin lesion of LE after UV radiation	Promotes B-cell differentiation into Ig-secreting plasma cells; stimulates Treg to Th17 cells[42]
IL-10	Suppresses inflammatory cells and sustains peripheral tolerance	Increased serum level in SLE patients, undecided role in murine model and cutaneous manifestation of LE	May be by the activation of B cells[6,11]
IL-12	Regulator of T cell via production of IFN-γ	Reduced expression of IL-12 in the skin lesions of MRL/lpr mice	Weakens apoptotic process in an IFN-dependent way[11]
IL-17	Important inflammatory factor	IL-17A is highly expressed in the skin lesion of SLE, SCLE and DLE, and serum of DLE and SCLE patients	Stimulates the Th17 pathways and IFN secretion[17]
IL-18	Belongs to IL-1 cytokine family, a Th1 type pro-inflammatory cytokine	IL-18 and IL-18 receptor are highly expressed in the skin lesion of CLE patients	Promotes Th1 response, stimulates the production of cytokines such as IFN and TNF[19]
CXCL9/10	Belong to Th1 type family of chemokines, mediates the Th1 pathways	CXCL9/10 expression are upregulated in SCLE and LET lesions when compared to chronic DLE	Recruits CXCR3+ cytotoxic T cells and pDCs, mediates a IFN-dependent inflammatory response, expression of CXCL9 may be related to a type 3 IFN-mediated immune response in the epidermis[42]
CXCL12/ CXCR4	Attract multiple leukocyte subsets and stimulate B cell production and myelopoeisis	CXCL12 is highly expressed in the skin of SLE patients	Attract T cells, B cells, pre-B cells, and monocytes to inflammatory sites[20]
CCL17/CCR4	Predominantly expressed by Th2 cells and stimulate Th2 pathway	CCR4/CCL17 expression is high in skin lesions and serum of CLE patients. Cytotoxic CD8+ T cells expressing CCR4+ are associated with CLE patients with scarring lesions	Recruit CCR4+ T cells to second lymphoid organs and inflammatory sites. Possible role in the forming of scar in CLE[21,23,55]
CXCL16/ CXCR6	Induce strong chemotactic response in activated T cells	The expression of CXCL16 is high in the serum of SLE patient and is associated with disease activity	Cause vascular injury via stimulating the production of IL-18, IFN-γ, and TNF-α; induce endothelial cell proliferation; and promote cellular adhension[56]

as self-nucleic acid and nucleic acid-containing immune complexes stimulate the generation of IFN-1 in a TLR-independent manner. Indeed, Meller et al. found that a number of IFN-inducible genes and proteins are upregulated in CLE lesions, including antiviral-MxA protein, a specific marker for the IFN-1 system, IRF7, Th1-associated chemokines CXCL9, CXCL10, and CXCL11, as well as their corresponding receptor CXCR3.[3,8,42] Because CXCR3 is predominantly expressed on the surface of IFN-producing Th1 cells and IFN-α/γ are potent inducers of CXCL9,10,11 in vitro and in vivo, it has been suggested that IFN-1 facilitate CXCL9 and CXL10 expression and orchestrate the recruitment of CXCR3[+] cytotoxic T cells into the lesions.[11] In turn, the recruitment of CXCR3[+] T cells may be responsible for enhanced IFN-γ and TNF-α production, which stimulates the secretion of CXCL9, 10, 11, thereby presenting an inflammatory feedback loop (Figure 3). The CXCR3[+] cytotoxic T cells invade the basal epidermal layer and induce apoptosis, which causes the appearance of an important histologic finding on CLE, termed *interface dermatitis*.[8]

Unlike IFN-1, whose role in LE is fairly certain, the involvement of another pro-inflammatory factor, TNF-α, is more controversial. The biological activities of TNF-α vary from Fas-associated death domain mediated apoptosis to TNF receptor-associated factor-2 (TRAF-2) activated cell survival and differentiation. A strongly positive distribution of TNF-α in refractory lesional skin tissue of SCLE patients has been documented and certain clinical manifestations such as malar rash, discoid rash, oral ulcers, serositis, and hematological disorders are associated with the polymorphism of the TNF-α promoter -308A in a Taiwanese cohort study.[40,48] TNF-α exerts its effect by binding to TNFRI and TNFRII. TNFR preligand assemble domain (PLAD) has been found to block the effects of TNF-α. During the process of lesion genesis, it is TNFRI but not TNFRII that is predominantly expressed in skin lesions of lupus, and TNFRI PLAD can significantly inhibit skin injury in MRL/lpr mouse model of lupus.[49,50] The effect of TNF-α is probably mediated by its upstream cytokine IL-18. IL-18, which is expressed in the epidermis of skin lesions of LE patients, induces epidermal production of the chemokine CXCL10, which favors the attraction of IFN-γ producing lymphocytes as mentioned. Furthermore, IL-18 results in the release of TNF-α from activated keratinocytes.[19] However, the proinflammatory role of TNF-α is controversial due to the fact that in some LE-prone murine models, such as NZB/W F1 mice, TNF-α was found to have a protective effect. Meanwhile, lupus-like syndrome of CLE induced by anti-TNF-α agents has been reported.[51]

Other Cytokines and Chemokines

Other cytokines, such as IL-1, IL-6, IL-10, IL-12, IL-17, and IL-18, have also been implicated in the pathogenesis

of CLE. Among them, IL-6, IL-17, and IL-18 have been reported to exacerbate the progress of skin damage of LE and correlate with disease activity, while IL-12 and IL-27 tend to provide a protective effect[3,6,9,11,15,17,19,42,43] (Table 1). As a major pro-inflammatory cytokine, IL-6 affects immune responses through the induction of B-cell maturation, immunoglobulin secretion, and cytotoxic T-cell differentiation. IL-17 is produced by Th17 T-helper cells. High serum concentrations of IL-6 and IL-17 are found in lupus-prone murine models and LE patients, respectively.[17] Moreover, the expression of IL-17 is positively correlated with the expression of IFN-1. IL-12 is thought to weaken the apoptotic process of keratinocytes in an IFN-dependent way. In MRL/lpr mice, reduced expression of IL-12 was found in skin lesions. Meanwhile, it was proposed that another pro-inflammatory interleukin, IL-18, can reduce IL-12 expression in hair-derived keratinocytes via TNF-α.[19]

The formation of skin inflammation in SLE is a process that involves the molecular regulation of immune cell homing to the skin. It has been demonstrated that naïve T cells expressing different intracellular adhesion molecules and chemokines can enter certain specific organs and tissues. Once activated by antigen-presenting cells in the inflamed dermis and epidermis of SLE patients, they proliferate, express activation and effector molecules, and transform to effector and memory T cells. The chemokines are a family of more than 40 distinct structurally related cytokines. They are classified into four groups—CC, CXC, XC, and CX3C—based on the amino acid motif present between the first two N-terminal cysteine residues.[52] CXCL9/10/11 are the typical chemokines taking part in the inflammatory process of cutaneous lupus.

Studies have highlighted the role of other chemokines, such as chemokine receptor 4 (CCR4) and its ligand thymus and activation-regulated chemokine (TARC/CCL17), CXCL12 and CXCL16, in the pathogenesis of skin lesion in LE. CXCL12, also known as stromal cell-derived factor (SDF-1), is highly expressed in SLE patients.[53] A common variant at position 801 in the 3′-untranslated region in CXCL12 gene (designated CXCL12-3′G801A) has been reported to be associated with skin damage in SLE patients in a Han Chinese population study.[54] CCR4 is predominantly expressed by Th2 cells.[55] Wenzel et al. found that the coexpression of CCR4 and cutaneous lymphocyte antigen (CLA), which drives effector T cells and memory T cells migration into inflamed skin, defines a subset of CLE patients characterized by disseminated scarring lesions.[55] CXCL16 is the sole ligand for the receptor CXCR6. It is present in two forms: a transmembrane multidomain molecule and a soluble form of CXCL16 (sCXCL16). CXCL16 can be selectively upregulated in a wide range of tissues in response to damage, and research has demonstrated that the level of serum sCXCL16 correlates with disease activity and organ damage in the kidney and skin of SLE and rheumatoid arthritis patients.[56] Other chemokines and chemokine receptors that have been reported to be increased in SLE include CCR1, CXCR2, CXCR3, MIP-1beta, MCP-1, IP-10, and RANTES. However, their roles in the pathogenesis of skin injury still need to be determined.[24,26]

The Genetic and Epigenetic Mechanisms for Skin Damage in CLE

LE is a heterogeneous autoimmune condition affecting multiple organs, including skin. Its etiology involves both genetic predisposition and environmental stimuli. Recently, Dey Rao et al. obtained genome-wide expression data from CCLE patients.[57] In the research, a subset of CCLE differentially expressed genes (DEGs) was found to overlap with SLE, including those linked to IFN and apoptosis, which are two major pathogenic pathways in CLE.[3,10,40] CCLE DEGs relate to IFN-1 pathways including IFN-α inducible genes (OAS1/2/L, IFIT1, and PLSCR1) and some key chemokines and their ligands, such as CXCL1. Significant upregulation of these genes have been correlated with previous results from quantitative reverse-transcriptase polymerase chain reaction in DLE patients.[58] In addition, dysregulated complement function (including C1R, C2, C1QB, C3AR1, CFB, CFD, and C4A/C4B) has been found in lesions, supporting their role in the clearing of cellular fragment debris generated by apoptosis. Other mediators of leukocyte chemotaxis, including FCGR3A, ITGAL, ITGB2, and NCF4, have also been reported to be dysregulated in CLE lesions.

Epigenetics serves as an essential component in modulating the pathophysiology of diseases, and recent work has stimulated great interest in its role in autoimmune diseases. Numerous data have demonstrated that, in patients with SLE, there are striking alterations of DNA methylation, histone modifications, and deregulated microRNA expression. However, studies of the relationship between epigenetics and cutaneous manifestations in LE have been lacking until recently. A research group from China studied the relationship of different epigenetic modifications with gene expression and disease phenotype in SLE CD4$^+$ T cells.[59] Hypomethylated differentially methylated regions (DMRs) that are associated with corresponding gene expression in SLE are enriched in gene regions relevant to the inflammatory response, regulation of immune system processes, and induction of apoptosis and regulation of cell migration. Some of them are well known for their undoubted pathogenic effects during the generation of skin damage in CLE, such as CXCL13, and TLR7.[10,41] Many genes encoding for TNF and TNF receptor family members have also been reported to be involved in this epigenetic regulation network. These encouraging results will surely promote further advances into the investigation of epigenetic modification in CLE pathogenesis.

REFERENCES

1. Gilliam JN, Sontheimer RD. Distinctive cutaneous subsets in the spectrum of lupus erythematosus. *J Am Acad Dermatol* 1981;**4**(4):471–5.
2. Tan EM, Cohen AS, Fries JF, Masi AT, McShane DJ, Rothfield NF, et al. The 1982 revised criteria for the classification of systemic lupus erythematosus. *Arthritis Rheum* 1982;**25**(11):1271–7.
3. Meller S, Winterberg F, Gilliet M, Muller A, Lauceviciute I, Rieker J, et al. Ultraviolet radiation-induced injury, chemokines, and leukocyte recruitment: an amplification cycle triggering cutaneous lupus erythematosus. *Arthritis Rheum* 2005;**52**(5):1504–16.
4. Kuhn A, Ruland V, Bonsmann G. Photosensitivity, phototesting, and photoprotection in cutaneous lupus erythematosus. *Lupus* 2010;**19**(9):1036–46.
5. Deng GM, Tsokos GC. Cholera toxin B accelerates disease progression in lupus-prone mice by promoting lipid raft aggregation. *J Immunol* 2008;**181**(6):4019–26.
6. Suarez A, Lopez P, Mozo L, Gutierrez C. Differential effect of IL10 and TNF{alpha} genotypes on determining susceptibility to discoid and systemic lupus erythematosus. *Ann Rheum Dis* 2005;**64**(11):1605–10.
7. Franz S, Gaipl US, Munoz LE, Sheriff A, Beer A, Kalden JR, et al. Apoptosis and autoimmunity: when apoptotic cells break their silence. *Curr Rheumatol Rep* 2006;**8**(4):245–7.
8. Wenzel J, Tuting T. An IFN-associated cytotoxic cellular immune response against viral, self-, or tumor antigens is a common pathogenetic feature in "interface dermatitis". *J Invest Dermatol* 2008;**128**(10):2392–402.
9. Kuhn A, Sontheimer RD. Cutaneous lupus erythematosus: molecular and cellular basis of clinical findings. *Curr Dir Autoimmun* 2008;**10**:119–40.
10. Gregorio J, Meller S, Conrad C, Di Nardo A, Homey B, Lauerma A, et al. Plasmacytoid dendritic cells sense skin injury and promote wound healing through type I interferons. *J Exp Med* 2010;**207**(13):2921–30.
11. Mikita N, Ikeda T, Ishiguro M, Furukawa F. Recent advances in cytokines in cutaneous and systemic lupus erythematosus. *J Dermatol* 2011;**38**(9):839–49.
12. Vermi W, Lonardi S, Morassi M, Rossini C, Tardanico R, Venturini M, et al. Cutaneous distribution of plasmacytoid dendritic cells in lupus erythematosus. Selective tropism at the site of epithelial apoptotic damage. *Immunobiology* 2009;**214**(9–10):877–86.
13. Kirchhof MG, Dutz JP. The immunopathology of cutaneous lupus erythematosus. *Rheum Dis Clin North Am* 2014;**40**(3):455–74, viii.
14. Abeler-Dorner L, Rieger CC, Berger B, Weyd H, Graf D, Pfrang S, et al. Interferon-alpha abrogates the suppressive effect of apoptotic cells on dendritic cells in an in vitro model of systemic lupus erythematosus pathogenesis. *J Rheumatol* 2013;**40**(10):1683–96.
15. Kuhn A, Herrmann M, Kleber S, Beckmann-Welle M, Fehsel K, Martin-Villalba A, et al. Accumulation of apoptotic cells in the epidermis of patients with cutaneous lupus erythematosus after ultraviolet irradiation. *Arthritis Rheum* 2006;**54**(3):939–50.
16. Yu C, Chang C, Zhang J. Immunologic and genetic considerations of cutaneous lupus erythematosus: a comprehensive review. *J Autoimmun* 2013;**41**:34–45.
17. Oh SH, Roh HJ, Kwon JE, Lee SH, Kim JY, Choi HJ, et al. Expression of interleukin-17 is correlated with interferon-alpha expression in cutaneous lesions of lupus erythematosus. *Clin Exp Dermatol* 2011;**36**(5):512–20.

18. Apostolidis SA, Lieberman LA, Kis-Toth K, Crispin JC, Tsokos GC. The dysregulation of cytokine networks in systemic lupus erythematosus. *J Interferon Cytokine Res* 2011;**31**(10):769–79.

19. Wittmann M, Macdonald A, Renne J. IL-18 and skin inflammation. *Autoimmun Rev* 2009;**9**(1):45–8.

20. Chong BF, Mohan C. Targeting the CXCR4/CXCL12 axis in systemic lupus erythematosus. *Expert Opin Ther Targets* 2009;**13**(10): 1147–53.

21. Okamoto H, Nishimura H, Kamatani N. A role for TARC/CCL17, a CC chemokine, in New Zealand mice. *Rheumatol Oxf* 2005;**44**(6): 819–20.

22. Gombert M, Dieu-Nosjean MC, Winterberg F, Bunemann E, Kubitza RC, Da Cunha L, et al. CCL1-CCR8 interactions: an axis mediating the recruitment of T cells and Langerhans-type dendritic cells to sites of atopic skin inflammation. *J Immunol* 2005;**174**(8):5082–91.

23. Yang PT, Kasai H, Zhao LJ, Xiao WG, Tanabe F, Ito M. Increased CCR4 expression on circulating CD4(+) T cells in ankylosing spondylitis, rheumatoid arthritis and systemic lupus erythematosus. *Clin Exp Immunol* 2004;**138**(2):342–7.

24. Sen Y, Chunsong H, Baojun H, Linjie Z, Qun L, San J, et al. Aberration of CCR7 CD8 memory T cells from patients with systemic lupus erythematosus: an inducer of T helper type 2 bias of CD4 T cells. *Immunology* 2004;**112**(2):274–89.

25. Okamoto H, Katsumata Y, Nishimura K, Kamatani N. Interferon-inducible protein 10/CXCL10 is increased in the cerebrospinal fluid of patients with central nervous system lupus. *Arthritis Rheum* 2004;**50**(11):3731–2.

26. Eriksson C, Eneslatt K, Ivanoff J, Rantapaa-Dahlqvist S, Sundqvist KG. Abnormal expression of chemokine receptors on T-cells from patients with systemic lupus erythematosus. *Lupus* 2003;**12**(10): 766–74.

27. Farkas L, Beiske K, Lund-Johansen F, Brandtzaeg P, Jahnsen FL. Plasmacytoid dendritic cells (natural interferon- alpha/beta-producing cells) accumulate in cutaneous lupus erythematosus lesions. *Am J Pathol* 2001;**159**(1):237–43.

28. Kuhn A, Landmann A. The classification and diagnosis of cutaneous lupus erythematosus. *J Autoimmun* 2014;**48-49**:14–9.

29. Sontheimer RD. Subacute cutaneous lupus erythematosus: 25-year evolution of a prototypic subset (subphenotype) of lupus erythematosus defined by characteristic cutaneous, pathological, immunological, and genetic findings. *Autoimmun Rev* 2005;**4**(5):253–63.

30. Arai S, Katsuoka K. Clinical entity of lupus erythematosus paniculitis/lupus erythematosus profundus. *Autoimmun Rev* 2009;**8**(6): 449–52.

31. Baltaci M, Fritsch P. Histologic features of cutaneous lupus erythematosus. *Autoimmun Rev* 2009;**8**(6):467–73.

32. Hochberg MC. Updating the American College of Rheumatology revised criteria for the classification of systemic lupus erythematosus. *Arthritis Rheum* 1997;**40**(9):1725.

33. Nyberg F, Hasan T, Puska P, Stephansson E, Hakkinen M, Ranki A, et al. Occurrence of polymorphous light eruption in lupus erythematosus. *Br J Dermatol* 1997;**136**(2):217–21.

34. Petri M, Orbai AM, Alarcon GS, Gordon C, Merrill JT, Fortin PR, et al. Derivation and validation of the Systemic Lupus International Collaborating Clinics classification criteria for systemic lupus erythematosus. *Arthritis Rheum* 2012;**64**(8):2677–86.

35. Coleman ML, Sahai EA, Yeo M, Bosch M, Dewar A, Olson MF. Membrane blebbing during apoptosis results from caspase-mediated activation of ROCK I. *Nat Cell Biol* 2001;**3**(4):339–45.

36. Lavrik IN, Krammer PH. Regulation of CD95/Fas signaling at the DISC. *Cell Death Differ* 2012;**19**(1):36–41.

37. Toberer F, Sykora J, Gottel D, Hartschuh W, Werchau S, Enk A, et al. Apoptotic signal molecules in skin biopsies of cutaneous lupus erythematosus: analysis using tissue microarray. *Exp Dermatol* 2013;**22**(10):656–9.

38. Martens HA, Zuurman MW, de Lange AH, Nolte IM, van der Steege G, Navis GJ, et al. Analysis of C1q polymorphisms suggests association with systemic lupus erythematosus, serum C1q and CH50 levels and disease severity. *Ann Rheum Dis* 2009;**68**(5):715–20.

39. Dall'era MC, Cardarelli PM, Preston BT, Witte A, Davis Jr JC. Type I interferon correlates with serological and clinical manifestations of SLE. *Ann Rheum Dis* 2005;**64**(12):1692–7.

40. Zampieri S, Alaibac M, Iaccarino L, Rondinone R, Ghirardello A, Sarzi-Puttini P, et al. Tumour necrosis factor alpha is expressed in refractory skin lesions from patients with subacute cutaneous lupus erythematosus. *Ann Rheum Dis* 2006;**65**(4):545–8.

41. Guiducci C, Tripodo C, Gong M, Sangaletti S, Colombo MP, Coffman RL, et al. Autoimmune skin inflammation is dependent on plasmacytoid dendritic cell activation by nucleic acids via TLR7 and TLR9. *J Exp Med* 2010;**207**(13):2931–42.

42. Gambichler T, Genc Z, Skrygan M, Scola N, Tigges C, Terras S, et al. Cytokine and chemokine ligand expression in cutaneous lupus erythematosus. *Eur J Dermatol* 2012;**22**(3):319–23.

43. Mendez-Reguera A, Perez-Montesinos G, Alcantara-Hernandez M, Martinez-Estrada V, Cazarin-Barrientos JR, Rojas-Espinosa O, et al. Pathogenic CCR6+ dendritic cells in the skin lesions of discoid lupus patients: a role for damage-associated molecular patterns. *Eur J Dermatol* 2013;**23**(2):169–82.

44. Mizui M, Koga T, Lieberman LA, Beltran J, Yoshida N, Johnson MC, et al. IL-2 protects lupus-prone mice from multiple end-organ damage by limiting CD4-CD8- IL-17-producing T cells. *J Immunol* 2014;**193**(5):2168–77.

45. Crispin JC, Tsokos GC. Human TCR-alpha beta+ CD4- CD8- T cells can derive from CD8+ T cells and display an inflammatory effector phenotype. *J Immunol* 2009;**183**(7):4675–81.

46. Koga T, Ichinose K, Mizui M, Crispin JC, Tsokos GC. Calcium/calmodulin-dependent protein kinase IV suppresses IL-2 production and regulatory T cell activity in lupus. *J Immunol* 2012;**189**(7):3490–6.

47. Zahn S, Rehkamper C, Kummerer BM, Ferring-Schmidt S, Bieber T, Tuting T, et al. Evidence for a pathophysiological role of keratinocyte-derived type III interferon (IFNlambda) in cutaneous lupus erythematosus. *J Invest Dermatol* 2011;**131**(1):133–40.

48. Werth VP, Zhang W, Dortzbach K, Sullivan K. Association of a promoter polymorphism of tumor necrosis factor-alpha with subacute cutaneous lupus erythematosus and distinct photoregulation of transcription. *J Invest Dermatol* 2000;**115**(4):726–30.

49. Deng GM, Liu L, Tsokos GC. Targeted tumor necrosis factor receptor I preligand assembly domain improves skin lesions in MRL/lpr mice. *Arthritis Rheum* 2010;**62**(8):2424–31.

50. Deng GM, Liu L, Kyttaris VC, Tsokos GC. Lupus serum IgG induces skin inflammation through the TNFR1 signaling pathway. *J Immunol* 2010;**184**(12):7154–61.

51. Moustou AE, Matekovits A, Dessinioti C, Antoniou C, Sfikakis PP, Stratigos AJ. Cutaneous side effects of anti-tumor necrosis factor biologic therapy: a clinical review. *J Am Acad Dermatol* 2009;**61**(3):486–504.

52. Griffith JW, Sokol CL, Luster AD. Chemokines and chemokine receptors: positioning cells for host defense and immunity. *Annu Rev Immunol* 2014;**32**:659–702.

53. Robak E, Kulczycka L, Sysa-Jedrzejowska A, Wierzbowska A, Robak T. Circulating proangiogenic molecules PIGF, SDF-1 and sVCAM-1 in patients with systemic lupus erythematosus. *Eur Cytokine Netw* 2007;**18**(4):181–7.

54. Wu FX, Luo XY, Wu LJ, Yang MH, Long L, Liu NT, et al. Association of chemokine CXCL12-3′G801A polymorphism with systemic lupus erythematosus in a Han Chinese population. *Lupus* 2012;**21**(6): 604–10.

55. Wenzel J, Henze S, Worenkamper E, Basner-Tschakarjan E, Sokolowska-Wojdylo M, Steitz J, et al. Role of the chemokine receptor CCR4 and its ligand thymus- and activation-regulated chemokine/CCL17 for lymphocyte recruitment in cutaneous lupus erythematosus. *J Invest Dermatol* 2005;**124**(6):1241–8.

56. Qin M, Guo Y, Jiang L, Wang X. Elevated levels of serum sCXCL16 in systemic lupus erythematosus; potential involvement in cutaneous and renal manifestations. *Clin Rheumatol* 2014;**33**(11):1595–601.

57. Dey-Rao R, Smith JR, Chow S, Sinha AA. Differential gene expression analysis in CCLE lesions provides new insights regarding the genetics basis of skin vs. systemic disease. *Genomics* 2014;**104**(2):144–55.

58. Arasappan D, Tong W, Mummaneni P, Fang H, Amur S. Meta-analysis of microarray data using a pathway-based approach identifies a 37-gene expression signature for systemic lupus erythematosus in human peripheral blood mononuclear cells. *BMC Med* 2011;**9**:65.

59. Zhao M, Liu S, Luo S, Wu H, Tang M, Cheng W, et al. DNA methylation and mRNA and microRNA expression of SLE CD4+ T cells correlate with disease phenotype. *J Autoimmun* 2014;**54**:127–36.

Chapter 36

Pathogenesis of Tissue Injury in the Brain in Patients with Systemic Lupus Erythematosus

Bruce T. Volpe

Biomedical Sciences, Feinstein Institute for Medical Research, Hofstra North Shore LIJ School of Medicine, Manhasset, NY, USA

INTRODUCTION

Systemic lupus erythematosus (SLE) is an autoimmune disease that affects many organs in the body, and it always includes the production of autoantibodies. The underlying mechanism for the nervous system involvement of patients with this dysregulated immune system is not a single process, and there are clinical syndromes caused by pathophysiology at the neuromuscular junction, peripheral and autonomic nerves, nerve roots, spinal cord, and the brain[1] (see Table 1). This chapter will focus on the established and emerging mechanisms of injury that occur in the brain of patients with SLE.

There is consensus that brain dysfunction in SLE patients leads to a bewildering array of reversible and irreversible symptoms that affect 40–90% of patients.[2] The challenge of attributing brain dysfunction to SLE is difficult because in patients with chronic waxing and waning autoimmune disease, brain dysfunction may also result from infection, hypertension, hyperlipidemia, metabolic derangement such as uremia, hormonal dysregulation, and acute and chronic side effects of medications used to treat SLE. The primary clinical responsibility, therefore, must always be to consider other causative pathophysiology before making the diagnosis of neuropsychiatric systemic lupus erythematosus (NPSLE).

Cognitive dysfunction, emotional disturbance, and headaches can be the initial symptoms or can be among the chronic symptoms that can wax and wane or be progressive. Stroke, seizures, and encephalopathy can also be symptoms of neurologic impairment in patients with SLE.[2,3] Evidence that better treatments are leading to longer life for patients with SLE[4] belies the accumulating disease burden of NPSLE as well as neuroradiologically defined structural and metabolic brain alterations.[5–8] Thus, morbidity from brain dysfunction presents an urgent challenge to define disease mechanisms and generate new therapies.

FOCAL BRAIN INJURY DEPENDS ON CEREBROVASCULAR STATE AND AN ACTIVATED ADAPTIVE IMMUNE RESPONSE

SLE patients sustain focal brain injury because the immunological activity that underlies the chronic inflammatory condition interrupts blood flow to the brain, either by antibody activity altering the coagulation process or the endothelial cells of the vessels or both. Rheological dysfunction results when antibodies that bind to soluble factors in the blood and trigger coagulation that blocks small and medium vessels with inflammation or emboli, and initiates brain ischemia and vasculitis that cause focal neurological disease. It has become abundantly clear that patients with SLE also have rapidly advancing atherosclerosis with large vessel obstruction that can cause brain infarction and stroke. Microemboli are more frequent in SLE patients with antiphospholipid antibodies: 30% of SLE patients will have antiphospholipid antibodies and 50% of patients with primary antiphospholipid syndrome will have SLE.[9,10] Many studies, but not all,[11] show a strong correlation between the presence of antiphospholipid antibodies and brain dysfunction.

Neuropathological analysis has demonstrated microvascular injury and widespread microinfarcts (35–70%), microhemorrhages (25–30%), vasculopathy with perivascular lymphocytic infiltrates, and endothelial cell proliferation (65–83%). Vasculitis with fibrinoid necrosis in the vessel wall and transmural neutrophilic infiltrate is less frequent (7–13%). Microinfarcts may result in stroke syndromes (10–25%) or seizures, but much of the cerebrovascular disease can be subclinical.[12–14] Patients with SLE do not have

TABLE 1 Neuropsychiatric Syndromes Observed in Systemic Lupus Erythematosus

Focal or multifocal brain disorder
Cerebrovascular disease
Seizures
Aseptic meningitis
Movement disorder
Diffuse brain disorder
Headache
Cognitive impairment
Mood disorder
Anxiety disorder
Psychosis
Acute confusional state
Spinal cord disorder
Myelopathy
Autonomic disorder
Peripheral nerve disorder
Cranial neuropathy
Polyradiculopathy
Plexopathy
Mono- or polyneuropathy
Motor nerve end plate disorder

a higher mortality from stroke; the incidence of stroke is, however, increased in those with attendant atherosclerosis, hypertension, valvular heart disease, and hypercoagulable states.[15]

The connection between premature atherosclerosis and SLE has been demonstrated by a high incidence of carotid plaques in female SLE patients across the age spectrum.[16] Studies confirm an increased stroke risk in patients with IgG or IgA anti-β2 glycoprotein 1, anticardiolipin, or the lupus anticoagulant.[15,17] The procoagulant effects of antiphospholipid antibodies include activating endothelial cells, inhibiting the action of β2-glycoprotein 1 and prothrombin, impairing function of several components of the protein C system, or annexin 5, tissue factor pathway inhibitor, and proteins of the fibrinolytic and coagulation cascade.[18,19] Antiphospholipid antibodies are also present in SLE patients who have headache, seizures, movement disorder, psychosis, and depression, and who may not have stroke.[20] Thus, focal and multifocal brain injury can result from an antibody-initiated inflammatory reaction that causes coagulation and vascular lumen blockade. Although seizures may result from microinfarcts, additional inflammatory mechanisms are likely involved.

DIFFUSE NEUROLOGICAL DISEASE

There is much nonfocal brain disease in SLE that lacks a mechanistic explanation. SLE patients sustain nonfocal or diffuse brain dysfunction characterized by seizures, encephalopathy with confusion, obtundation and coma, mood and behavioral abnormalities, and cognitive impairment. Likely candidate mechanisms for these brain disorders include activated B and T cells, dendritic cells, activated macrophages, and the inflammatory responses generated by their products—antibodies and cytokines. The blood–brain barrier (BBB) must be breached by either the immune active cells or their products to affect brain injury. Although active pathology in the brain for the nonfocal or diffuse disorders is elusive, the chronic effects are well documented.[21] An approach to investigate mechanisms for the diffuse brain dysfunction includes clues from animal experiments with attention to autoantibody fine specificity, mechanisms of penetration of the BBB, and recent clinical information from analysis of cerebrospinal fluid (CSF) in patients with diffuse brain injury.

ANIMAL MODELS ABET MECHANISM INVESTIGATION

There are murine models of SLE in which the animals spontaneously develop elevated anti-DNA antibodies, abnormal T cells, and autoimmune pathology early in life. The central defect of MRL^lpr mice is a spontaneous mutation, Fas, that results in massive accumulation of T-lymphocytes. Loss of function of the Fas receptor in old mice causes a deficit in apoptosis of self-reactive clones in the thymus. While these mutations have some similarity with autoimmune lymphoproliferative syndrome (ALPS), children with ALPS may have positive anti-DNA antibodies, but do not, for the most part, have brain disorders.[22] Nonetheless, the particular MRL/lpr spontaneous lupus prone mouse has provided important information about abnormal behaviors, including impaired maze exploration, enhanced emotional reactivity, and the associated brain changes, including increased apoptotic neuron loss during symptom development, atrophy, and focal loss of CA1 dendritic arborization.[23–25] Brain disease in this model apparently depends on brain reactive antibodies that are also found in the CSF.[26,27] This suggests that a model focused on cross-reactive brain antibodies, which penetrate the BBB and generate toxic conditions for neurons, might point to a mechanism of brain impairment in SLE.

Because the most common class of autoantibodies in SLE are anti-DNA antibodies, and these antibodies cause tissue damage in the kidney, investigators reasonably executed an extended search for their cross-reactivities using anti-DNA antibodies that bind to glomerular basement membrane or to cross-reactive renal antigen.[28] Investigators identified a consensus peptide sequence, DWEYS, for one glomerulotropic anti-DNA antibody.[29] Murine and human GluN2A and GluN2B, subunits of the N-methyl D aspartate receptor (NMDAR), contain the DWEYS consensus sequence. The NMDAR has a prominent role in learning and memory and is found at high density in the dendrites of the CA1 region of the hippocampus, although it exhibits wide distribution in the brain.[30,31] NMDARs and 5-methylisoxazole-4 propionic acid receptors (AMPARs) are critical for synaptic transmission in the brain and are required for long-term potentiation, the cellular basis for memory formation.[32]

Although the complex cognitive and behavioral abnormalities and nonfocal brain injury in SLE likely do not depend on one potential causative agent and are likely driven by multiple mediators of brain injury, the ability to investigate a single contributing component provides a unique opportunity to dissect mechanisms of disease. Murine and human anti-DNA, anti-GluN2 cross-reactive antibodies demonstrated neuronal toxicity when directly injected into mouse brain and when applied to human fetal brain cells.[33,34] Furthermore, studies of antibody-mediated neuronal toxicity showed the antibodies to be positive modulators of receptor function that, at low concentrations, enhanced the NMDAR-mediated excitatory postsynaptic potential, and, at high concentrations, enhanced mitochondrial permeability and promoted excitotoxicity, a well-described form of neuronal demise.[35] In fact, 10-fold lower concentrations of anti-DNA, anti-GluN2 were required to alter synaptic activity than were needed to mediate neuronal death. Perhaps most importantly, the concentrations of anti-DNA, anti-GluN2 antibody in these experiments were comparable to concentrations reported in CSF from SLE patients with brain impairment.[35,36] These data suggest that some symptoms that result from brain exposure to anti-DNA, anti-GluN2 antibodies might be reversible, transiently altering excitatory postsynaptic potentials, while other symptoms might be permanent, reflecting neuronal loss.

This model advanced when mice immunized with an octameric form of the consensus sequence developed anti-DNA, antipeptide antibodies that bound the NMDAR.[37] A competent BBB checked brain injury in mice harboring these antibodies. Both lipopolysaccharide (LPS) and epinephrine are well-established causes of transient impairment in the integrity of the BBB. Mice possessing anti-DNA, anti-peptide (DWEYS) antibodies that were treated with LPS or epinephrine sustained structural damage, focal metabolic derangement visualized in micro-positron emission tomography (PET) analyses, and demonstrated behavioral abnormalities compared to mice bearing nontoxic antibodies.[34,38,39]

Antibody-bearing animals treated with LPS had neuronal loss and metabolic disruption (18F-fluorodeoxyglucose micro-PET) restricted to the CA1 region of the hippocampus and exhibited cognitive abnormality limited to spatial memory impairment, whereas antibody-bearing animals treated with epinephrine exhibited neuronal loss and metabolic disruption in the amygdala, and exhibited abnormal behavior limited to impaired fear conditioning. Of note, the animals with hippocampal destruction had normal fear conditioning behavior and those with amygdala destruction had normal spatial memory. These data support two clinically relevant points: serum levels of toxic antibodies may be less informative about brain impairment than CSF levels, and a single antibody specificity may give rise to varying symptoms depending on the region of BBB penetration.

AUTOANTIBODY TOXICITY IN CLINICAL SLE

Studies of animal models that dissect antibody fine specificity, like anti-DNA, anti-GluN2 antibodies,[40] have been replicated for antiribosomal P autoantibodies[41,42] and antiphospholipid autoantibodies,[43] but in view of the burgeoning diversity of autoantibodies in SLE, and in order to make these animal models valuable, clinical data is needed. Currently, some clinical studies have recorded a significant association of serum anti-DNA, anti-GluN2 antibodies with depression[44,45] and memory disorders.[45] Other studies failed to find an association of the serum anti-DNA, antiGluN2 antibodies with cognitive impairment.[46–49] In patients with severe disorders of cognition and consciousness, from whom CSF samples were available, there appears to be a significant association between antibodies and symptoms, and in some patients the fluctuation of their clinical course mirrored the CSF anti-DNA, antiGluN2 antibody level[36,50–54] (reviewed in clinical detail[55]). In sum, the anti-DNA, anti-GluN2 antibodies are candidate toxic molecules responsible for the loss of neurons through nonvascular mechanisms of excitotoxicity and apoptosis, but this toxicity depends on access to the brain neuropil and penetration of the BBB.

The expanded investigation of antineuronal antibodies, as there are also nonautoimmune diseases that are currently considered to be mediated by toxic antibodies (for review[40] and contrasting point of view[56]), prompts the development of criteria that qualify an antibody to be considered pathogenetic, especially in SLE. To become clinically relevant, antibodies should recognize a defined cell-surface antigen and demonstrate activity in vivo and in vitro. The cell surface antigen should have relevance to the symptomatology of human disease. Some investigators assert that the antibody binding characteristics be confirmed in a cell-based system, although the cell-based system may well overlook fine specificity. For example, cell-based assay for the glutamate receptor requires co-transfection with GluN1 and GluN2 to produce viable cells; thus, differences between GluN1 and GluN2 antibodies would be obscured. Furthermore, antibody toxicity should be transmitted by passive transfer and through immunization strategies. Perhaps most importantly, the target antibody should be present in clinical disease and there should be a clinical response to antibody modulation.

In sum, the etiology for brain injury in SLE is multifactorial and reliance on a single toxic autoantibody ignores the contribution of cytokines, activated adaptive immune cells other than antibody secreting B cells, the contribution of brain-infiltrating myeloid cells, and the response of microglia and astrocytes, and other soluble factors, and ultimately the BBB.

BLOOD–BRAIN BARRIER

The endothelial BBB and the epithelial blood–cerebrospinal barrier form the outer walls in a recent analogy of BBB properties as a two-walled castle moat.[57] These walls prevent molecules and cells from passing freely between the blood and the brain. In mice, this barrier is fully formed by parturition, and specialized proteins, especially claudin-5, form tight junctions linking the endothelial cells. Barrier properties are most restrictive in the capillaries and weaker in the postcapillary venules. Pericytes are present in the postcapillary perivascular space where the BBB structure includes the glia limitans, and inner and outer basement membrane in close apposition on the brain side to astrocytic endfeet.[40] Mechanisms for crossing the barrier alter the integrity of the tight junctions allowing molecules and cells to pass between endothelial cells.[58] There are also mechanisms that affect the capacity of the endothelial cells to internalize molecules through receptor transmission or internalization, as in the transport of cytokines or chemokines. Generally, the entry of immunoglobulins into the brain is negligible under normal physiological conditions. There are measures to indicate penetration into the CSF space of immunoglobulin. For example, the IgG index [IgG index = (CSF IgG) × (serum albumin)/(CSF albumin) × (Serum IgG)] and Q-albumin [Q-albumin = (CSF albumin × 10³)/(serum albumin)] is a useful measure of immunoglobulin penetrating the BBB. Pathological conditions may lead to activation of endothelial cell receptors, Toll-like receptors, cytokine receptors, neurotransmitter receptors, and hormone receptors; all can alter the barrier function. In the perivascular compartment, macrophages can become activated to contribute to an inflammatory condition and also alter the barrier properties.

Modulators of BBB permeability include bacterial or viral infection, systemic inflammation, trauma, brain ischemia, and stress, and agonists to endothelial receptors such as nicotine, caffeine, and cocaine.[59,60] Other molecules, such as corticosteroids and interferon (IFN)-α and IFNβ, may preserve or increase BBB integrity. The circumventricular organs that include the posterior pituitary, the area postrema, the subcommissural organ, the pineal body, the subfornical organ, and the lamina terminalis act as sensory and secretory organs of the neuroendocrine system. With no formal barrier between blood and brain, these regions may function to initiate an inside out signaling process to modulate the BBB. There is also an inside-out system that depends on the neonatal Fc receptor (FcRn) that is resident on the luminal surface on most endothelial cells and permits immunoglobulins to leave the circulation and penetrate tissue; in the brain, it has the opposite polarity on endothelial cells and has been proposed to remove immunoglobulins from brain tissue cells.[61]

TRANSPORT OF MATERNAL IgG TO FETAL BRAIN

Considering the fetal receptor on endothelial cells at the BBB raises issues of intrauterine and perinatal exposure to maternal immunoglobulins. The transport of IgG from mother to fetus begins after the first trimester, and, by term, the IgG level in the newborn will often exceed the mother's level. Generally, the maternal antibodies confer protection, but in circumstances of neonatal lupus there is a toxic class of antibodies, anti-Ro,[62] that can cause complete heart block in the developing infant. Given the precedent for antibodies in autoimmune disease directly causing pathology in the developing fetus, it is instructive to consider the potential fetal risk conferred by anti-brain antibodies. Anti-DNA, anti-NMDA receptor antibodies will cause cognitive impairments and abnormal histopathological brain development in male offspring and a significant loss of viability of female fetuses.[63,64] Whether these data in animal models are borne out in the clinic has raised some controversy,[65] but it is worth a reexamination, in light of findings suggesting a high frequency of autism in the children of women with SLE.[66]

CYTOKINES AND OTHER SOLUBLE TOXIC MOLECULES

Cytokines are produced by many classes of cells of the innate and adaptive immune system to initiate and regulate the inflammatory state.[2,67] In the brain, astrocytes and microglia contribute to CNS production of cytokines. Currently, in patients with SLE, the role of cytokines in brain pathology is best defined in focal disease that depends on vasculopathy or vasculitis with thrombosis or embolic compromise of vessels. In cerebrovascular insufficiency or stroke, the sheer stress in the vessels initiates a pro-inflammatory response; while those forces may play a role in the amplification phase of inflammation and vessel obstruction in patients with SLE, antibodies are more likely to increase clotting and obstruct vessels in the initiation phase. Prominent in the catalog of cytokines participating in neuron injury after ischemia are the metalloproteases, particularly MM2, MM8, and MM9.[60] Ischemia and reperfusion brain injury with hypoxia have implicated cytokines and chemokines in a complex process that includes initiation, amplification, and resolution of brain injury. Interleukin (IL)-1β, IL-1α, tumor necrosis factor (TNF) are important in the initiation phase; IL-1, IL-6, IL-10; IL-17, IL-20 TNF are important in the amplification phase; and TGF β, IL-10, IL-17, IL-23 are important in the resolution phase.[60] Reactive oxygen species, nitric oxide, the complement system, induce cytotoxic T cells and NK cells to release perforin and granzyme and trigger apoptosis in tissue resident cells.[60] Neuron death releases antigens that activate pattern recognition receptors for danger-associated molecular patterns. This model is derived from animal experiments but the results strongly suggest therapeutic options that must be validated in clinical situations.

In patients with SLE and diffuse brain involvement, several pro-inflammatory cytokines have been identified in the CSF: INFα, TNF, fractalkine, IL-6, IL-8, IL-1, BAFF (B-cell activating factor), APRIL (a proliferation inducing ligand), and MMP9. Among the long list, IL-6 has been found in the CSF in patients with brain impairment and SLE. The association between CSF IL-6 and the IgG index suggests that IL-6 increases B-cell activation, a finding supported by increased BAFF and April in patients with diffuse and severe brain impairment, although other studies have not replicated this finding. IFNα plays a pivotal role in brain impairment in patients with SLE.[68] Major side effects from IFNα include depression and psychosis, although these patients had hepatitis. Together with IL-6, IFNα plays an interdependent role in sickness behaviors that are characterized by depression, anxiety, and confusion—symptoms common in patients with NPSLE. Although CSF levels of IFNα were significantly higher in patients with NPSLE who were confused, IFNα levels in other stressed patient populations and non-NPSLE groups have decreased its effectiveness as a biomarker.[69] Another candidate molecule that modulates sickness behaviors, TNF, also plays a prominent role in serum titers of patients with SLE. It is worth recounting the experience using anti-TNF treatment in rheumatoid arthritis in which the patients experience improved mood and outlook, despite little effect on progressive joint destruction.[70] Clearly, more clinical work needs to focus on the presence of the cytokines in relation to symptom initiation, flare, and resolution.

CONCLUSIONS

Focal injury to the brain depends on vascular pathology and occlusion because autoantibodies initiate clotting mechanisms or local endothelial inflammation. Nonfocal injury to the brain likely depends on a variety of mechanisms that include autoantibodies and inflammation. Metabolic dysregulation as in uremia, infection, and side effects of chronic toxic medicine may complicate the diagnosis of diffuse brain injury. In documented clinical situations and in preclinical experiments, toxic autoantibodies exert dose related effects and can be assayed in cell-based systems.[71] Also, the toxicity in vitro can be transferred passively and induced by active immunization. Data from preclinical models suggest toxic autoantibodies need access to the brain which is protected by the BBB. This finding has bearing for the clinical situation where there is often a weak or modest association of serum antibody assay with brain dysfunction symptoms; however, antibody levels in the CSF demonstrate a strong association with symptoms. The BBB apparently has nonuniform penetration capacity that can lead to regional brain toxicity. These candidate mechanisms can account for acute waxing and waning symptoms, but there is much to be learned about the cumulative pathology of the chronic progressive state.

ACKNOWLEDGMENT

This study was supported by National Institutes of Health grants 1P01AI073693-06 and 1P01 AI102852-01.

REFERENCES

1. The American College of Rheumatology nomenclature and case definitions for neuropsychiatric lupus syndromes. *Arthritis Rheum* 1999; **42**(4):599–608. http://dx.doi.org/10.1002/1529-0131(199904)42:4<599. AID-ANR2>3.0.CO;2-F.
2. Bertsias GK, Boumpas DT. Pathogenesis, diagnosis and management of neuropsychiatric SLE manifestations. *Nat Rev Rheumatol* 2010;**6**(6):358–67. http://dx.doi.org/10.1038/nrrheum.2010.62.
3. Hanly JG. Neuropsychiatric lupus. *Rheum Dis Clin North Am* 2005;**31**(2):273–98. http://dx.doi.org/10.1016/j.rdc.2005.01.007. vi.
4. Borchers AT, Keen CL, Shoenfeld Y, Gershwin ME. Surviving the butterfly and the wolf: mortality trends in systemic lupus erythematosus. *Autoimmun Rev* 2004;**3**(6):423–53. http://dx.doi.org/10.1016/j.autrev.2004.04.002.
5. Appenzeller S, Cendes F, Costallat LT. Cognitive impairment and employment status in systemic lupus erythematosus: a prospective longitudinal study. *Arthritis Rheum* 2009;**61**(5):680–7. http://dx.doi.org/10.1002/art.24346.
6. Mackay M, Bussa MP, Aranow C, Ulug AM, Volpe BT, Huerta PT, et al. Differences in regional brain activation patterns assessed by functional magnetic resonance imaging in patients with systemic lupus erythematosus stratified by disease duration. *Mol Med* 2011;**17**(11–12):1349–56. http://dx.doi.org/10.2119/molmed.2011.00185; 3321819.

7. Mackay M, Tang CC, Volpe BT, Aranow C, Mattis PJ, Korff RA, et al. Brain metabolism and autoantibody titres predict functional impairment in systemic lupus erythematosus. *Lupus Sci Med* 2015;**2**(1):e000074. http://dx.doi.org/10.1136/lupus-2014-000074; 4379887.

8. Urowitz MB, Gladman DD, Ibanez D, Fortin PR, Bae SC, Gordon C, et al. Evolution of disease burden over five years in a multicenter inception systemic lupus erythematosus cohort. *Arthritis Care Res* 2012;**64**(1):132–7. http://dx.doi.org/10.1002/acr.20648.

9. Cervera R, Piette JC, Font J, Khamashta MA, Shoenfeld Y, Camps MT, et al. Antiphospholipid syndrome: clinical and immunologic manifestations and patterns of disease expression in a cohort of 1000 patients. *Arthritis Rheum* 2002;**46**(4):1019–27.

10. Fujieda Y, Atsumi T, Amengual O, Odani T, Otomo K, Kato M, et al. Predominant prevalence of arterial thrombosis in Japanese patients with antiphospholipid syndrome. *Lupus* 2012;**21**(14):1506–14. http://dx.doi.org/10.1177/0961203312458469.

11. Sciascia S, Bertolaccini ML, Roccatello D, Khamashta MA, Sanna G. Autoantibodies involved in neuropsychiatric manifestations associated with systemic lupus erythematosus: a systematic review. *J Neurol* 2014;**261**(9):1706–14. http://dx.doi.org/10.1007/s00415-014-7406-8.

12. Ellis SG, Verity MA. Central nervous system involvement in systemic lupus erythematosus: a review of neuropathologic findings in 57 cases, 1955–1977. *Semin Arthritis Rheum* 1979;**8**(3):212–21.

13. Hanly JG, Walsh NM, Sangalang V. Brain pathology in systemic lupus erythematosus. *J Rheumatol* 1992;**19**(5):732–41.

14. Johnson RT, Richardson EP. The neurological manifestations of systemic lupus erythematosus. *Medicine* 1968;**47**(4):337–69.

15. Timlin H, Petri M. Transient ischemic attack and stroke in systemic lupus erythematosus. *Lupus* 2013;**22**(12):1251–8. http://dx.doi.org/10.1177/0961203313497416.

16. Hahn BH, Grossman J, Chen W, McMahon M. The pathogenesis of atherosclerosis in autoimmune rheumatic diseases: roles of inflammation and dyslipidemia. *J Autoimmun* 2007;**28**(2–3):69–75. http://dx.doi.org/10.1016/j.jaut.2007.02.004.

17. Mehrani T, Petri M. Association of IgA Anti-beta2 glycoprotein I with clinical and laboratory manifestations of systemic lupus erythematosus. *J Rheumatol* 2011;**38**(1):64–8. http://dx.doi.org/10.3899/jrheum.100568.

18. Palomo I, Segovia F, Ortega C, Pierangeli S. Antiphospholipid syndrome: a comprehensive review of a complex and multisystemic disease. *Clin Exp Rheumatol* 2009;**27**(4):668–77.

19. Salmon JE, de Groot PG. Pathogenic role of antiphospholipid antibodies. *Lupus* 2008;**17**(5):405–11. http://dx.doi.org/10.1177/0961203308090025; 2693020.

20. Sanna G, Bertolaccini ML, Cuadrado MJ, Laing H, Khamashta MA, Mathieu A, et al. Neuropsychiatric manifestations in systemic lupus erythematosus: prevalence and association with antiphospholipid antibodies. *J Rheumatol* 2003;**30**(5):985–92.

21. Appenzeller S, Pereira DA, Costallat LT. Greater accrual damage in late-onset systemic lupus erythematosus: a long-term follow-up study. *Lupus* 2008;**17**(11):1023–8. http://dx.doi.org/10.1177/0961203308089695.

22. Shah S, Wu E, Rao VK, Tarrant TK. Autoimmune lymphoproliferative syndrome: an update and review of the literature. *Curr Allergy Asthma Rep* 2014;**14**(9):462. http://dx.doi.org/10.1007/s11882-014-0462-4; 4148697.

23. Jeltsch-David H, Muller S. Neuropsychiatric systemic lupus erythematosus and cognitive dysfunction: the MRL-lpr mouse strain as a model. *Autoimmun Rev* 2014;**13**(9):963–73. http://dx.doi.org/10.1016/j.autrev.2014.08.015.

24. Sakic B, Szechtman H, Denburg JA, Gorny G, Kolb B, Whishaw IQ. Progressive atrophy of pyramidal neuron dendrites in autoimmune MRL-lpr mice. *J Neuroimmunol* 1998;**87**(1–2):162–70.

25. Sakic B, Szechtman H, Denburg S, Carbotte R, Denburg JA. Spatial learning during the course of autoimmune disease in MRL mice. *Behav Brain Res* 1993;**54**(1):57–66.

26. Sidor MM, Sakic B, Malinowski PM, Ballok DA, Oleschuk CJ, Macri J. Elevated immunoglobulin levels in the cerebrospinal fluid from lupus-prone mice. *J Neuroimmunol* 2005;**165**(1–2):104–13. http://dx.doi.org/10.1016/j.jneuroim.2005.04.022; 1635784.

27. Stanojcic M, Loheswaran G, Xu L, Hoffman SA, Sakic B. Intrathecal antibodies and brain damage in autoimmune MRL mice. *Brain Behav Immun* 2010;**24**(2):289–97. http://dx.doi.org/10.1016/j.bbi.2009.10.009.

28. Katz JB, Limpanasithikul W, Diamond B. Mutational analysis of an autoantibody: differential binding and pathogenicity. *J Exp Med* 1994;**180**(3):925–32. 2191646.

29. Gaynor B, Putterman C, Valadon P, Spatz L, Scharff MD, Diamond B. Peptide inhibition of glomerular deposition of an anti-DNA antibody. *Proc Natl Acad Sci USA* 1997;**94**(5):1955–60. 20024.

30. Huerta PT, Sun LD, Wilson MA, Tonegawa S. Formation of temporal memory requires NMDA receptors within CA1 pyramidal neurons. *Neuron* 2000;**25**(2):473–80.

31. O'Keefe J. *Hippocampal neurophysiology in the behaving animal.* New York: Oxford University Press; 2007.

32. Bliss TV, Lomo T. Long-lasting potentiation of synaptic transmission in the dentate area of the anaesthetized rabbit following stimulation of the perforant path. *J Physiol* 1973;**232**(2):331–56. 1350458.

33. DeGiorgio LA, Konstantinov KN, Lee SC, Hardin JA, Volpe BT, Diamond B. A subset of lupus anti-DNA antibodies cross-reacts with the NR2 glutamate receptor in systemic lupus erythematosus. *Nat Med* 2001;**7**(11):1189–93. http://dx.doi.org/10.1038/nm1101-1189.

34. Kowal C, Degiorgio LA, Lee JY, Edgar MA, Huerta PT, Volpe BT, et al. Human lupus autoantibodies against NMDA receptors mediate cognitive impairment. *Proc Natl Acad Sci USA* 2006;**103**(52):19854–9. http://dx.doi.org/10.1073/pnas.0608397104; 1702320.

35. Faust TW, Chang EH, Kowal C, Berlin R, Gazaryan IG, Bertini E, et al. Neurotoxic lupus autoantibodies alter brain function through two distinct mechanisms. *Proc Natl Acad Sci USA* 2010;**107**(43):18569–74. http://dx.doi.org/10.1073/pnas.1006980107; 2972998.

36. Fragoso-Loyo H, Cabiedes J, Orozco-Narvaez A, Davila-Maldonado L, Atisha-Fregoso Y, Diamond B, et al. Serum and cerebrospinal fluid autoantibodies in patients with neuropsychiatric lupus erythematosus. Implications for diagnosis and pathogenesis. *PLoS One* 2008;**3**(10):e3347.

37. Kowal C, DeGiorgio LA, Nakaoka T, Hetherington H, Huerta PT, Diamond B, et al. Cognition and immunity; antibody impairs memory. *Immunity* 2004;**21**(2):179–88. http://dx.doi.org/10.1016/j.immuni.2004.07.011.

38. Huerta PT, Kowal C, DeGiorgio LA, Volpe BT, Diamond B. Immunity and behavior: antibodies alter emotion. *Proc Natl Acad Sci USA* 2006;**103**(3):678–83. http://dx.doi.org/10.1073/pnas.0510055103; 1334673.

39. Vo A, Volpe BT, Tang CC, Schiffer WK, Kowal C, Huerta PT, et al. Regional brain metabolism in a murine systemic lupus erythematosus model. *J Cereb Blood Flow Metab* 2014;**34**(8):1315–20. http://dx.doi.org/10.1038/jcbfm.2014.85; 4126091.

40. Diamond B, Honig G, Mader S, Brimberg L, Volpe BT. Brain-reactive antibodies and disease. *Annu Rev Immunol* 2013;**31**:345–85. http://dx.doi.org/10.1146/annurev-immunol-020711-075041.

41. Bravo-Zehnder M, Toledo EM, Segovia-Miranda F, Serrano FG, Benito MJ, Metz C, et al. Anti-ribosomal P protein autoantibodies from patients with neuropsychiatric lupus impair memory in mice. *Arthritis Rheumatol* 2015;**67**(1):204–14. http://dx.doi.org/10.1002/art.38900.

42. Matus S, Burgos PV, Bravo-Zehnder M, Kraft R, Porras OH, Farias P, et al. Antiribosomal-P autoantibodies from psychiatric lupus target a novel neuronal surface protein causing calcium influx and apoptosis. *J Exp Med* 2007;**204**(13):3221–34. http://dx.doi.org/10.1084/jem.20071285; 2150977.

43. Katzav A, Ben-Ziv T, Blank M, Pick CG, Shoenfeld Y, Chapman J. Antibody-specific behavioral effects: intracerebroventricular injection of antiphospholipid antibodies induces hyperactive behavior while anti-ribosomal-P antibodies induces depression and smell deficits in mice. *J Neuroimmunol* 2014;**272**(1–2):10–5. http://dx.doi.org/10.1016/j.jneuroim.2014.04.003.

44. Lapteva L, Nowak M, Yarboro CH, Takada K, Roebuck-Spencer T, Weickert T, et al. Anti-N-methyl-D-aspartate receptor antibodies, cognitive dysfunction, and depression in systemic lupus erythematosus. *Arthritis Rheum* 2006;**54**(8):2505–14. http://dx.doi.org/10.1002/art.22031.

45. Omdal R, Brokstad K, Waterloo K, Koldingsnes W, Jonsson R, Mellgren SI. Neuropsychiatric disturbances in SLE are associated with antibodies against NMDA receptors. *Eur J Neurol* 2005;**12**(5):392–8. http://dx.doi.org/10.1111/j.1468-1331.2004.00976.x.

46. Hanly JG, Robichaud J, Fisk JD. Anti-NR2 glutamate receptor antibodies and cognitive function in systemic lupus erythematosus. *J Rheumatol* 2006;**33**(8):1553–8.

47. Hanly JG, Urowitz MB, Siannis F, Farewell V, Gordon C, Bae SC, et al. Autoantibodies and neuropsychiatric events at the time of systemic lupus erythematosus diagnosis: results from an international inception cohort study. *Arthritis Rheum* 2008;**58**(3):843–53. http://dx.doi.org/10.1002/art.23218.

48. Harrison MJ, Ravdin LD, Lockshin MD. Relationship between serum NR2a antibodies and cognitive dysfunction in systemic lupus erythematosus. *Arthritis Rheum* 2006;**54**(8):2515–22. http://dx.doi.org/10.1002/art.22030.

49. Kozora E, West SG, Maier SF, Filley CM, Arciniegas DB, Brown M, et al. Antibodies against N-methyl-D-aspartate receptors in patients with systemic lupus erythematosus without major neuropsychiatric syndromes. *J Neurol Sci* 2010;**295**(1–2):87–91. http://dx.doi.org/10.1016/j.jns.2010.04.016; 2920062.

50. Arinuma Y, Yanagida T, Hirohata S. Association of cerebrospinal fluid anti-NR2 glutamate receptor antibodies with diffuse neuropsychiatric systemic lupus erythematosus. *Arthritis Rheum* 2008;**58**(4):1130–5.

51. Gono T, Kawaguchi Y, Kaneko H, Nishimura K, Hanaoka M, Kataoka S, et al. Anti-NR2A antibody as a predictor for neuropsychiatric systemic lupus erythematosus. *Rheumatology* 2011;**50**(9):1578–85. http://dx.doi.org/10.1093/rheumatology/keq408.

52. Hirohata S, Arinuma Y, Yanagida T, Yoshio T. Blood–brain barrier damages and intrathecal synthesis of anti-N-methyl-D-aspartate receptor NR2 antibodies in diffuse psychiatric/neuropsychological syndromes in systemic lupus erythematosus. *Arthritis Res Ther* 2014;**16**(2):R77. http://dx.doi.org/10.1186/ar4518; 4060173.

53. Husebye ES, Sthoeger ZM, Dayan M, Zinger H, Elbirt D, Levite M, et al. Autoantibodies to a NR2A peptide of the glutamate/NMDA receptor in sera of patients with systemic lupus erythematosus. *Ann Rheum Dis* 2005;**64**(8):1210–3.

54. Steup-Beekman G, Steens S, van Buchem M, Huizinga T. Anti-NMDA receptor autoantibodies in patients with systemic lupus erythematosus and their first-degree relatives. *Lupus* 2007;**16**(5):329–34.

55. Lauvsnes MB, Omdal R. Systemic lupus erythematosus, the brain, and anti-NR2 antibodies. *J Neurol* 2012;**259**(4):622–9. http://dx.doi.org/10.1007/s00415-011-6232-5.

56. Hammer C, Stepniak B, Schneider A, Papiol S, Tantra M, Begemann M, et al. Neuropsychiatric disease relevance of circulating anti-NMDA receptor autoantibodies depends on blood–brain barrier integrity. *Mol Psychiatry* 2014;**19**(10):1143–9. http://dx.doi.org/10.1038/mp.2013.110.

57. Engelhardt B, Coisne C. Fluids and barriers of the CNS establish immune privilege by confining immune surveillance to a two-walled castle moat surrounding the CNS castle. *Fluids Barriers CNS* 2011;**8**(1):4. http://dx.doi.org/10.1186/2045-8118-8-4; 3039833.

58. Steiner O, Coisne C, Cecchelli R, Boscacci R, Deutsch U, Engelhardt B, et al. Differential roles for endothelial ICAM-1, ICAM-2, and VCAM-1 in shear-resistant T cell arrest, polarization, and directed crawling on blood–brain barrier endothelium. *J Immunol* 2010;**185**(8):4846–55. http://dx.doi.org/10.4049/jimmunol.0903732.

59. Banks WA. Blood–brain barrier transport of cytokines: a mechanism for neuropathology. *Curr Pharm Des* 2005;**11**(8):973–84.

60. Iadecola C, Anrather J. The immunology of stroke: from mechanisms to translation. *Nat Med* 2011;**17**(7):796–808. http://dx.doi.org/10.1038/nm.2399; 3137275.

61. Roopenian DC, Akilesh S. FcRn: the neonatal Fc receptor comes of age. *Nat Rev Immunol* 2007;**7**(9):715–25. http://dx.doi.org/10.1038/nri2155.

62. Buyon JP, Swersky SH, Fox HE, Bierman FZ, Winchester RJ. Intrauterine therapy for presumptive fetal myocarditis with acquired heart block due to systemic lupus erythematosus. Experience in a mother with a predominance of SS-B (La) antibodies. *Arthritis Rheum* 1987;**30**(1):44–9.

63. Lee JY, Huerta PT, Zhang J, Kowal C, Bertini E, Volpe BT. Neurotoxic autoantibodies mediate congenital cortical impairment of offspring in maternal lupus. *Nat Med* 2009;**15**:91–6.

64. Wang L, Zhou D, Lee J, Niu H, Faust TW, Frattini S. Female mouse fetal loss mediated by maternal autoantibody. *J Exp Med* 2012;**209**:1083–9.

65. Vinet E, Bernatsky S, Pineau CA, Clarke AE, Nashi EP, Scott S, et al. Increased male-to-female ratio among children born to women with systemic lupus erythematosus: comment on the article by Lockshin et al.. *Arthritis Rheum* 2013;**65**(4):1129. http://dx.doi.org/10.1002/art.37852.

66. Vinet E, Pineau CA, Clarke AE, Fombonne E, Platt RW, Bernatsky S. Neurodevelopmental disorders in children born to mothers with systemic lupus erythematosus. *Lupus* 2014;**23**(11):1099–104. http://dx.doi.org/10.1177/0961203314541691.

67. Jeltsch-David H, Muller S. Neuropsychiatric systemic lupus erythematosus: pathogenesis and biomarkers. *Nat Rev Neurol* 2014;**10**(10):579–96. http://dx.doi.org/10.1038/nrneurol.2014.148.

68. Santer DM, Yoshio T, Minota S, Moller T, Elkon KB. Potent induction of IFN-alpha and chemokines by autoantibodies in the cerebrospinal fluid of patients with neuropsychiatric lupus. *J Immunol* 2009;**182**(2):1192–201. 2745922.

69. Fragoso-Loyo H, Atisha-Fregoso Y, Nunez-Alvarez CA, Llorente L, Sanchez-Guerrero J. Utility of interferon-alpha as a biomarker in central neuropsychiatric involvement in systemic lupus erythematosus. *J Rheumatol* 2012;**39**(3):504–9. http://dx.doi.org/10.3899/jrheum.110983.

70. Siebert S, Tsoukas A, Robertson J, McInnes I. Cytokines as therapeutic targets in rheumatoid arthritis and other inflammatory diseases. *Pharmacol Rev* 2015;**67**(2):280–309. http://dx.doi.org/10.1124/pr.114.009639.

71. Chang EH, Volpe BT, Mackay M, Aranow C, Watson P, Kowal C, et al. Selective impairment of spatial cognition caused by autoantibodies to the *N*-methyl-d-aspartate receptor. *EBioMedicine* 2015;**2**(7):755–64. http://dx.doi.org/10.1016/j.ebiom.2015.05.027. eCollection 2015 Jul. PubMed PMID: 26286205; PubMed Central PMCID: PMC4534689.

Part IV

Clinical Aspects of the Disease

Chapter 37

Constitutional Symptoms and Fatigue in Systemic Lupus Erythematosus

Syahrul Shaharir[1,2], Caroline Gordon[1,3]

[1]Department of Rheumatology, City Hospital, Sandwell and West Birmingham Hospitals NHS Trust, Birmingham, UK; [2]Department of Internal Medicine, National University of Malaysia Medical Centre, Cheras, Kuala Lumpur, Malaysia; [3]Rheumatology Research Group, College of Medical and Dental Sciences, University of Birmingham, Edgbaston, Birmingham, UK

INTRODUCTION

Constitutional symptoms are very common in systemic lupus erythematosus (SLE) but are rather nonspecific; therefore, they are not taken into account in the classification criteria for SLE. Fatigue is the most common constitutional symptom associated with SLE, affecting up to 90% of patients. Other constitutional symptoms such as fever, anorexia, lymphadenopathy, and splenomegaly are less common.

The presence of constitutional symptoms may reflect ongoing active disease. It is one of the systems assessed in British Isles Lupus Assessment Group (BILAG) 2004 disease activity index, which includes the assessment of fever, anorexia, lymphadenopathy, and splenomegaly but not fatigue because attribution to lupus is difficult and fatigue is often multifactorial, as will be discussed later.[1,2] In the Systemic Lupus Erythematosus Disease Activity Index (SLE-DAI), fever is the only variable that is taken into account for disease activity scoring.[3] Clinicians should be aware that constitutional symptoms have an exhaustive list of differential diagnoses that need to be excluded before attributing the symptoms to the underlying lupus. Other differential diagnoses that need to be considered include infection, metabolic disorders, malignancy, primary hematological disorders, and other systemic rheumatic diseases.

This chapter discusses each of the constitutional symptoms that may occur in SLE in more detail, focusing the potential differential diagnosis and the potential underlying cause of the constitutional symptoms in lupus patients.

FATIGUE

Fatigue is defined as "an uncommon, abnormal or extreme whole bodily tiredness disproportionate or unrelated to activity or exertion."[4,5] It is one of the most common and often most disabling symptoms, affecting up to 80–90% of patients.[4] It causes significant morbidity with negative impact on quality of life (QoL). Studies have shown that fatigue correlates moderately or strongly with all components of the SF–36[6] and is a major component of vitality domain.

Fatigue is multifactorial[5–14] and is only related in part to lupus disease activity.[6] Even patients with quiescent lupus continue to experience marked fatigue.[7] A study has shown that there was a significant decrease in the deformability of the red blood cells membrane in SLE patients, thus reducing their ability to flow through small capillaries in the brain and muscle. This phenomenon was due to the C4d deposition and complement activation.[8] Hence, the defective oxygen delivery may partly explain the chronic fatigue experienced by SLE patients. Due to the various factors that are associated with fatigue in SLE, the underlying causes need to be investigated so that appropriate intervention can be initiated (see Figure 1).

Psychosocial variables have also been found to have compelling associations with fatigue levels.[7,12] It is associated with high scores on subscales for depression and hysteria on the Minnesota Multiphasic Personality Inventory-2, as well as with high scores in Beck Depression Inventory.[12]

Due to the substantial impact of fatigue on SLE patients, the Outcomes Measures in Rheumatology initiative recommended the measurement of fatigue in SLE clinical trials.[15] The American College of Rheumatology has published a systematic review of fatigue instruments that can be used to measure the severity and frequency of fatigue as a symptom and the impact of fatigue on functioning in SLE.[16] The working group and expert panel recommended the nine-item FSS for evaluating fatigue in SLE patients. This instrument was developed in patients with SLE, has a valid psychometric properties, and is commonly used in SLE studies.[16] Therefore, when evaluating patients with SLE in clinical trials and in clinical practice, it is important to measure not only disease activity and damage, but also patient-reported fatigue and other measure of QoL.

Besides disease activity and damage, psychosocial factors have emerged as one of the important predictors of poor

Systemic Lupus Erythematosus. http://dx.doi.org/10.1016/B978-0-12-801917-7.00037-1

317

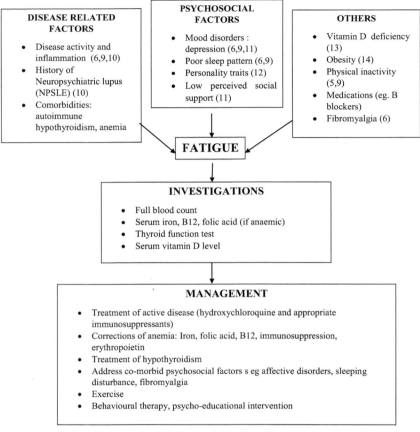

DISEASE RELATED FACTORS	PSYCHOSOCIAL FACTORS	OTHERS

- Disease activity and inflammation (6,9,10)
- History of Neuropsychiatric lupus (NPSLE) (10)
- Comorbidities: autoimmune hypothyroidism, anemia

- Mood disorders : depression (6,9,11)
- Poor sleep pattern (6,9)
- Personality traits (12)
- Low perceived social support (11)

- Vitamin D deficiency (13)
- Obesity (14)
- Physical inactivity (5,9)
- Medications (eg. B blockers)
- Fibromyalgia (6)

FATIGUE

INVESTIGATIONS

- Full blood count
- Serum iron, B12, folic acid (if anaemic)
- Thyroid function test
- Serum vitamin D level

MANAGEMENT

- Treatment of active disease (hydroxychloroquine and appropriate immunosuppressants)
- Corrections of anemia: Iron, folic acid, B12, immunosuppression, erythropoietin
- Treatment of hypothyroidism
- Address co-morbid psychosocial factors s eg affective disorders, sleeping disturbance, fibromyalgia
- Exercise
- Behavioural therapy, psycho-educational intervention

FIGURE 1 Factors and associations of fatigue in systemic lupus erythematosus.

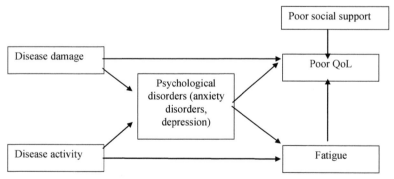

FIGURE 2 Association and relationship between psychosocial factors with fatigue and poor quality of life in SLE.

QoL in SLE (See Figure 2). Important factors include psychological disorders (anxiety, depression), which may be exacerbated by active disease and damage and lead to poor QoL (greater pain, helplessness and physical disability)[17] and poor social support[18] (see Chapter 6).

Management of Fatigue in SLE

Despite being the most frequent disabling symptom in SLE, there are very few clinical trials that have addressed both pharmacologic and nonpharmacologic management of fatigue. Aerobic exercise, muscle strengthening, or supervised exercise strategy has been shown to improve fatigue among SLE population.[19] Psychoeducational intervention has been used in a randomized clinical trial compared to placebo, with reported improvement in social support between patients and their partners, better self-efficacy, and lower fatigue after 1 year of therapy.[20]

The benefit of pharmacological treatment in fatigue is also weak. There is some evidence that stopping hydroxychloroquine results in increased fatigue.[21] The role of dehydroepiandrosterone in quiescent SLE patients with fatigue has been investigated in one randomized controlled trial, but unfortunately it showed no benefit over placebo.[22] Belimumab improved fatigue in the BLISS (Study of Belimumab in Subjects with Systemic Lupus Erythematosus) trials as assessed by the Functional Assessment of Chronic Illness Therapy Fatigue scale (secondary end point).[23] Improvement in QoL measured by Short Form-36 survey was observed in the randomized control trial of epratuzumab in SLE patients.[24] Unfortunately, the high cost and potential side effects of these new biologic agents limit their use for the exclusive treatment of fatigue in SLE.

There are many causes of fatigue in SLE patients, and most commonly many factors contribute to fatigue in lupus patients rather than a single factor. Therefore, the treatment strategy should be tailored to the individual's main underlying cause, and will include physical and psychosocial health factors and other comorbidities that are associated with fatigue in SLE.

FEVER

The prevalence of fever in lupus patients has declined over the years. Earlier reviews in the 1950s–1960s reported a prevalence of up to 86%.[25] However, it has declined to 41% in studies between 1980 and 1989.[26] In the Eurolupus cohort, fever was observed in 36% of patients at disease onset and in 52% during the course of the disease.[27] Although an earlier report postulated that the availability and use of nonsteroidal anti-inflammatory drugs and steroids were the reason behind the reducing frequency of fever among SLE patients, the phenomenon is most likely explained by the greater awareness among clinicians to exclude other causes of fever (i.e., infection and malignancy). Fever is more common in childhood-onset lupus as compared to adult-onset lupus,[28] and patients with late-onset lupus (onset of more than 50 years old) experienced much less fever, with the reported prevalence of 8% at presentation.[29]

Although fever is becoming less common in SLE, its presence has always been a challenge and often creates a clinical conundrum for the clinicians. This is particularly the case when the symptoms occur at disease onset, prior to the diagnosis of SLE. Apart from SLE, fever may indicate the presence of many other conditions, such as infections, malignancies, or drug reactions[30,31] (see Table 1). It is imperative to exclude these differential diagnoses because immunosuppressive treatment that is commonly used to treat SLE will cause detrimental effects to the patients in these situations. Careful history taking, physical examination and thorough investigations may help to identify the potential causes of fever, including atypical infections.

To further complicate matters, an infectious process may also trigger SLE, and the two can occur concomitantly. The features that favor infection include presence of chills/rigors, leukocytosis in the absence of steroid therapy,[31] neutrophilia with increased numbers of band forms or

TABLE 1 Possible Etiology of Fever in Systemic Lupus Erythematosus

Acute Lupus	Usually Associated with Other Manifestations of SLE
Infection	Viral
	Bacterial
	Mycobacterial
	Fungal
	Protozoal
	Nematodes
Malignancy	Lymphoma (Hodgkin's or non-Hodgkin's
	Primary carcinoma (e.g., renal)
	Metastatic carcinoma
	Myeloma

metamyelocytes[32] and high C-reactive protein (CRP).[32] The median level of CRP in patients with SLE flares without serositis appears to be around 1.4–1.6 mg/dl, with a range of 0–6 mg/dl.[33] Nevertheles, mild to moderately elevated serum CRP may also reflect an active disease, especially in serositis, synovitis, and lupoid hepatitis. Serum CRP levels above 6.0 mg/dl in febrile patients may occur with lupus serositis[33] and synovitis.[34]

Serum procalcitonin (PCT) may be a potential negative predictive value for bacterial infection in SLE patients in one study.[35] However, in this study, serum PCT level was also raised in active SLE patients with infection,[35] while other studies involved a very small number of SLE patients or found no correlation between serum PCT and infection in lupus.[36] Therefore, serum PCT is not routinely used in differentiating between active disease and bacterial infections in lupus.

The effect of corticosteroids in suppressing fever in SLE is not well studied. However, in a study of small cohort of 22 SLE patients with fever, 28 mg (20–40 mg) prednisone completely suppressed SLE fever, usually within 24 h.[37] In a study by Zhou et al., a prednisolone dose of ≤100 mg/d was able to suppress SLE fever in 80.6% of the patients within 1–5 days. When the maximum steroid dose was increased to ≥100 mg/d, only 5.3% of patients remained febrile.[30] Therefore, a refractory fever despite a very high dose of steroid or immunosuppressive treatment should prompt the clinicians to further investigate for other potential causes, especially infections, in immunosuppressed SLE patients. A persistent fever despite a higher dose of steroids (>150 mg/day) may be associated with lupus encephalopathy and hemophagocytosis.[30]

SLE patients are immunosuppressed due to the underlying disease and treatment, thus making them susceptible to various other less common pathogens, including opportunistic infections (see Table 1), such as tuberculosis, *Pneumocystis carinii*, fungal infections, viral infections, nematodes, toxoplasmosis, and other protozoal infections (see Chapter 45). Lupus patients are at increased risk of such infections because SLE patients often have antibodies to CD4+ T cells. Consequently, they can have low CD4+ T cell counts and reversed CD4:CD8 lymphocyte ratios, and they may even be misdiagnosed initially as suffering from human immunodeficiency virus (HIV; see Chapter 13).

Therefore, SLE patients with fever should be investigated thoroughly with multiple blood cultures, appropriate swabs of any potential sites of infection, and cultures and examination of urine, stool, and sputum. Further investigation may include white cell scans, ultrasound, and computed tomography or magnetic resonance imaging scans to exclude abscesses or cancers. Apart from infection, the possibility of malignancy and lymphoma should also be considered (see Table 1 and Figure 3). Studies have shown that there is a slightly increased risk

for malignancy in SLE patients, compared to the general population, particularly non-Hodgkin's lymphoma[38] (see Chapter 46).

After all of the possible nonlupus causes of pyrexia have been ruled out, the fever can be attributed to the underlying SLE and can be recorded as part of the disease activity assessment, using standardized disease activity indices.[2] However, it is important to note that different levels of fever are recorded in the various validated disease activity indices. The SLEDAI requires a documented temperature of more than 38 °C.[3] Meanwhile, the BILAG Index and the European Consensus Lupus Assessment Measure (ECLAM) record a documented fever of greater than 37.5 °C.[1,2] However, the ECLAM specifically requires that this should be the documented base or morning temperature.[2] In all cases, the temperature must have been documented and not estimated by the patient or doctor, and infection should have been excluded as a cause. Figure 3 illustrated the suggested approach and management of fever in SLE patients.[39,40]

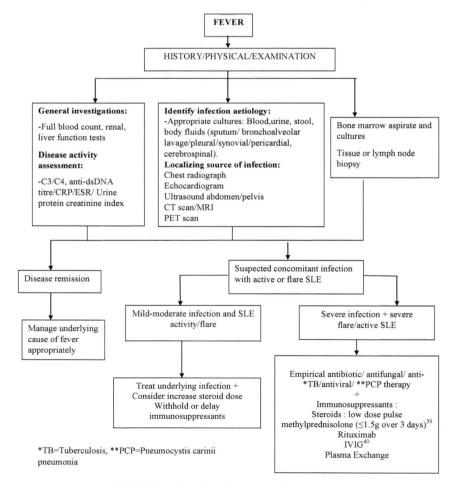

FIGURE 3 Algorithm of approach to fever in SLE.

LYMPHADENOPATHY

The estimated prevalence is between 5% and 7% at the onset of the disease, and 12–15% at any time during course of the disease.[41,42] Patients with lymphadenopathy are likely to have other constitutional symptoms, such as fever, weight loss, and lethargy.[43] Therefore, it is pivotal to exclude underlying infection and malignancy as well (as discussed above). Other common associated features of SLE patients with lymphadenopathy are more cutaneous and mucosal signs (malar rash, vasculitis, skin ulcers, mouth ulcers, discoid lesions, alopecia, and subcutaneous lupus erythematosus), higher rate of hepatomegaly and splenomegaly, increased anti-dsDNA antibodies titers, and decreased complement levels.[43]

Lymph nodes in SLE are usually soft, nontender, mobile, generalized, and of varying size.[44] Importantly, the size tends to fluctuate over time. In the BILAG Index palpable lymph nodes greater than 1 cm in diameter are recorded, providing that the cause is attributed to lupus.[1,2] However, other disease activity indices, such as SLEDAI, Systemic Lupus Activity Measure (SLAM), and ECLAM, do not record lymphadenopathy as part of their disease activity assessment.[2] Malignancy, particularly lymphoma, should be suspected if the nodes steadily increase in size. This is particularly important because SLE patients have almost up to fourfold increase risk of non-Hodgkin's lymphoma.[38]

Other infrequent infective causes of lymphadenopathy need to be excluded, including viral (cytomegalovirus [CMV], Epstein–Barr virus [EBV], parvovirus, varicella zoster virus [VZV], hepatitis, HIV), bacterial (brucellosis, syphilis, mycobacterial), fungal (histoplasmosis, toxoplasmosis, leishmaniosis), and rickettsial infection. A number of studies have confirmed a high frequency of previous EBV and CMV infection in SLE patients, but the role of these viruses in the lymphadenopathy and onset of lupus remains unclear. Clinical presentation of viral infections, especially CMV and EBV, may be difficult to distinguish from manifestations of active SLE[45] (see Chapter 45).

In case of significant lymphadenopathy, lymph node biopsy is indicated to rule out infections, especially tuberculosis, or malignancy. Lymphadenopathy secondary to SLE represents a benign finding, with a mononucleosis-like behavior.[46] Biopsy commonly shows reactive follicular hyperplasia, with or without atypical cells, and it is considered a nonspecific finding. Coagulative necrosis with hematoxylin bodies, which is a unique finding in SLE, is rarely seen.[47]

Lymph node lesions of SLE patients may also be similar to those of hyaline-vascular or intermediate types of Castleman's disease or T-zone dysplasia with hyperplastic follicles.[48] Kikuchi–Fujimoto syndrome is also one of the important differential diagnoses as it shares the typical features of SLE, such as fever, arthralgia, and leukopenia, and

TABLE 2 Histological Differences Between SLE and Kikuchi–Fujimoto Syndrome

Histological Features	SLE Lymphadenitis	Kikuchi–Fujimoto Syndrome
Necrosis	Present	Present
Hematoxylin bodies[a]	Present	Not present
Cytotoxic T cells (CD8+ lymphocytes)	Sparse	Abundant
Plasma cells	Abundant	Sparse

[a]Degenerated nuclei that have reacted with antinuclear antibodies, and the Azzopardi phenomenon (i.e., encrustation of blood vessel walls with nuclear material).

it commonly affects young women. Biopsy of the lymph nodes typically shows granulomatous necrotizing lymphadenitis and sometimes can be difficult to distinguish from with lupus lymphadenopathy.[48] In addition, about 30% of patients presenting with this form of necrotizing lymphadenitis have or go on to develop SLE or discoid lupus.[48] However, it may be possible to identify differences in the histology between those that are really SLE from the onset of lymphadenopathy and those that are true Kikuchi–Fujimoto syndrome[49] (see Table 2).

Lymphadenopathy appears to be most common in the first few years of lupus and is rare later in the disease course. The development of lymphadenopathy for the first time in a patient who has had SLE for more than 5 years should prompt further investigations due to broader differential diagnoses, including lymphoma.

SPLENOMEGALY

Splenomegaly occurs in 10–45% of patients, particularly during active disease. Mild to moderate splenomegaly may be recorded in the BILAG index but not in other indices, such as SLEDAI and ECLAM.[2] It usually develops as a result of lymphoid hyperplasia with enlarged white pulp lymphoid follicles, and a buildup of macrophages and plasma cells around the arterioles and cells of the red pulp.[50] Its occurrence is often associated with hepatomegaly and/or lymphadenopathy; therefore, it may herald many other differential diagnoses (see Table 3). However, the presence of splenomegaly is not necessarily associated with cytopenia.

WEIGHT LOSS

Unexplained weight loss of at least 5% body weight can be a manifestation of active disease. However, it is also a nonspecific finding of many other diseases, such as malignancy,

TABLE 3 Differential Diagnosis of Splenomegaly in SLE

Neoplastic and lymphoproliferative disease	• Lymphoma • Leukemia or hematological cytopathologies • Splenic tumors (primary splenic lymphoma/tumors, metastatic)
Hepatic	• Liver cirrhosis with portal hypertension (associated with autoimmune hepatitis, primary biliary cirrhosis, primary sclerosing cholangitis)
Vascular occlusive	• Splenic vein thrombosis • Portal vein thrombosis
Immunological	• Autoimmune hemolytic anemia • Immune thrombocytopenic purpura
Infection	• Viral (EBV, CMV, hepatitis virus) • Malaria • Endocarditis • Splenic abscess
Inherited hemoglobinopathies	• Thalassemia • Cytoskeletal defects: hereditary sphero- or elliptocytosis

TABLE 4 Differential Diagnosis of Weight Loss in SLE

Infection	Tuberculosis, fungal, opportunistic infections.
Malignancy	Lymphoma, solid tumors
Gastrointestinal	Nausea, vomiting, decreased appetite
	Malabsorption (celiac disease, fat malabsorption)
	Protein-losing enteropathy
	Dysphagia (overlapping features of scleroderma or CREST)
	Lupus enteritis (colitis or vasculitis)
	Pancreatitis
Organ damage	Uremia from renal failure
Medications	Mycophenolic acid or mycophenolate mofetil (GI side effects: diarrhea, nausea, abdominal pain)
	Nonsteroidal anti-inflammatory drugs

CREST: calcinosis, Raynaud's, esophageal dysmolitility, sclerodactyl, telangiectasia.

chronic infection, endocrinopathy (thyrotoxicosis), and other rheumatic diseases. The BILAG index records both anorexia and unintentional weight loss (>5%) under constitutional or general features.[1] In the SLAM-R Index,[51] weight loss can be recorded as mild if it is up to 10% of preexisting body weight, and it is recorded as severe if it is greater than 10% of body weight. SLEDAI and ECLAM do not record weight loss.[2,3,52]

Loss of appetite or anorexia usually precedes the development of weight loss. Apart from that, weight loss can be attributed to gastrointestinal (GI) disturbance, particularly nausea and vomiting. Anorexia, nausea, and vomiting are frequent and can affect up to 50% of patients with SLE.[53] They can occur as an early manifestation of new-onset lupus or lupus flare in the absence of GI features. Apart from disease activity, they may be due to the consequences of disease complications (e.g., uremia in lupus nephritis) or side effects of medication. Other rarer causes of weight loss in SLE include other GI involvement in SLE, such as malabsorption or gut vasculitis.

Specific investigations of the gastrointestinal tract may be required to exclude comorbid disease and to look for evidence of localized lupus involvement that is interfering with absorption of nutrients (see Table 4). Weight loss usually responds to treatment given for other manifestations of lupus, particularly when corticosteroids are involved. However, as with fever and lymphadenopathy, such treatment should not be given or increased until infection and malignancy have been excluded (see Chapter 44).

CONCLUSIONS

Constitutional features of SLE are common during the initial presentation and recurrence of active SLE flares. However, these clinical features are very nonspecific and have a broad differential diagnosis. As discussed in this chapter, it is essential to consider the differential diagnosis of each symptom and sign in turn. Only by having excluded other possibilities can the various features be attributed to lupus and treated as such.

Constitutional symptoms are the important features of the disease that need to be assessed and managed appropriately as they cause considerable distress to the patient. Immunosuppression and antimalarial therapy are important in the treatment of fever, weight loss, and lymphadenopathy due to lupus. However, because fatigue may not necessarily be attributed to the active disease, a careful search for and treatment of comorbid conditions including depression, fibromyalgia, and sleep disorders should be undertaken. Therefore, the treatment of fatigue may require additional measures, such as an aerobic exercise program, self-management plan, or psychoeducational intervention.

REFERENCES

1. Yee CS, Farewell V, Isenberg DA, Griffiths B, Teh LS, Bruce IN, et al. The BILAG-2004 index is sensitive to change for assessment of SLE disease activity. *Rheumatology (Oxford)* 2009;**48**(6):691–5.
2. Griffiths B, Mosca M, Gordon C. Assessment of patients with systemic lupus erythematosus and the use of lupus disease activity indices. *Best Pract Res Clin Rheumatol* 2005;**19**(5):685–708.
3. Gladman DD, Ibanez D, Urowitz MB. Systemic lupus erythematosus disease activity index 2000. *J Rheumatol* 2002;**29**(2):288–91.
4. Cleanthous S, Tyagi M, Isenberg DA, Newman SP. What do we know about self-reported fatigue in systemic lupus erythematosus? *Lupus* 2012;**21**(5):465–76.
5. Balsamo S, Santos-Neto LD. Fatigue in systemic lupus erythematosus: an association with reduced physical fitness. *Autoimmun Rev* 2011;**10**(9):514–8.
6. Tench CM, McCurdie I, White PD, D'Cruz DP. The prevalence and associations of fatigue in systemic lupus erythematosus. *Rheumatology (Oxford)* 2000;**39**(11):1249–54.
7. Zonana-Nacach A, Roseman JM, McGwin Jr G, Friedman AW, Baethge BA, Reveille JD, et al. Systemic lupus erythematosus in three ethnic groups. VI: Factors associated with fatigue within 5 years of criteria diagnosis. LUMINA Study Group. LUpus in MInority populations: NAture vs Nurture. *Lupus* 2000;**9**(2):101–9.
8. Ghiran IC, Zeidel ML, Shevkoplyas SS, Burns JM, Tsokos GC, Kyttaris VC. Systemic lupus erythematosus serum deposits C4d on red blood cells, decreases red blood cell membrane deformability, and promotes nitric oxide production. *Arthritis Rheum* 2011;**63**(2):503–12.
9. Da Costa D, Dritsa M, Bernatsky S, Pineau C, Menard HA, Dasgupta K, et al. Dimensions of fatigue in systemic lupus erythematosus: relationship to disease status and behavioral and psychosocial factors. *J Rheumatol* 2006;**33**(7):1282–8.
10. Kozora E, Ellison MC, West S. Depression, fatigue, and pain in systemic lupus erythematosus (SLE): relationship to the American College of Rheumatology SLE neuropsychological battery. *Arthritis Rheum* 2006;**55**(4):628–35.
11. Jump RL, Robinson ME, Armstrong AE, Barnes EV, Kilbourn KM, Richards HB. Fatigue in systemic lupus erythematosus: contributions of disease activity, pain, depression, and perceived social support. *J Rheumatol* 2005;**32**(9):1699–705.
12. Omdal R, Waterloo K, Koldingsnes W, Husby G, Mellgren SI. Fatigue in patients with systemic lupus erythematosus: the psychosocial aspects. *J Rheumatol* 2003;**30**(2):283–7.
13. Ruiz-Irastorza G, Egurbide MV, Olivares N, Martinez-Berriotxoa A, Aguirre C. Vitamin D deficiency in systemic lupus erythematosus: prevalence, predictors and clinical consequences. *Rheumatology (Oxford)* 2008;**47**(6):920–3.
14. Oeser A, Chung CP, Asanuma Y, Avalos I, Stein CM. Obesity is an independent contributor to functional capacity and inflammation in systemic lupus erythematosus. *Arthritis Rheum* 2005;**52**(11):3651–9.
15. Strand V, Gladman D, Isenberg D, Petri M, Smolen J, Tugwell P. Outcome measures to be used in clinical trials in systemic lupus erythematosus. *J Rheumatol* 1999;**26**(2):490–7.
16. Measurement of fatigue in systemic lupus erythematosus: a systematic review. *Arthritis Rheum* 2007;**57**(8):1348–57.
17. Seawell AH, Danoff-Burg S. Psychosocial research on systemic lupus erythematosus: a literature review. *Lupus* 2004;**13**(12):891–9.
18. Sutcliffe N, Clarke AE, Levinton C, Frost C, Gordon C, Isenberg DA. Associates of health status in patients with systemic lupus erythematosus. *J Rheumatol* 1999;**26**(11):2352–6.
19. Ayán C, Martín V. Systemic lupus erythematosus and exercise. *Lupus* 2007;**16**(1):5–9.
20. Karlson EW, Liang MH, Eaton H, Huang J, Fitzgerald L, Rogers MP, et al. A randomized clinical trial of a psychoeducational intervention to improve outcomes in systemic lupus erythematosus. *Arthritis Rheum* 2004;**50**(6):1832–41.
21. A randomized study of the effect of withdrawing hydroxychloroquine sulfate in systemic lupus erythematosus. *N. Engl J Med* 1991;**324**(3):150–4.
22. Hartkamp A, Geenen R, Godaert GL, Bijl M, Bijlsma JW, Derksen RH. Effects of dehydroepiandrosterone on fatigue and well-being in women with quiescent systemic lupus erythematosus: a randomised controlled trial. *Ann Rheum Dis* 2010;**69**(6):1144–7.
23. Strand V, Levy RA, Cervera R, Petri MA, Birch H, Freimuth WW, et al. Improvements in health-related quality of life with belimumab, a B-lymphocyte stimulator-specific inhibitor, in patients with autoantibody-positive systemic lupus erythematosus from the randomised controlled BLISS trials. *Ann Rheum Dis* 2013;**73**(5):838–44. http://dx.doi.org/10.1136/annrheumdis-2012-202865. Published Online First: 22 March 2013.
24. Strand V, Petri M, Kalunian K, Gordon C, Wallace DJ, Hobbs K, et al. Epratuzumab for patients with moderate to severe flaring SLE: health-related quality of life outcomes and corticosteroid use in the randomized controlled ALLEVIATE trials and extension study SL0006. *Rheumatology (Oxford)* 2014;**53**(3):502–11.
25. Dubois EL, Tuffanelli DL. Clinical manifestations of systemic lupus erythematosus. Computer analysis of 520 cases. *JAMA* 1964;**190**:104–11.
26. Pistiner M, Wallace DJ, Nessim S, Metzger AL, Klinenberg JR. Lupus erythematosus in the 1980s: a survey of 570 patients. *Semin Arthritis Rheum* 1991;**21**(1):55–64.
27. Font J, Cervera R, Ramos-Casals M, Garcia-Carrasco M, Sents J, Herrero C, et al. Clusters of clinical and immunologic features in systemic lupus erythematosus: analysis of 600 patients from a single center. *Semin Arthritis Rheum* 2004;**33**(4):217–30.
28. Livingston B, Bonner A, Pope J. Differences in clinical manifestations between childhood-onset lupus and adult-onset lupus: a meta-analysis. *Lupus* 2011;**20**(13):1345–55.
29. Lalani S, Pope J, de Leon F, Peschken C. Clinical features and prognosis of late-onset systemic lupus erythematosus: results from the 1000 faces of lupus study. *J Rheumatol* 2010;**37**(1):38–44.
30. Zhou WJ, Yang CD. The causes and clinical significance of fever in systemic lupus erythematosus: a retrospective study of 487 hospitalised patients. *Lupus* 2009;**18**(9):807–12.
31. Stahl NI, Klippel JH, Decker JL. Fever in systemic lupus erythematosus. *Am J Med* 1979;**67**(6):935–40.
32. Inoue T, Takeda T, Koda S, Negoro N, Okamura M, Amatsu K, et al. Differential diagnosis of fever in systemic lupus erythematosus using discriminant analysis. *Rheumatol Int* 1986;**6**(2):69–77.
33. ter Borg EJ, Horst G, Limburg PC, van Rijswijk MH, Kallenberg CG. C-reactive protein levels during disease exacerbations and infections in systemic lupus erythematosus: a prospective longitudinal study. *J Rheumatol* 1990;**17**(12):1642–8.
34. Gabay C, Roux-Lombard P, de Moerloose P, Dayer JM, Vischer T, Guerne PA. Absence of correlation between interleukin 6 and C-reactive protein blood levels in systemic lupus erythematosus compared with rheumatoid arthritis. *J Rheumatol* 1993;**20**(5):815–21.

35. Bador K, Intan S, Hussin S, Gafor A. Serum procalcitonin has negative predictive value for bacterial infection in active systemic lupus erythematosus. *Lupus* 2012;**21**(11):1172–7.

36. Lanoix J, Bourgeois A, Schmidt J, Desblache J, Salle V, Smail A, et al. Serum procalcitonin does not differentiate between infection and disease flare in patients with systemic lupus erythematosus. *Lupus* 2011;**20**(2):125–30.

37. Rovin BH, Tang Y, Sun J, Nagaraja HN, Hackshaw KV, Gray L, et al. Clinical significance of fever in the systemic lupus erythematosus patient receiving steroid therapy. *Kidney Int* 2005;**68**(2):747–59.

38. Bernatsky S, Boivin JF, Joseph L, Rajan R, Zoma A, Manzi S, et al. An international cohort study of cancer in systemic lupus erythematosus. *Arthritis Rheum* 2005;**52**(5):1481–90.

39. Badsha H, Kong KO, Lian TY, Chan SP, Edwards CJ, Chng HH. Low-dose pulse methylprednisolone for systemic lupus erythematosus flares is efficacious and has a decreased risk of infectious complications. *Lupus* 2002;**11**(8):508–13.

40. Karim MY, Pisoni CN, Khamashta MA. Update on immunotherapy for systemic lupus erythematosus–what's hot and what's not!. *Rheumatology (Oxford)* 2009;**48**(4):332–41.

41. Cervera R, Khamashta MA, Font J, Sebastiani GD, Gil A, Lavilla P, et al. Systemic lupus erythematosus: clinical and immunologic patterns of disease expression in a cohort of 1,000 patients. The European Working Party on Systemic Lupus Erythematosus. *Medicine (Baltimore)* 1993;**72**(2):113–24.

42. Pons-Estel BA, Catoggio LJ, Cardiel MH, Soriano ER, Gentiletti S, Villa AR, et al. The GLADEL multinational Latin American prospective inception cohort of 1,214 patients with systemic lupus erythematosus: ethnic and disease heterogeneity among "Hispanics". *Medicine (Baltimore)* 2004;**83**(1):1–17.

43. Shapira Y, Weinberger A, Wysenbeek AJ. Lymphadenopathy in systemic lupus erythematosus. Prevalence and relation to disease manifestations. *Clin Rheumatol* 1996;**15**(4):335–8.

44. Calguneri M, Ozturk MA, Ozbalkan Z, Akdogan A, Ureten K, Kiraz S, et al. Frequency of lymphadenopathy in rheumatoid arthritis and systemic lupus erythematosus. *J Int Med Res* 2003;**31**(4):345–9.

45. Sekigawa I, Nawata M, Seta N, Yamada M, Iida N, Hashimoto H. Cytomegalovirus infection in patients with systemic lupus erythematosus. *Clin Exp Rheumatol* 2002;**20**(4):559–64.

46. Melikoglu MA, Melikoglu M. The clinical importance of lymphadenopathy in systemic lupus erythematosus. *Acta Reumatol Port* 2008;**33**(4):402–6.

47. Kojima M, Motoori T, Asano S, Nakamura S. Histological diversity of reactive and atypical proliferative lymph node lesions in systemic lupus erythematosus patients. *Pathol Res Pract* 2007;**203**(6):423–31.

48. Santana A, Lessa B, Galrao L, Lima I, Santiago M. Kikuchi-Fujimoto's disease associated with systemic lupus erythematosus: case report and review of the literature. *Clin Rheumatol* 2005;**24**(1):60–3.

49. Bosch X, Guilabert A, Miquel R, Campo E. Enigmatic Kikuchi-Fujimoto disease: a comprehensive review. *Am J Clin Pathol* 2004;**122**(1):141–52.

50. Buskila D, Gladman DD, Hannah W, Kahn HJ. Primary malignant lymphoma of the spleen in systemic lupus erythematosus. *J Rheumatol* 1989;**16**(7):993–6.

51. Liang MH, Socher SA, Larson MG, Schur PH. Reliability and validity of six systems for the clinical assessment of disease activity in systemic lupus erythematosus. *Arthritis Rheum* 1989;**32**(9):1107–18.

52. Bencivelli W, Vitali C, Isenberg DA, Smolen JS, Snaith ML, Sciuto M, et al. Disease activity in systemic lupus erythematosus: report of the Consensus Study Group of the European Workshop for Rheumatology Research. III. Development of a computerised clinical chart and its application to the comparison of different indices of disease activity. The European Consensus Study Group for Disease Activity in SLE. *Clin Exp Rheumatol* 1992;**10**(5):549–54.

53. Sultan SM, Ioannou Y, Isenberg DA. A review of gastrointestinal manifestations of systemic lupus erythematosus. *Rheumatology (Oxford)* 1999;**38**(10):917–32.

Chapter 38

The Musculoskeletal System in Systemic Lupus Erythematosus

Diane Horowitz, Galina Marder, Richard Furie

North Shore LIJ Division of Rheumatology, Great Neck, NY, USA; Hofstra North Shore LIJ School of Medicine, Hofstra University, Hempstead, NY, USA

SUMMARY

Along with cutaneous disease, musculoskeletal manifestations are quite prevalent in systemic lupus erythematosus (SLE). Whereas some musculoskeletal complications, such as myositis and arthritis, reflect disease activity, others, such as osteonecrosis and osteoporosis, are typically adverse effects of treatment. In this chapter, we review the most common musculoskeletal manifestations that affect patients with SLE.

ARTHRITIS

Clinical trials confirmed the high prevalence of arthritis in systemic lupus erythematosus (SLE), with 60–65% of subjects entering BLISS (BeLimumab International SLE Study)-52 and BLISS-76 with musculoskeletal disease activity.[1–3] The ALMS (Aspreva Lupus Management Study) study, a trial restricted to lupus nephritis, documented a 16% frequency of BILAG (British Isles Lupus Activity Group) A or B musculoskeletal involvement.[4] Reviews of lupus arthropathy have been provided by Fernandez et al. as well as Zoma et al.[5,6] The patterns of lupus arthritis are described in this section.

Nonerosive Arthritis

The most common type of lupus arthritis has historically been described as nonerosive inflammatory arthritis. Insidious in onset, it is an early disease manifestation causing joint erythema, tenderness, and/or effusion. Usually symmetric with a predilection for hands, wrists, and knees, it can be confused with early rheumatoid arthritis (RA). Therefore, it is vital during the diagnostic evaluation of patients with inflammatory arthritis to include lupus serologies.

Patients with lupus arthritis do not develop voluminous synovial effusions. When obtained, the fluid is clear to mildly opaque, and viscosity may be normal or slightly reduced. The white cell count of synovial fluid is low, rarely exceeding 10,000 cells/ml.[7] Lymphocytes and monocytes predominate, although neutrophils may be abundant in fluids with marked leukocytosis. Serologic tests on synovial fluid are of no diagnostic value, but it is imperative to culture the fluid if circumstances warrant. Radiographs may demonstrate soft tissue swelling, but erosive changes and joint space narrowing are typically absent.[8]

The concept of nonerosive arthritis in lupus has been challenged with the advent of sensitive imaging techniques, such as high-resolution ultrasound (HRUS) with power Doppler or magnetic resonance imaging (MRI). Wright et al. examined 17 patients with SLE and hand involvement using HRU.[9] Sixteen (94%) patients had joint effusions or synovial hypertrophy in the wrist and 12 (71%) in the second or third metacarpophalangeal (MCP) joints. Eight (47%) patients had erosions at the second or third MCP joints. Eleven (65%) patients had tenosynovitis. In a meta-analysis performed by Lins and Santiago, a total of 1091 joints, representing 610 SLE patients, were studied by ultrasound.[10] Hands and wrists represented approximately 80% of the studies. Effusions were observed in 55% of joints, synovitis in 20%, tenosynovitis in 19%, synovial hypertrophy in 14%, and erosions in just 7%.

Yoon et al. utilized gray-scale ultrasound and power Doppler to identify subclinical inflammatory changes in the joints of 48 SLE patients without clinically overt musculoskeletal involvement.[11] Synovitis, found in 58.3% of patients, was noted at the wrist (33.3%), second MCP joint (29.2%), and the third MCP joint (31.3%). New musculoskeletal symptoms subsequently developed in 22.9% of patients, and among predictive risk factors was a higher baseline ultrasound synovitis index.

Chiara et al. reported MRI findings in 50 SLE patients with arthritis who underwent hand and wrist MRIs without contrast.[12] Bone marrow edema was observed in two (4%) patients in the hand (4%) and in 15 in the wrist (13%). Erosions were observed in hands in 24 patients (48%) and in wrists in 41 (82%) patients. They concluded that involvement of the wrist in SLE is similar to RA, but involvement of the hand in SLE is significantly lower compared to RA.

Systemic Lupus Erythematosus. http://dx.doi.org/10.1016/B978-0-12-801917-7.00038-3

In their study of 34 patients with SLE arthritis, Ball et al. demonstrated the presence of erosions at the wrist in 93% of subjects and at the MCPs in 61% using contrast-enhanced MRI.[13] Ninety-three percent of patients had at least grade 1 synovitis at one or more MCP joints, and wrist synovitis was present in all.

In contrast to RA, synovium from patients with lupus does not demonstrate exuberant inflammatory changes. Natour et al. examined 30 percutaneous synovial knee biopsies from lupus patients and noted: (1) synoviocyte hyperplasia, (2) scarce inflammatory infiltrates, (3) vascular proliferation, (4) edema and congestion, (5) fibrinoid necrosis and intimal fibrous hyperplasia of blood vessels, and (6) fibrin on the synovial surface.[14] Insight into the mechanism by which lupus patients with arthritis are generally spared from significant erosions was provided by Mensah et al.[15] They postulated that an interferon-rich milieu, as is seen in most lupus patients, supports the differentiation of myelomonocytic precursors to myeloid dendritic cells as opposed to osteoclasts.

Erosive Arthritis ("Rhupus")

An uncommon subset of lupus arthritis, referred to as "rhupus," is marked by articular features of RA, namely erosive arthritis, and serologic features of lupus.[16,17] Findings may include synovitis, synovial proliferation, rheumatoid nodules, and malalignment. Predictors for the development of erosive arthritis are poorly understood. Amezcua-Guerra et al. demonstrated a median C-reactive protein concentration in erosive arthritis of 14.5 mg/l compared to 0.8 in nonerosive arthritis. Anti-CCP antibodies were also significantly associated with erosive arthritis, but serum interleukin (IL)-6, interferon-gamma, IL-4, and IL-10, while numerically greater in erosive arthritis, were not statistically different.[18]

Similar observations were made by Chan et al. who categorized 104 SLE patients into one of three categories: (1) erosive arthritis (subdivided into minor and major erosions); (2) nonerosive arthritis; or (3) no arthritis. While only six patients had major erosive arthritis, four (67%) had anti-CCP2 antibodies; only four of the other 98 patients were CCP2 antibody positive. Kakumanu et al. compared the frequency of anti-CCP antibodies (>1.7 units) in patients with RA (68%) to those with SLE (17%). Their presence was over twofold higher in SLE patients with erosive arthritis (38%). Anti-CCP antibodies were less commonly observed (8.8%) in the SLE cohort described by Ball et al.[13]

Jaccoud's Arthropathy

Sigismond Jaccoud, a Swiss physician living in Paris in the 1800s, originally described an arthritis associated with rheumatic fever. Jaccoud's arthropathy is characterized by reducible deformities and the absence of erosions. Bleifeld and Inglis published their observations of the hands of 50 lupus patients.[19] Abnormalities included laxity (50%) and reducible deformities (38%), but radiographs failed to demonstrate erosive changes. Prevalence figures for Jaccoud's arthropathy from two SLE cohorts were 3.47% and 6.1%.[20,21] Santiago and Galvao noted the most frequently observed joint deformities were swan neck and thumb subluxation, followed by ulnar deviation and boutonniere deformity.[20] They found no differences in the clinical or laboratory features in SLE patients with or without Jaccoud's arthropathy.

Jaccoud's arthropathy could be mistaken for RA as the patient with advanced Jaccoud's arthropathy has ulnar deviation as well as subluxation at the MCPs. Features that distinguish Jaccoud's arthropathy from RA include reducibility of the deformities and the lack of erosions on X-ray. Severe Jaccoud's arthropathy may compromise hand function as a result of contractures or ulnar deviation. The pathogenesis of joint laxity in Jaccoud's arthropathy is not understood. Although rarely obtained, biopsy specimens have shown normal synovium. Whereas Jaccoud's arthropathy is generally observed in the hands, it has been reported in feet and knees.

Treatment

Arthritis activity dictates how aggressively the clinician will need to intervene. Nonsteroidal anti-inflammatory drugs and low-dose corticosteroid (e.g., prednisone 5–10 mg daily) are often effective for mild symptoms. For those failing minor interventions, hydroxychloroquine or immunosuppressives may be warranted. Wong and Esdaile noted inconsistent effects in their review of methotrexate in controlled and uncontrolled studies.[22] Fortin et al. demonstrated the steroid-sparing effects of methotrexate in a randomized, double-blind placebo-controlled study of 86 SLE patients.[23] While the study did not focus solely on articular manifestations, 90% of participants had musculoskeletal involvement at baseline. Azathioprine represents yet another treatment option.

A trial comparing the efficacy of mycophenolate to cyclophosphamide in lupus nephritis yielded data on extrarenal responses.[4] Of those with baseline BILAG A or B musculoskeletal domain scores, over 85% of the patients in both arms had improvements in their domain scores at 24 weeks. In a study of 27 patients with lupus arthritis, mycophenolate, administered to a target dose of 3 g daily, outperformed placebo in the achievement of a musculoskeletal domain BILAG C response.[24]

In post hoc analyses of phase 3 belimumab data, Manzi et al. published that those subjects who entered BLISS-52 and BLISS-76 studies with musculoskeletal domain activity had statistically significant improvement when belimumab, as opposed to placebo, was added to standard of care.[3] While most rheumatologists shy away from off-label use of tumor necrosis factor (TNF) inhibitors in lupus because of fear of disease exacerbations, anecdotal experience suggests that some patients with lupus arthritis benefit. It must be remembered that TNF inhibitors can promote the synthesis of anti-DNA antibodies, thus confusing the picture for those clinicians whose assessment of disease activity is guided by serologies.

Favorable effects on musculoskeletal disease activity, albeit not statistically significant, have been demonstrated with tocilizumab and abatacept.[25,26] Laquinimod, in development for multiple sclerosis, was studied in lupus arthritis; however, study results were never presented. Rituximab, while not approved for SLE, is favored by some for refractory arthritis.

Splints will correct the maligned digits in a patient with Jaccoud's arthropathy. However, it is the author's experience that deformities recur once splints are removed. Similarly, pharmacologic interventions, while capable of reducing inflammation in the more typical subset of lupus arthritis, do not affect deformities associated with Jaccoud's. On occasion, surgical intervention of the hand is required. Reported results have been variable.[27]

The traditional teaching that lupus arthritis is not associated with erosions has been contested with the introduction of sensitive imaging modalities. These findings further confound the classification of joint disease in SLE. Ball and Bell emphasized that lupus arthritis remains largely understudied in comparison to RA. It is this lack of understanding of SLE arthritis pathogenesis and classification that may thwart therapeutic advances for this disease.[28]

TENDON RUPTURE

Spontaneous tendon rupture, albeit rare, occurs in patients with lupus.[29] Ruptures may be acute and are sometimes bilateral, with the most commonly affected tendons being the patellar and Achilles tendons. Predisposing factors include trauma and steroids. Histology, reported in a limited number of cases, has shown variable degrees of inflammatory changes, ranging from no inflammation to exuberant synovial proliferation.

MYOSITIS

Clinical Features

Muscular involvement in SLE ranges from commonly seen myalgia to rarely observed inflammatory myopathy, or myositis. Clinical and laboratory features of lupus myositis are no different than idiopathic inflammatory myopathy (IIM) and include proximal muscle weakness with or without myalgia as well as elevated muscle enzymes, typically creatine phosphokinase (CPK).

In about 5% of SLE patients, myositis may be a first manifestation of lupus,[30] but more frequently, it is observed years after the diagnosis of SLE has been established. Raynaud's phenomena, anemia, alopecia, oral ulcers, erosive arthritis, and pulmonary disease were observed more frequently in SLE patients with myositis, whereas lupus nephritis was less often seen in patients with lupus myositis.[31] It has been suggested that serositis and lymphopenia are predictive of the subsequent development of myositis.[32]

Garton and Isenberg compared the clinical and laboratory features of lupus myositis to primary IIM. Relapsing and remitting courses were common in both, whereas monophasic disease was the least frequent pattern. There were no significant differences in muscle strength and serum CPK levels between groups of patients.[33] RNP antibodies are more prevalent in SLE patients with myositis as opposed to SLE patients without myositis.[30]

It was initially suggested that lupus myositis follows a much milder course than IIM. Foote et al. reported significantly lower mortality rates in patients with lupus myositis compared to those with polymyositis complicating scleroderma or RA (18% vs 47%).[34] However, Garton and Isenberg concluded lupus myositis can be as severe as in IIM with similar mortality rates.[33] Dayal and Isenberg later observed that mortality in lupus patients with myositis was no different from lupus patients without myositis; however, lupus patients with myositis at the time of their deaths were significantly younger than lupus patients without myositis (24.7 vs 51 years).[31] The prognosis of lupus patients with myositis depends on other manifestations of SLE.

Histologic Features

Histological findings from biopsy and autopsy series of lupus myositis include the following: (1) lymphocytic and plasma cell infiltrates in perivascular, perimysial, and endomysial locations; (2) mononuclear and lymphocytic vasculitis but rare vessel wall necrosis; (3) perifasicular atrophy; and (4) vacuolar myopathy (in the absence of corticosteroid or chloroquine exposure).[35,36] Oxenhandler et al. demonstrated immunoglobulin and complement deposition in the skeletal muscle of SLE patients, highlighting similar mechanisms of injury in lupus myositis as is described for cutaneous and renal involvement.[35] Moreover, histologic evidence of inflammatory myopathy was found even in clinically uninvolved muscles of lupus patients.[35] Furthermore, SLE patients with nonspecific arthralgia and myalgia were more likely to have type II fiber atrophy and vessel wall thickening on muscle biopsy than patients with fibromyalgia (87% vs 58%); lymphocytic vasculitis and myositis were reported in 38% of SLE patients with muscular symptoms in contrast to 0% in fibromyalgia.[36] Increased capillary basement membrane thickness associated with C3d-g deposition and endothelial microtubular inclusions were also observed.[37,38]

Differential Diagnosis

The differential diagnosis of muscle injury in SLE includes drug-induced myopathy. Although corticosteroids frequently cause weakness, they are not associated with muscle enzyme elevations. The characteristic histologic findings consist of type II myofiber atrophy without inflammation. Myotoxicity due to antimalarials is extremely rare. Renal failure is an important risk factor.[39] The presence of vacuolar myopathy with acid phosphatase positive vacuoles and curvilinear body formation on muscle biopsy is diagnostic of chloroquine and hydroxychloroquine myotoxicity. Timely recognition of drug-induced myopathy is important as the myopathic process is reversible once the drug is discontinued.

Treatment

Just as with designing treatment plans for other manifestations of lupus, the treatment regimen for myositis needs to be customized according to disease severity. Corticosteroids, the mainstay of therapy for lupus myositis, are used in doses that range from 0.5 to 1.5 mg/kg to intravenous "pulse" methylprednisolone. Even as our therapeutic arsenal expanded, there has been no consensus regarding an immunosuppressive regimen for induction or maintenance. Hence, for patients refractory to corticosteroids, azathioprine, methotrexate, or mycophenolate are often used. Rituximab has been reported to be useful in refractory cases of SLE myositis.[40]

Overexpression of the type I interferon signature in the serum and tissue of patients with either SLE or inflammatory myositis has been observed.[41] These findings suggest a common pathway in disease pathogenesis and may explain clinical similarities between the two diseases. A phase 1b clinical trial was designed to evaluate sifalimumab, a human anti-interferon-alpha monoclonal antibody in development for SLE, in adult subjects with myositis.[42] The interferon gene signature was suppressed by 50% in blood and in muscle specimens post-sifalimumab administration. These preliminary observations require confirmation in a larger trial powered to evaluate efficacy. With lupus clinical trial activity at unprecedented levels, the lupus community eagerly awaits the further development of targeted therapies.

OSTEONECROSIS

Introduction

Osteonecrosis, also known as ischemic necrosis of bone, avascular necrosis, osteochondriits dissecans, and aseptic necrosis, compromises the structural integrity of bone architecture. While there are numerous etiologies and varied clinical presentations of avascular necrosis, cell death due to interrupted blood supply to periarticular bone is the common pathogenic mechanism.[43,44] Osteonecrosis, which can cause substantial pain and disability, represents a significant challenge in the SLE patient.

Clinical Impact

Clinicians should view osteonecrosis as a spectrum ranging from the asymptomatic patient with abnormal findings on imaging to the patient with severe disease with pain and disability from advanced cortical destruction. Asymptomatic or silent osteonecrosis is usually found incidentally on imaging. While asymptomatic osteonecrosis is associated with less severe changes on imaging than symptomatic osteonecrosis, patients with asymptomatic disease have the potential to progress to symptomatic disease. A prospective study of hip MRIs in 23 SLE patients on glucocorticoids for SLE discovered asymptomatic osteonecrosis at baseline in 35% of subjects. At the 3-year follow up, 25% of subjects had progression of osteonecrosis on MRI, and 12.5% developed hip pain.[45] In a case–control study of 95 SLE patients, those with osteonecrosis had higher HAQ (Health Assessment Questionnaire) scores and lower scores on the physical functioning domain of the SF-20.[46]

Epidemiology

SLE is an independent risk factor for the development of osteonecrosis. The prevalence of symptomatic and asymptomatic osteonecrosis in patients with SLE is 5–15% and 50%, respectively.[46–54] While osteonecrosis has been reported in almost every bone, the most common site is the hip. The majority of patients will have multisite involvement.

Pathogenesis

There are three proposed mechanisms of ischemia in osteonecrosis[1]: intravascular occlusion,[2] diminished blood flow from increased extravascular pressure,[3] or inhibition of angiogenesis.[55–57] Intravascular occlusion can stem from thrombosis associated with inflammation-mediated elevations in homocysteine, anticardiolipin antibody activity, small vessel vasculitis, vasospasm, and fat emboli. Corticosteroids can increase adipocytes in the marrow, which can cause intracortical pressure leading to decreased blood flow in the cortical vessels. Lastly, the pro-inflammatory cytokine milieu induces osteoclast formation, decreases osteoblast activity, and reduces angiogenic factors.[55]

Risk Factors

While there is a strong association between corticosteroids and osteonecrosis, other factors such as disease activity, age at SLE onset, use of cytotoxic agents,[58,59] Raynaud's phenomenon,[60] vasculitis, and antiphospholipid antibodies[61,62] have been found to be risk factors in SLE.[53] Multiple studies have evaluated the pattern of steroid use in relation to the development of osteonecrosis. In a study of 539 patients, each 2-month exposure to high-dose prednisone conferred a 1.2-fold increased risk of developing osteonecrosis.[54] The development of osteonecrosis occurred in temporal proximity to high-dose steroid use.[62,63]

Susceptibility to osteonecrosis is not understood. There are patients that are treated with steroids who do not develop osteonecrosis. As with many conditions, it is likely there are genetic factors that contribute to susceptibility to corticosteroid-induced osteonecrosis. Polymorphisms in MDR1(ABCB1) have been shown to be associated with steroid-induced osteonecrosis in patients with SLE.[64,65]

Diagnosis

Symptomatic osteonecrosis presents with pain localized to the involved bone and is exacerbated by weight bearing. While computed tomography, MRI, radionucleotide bone scan, and radiographs are all used to detect osteonecrosis, radiographs are the least sensitive and MRI the most sensitive.[45] Radiographs are used for initial screening, but MRIs are ordered when radiographs are normal.

Treatment

Asymptomatic osteonecrosis is treated conservatively and by reducing modifiable risk factors, whereas symptomatic osteonecrosis can be treated conservatively or surgically. Conservative measures include modification of activity with restricted weight bearing, stimulation of repair with ultrasound or electrical signals, and pharmacologic treatment.[55,57] Convincing data are not available to support the routine use of pharmaceutical treatments other than to control pain. The prevention of osteonecrosis in lupus patients with statins, anticoagulants, or bisphosphonates have been studied in small studies. However, additional studies are needed prior to the adoption of these therapies.[63,66]

Surgical treatment of osteonecrosis is reserved for patients with severe symptoms and/or collapse on imaging. Options include joint replacement or joint-preserving procedures such as support of subchondral bone, vascularized and nonvascularized bone grafting, cementation, implantation of trabecular metal rods, core decompression, or osteotomy.[56,57]

Given the interest in stem cell therapy, a systematic review was performed by Lau et al. They noted that stem cell therapy was associated with a significant improvement in patient-reported outcomes, but there were no statistically significant changes in joint survival.[67]

OSTEOPOROSIS

Introduction

The importance of bone health in lupus has come into focus as both long-term survival rates in lupus increase and the diagnostic modalities to assess bone mineral density have become more refined. In addition to traditional risk factors, lupus patients have additional risk factors for low bone density. These risk factors are associated with disease activity and pharmacotherapy.[68,69]

Epidemiology of Osteopenia and Osteoporosis

According to the Centers for Disease Control and Prevention, data collected from 1988 to 1994 in men and women over the age of 50 revealed a prevalence of osteopenia of 16% in men and 40% in women and a prevalence of osteoporosis of 2% in men and 16% in women.[70] Studies of patients with lupus yielded prevalence figures for osteopenia as high as 50.8% and for osteoporosis as high as 23%.[71,72] In a study of 702 women with lupus followed over 5951 person-years, there was an almost fivefold increase in fracture risk seen in the subjects with lupus compared to the general female population.[73] In these studies, the average age was under 50, although the majority of patients were postmenopausal. Male lupus patients have a higher prevalence of osteopenia and osteoporosis than healthy males but a lower prevalence of osteopenia and osteoporosis than female lupus patients.[71,72,74] Children with juvenile systemic lupus erythematosus also have a significant risk of osteopenia, with a reported prevalence of approximately 40% in two studies.[75,76]

Pathophysiology of Bone Loss in Lupus and Risk Factors for Accelerated Bone Loss in Lupus

After peak bone mass is achieved between ages 20 and 30, bone is remodeled through a balance between osteoclastic and osteoblastic activities. In the general population, an imbalance caused by hormonal changes associated with menopause and aging leads to osteoporosis.[77–79] Inflammation, metabolic changes, and corticosteroid use are more detrimental to trabecular bone than cortical bone due to the higher turnover rate of trabecular bone. The ratio of trabecular bone to cortical bone is greater in the lumbar spine compared to the hip.[78–80]

Traditional risk factors that are more prevalent in the lupus population include female sex, premature menopause, low vitamin D levels, and sedentary lifestyle. Independent traditional risk factors include weight less than 58 kg, age 65 or greater, personal or family history of fractures as an adult, inadequate calcium intake, excessive alcohol use, and smoking. Lupus-related risk factors include inflammatory-mediated bone loss, glucocorticoid use, nonglucocorticoid medications, reduced mobility and corresponding decline in muscle mass, myopathy, renal disease, endocrine factors, amenorrhea, low plasma androgen levels, hyperprolactinemia, and chronic induction of bone-resorbing cytokines.[81]

Glucocorticoids

Bone loss associated with corticosteroid use is greatest in the first year of treatment, but it does continue throughout treatment.[82,83] Glucocorticoids are thought to adversely affect bone formation, bone resorption, and calcium metabolism (both vitamin D-dependent and vitamin D-independent).[84,85] Glucocorticoids decrease the number of functional osteoblasts.[86,87] Both the maximum daily dose and the cumulative dose of steroids have been associated with bone loss in lupus patients.[71,83]

Other Factors

There are risk factors other than corticosteroid exposure that contribute to the increased prevalence of osteopenia and osteoporosis in this population. Bone loss is stimulated by activation of RANKL-OPG (receptor activator of nuclear factor kappa B ligand-osteoprotegerin) and cytokines, such as IL-1, IL-6, and TNFα, vitamin D_3, and IL-11, are thought to affect RANKL-OPG. In addition, TNF also stimulates osteoclast maturation.[68,69,81] Hormonal factors such as amenorrhea, low androgen levels, premature menopause, and hyperprolactinemia have been associated with low bone mineral density in lupus.[68,88-91] Medications such as anticoagulants, cyclophosphamide, mycophenalate mofetil, and cyclosporine have been associated with reduced bone density.

Treatment

Patients should maintain adequate calcium intake, monitor vitamin D levels, avoid tobacco, avoid alcohol, and engage in muscle-building exercises. Multiple pharmacologic options are available for bone loss. Bisphosphonates, including etidronate, risedronate, and alendronate, have been shown to mitigate bone loss in both postmenopausal and glucocorticoid-induced osteoporosis.[69,81] The long half-life of bisphosphonates, which bind bone hydroxyapatite and inhibit osteoclastic activity, raises concerns about their use in premenopausal women desirous of future child-bearing.[78,79,92] Other pharmacologic interventions such as teriparitide, raloxifine, and denosumab have been shown to be effective in mitigation of bone loss, but there are no large clinical trials of these medications in lupus patients with osteoporosis.

REFERENCES

1. Navarra SV, Guzman RM, Gallacher AE, Hall S, Levy RA, Jimenez RE, et al. Efficacy and safety of belimumab in patients with active systemic lupus erythematosus: a randomised, placebo-controlled, phase 3 trial. *Lancet* 2011;**377**(9767):721–31.
2. Furie R, Petri M, Zamani O, Cervera R, Wallace DJ, Tegzova D, et al. A phase III, randomized, placebo-controlled study of belimumab, a monoclonal antibody that inhibits B lymphocyte stimulator, in patients with systemic lupus erythematosus. *Arthritis Rheum* 2011;**63**(12):3918–30.
3. Manzi S, Sanchez-Guerrero J, Merrill JT, Furie R, Gladman D, Navarra SV, et al. Effects of belimumab, a B lymphocyte stimulator-specific inhibitor, on disease activity across multiple organ domains in patients with systemic lupus erythematosus: combined results from two phase III trials. *Ann Rheum Dis* 2012;**71**(11):1833–8.
4. Ginzler EM, Wofsy D, Isenberg D, Gordon C, Lisk L, Dooley MA, et al. Nonrenal disease activity following mycophenolate mofetil or intravenous cyclophosphamide as induction treatment for lupus nephritis: findings in a multicenter, prospective, randomized, open-label, parallel-group clinical trial. *Arthritis Rheum* 2010;**62**(1):211–21.
5. Fernandez A, Quintana G, Matteson EL, Restrepo JF, Rondon F, Sanchez A, et al. Lupus arthropathy: historical evolution from deforming arthritis to rhupus. *Clin Rheumatol* 2004;**23**(6):523–6.
6. Zoma A. Musculoskeletal involvement in systemic lupus erythematosus. *Lupus* 2004;**13**(11):851–3.
7. Pekin Jr TJ, Zvaifler NJ. Synovial fluid findings in systemic lupus erythematosus (SLE). *Arthritis Rheum* 1970;**13**(6):777–85.
8. Weissman BN, Rappoport AS, Sosman JL, Schur PH. Radiographic findings in the hands in patients with systemic lupus erythematosus. *Radiology* 1978;**126**(2):313–7.
9. Wright S, Filippucci E, Grassi W, Grey A, Bell A. Hand arthritis in systemic lupus erythematosus: an ultrasound pictorial essay. *Lupus* 2006;**15**(8):501–6.
10. Lins CF, Santiago MB. Ultrasound evaluation of joints in systemic lupus erythematosus: a systematic review. *Eur Radiol* 2015;**25**(9):2688–92.
11. Yoon HS, Kim KJ, Baek IW, Park YJ, Kim WU, Yoon CH, et al. Ultrasonography is useful to detect subclinical synovitis in SLE patients without musculoskeletal involvement before symptoms appear. *Clin Rheumatol* 2014;**33**(3):341–8.
12. Chiara T, Dario D, Niccolo P, Andrea DS, Davide C, Stefano B, et al. MRI pattern of arthritis in systemic lupus erythematosus: a comparative study with rheumatoid arthritis and healthy subjects. *Skelet Radiol* 2015;**44**(2):261–6.
13. Ball EM, Tan AL, Fukuba E, McGonagle D, Grey A, Steiner G, et al. A study of erosive phenotypes in lupus arthritis using magnetic resonance imaging and anti-citrullinated protein antibody, anti-RA33 and RF autoantibody status. *Rheumatology* 2014;**53**(10):1835–43.
14. Natour J, Montezzo LC, Moura LA, Atra E. A study of synovial membrane of patients with systemic lupus erythematosus (SLE). *Clin Exp Rheumatol* 1991;**9**(3):221–5.
15. Mensah KA, Mathian A, Ma L, Xing L, Ritchlin CT, Schwarz EM. Mediation of nonerosive arthritis in a mouse model of lupus by interferon-alpha-stimulated monocyte differentiation that is nonpermissive of osteoclastogenesis. *Arthritis Rheum* 2010;**62**(4):1127–37.
16. Panush RS, Edwards NL, Longley S, Webster E. 'Rhupus' syndrome. *Archives Intern Med* 1988;**148**(7):1633–6.
17. Amezcua-Guerra LM, Springall R, Marquez-Velasco R, Gomez-Garcia L, Vargas A, Bojalil R. Presence of antibodies against cyclic citrullinated peptides in patients with 'rhupus': a cross-sectional study. *Arthritis Res Ther* 2006;**8**(5):R144.
18. Amezcua-Guerra LM, Marquez-Velasco R, Bojalil R. Erosive arthritis in systemic lupus erythematosus is associated with high serum C-reactive protein and anti-cyclic citrullinated peptide antibodies. *Inflamm Res* 2008;**57**(12):555–7.
19. Bleifeld CJ, Inglis AE. The hand in systemic lupus erythematosus. *J Bone Joint Surg Am* 1974;**56**(6):1207–15.
20. Santiago MB, Galvao V. Jaccoud arthropathy in systemic lupus erythematosus: analysis of clinical characteristics and review of the literature. *Medicine* 2008;**87**(1):37–44.

21. Skare TL, Godoi Ade L, Ferreira VO. Jaccoud arthropathy in systemic lupus erythematosus: clinical and serological findings. *Rev Assoc Med Bras* 2012;**58**(4):489–92.

22. Wong JM, Esdaile JM. Methotrexate in systemic lupus erythematosus. *Lupus* 2005;**14**(2):101–5.

23. Fortin PR, Abrahamowicz M, Ferland D, Lacaille D, Smith CD, Zummer M, et al. Steroid-sparing effects of methotrexate in systemic lupus erythematosus: a double-blind, randomized, placebo-controlled trial. *Arthritis Rheum* 2008;**59**(12):1796–804.

24. Merrill JTCF, Wilson SK, Kamp S, Hutcheson J, Rawdon J, Finley E, et al. Mycophenolate mofetil (MMF) for treatment of arthritis in patients with systemic lupus erythematosus (SLE). *Arthrit Rheum-Arthr* 2008.

25. Illei GG, Shirota Y, Yarboro CH, Daruwalla J, Tackey E, Takada K, et al. Tocilizumab in systemic lupus erythematosus: data on safety, preliminary efficacy, and impact on circulating plasma cells from an open-label phase I dosage-escalation study. *Arthritis Rheum* 2010;**62**(2):542–52.

26. Merrill JT, Burgos-Vargas R, Westhovens R, Chalmers A, D'Cruz D, Wallace DJ, et al. The efficacy and safety of abatacept in patients with non-life-threatening manifestations of systemic lupus erythematosus: results of a twelve-month, multicenter, exploratory, phase IIb, randomized, double-blind, placebo-controlled trial. *Arthritis Rheum* 2010;**62**(10):3077–87.

27. Nalebuff EA. Surgery of systemic lupus erythematosus arthritis of the hand. *Hand Clin* 1996;**12**(3):591–602.

28. Ball EM, Bell AL. Lupus arthritis–do we have a clinically useful classification? *Rheumatology* 2012;**51**(5):771–9.

29. Furie RA, Chartash EK. Tendon rupture in systemic lupus erythematosus. *Semin Arthritis Rheum* 1988;**18**(2):127–33.

30. Font J, Cervera R, Ramos-Casals M, Garcia-Carrasco M, Sents J, Herrero C, et al. Clusters of clinical and immunologic features in systemic lupus erythematosus: analysis of 600 patients from a single center. *Semin Arthritis Rheum* 2004;**33**(4):217–30.

31. Dayal NA, Isenberg DA. SLE/myositis overlap: are the manifestations of SLE different in overlap disease? *Lupus* 2002;**11**(5):293–8.

32. Jacobsen S, Petersen J, Ullman S, Junker P, Voss A, Rasmussen JM, et al. A multicentre study of 513 Danish patients with systemic lupus erythematosus. Disease manifestations and analyses of clinical subsets. *Clin Rheumatol* 1998;**17**(6):468–84.

33. Garton MJ, Isenberg DA. Clinical features of lupus myositis versus idiopathic myositis: a review of 30 cases. *Br J Rheum* 1997;**36**:1067–74.

34. Foot RA, Kimbrough SM, Stevens JC. Lupus myositis. *Muscle Nerve* 1982;**5**:65–8.

35. Oxenhandler R, Hart MN, Bickel J, Scearce D, Durham J, Irvin W. Pathologic features of muscle in systemic lupus erythematosus. *Hum Pathol* 1982;**13**:745–57.

36. Lim KL, Abdul-Wahab R, Lowe J, Powell RJ. Muscle biopsy abnormalities in systemic lupus erythematosus: correlation with clinical and laboratory parameters. *Ann Rheum Dis* 1994;**53**:178–82.

37. Pallis M, Lowe J, Powell R. An electron microscopic study of muscle capillary wall thickening in systemic lupus erythematosus. *Lupus* 1994;**3**(5):401–7.

38. Bronner IM, Hoogendijk JE, Veldman H, Ramkema M, van den Bergh Weerman MA, Rozemuller AJ, et al. Tubuloreticular structures in different types of myositis: implications for pathogenesis. *Ultrastruct Pathol* 2008;**32**(4):123–6.

39. Stein M, Bell MJ, Ang LC. Hydroxychloroquine neuromyotoxicity. *J Rheumatol* December 2000;**27**(12):2927–31.

40. Ramos-Casals M, Garcia-Hernandez FJ, de Ramon E, Callejas JL, et al. Off-label use of rituximab in 196 patients with severe, refractory systemic autoimmune diseases. *Clin Exp Rheumatol* 2010;**28**(4):468–76.

41. Walsh RJ, Kong SW, Yao Y, Jallal B, Kiener PA, Pinkus JL, et al. Type I interferon-inducible gene expression in blood is present and reflects disease activity in dermatomyositis and polymyositis. *Arthritis Rheum* 2007;**56**(11):3784–92.

42. Higgs BW, Zhu W, Morehouse C, White WI, Brohawn P, Guo X, et al. A phase 1b clinical trial evaluating sifalimumab, an anti-IFN-α monoclonal antibody, shows target neutralisation of a type I IFN signature in blood of dermatomyositis and polymyositis patients. *Ann Rheum Dis* 2014;**73**(1):256–62.

43. Zizic TM, Marcoux C, Hungerford DS, Stevens MB. The early diagnosis of ischemic necrosis of bone. *Arthritis Rheum* 1986;**29**(10):1177–86.

44. Assouline-Dayan Y, Chang C, Greenspan A, Shoenfeld Y, Gershwin ME. Pathogenesis and natural history of osteonecrosis. *Semin Arthritis Rheum* 2002;**32**(2):94–124.

45. Nagasawa K, Tsukamoto H, Tada Y, Mayumi T, Satoh H, Onitsuka H, et al. Imaging study on the mode of development and changes in avascular necrosis of the femoral head in SLE: long-term observations. *Br J Rheumatol* 1994;**33**:343–7.

46. Gladman DD, Chaudhry-Ahluwalia V, Ibañez D, Bogoch E, Urowitz MB. Outcomes of symptomatic osteonecrosis in 95 patients with SLE. *J Rheumatol* 2001;**28**:2226–9.

47. Abeles M, Urman JD, Rothfield NF. Aseptic necrosis of bone in SLE: relationship to corticosteroid therapy. *Arch Intern Med* 1978;**138**:750–4.

48. Petri M. Musculoskeletal complications of SLE in the Hopkins Lupus Cohort: an update. *Arthritis Rheum* 1995;**8**(3):137–45.

49. Urowitz MB, Gladman DD, Tom BDM, Ibañez D, Farewell VT. Changing patterns in mortality and disease outcomes for patients with SLE. *J Rheum* 2008;**35**(11):2152–8.

50. Zizic TM, Marcoux C, Hungerford DS, Dansereau JV, Stevens MB. Corticosteroid therapy associated with ischemic necrosis of bone in SLE. *Am J Med* 1985;**79**:596–604.

51. Joo YB, Sung YK, Shim JS, et al. Prevalence, incidence and associated factors of avascular necrosis in Korean patients with systemic lupus erythematosus: a nationwide epidemiologic study. *Rheumatology International* 2014;**35**(5):879–86.

52. Kunyakham W, Foocharoen C, Mahakkanukrauh A, et al. Prevalance and risk factor for symptomatic avascular necrosis development in Thai systemic lupus erythematosus patients. *Asian Pac J Allergy Immunol* 2012;**30**:152–7.

53. Sayarlioglu M, Yuzbasioglu N, Inanc M, et al. Risk factors for avascular bone necrosis in patients with systemic lupus erythematosus. *Rheumatol Int* 2012;**32**:177–82.

54. Zonana-Nacach A, Barr SG, Magder LS, Petri M. Damage in SLE and its association with corticosteroids. *Arthritis Rheum* 2000;**43**(8):1801–8.

55. Lane NE. Therapy insight: osteoporosis and osteonecrosis in SLE. *Nat Clin Pract Rheum* 2006;**2**(10):562–9.

56. Jones LC, Hungerford DS. Osteonecrosis: etiology, diagnosis, and treatment. *Curr Opin Rheumatol* 2004;**16**:443–9.

57. Mont MA, Jones LC. Management of osteonecrosis in SLE. *Rheum Dis Clin N Am* 2000;**26**(2):279–309.

58. Calvo-Alen J, McGwin G, Toloza S, Fernandez M, Roseman JM, Bastian HM, et al. Alarcon GSl. SLE in a multiethnic US cohory (LUMINA): XXIV. Cytotoxic treatment is an additional risk factor for the development of symptomatic osteonecrosis in lupus patients: results of a nested matched case-control study. *Ann Rheum Dis* 2006;**65**:785–90.

59. Sweet DL, Roth DG, Desser RK, et al. Avascular necrosis of the femoral head with combination therapy. *Ann Intern Med* 1976;**85**:67–8.

60. Rueda JC, Duque MA, Mantilla RD, Iglesias-Gamarra A. Osteonecrosis and antiphospholipid syndrome. *J Clin Rheumatol* 2009;**15**(3):130–2.

61. Tektonidiou MG, Malagari K, Vlachoyiannopoulos PG, et al. Asymptomatic avascular necrosis in patients with primary antiphospholipid syndrome in the absence of corticosteroid use. *Arthritis Rheum* 2003;**48**(3):732–6.

62. Oinuma K, Haradaa Y, Nawatab Y, Takabayashib K, Abea I, Kamikawaa K, et al. Osteonecrosis in patients with SLE develops very early after starting high dose corticosteroid treatment. *Ann Rheum Dis* 2001;**60**:1145–8.

63. Nagasawa K, Tada Y, Koarada S, et al. Prevention of steroid-induced osteonecrosis of femoral head in SLE by anti-coagulant. *Lupus* 2006;**15**:354–7.

64. Yang XY, Xu DH. MDR1(ABCB1) gene polymorphisms associated with steroid-induced osteonecrosis of femoral head in SLE. *Pharmazie* 2007;**62**(12):930–2.

65. Asano T, Takahashi KA, Fujioka M, et al. ABCB1 C3435T and G2677T/A polymorphism decreased the risk for steroid induced osteonecrosis of the femoral head after kidney transplantation. *Pharmacogenetics* 2003;**13**(11):675–82.

66. Lydon EJ, Schweitzer M, Godberg JD, Belmont HM. Atorvastatin to prevent avascular necrosis of bone in systemic lupus erythematosus. *Arthritis Rheum* 2008;**54**:S432. [abstract].

67. Lau RL, Perruccio AV, Evans HMK, et al. Stem cell therapy for the treatment of early stage avascular necrosis of the femoral head: a systematic review. *BMC Musculoskele Disord* 2014;**15**:156.

68. Di Munno O, Mazzantini M, Delle Sedie A, et al. Risk factors for osteoporosis in female patients with systemic lupus erythematosus. *Lupus* 2004;**13**:724–30.

69. Lee C, Ramsey-Goldman R. Bone health and systemic lupus erythematosus. *Current Rheumatology Reports* 2005;**7**:482–9.

70. National Health and Nutrition Survey. CDC/NHANES. http://www.cdc; 2001 [accessed 22.12.09].

71. Yee CS, Crabtree N, Skan J, et al. Prevalence and predictors of fragility fractures in systemic lupus erythematosus. *Ann Rheum Dis* 2005;**64**:111–3.

72. Almehed K, Forsblad d'Elia H, Kvist G, et al. Prevalence and risk factors for osteoporosis in female SLE patients – extended report. *Rheumatology* 2007;**46**:1185–90.

73. Ramsey-Goldman R, Dunn JE, Huang CE, et al. Frequency of fractures in women with systemic lupus erythematosus: comparison with United States population data. *Arthritis Rheum* 1999;**42**(5):882–90.

74. Mok CC, Yee SK, Ying Y, et al. Bone mineral density and body composition in men with systemic lupus erythematosus: a case control study. *Bone* 2008;**43**:327–31.

75. Lilleby V, Lien G, Frey Froslie K, et al. Frequency of osteopenia in children and young adults with childhood-onset systemic lupus erythematosus. *Arthritis Rheum* 2005;**52**:2051–9.

76. Compeyrot-Lacassagne S, Tyrrell PN, Atenafu E, et al. Prevalence and etiology of low bone mineral denisty in juvenile systemic lupus erythematosus. *Arthritis Rheum* 2007;**56**(6):1966–73.

77. Alele JD, Kamen DL. The importance of inflammation and vitamin D status in SLE-associated osteoporosis. *Autoimmun Rev* 2009;**9**(3):137–9.

78. Lane N. Osteoporosis: is there a rational approach to fracture prevention. *B Hosp Joint Dis Ort* 2006;**64**:67–71.

79. Lane NE. Therapy insight: osteoporosis and osteonecrosis in systemic lupus erythematosus. *Nat Clin Pract Rheum* 2006;**2**(10):562–9.

80. Lane NE, Rehman Q. Osteoporosis in the rheumatic disease patient. *Lupus* 2002;**11**:675–9.

81. Lee C, Ramsey-Goldman R. Osteoporosis in systemic lupus erythematosus mechanisms. *Rheum Dis Clin N Am* 2005;**31**:363–85.

82. Lo Cascio V, Bonucci E, Imbimbo B, et al. Bone loss in response to long-term glucocorticoid therapy. *Bone Miner* 1990;**8**:39–51.

83. Jardinet D, Lefebvre C, Depresseux G. Longitudinal analysis of bone mineral density in pre-menopausal female systemic lupus erythematosus patients: deleterious role of glucocorticoid therapy at the lumbar spine. *Rheumatology* 2000;**39**:389–92.

84. Reid IR. Glucocorticoid osteoporosis – mechanisms and management. *Eur J Endocrinol* 1997;**137**:209–17.

85. Klein RG, Arnaud SB, Gallagher JC, et al. Intestinal calcium absorption in exogenous hypercortisolism. Role of 25-hydroxyvitamin D and corticosteroid dose. *J Clin Invest* 1977;**60**:253–9.

86. Manolagas SC, Weinstein RS. New developments in pathogenesis and teratment of steroid induced osteoporosis. *J Bone Miner Res* 1999;**14**:1061–6.

87. Weinstein RS, Jilka RL, Parfitt AM, et al. Inhibition of osteoblastogenesis and promotion of apoptosis of osteopblasts and osteocytes by glucocorticoids. *J Clin Invest* 1998;**102**:274–82.

88. Sinigaglia L, Varenna M, Binelli L, et al. Bone mass in systemic lupus erythematosus. *Clin Exp Rheumatol* 2000;**18**(2). 19:S27.

89. Lahita RG, Bradlow HL, Ginzler E, et al. Low plasma androgens in women with systemic lupus erythematosus. *Arthritis Rheum* 1987;**30**:241–8.

90. Lahita RG. Sex hormones and systemic lupus ertythematosus. *Rheum Dis Clin N Am* 2000;**26**(4):951–68.

91. Shabanova SS, Ananieva LP, Alekberova ZS, Guzov II. Ovarian function and disease activity in patients with systemic lupus erythematosus. *Clin Exp Rheumatol* 2008;**26**(3):436–41.

92. Saag KG, Zanchetta JR, Devogelaer JP, et al. Effects of teriparatide versus alendronate for treating glucocorticoid-induced osteoporosis. *Arthritis Rheum* 2009;**60**(11):3346–55.

Chapter 39

Cutaneous Lupus Erythematosus

Annegret Kuhn[1,2], Aysche Landmann[2], Gisela Bonsmann[3]

[1]Interdisciplinary Center for Clinical Trials (IZKS), University Medical Center Mainz, Mainz, Germany; [2]Division of Immunogenetics, Tumor Immunology Program, German Cancer Research Center (DKFZ), Heidelberg, Germany; [3]Department of Dermatology, University of Muenster, Muenster, Germany

EPIDEMIOLOGY

Cutaneous manifestations occur in approximately 75% of patients with systemic lupus erythematosus (SLE) during the course of the disease and are the first sign in about 25% of patients.[1] Epidemiological data of the different subtypes of cutaneous lupus erythematosus (CLE) have rarely been investigated, as most studies rather evaluate the incidence of SLE.[2] In 2007, a study from Stockholm County, Sweden, reported that subacute cutaneous lupus erythematosus (SCLE) with anti-Ro/SSA antibodies has an incidence of 0.7 per 100,000 persons per year compared with an incidence of SLE of 4.8 per 100,000 persons per year.[3]

CLASSIFICATION CRITERIA FOR SLE

The criteria developed by the American College of Rheumatology (ACR) for the classification of SLE comprise 11 clinical and laboratory features and provide some degree of uniformity to the patient population of clinical studies.[4] However, 4 of the 11 ACR criteria include mucocutaneous manifestations (malar rash, discoid lesions, photosensitivity, and oral ulcers) and therefore may result in an overestimation of SLE.[5] In particular, the ACR criteria poorly define photosensitivity as "a result of an unusual reaction to sunlight by patient's history or physician's observation."[4] Furthermore, photosensitivity is not specific for SLE, as it is also observed in other photodermatoses, such as polymorphous light eruption.[5]

To improve the clinical relevance and to incorporate new knowledge in SLE immunology, the Systemic Lupus Collaborating Clinics (SLICC) revised the ACR criteria in 2012.[6] The SLICC criteria include 11 clinical criteria (e.g., nonscarring alopecia or synovitis) and 6 immunological criteria (e.g., decreased complement and antiphospholipid antibodies), whereas photosensitivity is no longer listed. The SLICC criteria have still to be assessed in routine clinical practice, and it is unclear how much impact these criteria will have on the validity of the diagnosis of SLE.

PHOTOSENSITIVITY

The importance of photosensitivity as one of the most common environmental triggers in lupus erythematosus (LE) has been outlined by different groups from Europe, Japan, and the United States.[7-11] In SLE patients, even induction of systemic organ involvement, such as lupus nephritis, has been reported as a result of extensive sun exposure.[10,12] Moreover, consistent sunscreen protection in patients with SLE is associated with better clinical outcomes, as well as a decreased need for immunosuppressive agents.[13] In addition, several studies with a high number of CLE patients have been performed to show a clear relationship between ultraviolet (UV) radiation and disease-specific skin manifestations using a standardized photoprovocation protocol.[14-16] Meanwhile, photoprovocation has been accepted as a diagnostic procedure to evaluate photosensitivity in CLE.[17] In two retrospective studies of more than 400 patients with different subtypes of CLE, skin lesions induced by UVA and/or UVB radiation were observed in 54.0% and 61.7% of patients, respectively.[15,18] The more recent analysis suggests that the reaction to UV light may change during the course of the disease and that photosensitivity should not be defined only on the basis of patients' history.[18] Moreover, a randomized, vehicle-controlled, intraindividual, comparative, double-blind study demonstrated that the application of a broad-spectrum sunscreen with a high protection factor prevented the appearance of disease-specific skin lesions in all tested patients with photosensitive CLE.[14] A further study confirmed these results.[19] In addition, immunohistological analysis of skin biopsy specimens taken from patients with CLE after UV exposure demonstrated that sunscreen protection reduces lesional tissue damage and inhibits the typical interferon-driven inflammatory response.[20] The published studies imply that patients with CLE should receive thorough advice (i.e., information that UVA passes window glass) and instructions on photoprotective measures (i.e., information on suitable clothing).[14,19-21] Sunscreens with a high sun protection factor ($\geq$50) should be applied in a sufficient amount (2 mg/cm^2) 20–30 minutes before sun exposure.[22]

Systemic Lupus Erythematosus. http://dx.doi.org/10.1016/B978-0-12-801917-7.00039-5

CUTANEOUS MANIFESTATIONS

Skin lesions associated with LE show great heterogeneity and have led to the differentiation into LE-specific and LE-nonspecific manifestations by clinical parameters and histological analysis of skin biopsy specimens.[23] LE-nonspecific cutaneous manifestations, which may also appear in other diseases, are preferably associated with higher disease activity in SLE.[24,25] These include cutaneous vascular lesions, such as periungual telangiectasia, red lunula, livedo racemosa, Raynaud's phenomenon, acral occlusive vasculopathy, thrombophlebitis, and leukocytoclastic vasculitis, which can occur as palpable purpura or urticarial vasculitis (especially hypocomplementemic urticarial vasculitis). Other nonspecific skin lesions include papular mucinosis, calcinosis cutis, nonscarring alopecia (i.e., "lupus hair"), and erythema multiforme, among others.[26]

LE-specific cutaneous manifestations comprise the different subtypes of CLE, which are defined by a constellation of clinical and histological features, serological parameters, such as antinuclear antibodies, and the course of the disease.[23] Since the first classification system of Gilliam including acute CLE (ACLE), SCLE, and chronic CLE (CCLE) more than three decades ago, several approaches have been made to further develop this system and to present a more detailed classification of the different CLE subtypes.[23,27–29] For example, the subtype named LE tumidus (LET) with specific clinical, histological, and photobiological features has been analyzed and defined as a separate entity of CLE in the past years.[30–32] Its course and prognosis is generally more favorable compared to other subtypes of CLE; therefore, a revised classification system, including LET as the intermittent, non-chronic subtype of CLE, was suggested as the "Duesseldorf Classification" (Table 1).[27,33]

In 2004, the European Society of Cutaneous Lupus Erythematosus (EUSCLE) was founded to further differentiate and assess the various subtypes of CLE and to achieve a general consensus concerning evidence-based clinical standards for disease evaluation. A study group of EUSCLE defined a core set of variables for the evaluation of the characteristic features of the disease and developed the EUSCLE Core Set Questionnaire, which includes various parameters considered the most relevant features of CLE.[34,35] Data of 1002 patients with CLE from 30 centers in Europe were collected using the EUSCLE Core Set Questionnaire, and statistical analysis of clinical and laboratory features, as well as an evaluation of treatment options and their efficacies was performed.[36,37] In addition, an analysis of the smoking behavior and the efficacy of antimalarials in part of the study population suggests that smoking is a risk factor for the disease, in particular for LET, and negatively influences CLE disease activity and the efficacy of antimalarial treatment.[38]

TABLE 1 Subtypes of Cutaneous Lupus Erythematosus (CLE)[a]

Acute cutaneous lupus erythematosus (ACLE)
Localized
Generalized
Subacute cutaneous lupus erythematosus (SCLE)
Annular
Papulosquamous/psoriasiform
Chronic cutaneous lupus erythematosus (CCLE)
Discoid lupus erythematosus (DLE)
Localized
Disseminated
Lupus erythematosus profundus/panniculitis (LEP)
Chilblain lupus erythematosus (CHLE)
Intermittent cutaneous lupus erythematosus (ICLE)
Lupus erythematosus tumidus (LET)

[a]Modified after.[27]

SCORES IN CUTANEOUS LUPUS ERYTHEMATOSUS

To determine disease activity in everyday clinical practice and during clinical trials, several disease activity scores Systemic Lupus Erythematosus Disease Activity Index (SLEDAI); European Consensus Lupus Activity Measurement (ECLAM); British Isles Lupus Assessment Group (BILAG) have been established for SLE.[39,40] In addition, the damage should be assessed once a year by the SLICC/ACR Damage Index.[41] Although these scores include dermatological manifestations (e.g., butterfly rash, generalized erythema, oral ulcers), they are not suitable for evaluating the activity and damage of the different CLE subtypes. Therefore, the scoring system Cutaneous Lupus Erythematosus Disease Area and Severity Index (CLASI) has been developed for patients with cutaneous manifestations to assess disease activity and damage, taking into account anatomical regions (e.g., face, chest, arms) and morphological aspects (e.g., erythema, edema, infiltration, scarring, atrophy).[42] By increasing the accuracy of existing parameters, such as scaling/hypertrophy and dyspigmentation, and by including several new parameters, such as edema/infiltration and subcutaneous nodule/plaque, the CLASI was revised in 2010.[43] Thus, the revised CLASI is a validated scoring system for the clinical evaluation of activity and damage in different CLE subtypes, and is currently applied in several clinical trials.

SUBTYPES OF CUTANEOUS LUPUS ERYTHEMATOSUS

Acute Cutaneous Lupus Erythematosus

Acute cutaneous lupus erythematosus (ACLE) may occur as a localized, occasionally transient, or generalized widespread form.[44] Most common is localized ACLE, which presents as a malar rash ("butterfly rash") in approximately 50% of patients during the course of SLE (Figure 1).[25] The erythema symmetrically affects the bridge of the nose and cheeks, typically sparing the nasolabial folds, and can be misdiagnosed as sunburn. It commonly starts with discrete small, erythematous macules or papules, which subsequently become confluent. Generalized ACLE is less common and often occurs concomitantly with systemic disease activity. The erythematous to violaceous, maculopapular widespread exanthema symmetrically involves the trunk and extremities, in particular UV-exposed areas (V-area of the neck and extensor aspects of the arms). On the hands, the knuckles are typically spared; telangiectasia and periungual erythema occur at the nail fold and may be associated with a red lunula. Skin lesions in ACLE usually heal without scarring or dyspigmentation. Diffuse thinning of the hair ("lupus hair") along the hairline is frequently associated with ACLE.[45] Superficial mucosal ulcers may affect the hard palate, but they may also be found anywhere in the oral cavity, on the lips, and in the nose. However, the highly acute form of generalized ACLE characterized by toxic epidermal necrolysis (TEN)-like lesions and described as "Acute Syndrome of Apoptotic Panepidermolysis" is rarely seen in patients with the disease.[46]

Subacute Cutaneous Lupus Erythematosus (SCLE)

In the cohort evaluated by EUSCLE, SCLE was diagnosed in 236 of 1002 patients and was associated with discoid LE (DLE) in 53 patients.[36] Drug-induced CLE was found in 6% of the 1002 patients, with the highest prevalence of drug-induced SCLE (31 of 236 patients). In annular SCLE, the lesions are characterized by a ring-shaped erythema with peripheral collarette scaling at the inner border, central clearing, and polycyclic confluence of the annular lesions (Figure 2).[47] In rare cases, vesiculobullous lesions develop at the periphery of annular SCLE lesions. The papulosquamous/psoriasiform SCLE shows psoriasis- or eczema-like lesions. Both forms, the annular and the papulosquamous/psoriasiform type of SCLE, can be concurrently present in the same patient. The recurrent, non-scarring skin lesions of SCLE usually appear in a symmetric distribution on sun-exposed areas, such as the V-area of the neck (often sparing the area under the chin), the upper ventral and/or the dorsal part of the trunk and extensor aspects of the extremities; face and scalp are rarely involved.

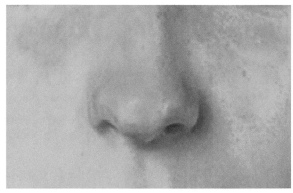

FIGURE 1   ACLE: butterfly rash with symmetrical erythema on malar areas and back of the nose sparing the nasolabial folds.

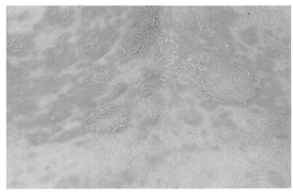

FIGURE 2   SCLE: polycyclic confluence of the annular lesions with central clearing and collarette staining at the inner border of the lower back.

A diagnostic "clue" of this subtype can be the healing with vitiligo-like, sometimes permanent hypopigmentation, especially if treatment is delayed.[45] Patients with SCLE are typically photosensitive and UV radiation can induce and/or exacerbate skin manifestations.[15] Similar to ACLE, a TEN-like picture can rarely occur in patients with SCLE, especially after exposure to UV light.[46] In particular in genetically susceptible individuals, SCLE can be triggered by different drugs, such as anti-diuretics/anti-hypertensives (i.e., hydrochlorothiazide, calcium channel blockers, ACE inhibitors) and anti fungals (up to now, terbinafine is considered the most common cause of drug-induced SCLE).[48,49] SCLE shows a characteristic immunogenetic disposition and is associated with the HLA-A1, -B8, -DR3 haplotype and the -308A TNF promoter polymorphism.[50] Characteristic serological features of SCLE are anti-Ro/SSA (in 70–90%) and anti-La/SSB antibodies (in 30–50%, nearly always together with anti-Ro/SSA antibodies).[51–53] SLE with often milder course will develop in 10–15% of SCLE patients.[47] The immunogenetic background of SCLE is similar to Sjögren's syndrome; therefore, patients with SCLE are reported to be at higher risk to develop features of Sjögren's syndrome in the course of the disease.[47,54]

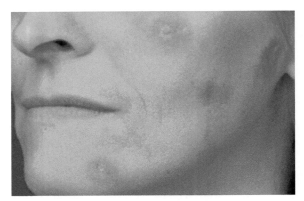

FIGURE 3   DLE: several active discoid lesions with erythematous border and white hyperkeratotic center on the left part of the face.

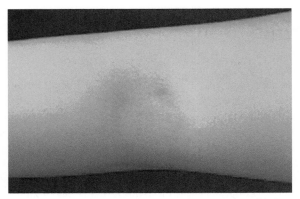

FIGURE 4   LEP: typical deep lipatrophy after resolution of lesions on the upper right arm.

Chronic Cutaneous Lupus Erythematosus (CCLE)

CCLE includes three different forms: discoid LE (DLE), LE profundus/LE panniculitis (LEP), and chilblain LE (CHLE).

Discoid Lupus Erythematosus (DLE)

In the study published by EUSCLE, DLE was diagnosed in 397 of 1002 patients.[36] DLE is the most common form of CCLE and occurs as localized form (ca. 80%) with lesions on the face and scalp, especially the cheeks, forehead, ears, nose, and upper lip or as disseminated/generalized form (ca. 20%) with lesions involving the upper part of the trunk and the extensor aspects of the extremities.[44] The lesions of DLE develop unilaterally or bilaterally and consist of sharply-demarcated, coin-shaped ("discoid") indurated erythematous plaques with adherent follicular hyperkeratosis (Figure 3). Removal of the keratotic spikes causes pain and is termed "carpet tack sign."[45] Slowly, the lesions expand at the periphery with an active erythematous border and hyperpigmentation, resulting in atrophy, scarring, telangiectasia and hypopigmentation in the center of the lesions. At the scalp, eyebrows and bearded regions of the face, DLE can progress to total, irreversible scarring alopecia. In the perioral region, DLE lesions can lead to characteristic pitted acneiform ("vermicular") scarring.[55] Mucosal DLE with chronic buccal plaques, presenting typically as roundish lesions with peripheral white hyperkeratotic striae and central atrophy, erosion or ulceration, has to be differentiated from lichen planus.[45] In anatomically specific regions (for example ear, tip of the nose, margin of eyelid), mutilations can occur resulting in high burden of the disease. Palmoplantar involvement can present as discoid and erythematous scaly plaques or rarely painful erosions. Exposure to the sun or irritating stimuli ("Koebner phenomenon" or "isomorphic response"), such as trauma, tattoos, scratching, and various types of dermatitis, can provoke or exacerbate the disease.[56,57] DLE lesions occur in approximately 15–25% in the course of SLE, but more than 95% of patients with DLE lesions suffer from cutaneous lesions only. Disseminated DLE has an increased risk to develop systemic organ manifestations.[25,44,58]

Lupus Erythematosus Profundus/Panniculitis (LEP)

LEP is a rare variant of CCLE and is associated with DLE in 70% of patients,[44] but is rarely (less than 3%) present in the context of SLE.[25,44] This subtype clinically presents with single or multiple well-defined, persistent asymptomatic and sometimes painful indurated subcutaneous nodules and plaques, which may later firmly adhere to the overlying skin. The surface of the LEP lesions may appear without clinical changes or can show signs of DLE. In the course of the disease, the nodules develop into deep, asymptomatic lipatrophy or deep retracted scars; ulceration is rare (Figure 4). Skin lesions of LEP are typically located in areas of increased fat deposition, such as the gluteal region, the thighs or the upper and lower extremities, but face, scalp, and chest can also be involved. Rarely, periorbital edema may be an initial presenting symptom prior to the development of typical skin changes.[45] LEP can also be induced by irritative stimuli but usually not by UV exposure.[44]

Chilblain Lupus Erythematosus (CHLE)

CHLE is a further manifestation of CCLE, which is influenced by environmental factors, such as cold, damp weather or a critical drop in temperature, and often clinically and histologically difficult to distinguish from frostbites ("chilblains"). Association of CHLE with other CLE subtypes, such as DLE, has been described in the literature; in up to 20% of patients, CHLE is associated with SLE.[59–61] This subtype is characterized by symmetrically distributed, circumscribed pruriginous or painful bluish plaques and nodules.[45] Edematous plaques and nodules may develop central erosions or ulcerations, which affect the acral surfaces,

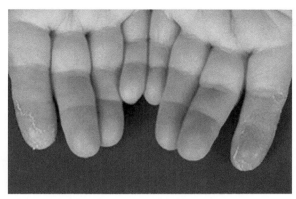

FIGURE 5   CHLE: erythematous inflammation with scaling and hyper-keratosis at finger tips and palmar sites of D2.

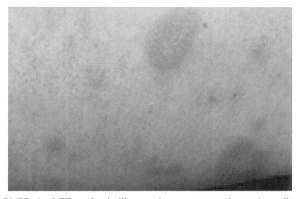

FIGURE 6   LET: urticaria-like, erythematous, annular and semilunar plaques and papules on the upper arm.

especially fingers, toes, heels, nose, ears, elbows, knees, and calves (Figure 5).[62] The description of a monogenic autosomal dominant, inherited familial chilblain lupus presenting in early childhood and usually caused by mutations in TREX-1, has provided novel insights into the molecular pathogenesis and on our understanding of the disease.[63–65] Recently, associations with mutations in TREX-1 have also been described in single SLE patients.[65]

Intermittent Cutaneous Lupus Erythematosus (ICLE)

Lupus Erythematosus Tumidus (LET)

LET is characterized by sharply-bordered, "succulent," urticaria-like, single or multiple erythematous papules and plaques with a smooth surface without epidermal involvement (Figure 6).[66] In the course of the disease, the lesions may be semilunar or annular with swelling in the periphery and flattening in the center.[30] In contrast to annular SCLE, the lesions of LET show no scaling and resolve without residual defects, such as scarring or dyspigmentation. The lesions of LET patients are typically found in sun-exposed areas (e.g., face, upper back, upper chest, extensor aspects of the upper arms), but rare reports exist describing LET below the waist.[67] LET is the most photosensitive subtype of CLE, as skin lesions can be experimentally induced by UV radiation in more than 70% of patients.[10,68] The analysis of 1002 patients by EUSCLE revealed that smoking is a risk factor for the development of this subtype.[38] Association with SLE seems to be extremely rare in patients with LET, only a few cases have been reported.[31] Therefore, this subtype has a good prognosis with a variable course of the disease in the majority of patients.[30] The identification of the specific clinical, histological, and photobiological criteria has resulted in the definition of LET as a distinct entity and has therefore been included in the "Duesseldorf Classification" as "intermittent cutaneous LE" (ICLE).[27]

CONCLUSION

Skin manifestations are one of the most frequent symptoms in patients with SLE, can develop at any stage of the disease and are the first sign in approximately 25% of patients. To differentiate SLE from other connective tissue diseases, the 11 ACR criteria can be helpful, but the comparative high number of dermatological criteria (malar rash, discoid lesions, photosensitivity, and oral ulcers) may result in an overestimation of SLE.[4,5] The recently developed SLICC criteria have still to be evaluated in everyday clinical practice. Skin manifestations in SLE are divided in LE-nonspecific manifestations, such as urticarial vasculitis, and LE-specific manifestations comprising the four CLE subtypes including ACLE, SCLE, CCLE, and ICLE. Patients should be advised that UV exposure can induce and exacerbate existing skin lesions. Sun protection, such as protective clothing and daily application of broad spectrum sunscreens, continuous avoidance of the sun, and elimination of potentially photosensitizing drugs are of high importance in the prevention of the disease.

ACKNOWLEDGMENT

The figures were kindly provided by the Photographic Laboratory (with thanks to J. Bueckmann and P. Wissel), Department of Dermatology, University of Muenster, Germany.

REFERENCES

1. Jimenez S, Cervera R, Ingelmo M, Font J. The epidemiology of cutaneous lupus erythematosus. In: Kuhn A, Lehmann P, Ruzicka T, editors. *Cutaneous lupus erythematosus.* Berlin: Springer-Verlag; 2004. p. 45–52.
2. Tebbe B, Orfanos CE. Epidemiology and socioeconomic impact of skin disease in lupus erythematosus. *Lupus* 1997;**6**:96–104.
3. Popovic K, Nyberg F, Wahren-Herlenius M. A serology-based approach combined with clinical examination of 125 Ro/SSA-positive patients to define incidence and prevalence of subacute cutaneous lupus erythematosus. *Arthritis Rheum* 2007;**56**:255–64.

4. Tan EM, Cohen AS, Fries JF, et al. The 1982 revised criteria for the classification of systemic lupus erythematosus. *Arthritis Rheum* 1982;**25**:1271–7.

5. Albrecht J, Berlin JA, Braverman IM, et al. Dermatology position paper on the revision of the 1982 ACR criteria for systemic lupus erythematosus. *Lupus* 2004;**13**:839–49.

6. Petri M, Orbai AM, Alarcon GS, et al. Derivation and validation of the Systemic Lupus International Collaborating Clinics classification criteria for systemic lupus erythematosus. *Arthritis Rheum* 2012;**64**:2677–86.

7. Kuhn A, Beissert S. Photosensitivity in lupus erythematosus. *Autoimmunity* 2005;**38**:519–29.

8. Scheinfeld N, Deleo VA. Photosensitivity in lupus erythematosus. *Photodermatol Photoimmunol Photomed* 2004;**20**:272–9.

9. Furukawa F. Photosensitivity in cutaneous lupus erythematosus: lessons from mice and men. *J Dermatol Sci* 2003;**33**:81–9.

10. Kuhn A, Ruland V, Bonsmann G. Photosensitivity, phototesting, and photoprotection in cutaneous lupus erythematosus. *Lupus* 2010;**19**:1036–46.

11. Foering K, Chang AY, Piette EW, et al. Characterization of clinical photosensitivity in cutaneous lupus erythematosus. *J Am Acad Dermatol* 2013;**69**:205–13.

12. Schmidt E, Tony HP, Brocker EB, Kneitz C. Sun-induced life-threatening lupus nephritis. *Ann N Y Acad Sci* 2007;**1108**:35–40.

13. Vila LM, Mayor AM, Valentin AH, et al. Association of sunlight exposure and photoprotection measures with clinical outcome in systemic lupus erythematosus. *P R Health Sci J* 1999;**18**:89–94.

14. Kuhn A, Gensch K, Haust M, et al. Photoprotective effects of a broad-spectrum sunscreen in ultraviolet-induced cutaneous lupus erythematosus: a randomized, vehicle-controlled, double-blind study. *J Am Acad Dermatol* 2011;**64**:37–48.

15. Kuhn A, Sonntag M, Richter-Hintz D, et al. Phototesting in lupus erythematosus: a 15-year experience. *J Am Acad Dermatol* 2001;**45**:86–95.

16. Sanders CJ, Van Weelden H, Kazzaz GA, et al. Photosensitivity in patients with lupus erythematosus: a clinical and photobiological study of 100 patients using a prolonged phototest protocol. *Br J Dermatol* 2003;**149**:131–7.

17. Kuhn A, Wozniacka A, Szepietowski JC, et al. Photoprovocation in cutaneous lupus erythematosus: a multicenter study evaluating a standardized protocol. *J Invest Dermatol* 2011;**131**:1622–30.

18. Ruland V, Haust M, Stilling RM, et al. Updated analysis of standardised photoprovocation in patients with cutaneous lupus erythematosus. *Arthritis Care Res* 2012;**65**:767–76.

19. Patsinakidis N, Wenzel J, Landmann A, et al. Suppression of UV-induced damage by a liposomal sunscreen: a prospective, open-label study in patients with cutaneous lupus erythematosus and healthy controls. *Exp Dermatol* 2012;**21**:958–61.

20. Zahn S, Graef M, Patsinakidis N, et al. Ultraviolet light protection by a sunscreen prevents interferon-driven skin inflammation in cutaneous lupus erythematosus. *Exp Dermatol* 2014;**23**:516–8.

21. Gutmark EL, Lin DQ, Bernstein I, Wang SQ, Chong BF. Sunscreen use in cutaneous lupus erythematosus patients. *Br J Dermatol* 2015;**173**:831–4.

22. Faurschou A, Wulf HC. The relation between sun protection factor and amount of suncreen applied in vivo. *Br J Dermatol* 2007;**156**:716–9.

23. Gilliam JN, Sontheimer RD. Distinctive cutaneous subsets in the spectrum of lupus erythematosus. *J Am Acad Dermatol* 1981;**4**:471–5.

24. Uva L, Miguel D, Pinheiro C, et al. Cutaneous manifestations of systemic lupus erythematosus. *Autoimmune Dis* 2012;**2012**:834291.

25. Obermoser G, Sontheimer RD, Zelger B. Overview of common, rare and atypical manifestations of cutaneous lupus erythematosus and histopathological correlates. *Lupus* 2010;**19**:1050–70.

26. Provost TT. Nonspecific cutaneous manifestations of systemic lupus erythematosus. In: Kuhn A, Lehmann P, Ruzicka T, editors. *Cutanoeus lupus erythematosus.* Heidelberg: Springer; 2004. p. 93–106.

27. Kuhn A, Ruzicka T. Classification of cutaneous lupus erythematosus. In: Kuhn A, Lehmann P, Ruzicka T, editors. *Cutaneous lupus erythematosus.* Heidelberg: Springer; 2004. p. 53–8.

28. Werth VP. Cutaneous lupus: insights into pathogenesis and disease classification. *Bull NYU Hosp Jt Dis* 2007;**65**:200–4.

29. Sontheimer RD. The lexicon of cutaneous lupus erythematosus - a review and personal perspective on the nomenclature and classification of the cutaneous manifestations of lupus erythematosus. *Lupus* 1997;**6**:84–95.

30. Schmitt V, Meuth AM, Amler S, et al. Lupus erythematosus tumidus is a separate subtype of cutaneous lupus erythematosus. *Br J Dermatol* 2010;**162**:64–73.

31. Kuhn A, Bein D, Bonsmann G. The 100th anniversary of lupus erythematosus tumidus. *Autoimmun Rev* 2009b;**8**:441–8.

32. Rodriguez-Caruncho C, Bielsa I. Lupus erythematosus tumidus: a clinical entity still being defined. *Actas Dermosifiliogr* 2011;**102**:668–74.

33. Kuhn A, Landmann A. The classification and diagnosis of cutaneous lupus erythematosus. *J Autoimmun* 2014;**48-49**:14–9.

34. Kuhn A, Kuehn E, Meuth AM, et al. Development of a core set questionnaire by the European Society of Cutaneous Lupus Erythematosus (EUSCLE). *Autoimmun Rev* 2009;**8**:702–12.

35. Kuhn A, Patsinakidis N, Bonsmann G. The impact of the EUSCLE Core Set Questionnaire for the assessment of cutaneous lupus erythematosus. *Lupus* 2010;**19**:1144–52.

36. Biazar C, Sigges J, Patsinakidis N, et al. Cutaneous lupus erythematosus: first multicenter database analysis of 1002 patients from the European Society of Cutaneous Lupus Erythematosus (EUSCLE). *Autoimmun Rev* 2013;**12**:444–54.

37. Sigges J, Biazar C, Landmann A, et al. Therapeutic strategies evaluated by the European Society of Cutaneous Lupus Erythematosus (EUSCLE) Core Set Questionnaire in more than 1000 patients with cutaneous lupus erythematosus. *Autoimmun Rev* 2013;**12**:694–702.

38. Kuhn A, Sigges J, Biazar C, et al. Influence of smoking on disease severity and antimalarial therapy in cutaneous lupus erythematosus: analysis of 1002 patients from the EUSCLE database. *Br J Dermatol* 2014;**171**:571–9.

39. Griffiths B, Mosca M, Gordon C. Assessment of patients with systemic lupus erythematosus and the use of lupus disease activity indices. *Best Pract Res Clin Rheumatol* 2005;**19**:685–708.

40. Ward MM, Marx AS, Barry NN. Comparison of the validity and sensitivity to change of 5 activity indices in systemic lupus erythematosus. *J Rheumatol* 2000;**27**:664–70.

41. Gladman D, Ginzler E, Goldsmith C, et al. The development and initial validation of the Systemic Lupus International Collaborating Clinics/American College of Rheumatology damage index for systemic lupus erythematosus. *Arthritis Rheum* 1996;**39**:363–9.

42. Albrecht J, Taylor L, Berlin JA, et al. The CLASI (Cutaneous Lupus Erythematosus Disease Area and Severity Index): an outcome instrument for cutaneous lupus erythematosus. *J Invest Dermatol* 2005;**125**:889–94.

43. Kuhn A, Meuth AM, Bein D, et al. Revised Cutaneous Lupus Erythematosus Disease Area and Severity Index (RCLASI): a modified outcome instrument for cutaneous lupus erythematosus. *Br J Dermatol* 2010;**163**:83–92.

44. Costner MI, Sontheimer RD, Provost TT. Lupus erythematosus. In: Sontheimer RD, Provost TT, editors. *Cutaneous manifestations of rheumatic diseases*. Philadelphia: Williams & Wilkins; 2003. p. 15–64.

45. Kuhn A, Sticherling M, Bonsmann G. Clinical manifestations of cutaneous lupus erythematosus. *J Dtsch Dermatol Ges* 2007;**5**:1124–37.

46. Ting W, Stone MS, Racila D, Scofield RH, Sontheimer RD. Toxic epidermal necrolysis-like acute cutaneous lupus erythematosus and the spectrum of the acute syndrome of apoptotic pan-epidermolysis (ASAP): a case report, concept review and proposal for new classification of lupus erythematosus vesiculobullous skin lesions. *Lupus* 2004;**13**:941–50.

47. Sontheimer RD. Subacute cutaneous lupus erythematosus: 25-year evolution of a prototypic subset (subphenotype) of lupus erythematosus defined by characteristic cutaneous, pathological, immunological, and genetic findings. *Autoimmun Rev* 2005;**4**:253–63.

48. Sontheimer RD, Henderson CL, Grau RH. Drug-induced subacute cutaneous lupus erythematosus: a paradigm for bedside-to-bench patient-oriented translational clinical investigation. *Arch Dermatol Res* 2009;**301**:65–70.

49. Gronhagen CM, Fored CM, Linder M, Granath F, Nyberg F. Subacute cutaneous lupus erythematosus and its association with drugs: a population-based matched case-control study of 234 patients in Sweden. *Br J Dermatol* 2012;**167**:296–305.

50. Werth VP, Zhang W, Dortzbach K, Sullivan K. Association of a promoter polymorphism of tumor necrosis factor-alpha with subacute cutaneous lupus erythematosus and distinct photoregulation of transcription. *J Invest Dermatol* 2000;**115**:726–30.

51. Sontheimer RD, Maddison PJ, Reichlin M, et al. Serologic and HLA associations in subacute cutaneous lupus erythematosus, a clinical subset of lupus erythematosus. *Ann Intern Med* 1982;**97**:664–71.

52. Chlebus E, Wolska H, Blaszczyk M, Jablonska S. Subacute cutaneous lupus erythematosus versus systemic lupus erythematosus: diagnostic criteria and therapeutic implications. *J Am Acad Dermatol* 1998;**38**:405–12.

53. Lee LA, Roberts CM, Frank MB, McCubbin VR, Reichlin M. The autoantibody response to Ro/SSA in cutaneous lupus erythematosus. *Arch Dermatol* 1994;**130**:1262–8.

54. Black DR, Hornung CA, Schneider PD, Callen JP. Frequency and severity of systemic disease in patients with subacute cutaneous lupus erythematosus. *Arch Dermatol* 2002;**138**:1175–8.

55. Chang YH, Wang SH, Chi CC. Discoid lupus erythematosus presenting as acneiform pitting scars. *Int J Dermatol* 2006;**45**:944–5.

56. Ueki H. Koebner phenomenon in lupus erythematosus with special consideration of clinical findings. *Autoimmun Rev* 2005;**4**:219–23.

57. Kuhn A, Aberer E, Barde C, et al. Leitlinien kutaner lupus erythematodes (Entwicklungsstufe 1). In: Korting HCCR, Reusch M, Schlaeger M, Sterry W, editors. *Dermatologische qualitätssicherung: leitlinien und empfehlungen*. Berlin: ABW Wissenschaftsverlag GmbH; 2009. p. 214–57.

58. Tebbe B, Mansmann U, Wollina U, et al. Markers in cutaneous lupus erythematosus indicating systemic involvement. A multicenter study on 296 patients. *Acta Derm Venereol* 1997;**77**:305–8.

59. Viguier M, Pinquier L, Cavelier-Balloy B, et al. Clinical and histopathologic features and immunologic variables in patients with severe chilblains. A study of the relationship to lupus erythematosus. *Medicine* 2001;**80**:180–8.

60. Hedrich CM, Fiebig B, Hauck FH, et al. Chilblain lupus erythematosus–a review of literature. *Clin Rheumatol* 2008;**27**:949–54.

61. Millard LG, Rowell NR. Chilblain lupus erythematosus (Hutchinson). A clinical and laboratory study of 17 patients. *Br J Dermatol* 1978;**98**:497–506.

62. Helm TN, Jones CM. Chilblain lupus erythematosus lesions precipitated by the cold. *Cutis* 2002;**69**:183–4.

63. Lee-Kirsch MA, Gong M, Schulz H, et al. Familial chilblain lupus, a monogenic form of cutaneous lupus erythematosus, maps to chromosome 3p. *Am J Hum Genet* 2006;**79**:731–7.

64. Gunther C, Berndt N, Wolf C, Lee-Kirsch MA. Familial chilblain lupus due to a novel mutation in the exonuclease III domain of 3′ repair exonuclease 1 (TREX1). *JAMA Dermatol* 2015;**151**:426–31.

65. Rice GI, Rodero MP, Crow YJ. Human disease phenotypes associated with mutations in TREX1. *J Clin Immunol* 2015;**35**:235–43.

66. Kuhn A, Richter-Hintz D, Oslislo C, et al. Lupus erythematosus tumidus - a neglected subset of cutaneous lupus erythematosus: report of 40 cases. *Arch Dermatol* 2000;**136**:1033–41.

67. Stead J, Headley C, Ioffreda M, Kovarik C, Werth V. Coexistence of tumid lupus erythematosus with systemic lupus erythematosus and discoid lupus erythematosus: a report of two cases of tumid lupus. *J Clin Rheumatol* 2008;**14**:338–41.

68. Kuhn A, Sonntag M, Richter-Hintz D, et al. Phototesting in lupus erythematosus tumidus-review of 60 patients. *Photochem Photobiol* 2001;**73**:532–6.

Chapter 40

The Clinical Evaluation of Kidney Disease in Systemic Lupus Erythematosus

Brad H. Rovin, Isabelle Ayoub

Division of Nephrology, Ohio State University Wexner Medical Center, Columbus, OH, USA

INTRODUCTION

Kidney disease is common in patients with systemic lupus erythematosus (SLE). This is most often due to lupus nephritis (LN). In LN, immune complexes accumulate in glomeruli and initiate an inflammatory response that can also involve the renal interstitium. This process may result in injury to the entire kidney parenchyma (see Chapter 33). Besides LN, other mechanisms may lead to kidney damage in SLE, such as thrombotic microangiopathy. LN is one of the major causes of morbidity and mortality in SLE patients and is associated with poorer outcomes than in those patients with no kidney involvement.[1,2] This poor prognosis is explained only in part by the risk of chronic kidney disease (CKD) and end-stage renal disease (ESRD), suggesting that LN is a manifestation of a more severe form of SLE.

LN is often treatable. The best outcomes occur with early recognition and prompt treatment. Early recognition requires a high index of suspicion and the appropriate use of screening tests for kidney involvement followed by confirmatory tests and a kidney biopsy.

THE SCOPE OF LUPUS NEPHRITIS

Examination of kidney tissue from SLE patients who had no clinical signs of kidney disease suggested that LN may be present in up to 90% of lupus patients.[3,4] Most of this clinically silent LN was associated with very mild histologic changes, but about 15% of patients had moderate to severe pathology, many of whom did eventually develop proteinuria, an abnormal urine sediment, or renal insufficiency. Silent LN may represent the earliest stage in the natural history of LN.[5]

The incidence of clinically overt kidney disease in all lupus populations is about 38%, but this varies greatly among racial and ethnic groups. The incidence of LN in nonwhite SLE patients is 50% or more, whereas only 12–33% of white patients (European, European Americans) develop LN.[6]

LN is reported in 40–69% of black patients (African American, Afro-Caribbean) and 47–53% of Asian patients, and occurs frequently (36–61%) in Hispanic patients.[6]

Adverse kidney outcomes, such as ESRD or doubling of serum creatinine (a surrogate marker of ESRD) are also more frequent in black and Hispanic patients as compared to white patients.[7] The incidence of ESRD attributed to LN in adults is 4.9 cases per million in the general population, but is 17–20 per million in black patients and 6 per million in Hispanics compared to 2.5 per million in white patients.[6] According to the 2014 United States Renal Data System report, about 2% of the prevalent patients receiving renal replacement therapy have ESRD attributable to LN.

Beyond ESRD, the prevalence of CKD in patients with LN is difficult to quantify. However, if it is assumed that, at a minimum, a complete clinical renal response after treatment is needed to prevent CKD from developing, the prevalence of CKD is likely to be high, as many LN patients achieve only a partial renal response (Chapters 5 and 62). CKD in LN is important not only because it may progress to ESRD, but also because it is a nontraditional risk factor for cardiovascular morbidity, as is lupus itself.[8,9] The highest mortality in LN is seen in patients with chronic kidney damage.[1,2]

THE DIAGNOSIS OF LUPUS NEPHRITIS

The early diagnosis and treatment of LN is critical to preserve kidney function.[10–12] The key to early diagnosis is maintaining a high index of suspicion for renal involvement in every SLE patient. Patients who present with LN when SLE is first diagnosed have higher rates of prolonged remission and a lower frequency of chronic kidney damage than those whose LN presents later. This may be because of early recognition, but only about half of LN patients have evidence of kidney disease at the initial presentation of SLE.[13,14] An algorithm to identify kidney involvement in SLE patients is shown in Figure 1.

Systemic Lupus Erythematosus. http://dx.doi.org/10.1016/B978-0-12-801917-7.00040-1

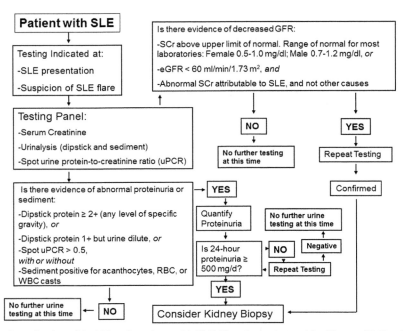

FIGURE 1 An algorithm for the evaluation of the kidney in patients with SLE. Note that patients with a history of LN and previous kidney biopsy may not need a repeat biopsy (see Figure 4). Kidney biopsy should be done for new diagnoses of kidney involvement. Acanthocytes are dysmorphic red blood cells specific for glomerular bleeding (see Figure 2). Abbreviations: SCr, serum creatinine; GFR, glomerular filtration rate; uPCR, protein-to- creatinine ratio in a urine sample.

Evaluation of Kidney Function

Kidney function should be assessed during the initial evaluation of SLE, during SLE flares, and whenever a renal flare is suspected. Traditionally, renal function has been evaluated by the serum creatinine level or by calculating creatinine clearance from a 24-h urine collection. Because it is difficult to reliably determine the completeness of a 24-h urine collection, equations to estimate creatinine clearance and, more recently, the glomerular filtration rate (GFR) have been incorporated into clinical practice. Nonetheless, all methods used to estimate kidney function in place of measuring GFR (which is not clinically practical) have limitations that affect their interpretation (Table 1).

Creatinine production is proportional to muscle mass. Individuals with small to moderate muscle mass, like many women with SLE, may normally have low serum creatinine levels (even below the lower limit of the clinical laboratory's range). In such individuals, a serum creatinine that falls at the clinical laboratory's upper limit may reflect impaired renal function. Conversely, individuals with high muscle mass may have normal kidney function despite a serum creatinine that is above the clinical laboratory's upper limit. Additionally, tubular secretion of creatinine increases in hypoalbuminemic nephrotic patients, lowering serum creatinine and giving the impression that GFR is better than it really is.[15] Finally, muscle metabolism can be affected by the high-dose glucocorticoids used in the treatment of LN, and this may acutely increase serum creatinine

levels.[16] Although cystatin C has been suggested as a superior endogenous marker of GFR than serum creatinine, it too can be affected by medications used to treat LN, such as corticosteroids and cyclosporine A.[17]

The Cockcroft-Gault formula has been used to estimate creatinine clearance for years. Now, however, many clinical laboratories provide an estimated GFR (eGFR) value whenever serum creatinine is measured. The eGFR is calculated using serum creatinine, sex, race, and age in equations derived from the Modification of Diet in Renal Disease (MDRD) study or the Chronic Kidney Disease Epidemiology Collaboration (CKD-Epi). CKD-Epi is more accurate than MDRD at eGFR >60 ml/min and is now the preferred GFR estimating equation for patients with CKD.[18]

GFR estimating equations have several limitations. All estimating equations assume that patients of a given serum creatinine, sex, race, and age have similar body surface areas and rates of creatinine production.[19] None of the equations were developed using a typical SLE population of young women. Two studies compared the accuracy and precision of the Cockcroft-Gault and MDRD equations to directly measured creatinine clearance, one in Chinese patients with LN[20] and the other in Caucasian and African American patients with LN.[21] In Asian patients with impaired kidney function, the MDRD equation was a modestly better estimate of creatinine clearance than Cockcroft-Gault, but the opposite was found in Caucasian and African American patients.

TABLE 1 Comparison of Methods for Estimating GFR

Method	Rationale	Strengths	Weaknesses
(1) Serum creatinine (SCr)	Creatinine is usually produced at a constant rate, excreted almost entirely by the kidney, and mainly by glomerular filtration. Thus, usually changes in SCr reflect change in GFR.	Simple and relatively inexpensive.	There are many conditions that can increase or decrease SCr independent of GFR. The most common are: • Changes in intake of cooked meat (cooking converts creatine to creatinine). SCr is about 25% lower on a vegetarian diet. • Drugs that decrease tubular secretion of creatinine (trimethoprim and cimetidine) raise SCr by 10–30%. • Hypoalbuminemia in severely nephrotic patients is associated with an increase in tubular secretion of creatinine. • Drugs that affect muscle metabolism Small changes in SCr (e.g., ±0.3 mg/dl) when SCr is in the normal range correspond to very large changes in GFR (about ±20%). Confounding this interpretation is that the 95% confidence intervals of the measurement of SCr are also about ±0.2 mg/dl for SCr values around the normal range. Thus, often it is necessary to measure SCr 2 or 3 times to assess whether a real change in GFR has occurred versus a spontaneous laboratory variation.
(2) Creatinine clearance (C$_{Cr}$)	C$_{Cr}$ refers to the renal clearance of creatinine, which is usually a close estimate of GFR. C$_{Cr}$ = (amount of creatinine in a complete 24-hr urine collection)/(average SCr during the period that the urine was collected). In most patients SCr is stable. Thus, SCr measured at the start or end of the 24-hr collection reflects the average SCr during the urine collection. If SCr is changing (as in acute renal failure), the SCr measured at the midpoint of the collection is a good estimate of the average SCr during the collection.	C$_{Cr}$ estimate of GFR is not affected by changes in creatinine production so long as the patient is in a steady state (serum creatinine is stable).	An accurate estimate of C$_{Cr}$ is dependent on a complete 24-hr collection. Thus, the error in estimating GFR from C$_{Cr}$ is directly proportional to the completeness of the intended 24-hr collection. • C$_{Cr}$ underestimates GFR if the patient is receiving trimethoprim or cimetidine. See weaknesses of SCr (above). • At low GFR (e.g., <30% of normal), C$_{Cr}$ overestimates GFR by 10–50%.
Cockroft-Gault (C-G)	C-G estimates creatinine clearance from patients' age, sex, race, ideal body weight (IBW), and serum creatinine. C-G = (140-age) × IBW kg (×0.85 if female)/72 × SCr, mg/dl (×1.21 if black) = ml/min.	C-G takes into account the most common reasons for variation in serum creatinine: variation in body size, sex, and race.	C-G does not take into account the factors that change SCr independent of change in GFR. See weaknesses of SCr (above). • In advanced renal failure, creatinine clearance can be 10–50% higher than GFR.

Continued

TABLE 1 Comparison of Methods for Estimating GFR—cont'd

Method	Rationale	Strengths	Weaknesses
MDRD-4	MDRD-4 GFR (eGFR) is estimated from a complex formula based on the patient's age, sex, race, and serum creatinine. The eGFR equation was calculated from a large number of patients whose GFR was directly measured (usually by iothalamate clearance, see below) and whose age, sex, race, and serum creatinine were known.	The MDRD-4 eGFR provides a quantitative estimate of GFR level that is not intuitively obvious from the serum creatinine level because of the hyperbolic relationship between serum creatinine and GFR.	MDRD-4 eGFR has poor precision at GFR >60ml/min/1.73 m². Thus, a single measure in patients with serum creatinine at or near the normal range is not a reliable measure of GFR. Multiple measures, however, improve precision. The MDRD-4 eGFR assumes everyone of the same age, race, and sex has the same rate of creatinine production. Thus, MDRD-4 underestimates GFR in large persons (or those with other mechanisms of increased creatinine production) and overestimates GFR in those with low creatinine production. MDRD-4 eGFR also suffers from confounding by all of the other factors that influence SCr, independent of GFR. See weaknesses, SCr (above). The MDRD-4 eGFR is most useful in comparing GFR between large populations where the influence of body size, diet, etc. can be expected to be similar in the groups being compared.
CKD-EPI	This is the latest version of eGFR. It is calculated from a complex formula similar to that of MDRD-4 eGFR. However, CKD-Epi used a larger and more diverse data set.	CKD-EPI eGFR is somewhat more accurate than MDRD-4 eGFR in those with GFR >60ml/min/1.73 m².	The weaknesses are the same as MDRD-4 eGFR.
Iothalamate clearance (C_{Iotha}) Inulin clearance (C_{In}), Iohexol clearance (C_{Iohex})	These molecules are true markers of glomerular filtration. They are freely filtered at the glomerulus and there is little or no tubular secretion or absorption of these markers. Thus, their renal clearance reflects GFR.	C_{Iotha}, C_{In} and C_{Iohex} are true measures of GFR.	A single measure is not a reliable estimate of the patient's prevailing GFR, particularly in those with GFR >60ml/min/1.73 m². • Expensive. Time consuming. • Not useful in individual patients to decide whether GFR is normal based on a single measure.

A third study compared creatinine clearance and several estimating equations to CKD-Epi in an LN cohort and recommended CKD-Epi.[22] However, none of the studies compared calculated and measured eGFR, so none of the GFR equations have truly been compared to a gold standard GFR measurement in SLE patients.

In summary, serial serum creatinine measurements remain useful in the management of individual patients. For individuals who are obese, have extremes of muscle mass, or have skewed diets (vegetarian, high meat intake), the Cockcroft-Gault formula adjusted for actual body surface area is a better estimate of GFR than the creatinine-based equations that do not include body weight and size.[23] After determining that a lupus patient has impaired GFR, other common causes of acute kidney injury (Table 2) should be excluded to attribute the reduced function to LN.

TABLE 2 Etiologies of Acute Renal Insufficiency in SLE Other than LN

Infections including bacteriemia and sepsis

Volume depletion

Hypotension

Nephrotoxin exposure (e.g., radiographic contrast)

Hemolysis

Thrombosis

Cardiac failure

Commonly prescribed medications:

    Nonsteroidal anti-inflammatory drugs

    Angiotensin-converting enzyme inhibitors/angiotensin receptor blockers

Allergic interstitial nephritis (e.g., from antibiotics)

Other, nonlupus glomerular diseases

Evaluation of the Urine

A comprehensive urinalysis should be done in all SLE patients at initial diagnosis, whenever renal involvement is suspected because of other symptoms or signs, such as edema, and at every extrarenal flare. While the clinical laboratory may be used for reporting the urine dipstick, urine microscopy should be done by a qualified individual. The urine dipstick is a commonly used screening test, and kidney involvement in SLE should be considered if the dipstick is positive for blood and/or protein. A positive test for blood is usually the result of hematuria. However, if the test for blood is strongly positive but there are only rare red blood cells in the urine sediment, the patient may have hemoglobinuria or myoglobinuria. If the urine is very dilute (e.g., specific gravity of 1.005 or less), red cells will lyse, mimicking hemoglobinuria.

Hematuria may be due to several conditions unrelated to LN. For example, in the SLE population, menstruation is an important consideration. The urine sediment should be examined to verify the source of hematuria. Glomerular bleeding, which is expected to be present in a glomerulonephritis like LN, is suggested by the morphology of the urine red blood cells. Red cells indicative of glomerular bleeding are called acanthocytes and are dysmorphic cells that show cell-membrane blebs (Figure 2). In addition to acanthocytes, red blood cell casts, as well as white blood cells and white blood cell casts in the absence of infection, are indicative of glomerulonephritis (Figure 2). Glomerular hematuria in the absence of proteinuria and/or renal insufficiency does not require an immediate kidney biopsy for evaluation, but it needs to be followed closely for accompanying changes in kidney function and protein excretion.

Evaluation of Proteinuria

At present, the most sensitive indicator of kidney involvement in SLE is proteinuria, and its magnitude is a key biomarker of relapse and response to treatment. Therefore,

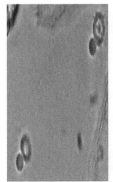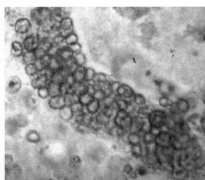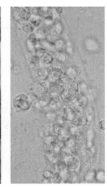

FIGURE 2   Urine sediment findings in LN. Two acanthocytes under brightfield microscopy are shown in the left frame. A red blood cell cast is shown in the middle frame. A white blood cell cast is shown in the right frame.

accurate measurement of proteinuria is crucial to the optimal management of LN. The gold standard for estimating the magnitude of proteinuria is the protein content of a 24-h urine collection. However, 24-h urines are often over- or undercollected, with a strong bias toward undercollection.[24]

Because of these issues with 24-h urine collections, the random spot urine protein-to-creatinine ratio (uPCR) is endorsed by nephrology and rheumatology societies to estimate and monitor 24-h proteinuria in clinical practice.[25,26] However, random spot uPCR has hour-to-hour variability mainly attributed to changes in urine protein excretion rates.[24,27] A study comparing random spot uPCR variability to 24-h urine PCR in LN and CKD cohorts found that, especially in LN with subnephrotic proteinuria (the most common level of proteinuria), random spot uPCR is unreliable.[28] In contrast to random spot uPCR, a uPCR from a first morning void urine provides an accurate estimate of 24-h urine PCR.[29]

A reasonable and straightforward approach to assessing proteinuria in individual patients is to follow trends in the first morning void uPCR (Figure 3). If a change in first morning void uPCR is observed that would warrant a change in therapy, the magnitude of proteinuria should be verified in a 24-h urine collection. Similarly, a 24-h collection should be used to declare a renal remission or diagnose a renal flare in an individual. To correct for over- and undercollections, the uPCR of the intended 24-h urine collection should be multiplied by the individual's expected 24-h urine creatinine excretion (Figure 3).[30]

THE KIDNEY BIOPSY

A kidney biopsy is essential to plan the management of kidney disease in SLE. A kidney biopsy should be considered if proteinuria above 500 mg/day is confirmed, especially in the presence of hematuria or abnormal urine sediment. Survey studies of SLE kidney biopsies have shown significant kidney pathology with levels of proteinuria in this range.[31,32]

The main reasons to perform a biopsy are to establish the correct diagnosis and determine the activity of the kidney disease. In this regard, the clinical utility of the kidney biopsy depends on obtaining an adequate sample of renal cortex so the clinician and renal pathologist are confident that the histology is representative of what is occurring globally within the kidney.[33] An algorithm for using the kidney biopsy in LN is shown in Figure 4.

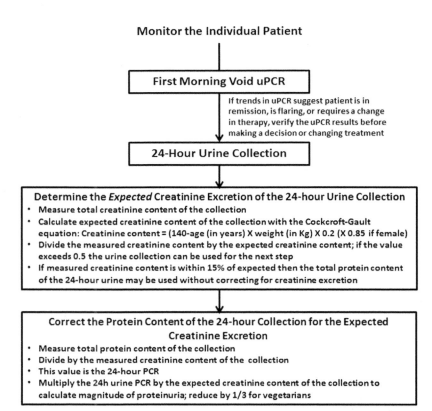

FIGURE 3 An approach to monitoring proteinuria in lupus nephritis. Individual patients can be followed with the urine protein-to-creatinine ratio (uPCR) of first morning void urine specimens. Trends in the uPCR that would warrant a change in therapy, such as a decline in proteinuria consistent with remission, or a worsening of proteinuria consistent with renal flare should be verified with a 24-h urine collection. To avoid over- or under-estimating proteinuria because of incomplete collection or overcollection of the 24-h specimen, the protein content of the 24-h urine should be corrected for the expected 24-h creatinine excretion of the individual.

Although the findings of proteinuria and glomerular hematuria, with or without red or white blood cell casts, are highly suggestive of LN in a patient with SLE, not all kidney disease in lupus is classic, immune-complex-mediated glomerulonephritis. Other glomerular diseases do occur, and they often require therapies distinct from those used in LN. In a series of 252 SLE patients, 5% were found to have pathologies such as focal segmental glomerulosclerosis, minimal change disease, thin glomerular basement membrane disease, hypertensive nephrosclerosis, and amyloidosis.[34] Minimal change disease and focal segmental glomerulosclerosis are considered diseases of the podocyte and are called podocytopathies. The incidence of podocytopathies in LN appears to be higher than the general population.[35] Differentiating these glomerulopathies from LN is important for treatment decisions.

Additionally, there are other important kidney lesions found in SLE patients. For example, patients with antiphospholipid antibodies who are hypercoagulable can develop glomerular thrombi that lead to insidious and progressive renal insufficiency.[36,37] Antiphospholipid syndrome (APS) nephropathy may occur in the presence or absence of LN, and it is not infrequent. APS nephropathy is discussed later, but identifying it by kidney biopsy is critical because treatment requires anticoagulation and not immunosuppression.

Lupus can also cause a predominantly interstitial nephritis without glomerulonephritis. Although pure interstitial nephritis is rare, it can be associated with an active urine sediment and renal insufficiency.[38]

Not all LN needs to be treated with aggressive immunosuppression. The kidney biopsy assesses the degree of active and chronic kidney injury. Clinical findings, including GFR, amount of proteinuria, urine sediment abnormalities, complement levels, and serologies cannot predict the underlying kidney histology.[39] In contrast to active lesions (e.g., cellular proliferation, glomerular crescents, interstitial inflammation), chronic renal injury—which is recognized as glomerular sclerosis, tubular atrophy, and interstitial fibrosis—does not respond to immunosuppression.

The kidney biopsy can thus be used to tailor immunosuppressive therapy to the activity and severity of an individual's disease process. If, however, scarring is the dominant finding on biopsy, even with some areas of active inflammation, the risk of immunosuppression may outweigh its benefits in terms of renal survival. Such patients may be more appropriately treated with kidney-protective therapies.[40]

There are no established recommendations for when kidney biopsies should be repeated in lupus patients. A repeat biopsy may be helpful in patients who have not responded as expected to one or more therapeutic regimens, patients who flare after a period of disease quiescence and there is concern that histology may have changed, or to differentiate between active disease and chronic injury. Several studies have shown that patients may have ongoing histologic activity despite no clinical activity.[33] A repeat kidney biopsy may be useful to identify such patients when there is consideration of discontinuing maintenance immunosuppressive therapy.

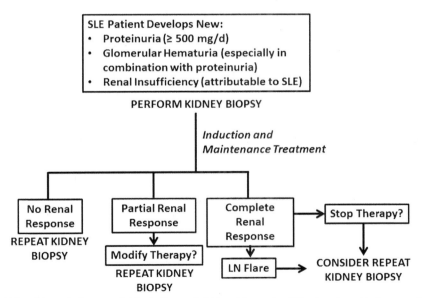

FIGURE 4   Algorithm for kidney biopsy in lupus nephritis. A diagnostic kidney biopsy should be done to guide therapy when a lupus patient presents with clinical evidence of new kidney injury. A repeat biopsy could be considered to confirm complete histologic remission in patients who have achieved complete clinical renal response so maintenance immunosuppression may be stopped. A repeat biopsy should be considered to guide changes in therapy for patients who have incompletely responded. A repeat kidney biopsy should be considered at LN flare if there is suspicion that histology changed and therapy may need to be modified.

ANTIPHOSPHOLIPID SYNDROME AND THE KIDNEY

APS (Chapters 56–58) can result in kidney injury by causing noninflammatory occlusions of renal blood vessels, including the intrarenal microvasculature. APS is seen in about 30% of patients with SLE, often (but not always) accompanied by LN and antiphospholipid antibodies such as anticardiolipin and anti-β2-glycoprotein I antibodies, or lupus anticoagulants.[41] It is important to consider the diagnosis of renal APS and verify with a kidney biopsy, because the usual immunosuppression used for LN does not treat renal APS, which requires anticoagulation. Failure to treat APS can lead to CKD or ESRD.

PREGNANCY AND LUPUS NEPHRITIS

Pregnancy is an important consideration for patients with SLE and is discussed in detail elsewhere (Chapter 50). LN can significantly compromise a pregnancy and pregnancy can adversely affect the kidneys in LN patients. To protect the fetus and the kidneys, it is recommended that SLE patients with LN wait at least 6 months after complete renal remission before trying to become pregnant. This recommendation is based on a fetal loss rate of 8–13% in quiescent LN, but which is as high as 35% in active LN.[42,43] Additionally, renal flare rates of 10–69% have been reported during or after pregnancy, and risk of renal flare or progressive renal impairment appears to be higher in patients who have achieved only a partial renal remission.[42–44]

CHILDHOOD LUPUS NEPHRITIS

About 15% of all SLE is diagnosed before the age of 16.[45] Childhood LN is discussed in detail in Chapter 53. Briefly, the incidence of LN in pediatric SLE patients appears to be between 64% and 87%, and children tend to have more proliferative LN than adults.[46–48] In pediatric LN, the incidence of CKD ranges from 16% to 45%, and ESRD from 4% to 19%.[45,47,48] In multivariate analyses unfavorable prognostic factors for renal survival in children with LN were male sex, hypertension, and inability to achieve remission, but not class IV LN.[45,48,49]

CONCLUSION

LN is a severe manifestation of SLE and is associated with significant morbidity and mortality. To improve outcomes, early evaluation and treatment of patients with LN is necessary. This requires the treating physician to maintain a high level of suspicion for kidney involvement, both at the time of initial diagnosis of SLE and during follow-up. When LN is diagnosed, consultation with a nephrologist experienced in autoimmune diseases is appropriate, and a comanagement approach for patient care should be initiated.

REFERENCES

1. Reich HN, Gladman DD, Urowitz MB, Bargman JM, Hladunewich MA, Lou W, et al. Persistent proteinuria and dyslipidemia increase the risk of progressive chronic kidney disease in lupus erythematosus. *Kidney Int* 2011;**79**(8):914–20.
2. Mok CC, Kwok RC, Yip PS. Effect of renal disease on the standardized mortality ratio and life expectancy of patients with systemic lupus erythematosus. *Arthritis Rheum* 2013;**65**(8):2154–60.
3. Gonzalez-Crespo MR, Lopez-Fernandez JI, Usera G, Poveda MJ, Gomez-Reino JJ. Outcome of silent lupus nephritis. *Semin Arthritis Rheum* 1996;**26**(1):468–76.
4. Valente de Almeida R, Rocha de Carvalho JG, de Azevedo VF, Mulinari RA, Ioshhi SO, da Rosa Utiyama S, et al. Microalbuminuria and renal morphology in the evaluation of subclinical lupus nephritis. *Clin Neprol* 1999;**52**:218–29.
5. Zabaleta-Lanz ME, Munoz LE, Tapanes FJ, Vargas-Arenas RE, Daboin I, Barrios Y, et al. Further description of early clinically silent lupus nephritis. *Lupus* 2006;**15**(12):845–51.
6. Rovin BH, Stillman IE. The kidney in systemic lupus erythematosus. In: Lahita RG, editor. *Systemic lupus erythematosus*. 5th ed. London: Academic Press; 2011. p. 769–814.
7. Contreras G, Pardo V, Cely C, Borja E, Hurtado A, De La Cuesta C, et al. Factors associated with poor outcomes in patients with lupus nephritis. *Lupus* 2005;**14**(11):890–5.
8. Sinicato NA, da Silva PA, Appenzeller S. Risk factors in cardiovascular disease in systemic lupus erythematosus. *Curr Cardiol Rev* 2013;**9**:15–9.
9. Sozeri B, Deveci M, Dincel N, Mir S. The early cardiovascular changes in pediatric patients with systemic lupus erythematosus. *Pediatr Nephrol* 2013;**28**(3):471–6.
10. Faurschou M, Starklint H, Halbert P, Jacobsen S. Prognosis factors in lupus nephritis: diagnostic and therapeutic delay increases the risk of terminal renal failure. *J Rheumatol* 2006;**33**(8):1563–9.
11. Fiehn C. Early diagnosis and treatment in lupus nephritis: how we can influence the risk for terminal renal failure. *J Rheumatol* 2006;**33**(8):1464–6.
12. Fiehn C, Hajjar Y, Mueller K, Waldherr R, Ho AD, Andrassy K. Improved clinical outcome of lupus nephritis during the past decade: importance of early diagnosis and treatment. *Ann Rheum Dis* 2003;**62**:435–9.
13. Bastian HM, Roseman JM, McGwin Jr G, Alarcon GS, Friedman AW, Fessler BJ, et al. Systemic lupus erythematosus in three ethnic groups. XII. Risk factors for lupus nephritis after diagnosis. *Lupus* 2002;**11**(3):152–60.
14. Seligman VA, Lum RF, Olson JL, Li H, Criswell LA. Demographic differences in the development of lupus nephritis: a retrospective analysis. *Am J Med* 2002;**112**:726–9.
15. Branten AJW, Vervoort G, Wetzels JFM. Serum creatinine is a poor marker of GFR in nephrotic syndrome. *Nephrol Dial Transplant* 2005;**20**:707–11.
16. van Acker BA, Prummel MF, Weber JA, Wiersinga WM, Arisz L. Effect of prednisone on renal function in man. *Nephron* 1993;**65**(2):254–9.
17. Risch L, Herklotz R, Blumberg A, Huber AR. Effects of glucocorticoid immunosuppression on serum cystatin C concentrations in renal transplant patients. *Clin Chem* 2001;**47**(11):2055–9.
18. Levey AS, Inker LA, Coresh J. GFR estimation: from physiology to public health. *Am J Kidney Dis* 2014;**63**(5):820–34.
19. Hebert LA, Nori U, Hebert PL. Measured and estimated glomerular filtration rate. *N Engl J Med* 2006;**355**(10):1068. author reply 1069–70.

20. Leung YY, Lo KM, Tam LS, Szeto CC, Li EK, Kun EW. Estimation of glomerular filtration rate in patients with systemic lupus erythematosus. *Lupus* 2006;**15**(5):276–81.

21. Kasitanon N, Fine DM, Haas M, Magder LS, Petri M. Estimating renal function in lupus nephritis: comparison of the Modification of Diet in Renal Disease and Cockcroft-Gault equations. *Lupus* 2007;**16**:887–95.

22. Martinez-Martinez MU, Borjas-Garcia JA, Magana-Aquino M, Cuevas-Orta E, Llamazares-Azuara L, Abud-Mendoza C. Renal function assessment in patients with systemic lupus erythematosus. *Rheumatol Int* 2012;**32**(8):2293–9.

23. Hebert PL, Nori US, Bhatt UY, Hebert LA. A modest proposal for improving the accuracy of creatinine-based GFR-estimating equations. *Nephrol Dial Transplant* 2011;**26**(8):2426–8.

24. Birmingham DJ, Rovin BH, Shidham G, Nagaraja HN, Zou X, Bissell M, et al. Spot urine protein/creatinine ratios are unreliable estimates of 24 h proteinuria in most systemic lupus erythematosus nephritis flares. *Kidney Int* 2007;**72**(7):865–70.

25. Levey AS, Coresh J, Balk E, Kausz AT, Levin A, Steffes MW, et al. National Kidney Foundation practice guidelines for chronic kidney disease: evaluation, classification, and stratification. *Ann Intern Med* 2003;**139**(2):137–47.

26. Hahn BH, McMahon MA, Wilkinson A, Wallace WD, Daikh DI, Fitzgerald JD, et al. American College of Rheumatology guidelines for screening, treatment, and management of lupus nephritis. *Arthritis Care Res* 2012;**64**(6):797–808.

27. Hebert LA, Birmingham DJ, Shidham G, Rovin B, Nagaraja HN, Yu CY. Random spot urine protein/creatinine ratio is unreliable for estimating 24-hour proteinuria in individual systemic lupus erythematosus nephritis patients. *Nephron Clin Pract* 2009;**113**(3):c177–82.

28. Birmingham DJ, Shidham G, Perna A, Fine DM, Bissell M, Rodby R, et al. Spot PC ratio estimates of 24-hour proteinuria are more unreliable in lupus nephritis than in other forms of chronic glomerular disease. *Ann Rheum Dis* 2014;**73**(2):475–6.

29. Fine DM, Ziegenbein M, Petri M, Han E, McKinley A, Chellini J, et al. A prospective study of 24-hour protein excretion in lupus nephritis: adequacy of short-interval timed urine collections. *Kidney Int* 2009;**76**:1284–8.

30. Glassock RJ, Fervenza FC, Hebert L, Cameron JS. Nephrotic syndrome redux. *Nephrol Dial Transplant* 2015;**30**(1):12–7.

31. Grande JP, Balow JE. Renal biopsy in lupus nephritis. *Lupus* 1998;**7**(9):611–7.

32. Christopher-Stine L, Siedner MJ, Lin J, Haas M, Parekh H, Petri M, et al. Renal biopsy in lupus patients with low levels of proteinuria. *J Rheumatol* 2007;**34**:332–5.

33. Rovin BH, Parikh SV, Alvarado A. The kidney biopsy in lupus nephritis: is it still relevant? In: Ginzler EM, Dooley MA, editors. *Systemic lupus erythematosus. Rheumatic Disease Clinics of North America*, vol. 40. Philadelphia: Elsevier; 2014. p. 537–52.

34. Baranowska-Daca E, Choi Y-J, Barrios R, Nassar G, Suki WN, Truong LD. Non-lupus nephrritides in patients with systemic lupus erythematosus: a comprehensive clinicopathologic study and review of the literature. *Hum Pathol* 2001;**32**:1125–35.

35. Kraft SW, Schwartz MM, Korbet SM, Lewis EJ. Glomerular podocytopathy in patients with systemic lupus erythematosus. *J Am Soc Nephrol* 2005;**16**(1):175–9.

36. Tektonidou MG, Sotsiou F, Moutsopoulos HM. Antiphospholipid syndrome nephropathy in catastrophic, primary, and systemic lupus erythematosus-related APS. *J Rheumatol* 2008;**35**:1983–8.

37. Daugas E, Nochy D, Huong DL, Duhaut P, Beaufils H, Caudwell V, et al. Antiphospholipid syndrome nephropathy in systemic lupus erythematosus. *J Am Soc Nephrol* 2002;**13**(1):42–52.

38. Mori Y, Kishimoto N, Yamahara H, Kijima Y, Nose A, Uchiyama-Tanaka Y, et al. Predominant tubulointerstitial nephritis in a patient with systemic lupus nephritis. *Clin Exp Nephrol* 2005;**9**(1):79–84.

39. Alvarado A, Malvar A, Lococo B, Alberton V, Toniolo F, Nagaraja H, et al. The value of repeat kidney biopsy in quiescent Argentinian lupus nephritis patients. *Lupus* 2014;**23**(8):840–7.

40. Neusser MA, Lindenmeyer MT, Edenhofer I, Gaiser S, Kretzler M, Regele H, et al. Intrarenal production of B-cell survival factors in human lupus nephritis. *Mod Pathol* 2011;**24**(1):98–107.

41. Tektonidou MG. Renal involvement in the antiphospholipid syndrome (APS)-APS nephropathy. *Clin Rev Allergy Immunol* 2009;**36**(2–3):131–40.

42. Imbasciati E, Tincani A, Gregorini G, Doria A, Moroni G, Cabiddu G, et al. Pregnancy in women with pre-existing lupus nephritis: predictors of fetal and maternal outcome. *Nephrol Dial Transplant* 2009;**24**(2):519–25.

43. Wagner SJ, Craici I, Reed D, Norby S, Bailey K, Wiste HJ, et al. Maternal and fetal outcomes in pregnant patients with active lupus nephritis. *Lupus* 2009;**18**(4):342–7.

44. Tandon A, Ibanez D, Gladman D, Urowitz M. The effect of pregnancy on lupus nephritis. *Arthritis Rheum* 2004;**50**:3941–6.

45. Hagelberg S, Lee Y, Bargman J, Mah G, Schneider R, Laskin C, et al. Longterm followup of childhood lupus nephritis. *J Rheumatol* 2002;**29**(12):2635–42.

46. Brunner HI, Gladman DD, Ibanez D, Urowitz MD, Silverman ED. Difference in disease features between childhood-onset and adult-onset systemic lupus erythematosus. *Arthritis Rheum* 2008;**58**(2):556–62.

47. Tucker LB, Uribe AG, Fernandez M, Vila LM, McGwin G, Apte M, et al. Adolescent onset of lupus results in more aggressive disease and worse outcomes: results of a nested matched case-control study within LUMINA, a multiethnic US cohort (LUMINA LVII). *Lupus* 2008;**17**(4):314–22.

48. Lee BS, Cho HY, Kim EJ, Kang HG, Ha IS, Cheong HI, et al. Clinical outcomes of childhood lupus nephritis: a single center's experience. *Pediatr Nephrol* 2007;**22**(2):222–31.

49. Vachvanichsanong P, Dissaneewate P, McNeil E. Diffuse proliferative glomerulonephritis does not determine the worst outcome in childhood-onset lupus nephritis: a 23-year experience in a single centre. *Nephrol Dial Transplant* 2009;**24**(9):2729–34.

Chapter 41

The Pathology of Lupus Nephritis

Isaac Ely Stillman

Beth Israel Deaconess Medical Center, Boston, MA, USA

INTRODUCTION

The kidney, an "innocent bystander" in the pathogenesis of systemic lupus erythematosus (SLE), nevertheless bears the brunt of the morbidity and mortality of the disease. Indeed, the majority of patients with lupus eventually develop some degree of renal involvement, which in some cases precedes (occasionally by years) the diagnosis of SLE. This clinically oriented chapter will focus on the varied expressions of SLE-associated renal disease, their classification, and their relationship to treatment.

INTRODUCTION TO NEPHROPATHOLOGY

The diagnostic utility of the renal biopsy is a direct function of the skills of those procuring and interpreting the sample, as well as the communication between them.[1] The nephrologist and nephropathologist should review the findings together to ensure that clinical concerns have been addressed and that the biopsy has been appropriately interpreted.

Biopsies are evaluated using three techniques: light microscopy (LM, typically formalin fixed), immunofluorescence microscopy (IF, performed on fresh frozen tissue), and electron microscopy (EM, typically glutaraldehyde fixed). These complementary techniques should be evaluated by the same nephropathologist to maximize the integration of all findings. The bedrock of pathologic evaluation is LM, performed on 2-μm serial sections, suitably stained with hematoxylin and eosin (H&E), as well as the "special" stains that supplement it: periodic acid–Schiff reaction (PAS), Masson trichrome (MT), and Jones (methenamine silver-periodic acid; Figure 1). Most laboratories in North America continue to use the IF technique (in contrast to immunohistochemistry on the paraffin block) because it remains more sensitive, reliable, and reproducible. Frozen tissue is routinely stained for IgG, IgA, IgM, C3, C1q, fibrin (including fibrinogen and breakdown products), kappa and lambda (light chains), and albumin (which serves as a control) using fluorescein isothiocyanate-conjugated antibodies. An important limitation of EM is sample size (far smaller than LM and IF); ultrastructural findings must always be interpreted in context.

INTRODUCTION TO THE NEPHROPATHOLOGY OF SLE

The pathogenesis of autoantibody formation and immune complex (IC) formation and deposition in SLE and lupus nephritis (LN) is addressed elsewhere in this book, and its nephropathology has been detailed in two references—one encyclopedic[2] and the other diagnostic.[3] LN is by definition an IgG dominant IC disease and the pattern/location of the deposition determines the resulting histopathological pattern. The pathologic pleomorphism that is the hallmark of LN reflects the multiple possible patterns of deposition, themselves a function of the diversity of the autoantibodies/complexes involved and their deposition kinetics. While many autoantibodies have been eluted from LN renal tissue, anti-dsDNA antibodies directed against nucleosomes are thought to predominate.[4] Autoantibodies may form in situ with endogenous or exogenous antigens or, alternatively, deposit from the circulation as preformed IC. Factors determining the location of deposition include immunoglobulin class and subclass, the ability to activate complement and/or cellular immunity, avidity, charge, size, ratio of antibody to antigen, as well as specificity and rate of production and clearance. Relatively small amounts of IC may deposit in the mesangium alone, whereas larger amounts may progress to subendothelial deposits. Low avidity cationic deposits may be more likely to transverse the anionic glomerular basement membrane (GBM) and accumulate in the subepithelial space. Thus, while the overwhelming majority of lesions seen in SLE are due to one process—IC deposition (primarily but not exclusively glomerular)—the range of lesions produced is extraordinarily varied.

While LM is the primary technique for evaluating lesions resulting from IC deposition, it is not ideal at identifying the deposits themselves, particularly when they are small. Eosin stains cytoplasm, membranes, and IC alike. In contrast, the "special stains" PAS and Jones delineate both basement membranes and mesangial matrix (they are biochemically similar) but not cytoplasm (Figure 2). Small ICs are also usually negative and may be appreciated by their "spaces" within the tissue. In contrast, larger deposits may be identified by their glassy ("hyaline") appearance on H&E and are visible

Systemic Lupus Erythematosus. http://dx.doi.org/10.1016/B978-0-12-801917-7.00041-3

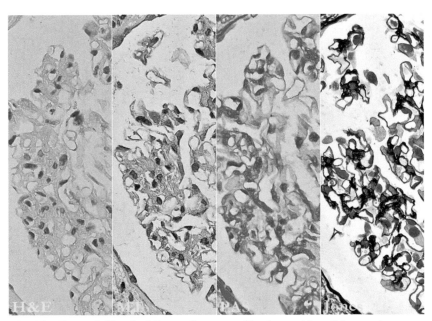

FIGURE 1   Normal glomerulus (class I pattern). Note the delicate and patent capillary loops with a mildly conspicuous mesangium. There is no hyper-cellularity (proliferation) within the tuft of capillaries or in the open urinary space. The montage demonstrates the difference between routine H&E (starting on left), Masson trichrome, and the matrix stains PAS and the higher contrast Jones (right) which both highlight mesangial matrix and basement membranes (glomerular and tubular). Original magnification: 40×.

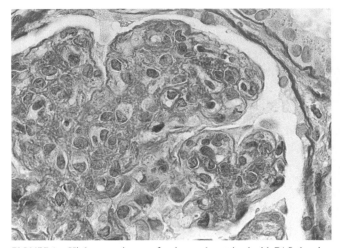

FIGURE 2   High-power image of a glomerulus stained with PAS showing endocapillary proliferation (occlusion of capillary lumens). Note that the cytoplasm is PAS negative, as are the immune complexes, seen as mottled areas within the mesangial matrix. Basement membranes are PAS positive. Tubule in upper right corner shows some cytoplasmic PAS positive protein resorption droplets. Original magnification: 100×.

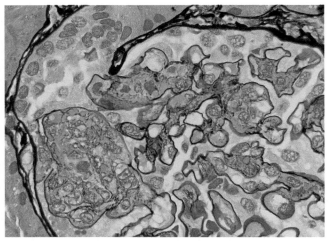

FIGURE 3   High-power image of a glomerulus stained with Jones (methe-namine silver) showing segmental endocapillary proliferation (occlusion of capillary lumens) protruding across the urinary pole. Note that cytoplasm is silver negative, as are the immune complexes, which are seen as hype-reosinophilic endocapillary deposits within the mesangium and along the silver positive (black) capillary membranes (in the subendothelial zone). Within the urinary space podocyte nuclei show reactive changes secondary to injury. Original magnification: 100×.

on special stains as PAS positive (particularly when IgM rich), red (MT), or pink (Jones) deposits (Figure 3). MT stains fibrin and necrosis intensely red and is especially helpful in assessing chronicity by highlighting interstitial collagen blue.

IF defines the nature of the deposits and, to a lesser degree, their location. While IgG is dominant in LN, other immunoglobulins are frequently codeposited. The "full house pattern" consisting of all three (IgG, IgA, and IgM), as well as two complement fractions (C1q and C3) is classic

for LN. When IgG and IgA are codominant, the possibility of IgA nephropathy must be considered. C1q implies acti-vation of the classic complement pathway; when strongly present, it suggests LN.[5] IC staining in LN is typically granular or confluent and is graded from 0 to 4+. The loca-tion of glomerular deposition is described: urinary space, mesangial, and capillary wall (deposits with a smooth outer

(A) (B)

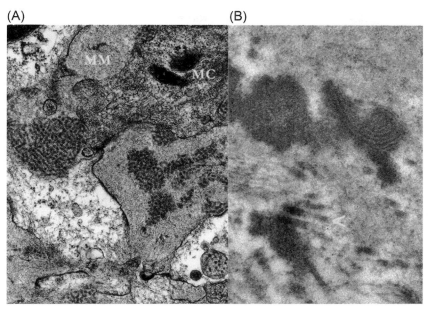

FIGURE 4 Transmission electron microscopy of deposits with substructure. A. Short curved cylindrical structures with the typical appearance of cryoglobulins (usually Type III, mixed in LN) deposited within the mesangial matrix (MM), which is surrounded by membrane-bound mesangial cell cytoplasm (MC). Original magnification: 25,000×. B. Tubular basement membrane "fingerprint deposits" with curved parallel arrays, arising out of amorphous granular deposits that are typical of immune complexes. This substructure is highly suggestive of LN; their relationship to cryoglobulins is uncertain. Arrowhead points to a type III collagen bundle, present in the renal interstitium. Original magnification: 50,000×.

contour are more likely to be subendothelial as they lay against the GBM as opposed to the more ragged edges of subepithelial deposits). Another distinctive feature of LN is the presence of vascular, interstitial, and tubular basement membrane staining for IgG.

EM complements IF, as it excels at precisely localizing deposits and their accompanying ultrastructural lesions, but it is poor at defining their nature (they all appear similarly granular and amorphous).[6] IC deposition is extracellular—the electron-dense deposits appear within matrix or membranes, never membrane bound (intracytoplasmic). Their location is described as mesangial, subendothelial, intramembranous, and subepithelial. The simultaneous presence of deposits in multiple sites is suggestive of LN. On occasion, foci within otherwise typical granular deposits show varying degrees of substructure, such as alternating bands measuring 10–15 nm in a crystalline pattern, which may be curved ("fingerprinting"), tubular, or straight (Figure 4). Some deposits are similar to those seen with cryoglobulinemia (typically Type III–mixed), and indeed such antibodies are common in lupus patients.

RENAL BIOPSY AND SLE

The renal biopsy plays a fundamental role in the diagnosis of both SLE and LN.[7] It provides information regarding the activity and chronicity of renal lesions that is otherwise unobtainable but required to determine therapy and prognosis. Guidelines for biopsy indications are discussed elsewhere. Given the variation in glomerular involvement, at least 20 glomeruli may be necessary for reproducible classification.[8]

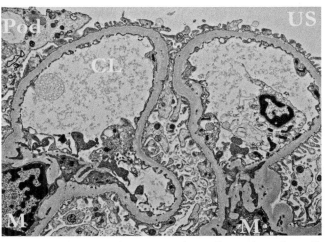

FIGURE 5 Ultrastructural appearance of two adjacent glomerular capillary loops that are within normal limits. Note that the mesangium (M) is continuous with the subendothelial space. The peripheral capillary wall is comprised of the fenestrated endothelium, the glomerular basement membrane and the podocyte (Pod) foot processes. CL, capillary lumen; US, urinary space. Original magnification: 8,000×.

Given the plasticity of lesions, repeat biopsy (uncommon in other diseases) plays an important role (see below).

THE LESIONS OF LUPUS NEPHRITIS

Glomeruli

A normal glomerulus (Figures 1 and 5) shows delicate patent capillary loops, and a mesangium that is no more than mildly conspicuous. LM evaluation begins with an assessment of

TABLE 1 Glossary of Pathologic Terms

Crescent: Extracapillary proliferation of cells in the urinary space, initially seen in association with fibrin/necrosis, over time undergoes organization (fibrosis)

Diffuse: A lesion involving most (≥50%) glomeruli

Double contours: Thickened glomerular capillary walls with duplication of the basement membrane due to the growth of an inner neomembrane; usually in response to chronic subendothelial deposition

Endocapillary proliferation: Endocapillary hypercellularity due to increased number of mesangial cells, endothelial cells, and infiltrating monocytes, and causing narrowing of the glomerular capillary lumina

Extracapillary proliferation or cellular crescent: Extracapillary cell proliferation of more than two cell layers occupying one-fourth or more of the glomerular capillary circumference

Focal: A lesion involving <50% of glomeruli

Fibrinoid necrosis: Hypereosinophilic focus of necrosis associated with fibrin/denatured proteins

Fibrous crescent: Organized (previously cellular) crescent of fibrous tissue in urinary space

Global: A lesion involving more than half of the glomerular tuft

Hyaline thrombus: Intracapillary eosinophilic material of a homogenous consistency, which immunofluorescence demonstrates to consist of immune deposits

Intramembranous: Within the lamina densa of the glomerular basement membrane

Karyorrhexis: Presence of apoptotic, pyknotic, and fragmented nuclei

Membranoproliferative: Glomerular pattern with prominent double contour formation

Mesangial hypercellularity (proliferation): At least three mesangial cells per mesangial region in a 3-μm thick section

Mesangial interposition: Extension of cytoplasm into the subendothelial space associated with double contours

Necrosis: Characterized by fragmentation of nuclei or disruption of the glomerular basement membrane, often associated with the presence of fibrin-rich material

Proportion of involved glomeruli: Intended to indicate the percentage of total glomeruli affected by LN, including the glomeruli that are sclerosed due to LN, but excluding ischemic glomeruli with inadequate perfusion due to vascular pathology separate from LN

Sclerosis: Glomerular scarring by expansion of matrix and loss of normal architecture

Segmental: A lesion involving less than half of the glomerular tuft (i.e., at least half of the glomerular tuft is spared)

Subendothelial: Space between the endothelium and the glomerular basement membrane

Subepithelial (epimembranous): Space between the visceral epithelial cell (podocyte) and the glomerular basement membrane

Wire loops: Thickened hypereosinophilic segment of glomerular capillary wall composed of large subendothelial immune deposits

Terms in bold, as defined by the ISN/RPS Classification.

glomerular cellularity. Increased glomerular cellularity (historically, but somewhat inaccurately called "proliferation") may be due to both an increase in native cells as well as exogenous inflammatory cells. Proliferation may be noted in the mesangial, endocapillary, or extracapillary (crescent) zones. The distribution of glomerular lesions is described within individual glomeruli (segmental vs global) as well as their total population (focal vs diffuse). Table 1 contains a glossary of basic pathological terminology.

The fundamental lesion of LN is mesangial IC deposition, with all other glomerular lesions superimposed on it. Mesangial IC deposition is identified by IF and EM (Figures 6 and 7) and is usually associated with mesangial

proliferation and matrical increase (three or more cells in a region away from the vascular pole) best recognized on LM (Figure 8). The correlation between the extent of mesangial proliferation and immunodeposition may be poor. Mesangial processes are typically expressed by hematuria, although the mechanism for this remains unclear. Mesangial hypercellularity, by definition, does not involve the capillaries, whose lumens remain patent and normocellular.

The term "proliferative glomerulonephritis" in the context of LN refers to endocapillary proliferation, which is recognized by hypercellular occlusion of the capillary lumens. The cells are typically a mixture of proliferating

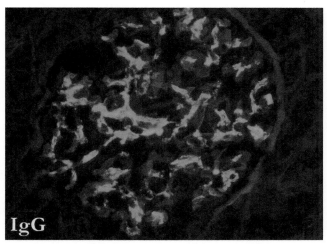

FIGURE 6   Mesangial immune complex deposition. Capillary walls are predominantly negative with patent lumens. Very rare granules are seen along the capillary wall, likely representing isolated subepithelial deposits that are still consistent with a class I or II pattern. IF, anti-IgG; original magnification: 40×.

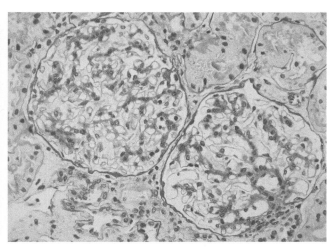

FIGURE 8   Mild mesangial proliferation (class II Pattern). Note that the capillary lumens are patent and normocellular. The vascular pole/macula densa is seen at five o'clock of the glomerulus on the right. Surrounding proximal tubules are healthy with intact apical brush borders. PAS, original magnification: 40×.

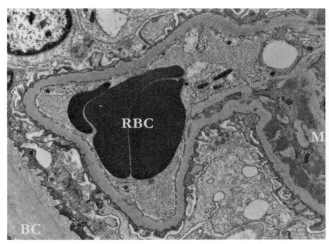

FIGURE 7   Extensive granular mesangial electron dense deposits (class I or II pattern). The capillary lumen shows incidental circulating red blood cells (RBC) but no deposits are seen there. Note that the mesangial region (M) is separated from the capillary lumen by endothelium alone, without a basement membrane dividing it from the circulation. Only focal podocyte (Pod) foot process effacement is seen along a capillary wall that shows isolated small subepithelial deposits. BC, Bowman's capsule. EM, original magnification: 10,000×.

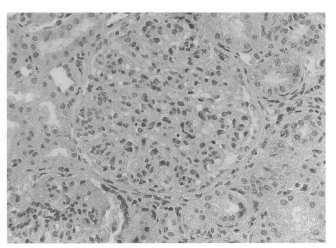

FIGURE 9   Global endocapillary proliferation (class III or IV pattern). Capillary lumens are occluded by the hypercellularity, which obscures the distinction between mesangium and capillary lumen. A second glomerulus is partially seen in the lower left corner and also shows hyperreosinophilic areas representing confluent IC deposition. H&E, original magnification: 40×.

native (mesangial and endothelial) cells in conjunction with infiltrating leukocytes (Figure 9). Endocapillary proliferation can be variable and its distribution throughout the sample must be quantitated. Copious IC deposition, particularly involving the subendothelial space, is common in this setting (Figure 10). Subendothelial deposits are the most accessible to the circulation and are therefore most able to activate complement, generate chemoattractants, and generate the influx of leukocytes. These deposits are therefore associated with more damaging forms of

the disease. When large, such deposits may be seen on LM as capillary wall thickening and are referred to as "wire loops" (Figure 11). Interestingly, glomeruli with such deposits often show less proliferation than ones without. Endolumenal IC plugs (so-called fibrin thrombi, although they are neither) are actually projections in continuity with subendothelial deposits (Figure 12). True fibrin thrombi may be seen as a result of complement activation or when a thrombotic microangiopathy (TMA) is superimposed. Hematoxylin bodies are the tissue equivalent of the LE body and are comprised of basophilic nuclei coated with

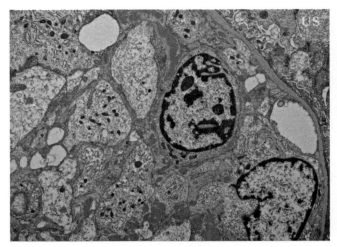

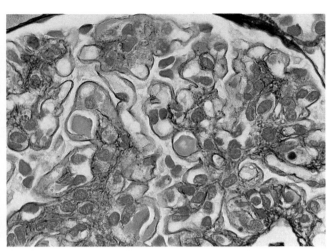

FIGURE 10 Endocapillary proliferation with electron dense deposits representing IC present throughout the distorted mesangial matrix and along the attenuated glomerular basement membrane in the subendothelial zone. US, urinary space. EM, original magnification: 8,000×.

FIGURE 12 "Hyalin thrombi" by LM (class III or IV pattern). Large plugs of immune complexes are seen within capillary lumens, some of them in approximation with subendothelial deposits. There is focal "double contour" formation, and mesangial deposits are visible. Interestingly, areas with massive deposition tend to show less proliferation, as demonstrated here. Jones, original magnification: 40×.

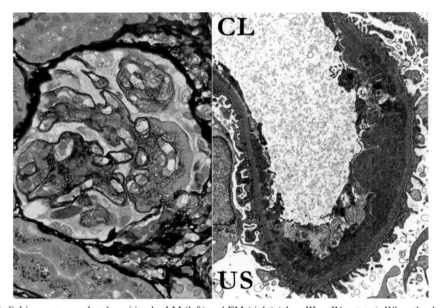

FIGURE 11 Subendothelial immune complex deposition by LM (left) and EM (right) (class III or IV pattern). When the deposits are large, they can be visualized by LM, here on Jones as hypereosinophilic deposits, where they thicken the capillary wall ("wire loops"). The GBM stains black and is attenuated in the region of deposition. The lobule above it shows "double contour" formation, secondary to chronic subendothelial deposition. Original magnification: 40×. EM localizes the amorphous granular deposits to the subendothelial space (underneath the mildly swollen/injured endothelium) with a smooth outer contour where they abut the glomerular basement membrane. CL, capillary lumen; US, urinary space. Original magnification: 12,000×.

antinuclear antibodies. Although highly specific for SLE, they are also very rare (Figure 13).

Proliferative lesions are most associated with "active lesions" and particularly necrosis of the glomerular tuft. (Figures 14 and 15) Necrosis is usually segmental and is identified by the presence of fibrin, neutrophilic exudation, apoptosis, karyorrhexis, and/or fragmentation of the basement membrane (Figure 16). Severe inflammation, and especially fibrinoid necrosis, results in glomerular capillary rupture with hemorrhage into Bowman's space and formation of cellular crescents (extracapillary proliferation; Figure 17). Cellular crescents (a combination of proliferating epithelial cells and infiltrating leukocytes) indicate severe glomerular injury and when persistent organize into fibrocellular and then fibrous crescents (often seen with glomerular obsolescence; Figure 18).

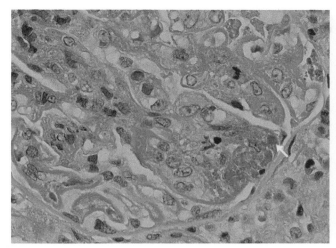

FIGURE 13 Glomerulus with extensive hypereosinophilic immune complex deposition in the mesangium and along capillary walls. Podocytes show protein resorption droplets (2–3 o'clock). The arrow points to a hematoxylin body (tissue equivalent of LE body). A rare finding, usually seen in association with necrosis, they may be the only lesion that is pathognomonic for lupus. H&E, original magnification: 40×.

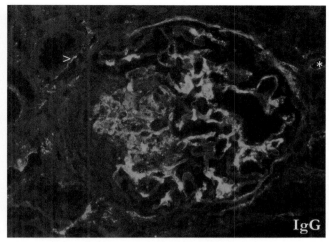

FIGURE 15 Segmental endocapillary immune complex deposition (class III or IV-S pattern). The endocapillary deposits are seen from 8 to 10 o'clock; the remainder of the tuft shows global mesangial deposits. Some of the capillary loops show small granular deposits representing isolated subepithelial deposits or protein resorption droplets within podocytes. Surrounding tubules show deposition (>) along their basement membranes, a common finding in LN. A peri-tubular capillary (*) also shows deposits. IF, anti-IgG, original magnification: 40×.

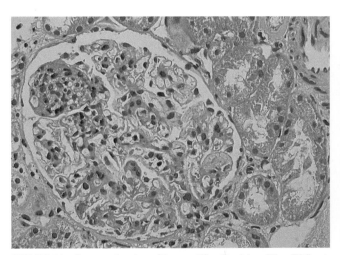

FIGURE 14 Segmental endocapillary proliferation (class III or IV-S pattern). The hypercellularity occludes the capillary lumen and obscures the mesangial/capillary lumen architecture, but is bounded by the peripheral capillary wall. These lesions are often (but not always) seen in association with overt segmental necrosis. The other glomerular lobules show mesangial prominence. H&E, original magnification: 40×.

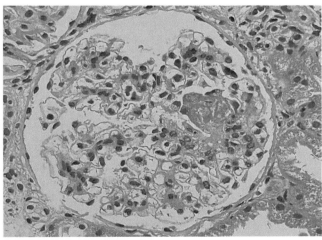

FIGURE 16 Segmental fibrinoid necrosis (class III or IV-S pattern). This lesion typically incites cellular crescent formation. The other glomerular lobules show only mesangial prominence (class II pattern). H&E, original magnification: 40×.

Despite their association, both segmental necrosis and cellular crescents may be seen alone.

Chronic subendothelial deposition may result in a membranoproliferative pattern, reflecting reactive basement membrane/"double contour" formation (Figure 19). In addition to a neomembrane covering the subendothelial deposits, EM may reveal cells in that space, in continuity with the mesangium (so-called "mesangial interposition," although they might be leukocytes; Figure 20).

Scattered subepithelial IC deposition is common in LN and may be associated with reactive changes of the lamina

densa. Such "membranous" changes are best identified on IF and EM, and when more extensive on Jones stain (Figure 21). Deposits in this "protected" location (walled off from the circulation) may activate complement, but they are not associated with inflammatory cell influx (proliferation). When this pattern dominates, the appearance may suggest idiopathic membranous glomerulonephritis (GN). Often, however, subepithelial deposition is combined with endocapillary proliferation due to deposits at other sites.

The active changes noted above (immune deposition, proliferation, necrosis, etc.) may progress to chronic scarring. Serial biopsies suggest that segmental necrosis heals as segmental scars (sclerosis; Figure 22). More severe glomerular injury or crescent formation may result in global sclerosis. The percentage of sclerotic glomeruli (global and segmental) is an important metric of chronicity. Similar chronic changes may also result from unrelated processes, such as hypertension and aging. Only glomerulosclerosis that can be attributed to postinflammatory scarring is classified as LN involvement. Unfortunately, that distinction may be difficult to make on morphologic grounds.

EM usually shows frequent tubuloreticular structures (or inclusions), most commonly in glomerular endothelial cells (Figure 23). These 24-nm interanastamosing structures located within endoplasmic reticulum are associated with elevated levels of circulating interferon and can also be seen in viral infections. Their association with LN underscores the central role of interferon in this disease.[9] Their presence in a case of otherwise primary membranous GN may portend the subsequent development of SLE.

Tubulointerstitium

Tubules and interstitium share a tight anatomical association and their lesions (either acute or chronic) are often considered together. Interstitial edema (appearing as clear space) and inflammation, predominantly comprised of mononuclear cells (lymphocytes, plasma cells, and macrophages), are acute changes seen to varying degrees in LN and in association with tubulitis and other forms of acute tubular injury (degenerative and regenerative), including red cell and/or "pus" casts. While interstitial infiltrates are rarely seen alone, the extent of inflammation usually parallels the severity of glomerular disease. The degree of inflammation has been correlated with both reduction in glomerular filtration rate (GFR) and serologic activity.[10] Studies immunophenotyping the infiltrates have not yielded consistent results, but it seems that most are T-cells and that

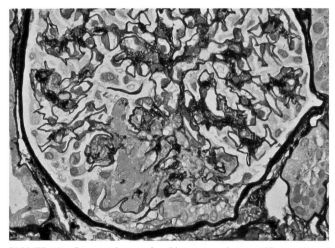

FIGURE 17 Segmental necrosis with rupture of the capillary wall and release of fibrin and other inflammatory mediators into the urinary space (class III or IV pattern). An early cellular crescent is seen at 5–6 o'clock. The remainder of the glomerulus is intact. These active lesions may heal as segmental sclerosis. Jones, original magnification: 40×.

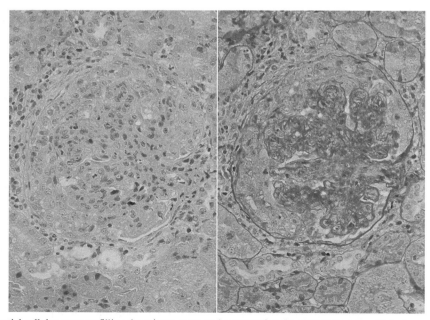

FIGURE 18 Circumferential cellular crescent filling the urinary space and compressing the glomerular tuft, which shows endocapillary proliferation (class III or IV pattern). The PAS (right) by delineating the membranes, allows easier discrimination between the positive tuft and the negative cells in the urinary space than H&E (left). Comprised primarily of native glomerular epithelium, macrophages, and lymphocytes, cellular crescents may completely resolve in response to therapy. With time however, these crescents scar and lead to glomerulosclerosis. Original magnification: 40×.

CD8+ cells are more common than in other types of GN. Macrophage infiltration may correlate with current and future renal function.[11]

IF and EM often reveal deposits (most commonly IgG) along tubular basement membranes (always suggestive of LN) and even within the interstitium (Figure 24). While tubulointerstitial deposits can rarely be seen in the absence of glomerular deposition, typically their extent parallels glomerular proliferation.[12] Nuclei may show staining for IgG on IF ("tissue ANA," perhaps an artifact of tissue sectioning), which when strong may obscure other deposits (Figure 24 (left)).

Evaluation of interstitial fibrosis (and tubular atrophy) is critical to define the extent of chronic injury. It is best assessed on MT, where expansion of the normally

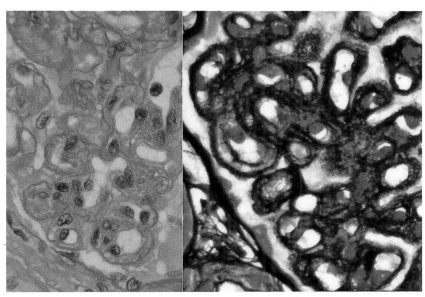

FIGURE 19 Membranoproliferative pattern of glomerular injury by PAS (left) and Jones (right) (class III or IV pattern). In the context of LN, this pattern results from chronic subendothelial immuno-deposits, inciting the formation by the endothelial cells of an inner neomembrane and the resultant "double contour" or "tram track" lesion. The space between the membranes appears clear because the cytoplasm and deposits present there do not stain. Original magnification: 100×.

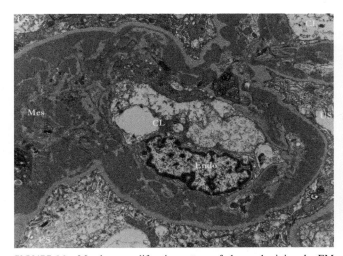

FIGURE 20 Membranoproliferative pattern of glomerular injury by EM (class III or IV pattern). Subendothelial granular electron dense deposits are seen within a markedly thickened capillary wall, and in continuity with the mesangium (Mes). Cellular elements are also embedded within the deposits and interposed between the outer basement membrane and neomembrane (seen on LM as "double contours"). Endothelial cells (Endo) encircle a reduced capillary lumen (CL). US, urinary space. Original magnification: 8,000×.

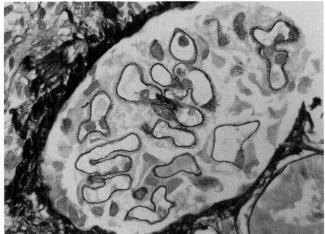

FIGURE 21 Membranous changes involving the glomerular basement membranes to varying degrees. Areas of reactive changes, with growth of the lamina densa (of the basement membrane) in between the subepithelial deposits are seen as "spikes" and "holes," as the deposits themselves are sliver negative. Some of the membranes appear uninvolved, a finding more typical of a lupus rather than primary membranous pattern. No proliferation is present. The epithelial cells (podocytes) show reactive changes suggestive of acute injury. Jones, original magnification: 100×.

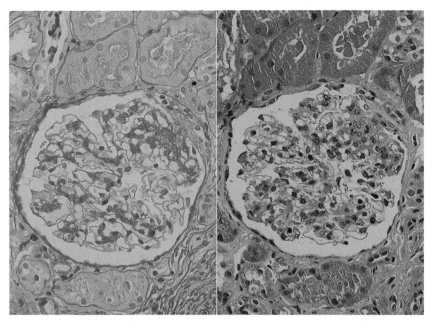

FIGURE 22 Segmental sclerosis by PAS (left) and MT (right). There is segmentally increased PAS positive matrix effacing the glomerular capillary architecture and forming an adhesion to a small fibrous crescent (1–2 o'clock). This scar, likely the sequel of prior necrosis and crescent formation, is incompatible with a class II designation, and is indicative of class III or IV (C). This lesion will not respond to anti-inflammatory therapy. Original magnification: 40×.

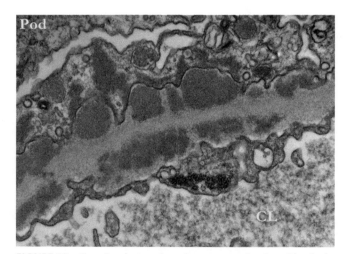

FIGURE 23 Granular electron dense immune complex deposition in the glomerular capillary wall. CL, capillary lumen; Pod, podocyte cell body. A tubuloreticular inclusion is present within a glomerular endothelial cell. These 24 nm structures, relating to the rough endoplasmic reticulum, are associated with elevated levels of circulating interferon, and their frequent occurrence in LN underscores the central role of interferon in this disease. Subendothelial deposits are seen to connect through the lamina densa to subepithelial deposits, a pattern of deposition suggestive of LN. Podocytes show injury with widespread foot process effacement. The simultaneous presence of extensive subepithelial and subendothelial immune deposits warrants the addition of class III or IV (focal or diffuse LN) to the class V (membranous) designation. EM may be necessary to identify such cases, which have a significantly worse prognosis than pure class V. EM, original magnification: 30,000×.

inconspicuous interstitium appears as varying intensities of blue, reflecting the density of collagen deposition (Figure 25). As in other renal diseases, the degree of tubulointerstitial scarring is the histologic parameter that best correlates with current and future renal function. Morphometric evaluation has been shown to improve the assessment, but it has not been adopted in clinical practice.[13] As tubules progress from acute injury to chronic atrophy, they undergo changes that result in diminished cytoplasm and diameter, thickening of basement membranes (best seen on PAS stain), and cast formation. Like interstitial fibrosis, these processes are thought to be irreversible.

Vessels

Nonspecific chronic lesions (secondary to hypertension, aging, etc.) are the most common changes seen. Lesions specific to SLE receive insufficient attention, in part because they (like tubulointerstitial changes) are absent from LN classifications and their terminology has not been standardized. Their clinical significance ranges from trivial to profound. A schema is presented in Table 2.[14] The most common lesion, uncomplicated vascular immune deposits, is recognized by irregular deposition of immunoreactants (most commonly IgG, although other immunoglobulins and complement components may be present) in vessel walls (predominantly small arteries and arterioles) as seen by IF (Figure 26). The presence of IgM and/or complement alone may reflect nonspecific injury and is not diagnostic of a

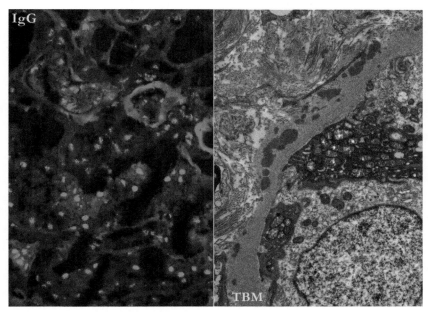

FIGURE 24 Left: Nuclei of tubular epithelium showing diffuse coating by IgG ("tissue ANA"). This finding confirms the presence of autoantibodies. IF, anti-IgG, original magnification: 40×. Right: Granular immune complex deposition along tubular basement membranes. This finding is highly suggestive of LN. EM, original magnification: 8,000×.

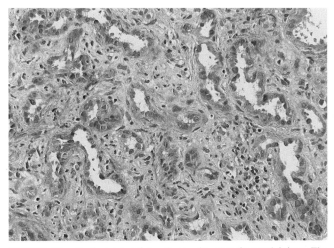

FIGURE 25 Cortical tubulointerstitum with chronic renal injury. The normally inconspicuous interstitium is markedly expanded by fibrosis (blue). Some proximal tubules show dilation and cytological features of acute injury. Others show atrophy and thickened basement membranes. The condition of the tubulointerstitium is the histological feature that best correlates with current and future GFR. MT, original magnification: 40×.

TABLE 2 Vascular Lesions
Lupus Specific
Uncomplicated immune complex deposition   Lupus vasculopathy
Lupus Related

Necrotizing arteritis (? ANCA associated)
   Thrombotic microangiopathy
   HUS/TTP
   Scleroderma
   Lupus anticoagulant/antiphospholipid syndrome
   Malignant hypertension

Non-lupus Related
Arteriosclerosis   Arteriolarsclerosis

lupus-related process. Vessel walls may display IC on LM but the lumen is not compromised by them. EM localizes the deposits to the intimal basement membrane and medial matrix. The degree of deposition roughly correlates with glomerular proliferation and tubulointerstitial deposition. These deposits are usually clinically silent and do not carry negative prognostic implications.[15]

Lupus vasculopathy (noninflammatory necrotizing vasculopathy), in contrast, is far less common and is associated with a poor prognosis.[16] Seen most commonly in the setting of severe proliferative LN, vessels (usually arterioles) show lumenal narrowing by IC deposition accompanied by endothelial and medial injury. Fibrinoid and necrosis may be present but inflammation (by definition) is absent (Figure 27).

Literal vasculitis—fibrinoid necrosis of the vessel wall with associated inflammation—is a very rare finding in LN. Its histologic appearance is indistinguishable from a systemic vasculitis of the antineutrophil cytoplasmic antibodies (ANCA) type, and it may represent the simultaneous occurrence of an unrelated systemic or "renal limited" vasculitis.

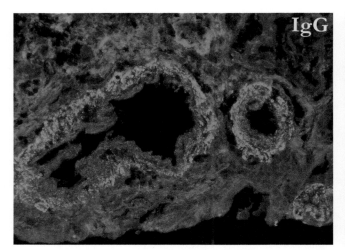

FIGURE 26 Uncomplicated immune complex deposition in the intima and media of an arteriole (lower right) and artery (left). The lumen is not compromised. This finding is highly suggestive of LN but does not carry an adverse prognosis. IF, anti-IgG, original magnification: 40×.

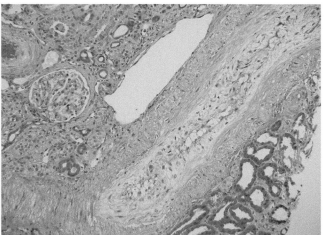

FIGURE 28 Thrombotic microangiopathy. Artery in longitudinal section shows marked mucoid intimal hyperplasia, a smaller vessel in upper left shows a thrombus. While the tubulointerstitium on the right is relatively preserved, the glomerulus shows signs of hypoperfusion and the tubules show atrophy suggestive of ischemia. Immune complex deposition is not a part of this lesion. MT, original magnification: 40×.

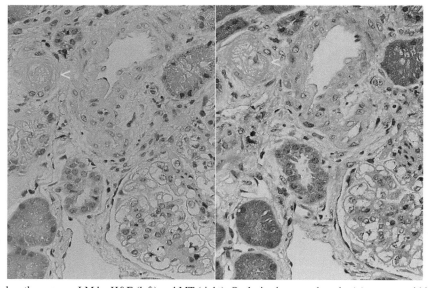

FIGURE 27 Lupus vasculopathy, seen on LM by H&E (left) and MT (right): Occlusive immune deposits (<) are seen within the lumen of an arteriole that has branched off of the artery seen in longitudinal section. The deposits are hypereosinophilic and stain light blue on MT. Seen most commonly in the setting of proliferative LN, this finding is associated with a poor prognosis. In this case, the glomerulus shows a class V (membranous) pattern. The artery also shows deposits (6–8 o'clock), but they are not overtly occlusive. Original magnification, 40×.

Thrombotic microangiopathy (TMA) in the lupus setting may be seen in association with any of its related clinical entities (e.g., malignant hypertension, systemic sclerosis, hemolytic–uremic syndrome/thrombotic thrombocytopenic purpura (HUS/TTP)), or with antiphospholipid antibody nephropathy/lupus anticoagulant syndrome. However, TMA can be present without any systemic syndrome. Small arteries and arterioles may show thrombosis, fibrinoid necrosis, and mucoid intimal hyperplasia ("onion skinning") (Figure 28). As opposed to lupus vasculopathy, lesions show no significant IgG immune deposition (IgM and C3 may be present, secondary to vascular injury). Glomeruli show typical TMA changes such as thrombosis, mesangiolysis, and double contour formation, which may be superimposed on other glomerular changes of LN.

Antiphospholipid antibody syndrome may be primary or lupus (or "lupus-like") associated. It is a clinically important cause of systemic and renal thrombosis, resulting in systemic and renal infarctions and subsequent organization and

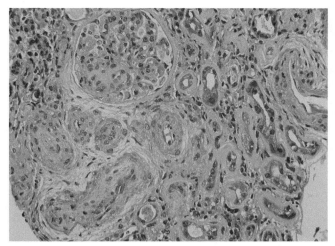

FIGURE 29 Chronic thrombotic microangiopathy, in a patient with LN and multiple pregnancy losses secondary to antiphospholipid autoantibody syndrome. The vessels are prominent and show chronic injury with marked medial and intimal fibrosis. Endothelial cells show reactive changes. The tubulointerstitium shows diffuse scarring with marked tubular atrophy and thickened basement membranes. The glomerulus also shows signs of chronic ischemia—hypoperfusion and segmental sclerosis (6–8 o'clock). MT, original magnification: 40×.

recanalization of the vessels.[17] The SLE-associated variant is more likely to also involve smaller vessels and display more typical findings of TMA (Figure 29). TMA lesions are significantly more common in lupus patients with antiphospholipid antibodies.[18] However, many patients may be antibody positive without demonstrating the syndrome.

CLASSIFICATION OF LUPUS NEPHRITIS

The wide spectrum of lesions seen in LN has served as both a stimulus for and challenge to efforts at a comprehensive classification. Indeed, the history of LN classification is coincident with the history of the development of the specialties of both nephrology and nephropathology. The introduction of the renal biopsy, and the subsequent application of IF and EM, has improved the understanding of the nature of SLE and led to a pioneering period of characterization and early classification in the 1950s–1960s.[19]

The "modern" era of classification began in 1974 with the formulation of what came to be known as the World Health Organization (WHO) classification of LN.[20,21] Widely adopted, it served as the framework for many subsequent modifications. Over time, a rather confusing situation developed, defeating the primary purpose of having a classification system. Consequently, the International Society of Nephrology/Renal Pathology Society (ISN/RPS) convened a consensus conference in 2002 that produced an updated system with guidelines for biopsy adequacy, standard definitions, and well-defined classes emphasizing "clinically relevant lesions" and encouraging "uniform and

TABLE 3 Abbreviated International Society of Nephrology/Renal Pathology Society (ISN/RPS) Classification of Lupus Nephritis (2003)

Class I: minimal mesangial lupus nephritis
Class II: mesangial proliferative lupus nephritis
Class III: focal lupus nephritis[a]
Class IV: diffuse segmental (IV-S) or global (IV-G) lupus nephritis[b]
Class V: membranous lupus nephritis[c]
Class VI: advanced sclerosing lupus nephritis

Indicate and grade (mild, moderate, severe) tubular atrophy, interstitial inflammation and fibrosis, severity of arteriosclerosis or other vascular lesions.
[a]Indicate the proportion of glomeruli with active and with sclerotic lesions.
[b]Indicate the proportion of glomeruli with fibrinoid necrosis and cellular crescents.
[c]Class V may occur in combination with class III or IV, in which case both will be diagnosed.

reproducible reporting between centers." As in all prior systems, classification was entirely glomerulocentric. The new system was widely supported, as attested to by its simultaneous appearance in two of the most prominent renal journals, and has been rapidly and widely adopted, replacing all others.[22] An understanding of prior systems remains important only to those translating historical studies to the present.

An overview of the classification is provided in Table 3, with details in Table 4. The system requires the characterization of each glomerulus in the sample based on the integration of both LM and IF findings. To facilitate worldwide adoption, it was designed to be (at least theoretically) EM independent. Nevertheless, a minority of cases require EM to define the glomerular lesions used in classification. The word "proliferative" is not used in classes III/IV, in recognition of the pathogenetic centrality of subendothelial deposits, even in the absence of endocapillary hypercellularity. The system affixes a mnemonic within each class to designate the nature of its lesions: purely active (A) or chronic lesions (C), or any combination (A/C), as defined in Table 5. The classification also requires the separate enumeration and grading of tubular atrophy, interstitial inflammation and fibrosis, and vascular lesions, together with all other pathologic processes, glomerular or otherwise, in the diagnosis.

Class I (Minimal Mesangial LN)

Clinical: These patients may have active systemic SLE, but urinary findings are minimal.

Pathology: The glomeruli are essentially normal by LM, with mesangial immune deposits seen by IF and EM. No deposits are seen along the capillary walls.

TABLE 4 International Society of Nephrology/Renal Pathology Society (ISN/RPS) 2003 Classification of Lupus Nephritis

Class I: Minimal Mesangial Lupus Nephritis

Normal glomeruli by light microscopy, but mesangial immune deposits by immunofluorescence

Class II: Mesangial Proliferative Lupus Nephritis

Purely mesangial hypercellularity of any degree or mesangial matrix expansion by light, microscopy, with mesangial immune deposits

May be a few isolated subepithelial or subendothelial deposits visible by immunofluorescence or, electron microscopy, but not by light microscopy

Class III: Focal Lupus Nephritis[a]

Active or inactive focal, segmental or global endo- or extracapillary glomerulonephritis involving <50% of all glomeruli, typically with focal subendothelial immune deposits, with or without mesangial alterations

Class III (A) Active lesions: focal proliferative lupus nephritis

Class III (A/C) Active and chronic lesions: focal proliferative and sclerosing lupus nephritis

Class III (C) chronic inactive lesions with glomerular scars: focal sclerosing lupus nephritis

Class IV: Diffuse Lupus Nephritis[b]

Active or inactive diffuse, segmental or global endo- or extracapillary glomerulonephritis, involving ≥50% of all glomeruli, typically with diffuse subendothelial immune deposits, with or, without mesangial alterations. This class is divided into diffuse segmental (IV-S) lupus nephritis when ≥50% of the involved glomeruli have segmental lesions, and diffuse global (IV-G) lupus nephritis when ≥50% of the involved glomeruli have global lesions. Segmental is defined as a glomerular lesion that involves less than half of the glomerular tuft. This class includes cases with diffuse wire loop deposits but with little or no glomerular proliferation

Class IV-S (A) Active lesions: Diffuse segmental proliferative lupus nephritis

Class IV-G (A) Active lesions: Diffuse global proliferative lupus nephritis

Class IV-S (A/C) Active and chronic lesions: Diffuse segmental proliferative and sclerosing lupus nephritis

Class IV-G (A/C) Active and chronic lesions: Diffuse global proliferative and sclerosing lupus nephritis

Class IV-S (C) chronic inactive lesions with scars: Diffuse segmental sclerosing lupus nephritis

Class IV-G (C) chronic inactive lesions with scars: Diffuse global sclerosing lupus nephritis

Class V: Membranous Lupus Nephritis

Global or segmental subepithelial immune deposits or their morphologic sequelae by light, microscopy and by immunofluorescence or electron microscopy, with or without mesangial, alterations

Class V lupus nephritis may occur in combination with class III or IV in which case both will be diagnosed

Class V lupus nephritis show advanced sclerosis

Class VI: Advanced Sclerosis Lupus Nephritis

≥90% of glomeruli globally sclerosed without residual activity

Indicate and grade (mild, moderate, severe) tubular atrophy, interstitial inflammation and fibrosis, severity of arteriosclerosis or other vascular lesions.
[a]Indicate the proportion of glomeruli with active and with sclerotic lesions.
[b]Indicate the proportion of glomeruli with fibrinoid necrosis and/or cellular crescents.

Class II (Mesangial Proliferative LN)

Clinical: Mild proteinuria (<1 g) and/or hematuria may be seen; even mildly reduced GFR is uncommon. This lesion may be stable for years. Increasing renal dysfunction suggests transformation to a higher class or superimposition of another renal disease.

Pathology: Glomerular changes by LM are limited to mesangial proliferation/matrical increase of any degree and distribution. Mesangial deposits are rarely visible by

LM, but they are easily seen on IF and EM. Identification of subendothelial deposits by LM indicates class III or IV. However, small subendothelial deposits seen by IF, or more usually by EM, may be seen, particularly in continuity with the mesangium. Whether this finding suggests a more ominous prognosis is unclear. The presence of segmental or global sclerosis that is interpreted to represent the scars of prior proliferative, necrotizing, or crescentic lesions is incompatible with this class and represents the chronic lesions of class III or IV. For example, a biopsy where all

TABLE 5 Active and Chronic Glomerular Lesions: ISN/RPS Classification of Lupus Nephritis (2003)

Active Lesions

  Endocapillary hypercellularity with or without leukocyte
  infiltration and with substantial luminal reduction
  Karyorrhexis
  Fibrinoid necrosis
  Rupture of glomerular basement membrane
  Crescents, cellular or fibrocellular
  Subendothelial deposits identifiable by light microscopy (wire
  loops)
  Intralumenal immune aggregates (hyaline thrombi)

Chronic lesions

  Glomerular sclerosis (segmental, global)
  Fibrous adhesions
  Fibrous crescents

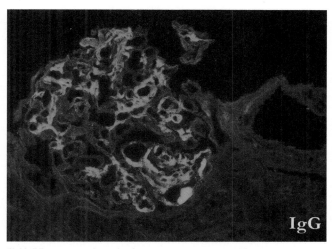

FIGURE 31 Multiple site immune complex deposition. The dominant pattern is mesangial deposition. In some areas, segmental mural staining of the capillary wall is seen, with two endoluminal deposits present at four to five o'clock. Some capillary loops are entirely negative, and others show only occasional granules suggestive of subepithelial deposits (e.g., 11–12 o'clock). The large vessel on the right shows focal mural IgG. IF, anti-IgG, original magnification: 40×.

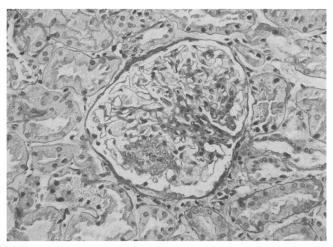

FIGURE 30 Segmental endocapillary proliferation may be seen in class III or IV-S. This lesion (6–8 o'clock) will heal as segmental sclerosis. Note that the remainder of the tuft shows only mesangial prominence. When lesions are focal and small, they may be missed due to limited tissue sampling, leading to a false class II designation. Surrounding tubules are intact. PAS, original magnification: 40×.

intact glomeruli show exclusively mesangial lesions would still be classed as III or IV if glomerulosclerosis due to prior activity is present. Lesions in other renal compartments are unusual for this class and suggest another process.

Class III (Focal LN)

Clinical: The picture parallels the variability of the histopathology. About 50% of these patients have an "active urinary sediment" (less so when lesions are predominantly chronic). Proteinuria is common (up to one-third have nephrotic syndrome), while the nephritic syndrome is not.

Pathology: Classes III and IV (habitually called "proliferative") are distinguished by the percentage of glomeruli

involved by "active" and/or "chronic" lesions (Table 5). Focal or diffuse mesangial proliferation is typically superimposed. Typical active lesions include endocapillary and/or extracapillary proliferation, as well as necrosis, wire loops, hyaline thrombi, and a membranoproliferative pattern. Glomerular necrosis is indicative of Class III or IV, and is incompatible with other classes. Chronic lesions include segmental or global glomerulosclerosis secondary to LN. Both A and C lesions may be segmental (S) or global (G). Focal lesions may be missed, particularly with limited sampling, leading to the inappropriate designation as class II (Figure 30).

As the term "focal" implies, class III glomerular changes (acute and/or chronic) involve less than 50% of sampled glomeruli and are primarily segmental. Cases with glomerular involvement approaching 50%, particularly those with necrosis, may behave more like class IV. IF and EM display widespread mesangial deposits accompanied by variable subendothelial deposition (paralleling the LM findings). As subendothelial deposits may be focal and mesangial deposits diffuse, limited IF and EM sampling may falsely suggest class II (Figure 31). A minor component of subepithelial deposits may be present—widespread deposition warrants an additional class V designation. A subset of patients with focal GN show segmental necrotizing lesions and crescents in association with limited IC deposition. This pattern raises the possibility of a pauci-immune glomerular disease similar to ANCA-positive vasculitis.[23]

LN is a recurring condition that often results in the simultaneous presence of both active and sclerosing lesions. The presence of sclerosing lesions in an initial biopsy suggests prior, perhaps subclinical, flares. Class III biopsies usually show some degree of acute and/or chronic tubulointerstitial injury.

Class IV (Diffuse LN)

Clinical: These patients typically have the most severe renal dysfunction. Consequently, this class is the largest in biopsy series. Patients with a membranoproliferative pattern tend to have more severe proteinuria and hypocomplementemia.

Pathology: By definition, a majority of the glomeruli are involved by lupus lesions. Whether classes III and IV represent a continuum of disease or reflect pathogenetically different processes is an ongoing debate. Nevertheless, in class IV, the histopathology of active LN finds its fullest expression (Figure 32). Almost all cases exhibit some endocapillary proliferation, but extensive subendothelial deposits and/or a membranoproliferative pattern alone is sufficient (Figure 33). Cases are further subclassed (discussed below) based on whether the lesions are predominantly segmental (S) or global (G). In contrast to class III, most cases are (G). The percentage of glomeruli with crescents and/or necrotizing lesions is recorded. Lupus-related vascular disease is most commonly found in this class but involves a minority of cases. In contrast, tubulointerstitial disease is common.

Class V (Membranous LN)

Clinical: As expected, the dominant finding is proteinuria, usually nephrotic range, although hematuria is frequent. Activity in the urinary sediment suggests the copresence of classes III or IV. This class is notorious for presenting prior to the clinical diagnosis of SLE.

Pathology: As scattered subepithelial deposits are common, class V requires involvement (continuous subepithelial deposition and/or associated basement membrane changes) of the majority of the membranes of the majority of glomeruli (Figure 34). As in "idiopathic" membranous GN, the basement membrane changes visible by LM primarily represent reaction to the deposits, not the immunodeposits themselves. Thus, in "early" stages, subepithelial

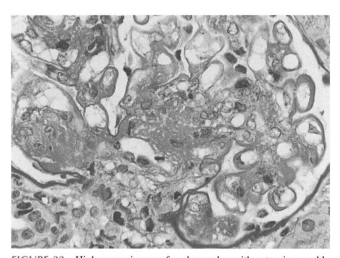

FIGURE 33 High-power image of a glomerulus with extensive weakly PAS-positive immune complex deposition that is confluent in the mesangium and prominent in the capillary walls in the subendothelial zone, up against the strongly staining membranes. Occasional early double-contour formation is seen, suggesting chronicity. This pattern is indicative of class III or IV, even though there is no proliferation, in recognition of the pathogenic centrality of subendothelial deposition. PAS, original magnification: 100×.

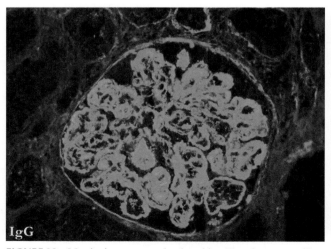

FIGURE 32 Massive immune complex deposition. There is strong capillary wall deposition with a sharp outer contour, suggestive of subendothelial deposition. In areas (9–11 o'clock), an endocapillary pattern is also seen. Some foci show confluent deposition involving all zones. Two "hyalin thrombi" are also seen. Note the extensive deposition along Bowman's capsule and tubular basement membranes. IF, anti-IgG, original magnification: 40×.

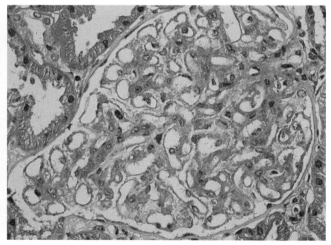

FIGURE 34 Membranous pattern with some mesangial and no endocapillary proliferation (pure class V pattern). The capillary loops, while patent and normocellular, show thickened walls, with granular subepithelial fuchsinophilic (red) IC deposits seen (as well as in the mesangium). The vascular pole is seen at 2 o'clock. Surrounding proximal tubules are healthy and show intact light blue brush borders. MT, original magnification: 100×.

deposits may only be visible by IF and EM (Figures 35 and 36). The presence of significant subendothelial deposits or endocapillary proliferation warrants the addition of class III/IV. With evolution, classic membranous changes (thickening, "spikes," and vacuolation) appear, particularly on PAS and Jones. With time, the deposits become incorporated into the membranes and may lose their antigenicity, and/or become electron lucent. Segmental or global glomerulosclerosis may result. However, as always, the

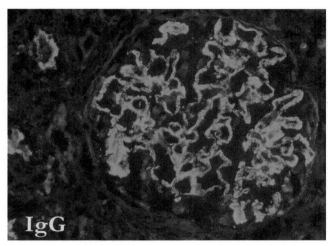

FIGURE 35 Membranous pattern of global subepithelial granular deposition (class V pattern). The capillary loops are patent, but some mesangial regions with deposits are identifiable. Adjacent atrophic tubules show irregular and thickened membranes with deposits. IF, anti-IgG, original magnification: 400×.

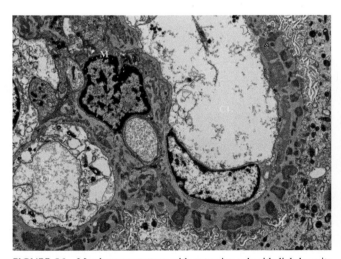

FIGURE 36 Membranous pattern with extensive subepithelial deposits (class V pattern). Some of the deposits show adjacent reactive "spike" formation by the basement membranes; most of the deposits have been "roofed over," implying some duration. Transmembranous (^), as well as extensive mesangial (M) deposition is also seen. The loop on the right also shows prominent subendothelial deposition that warrants an additional Class III or IV designation. Podocytes show diffuse injury. This pattern of multizone deposition is strongly suggestive of LN and is inconsistent with a primary membranous glomerulonephritis. EM, original magnification: 6,000×.

presence of glomerular scars judged to be the sequela of prior activity warrants an additional class III/IV.

Pure class V patients may have no extrarenal signs of SLE (ANA negative) and may present with renal disease years before the clinical diagnosis of SLE. Distinguishing class V LN from idiopathic membranous GN is therefore an ongoing challenge. The presence of any of the following suggests membranous GN secondary to SLE: mesangial hypercellularity, mesangial IC, "full house" positivity or significant C1q positivity, subendothelial deposits, vascular, tubular or interstitial immune deposits, tissue ANA, and tubuloreticular structures.[24] Significant staining for PLA2R points away from LN.[25]

Class V patients are at increased risk for the development of renal vein thrombosis. Acute thrombosis may result in interstitial edema and or hemorrhage, as well as glomerular congestion, thrombosis, and neutrophil margination. Chronic thrombosis is suggested by interstitial fibrosis and tubular atrophy that is out of proportion to glomerulosclerosis.

Class VI (Advanced Sclerosing LN)

Clinical: Patients may have inactive serologies and the dominant picture is advanced renal insufficiency. Most of these cases represent "burnt out" focal or diffuse LN.

Pathology: At least 90% of the glomeruli show sclerosis, usually global, accompanied by marked interstitial fibrosis and tubular atrophy, as well as chronic vascular injury. There must be no signs of activity. Sclerotic glomeruli may lose their immunoreactivity and appear IF negative. End-stage changes may be so nonspecific that the diagnosis of LN rests on clinical context or prior biopsy findings (Figure 37).

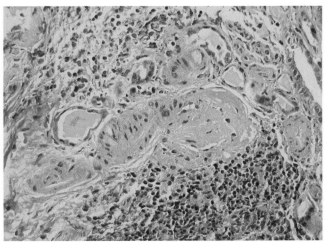

FIGURE 37 Cortex with end-stage renal injury (class VI pattern). There is extensive interstitial fibrosis and tubular atrophy, accompanied by mononuclear inflammation. A globally sclerotic glomerulus with its fibrotic arteriole is noted. This scarring is so advanced and nonspecific that only clinical context or prior biopsy findings may enable this to be attributed to LN. MT, original magnification: 40×.

SELECTED TOPICS IN CLASSIFICATION

Distinction Between Classes IV-S and IV-G

The distinction between classes IV-S and IV-G, undoubtedly the most controversial aspect of the system, was introduced based on a prospective study reporting that, despite similar clinical and serological parameters and treatment, IV-S (retrospectively classified) had both lower remission rates and 10 year renal survival compared to IV-G.[26] The authors speculated that segmental necrotizing lesions with a relative absence of subendothelial deposits might be pathogenetically different from IV-G (akin to "pauci-immune" crescentic GN although ANCA results were not reported), and thus the two subclasses are not a single disease continuum. Subsequent studies have identified some clinical and pathological differences between the subgroups. Not surprisingly, repeat biopsies have documented the "transformation" of IV-S to IV-G[27] Meta-analysis of eight such studies concluded that there was no difference in outcome (the rate of doubling of serum creatinine (SCr) or of end-stage renal disease) between the two subgroups.[28] Thus, the prognosis for the continued existence of these subgroups is guarded.

Glomerulosclerosis

The ISN/RPS system mandates that sclerotic glomeruli be counted to assign class only when they are thought to be the sequela of prior active glomerular lesions. While this distinction is (theoretically) reasonable, its application in the "real world" is difficult as there are limited histologic criteria to determine the etiology of glomerulosclerosis. Nephropathologists tend to attribute sclerosis to LN in young patients, as they often have less renal comorbidities. Including globally sclerotic glomeruli seems to increase the percentage of class III and IV biopsies.[29] The percentage of global and segmental glomerulosclerosis (independent of cause) is an important quantitation of parenchymal scarring.

Reproducibility of Classification

Two studies have demonstrated the superior reproducibility of the ISN/RPS versus WHO classifications.[30] Furness and Taub performed the best real-world comparison by using the same biopsies.[29] Reproducibility of the A/C designations was less robust than class but still within usual ranges. Interestingly, the ISN/RPS classification tended to produce more class IV (and less class III and V) than the WHO, attributed by the authors to increased recognition of capillary immune deposition unrelated to proliferation.

TREATMENT AND TRANSFORMATION

The lesions of LN are notoriously dynamic, as evidenced by the frequent occurrence of relapses and transformations (both spontaneous and treatment related) in class.[31] Recognition of these transformations is a function of how closely patients are monitored (clinically and pathologically, usually in the context of a flare). The most commonly reported transformation is class III to IV (hardly surprising, given that they likely represent a continuum), seen in about one-third of class III patients studied, with the presence of extensive subendothelial deposits being a possible risk factor.[32] A retrospective study found clinically relevant class transformation to be frequent in patients whose initial biopsy was "nonproliferative." In contrast, when the reference biopsy was "proliferative," transformation to "nonproliferative" was rare.[33]

Consensus regarding indications for repeat biopsy is limited. The new onset of laboratory findings unusual for the patient's known class is a common consideration. In contrast, the utility of rebiopsy in a patient with documented class IV who presents again with active sediment is limited. Other indications include rapid decline in renal function (crescentic disease) or the possibility of non-LN disease. Assessment of treatment efficacy or the extent of chronic injury prior to further toxic therapy is a common reason (see below). A common scenario is increasing proteinuria (potentially from either activity or chronicity), with one study showing 77% of biopsies resulting in a treatment change.[34] Finally, a high index of suspicion and experienced clinical judgment are essential, as the correlations between clinical findings and biopsy class are imperfect.[35] Furthermore, significant progression of chronicity can occur silently, as documented by a study showing relatively stable GFR over 36 months, despite an increase in global glomerulosclerosis from 15% to 60%.[36]

Activity, Chronicity, Plasticity, and Prognosis

Immunosuppression is primarily effective against active lesions, involves considerable toxicity, and has minimal effect on scarring. Treatment decisions, a function of the risk–benefit ratio, are predominantly determined by the degree of activity (reversible) and chronicity (irreversible) in the biopsy. Moreover, activity and chronicity can be quite variable within a particular class (especially III/IV) and poorly expressed by the A/C designations. For example, a biopsy with 51% of glomeruli showing endocapillary proliferation alone is designated the same class IV-A as one with 100% of the glomeruli showing necrosis and crescents, yet most clinicians would approach the latter differently. This underscores the importance of communication with the nephropathologist and explains why many nephrologists continue to find semiquantitative scoring of activity and chronicity useful in conveying a snapshot of current disease and for comparison with subsequent biopsies.

Austin et al. devised the widely adopted National Institutes of Health (NIH) scheme,[37] as shown in Table 6. Activity is scored from 0 to 24 using six histological parameters,

TABLE 6 NIH Activity and Chronicity Indexes

Activity Index (0–24)

  Endocapillary hypercellularity: 0–3
  Glomerular neutrophils (>2 per glomerulus): 0–3
  Karyorrhexis/fibrinoid necrosis: (0–3)×2
  Cellular crescents: (0–3)×2
  Hyaline deposits (thrombi or wire loops: 0–3)
  Interstitial inflammation: 0–3

Chronicity Index (0–12)

  Glomerular sclerosis: 0–3
  Fibrous crescents: 0–3
  Tubular atrophy: 0–3
  Interstitial fibrosis: 0–3

Scale of glomerular involvement: none=0, <25%=1, 25–50%=2, and >50% of glomeruli=3.
Neutrophil exudation and Interstitial Involvement: none=0, mild=1, moderate=2, and severe=3.

each semiquantitatively graded from 0 to 3. The numerical weight of cellular crescents and glomerular necrosis are doubled to reflect their clinical severity. Chronicity is scored from 0 to 12 using four semiquantitatively graded parameters. These criteria are somewhat different from those in the ISN/RPS classification (Table 5) and tubulointerstitial findings play a greater role in determining chronicity than activity. Vascular lesions are entirely ignored in both indices.

As with all schema, the reproducibility of these scores and their prognostic ability are controversial.[38] Correlation with outcomes may improve with higher scores: activity >7 and chronicity >3.[39] The findings on repeat biopsy, following 6 months of treatment, are often more prognostically significant than initial values.[40] The CI is generally thought to be more predictive of outcome than the AI or class.[41] Newer systems may be more prognostically powerful but remain too cumbersome for routine use.[42] Despite these concerns, most continue to find these indices useful in guiding therapy, and they function as a concise method of comparing sequential biopsies.

Traditional pathologic findings of prognostic significance include class on initial biopsy and progression to a higher class on repeat biopsy.[8] Patients with combined membranous and proliferative LN also tend to do worse.[43] The prognostic significance of class alone improved by the addition of extraglomerular findings, such as vasculopathy.[44] A single-center study in children showed no difference in patient or renal survival between those with and without proliferative disease (class II vs class IV), with gender (male) being the only independent risk factor for mortality.[45] A retrospective study suggests that patients with the synchronous onset of LN with SLE have higher rates of prolonged remissions and a lower frequency of chronic

renal damage than those with delayed onset of LN, despite similar rates of class IV lesions.[46]

SELECTED CLINCOPATHOLOGIC TOPICS

"Silent" LN

Histopathological LN without clinical renal disease may be more common than generally recognized.[47] Its frequency is a function of how rigorously the "silence" is defined (SCr vs other renal parameters vs serologic positivity). While much of the literature describes a benign course, comparative studies suggest that silent LN represents the earliest stage in the natural history of LN (Zabaleta-Lanz et al., 2006).[48]

ANCA, Crescentic GN, and LN

Approximately 20% of patients with SLE are ANCA (overwhelmingly p-ANCA) positive by indirect IF. Some studies suggest a correlation between ANCA positivity and LN activity. An initial series reports 10 cases of necrotizing and crescentic LN, all with associated ANCA positivity.[23] More data are necessary to explore this association; ANCA testing in cases of LN with crescents and necrosis out of proportion to the degree of proliferation and subendothelial deposition merits consideration. Myeloperoxidase-ANCAs are particularly common in patients with drug-induced SLE.[49]

Other Renal Diseases and SLE

Renal disease in SLE patients cannot be assumed to represent LN. Biopsy may reveal another process, either alone or superimposed on LN. Virtually every disease has appeared as a case report.[50] There is increasing recognition of the occurrence of SLE-associated "podocytopathies" (minimal change/focal and segmental glomerulosclerosis and its collapsing variant) that tend to be highly steroid-responsive. Their incidence appears to be greater than in the general population, suggesting a causal link to the immune dysregulation of SLE.[51] APOL1 risk alleles strongly associate with collapsing GN in African–American SLE patients.[52]

Drug-induced lupus is relatively common; fortunately, renal involvement is not. Many drugs have been implicated and all classes have been noted. A high index of suspicion is warranted as there are no specific histologic features suggesting a drug-related process.

Patients with both HIV and SLE may show lesions related to either or both entities. In contrast, HIV-associated "lupus-like" IC GN shows multiple site deposits and other morphologic features of LN without positive lupus serologies.[53]

The glomerular lesions of mixed connective tissue disease may be indistinguishable from LN. Vessels may display TMA changes similar to systemic sclerosis. Patients with both SLE and Sjogren's syndrome may have milder renal disease than those with SLE alone.[54]

Transplantation

Studies suggest that both patient and allograft survival are comparable to nonlupus cohorts.[55] The rate of detection of recurrent disease is a direct function of the use of IF and EM on allograft biopsies. A study suggested that it may be more common than previously thought, although most recurrences are subclinical.[56]

REFERENCES

1. Walker PD. The renal biopsy. *Arch Pathol Lab Med* February 2009;**133**(2):181–8. PubMed PMID: 19195962. Epub 07.02.09 eng.

2. Jennette JC, Olson JL, Silva FG, D'Agati VD. Heptinstall's pathology of the kidney. 7th ed. ; 2015. 2 volumes (various pagings) p.

3. Colvin RB. *Diagnostic pathology. Kidney diseases.* 1st ed. Salt Lake City, Utah: Amirsys; 2011.

4. Mannik M, Merrill CE, Stamps LD, Wener MH. Multiple autoantibodies form the glomerular immune deposits in patients with systemic lupus erythematosus. *J Rheumatol* July 2003;**30**(7):1495–504. PubMed PMID: 12858447. Epub 15.07.03 eng.

5. Williams DG, Peters DK, Fallows J, Petrie A, Kourilsky O, Morel-Maroger L, et al. Studies of serum complement in the hypocomplementaemic nephritides. *Clin Exp Immunol* November 1974;**18**(3):391–405. PubMed PMID: 4219908. PMCID: 1537992. Epub 01.11.74 eng.

6. Herrera GA. The value of electron microscopy in the diagnosis and clinical management of lupus nephritis. *Ultrastruct Pathol* 1999;**23**(2).

7. Kashgarian M. Lupus nephritis: lessons from the path lab. *Kidney Int* March 1994;**45**(3):928–38. PubMed PMID: 8196299.

8. Lewis EJ, Kawala K, Schwartz MM. Histologic features that correlate with the prognosis of patients with lupus nephritis. *Am J Kidney Dis* September 1987;**10**(3):192–7. PubMed PMID: 3631068.

9. Ronnblom L, Alm GV, Eloranta ML. Type I interferon and lupus. *Curr Opin Rheumatol* September 2009;**21**(5):471–7. PubMed PMID: 19525849. Epub 16.06.09 eng.

10. Park MH, D'Agati V, Appel GB, Pirani CL. Tubulointerstitial disease in lupus nephritis: relationship to immune deposits, interstitial inflammation, glomerular changes, renal function, and prognosis. *Nephron* 1986;**44**(4):309–19. PubMed PMID: 3540691. Epub 01.01.86. eng.

11. Hill GS, Delahousse M, Nochy D, Mandet C, Bariety J. Proteinuria and tubulointerstitial lesions in lupus nephritis. *Kidney Int* November 2001;**60**(5):1893–903. PubMed PMID: 11703608.

12. Mori Y, Kishimoto N, Yamahara H, Kijima Y, Nose A, Uchiyama-Tanaka Y, et al. Predominant tubulointerstitial nephritis in a patient with systemic lupus nephritis. *Clin Exp Nephrol* March 2005;**9**(1):79–84. PubMed PMID: 15830279. Epub 15.04.05. eng.

13. Hunter MG, Hurwitz S, Bellamy CO, Duffield JS. Quantitative morphometry of lupus nephritis: the significance of collagen, tubular space, and inflammatory infiltrate. *Kidney Int* January 2005;**67**(1):94–102. PubMed PMID: 15610232. Epub 22.12.04. eng.

14. Appel GB, Pirani CL, D'Agati V. Renal vascular complications of systemic lupus erythematosus. *J Am Soc Nephrol* February 1994;**4**(8):1499–515. PubMed PMID: 8025223. Epub 01.02.94. eng.

15. Descombes E, Droz D, Drouet L, Grunfeld JP, Lesavre P. Renal vascular lesions in lupus nephritis. *Med Baltim* September 1997;**76**(5):355–68. PubMed PMID: 9352738. Epub 14.11.97. eng.

16. Banfi G, Bertani T, Boeri V, Faraggiana T, Mazzucco G, Monga G, et al. Renal vascular lesions as a marker of poor prognosis in patients with lupus nephritis. Gruppo Italiano per lo Studio della Nefrite Lupica (GISNEL). *Am J Kidney Dis* August 1991;**18**(2):240–8. PubMed PMID: 1867181. Epub 01.08.91. eng.

17. Tektonidou MG. Renal involvement in the antiphospholipid syndrome (APS)-APS nephropathy. *Clin Rev Allergy Immunol* June 2009;**36**(2–3):131–40. PubMed PMID: 19048414. Epub 03.12.08. eng.

18. Tektonidou MG, Sotsiou F, Nakopoulou L, Vlachoyiannopoulos PG, Moutsopoulos HM. Antiphospholipid syndrome nephropathy in patients with systemic lupus erythematosus and antiphospholipid antibodies: prevalence, clinical associations, and long-term outcome. *Arthritis Rheum* August 2004;**50**(8):2569–79. PubMed PMID: 15334471.

19. Pollak VE, Pirani CL, Schwartz FD. The natural history of the renal manifestations of systemic lupus erythematosus. *J Lab Clin Med* April 1964;**63**:537–50. PubMed PMID: 14155443. Epub 01.04.64. eng.

20. Sommers SC, Bernstein J. *Kidney pathology decennial, 1966–1975.* New York: Appleton-Century-Crofts; 1975. x, 687 pp. 2 leaves of plates p.

21. Appel GB, Silva FG, Pirani CL, Meltzer JI, Estes D. Renal involvement in systemic lupud erythematosus (SLE): a study of 56 patients emphasizing histologic classification. *Med Baltim* September 1978;**57**(5):371–410. PubMed PMID: 682942. Epub 01.09.78. eng.

22. Weening JJ, D'Agati VD, Schwartz MM, Seshan SV, Alpers CE, Appel GB, et al. The classification of glomerulonephritis in systemic lupus erythematosus revisited. *J Am Soc Nephrol* February 2004;**15**(2):241–50. PubMed PMID: 14747370. Epub 30.01.04. eng.

23. Nasr SH, D'Agati VD, Park HR. Necrotizing and crescentic lupus nephritis with antineutrophil cytoplasmic antibody seropositivity. *Clin J Am Soc Nephrol* 2008;**3**:682–90.

24. Jennette JC, Iskandar SS, Dalldorf FG. Pathologic differentiation between lupus and nonlupus membranous glomerulopathy. *Kidney Int* September 1983;**24**(3):377–85. PubMed PMID: 6358633. Epub 01.09.83. eng.

25. Larsen CP, Messias NC, Silva FG, Messias E, Walker PD. Determination of primary versus secondary membranous glomerulopathy utilizing phospholipase A2 receptor staining in renal biopsies. *Mod Pathol* May 2013;**26**(5):709–15. PubMed PMID: 23196797.

26. Najafi CC, Korbet SM, Lewis EJ, Schwartz MM, Reichlin M, Evans J, et al. Significance of histologic patterns of glomerular injury upon long-term prognosis in severe lupus glomerulonephritis. *Kidney Int* 2001;**59**(6):2156–63.

27. Mittal B, Hurwitz S, Rennke H, Singh AK. New subcategories of class IV lupus nephritis: are there clinical, histologic, and outcome differences? *Am J Kidney Dis* December 2004;**44**(6):1050–9. PubMed PMID: 15558526. Epub 24.11.04. eng.

28. Haring CM, Rietveld A, van den Brand JA, Berden JH. Segmental and global subclasses of class IV lupus nephritis have similar renal outcomes. *J Am Soc Nephrol* January 2012;**23**(1):149–54. PubMed PMID: 22034639. PMCID: 3269930.

29. Furness PN, Taub N. Interobserver reproducibility and application of the ISN/RPS classification of lupus nephritis-a UK-wide study. *Am J Surg Pathol* August 2006;**30**(8):1030–5. PubMed PMID: 16861976. Epub 25.07.06. eng.

30. Yokoyama H, Wada T, Hara A, Yamahana J, Nakaya I, Kobayashi M, et al. The outcome and a new ISN/RPS 2003 classification of lupus nephritis in Japanese. *Kidney Int* December 2004;**66**(6):2382–8. PubMed PMID: 15569330. Epub 01.12.04. eng.

31. Lu J, Tam LS, Lai FM, Kwan BC, Choi PC, Li EK, et al. Repeat renal biopsy in lupus nephritis: a change in histological pattern is common. *Am J Nephrol* 2011;**34**(3):220–5. PubMed PMID: 21791918.

32. Moroni G, Pasquali S, Quaglini S, Banfi G, Casanova S, Maccario M, et al. Clinical and prognostic value of serial renal biopsies in lupus nephritis. *Am J Kidney Dis* September 1999;**34**(3):530–9. PubMed PMID: 10469865. Epub 02.09.99 eng.

33. Daleboudt GMN, Bajema IM, Goemaere NNT, van Laar JM, Bruijn JA, Berger SP. The clinical relevance of a repeat biopsy in lupus nephritis flares. *Nephrol Dial Transpl* July 21, 2009;**2009**. gfp.359.

34. Bajaj S, Albert L, Gladman DD, Urowitz MB, Hallett DC, Ritchie S. Serial renal biopsy in systemic lupus erythematosus. *J Rheumatol* December 2000;**27**(12):2822–6. PubMed PMID: 11128670.

35. Christopher-Stine L, Siedner M, Lin J, Haas M, Parekh H, Petri M, et al. Renal biopsy in lupus patients with low levels of proteinuria. *J Rheumatol* February 2007;**34**(2):332–5. PubMed PMID: 17183619. Epub 22.12.06. eng.

36. Chagnac A, Kiberd BA, Farinas MC, Strober S, Sibley RK, Hoppe R, et al. Outcome of the acute glomerular injury in proliferative lupus nephritis. *J Clin Invest* September 1989;**84**(3):922–30. PubMed PMID: 2760219. PMCID: 329737.

37. Austin 3rd HA, Muenz LR, Joyce KM, Antonovych TT, Balow JE. Diffuse proliferative lupus nephritis: identification of specific pathologic features affecting renal outcome. *Kidney Int* April 1984;**25**(4):689–95. PubMed PMID: 6482173. Epub 01.04.84. eng.

38. Schwartz MM, Lan SP, Bernstein J, Hill GS, Holley K, Lewis EJ. Irreproducibility of the activity and chronicity indices limits their utility in the management of lupus nephritis. Lupus nephritis collaborative study group. *Am J Kidney Dis* April 1993;**21**(4):374–7. PubMed PMID: 8465815. Epub 01.04.93. eng.

39. Austin 3rd HA, Boumpas DT, Vaughan EM, Balow JE. Predicting renal outcomes in severe lupus nephritis: contributions of clinical and histologic data. *Kidney Int* February 1994;**45**(2):544–50. PubMed PMID: 8164443. Epub 01.02.94. eng.

40. Hill GS, Delahousse M, Nochy D, Remy P, Mignon F, Mery JP, et al. Predictive power of the second renal biopsy in lupus nephritis: significance of macrophages. *Kidney Int* January 2001;**59**(1):304–16. PubMed PMID: 11135084. Epub 03.01.01. eng.

41. Hiramatsu N, Kuroiwa T, Ikeuchi H, Maeshima A, Kaneko Y, Hiromura K, et al. Revised classification of lupus nephritis is valuable in predicting renal outcome with an indication of the proportion of glomeruli affected by chronic lesions. *Rheumatol Oxf* May 2008;**47**(5):702–7. PubMed PMID: 18390590. Epub 09.04.08. eng.

42. Hill GS, Delahousse M, Nochy D, Tomkiewicz E, Remy P, Mignon F, et al. A new morphologic index for the evaluation of renal biopsies in lupus nephritis. *Kidney Int* September 2000;**58**(3):1160–73. PubMed PMID: 10972679. Epub 06.09.2000. eng.

43. Pasquali S, Banfi G, Zucchelli A, Moroni G, Ponticelli C, Zucchelli P. Lupus membranous nephropathy: long-term outcome. *Clin Nephrol* April 1993;**39**(4):175–82. PubMed PMID: 8491046. Epub 01.04.93. eng.

44. Wu LH, Yu F, Tan Y, Qu Z, Chen MH, Wang SX, et al. Inclusion of renal vascular lesions in the 2003 ISN/RPS system for classifying lupus nephritis improves renal outcome predictions. *Kidney Int* April 2013;**83**(4):715–23. PubMed PMID: 23302713.

45. Vachvanichsanong P, Dissaneewate P, McNeil E. Diffuse proliferative glomerulonephritis does not determine the worst outcome in childhood-onset lupus nephritis: a 23-year experience in a single centre. *Nephrol Dial Transpl* September 2009;**24**(9):2729–34. PubMed PMID: 19395731. Epub 28.04.09. eng.

46. Takahashi Y, Mizoue T, Suzuki A, Yamashita H, Kunimatsu J, Itoh K, et al. Time of initial appearance of renal symptoms in the course of systemic lupus erythematosus as a prognostic factor for lupus nephritis. *Mod Rheumatol* 2009;**19**(3):293–301. PubMed PMID: 19277827. Epub 12.03.09. eng.

47. Wakasugi D, Gono T, Kawaguchi Y. Frequency of class III and IV nephritis in systemic lupus erythematosus without clinical renal involvement: an analysis of predictive measures. *J Rheumatol* 2012;**39**:79–85.

48. Zabaleta-Lanz ME., Muñoz LETapanes FJ, Vargas-Arenas RE, Tapanes FJ, Daboin I, Barrios I, et al. Further description of early clinically silent lupus nephritis. *Lupus* 2006;**15**(12):845–51. PubMed PMID: 17211989

49. Sen D, Isenberg DA. Antineutrophil cytoplasmic autoantibodies in systemic lupus erythematosus. *Lupus* 2003;**12**(9):651–8. PubMed PMID: 14514126. Epub 30.09.03. eng.

50. Baranowska-Daca E, Choi YJ, Barrios R, Nassar G, Suki WN, Truong LD. Nonlupus nephritides in patients with systemic lupus erythematosus: a comprehensive clinicopathologic study and review of the literature. *Hum Pathol* October 2001;**32**(10):1125–35. PubMed PMID: 11679948. Epub 27.10.01. eng.

51. Kraft SW, Schwartz MM, Korbet SM, Lewis EJ. Glomerular podocytopathy in patients with systemic lupus erythematosus. *J Am Soc Nephrol* January 2005;**16**(1):175–9. PubMed PMID: 15548564. Epub 19.11.04. eng.

52. Larsen CP, Beggs ML, Saeed M, Walker PD. Apolipoprotein L1 risk variants associate with systemic lupus erythematosus-associated collapsing glomerulopathy. *J Am Soc Nephrol* April 2013;**24**(5):722–5. PubMed PMID: 23520206. PMCID: 3636799.

53. Haas M, Kaul S, Eustace JA. HIV-associated immune complex glomerulonephritis with "lupus-like" features: a clinicopathologic study of 14 cases. *Kidney Int* April 2005;**67**(4):1381–90. PubMed PMID: 15780090.

54. Baer AN, Maynard JW, Shaikh F, Magder LS, Petri M. Secondary Sjogren's syndrome in systemic lupus erythematosus defines a distinct disease subset. *J Rheumatol* June 2010;**37**(6):1143–9. PubMed PMID: 20360189.

55. Burgos PI, Perkins EL, Pons-Estel GJ, Kendrick SA, Liu JM, Kendrick WT, et al. Risk factors and impact of recurrent lupus nephritis in patients with systemic lupus erythematosus undergoing renal transplantation: data from a single US institution. *Arthritis Rheum* September 2009;**60**(9):2757–66. PubMed PMID: 19714623. PMCID: 2771574.

56. Norby GE, Strom EH, Midtvedt K, Hartmann A, Gilboe IM, Leivestad T, et al. Recurrent lupus nephritis after kidney transplantation: a surveillance biopsy study. *Ann Rheum Dis* August 2010;**69**(8):1484–7. PubMed PMID: 20498208.

Chapter 42

Cardiovascular Disease in Systemic Lupus Erythematosus

Susan Manzi

Department of Medicine, Lupus Center of Excellence, Allegheny Health Network, Pittsburgh, PA, USA

INTRODUCTION

In 2011, the American Heart Association (AHA) first acknowledged that systemic lupus erythematosus is a unique risk factor for cardiovascular disease (CVD), in part due to a 1997 study that demonstrated a 50-fold higher relative risk of myocardial infarction in premenopausal women with lupus.[1–3] As newer therapies have prolonged the lives of lupus patients, their risk for CVD has increased at a rate that traditional CVD risk factors alone cannot explain.[4] It is estimated that there are over 1.5 million patients with some form of lupus in the United States; approximately 90% of them are women, and nearly half of all lupus patient autopsies reveal hallmarks of atherosclerosis.[5] Research suggests that longer lupus disease duration is associated with greater risk for CVD.[4]

Cutting-edge imaging techniques have provided a greater window inside the development of CVD in lupus patients, highlighting manifestations of disease long before symptoms may be reported.[6] Carotid ultrasound has revealed more carotid plaques, a sign of atherosclerosis, in lupus patients versus controls, independent of other traditional CVD risk factors and regardless of age group.[7] Electron beam computed tomography has demonstrated that coronary artery calcification (CAC) is significantly more common in lupus patients than controls and that the age of atherosclerosis onset is younger in the lupus population.[8,9] Carotid intima media thickness (IMT), a measurement of the inner layers of the arterial wall, and presence of carotid plaque have been reported to increase the risk of a future CV event in patients with lupus.[10,11] This suggests that imaging may play a role in risk stratification. Collectively, these findings prove CVD to be an urgent and growing problem, requiring a focused effort on defining pathogenesis, identifying risk factors, and evaluating management strategies in well-designed, randomized, controlled trials.

Although this discussion will touch upon the most recent advances and therapeutic approaches for common cardiac manifestations of lupus, we will focus primarily on the advances and therapeutic paradigms involving atherosclerotic CVD, as this disorder has the greatest impact on patient mortality and morbidity. We will not discuss cerebrovascular disease, which is a unique manifestation and beyond the scope of this chapter.

TRADITIONAL RISK FACTORS FOR CVD IN LUPUS

Consensus holds that CVD in lupus is caused by multifactorial processes that include traditional risk factors and disease-specific immune and inflammatory factors.[12] The traditional risk factors of obesity, smoking, a sedentary lifestyle, and advancing age that raise the general population's risk for CVD also affect patients with lupus.[13,14] This unique population of women has a significantly higher rate of hypertension and reduced vascular elasticity than healthy controls, which research suggests might be tied to their chronic use of corticosteroids.[15] Low-density lipoprotein (LDL) is a firmly established risk factor for CVD. After oxidation, LDL becomes more antigenic and plays a primary role in development of atherosclerosis. Lupus patients demonstrate aspects of dyslipidemia with higher percentages of oxidized low-density lipoproteins (oxLDL), elevated free fatty acid and triglyceride levels, and higher degrees of inflammation and endothelial activation.[16,17] In a study comparing lupus to rheumatoid arthritis (RA), the oxLDL percentage of total LDL was significantly higher in lupus patients compared to patients with RA ($p = 0.0311$), and significantly higher in lupus patients with carotid plaque than in those without plaque ($p < 0.001$)[16].

In the general population, high-density lipoproteins (HDLs) are considered protective against atherogenesis, in part by preventing oxidation of LDL, a critical step in the development of plaque.[18] This protective effect depends on both the quantity of HDL and its function. HDL particles

Systemic Lupus Erythematosus. http://dx.doi.org/10.1016/B978-0-12-801917-7.00042-5

are anti-inflammatory, but in chronic inflammatory diseases such as lupus, HDL can become oxidized and thus proinflammatory (piHDL). piHDLs fail to prevent the oxidation of LDL, and instead promote the oxidation of LDL. Women with lupus have been shown to have higher frequencies of piHDL compared to healthy controls and those with piHDL have more carotid plaques.[18]

Metabolic syndrome is a disorder of energy storage and usage characterized by high cholesterol levels, increased abdominal fat, and increased blood pressure.[19] The disorder is a predominant feature in lupus and may in fact be driven by the enhanced amounts of inflammation seen in these individuals.[19]

One of the most effective and commonly used therapies for lupus, corticosteroids, has been implicated in promoting CVD.[9] Although corticosteroids have been found to reduce overall inflammation and lupus disease activity, a study confirmed previous reports that longer duration of use and higher cumulative dosing were associated with a greater risk for atherosclerosis.[20] This risk can be explained in part by the adverse effects of steroids including weight gain, blood pressure elevation, dyslipidemia, and hyperglycemia. A 2012 study revealed that even short-term corticosteroid use of 20 mg/day or more resulted in a greater risk of cardiovascular event.[21] These findings reinforce the concept of limiting corticosteroid exposure in favor of other therapeutics, including antimalarials and immunoregulatory agents.[22,23]

NOVEL MECHANISMS AND AREAS OF INVESTIGATION

Research into the mechanisms of CVD development in lupus patients is ongoing and some of the current topics of investigation are discussed here. In the areas of inflammation and immune function, factors such as complement activation, resistin, adipokines, cytokines, T cells, and type I interferons are subjects of recent scrutiny. Atherosclerosis commences when inflammatory cells, such as T cells, are drawn to the endothelial surface, prompting a proinflammatory cycle of downstream events. Adhesion molecules, which are increased in states of inflammation, recruit immune cells to the endothelial surface and have been found to be upregulated in lupus patients, especially during disease flare-ups.[9]

Cytokines such as tumor necrosis factor (TNF)-α and interleukin (IL)-1 are significantly increased in lupus patients with CVD compared to those without CVD, and these cytokines promote adhesion molecule expression.[3,9] When immune cells are recruited to the endothelial surface, complement activation occurs. That activation further promotes atherosclerosis by increasing endothelial cell proliferation, recruiting additional immune cells to the site, and triggering greater amounts of procoagulant tissue factor.[3,9]

Leptin is an adipokine that regulates satiety and fat stores and is associated with endothelial dysfunction. Leptin levels have been independently associated with carotid plaques and positively correlated with piHDL and oxidized phospholipids in patients with lupus.[24] Resistin, also known as adipose tissue-specific secretary factor, participates in the inflammatory response by upregulating adhesion molecules, increasing expression of proinflammatory cytokines such as IL-1, IL-6, and TNF-α. Resistin may also play a role in insulin resistance associated with increased adiposity. Researchers have found that lupus patients with larger degrees of CAC demonstrated higher levels of resistin than those patients without CAC.[25]

Type I interferons, a family of secreted proteins that alert the immune system to the presence of pathogens, have gotten significant attention as key factors in lupus pathogenesis. This recognition led to the development of agents that target type I interferons as therapeutic alternatives in lupus. Type I interferons have also been linked with endothelial dysfunction and the progression of CVD in lupus patients, even in those without any other risk factors for vascular disease. These observations have resulted in recommendations that vascular end points be considered as secondary outcomes for future trials of antiinterferon therapies in lupus.[26–28]

Autoantibodies are a hallmark of lupus and have been useful biomarkers for diagnosis and prognosis. Some autoantibodies have been linked to thrombotic events, while others have been associated with atherogenesis. The most notable of these antibodies are antiphospholipid antibodies (aPLs). The link between aPLs and thrombosis is firmly established, and yet the association between these antibodies and the risk of atherosclerosis remains controversial, with some studies reporting positive, and others negative, correlations.[29] Because aPLs have been shown to predict both future arterial events and mortality, measuring these antibodies even in patients with no clinical CVD is recommended.[14,30] There are data to support aPLs as contributors to atherosclerosis.[31,32] One type of aPL specifically targets beta 2 glycoprotein I (B2GPI).[32,33] B2GPI is an apolipoprotein that can bind to phospholipids as well as cell membranes of platelets and endothelial cells, resulting in endothelial activation and atheroma formation.[33] The association between B2GPI and aPLs may provide one link between autoimmune disease and endothelial dysfunction.[33] aPLs in combination with other inflammatory and endothelial markers may serve as valuable indicators of CVD risk.[34]

Naturally occurring immunoglobulin (Ig) M autoantibodies to phosphorylcholine (IgM-anti-PC) can enhance apoptotic clearance and promote anti-inflammatory pathways.[35,36] Higher levels of IgM-anti-PC have been associated with lower frequency of CVD events and carotid plaque, independent of other traditional risk factors. This protective association was not seen with other IgM or IgG autoantibodies, suggesting that IgM-anti-PC may serve as a biomarker for CVD in lupus.[35,36]

Endothelial progenitor cells, a population of circulating stem cells that contributes to the repair of blood vessels, may serve as potential biomarkers to identify those patients at risk for CVD progression. In one study, lupus patients with lower circulating levels of progenitor cells had increased arterial stiffness and a higher prevalence of cardiovascular risk factors, such as tobacco use and metabolic syndrome.[37] A reduction in circulating endothelial progenitor cells may be an effective marker for vascular disease in its earliest stages.[37]

Deficiency in vitamin D is a common feature in lupus, particularly pediatric lupus, and has been linked to inflammatory markers that predict vascular disease.[38] Independent of traditional CVD risk factors, vitamin D deficiency has been associated with increased aortic stiffness, an early marker of vascular dysfunction.[39] A 2014 study reported that pediatric lupus patients whose vitamin D levels were greater than 20 ng/ml had less atherosclerotic progression, measured by carotid IMT, in response to atorvastatin treatment than those with lower vitamin D levels. This interesting observation suggests that vitamin D supplementation may be beneficial in combination with statins in CVD prevention.[40]

Genetic factors have long been implicated in the propensity for development of CVD. The concept that genes linked to CVD may also be linked to autoimmune disease predisposition has been explored by a number of investigators. A study from Vanderbilt University reported that 20 polymorphisms in 152 candidate genes linked to CVD and/or autoimmune diseases were associated with significant increases in CAC.[41] Furthermore, genes that play a role in the differentiation of monocytes to macrophages, key cells in the earliest components of atheroma, were found to be differentially regulated in lupus patients as compared to healthy controls and could differentiate lupus patients with and without subclinical atherosclerosis.[42] During atherogenesis, inflammatory monocytes differentiate into macrophages and contribute to the formation of atherosclerotic lesions by ingesting oxLDL and forming foam cells, the earliest component of plaque.[43] Monocytes from patients with lupus may be programmed to differentiate into macrophages with enhanced potential to form atheroma. Macrophage activation may also be mediated by interferon regulatory factors, a family of transcription factors that play a role in innate immunity and immune cell differentiation. Interferon regulatory factor (IRF)-8 allele has been identified as a possible genetic contributor to heart disease in lupus patients and has been associated with carotid plaque and increased IMT.[44]

Lupus is a complex and heterogeneous disease that is unpredictable and potentially fatal. For these reasons, the field of biomarker discovery is exploding and a significant effort has been focused on identification of patients at highest risk for comorbidities such as premature CVD.

THERAPEUTIC PARADIGMS FOR ATHEROSCLEROSIS

There is a paucity of randomized clinical trials to evaluate interventions in preventing or treating CVD in lupus. The following tables summarize recent randomized clinical trials and observational cohort studies of statins (Table 1), immunosuppressants (Table 2), antimalarial drugs (Table 3), antioxidants (Table 4), and oral hypoglycemic agents (Table 5).

There are conflicting findings in terms of benefits of statins on cardiovascular risk, with some studies reporting less progression of coronary calcification and reduction in CVD events and others showing no benefit. The randomized trials, however, uniformly demonstrate that statins are well tolerated, effectively reduce lipid levels, and have no significant effect on disease activity. In addition, statins have shown a favorable impact on biomarkers, such as high-sensitivity C reactive protein (hsCRP). There are little data from clinical trials to address the role of immunosuppressive therapies and biologics on development of atherosclerosis. Animal studies support the role of mycophenolate mofetil (MMF) in reducing CVD progression; however, in a human study, MMF did not improve either Carotid Intima Media Thickness or CAC progression over a 2-year period in a prospectively followed lupus cohort randomized to atorvastatin or placebo. Only 25 of the 187 patients were on MMF, underscoring a common limitation of small sample size in many of the therapeutic trials of CVD in lupus.[45]

The story with antimalarials has been evolving. A mainstay therapeutic in lupus for decades, more recently these agents have been shown to have benefits beyond disease activity. Antimalarial use has been associated with lower lipid levels, reduced vascular stiffness, improved glucose metabolism, less thrombovascular events, and improved survival in multiethnic lupus cohorts. The interest in antimalarials is now extending beyond autoimmune diseases, and several trials are evaluating the benefit of these agents in improving glycemic control and insulin sensitivity in diabetes.

While oxidative stress has been identified as critical in the pathophysiology of atherosclerosis and acute thrombosis, pooled data from large randomized trials of vitamin E, vitamin C, or beta carotene in CVD risk reduction in the general population have been disappointing.[46] Similarly, in one small trial in lupus, there was no significant effect on endothelial function after 12 weeks of vitamin C and vitamin E therapy. On the other hand, omega-3 fatty acids, which exert favorable pleiotropic, cardiometabolic effects on the cardiovascular system, have demonstrated benefit and are recommended in current guidelines for CVD risk reduction. Supplementation of up to

TABLE 1 Randomized Statin Trials

Drug	Study Design	Year	Authors	Results	Conclusions
Fluvastatin	Randomized, double blind, placebo controlled, 7–8 year follow-up trial in renal transplant recipients with lupus; n=33 (10 placebo and 23 drug treated) out of total 2102 in ALERT cohort 1° outcome: major cardiac event	2009	Norby et al.[a]	29% reduction in LDL levels, 73% reduction in time to first major cardiac event	No safety concerns. Fluvastatin in kidney transplant patients with lupus reduces major cardiac events. Note: small sample size and post-hoc analysis
Atorvastatin	Randomized, placebo-controlled, 2-year follow-up; n=200 lupus; 1° outcome: CAC, 2° outcomes: carotid IMT/plaque and biomarkers	2011	Petri et al.[b]	Total cholesterol declined 17% in drug treated group. No significant difference in CAC, plaque, IMT, disease activity, or measures of inflammation	Minor elevations in liver function tests. Atorvastatin did not impact progression of CAC over 2 years
Atorvastatin	Randomized, placebo-controlled, 1-year follow-up; n=60 lupus, 1° outcomes: MDCT-coronary calcium, and SPECT-myocardium perfusion, 2° outcomes: biomarkers, lupus disease activity	2011	Plazak et al.[c]	Less progression in coronary calcium scores and significant reductions in serum lipids, and CRP. No change in myocardium perfusion or disease activity	Atorvastatin reduces progression of coronary calcium over 1 year. Well tolerated. Note: small sample size
Rosuvastatin	Randomized, double blind, placebo controlled; 2-year follow-up (treatment unblinded after 12 months); n=72 lupus (1/2 in each arm received low dose ASA). Outcomes: biomarkers at 1 year and carotid IMT at 2 years	2011	Mok et al.[d]	At 12 months, significant decreases in LDL and hsCRP. No significant change in homocysteine. At 24 months, IMT decreased in drug treated patients, not significant	No adverse drug effects. Rosuvastatin treatment with trends in reducing progression of carotid IMT over 2 years

Statins are well tolerated and do show reduction in LDL and hsCRP in most trials. Downward trends in coronary calcium and IMT progression. No impact on disease activity, however most trials included patients with low lupus disease activity.

ALERT, Assessment of lescol in renal transplantation; ASA, aspirin; CAC, coronary artery calcification; CVD, cardiovascular disease; hsCRP, high-sensitivity C reactive protein; IMT, intima media thickness; LDL, low-density lipoprotein; MDCT, multidetector computed tomography; MI, myocardial infarction; SPECT, single-photon emission computed tomography; TPA, tissue plasminogen activator.
[a]Norby GE, Holme I, Fellstrom B, Jardine A, Cole E, Abedini S, et al. Effect of fluvastatin on cardiac outcomes in kidney transplant patients with systemic lupus erythematosus: a randomized placebo-controlled study. Arthritis Rheum 2009;**60**(4):1060–4.
[b]Petri MA, Kiani AN, Post W, Christopher-Stine L, Magder LS. Lupus atherosclerosis prevention study (LAPS). Ann Rheum Dis 2011;**70**(5):760–5.
[c]Plazak W, Gryga K, Dziedzic H, Tomkiewicz-Pajak L, Konieczynska M, Podolec P, et al. Influence of atorvastatin on coronary calcifications and myocardial perfusion defects in systemic lupus erythematosus patients: a prospective, randomized, double-masked, placebo-controlled study. Arthritis Res Ther 2011;**13**(4):R117.
[d]Mok CC, Wong CK, To CH, Lai JP, Lam CS. Effects of rosuvastatin on vascular biomarkers and carotid atherosclerosis in lupus: a randomized, double-blind, placebo-controlled trial. Arthritis Care Res (Hoboken) 2011;**63**(6):875–83.

1 g daily is generally well tolerated and encouraged in populations at high risk for CVD events. Similar benefits were noted in a small study of patients with lupus, where omega-3 fatty acids improved flow mediated vasodilation after 24 weeks.

In the absence of large, randomized, controlled trials in lupus, the 2011 AHA guidelines for prevention of CVD in women provide a roadmap for clinicians to follow. The AHA guidelines, updated from 2007 and with international applicability, acknowledged for the first time that lupus is an unrecognized risk factor for CVD, noting that lupus patients had a significantly increased relative risk for CVD.[2]

The updated guidelines recommend that all women with lupus be screened for CVD, even in the absence of symptoms, and—somewhat surprisingly—they recommend that women with prior CVD events be screened for lupus. The expert panel strongly considered effectiveness (benefits and risks observed in clinical practice), as well as evidence from clinical trials for the new prevention guidelines. Treatments that are considered not useful or effective for prevention of myocardial infarction include menopausal therapy (hormone therapy and selective estrogen-receptor modulators), antioxidant supplements (vitamins E, C, and beta-carotene),

TABLE 2 Immunosuppressant Studies

Drug	Study Design	Year	Authors	Conclusions
Cyclosporine A	Cross-sectional study of lupus nephritis patients; n = 82 outcome: carotid IMT	2011	Sazliyana et al.[a]	Higher cumulative cyclosporine A dose was independently associated with lower carotid IMT, controlling for traditional and other lupus related risk factors.
MMF	Posthoc analysis from a randomized trial of atorvastatin in lupus n = 187 n = 25 on MMF during the 2-year follow-up. Outcomes: CAC and carotid IMT	2012	Kiani et al.[b]	MMF did not impact progression of CAC and carotid IMT.
MMF	7-week-old gld.apoE mice fed high cholesterol diet with or without MMF.	2013	Richez et al.[c]	Those on MMF demonstrated less atherosclerotic lesion area and improved lupus activity than controls.

Data suggest that immunosuppressants may be beneficial in CVD risk reduction, but randomized trials are needed.

CAC, coronary artery calcification; CVD, cardiovascular disease; IMT, intima media thickness; LN, lupus nephritis; MMF, mycophenolate mofetil.
[a]Sazliyana S, Mohd Shahrir MS, Kong CT, Tan HJ, Hamidon BB, Azmi MT. Implications of immunosuppressive agents in cardiovascular risks and carotid intima media thickness among lupus nephritis patients. Lupus 2011;**20**(12):1260–6.
[b]Kiani AN, Magder LS, Petri M. Mycophenolate mofetil (MMF) does not slow the progression of subclinical atherosclerosis in SLE over 2 years. Rheumatol Int 2012;**32**(9):2701–5.
[c]Richez C, Richards RJ, Duffau P, Weitzner Z, Andry CD, Rifkin IR, et al. The effect of mycophenolate mofetil on disease development in the gld.apoE (−/−) mouse model of accelerated atherosclerosis and systemic lupus erythematosus. PLoS One 2013;**8**(4):e61042.

folic acid supplementation, and routine use of aspirin therapy for women <65 years.[2] The recommendation on routine aspirin therapy did not take into account those patients at high risk for thrombotic events, such as those with lupus and antiphospholipid syndrome. In addition, these guidelines focused on cardiovascular, not cerebrovascular, disease prevention.

The AHA and other supporting research in lupus strongly recommend lifestyle changes as first-line preventive strategies with pharmacologic interventions when needed, including cessation of cigarette smoking, moderate exercise, a diet rich in fruits and vegetables, weight maintenance or reduction, blood pressure monitoring, omega-3 supplementation, and lipid monitoring, as well as statins, beta blockers, aldosterone blockers, and angiotensin-converting enzyme (ACE) inhibitors where indicated.[2,22,47–49] Conducting randomized, placebo-controlled trials of these proposed interventions in lupus, with adequate power to determine efficacy, is a major undertaking and would require multicenter collaboration and significant financial support. Until studies of this scope are possible, there is no reason not to adopt the AHA prevention guidelines for at-risk populations to benefit patients with lupus.

OTHER CARDIAC MANIFESTATIONS OF LUPUS

Additional cardiac manifestations of lupus (pericarditis, myocardial dysfunction [heart failure], conduction abnormalities, and valvular disorders), their diagnosis, frequency, and recommended treatments are summarized in Table 6.

CONCLUSIONS AND FUTURE DIRECTIONS

In summary, the AHA has now recognized lupus as an at-risk population for CVD and recommends screening these patients for risk factors, even without clinically evident CVD. They even suggest screening women with prior CVD events for autoimmune conditions such as lupus. This is a major advance since the previous 2007 guidelines. This recognition now comes with a heightened responsibility. Many patients with lupus are young women and although the relative risk of CVD is high, the absolute risk is low. This dilemma has fueled the investigation of biomarker discovery, including imaging modalities, to identify those patients at highest risk. Given the complexity of lupus, it is unlikely that any one biomarker will be sufficient.

Efforts are now underway to develop biomarker panels that include traditional risk factors, adipokines, inflammatory markers, autoantibodies, cytokines, genetic markers, and imaging techniques to risk stratify and identify those patients with the highest likelihood of CVD progression. Until we have sufficient evidence-based intervention and prevention strategies from large clinical trials in lupus, we must rely on treatment guidelines developed for similar at-risk populations.

TABLE 3 Antimalarial Studies

Drug	Study Design	Year(s)	Authors	Results	Conclusions
Hydroxy-chloroquine (HCQ)	LUMINA cohort established in 1994, comprised of Hispanic, Caucasian, African American; case-controlled study of risk factors for mortality, n=608	2007	Alarcon et al.[a]	HCQ associated with improved survival after adding propensity score OR 0.319 (95% CI 0.118–0.864)	HCQ had a protective effect on survival even after adjusting for factors related to treatment decisions.
	GLADEL inception cohort established in 1997, multicenter cohort in 9 Latin American countries: observational study, n=1480, to evaluate the beneficial effect of HCQ on survival for those on drug ≥6 consecutive months (users) versus those <6 consecutive months or never used (nonusers)	2010	Shinjo et al.[b]	Lower mortality rate in users compared to nonusers 4.4% versus 11.5%, p<0.001). Improved survival with longer duration of use ≥24 mos.	Antimalarials associated with lower mortality with a duration of use effect.
	Nested case–control 2-year study Univ. Toronto, 54 cases with lupus identified with TEs (22 venous and 32 arterial) paired with 2 controls/case with lupus without TEs	2010	Jung et al.[c]	Ever use of antima-larials protective against TE. OR 0.32 (0.14–0.74) p<0.01	Antimalarial use associated with less thrombotic events.
	Longitudinal observation study, n=24, lipids measured before and after 3 months of treatment	2012	Cairoli et al.[d]	Significant reduction in TC and LDL	Antimalarials had a beneficial effect on reduction in lipid levels after only 3 months of treatment.
	Cross-sectional study, n=220, risk factors associated with PWV, a measure of aortic stiffness an early marker of CVD	2001	Selzer, et al.[e]	HCQ use associated with less aortic stiffness after controlling for other risk factors	Antimalarials may be protective against vascular stiffness and early CVD

Reduced mortality, vascular events, lipid levels, aortic vascular stiffness.

ACR, American College of Rheumatology; CVD, cardiovascular disease; HCQ, hydroxychloroquine; LDL, low-density lipoprotein; PWV, pulse wave velocity; TC, total cholesterol; TE, thrombovascular event.
[a]Alarcon GS, McGwin G, Bertoli AM, Fessler BJ, Calvo-Alen J, Bastian HM, et al. Effect of hydroxychloroquine on the survival of patients with systemic lupus erythematosus: data from LUMINA, a multiethnic US cohort (LUMINA L). Ann Rheum Dis 2007;**66**(9):1168–72.
[b]Shinjo SK, Bonfa E, Wojdyla D, Borba EF, Ramirez LA, Scherbarth HR, et al. Antimalarial treatment may have a time-dependent effect on lupus survival: data from a multinational Latin American inception cohort. Arthritis Rheum 2010;**62**(3):855–62.
[c]Jung H, Bobba R, Su J, Shariati-Sarabi Z, Gladman DD, Urowitz M, et al. The protective effect of antimalarial drugs on thrombovascular events in systemic lupus erythematosus. Arthritis Rheum 2010;**62**(3):863–8.
[d]Cairoli E, Rebella M, Danese N, Garra V, Borba EF. Hydroxychloroquine reduces low-density lipoprotein cholesterol levels in systemic lupus erythematosus: a longitudinal evaluation of the lipid-lowering effect. Lupus 2012;**21**(11):1178–82.
[e]Selzer F, Sutton-Tyrrell K, Fitzgerald S, Tracy R, Kuller L, Manzi S. Vascular stiffness in women with systemic lupus erythematosus. Hypertension 2001;**37**(4):1075–82.

TABLE 4 Antioxidant Trials

Chemical(s)	Study Design	Year	Authors	Conclusions
Vitamins C and E	Randomized, placebo-controlled study, 12 week follow-up; n=39 female lupus patients, outcomes: change in MDA (oxidative stress), antioxidants, vWF, PAI-1 and FMD.	2005	Tam et al.[a]	Well tolerated, most subjects demonstrated reduced serum peroxidation (MDA) but no effects on other markers of oxidative stress or endothelial function.
Omega-3 fatty acids	Randomized, double blind, placebo-controlled study, 24 week follow-up; n=60 lupus patients outcomes: lupus disease activity and FMD.	2008	Wright et al.[b]	Reductions in oxidative stress and disease activity with improvements in FMD. omega-3 fatty acids may provide cardiovascular benefits.

No role for vitamin C or vitamin E in CVD risk reduction, but omega-3 fatty acids may have potential benefit.

FMD, flow-mediated dilation; MDA, malondialdehyde; MI, myocardial infarction; PAI-1, plasminogen activator inhibitor; vWF, vonWillebrand factor.
[a]Tam LS, Li EK, Leung VY, Griffith JF, Benzie IF, Lim PL, et al. Effects of vitamins C and E on oxidative stress markers and endothelial function in patients with systemic lupus erythematosus: a double blind, placebo controlled pilot study. J Rheumatol 2005;**32**(2):275–82.
[b]Wright SA, O'Prey FM, McHenry MT, Leahey WJ, Devine AB, Duffy EM, et al. A randomised interventional trial of omega-3 polyunsaturated fatty acids on endothelial function and disease activity in systemic lupus erythematosus. Ann Rheum Dis 2008;**67**(6):841–8.

TABLE 5 Thiazolidinedione Trial

Chemical	Study Design	Year	Authors	Conclusions
Pioglitazone	Randomized, double-blind, placebo controlled study, 3 month follow-up; n=30 lupus patients outcomes: plasma HDL, insulin, inflammatory markers	2012	Juarez-Rojas et al.[a]	Fasting insulin, CRP, and serum amyloid significantly reduced and HDL increased on drug versus placebo. Trial suggests a potential benefit in reducing CVD risk.

Early data show promise but more randomized trials are needed.

CRP, C-reactive protein; CVD, cardiovascular disease; HDL, high-density lipoprotein.

[a]Juarez-Rojas, JG, Medina-Urrutia, AX, Jorge-Galarza, E, Caracas-Portilla, NA, Posadas-Sanchez, R, Cardoso-Saldana, GC et al. Pioglitazone improves the cardiovascular profile in patients with uncomplicated systemic lupus erythematosus: a double-blind randomized clinical trial. Lupus 2012;**21**(1):27–35.

TABLE 6 Other Cardiac Manifestations in Lupus

Disorder	Manifestations	Preferred Diagnostic Methodology	Frequency	Treatment
Pericarditis	Pleuritic chest pain, weakness, palpitations, difficulty breathing, coughing	ECG, echocardiogram, chest X-ray. Pericardial fluid may not be visible with acute pericarditis[a]	May be presenting manifestation of lupus[b]; estimated between 11% and 54% of lupus patients[c]	NSAIDs and/or corticosteroids, and colchicine[a,d]
Myocardial dysfunction (heart failure)	Chest pain, shortness of breath, light headedness, nausea, palpitations	MRI to detect and guide therapies (even without symptoms, dysfunction has been found)[e,f,g]	Clinical detection ranges from 3% to 15% of lupus patients[c]	Beta blockers, calcium channel blockers, ACE inhibitors, aldosterone antagonists, diuretics[h]
Conduction abnormalities	Arrhythmia – fragmented QRS complexes have been reported in lupus patients[i]; sinus tachycardia, atrial fibrillation, and ectopic beats are the most common arrhythmias in lupus patients[j]	ECG, stress test	Large-scale arrhythmia-specific studies in lupus are lacking[k]	Beta blockers, atropine, defibrillator placement[j]
Valvular disease	Heart murmur, fatigue, swelling in extremities, chest pain, heart fluttering; Libman Sacks (LS) endocarditis is a cardiac manifestation of lupus and antiphospholipid antibody syndrome that affects all four heart valves[l]	Echocardiogram, ECG, chest X-ray, stress test, heart catheterization[m,n,o]	Approximately 1 in 10 lupus patients[p]	Valve surgical replacement which is rare but is an option for stenosis caused by LS, conservative treatment with anticoagulants and immunosuppressants[l]

ECG, electrocardiogram; NSAIDs, nonsteroidal anti-inflammatory drugs; MRI, magnetic resonance imaging.

[a]Khandaker MH, Espinosa RE, Nishimura RA, Sinak LJ, Hayes SN, Melduni RM, et al. Pericardial disease: diagnosis and management. Mayo Clin Proc 2010;**85**(6):572–93.

[b]Chen PY, Chang CH, Hsu CC, Liao YY, Chen KT. Systemic lupus erythematosus presenting with cardiac symptoms. Am J Emerg Med 2014;**32**(9):1117–9.

[c]Tincani A, Rebaioli CB, Taglietti M, Shoenfeld Y. Heart involvement in systemic lupus erythematosus, anti-phospholipid syndrome and neonatal lupus. Rheumatology (Oxford) 2006;**45**(Suppl. 4):iv8–13.

[d]Imazio M, Brucato A, Cemin R, Ferrua S, Maggiolini S, Beqaraj F, et al. A randomized trial of colchicine for acute pericarditis. N Engl J Med 2013;**369**(16):1522–8.

[e]Puntmann VO, D'Cruz D, Smith Z, Pastor A, Choong P, Voigt T, et al. Native myocardial T1 mapping by cardiovascular magnetic resonance imaging in subclinical cardiomyopathy in patients with systemic lupus erythematosus. Circ Cardiovasc Imaging 2013;**6**(2):295–301.

[f]Mavrogeni S, Sfikakis PP, Gialafos E, Bratis K, Karabela G, Stavropoulos E, et al. Cardiac tissue characterization and the diagnostic value of cardiovascular magnetic resonance in systemic connective tissue diseases. Arthritis Care Res (Hoboken) 2014;**66**(1):104–12.

[g]Zhang Y, Corona-Villalobos CP, Kiani AN, Eng J, Kamel IR, Zimmerman SL, et al. Myocardial T2 mapping by cardiovascular magnetic resonance reveals subclinical myocardial inflammation in patients with systemic lupus erythematosus. Int J Cardiovasc Imaging 2014.

[h]Nonaka M, Morimoto S. Experimental models of inherited cardiomyopathy and its therapeutics. World J Cardiol 2014;**6**(12):1245–51.

[i]Demir K, Avci A, Yilmaz S, Demir T, Ersecgin A, Altunkeser BB. Fragmented QRS in patients with systemic lupus erythematosus. Scand Cardiovasc J 2014;**48**(4):197–201.

[j]Seferovic PM, Ristic AD, Maksimovic R, Simeunovic DS, Ristic GG, Radovanovic G, et al. Cardiac arrhythmias and conduction disturbances in autoimmune rheumatic diseases. Rheumatology (Oxford) 2006;**45**(Suppl. 4):iv39–42.

[k]Teixeira RA, Borba EF, Bonfa E, Martinelli Filho M. Arrhythmias in systemic lupus erythematosus. Rev Bras Reumatol 2010;**50**(1):81–9.

[l]Foroughi M, Hekmat M, Ghorbani M, Ghaderi H, Majidi M, Beheshti M. Mitral valve surgery in patients with systemic lupus erythematosus. Scientific World Journal 2014;**2014**:216291.

[m]Czarny MJ, Resar JR. Diagnosis and management of valvular aortic stenosis. Clin Med Insights Cardiol 2014;**8**(Suppl. 1):15–24.

[n]How is heart valve disease diagnosed?: National Heart, Lung, and Blood Institute; 2011 [updated November 16, 2011; March 18, 2015]. Available from: http://www.nhlbi.nih.gov/health/health-topics/topics/hvd/diagnosis.

[o]Testing for heart valve problems: American Heart Association; 2014 [updated April 2, 2014; March 18, 2015]. Available from: http://www.heart.org/HEARTORG/Conditions/More/HeartValveProblemsandDisease/Testing-for-Heart-Valve-Problems_UCM_450776_Article.jsp.

[p]Moyssakis I, Tektonidou MG, Vasilliou VA, Samarkos M, Votteas V, Moutsopoulos HM. Libman-Sacks endocarditis in systemic lupus erythematosus: prevalence, associations, and evolution. Am J Med 2007;**120**(7):636–42.

REFERENCES

1. Manzi S, Meilahn EN, Rairie JE, Conte CG, Medsger Jr TA, Jansen-McWilliams L, et al. Age-specific incidence rates of myocardial infarction and angina in women with systemic lupus erythematosus: comparison with the Framingham Study. *Am J Epidemiol* 1997;**145**(5):408–15.

2. Mosca L, Benjamin EJ, Berra K, Bezanson JL, Dolor RJ, Lloyd-Jones DM, et al. Effectiveness-based guidelines for the prevention of cardiovascular disease in women–2011 update: a guideline from the American heart association. *Circulation* 2011;**123**(11):1243–62.

3. Kahlenberg JM, Kaplan MJ. The interplay of inflammation and cardiovascular disease in systemic lupus erythematosus. *Arthritis Res Ther* 2011;**13**(1):203.

4. Hak AE, Karlson EW, Feskanich D, Stampfer MJ, Costenbader KH. Systemic lupus erythematosus and the risk of cardiovascular disease: results from the nurses' health study. *Arthritis Rheum* 2009;**61**(10):1396–402.

5. Haider YS, Roberts WC. Coronary arterial disease in systemic lupus erythematosus; quantification of degrees of narrowing in 22 necropsy patients (21 women) aged 16 to 37 years. *Am J Med* 1981;**70**(4):775–81.

6. Croca SC, Rahman A. Imaging assessment of cardiovascular disease in systemic lupus erythematosus. *Clin Dev Immunol* 2012;**2012**: 694143.

7. Roman MJ, Shanker BA, Davis A, Lockshin MD, Sammaritano L, Simantov R, et al. Prevalence and correlates of accelerated atherosclerosis in systemic lupus erythematosus. *N Engl J Med* 2003;**349**(25): 2399–406.

8. Asanuma Y, Oeser A, Shintani AK, Turner E, Olsen N, Fazio S, et al. Premature coronary-artery atherosclerosis in systemic lupus erythematosus. *N Engl J Med* 2003;**349**(25):2407–15.

9. Agarwal S, Elliott JR, Manzi S. Atherosclerosis risk factors in systemic lupus erythematosus. *Curr Rheumatol Rep* 2009;**11**(4):241–7.

10. Belibou C, Ancuta C, Ancuta E, Filos C, Chirieac R. Carotid intima-media thickness and plaque as surrogate biomarkers of atherosclerosis among consecutive women with systemic lupus erythematosus. *Rom J Morphol Embryol* 2012;**53**(1):29–34.

11. Kao AH, Lertratanakul A, Elliott JR, Sattar A, Santelices L, Shaw P, et al. Relation of carotid intima-media thickness and plaque with incident cardiovascular events in women with systemic lupus erythematosus. *Am J Cardiol* 2013;**112**(7):1025–32.

12. McMahon M, Hahn BH, Skaggs BJ. Systemic lupus erythematosus and cardiovascular disease: prediction and potential for therapeutic intervention. *Expert Rev Clin Immunol* 2011;**7**(2):227–41.

13. Amaya-Amaya J, Sarmiento-Monroy JC, Caro-Moreno J, Molano-Gonzalez N, Mantilla RD, Rojas-Villarraga A, et al. Cardiovascular disease in latin american patients with systemic lupus erythematosus: a cross-sectional study and a systematic review. *Autoimmune Dis* 2013;**2013**:794383.

14. Frostegard J. Prediction and management of cardiovascular outcomes in systemic lupus erythematosus. *Expert Rev Clin Immunol* 2015;**11**(2):247–53.

15. Sacre K, Escoubet B, Pasquet B, Chauveheid MP, Zennaro MC, Tubach F, et al. Increased arterial stiffness in systemic lupus erythematosus (SLE) patients at low risk for cardiovascular disease: a cross-sectional controlled study. *PLoS One* 2014;**9**(4):e94511.

16. Ahmad HM, Sarhan EM, Komber U. Higher circulating levels of OxLDL % of LDL are associated with subclinical atherosclerosis in female patients with systemic lupus erythematosus. *Rheumatol Int* 2014;**34**(5):617–23.

17. Ormseth MJ, Swift LL, Fazio S, Linton MF, Raggi P, Solus JF, et al. Free fatty acids are associated with metabolic syndrome and insulin resistance but not inflammation in systemic lupus erythematosus. *Lupus* 2013;**22**(1):26–33.

18. McMahon M, Skaggs BJ, Grossman JM, Sahakian L, Fitzgerald J, Wong WK, et al. A panel of biomarkers is associated with increased risk of the presence and progression of atherosclerosis in women with systemic lupus erythematosus. *Arthritis Rheumatol* 2014;**66**(1):130–9.

19. Parker B, Urowitz MB, Gladman DD, Lunt M, Donn R, Bae SC, et al. Impact of early disease factors on metabolic syndrome in systemic lupus erythematosus: data from an international inception cohort. *Ann Rheum Dis* 2014;**74**(8).

20. Sazliyana S, Mohd Shahrir MS, Kong CT, Tan HJ, Hamidon BB, Azmi MT. Implications of immunosuppressive agents in cardiovascular risks and carotid intima media thickness among lupus nephritis patients. *Lupus* 2011;**20**(12):1260–6.

21. Magder LS, Petri M. Incidence of and risk factors for adverse cardiovascular events among patients with systemic lupus erythematosus. *Am J Epidemiol* 2012;**176**(8):708–19.

22. Iaccarino L, Bettio S, Zen M, Nalotto L, Gatto M, Ramonda R, et al. Premature coronary heart disease in SLE: can we prevent progression? *Lupus* 2013;**22**(12):1232–42.

23. Lertratanakul A, Wu P, Dyer AR, Kondos G, Edmundowicz D, Carr J, et al. Risk factors in the progression of subclinical atherosclerosis in women with systemic lupus erythematosus. *Arthritis Care Res Hob* 2014;**66**(8):1177–85.

24. McMahon M, Skaggs BJ, Sahakian L, Grossman J, FitzGerald J, Ragavendra N, et al. High plasma leptin levels confer increased risk of atherosclerosis in women with systemic lupus erythematosus, and are associated with inflammatory oxidised lipids. *Ann Rheum Dis* 2011;**70**(9):1619–24.

25. Baker JF, Morales M, Qatanani M, Cucchiara A, Nackos E, Lazar MA, et al. Resistin levels in lupus and associations with disease-specific measures, insulin resistance, and coronary calcification. *J Rheumatol* 2011;**38**(11):2369–75.

26. Knight JS, Kaplan MJ. Cardiovascular disease in lupus: insights and updates. *Curr Opin Rheumatol* 2013;**25**(5):597–605.

27. Somers EC, Zhao W, Lewis EE, Wang L, Wing JJ, Sundaram B, et al. Type I interferons are associated with subclinical markers of cardiovascular disease in a cohort of systemic lupus erythematosus patients. *PLoS One* 2012;**7**(5):e37000.

28. Thacker SG, Zhao W, Smith CK, Luo W, Wang H, Vivekanandan-Giri A, et al. Type I interferons modulate vascular function, repair, thrombosis, and plaque progression in murine models of lupus and atherosclerosis. *Arthritis Rheum* 2012;**64**(9):2975–85.

29. Gustafsson JT, Svenungsson E. Definitions of and contributions to cardiovascular disease in systemic lupus erythematosus. *Autoimmunity* 2014;**47**(2):67–76.

30. Drakoulogkona O, Barbulescu AL, Rica I, Musetescu AE, Ciurea PL. The outcome of patients with lupus nephritis and the impact of cardiovascular risk factors. *Curr Health Sci J* 2011;**37**(2):70–4.

31. Motoki Y, Nojima J, Yanagihara M, Tsuneoka H, Matsui T, Yamamoto M, et al. Anti-phospholipid antibodies contribute to arteriosclerosis in patients with systemic lupus erythematosus through induction of tissue factor expression and cytokine production from peripheral blood mononuclear cells. *Thromb Res* 2012;**130**(4):667–73.

32. Murthy V, Willis R, Romay-Penabad Z, Ruiz-Limon P, Martinez-Martinez LA, Jatwani S, et al. Value of isolated IgA anti-beta2 -glycoprotein I positivity in the diagnosis of the antiphospholipid syndrome. *Arthritis Rheum* 2013;**65**(12):3186–93.

33. Conti F, Spinelli FR, Alessandri C, Pacelli M, Ceccarelli F, Marocchi E, et al. Subclinical atherosclerosis in systemic lupus erythematosus and antiphospholipid syndrome: focus on beta2GPI-specific T cell response. *Arterioscler Thromb Vasc Biol* 2014;**34**(3):661–8.

34. Gustafsson JT, Simard JF, Gunnarsson I, Elvin K, Lundberg IE, Hansson LO, et al. Risk factors for cardiovascular mortality in patients with systemic lupus erythematosus, a prospective cohort study. *Arthritis Res Ther* 2012;**14**(2):R46.

35. Gronwall C, Akhter E, Oh C, Burlingame RW, Petri M, Silverman GJ. IgM autoantibodies to distinct apoptosis-associated antigens correlate with protection from cardiovascular events and renal disease in patients with SLE. *Clin Immunol* 2012;**142**(3):390–8.

36. Gronwall C, Reynolds H, Kim JK, Buyon J, Goldberg JD, Clancy RM, et al. Relation of carotid plaque with natural IgM antibodies in patients with systemic lupus erythematosus. *Clin Immunol* 2014;**153**(1):1–7.

37. Castejon R, Jimenez-Ortiz C, Valero-Gonzalez S, Rosado S, Mellor S, Yebra-Bango M. Decreased circulating endothelial progenitor cells as an early risk factor of subclinical atherosclerosis in systemic lupus erythematosus. *Rheumatology* 2014;**53**(4):631–8.

38. Robinson AB, Tangpricha V, Yow E, Gurion R, McComsey GA, Schanberg LE, et al. Vitamin D deficiency is common and associated with increased C-reactive protein in children and young adults with lupus: an Atherosclerosis Prevention in Pediatric Lupus Erythematosus substudy. *Lupus Sci Med* 2014;**1**(1):e000011.

39. Reynolds JA, Haque S, Berry JL, Pemberton P, Teh LS, Ho P, et al. 25-Hydroxyvitamin D deficiency is associated with increased aortic stiffness in patients with systemic lupus erythematosus. *Rheumatology* 2012;**51**(3):544–51.

40. Robinson AB, Tangpricha V, Yow E, Gurion R, Schanberg LE, McComsey GA, et al. Vitamin D status is a determinant of atorvastatin effect on carotid intima medial thickening progression rate in children with lupus: an Atherosclerosis Prevention in Pediatric Lupus Erythematosus (APPLE) substudy. *Lupus Sci Med* 2014;**1**(1):e000037.

41. Chung C, Solus J, Oeser A, Li C, Raggi P, Smith J, et al. Genetic variation and coronary atherosclerosis in patients with systemic lupus erythematosus. *Lupus* 2014;**23**(9):876–80.

42. Korman BD, Huang CC, Skamra C, Wu P, Koessler R, Yao D, et al. Inflammatory expression profiles in monocyte-to-macrophage differentiation in patients with systemic lupus erythematosus and relationship with atherosclerosis. *Arthritis Res Ther* 2014;**16**(4):R147.

43. Ley K, Miller YI, Hedrick CC. Monocyte and macrophage dynamics during atherogenesis. *Arterioscler Thromb Vasc Biol* 2011;**31**(7):1506–16.

44. Leonard D, Svenungsson E, Sandling JK, Berggren O, Jonsen A, Bengtsson C, et al. Coronary heart disease in systemic lupus erythematosus is associated with interferon regulatory factor-8 gene variants. *Circ Cardiovasc Genet* 2013;**6**(3):255–63.

45. Kiani AN, Magder LS, Petri M. Mycophenolate mofetil (MMF) does not slow the progression of subclinical atherosclerosis in SLE over 2 years. *Rheumatol Int* 2012;**32**(9):2701–5.

46. Pashkow FJ. Oxidative stress and inflammation in heart disease: do antioxidants have a role in treatment and/or prevention? *Int J Inflam* 2011;**2011**:514623.

47. Barnes JN, Tanaka H. Cardiovascular benefits of habitual exercise in systemic lupus erythematosus: a review. *Phys Sportsmed* 2012;**40**(3):43–8.

48. Elkan AC, Anania C, Gustafsson T, Jogestrand T, Hafstrom I, Frostegard J. Diet and fatty acid pattern among patients with SLE: associations with disease activity, blood lipids and atherosclerosis. *Lupus* 2012;**21**(13):1405–11.

49. Tselios K, Koumaras C, Urowitz MB, Gladman DD. Do current arterial hypertension treatment guidelines apply to systemic lupus erythematosus patients? a critical appraisal. *Semin Arthritis Rheum* 2014;**43**(4):521–5.

Chapter 43

The Lung in Systemic Lupus Erythematosus

Sandra Chartrand[1], Aryeh Fischer[2], Roland M. du Bois[3]

[1]Hôpital Maisonneuve-Rosemont affiliated to Université de Montréal, Montréal, QC, Canada; [2]University of Colorado School of Medicine, Aurora, CO, USA; [3]Imperial College, London, UK

INTRODUCTION

Lung disease is common in systemic lupus erythematosus (SLE) and any of the respiratory compartments can be impacted (Table 1). The incidence of respiratory system involvement in SLE varies, depending on the sensitivity of the tools used to detect disease and the populations studied, but it likely occurs in more than half of SLE patients at some time during the course of their disease.[1,2] Clinical severity varies from asymptomatic imaging or pulmonary function test (PFT) abnormalities to fulminant, life-threatening disease. Lung disease in SLE has been associated with an increased risk of mortality.[3] Little is known about the natural history of, or predispositions to, SLE lung disease or how to best manage its various manifestations. In this chapter, we provide a focused review of the pulmonary manifestations associated with SLE.

PREVALENCE OF LUNG INVOLVEMENT IN SLE

Lung involvement in SLE is frequently identified. In a cohort of 110 SLE patients, 91.5% had either respiratory symptoms or evidence of pulmonary physiologic impairment, 57.3% reported dyspnea, and 31.8% had pleuritic chest pain.[4] PFT abnormalities were noted in 66.4%. The forced vital capacity (FVC) was abnormal in 31.8% of patients and the diffusing capacity of the lung for carbon monoxide (DL_{CO}) was abnormal in 45.9%.

PFT abnormalities are common even among asymptomatic SLE individuals,[1,5] with decreased DL_{CO} being the most common finding.[5,6] In this regard, in one study of 70 non-smoking SLE patients without respiratory symptoms and with normal chest radiography, abnormal PFT were found in 63% of patients (compared with 17% of controls), with isolated decreased DL_{CO} being found in 31% SLE patients (vs none in controls).[6] Small airway disease was relatively common in both groups (SLE 24% vs controls 17%). None of the 70 asymptomatic SLE patients had chest radiograph abnormalities.

In a study of 43 symptomatic SLE patients, abnormal chest radiographic features were observed in 23%.[5] Pleural changes appear to be the most common abnormality in SLE patients.[7] Thoracic high-resolution computed tomography (HRCT) scan abnormalities (including traction bronchiectasis, interstitial lung disease (ILD), lymphadenopathy, and pleuro-pericardial abnormalities) are seen in the majority of SLE patients, even in the absence of respiratory symptoms or impairment on PFT.[8] In the cohort of 110 SLE patients mentioned earlier, among the 95 patients who had a chest radiograph, 25.3% had an abnormal finding (7.4% with possible or definite interstitial infiltrates; 4.2% with pleural thickening). Among the 80 patients who had a chest CT scan, 18.8% displayed interstitial infiltrates, and 11.0% had pleural involvement.[4]

PULMONARY INFECTION

Of all the pulmonary manifestations in SLE, infection is the most common and needs to be excluded. Infection can mimic lung disease, which is part of the connective tissue disease (CTD) process and often requires immunosuppressive therapy; also, infection is associated with appreciable morbidity and mortality.[9] Both typical and atypical pathogenic organisms, including fungal and mycobacterial species, may be the cause.[9] Due to a patient's immunocompromised state, the clinical presentation may be insidious, particularly if opportunistic organisms are the culprit. Rigorous evaluation that often includes bronchoalveolar lavage (BAL) to exclude infection in SLE patients with any suggestive or unexplained pulmonary abnormality is mandatory. (See Chapter 45 for a thorough review of infectious complications associated with SLE.)

NONPULMONARY INVOLVEMENT AS A CAUSE OF RESPIRATORY SYMPTOMS

A comprehensive evaluation is needed to exclude nonrespiratory causes of dyspnea and/or cough. For example, cardiac ischemia, cardiomyopathy, valvular heart disease,

Systemic Lupus Erythematosus. http://dx.doi.org/10.1016/B978-0-12-801917-7.00043-7

TABLE 1 Pulmonary Manifestations Associated with SLE

Infection

Adverse Effects of Drugs Used to Treat Systemic Disease

Non Pulmonary Causes of Respiratory Symptoms
   Thoracic chondritis
   Lupus myositis
   Anemia
   Cardiac ischemia, valvular heart disease and cardiomyopathies
   Pericardial disease
   Deconditioning
   Gastro-esophageal reflux disease/aspiration

Pleural Disease
   Pleuritis
   Pleural effusion

Parenchymal
   Acute lupus pneumonitis
   Chronic interstitial lung disease
   Diffuse alveolar hemorrhage
   Acute reversible hypoxemia

Shrinking Lung Syndrome

Pulmonary Vascular Disease
   Pulmonary hypertension
   Thromboembolism
   Lung vasculitis

Airways Disease
   Upper airways (e.g., cricoarytenoid arthritis)
   Lower airways (small airways disease)

pericardial disease, anemia, and deconditioning are important etiologies to consider and need to be excluded. Cough may be more likely due to gastroesophageal reflux disease, esophageal dysmotility, or aspiration; these frequently-encountered comorbid conditions require thorough assessment and appropriate management.

PLEURAL DISEASE

Of all of the intrathoracic presentations of SLE, pleural abnormalities are seen most commonly,[9,10] and occur more frequently in SLE than in any other CTD.[11] Depending upon the population evaluated and the mode of detection, its prevalence varies greatly. Autopsy studies have reported pleural abnormalities in 78–93% of cases.[9,12] In large non-autopsy studies, a cumulative incidence of 36% (either pleural or pericardial involvement) was identified among a cohort of 1000 SLE patients[13]; in a large cohort of 520 SLE patients pleurisy was reported in 45% and pleural effusion in 30%.[14] Pleural abnormalities appear to be more common in men[13] and in African-Americans.[15] Pleural disease may rarely be the presenting manifestation of SLE,[16] and it may be unilateral or bilateral.[17]

Pleuritic pain can herald an SLE flare, can last for several weeks, and can be associated with fever, dyspnea, cough,

and/or pain, mostly at the costo-phrenic angle.[2] Pleuritic chest pain should prompt evaluation to exclude thrombo-embolism and evidence of pleural effusion requires investigation to exclude infection, states of volume overload, and malignancy. Pleural effusions are typically small to moderate in size, bilateral, and exudative.[17] Pleural glucose level is usually >70 mg/dL, lactate dehydrogenase <500 IU/L, and pH > 7.2.[17,18] The role of testing for pleural fluid ANA is not clear.[19]

There are no evidence-based recommendations for treatment of pleural disease, but we have found that pleurisy often responds rapidly to nonsteroidal anti-inflammatory drugs or corticosteroids (CS) in moderate doses (20–30 mg/day of prednisone equivalent). Pleural effusions often mandate a more protracted treatment course. In more severe or refractory cases, a CS-sparing agent such as azathioprine (AZA) or methotrexate may be needed.[20] Rarely, pleural disease requires intercostal steroid injection, pleurodesis, or pleurectomy.[21,22]

PARENCHYMAL DISEASE

Acute Lupus Pneumonitis

Acute lupus pneumonitis has a similar clinical presentation to infectious pneumonia[23] and may be seen in up to 9% of SLE cohorts[1,13]: acute onset of fever, cough, dyspnea, tachypnea, and hypoxemia are typical. Chest radiograph and thoracic HRCT scan usually demonstrate bilateral diffuse patchy alveolar infiltrates, which may involve all lung zones but favors the lower zones.[11] Given its clinical similarity with infectious pneumonia and their common co-existence,[23] a thorough diagnostic evaluation for an infectious etiology is indicated. Bronchoscopy is typically performed and surgical lung biopsy may be required to provide diagnostic certainty. Histopathology demonstrates diffuse alveolar damage (DAD) in the absence of vasculitis, capillaritis or hemorrhage, and the presence of interstitial edema and intra-alveolar hyaline membrane formation.[10] The prognosis is variable but with lethal potential (8–50%).[24]

Corticosteroids are first-line therapy, but more severe cases may require further immunosuppression with AZA,[25] cyclophosphamide (CYC),[26] or other immunosuppressive agents to reduce the likelihood of recurrent pneumonitis or to help effectively taper the CS dose. In more fulminant, life-threatening scenarios, plasmapheresis should be considered.[26]

Pulmonary Hemorrhage/Diffuse Alveolar Hemorrhage

Diffuse alveolar hemorrhage (DAH) is arguably the most debilitating pulmonary manifestation of SLE. Reliable estimates of the prevalence of DAH in SLE are lacking, but some data suggest a prevalence as high as 2% and

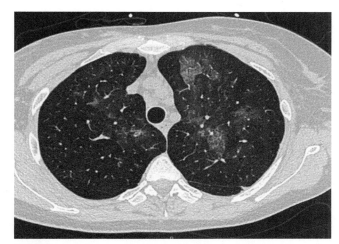

FIGURE 1   **Diffuse alveolar hemorrhage.** Chest CT scan shows patchy ground glass attenuation in a bronchocentric distribution, consistent with intra-alveolar blood. *Reproduced from Ref. 20, p. 853.*

accounting for roughly 3% of all SLE-related hospitalizations, and approximately 20% of hospitalizations for all SLE-associated lung disease.[2,27–29] Clinical presentation ranges from mild and insidious to fulminant and life-threatening disease. Presentation may be nonspecific, including acute onset of dyspnea, cough and fever, but with hemoptysis in only around 65% of patients.[2,29] DAH most often occurs in younger women with pre-existing SLE, especially with multisystem disease.[29] The clinical course is often one of rapid respiratory deterioration.[2,24,29]

With massive hemorrhage, hemoglobin and hematocrit will drop precipitately. Chest radiograph shows bilateral nonspecific peripheral infiltrates and thoracic HRCT scan reveals diffuse fluffy or nodular ground glass opacification changes due to alveolar filling admixed with areas of consolidation (Figure 1). Co-existent acute respiratory infection may be seen in 13–57% of cases.[29] Exclusion of infection and confirmation of the diagnosis of SLE-associated DAH requires bronchoscopy with BAL, demonstrating the presence of blood within the large airways and increasingly bloody returns from successive aliquots. The presence of hemosiderin-laden macrophages in the BAL fluid is a clue to insidious alveolar hemorrhage. Surgical lung biopsy is not usually needed to confirm the diagnosis of DAH but, when performed, histopathology reveals hemosiderin-laden macrophages, diffuse intra-alveolar hemorrhage, co-existent capillaritis, DAD, alveolar edema and necrosis, microvascular thrombi, and vascular intimal proliferative changes.[2,29,30]

DAH can lead to respiratory failure necessitating mechanical ventilatory support. Therapeutic intervention is based on anecdotal evidence and small case series and typically include pulse-high dose CS[27] with early addition of intravenous CYC[31,32]; plasmapheresis may improve chances of survival but also increases the risk of serious infection.[31,32] Even with such intensive regimens,

the overall prognosis is dismal, with a reported overall mortality between 70 and 90%, half dying during their hospitalization.[2,27,29]

Chronic Interstitial Lung Disease

Although chronic interstitial lung disease (ILD) is common in patients with other CTDs, it rarely occurs in SLE; its estimated prevalence is only about 3%.[33] Although ILD may be the presenting manifestation of SLE, it typically occurs with long-standing and multisystem disease and is characterized by an insidious onset of cough, exertional dyspnea, and bibasilar crackles.

PFT reveals reduced lung volumes, restriction on spirometry (proportionate reduction in forced expiratory volume in 1 second and FVC), and impaired gas exchange (reduced DL_{CO}). BAL shows a mixed neutrophil/eosinophil increase, but a lymphocyte increase may be seen in more cellular disease.[34] Whether the underlying histopathologic pattern has prognostic significance in SLE-ILD has yet to be determined.[35] Nearly all of the histopathologic patterns encountered in those with idiopathic interstitial pneumonia (IIP) have been encountered in SLE.[36] Nonspecific interstitial pneumonia (NSIP) is the most common pattern in SLE (Figure 2); less frequently encountered patterns include organizing pneumonia (OP) (Figure 3), lymphocytic interstitial pneumonia (LIP) (Figure 4), the DAD found in acute lupus pneumonitis (Figure 2), and more rarely usual interstitial pneumonia (UIP). Often the pattern contains a combination of features, commonly including co-existing pleural disease, and may not exhibit the classical features of any of the individual chronic ILD. At present, the precise role of surgical lung biopsy in SLE-ILD remains to be determined.[37] In our experience, the decision whether to pursue a surgical lung biopsy is made on a case-by-case basis and should be considered when there is an atypical or unclassifiable radiologic pattern or concerns for an alternative etiology to account for the ILD.

Patients with SLE-ILD do not always require pharmacologic treatment.[38,39] The decision to treat rests upon (1) whether the patient is clinically impaired by the ILD, (2) whether the ILD is progressive, and (3) what contraindications or mitigating factors exist. Therapy for SLE-associated ILD is generally reserved for those patients with clinically significant, progressive disease, based upon a combination of clinical assessment tools, including both subjective and objective measures of respiratory impairment.[38,39] There are limited data available to guide the choice of specific pharmacologic agents for the treatment of CTD-ILD as a group, and no controlled data for SLE-ILD.[39] Data from small uncontrolled trials in systemic sclerosis (SSc)-ILD and other CTD-ILD[39] and from three controlled trials in SSc-ILD[40–42] provide support for the use of CYC in SLE-ILD. Retrospective data suggest that AZA or mycophenolate mofetil (MMF) may be effective in CTD-ILD.[43] Two retrospective studies

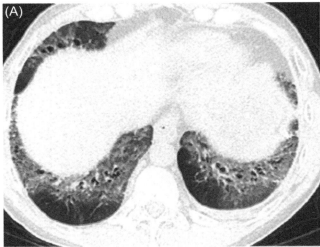

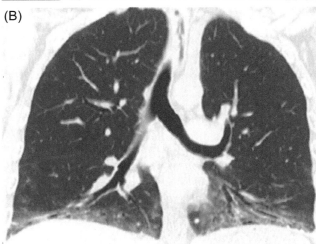

FIGURE 2 **Nonspecific interstitial pneumonia (NSIP) pattern.** (A) Chest CT scan at the lung bases shows widespread ground glass attenuation with traction bronchiectasis and subpleural sparing, compatible with a fibrotic NSIP histopathological pattern. Note the absence of honeycombing. (B) Coronal view showing the basal predominance of disease.

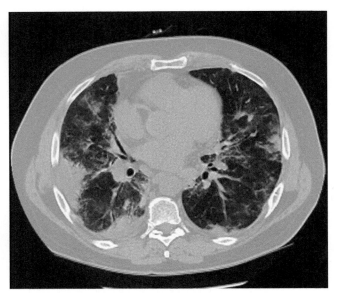

FIGURE 3 **Organizing pneumonia (OP) pattern.** Chest CT scan below the level of the carina shows patchy consolidation and some ground glass attenuation compatible with an OP histopathological pattern.

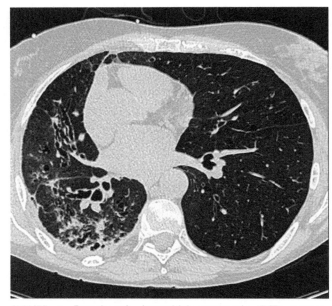

FIGURE 4 **Lymphocytic interstitial pneumonia (LIP) pattern.** Chest CT scan shows marked volume loss in the right lung with pleural thickening and an extensive reticular pattern consistent with diffuse established fibrosis. There are also widespread centrilobular nodules in both lungs, with some low attenuation areas throughout the left lung consistent with small cysts/bullae; both features are compatible with an LIP histopathological pattern.

demonstrated that MMF was associated with effective CS dose tapering and with longitudinal improvements in FVC and DL_{CO} in a diverse spectrum of CTD-ILD.[44,45] It is not known whether we can extrapolate from these data to SLE-ILD. Our usual regimen for SLE-ILD includes the use of CS at a moderate to high dose (30–60 mg/day of prednisone equivalent) combined with CYC for the most severe or progressive cases, or with AZA or MMF for less severe disease.[39]

SHRINKING LUNG SYNDROME

Shrinking lung syndrome (SLS) is characterized by unexplained dyspnea and restrictive pulmonary physiology the severity of which are disproportionate to the extent of parenchymal radiographic abnormalities. In our experience, SLE patients with SLS often have long-standing or recurrent symptoms of pleurisy. Elevation of the diaphragms together with bibasilar atelectasis are the hallmark radiographic features.[46] Among 110 SLE patients, 10.0% were found to meet the definition of SLS, with increased disease duration, RNP positivity and history of serositis being significant associations.[4] The precise pathogenesis remains to be determined. It is usually not progressive, but it is associated with chronic and persistent dyspnea. Inhaled β-agonist or theophylline therapy may favorably impact SLS.[47,48] Alternatively, CS or immunosuppressive agents such as AZA, methotrexate, CYC, or rituximab may improve the condition.[49]

PULMONARY VASCULAR DISEASE

Pulmonary Hypertension

Patients with SLE are at risk for developing several types of pulmonary hypertension (PH): pulmonary arterial hypertension (PAH), PH due to left heart disease, PH due to chronic ILD or chronic thromboembolic-associated PH (CTEPH).[50] Severe PH is relatively rare.[51] Mild, subclinical PH, however, is relatively common with a reported prevalence of 0.5–14%.[50] SLE-PH presents with exertional fatigue and dyspnea and more severe disease manifests with characteristic features of right-heart failure. Clues to the presence of PH may include a disproportionate reduction in the DL_{CO}, exertional hypoxemia or an elevated brain natriuretic peptide (BNP) level in those with more advanced disease. Echocardiography is the best noninvasive tool for PH assessment but is neither sensitive nor specific, and a right-heart catheterization must be performed for accurate measurement of cardiac hemodynamic parameters and to confirm a diagnosis of PH.[50] The pathophysiologic mechanisms of SLE-PAH are not known but prevailing theories include pulmonary circulatory vasospasm, intrinsic vasculopathy, in situ thrombosis, and endothelial dysfunction as possible causes.[50]

In general, the approach to managing SLE-PAH is similar to that of idiopathic PAH and includes monotherapy or combination therapy with oral endothelin receptor antagonists, phosphodiesterase-type 5 inhibitors, guanylate cyclase stimulators, parenteral or inhaled prostanoids and is optimized by a multidisciplinary approach that includes an experienced PH-treating cardiologist or pulmonologist. PAH in SLE is unique in that there have been reports in small series suggesting that immunosuppressive therapies (including high-dose CS and CYC) may be useful in selected cases, typically those with more of an inflammatory vasculopathy.[52,53] The prognosis of SLE-PAH is better than SSc-PAH.[54]

Pulmonary Thromboembolism

New-onset pleuritic chest pain or acute dyspnea requires evaluation for pulmonary embolism in any SLE patient. Thromboembolism occurs in up to 25% of SLE patients and is a major cause of morbidity and mortality[2]; the presence of antiphospholipid syndrome-associated antibodies increases the risk of thromboembolism.[55,56] In one study,

antiphospholipid antibody positivity was associated with a more than sixfold risk of thromboembolism[55]; in another study, lupus anticoagulant positivity carried a fivefold risk.[56] Evaluation for pulmonary embolism starts with noninvasive assessment that usually includes ventilation/perfusion (V/Q) scan or CT angiography but may require pulmonary angiography for a definitive diagnosis. D-dimer level appears to have limited utility in SLE because nonspecific increase is noted with disease flares, infections, and may be positive in 50% of those without thromboembolism.[57] The mainstay of therapy is anticoagulation with heparin followed by warfarin. SLE patients with thromboembolism and positive antiphospholipid syndrome-associated antibodies usually require lifelong anticoagulation.[58] (See Chapters 56–58 and 63 for a thorough review of antiphospholipid syndrome in SLE.)

ACUTE REVERSIBLE HYPOXIA SYNDROME

A novel syndrome of acute reversible hypoxemia affecting six SLE patients presenting with dyspnea and pleurisy, acute and reversible hypoxemia, absence of chest radiographic abnormalities, and a wide alveolar-arterial gradient that improved with CS treatment was reported in 1991.[59] In 1995, a similar clinical picture was reported in four SLE patients.[60] Complement-mediated aggregation and activation of neutrophils within the pulmonary vasculature or increased surface expression of adhesion molecules and a resultant leuko-occlusive pulmonary vasculopathy have been suggested as possible pathophysiologic mechanisms of disease.[59,60] Treatment is typically supportive, includes supplemental oxygen, and occasionally mandates a short-term course of CS.

AIRWAY DISEASE

Airflow limitation involving both the upper and lower airways, as defined by obstructive physiology on PFT, has been observed in patients with SLE, but its clinical significance is not known.[6] In a prospective study assessing thoracic HRCT scans from 34 patients with SLE (23% with symptoms), 21% of the scans showed bronchiectasis and bronchial wall thickening.[8] Symptomatic obstructive lung ("airways") disease is uncommon.

CLINICIANS SHOULD SCREEN FOR LUNG DISEASE IN SLE

Given the prevalence and wide range of lung diseases that can be seen in SLE, we would suggest that some degree of screening for lung disease in SLE is indicated, especially to establish a baseline when dealing with a disease in which some form of pulmonary manifestation may occur during the course of the disease. In our opinion, it would seem reasonable to perform chest radiography and PFT at first presentation. We also suggest careful assessment for respiratory symptoms or physical examination signs of impairment at each clinical encounter. Any abnormality detected, even if only mild or subtle, will prompt further investigation. In other words, although we cannot advocate wide-scale screening for lung disease for all SLE patients, we do highlight the importance of clinical vigilance in this situation while maintaining a low threshold to proceed with pulmonary evaluation given the potentially devastating manifestations of lung disease that can occur in SLE.

SUMMARY

Lung manifestations in SLE are diverse and can range from asymptomatic physiologic and radiographic abnormalities to severe, life-threatening disease. Given that lung disease is highly prevalent and can be associated with significant morbidity, clinicians should be vigilant about identifying possible lung disease in all patients with SLE. Patients with SLE and respiratory symptoms require a thorough evaluation to assess for both intra- and extrathoracic causes and respiratory infection must be rigorously excluded. Although treatment is not evidence-based, the general approach to management includes early detection and prompt initiation of immunosuppressive therapies for SLE-associated lung disease.

REFERENCES

1. Grigor R, Edmonds J, Lewkonia R, Bresnihan B, Hughes GR. Systemic lupus erythematosus. A prospective analysis. *Ann Rheum Dis* 1978;**37**(2):121–8.
2. Murin S, Wiedemann HP, Matthay RA. Pulmonary manifestations of systemic lupus erythematosus. *Clin Chest Med* 1998;**19**(4):641–65. viii.
3. Bertoli AM, Vila LM, Apte M, Fessler BJ, Bastian HM, Reveille JD, et al. Systemic lupus erythematosus in a multiethnic US Cohort LUMINA XLVIII: factors predictive of pulmonary damage. *Lupus* 2007;**16**(6):410–7.
4. Allen D, Fischer A, Bshouty Z, Robinson DB, Peschken CA, Hitchon C, et al. Evaluating systemic lupus erythematosus patients for lung involvement. *Lupus* 2012;**21**(12):1316–25.
5. Silberstein SL, Barland P, Grayzel AI, Koerner SK. Pulmonary dysfunction in systemic lupus erythematosus:prevalence classification and correlation with other organ involvement. *J Rheumatol* 1980;**7**(2):187–95.
6. Andonopoulos AP, Constantopoulos SH, Galanopoulou V, Drosos AA, Acritidis NC, Moutsopoulos HM. Pulmonary function of nonsmoking patients with systemic lupus erythematosus. *Chest* 1988;**94**(2):312–5.
7. Bulgrin JG, Dubois EL, Jacobson G. Chest roentgenographic changes in systemic lupus erythematosus. *Radiology* 1960;**74**:42–9.
8. Fenlon HM, Doran M, Sant SM, Breatnach E. High-resolution chest CT in systemic lupus erythematosus. *AJR Am J Roentgenol* 1996;**166**(2):301–17.
9. Quadrelli SA, Alvarez C, Arce SC, Paz L, Sarano J, Sobrino EM, et al. Pulmonary involvement of systemic lupus erythematosus: analysis of 90 necropsies. *Lupus* 2009;**18**(12):1053–60.
10. Keane MP, Lynch 3rd JP. Pleuropulmonary manifestations of systemic lupus erythematosus. *Thorax* 2000;**55**(2):159–66.
11. Wiedemann HP, Matthay RA. Pulmonary manifestations of systemic lupus erythematosus. *J Thorac Imaging* 1992;**7**(2):1–18.
12. Memet B, Ginzler EM. Pulmonary manifestations of systemic lupus erythematosus. *Semin Respir Crit Care Med* 2007;**28**(4):441–50.
13. Cervera R, Khamashta MA, Font J, Sebastiani GD, Gil A, Lavilla P, et al. Systemic lupus erythematosus: clinical and immunologic patterns of disease expression in a cohort of 1,000 patients. The European Working Party on Systemic Lupus Erythematosus. *Medicine (Baltimore)* 1993;**72**(2):113–24.
14. Dubois EL, Tuffanelli DL. Clinical manifestations of systemic lupus erythematosus. Computer analysis of 520 cases. *JAMA* 1964;**190**:104–11.
15. Ward MM, Studenski S. Clinical manifestations of systemic lupus erythematosus. Identification of racial and socioeconomic influences. *Arch Intern Med* 1990;**150**(4):849–53.
16. Winslow WA, Ploss LN, Loitman B. Pleuritis in systemic lupus erythematosus: its importance as an early manifestation in diagnosis. *Ann Intern Med* 1958;**49**(1):70–88.
17. Good Jr JT, King TE, Antony VB, Sahn SA. Lupus pleuritis. Clinical features and pleural fluid characteristics with special reference to pleural fluid antinuclear antibodies. *Chest* 1983;**84**(6):714–8.
18. Carr DT, Lillington GA, Mayne JG. Pleural-fluid glucose in systemic lupus erythematosus. *Mayo Clin Proc* 1970;**45**(6):409–12.
19. Khare V, Baethge B, Lang S, Wolf RE, Campbell Jr GD. Antinuclear antibodies in pleural fluid. *Chest* 1994;**106**(3):866–71.
20. Fischer A, du Bois RM. Lung. In: Lahita RG, Tsokos G, Buyon J, Koike T, editors. *Systemic lupus erythematosus.* 5th ed. London (UK): Academic Press; 2011. p. 847–64.
21. Elborn JS, Conn P, Roberts SD. Refractory massive pleural effusion in systemic lupus erythematosus treated by pleurectomy. *Ann Rheum Dis* 1987;**46**(1):77–80.
22. Kaine JL. Refractory massive pleural effusion in systemic lupus erythematosus treated with talc poudrage. *Ann Rheum Dis* 1985;**44**(1):61–4.
23. Swigris JJ, Fischer A, Gillis J, Meehan RT, Brown KK. Pulmonary and thrombotic manifestations of systemic lupus erythematosus. *Chest* 2008;**133**(1):271–80.
24. Matthay RA, Schwarz MI, Petty TL, Stanford RE, Gupta RC, Sahn SA, et al. Pulmonary manifestations of systemic lupus erythematosus: review of twelve cases of acute lupus pneumonitis. *Medicine (Baltimore)* 1975;**54**(5):397–409.
25. Matthay RA, Hudson LD, Petty TL. Acute lupus pneumonitis: response to azathioprine therapy. *Chest* 1973;**63**(1):117–20.
26. Isbister JP, Ralston M, Hayes JM, Wright R. Fulminant lupus pneumonitis with acute renal failure and RBC aplasia. Successful management with plasmapheresis and immunosuppression. *Arch Intern Med* 1981;**141**(8):1081–3.
27. Barile LA, Jara LJ, Medina-Rodriguez F, Garcia-Figueroa JL, Miranda-Limon JM. Pulmonary hemorrhage in systemic lupus erythematosus. *Lupus* 1997;**6**(5):445–8.
28. Santos-Ocampo AS, Mandell BF, Fessler BJ. Alveolar hemorrhage in systemic lupus erythematosus: presentation and management. *Chest* 2000;**118**(4):1083–90.
29. Zamora MR, Warner ML, Tuder R, Schwarz MI. Diffuse alveolar hemorrhage and systemic lupus erythematosus. Clinical presentation, histology, survival, and outcome. *Medicine (Baltimore)* 1997;**76**(3):192–202.

30. Mintz G, Galindo LF, Fernandez-Diez J, Jimenez FJ, Robles-Saavedra E, Enriquez-Casillas RD. Acute massive pulmonary hemorrhage in systemic lupus erythematosus. *J Rheumatol* 1978;**5**(1):39–50.

31. Erickson RW, Franklin WA, Emlen W. Treatment of hemorrhagic lupus pneumonitis with plasmapheresis. *Semin Arthritis Rheum* 1994;**24**(2):114–23.

32. Euler HH, Schroeder JO, Harten P, Zeuner RA, Gutschmidt HJ. Treatment-free remission in severe systemic lupus erythematosus following synchronization of plasmapheresis with subsequent pulse cyclophosphamide. *Arthritis Rheum* 1994;**37**(12):1784–94.

33. Weinrib L, Sharma OP, Quismorio Jr FP. A long-term study of interstitial lung disease in systemic lupus erythematosus. *Semin Arthritis Rheum* 1990;**20**(1):48–56.

34. Greene NB, Solinger AM, Baughman RP. Patients with collagen vascular disease and dyspnea. The value of gallium scanning and bronchoalveolar lavage in predicting response to steroid therapy and clinical outcome. *Chest* 1987;**91**(5):698–703.

35. Park JH, Kim DS, Park IN, Jang SJ, Kitaichi M, Nicholson AG, et al. Prognosis of fibrotic interstitial pneumonia: idiopathic versus collagen vascular disease-related subtypes. *Am J Respir Crit Care Med* 2007;**175**(7):705–11.

36. American Thoracic Society, European Respiratory Society. American Thoracic Society/European Respiratory Society International Multidisciplinary Consensus Classification of the Idiopathic Interstitial Pneumonias. This joint statement of the American Thoracic Society (ATS), and the European Respiratory Society (ERS) was adopted by the ATS board of directors, June 2001 and by the ERS Executive Committee, June 2001. *Am J Respir Crit Care Med* 2002;**165**(2):277–304.

37. Antoniou KM, Margaritopoulos G, Economidou F, Siafakas NM. Pivotal clinical dilemmas in collagen vascular diseases associated with interstitial lung involvement. *Eur Respir J* 2009;**33**(4):882–96.

38. Fischer A, Richeldi L. Cross-disciplinary collaboration in connective tissue disease-related lung disease. *Semin Respir Crit Care Med* 2014;**35**(2):159–65.

39. Solomon JJ, Chartrand S, Fischer A. Current approach to connective tissue disease-associated interstitial lung disease. *Curr Opin Pulm Med* 2014;**20**(5):449–56.

40. Hoyles RK, Ellis RW, Wellsbury J, Lees B, Newlands P, Goh NS, et al. A multicenter, prospective, randomized, double-blind, placebo-controlled trial of corticosteroids and intravenous cyclophosphamide followed by oral azathioprine for the treatment of pulmonary fibrosis in scleroderma. *Arthritis Rheum* 2006;**54**(12):3962–70.

41. Tashkin DP, Elashoff R, Clements PJ, Goldin J, Roth MD, Furst DE, et al. Cyclophosphamide versus placebo in scleroderma lung disease. *N Engl J Med* 2006;**354**(25):2655–66.

42. Tashkin DP, Elashoff R, Clements PJ, Roth MD, Furst DE, Silver RM, et al. Effects of 1-year treatment with cyclophosphamide on outcomes at 2 years in scleroderma lung disease. *Am J Respir Crit Care Med* 2007;**176**(10):1026–34.

43. Dheda K, Lalloo UG, Cassim B, Mody GM. Experience with azathioprine in systemic sclerosis associated with interstitial lung disease. *Clin Rheumatol* 2004;**23**(4):306–9.

44. Swigris JJ, Olson AL, Fischer A, Lynch DA, Cosgrove GP, Frankel SK, et al. Mycophenolate mofetil is safe, well tolerated, and preserves lung function in patients with connective tissue disease-related interstitial lung disease. *Chest* 2006;**130**(1):30–6.

45. Fischer A, Brown KK, Du Bois RM, Frankel SK, Cosgrove GP, Fernandez-Perez ER, et al. Mycophenolate mofetil improves lung function in connective tissue disease-associated interstitial lung disease. *J Rheumatol* 2013;**40**(5):640–6.

46. Gibson CJ, Edmonds JP, Hughes GR. Diaphragm function and lung involvement in systemic lupus erythematosus. *Am J Med* 1977;**63**(6):926–32.

47. Munoz-Rodriguez FJ, Font J, Badia JR, Miret C, Barbera JA, Cervera R, et al. Shrinking lungs syndrome in systemic lupus erythematosus: improvement with inhaled beta-agonist therapy. *Lupus* 1997;**6**(4):412–4.

48. Van Veen S, Peeters AJ, Sterk PJ, Breedveld FC. The "shrinking lung syndrome" in SLE, treatment with theophylline. *Clin Rheumatol* 1993;**12**(4):462–5.

49. Oud KT, Bresser P, ten Berge RJ, Jonkers RE. The shrinking lung syndrome in systemic lupus erythematosus: improvement with corticosteroid therapy. *Lupus* 2005;**14**(12):959–63.

50. Pope J. An update in pulmonary hypertension in systemic lupus erythematosus - do we need to know about it? *Lupus* 2008;**17**(4):274–7.

51. Prabu A, Patel K, Yee CS, Nightingale P, Situnayake RD, Thickett DR, et al. Prevalence and risk factors for pulmonary arterial hypertension in patients with lupus. *Rheumatology (Oxford)* 2009;**48**(12):1506–11.

52. Gonzalez-Lopez L, Cardona-Munoz EG, Celis A, Garcia-de la Torre I, Orozco-Barocio G, Salazar-Paramo M, et al. Therapy with intermittent pulse cyclophosphamide for pulmonary hypertension associated with systemic lupus erythematosus. *Lupus* 2004;**13**(2):105–12.

53. Sanchez O, Sitbon O, Jais X, Simonneau G, Humbert M. Immunosuppressive therapy in connective tissue diseases-associated pulmonary arterial hypertension. *Chest* 2006;**130**(1):182–9.

54. Condliffe R, Kiely DG, Peacock AJ, Corris PA, Gibbs JS, Vrapi F, et al. Connective tissue disease-associated pulmonary arterial hypertension in the modern treatment era. *Am J Respir Crit Care Med* 2009;**179**(2):151–7.

55. Wahl DG, Guillemin F, de Maistre E, Perret C, Lecompte T, Thibaut G. Risk for venous thrombosis related to antiphospholipid antibodies in systemic lupus erythematosus–a meta-analysis. *Lupus* 1997;**6**(5):467–73.

56. Somers E, Magder LS, Petri M. Antiphospholipid antibodies and incidence of venous thrombosis in a cohort of patients with systemic lupus erythematosus. *J Rheumatol* 2002;**29**(12):2531–6.

57. Wu H, Birmingham DJ, Rovin B, Hackshaw KV, Haddad N, Haden D, et al. D-dimer level and the risk for thrombosis in systemic lupus erythematosus. *Clin J Am Soc Nephrol* 2008;**3**(6):1628–36.

58. Cohen D, Berger SP, Steup-Beekman GM, Bloemenkamp KW, Bajema IM. Diagnosis and management of the antiphospholipid syndrome. *BMJ* 2010;**340**. c2541.

59. Abramson SB, Dobro J, Eberle MA, Benton M, Reibman J, Epstein H, et al. Acute reversible hypoxemia in systemic lupus erythematosus. *Ann Intern Med* 1991;**114**(11):941–7.

60. Martinez-Taboada VM, Blanco R, Armona J, Fernandez-Sueiro JL, Rodriguez-Valverde V. Acute reversible hypoxemia in systemic lupus erythematosus: a new syndrome or an index of disease activity? *Lupus* 1995;**4**(4):259–62.

Chapter 44

Gastrointestinal, Hepatic, and Pancreatic Disorders in Systemic Lupus Erythematosus

Chi Chiu Mok

Department of Medicine, Tuen Mun Hospital, New Territories, Hong Kong

INTRODUCTION

Gastrointestinal (GI) manifestations of systemic lupus erythematosus (SLE) are protean (Table 1). Clinical features are noncharacteristic and must be distinguished from infective, thrombotic, therapy-related, and non-SLE causes. Appropriate imaging investigations, endoscopic procedures, and biopsies are indicated. Early recognition and intervention help reduce mortality and morbidity.

The prevalence of GI lupus varies widely. Oral symptoms and mucosal lesions are most frequent, whereas acute abdominal pain is most sinister. GI manifestations are likely to be underestimated in SLE because some of these features are indistinct and not gauged by disease activity indices. In the literature, GI lupus appears to be more common in Asian patients.[1]

THE GASTROINTESTINAL TRACT IN SLE

Buccal Cavity

Oral ulceration is common in SLE.[2] Typically, these ulcers are superficial, painless, and mostly found on the hard palate, buccal cavity, and vermiform border. Oral ulceration is a marker for disease activity[3] and remains one of the 2012 revised classification criteria for SLE by the SLICC group of investigators.[4] However, painful oral ulcers and mucositis in SLE may be secondary to herpes simplex and candida infection, as well as treatment with cyclophosphamide and methotrexate.

Chronic discoid lupus erythematosus (DLE) may develop in the oral cavity.[5] It is frequently found in the buccal mucosa but the palate and tongue may also be involved. Lesion usually begins as a painless, erythematosus patch and slowly matures into a chronic plaque-like lesion. Mucosal DLE lesions can be severely painful and may be confused with lichen planus or leukoplakia. Tissue biopsy may show lupus-specific histopathology. Topical corticosteroids and the antimalarials are the main treatment but

intralesional corticosteroid, azathioprine, thalidomide, dapsone, retinoids, and mycophenolate mofetil (MMF) may be required in refractory cases.[5]

Secondary Sjogren's syndrome is reported in 9.2% of SLE patients.[6] Dry mouth can be alleviated by air humidification, stimulation of salivary flow by sugarless mints or chewing gums, and artificial saliva preparations. The muscarinic receptor agonists such as pilocarpine and cevimeline may also be considered.

SLE patients are prone to have poor dental health because of multiple factors that include mucosal ulceration, reduced salivary flow, bleeding diathesis, and medications such as corticosteroids (gingival infection), nonsteroidal anti-inflammatory drugs (NSAIDs) (platelet dysfunction), cyclosporin A (gingivitis, gingival hypertrophy), methotrexate (stomatitis and mucositis), antiepileptic agents (gum hypertrophy), and tricyclic antidepressants (worsen sicca). Case–control studies report a higher incidence of aphthous ulcers, erythema, dental plaques, gingival overgrowth and bleeding, and temporomandibular joint dysfunction in SLE patients.[7] Because of the association of periodontal disease with atherosclerosis,[8] impaired dental health in SLE patients may further aggravate their cardiovascular risk. SLE patients should receive regular dental checkups and treatment of periodontitis.

Esophagus

Dysphagia and heartburn in SLE patients may be caused by mucosal dryness, esophageal hypomotility, esophagitis, and esophageal ulceration. Manometry studies reveal functional abnormalities of the esophagus (aperistalsis or hypoperistalsis) in 10–32% of SLE patients, usually in the upper third.[9] Skeletal muscle fiber atrophy, inflammation of the esophageal muscles, and ischemic or vasculitic damage of the Auerbach's plexus have been postulated to be the mechanisms of impaired esophageal mobility.

Systemic Lupus Erythematosus. http://dx.doi.org/10.1016/B978-0-12-801917-7.00044-9

TABLE 1 Gastrointestinal and Hepatic Manifestations of Lupus

Oral cavity	Oral ulceration
	Mucosal discoid lupus
	Sicca symptoms
	Chronic periodontitis
Esophagus	Hypomotility
	Esophageal reflux/ulceration
Stomach	Gastritis, gastric ulceration
	Pernicious anemia
	Gastric antral vascular ectasia
Small bowel and peritoneum	Intestinal vasculitis (enteritis)
	Mesenteric insufficiency
	Intestinal pseudo-obstruction
	Protein-losing gastroenteropathy
	Peritonitis/ascites (serositis)
	Eosinophilic enteritis
	Malabsorption
Large bowel	Colitis
	Inflammatory bowel diseases
	Collagenous colitis
Liver	Subclinical hepatitis
	Autoimmune hepatitis (lupus hepatitis)
	Hemangioma
	Nodular regenerative hyperplasia
	Hepatic vein thrombosis
	Veno-occlusive disease
	Hepatic arteries and infarction
Biliary tract	Acalculous cholecystitis
	Primary biliary cirrhosis
	Autoimmune cholangiopathy
	Sclerosing cholangitis
Pancreas	Pancreatitis

Esophageal ulceration occurs in 3–5% of SLE patients[2] and is often caused by gastroesophageal reflux or infections such as candidia, herpes simplex, and cytomegalovirus (CMV). Vasculitis leading to ulceration is rare. Medications such as the NSAIDs and the oral bisphosphonates are occasionally associated with esophagitis and bleeding esophageal ulcers. Esophageal symptoms in SLE patients are treated with high-dose H_2 blockers, proton pump inhibitors, and prokinetic agents.

Stomach

Gastritis, gastric erosion, and ulceration in SLE patients may result from treatment with high-dose corticosteroids, NSAIDs, and the bisphosphonates. CMV infection rarely causes gastritis and gastric ulceration that may lead to bleeding and perforation.[10] Perforated peptic ulcer is diagnosed in 6–8% of SLE patients who present with acute abdomen.[11] Vasculitis of the gastric mucosa causing ulceration and bleeding is exceedingly rare. Recently, a link between *Helicobacter pylori* infection of the stomach and autoimmunity has been proposed.[12] However, the prevalence of antibodies to *H. pylori* is not higher in SLE than matched controls and the role of *H. pylori* infection in SLE remains to be elucidated.

Gastric antral vascular ectasia (GAVE) is a rare vascular malformation in the stomach that may cause acute or chronic bleeding. The characteristic endoscopic appearance is a collection of red spots of ectatic vessels arranged in stripes along the antral rugal folds. GAVE is mostly found in scleroderma but has been reported in SLE.[13] Endoscopic treatment or open surgery is indicated for persistent bleeding.

Pernicious anemia has been reported in 3% of patients with SLE, characterized by low serum cobalamin level, macrocytic anemia, and the presence of antibody against intrinsic factor.[14] A recent study showed a prevalence of antigastric parietal cell antibody in 3.6% of SLE patients, but clinical pernicious anemia developed only in 0.5% of patients.[15]

Small Intestine

Mesenteric/Intestinal Vasculitis/Lupus Enteritis

The prevalence of intestinal vasculitis in SLE patients ranges from 0.2% to 9.7%[16] and among those who present with acute abdominal pain, intestinal vasculitis is diagnosed in 29–65% of patients.[11,17] This manifestation is more commonly observed in Asian patients.

Symptoms of mesenteric vasculitis range from mild abdominal bloating with a variable degree of nausea, vomiting, fever, and loose stool to intestinal perforation which manifests as severe diffuse abdominal pain, abdominal distension, rebound tenderness, and paralytic ileus. In serious cases, mucosal ulceration leading to extensive GI bleeding, intussusception, and bowel gangrene may develop.[1,2,18] Serological and clinical disease activity in other organs is usually present.

An accurate and timely diagnosis of mesenteric vasculitis is essential. Other SLE and non-SLE-related causes of abdominal pain must be excluded. Plain radiograph of the abdomen is insensitive for diagnosing lupus mesenteric vasculitis at its early stage. In established disease, X-rays may demonstrate pseudo-obstruction, ileus or dilatation of the bowel loops, effacement of the mucosal folds, submucosal edema as a result of bowel ischemia (thumbprinting appearance), and uncommonly pneumatosis cystoids intestinalis (gas cysts within the submucosa or subserosa of the intestine).[1] Intraabdominal free gas may be seen after intestinal perforation.

Computer tomography (CT) scan of the abdomen is the most useful diagnostic tool for mesenteric vasculitis.[1,19] Apart from excluding other intraabdominal pathologies such as abscesses and collections, cholecystitis, and pancreatitis with or without pseudocyst formation, a contrast CT scan may demonstrate focal or diffuse bowel wall thickening with double halo or target sign (enhancing outer and inner rim with hypoattenuation in the center), prominent mesenteric vessels with palisade pattern or comb-like appearance supplying focally or diffusely dilated bowel loops, and ascites.[1,19,20] Segmental or multifocal involvement of the small and large bowel loops is highly suggestive of ischemic changes due to vasculitis. Early CT findings of lupus enteritis are reversible on immunosuppressive treatment.[20] Besides, CT angiography may help in differentiating lupus enteritis with thrombosis of the major mesenteric vessels.

Upper and lower endoscopies in lupus enteritis may show signs of ischemia and mucosal ulceration. The typical histopathological findings are usually observed in the arterioles and venules of the submucosa of the bowel wall rather than the medium-sized mesenteric arteries. Vasculitic lesions tend to be segmental and focal. Immunohistochemical staining of the tunica adventitia and media may reveal immune complex, C3 complement, and fibrinogen deposition. Fibrinoid necrosis, intraluminal thrombosis of affected vessels, acute or chronic inflammatory infiltrates consisting of lymphocytes, plasma cells, histiocytes, and neutrophils may also be demonstrated.[21]

Although any vessels can be involved, the territory of the superior mesenteric artery (jejunum and ileum) is most frequently affected by lupus enteritis.[1,19] The pathogenesis of lupus enteritis remains elusive. Immune complex-mediated vasculitis with complement activation that induces inflammation, microvascular injury, ischemia, and edema of the bowel wall, leading to increase in vascular permeability, is thought to be the mechanism.[22]

The mortality of lupus enteritis is high, depending on the extent of vascular involvement and the rapidity of diagnosis and treatment.[1,18] Aggressive immunosuppressive therapy with high-dose intravenous pulse methylprednisolone should be given early. Patients should be monitored closely and surgical intervention is indicated when a rapid clinical response is not achieved or there is clinical and radiological suspicion of bowel perforation. Lupus enteritis may recur in more than half of patients, especially in those with a bowel wall thickness of >9 mm at presentation.[23] Intravenous pulse cyclophosphamide has been used with success in refractory lupus enteritis[24] and reducing recurrence.[23]

Mesenteric Insufficiency

Atherosclerosis of the mesenteric arteries should be considered in SLE patients who present with chronic intermittent abdominal pain ("intestinal angina"). Symptoms usually start in the postprandial state and persist for several hours. Symptoms may worsen over time and weight loss may develop for fear of eating. Concomitant atherosclerotic disease in the coronary and carotid vessels supports the diagnosis. SLE patients with long-standing disease, traditional vascular risk factors, renal insufficiency, persistent proteinuria, antiphospholipid antibodies, and chronic corticosteroid therapy are at risk.

The diagnosis of chronic mesenteric insufficiency relies on a high index of suspicion. Conventional angiography is the gold standard imaging procedure. Digital subtraction angiography and magnetic resonance angiography are adjunctive diagnostic modalities.[25]

Acute mesenteric ischemia can result from thrombosis of the mesenteric arterial or venous systems. Classically, abdominal pain is persistent and disproportionately severe relative to physical signs. Bowel infarction and perforation may manifest as acute surgical abdomen, fever, bloody diarrhea, melena, and hypotension. SLE patients with underlying chronic mesenteric insufficiency or the antiphospholipid antibodies are prone to acute intestinal ischemia, which may be precipitated by hypoperfusion states.

Surgical revascularization and percutaneous transluminal mesenteric angioplasty with or without a stent are treatment options for patients with chronic mesenteric ischemia.[25] Acute mesenteric thrombosis causing bowel gangrene should be treated by surgical exploration and embolectomy. Long-term anticoagulation should be given to patients who qualify with the antiphospholipid syndrome.

Intestinal Pseudo-Obstruction

Intestinal pseudo-obstruction (IPO) is a syndrome characterized by impaired intestinal motility leading to features of a mechanical bowel obstruction. This condition is rare but more commonly reported in Asian patients with SLE. IPO may be the initial presentation of SLE and usually occurs in the setting of an active lupus.[1,2,26] The small bowel is more commonly affected than the large bowel.

Common presenting symptoms of IPO are subacute onset of abdominal pain, nausea, vomiting, abdominal distension, and constipation. The abdomen is diffusely tender with sluggish or absent bowel sounds. Rebound tenderness

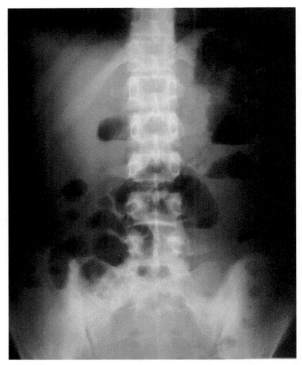

FIGURE 1   An SLE patient presented with intestinal pseudo-obstruction. Plain radiograph of the abdomen shows multiple dilated bowel loops with fluid level.

is usually absent unless there is bowel perforation. X-ray and CT examination may demonstrate multiple dilated bowel loops with fluid level and thickened bowel wall (Figure 1). Mechanical causes for intestinal obstruction should be excluded, preferably by nonsurgical means but laparotomy may be necessary in some patients.

Manometry motility studies in patients with IPO may demonstrate esophageal aperistalsis and intestinal hypomotility.[27] Interestingly, more than two-thirds of the reported cases of SLE-related IPO had concomitant ureterohydronephrosis and contracted/thickened urinary bladder, with the majority demonstrating histological features of chronic interstitial cystitis.[1,2,26]

The coexistence of ureterohydronephrosis in many patients with SLE-related IPO and dilatation of the biliary tract (megacholedochus) in occasional patients indicates that the basic pathophysiology is dysmotility of the intestinal musculature. The association with autoimmune cystitis and the demonstration of antibodies against proliferating cell nuclear antigen in some patients[28] suggest that immune complex-mediated vasculitis may be a mechanism for inflammation and subsequent damage of the visceral smooth muscles, leading to atrophy, fibrosis, and loss of function of the bowel wall. Other postulated mechanisms for visceral smooth muscle dysfunction include a primary myopathy of the bowel musculature, neuropathy of the enteric nerves or the visceral autonomic nervous system,

and direct cytotoxicity of antibodies directed against the smooth muscle of the gut wall.

SLE-related IPO often responds to high-dose corticosteroids.[1,2,18] Additional immunosuppressive agents such as azathioprine, cyclosporin A, and cyclophosphamide have been used with success in some reports.[29,30] Other adjunctive therapies for IPO are nasogastric tube insertion, intravenous fluid, parental nutrition, broad spectrum antibiotics, and prokinetic agents such as erythromycin, metoclopramide, and octreotide (a long-acting somatostatin analog).[30] Early recognition of IPO in SLE patients and timely initiation of immunosuppressive therapy are important because the condition is potentially reversible with nonsurgical measures. However, some patients may have a relapsing course despite maintenance immunosuppressive treatment.

Malabsorption and Celiac Disease

Malabsorption is reported to occur in 2/21 (9.5%) patients with SLE by standard screening tests.[31] In one of these patients, histologic examination revealed flattened and deformed villi with an inflammatory infiltrate. Up to 23% of patients with SLE have been tested positive for IgA or IgM anti-gliadin antibodies[32] and 5.7% of patients have positive IgA anti-endomysium antibodies.[15] However, biopsy proven celiac disease (gluten-sensitive enteropathy) in SLE patients is extremely rare.[33]

Protein-Losing Gastroenteropathy

Protein-losing gastroenteropathy (PLGE) is a condition characterized by hypoalbuminemia secondary to loss of protein from the GI tract. It is usually identified by an elevated clearance of stool $\alpha 1$-antitrypsin or the technetium-99m-labeled human serum albumin scan. A variety of pathologies from the stomach down to the colon may be responsible for protein loss. Significant proteinuria should be ruled out. Investigations into the causes of PLGE such as gastrointestinal lymphoma, malabsorption state, bacterial overgrowth, inflammatory bowel disease, chronic infection, polyposis, and lymphatic obstruction are essential. Endoscopic examination with mucosal biopsies, barium studies, radiologic examinations, and absorption tests are required.

PLGE is an uncommon manifestation of SLE, with an estimated point prevalence of 1.9% to 3.2%.[2,34,35] Two-thirds of the reported cases in the literature are in Asian patients and in 49% of patients, PLGE is the presenting feature of SLE.[36] Disease activity of SLE in other systems is usually present. The most common presenting symptoms of PLGE are generalized or dependent edema (80%), and abdominal symptoms such as pain (27%), nonbloody diarrhea (46%), nausea (22%), and vomiting (19%). Ascites (48%), pleural effusion (38%), and pericardial effusion (21%) related to hypoalbuminemia (96%) may also be present. Protein leakage occurs more frequently from the small bowel (84%) than the large bowel (29%).

Investigation findings in SLE-related PGLE are often nonspecific. The most common endoscopic appearance is mucosal edema (50%). Biopsy is either unremarkable or reveals thickened mucosa, submucosal edema, villous atrophy, dilated lacteals, or inflammatory infiltrates.[37] Definite lymphangiectasia, vasculitis, or C3 deposition in the capillary walls of the lamina propriae of villi is uncommon. Contrast CT of the abdomen may show ascites, bowel wall thickening, and edema.

The exact pathogenesis of PLGE is unknown. Mucosal disruption, increase in mucosal capillary permeability as a result of complement- or cytokine-mediated damage, mesenteric venulitis, and dilated/ruptured mucosal lacteals have been postulated.[34]

PLGE in SLE often responds to corticosteroid treatment. No controlled trials are available regarding the additional benefit of azathioprine. Our own experience shows that an initial regimen of high-dose prednisolone and azathioprine is well tolerated and effective in most patients with SLE-related PLGE.[36] Relapse is uncommon (6%) with low-dose prednisolone and azathioprine maintenance treatment.[34] Intravenous pulse cyclophosphamide, cyclosporine A, and azathioprine may be considered in patients with refractory disease. Albumin infusion, diuretics, and nutritional support may help to reduce symptoms of edema. Prophylaxis for thromboembolic complications should be considered in patients with severe and persistent protein loss, especially if the antiphospholipid antibodies are present.

Infective and Eosinophilic Enteritis

Infective enteritis should be considered in SLE patients presenting with abdominal symptoms. Bacterial enteritis is the most common, with nontyphoidal *Salmonella* infection being most frequently reported. *Campylobacter jejuni* infection and CMV enteritis may lead to ileal perforation.

Eosinophilic gastroenteritis is a rare condition characterized by eosinophilic infiltration of the deep layers of the intestinal wall,[18] leading to abdominal pain, nausea, vomiting, and diarrhea. Peripheral eosinophilia is usually present. Four cases of eosinophilic enteritis have been reported in patients with SLE. High-dose prednisolone treatment is usually effective and refractory cases may respond to intravenous immunoglobulin.

Ascites and Peritonitis

Acute peritonitis in SLE may be caused by mesenteric vasculitis, bowel infarction, perforated viscera, pancreatitis, intraabdominal infection, or serositis related to active SLE (lupus peritonitis). Subacute or chronic peritoneal effusion can result from lupus peritonitis, any causes of hypoalbuminemia, right heart failure, hepatic venous thrombosis, malignancy, and more indolent infections such as tuberculosis.

About 30% of serositis episodes in patients with SLE are caused by inflammatory peritonitis.[38] Abdominal pain is the usual presenting symptom, which may be severe enough to mimic acute surgical abdomen that leads to negative laparotomy. On the other hand, physical signs of peritonitis or ascites may not necessarily be present in mild cases of lupus peritonitis.

Lupus peritonitis often responds rapidly to moderate doses of corticosteroids. In patients with massive or refractory ascites, intravenous pulse methylprednisolone and additional immunosuppressive agents such as azathioprine, cyclosporin A, and cyclophosphamide may be needed.

Large Intestine

Lupus Colitis and Inflammatory Bowel Disease

The large bowel may occasionally be involved in lupus enteritis, leading to colitis and perforation.[11] Active SLE in other organs is often present and the mortality is high.

Crohn's disease and ulcerative colitis (UC) are rarely reported in SLE patients. The prevalence of UC in SLE patients is around 0.4%.[39] Clinically and pathologically, lupus colitis may be indistinguishable from UC. Symptoms include lower abdominal discomfort, per rectal bleeding, and persistent diarrhea that may be bloody. Cases of Crohn's disease presenting with persistent GI bleeding have been reported in patients with SLE.[40]

Infective and Collagenous Colitis

Colonic infections should be considered in SLE patients presenting with lower GI symptoms. CMV and amoebic colitis have been reported in patients with SLE.[2] Collagenous colitis is a disorder characterized by colonic intraepithelial lymphocytosis, expansion of the lamina propria with acute and chronic inflammatory cells, and a thickened subepithelial collagen band. Patients usually present with chronic watery diarrhea despite normal radiologic and endoscopic findings. Collagenous colitis has been reported in discoid and systemic lupus.[2]

THE LIVER IN SLE

Subclinical Liver Disease

Liver function abnormalities are common in patients with SLE. Multiple factors such as the use of aspirin, NSAIDs, azathioprine, and methotrexate, fatty infiltration of liver as a result of corticosteroid treatment, diabetes mellitus, or obesity as well as viral hepatitis and alcoholism may contribute. Persistent and severe liver function abnormalities require

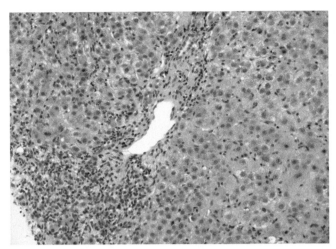

FIGURE 2   Liver biopsy in an SLE patient showing active interface hepatitis with prominent portal lymphoplasmacytic infiltrates (H&E stain).

further investigations such as ultrasonography and liver biopsy to delineate the underlying causes.

Elevation of liver enzymes occurs in 23–60% of SLE patients during the course of the illness but significant liver disease is not common.[41–43] No identifiable cause other than SLE itself is found in around one-third of patients.[43] In 80% of cases of persistent "unexplained" liver function derangement, the serial change in liver transaminases correlates with SLE activity.[43] Liver biopsy in SLE patients commonly reveals steatotic hepatitis, portal inflammatory infiltrates, and chronic active hepatitis.[41,42] Other reported pathologies include chronic granulomatous hepatitis, centrilobular necrosis, chronic persistent hepatitis, and microabscesses (6%).

Autoimmune Hepatitis

Autoimmune hepatitis (AIH) is characterized histologically by portal and periportal lymphoplasmacytic infiltration and extension of the infiltrates into the lobule (interface hepatitis) and hepatocyte rosette formation (Figure 2). As the disease progresses, evidence of hepatic injury such as bridging necrosis, panlobular necrosis, multilobular necrosis, and cirrhosis may develop. Hypergammaglobulinemia and a variety of autoantibodies that direct against hepatic antigens or liver–kidney microsomal proteins such as ANA, anti-smooth muscle antibodies (SMA), and anti-liver/kidney microsomal (LKM) antibodies may be present. AIH is classified into three types: (1) Type I AIH (the classical "lupoid hepatitis" described in the 1950s) is the most common form worldwide and is associated with ANA and/or SMA; (2) Type II AIH is associated with anti-LKM1 antibody; and (3) Type III AIH is associated with anti-soluble liver/liver pancreas antigen (SLA/LP) antibodies.

Patients with AIH commonly present with insidious onset of nonspecific symptoms such as fatigue, malaise, and anorexia. Liver enlargement, jaundice, and ascites may be present in severe cases. AIH is associated with SLE-like features such as arthritis, serositis, thrombocytopenia, hypergammaglobulinemia, and positive ANA and anti-dsDNA,[44] but only 10–23% of AIH patients fulfill the ACR criteria for SLE.[45]

The incidence of coexisting AIH in SLE patients is unclear as not all patients will undergo liver biopsy for liver derangement and mild AIH may respond completely to corticosteroids. Differentiation between AIH/SLE overlap and SLE-associated hepatitis can be difficult in the absence of histological information. Lupus-associated hepatitis runs a more benign course with predominant lobular involvement and mild lobular inflammation without piecemeal necrosis on liver histology.[45] Anti-ribosomal P antibody is more commonly found in SLE patients with hepatitis than in those without.[46] Features of lupus-associated hepatitis and SLE/AIH overlap are contrasted in Table 2.

High-dose prednisone alone or a lower dose of prednisone in conjunction with azathioprine is the main stay of treatment for AIH. Remission can be achieved in the majority of patients in the first 3 years of diagnosis. The use of azathioprine may reduce relapses and is corticosteroid sparing. Maintenance therapy with low-dose prednisone and azathioprine is preferred for patients with multiple relapses. MMF, cyclosporin A, or tacrolimus is reserved for refractory cases of AIH.

Viral and Drug-Induced Hepatitis

The prevalence of chronic hepatitis B virus (HBV) infection does not seem to be higher in patients with SLE as compared to the age- and sex-matched general population, even in endemic areas.[47] Some studies have reported a higher prevalence of chronic hepatitis C (HCV) infection in SLE patients compared to healthy controls.[48] SLE patients with HCV infection were less likely to have cutaneous disease and anti-dsDNA, but more likely to have hepatic dysfunction, low complement levels, and cryoglobulinemia than those without.

Aspirin, NSAIDs, methotrexate, and leflunomide may cause elevation of parenchymal liver enzymes. Corticosteroid may induce fatty liver disease (steatotic hepatitis), which is one of the more common histological findings from liver biopsy of SLE patients.[41,49] Azathioprine, hydroxychloroquine, and the statins may occasionally cause hepatitis.

Nodular Regenerative Hyperplasia

Nodular regenerative hyperplasia (NRH) is characterized by diffuse nodularity of the liver with little or no fibrosis. It is a cause of noncirrhotic portal hypertension and may lead to ascites and variceal bleeding. NRH has been described

TABLE 2 Main Features of Lupus-Associated Hepatitis and Idiopathic Autoimmune Hepatitis (AIH)

Features	SLE-Associated Hepatitis	AIH
Histology	Lobular, rarely periportal	Portal and periportal, piecemeal necrosis
ACR criteria for SLE	100%	10–23%
Elevated serum IgG	Common	Common
Complements (C3/4)	Normal or depressed	Often normal unless liver failure
ANA	>99%	80% in type I AIH
Anti-dsDNA	60–70%	20–50%, low titer
Anti-Ro	30–60%	11–14%
Anti-ribosomal P	70%	<10%
Anti-SMA	30%	60–80%
Anti-LKM-1	Negative	Diagnostic of type 2 AIH
Anti-LC-1	Negative	Diagnostic of type 2 AIH
Anti-SLA/LP	Negative	Diagnostic of AIH
Response to corticosteroids	Usually favorable	Generally favorable
Prognosis	Good	May progress to cirrhosis and liver failure

ACR, American College of Rheumatology; SLE, systemic lupus erythematosus; SMA, smooth muscle antibody; LKM, liver/kidney–microsomal; LC, liver cytosol; SLA/LP, soluble liver/liver pancreas antigen.

in patients with SLE and the primary antiphospholipid syndrome.[50] The association with the antiphospholipid antibodies suggests that NRH may result from liver regeneration to maintain its functional capacity after ischemia-induced injury. Another postulation is immune complex-mediated vasculitis leading to obliterative venopathy and impaired hepatic venous drainage.[51,52]

More than 70% of histologically confirmed cases of NRH are found in patients with SLE.[51] NRH should be suspected in SLE patients with unexplained portal hypertension and the diagnosis must be confirmed by liver biopsy. Hepatic nodules in NRH may be visualized with magnetic resonance imaging (MRI) of the liver.[50] Many patients with NRH of the liver are asymptomatic with normal liver function. Treatment should target at control of portal hypertension and its related complications.

Other Liver Diseases

Thromboembolic disorders of the liver may occur in patients with SLE, especially in the presence of the antiphospholipid antibodies. Budd-Chiari syndrome, a disease caused by occlusion of the hepatic veins, hepatic veno-occlusive disease, and hepatic infarction have been reported in patients with SLE and secondary antiphospholipid syndrome.[53] Finally, SLE is associated with a fourfold increase in the incidence of liver hemangioma compared to the general population.[53,54] While the explanation is unclear,

an increase in circulating estrogen metabolites and angiogenic factors in SLE patients might contribute to the development of hemangioma.[54]

BILIARY TRACT DISEASE IN SLE

Gallbladder disease appears to be no more frequent in SLE patients than in the general population. Cholecystitis in SLE may be confused with serositis. Acute acalculous cholecystitis has been described in patients with SLE.[55] Patients usually present with acute abdomen and cholecystectomy specimens may reveal vasculitis of the gall bladder. Contrast CT scan may demonstrate enhancement of the gall bladder wall and the presence of pericholecystic fluid. Although successful conservative treatment with corticosteroid has been reported, the condition is diagnosed after surgical treatment in most patients, especially if there is evidence of septicemia.

Primary biliary cirrhosis (PBC), autoimmune cholangiopathy (anti-mitochondrial antibody negative PBC), and primary sclerosing cholangitis have also been reported in patients with SLE.[2]

THE PANCREAS IN SLE

Acute pancreatitis is an uncommon manifestation of SLE, occurring in 1.3–3.5% of patients.[2,56] Pancreatitis is the initial presentation of SLE in 28% of cases.[56] Subclinical

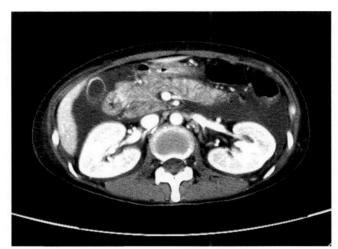

FIGURE 3   An SLE patient presented with a major disease flare with severe hemolysis, proteinuria, and acute abdominal pain (elevated amylase level). A contrast CT of the abdomen revealed a diffusely swollen pancreas and ascites. She was not a drinker and there was no evidence of choledocholithiasis. Her pancreatitis responded to high-dose prednisone and IVIG therapy.

pancreatitis with hyperamylasemia is probably common in patients with SLE. Medications such as corticosteroids, azathioprine, and thiazide diuretics and infection with CMV have been attributed to cause pancreatitis in some cases.

Acute pancreatitis appears to be more common in SLE than in non-SLE patients.[57] Around one-third of the episodes of acute pancreatitis in SLE patients are considered "idiopathic." SLE disease activity scores are usually higher in idiopathic cases of pancreatitis than those with identifiable causes such as alcoholism and choledocholithiasis (Figure 3).[57,58] Idiopathic pancreatitis often improves with corticosteroid treatment.[58] Taken together, pancreatitis is likely a distinct entity in SLE and possibly caused by vasculitis. In fact, in the presteroid era, cases of pancreatic vasculitis have been documented histopathologically. Autopsy studies have also demonstrated vascular damage consisting of severe intimal proliferation in the pancreatic vessels in patients with lupus pancreatitis.[59] Other postulated mechanisms for pancreatitis in SLE include vascular ischemia, microthrombi, and circulatory anti-pancreatic antibodies.

Common symptoms of lupus pancreatitis are abdominal pain (98%), nausea or vomiting (68%), and fever (58%). Diagnosis is based on raised pancreatic enzymes (amylase and lipase) and imaging findings. Contrast CT scan is the most useful investigation, which may demonstrate pancreatic enlargement and fat stranding, intraabdominal fluid collection and associated pleural effusion. CT scan also helps to exclude other causes of abdominal pain and detect complications of pancreatitis such as pancreatic necrosis, hemorrhage, pseudocysts, abscess formation, and pancreatic duct strictures. Other imaging options for acute pancreatitis include MRI of the abdomen.

A recent study compared the presentation and prognosis of acute pancreatitis between childhood and adult-onset SLE patients and reported a much higher prevalence of pancreatitis in pediatric patients (5.2% vs 1%).[56] The severity of pancreatitis, concomitant SLE activity, and mortality is also significantly greater in childhood-onset SLE patients.

IgG4-related disease (IgG4-RD) is an emerging multi-organ immune-mediated disease associated with abundant infiltration of IgG4-positive lymphoplasmacytic cells.[60] GI manifestations of IgG4-RD include mesenteritis, hepatopathy, cholecystitis, sclerosing cholangitis, pancreatitis, and pancreatic mass. However, coexistence of SLE and IgG4-RD with pancreatitis or other GI manifestations has not yet been described.

Management of pancreatitis in SLE patients includes fluid resuscitation, bowel resting, discontinuation of non-essential but potentially offending drugs, and the use of antibiotics if necessary. Secondary causes of pancreatitis such as cholelithiasis, alcoholism, and hypertriglyceridemia must be excluded. Close observation and serial contrast CT scan of the abdomen are needed to monitor for the progress of pancreatitis and its complications. Corticosteroid should be considered in idiopathic cases of pancreatitis, particularly if SLE is active in other systems.

ACUTE ABDOMINAL PAIN IN SLE

Depending on the setting in which patients are assessed, abdominal pain is reported in 8–37% of patients with SLE,[2] which can be due to SLE-related, treatment-related or non-SLE-related causes (Table 3).

In SLE patients who undergo exploratory laparotomy for acute abdomen, intestinal vasculitis (34%), intraabdominal thrombosis (5%), and serositis (3%) are the most common diagnoses.[11,61] More active SLE and a delay in surgical exploration are associated with higher mortality. In a recent study of 213 SLE Chinese patients presenting with acute abdominal pain, the most common SLE-related diagnoses are lupus enteritis (74%) and pancreatitis (17%).[62] Non-SLE-related causes of abdominal pain are more frequent in patients with inactive disease. This is concordant with the findings of a Mexican study in which pancreatitis (29%), intestinal ischemia (16%), gallbladder disease (15%), and appendicitis (14%) are the most common causes of acute abdomen in SLE patients.[6]

Abdominal pain in SLE patients may precede an intraabdominal catastrophe. Peritoneal signs may be masked by the immunosuppressive drugs. Acute, persistent, or severe abdominal symptoms in patients with SLE should be promptly investigated. Endoscopy, paracentesis, ultrasound scan, contrast CT scan, MRI, gallium scan, and angiography should be performed as indicated. A surgical opinion is required and exploratory laparotomy should be considered

TABLE 3 Differential Diagnoses of Abdominal Pain in Patients with SLE

Disease-Related	Therapy-Related	Non-SLE Etiologies
Serositis	Gastritis, duodenitis	Infective gastroenteritis
Intestinal vasculitis/colitis	Peptic ulcer ± perforation	Inflammatory bowel disease
Malabsorption	Pancreatitis	Cholecystitis/cholangitis
Intestinal pseudo-obstruction	Intraabdominal sepsis	Pancreatitis
Protein-losing gastroenteropathy	Infective enteritis	Viral hepatitis
Ischemic bowel disease	Infective colitis	Eosinophilic enteritis (rare)
Mesenteric thrombosis	Bacterial peritonitis	Celiac disease (rare)
Hepatic vein thrombosis		Surgical adhesions
Hepatitis		Appendicitis
Pancreatitis		Diverticulitis
Acalculous cholecystitis (rare)		Intussusception
		Gynecological conditions
		Rupture of vascular aneurysms (rare)

in patients with clinical and radiological suspicion of visceral perforation or intraabdominal collections.

CONCLUSIONS

The gastrointestinal and hepatic manifestations of SLE are heterogeneous. Despite the advances in imaging techniques, the diagnosis of GI lupus remains by exclusion. Because of the lack of controlled trials, treatment of GI lupus is largely based on anecdotal experience. Acute abdominal symptoms in SLE should be promptly evaluated. When infection and other important causes have been ruled out, immunosuppressive treatment should be commenced, preferably under coverage with broad spectrum antibiotics. Anticoagulation should be considered when thrombosis is the underlying mechanism. Refractory manifestations may require treatment with cyclophosphamide and other immunosuppressive agents. Early surgical intervention should be instituted when conservative management fails. Newer tools to quantify the activity and treatment response of GI lupus and randomized controlled therapeutic trials are needed in the future.

REFERENCES

1. Chng HH, Tan BE, Teh CL, Lian TY. Major gastrointestinal manifestations in lupus patients in Asia: lupus enteritis, intestinal pseudo-obstruction, and protein-losing gastroenteropathy. *Lupus* 2010;**19**:1404–13.
2. Mok CC. Investigations and management of gastrointestinal and hepatic manifestations of systemic lupus erythematosus. *Best Pract Res Clin Rheumatol* 2005;**19**:741–66.
3. Gladman DD, Ibañez D, Urowitz MB. Systemic lupus erythematosus disease activity index 2000. *J Rheumatol* 2002;**29**:288–91.
4. Petri M, Orbai AM, Alarcón GS, Gordon C, Merrill JT, Fortin PR, et al. Derivation and validation of the Systemic Lupus International Collaborating Clinics classification criteria for systemic lupus erythematosus. *Arthritis Rheum* 2012;**64**:2677–86.
5. Okon LG, Werth VP. Cutaneous lupus erythematosus: diagnosis and treatment. *Best Pract Res Clin Rheumatol* 2013;**27**:391–404.
6. Manoussakis MN, Georgopoulou C, Zintzaras E, Spyropoulou M, Stavropoulou A, Skopouli FN, et al. Sjogren's syndrome associated with systemic lupus erythematosus: clinical and laboratory profiles and comparison with primary Sjogren's syndrome. *Arthritis Rheum* 2004;**50**:882–91.
7. Fernandes EG, Savioli C, Siqueira JT, Silva CA. Oral health and the masticatory system in juvenile systemic lupus erythematosus. *Lupus* 2007;**16**:713–9.
8. Lockhart PB, Bolger AF, Papapanou PN, Osinbowale O, Trevisan M, Levison ME, et al. Periodontal disease and atherosclerotic vascular disease: does the evidence support an independent association?: a scientific statement from the American Heart Association. *Circulation* 2012;**125**:2520–44.
9. Lapadula G, Muolo P, Semeraro F, Covelli M, Brindicci D, Cuccorese G, et al. Esophageal motility disorders in the rheumatic diseases: a review of 150 patients. *Clin Exp Rheumatol* 1994;**12**:515–21.
10. Ozaki T, Yamashita H, Kaneko S, Yorifuji H, Takahashi H, Ueda Y, et al. Cytomegalovirus disease of the upper gastrointestinal tract in patients with rheumatic diseases: a case series and literature review. *Clin Rheumatol* 2013;**32**:1683–90.
11. Medina F, Ayala A, Jara LJ, Becerra M, Miranda JM, Fraga A. Acute abdomen in systemic lupus erythematosus: the importance of early laparotomy. *Am J Med* 1997;**103**:100–5.
12. Smyk DS, Koutsoumpas AL, Mytilinaiou MG, Rigopoulou EI, Sakkas LI, Bogdanos DP. Helicobacter pylori and autoimmune disease: cause or bystander. *World J Gastroenterol* 2014;**20**:613–29.

13. Fuccio L, Mussetto A, Laterza L, Eusebi LH, Bazzoli F. Diagnosis and management of gastric antral vascular ectasia. *World J Gastrointest Endosc* 2013;**5**:6–13.

14. Junca J, Cuxart A, Olive A, Tural C. Anti-intrinsic factor antibodies in systemic lupus erythematosus. *Lupus* 1993;**2**:111–4.

15. Picceli VF, Skare TL, Nisihara R, Kotze L, Messias-Reason I, Utiyama SR. Spectrum of autoantibodies for gastrointestinal autoimmune diseases in systemic lupus erythematosus patients. *Lupus* 2013;**22**:1150–5.

16. Ju JH, Min JK, Jung CK, Oh SN, Kwok SK, Kang KY, et al. Lupus mesenteric vasculitis can cause acute abdominal pain in patients with SLE. *Nat Rev Rheumatol* 2009;**5**:273–81.

17. Kwok SK, Seo SH, Ju JH, Park KS, Yoon CH, Kim WU, et al. Lupus enteritis: clinical characteristics, risk factor for relapse and association with anti-endothelial cell antibody. *Lupus* 2007;**16**:803–9.

18. Tian XP, Zhang X. Gastrointestinal involvement in systemic lupus erythematosus: insight into pathogenesis, diagnosis and treatment. *World J Gastroenterol* 2010;**16**:2971–7.

19. Goh YP, Naidoo P, Ngian GS. Imaging of systemic lupus erythematosus. Part II: gastrointestinal, renal, and musculoskeletal manifestations. *Clin Radiol* 2013;**68**:192–202.

20. Ko SF, Lee TY, Cheng TT, Ng SH, Lai HM, Cheng YF, et al. CT findings at lupus mesenteric vasculitis. *Acta Radiol* 1997;**38**:115–20.

21. Weiser MM, Andres GA, Brentjens JR, Evans JT, Reichlin M. Systemic lupus erythematosus and intestinal venulitis. *Gastroenterology* 1981;**81**:570–9.

22. Kishimoto M, Nasir A, Mor A, Belmont HM. Acute gastrointestinal distress syndrome in patients with systemic lupus erythematosus. *Lupus* 2007;**16**:137–41.

23. Kim YG, Ha HK, Nah SS, Lee CK, Moon HB, Yoo B. Acute abdominal pain in systemic lupus erythematosus: factors contributing to recurrence of lupus enteritis. *Ann Rheum Dis* 2006;**65**:1537–8.

24. Yuan S, Ye Y, Chen D, Qiu Q, Zhan Z, Lian F, et al. Lupus mesenteric vasculitis: clinical features and associated factors for the recurrence and prognosis of disease. *Semin Arthritis Rheum* 2014;**43**:759–66.

25. Matsuda M, Miyazaki D, Tojo K, Tazawa K, Shimojima Y, Kurozumi M, et al. Intestinal angina due to atherosclerosis in a 45-year-old systemic lupus erythematosus patient. *Intern Med* 2010;**49**:2175–8.

26. Zhang J, Fang M, Wang Y, Mao J, Sun X. Intestinal pseudo-obstruction syndrome in systemic lupus erythematosus. *Lupus* 2011;**20**:1324–8.

27. Perlemuter G, Chaussade S, Wechsler B, Cacoub P, Dapoigny M, Kahan A, et al. Chronic intestinal pseudo-obstruction in systemic lupus erythematosus. *Gut* 1998;**43**:117–22.

28. Nojima Y, Mimura T, Hamasaki K, Furuya H, Tanaka G, Nakajima A, et al. Chronic intestinal pseudoobstruction associated with autoantibodies against proliferating cell nuclear antigen. *Arthritis Rheum* 1996;**39**:877–9.

29. Khairullah S, Jasmin R, Yahya F, Cheah TE, Ng CT, Sockalingam S. Chronic intestinal pseudo-obstruction: a rare first manifestation of systemic lupus erythematosus. *Lupus* 2013;**22**:957–60.

30. Ceccato F, Salas A, Góngora V, Ruta S, Roverano S, Marcos JC, et al. Chronic intestinal pseudo-obstruction in patients with systemic lupus erythematosus: report of four cases. *Clin Rheumatol* 2008;**27**:399–402.

31. Mader R, Adawi M, Schonfeld S. Malabsorption in systemic lupus erythematosus. *Clin Exp Rheumatol* 1997;**15**:659–61.

32. Rensch MJ, Szyjkowski R, Shaffer RT, Fink S, Kopecky C, Grissmer L, et al. The prevalence of celiac disease autoantibodies in patients with systemic lupus erythematosus. *Am J Gastroenterol* 2001;**96**:1113–5.

33. Gupta D, Mirza N. Systemic lupus erythematosus, celiac disease and antiphospholipid antibody syndrome: a rare association. *Rheumatol Int* 2008;**28**:1179–80.

34. Mok CC, Ying KY, Mak A, To CH, Szeto ML. Outcome of protein losing gastroenteropathy in systemic lupus erythematosus treated with prednisolone and azathioprine. *Rheumatology (Oxford)* 2006;**45**:425–9.

35. Zheng WJ, Tian XP, Li L, Jing HL, Li F, Zeng XF, et al. Protein-losing enteropathy in systemic lupus erythematosus: analysis of the clinical features of fifteen patients. *J Clin Rheumatol* 2007;**13**:313–6.

36. Al-Mogairen SM. Lupus protein-losing enteropathy (LUPLE): a systematic review. *Rheumatol Int* 2011;**31**:995–1001.

37. Kobayashi K, Asakura H, Shinozawa T, Yoshida S, Ichikawa Y, Tsuchiya M, et al. Protein-losing enteropathy in systemic lupus erythematosus. Observations by magnifying endoscopy. *Dig Dis Sci* 1989;**34**:1924–8.

38. Man BL, Mok CC. Lupus-related serositis: prevalence and outcome. *Lupus* 2005;**14**:822–6.

39. Medeiros DA, Isenberg DA. Systemic lupus erythematosus and ulcerative colitis. *Lupus* 2009;**18**:762–3.

40. Yamashita H, Ueda Y, Kawaguchi H, Suzuki A, Takahashi Y, Kaneko H, et al. Systemic lupus erythematosus complicated by Crohn's disease: a case report and literature review. *BMC Gastroenterol* 2012;**12**:174.

41. Runyon BA, LaBrecque DR, Anuras S. The spectrum of liver disease in systemic lupus erythematosus. Report of 33 histologically-proved cases and review of the literature. *Am J Med* 1980;**69**:187–94.

42. Gibson T, Myers AR. Subclinical liver disease in systemic lupus erythematosus. *J Rheumatol* 1981;**8**:752–9.

43. Miller MH, Urowitz MB, Gladman DD, Blendis LM. The liver in systemic lupus erythematosus. *Q J Med* 1984;**53**:401–9.

44. Onder FO, Yürekli OT, Oztaş E, Kalkan IH, Köksal AS, Akdoğan M, et al. Features of systemic lupus erythematosus in patients with autoimmune hepatitis. *Rheumatol Int* 2013;**33**:1581–5.

45. Kaw R, Gota C, Bennett A, Barnes D, Calabrese L. Lupus-related hepatitis: complication of lupus or autoimmune association? Case report and review of the literature. *Dig Dis Sci* 2006;**51**:813–8.

46. Ohira H, Takiguchi J, Rai T, Abe K, Yokokawa J, Sato Y, et al. High frequency of anti-ribosomal P antibody in patients with systemic lupus erythematosus-associated hepatitis. *Hepatol Res* 2004;**28**:137–9.

47. Zhao J, Qiu M, Li M, Lu C, Gu J. Low prevalence of hepatitis B virus infection in patients with systemic lupus erythematosus in southern China. *Rheumatol Int* 2010;**30**:1565–70.

48. Ramos-Casals M, Font J, Garcia-Carrasco M, Cervera R, Jiménez S, Trejo O, et al. Hepatitis C virus infection mimicking systemic lupus erythematosus: study of hepatitis C virus infection in a series of 134 Spanish patients with systemic lupus erythematosus. *Arthritis Rheum* 2000;**43**:2801–6.

49. Bessone F, Poles N, Roma MG. Challenge of liver disease in systemic lupus erythematosus: clues for diagnosis and hints for pathogenesis. *World J Hepatol* 2014;**6**:394–409.

50. Horita T, Tsutsumi A, Takeda T, Yasuda S, Takeuchi R, Amasaki Y, et al. Significance of magnetic resonance imaging in the diagnosis of nodular regenerative hyperplasia of the liver complicated with systemic lupus erythematosus: a case report and review of the literature. *Lupus* 2002;**11**:193–6.

51. Matsumoto T, Kobayashi S, Shimizu H, Nakajima M, Watanabe S, Kitami N, et al. The liver in collagen diseases: pathologic study of 160 cases with particular reference to hepatic arteritis, primary biliary cirrhosis, autoimmune hepatitis and nodular regenerative hyperplasia of the liver. *Liver* 2000;**20**:366–73.

52. Uthman I, Khamashta M. The abdominal manifestations of the antiphospholipid syndrome. *Rheumatology (Oxford)* 2007;**46**:1641–7.

53. Grover S, Rastogi A, Singh J, Rajbongshi A, Bihari C. Spectrum of histomorphologic findings in liver in patients with SLE: a review. *Hepat Res Treat* 2014;**2014**:562979.

54. Berzigotti A, Frigato M, Manfredini E, Pierpaoli L, Mulè R, Tiani C, et al. Liver hemangioma and vascular liver diseases in patients with systemic lupus erythematosus. *World J Gastroenterol* 2011;**17**:4503–8.

55. Basiratnia M, Vasei M, Bahador A, Ebrahimi E, Derakhshan A. Acute acalculous cholecystitis in a child with systemic lupus erythematosus. *Pediatr Nephrol* 2006;**21**:873–6.

56. Wang CH, Yao TC, Huang YL, Ou LS, Yeh KW, Huang JL. Acute pancreatitis in pediatric and adult-onset systemic lupus erythematosus: a comparison and review of the literature. *Lupus* 2011;**20**:443–52.

57. Pascual-Ramos V, Duarte-Rojo A, Villa AR, Hernández-Cruz B, Alarcón-Segovia D, Alcocer-Varela J, et al. Systemic lupus erythematosus

as a cause and prognostic factor of acute pancreatitis. *J Rheumatol* 2004;**31**:707–12.

58. Derk CT, DeHoratius RJ. Systemic lupus erythematosus and acute pancreatitis: a case series. *Clin Rheumatol* 2004;**23**:147–51.

59. Serrano Lopez MC, Yebra Bango M, Lopez Bonet E, Sanchez Vegazo I, Albarrán Hernández F, Manzano Espinosa L, et al. Acute pancreatitis and systemic lupus erythematosus: necropsy of a case and review of the pancreatic vascular lesions. *Am J Gastroenterol* 1991;**86**:764–7.

60. Kamisawa T, Zen Y, Pillai S, Stone JH. IgG4-related disease. *Lancet* December 3, 2014;**385**(9976):1460–71. [Epub ahead of print].

61. Zizic TM, Classen JN, Stevens MB. Acute abdominal complications of systemic lupus erythematosus and polyarteritis nodosa. *Am J Med* 1982;**73**:525–31.

62. Yuan S, Lian F, Chen D, Li H, Qiu Q, Zhan Z, et al. Clinical features and associated factors of abdominal pain in systemic lupus erythematosus. *J Rheumatol* 2013;**40**:2015–22.

Chapter 45

Systemic Lupus Erythematosus and Infections

Amy Devlin, Robert Shmerling

Beth Israel Deaconess Medical Center, Division of Rheumatology, Boston, MA, USA

INTRODUCTION

Infections, including those due to common and rarer, opportunistic organisms, remain a significant contributor to morbidity and death among patients with systemic lupus erythematosus (SLE). In addition to inherent immune system dysfunction, standard immunosuppressive treatments (including corticosteroids) also render patients more vulnerable to attack from pathogens. Patients with SLE also face separate challenges related to accrued end-organ damage, functional hyposplenism, and reticuloendothelial system dysfunction. These further hamper their ability to defend against infections. As infections may trigger lupus flares, clinicians are frequently faced with the challenge of diagnosing active lupus, infection, or the combination of both. Thus, the diagnostic approach to the infected SLE patient must be thoughtful and thorough. In addition, vigilance is warranted regarding preventive strategies for SLE patients to mitigate the risk of infection.

EPIDEMIOLOGY OF SLE INFECTIONS

The largest cited epidemiologic lupus studies examining rates of deaths due to infection have found wide variation, ranging from 5% to 67% in larger cohorts (Table 1). Most studies examining the incidence of infection and related mortality among patients with lupus have used inpatient data. This likely presents a skewed perspective as inpatients have higher disease burden and nosocomial infections. The largest population-based study comparing infection-related mortality between SLE and non-SLE revealed that the highest mortality rates were among patients with opportunistic infections and those with mechanical ventilation requirements for pneumonia or sepsis.[1] The trend in hospitalization rates for serious infections in SLE increased substantially between 1996 and 2011, nearly 12 times higher than non-SLE patients.[1]

While SLE is a chronic illness with a lifelong risk of infection, the causes of death tend to vary by age and duration of disease. Deaths due to complications of SLE or infection are more common during the first 5 years of disease while deaths due to cardiac complications and thrombotic events are more common over subsequent decades.[2,3] Infections remain the most frequent cause of death within the first year of SLE onset.[4] A study of SLE with disease onset after age 50 found that infection was the major cause of death in this subgroup.[5]

Predictors associated with higher rates of infection among lupus patients include treatment with cyclophosphamide and/or corticosteroids and high disease activity.[6,7] One prospective cohort study including 249 patients with SLE found a lower infection rate among those taking antimalarial medications, while highest infection rates were correlated with prednisone use (even at moderate doses).[8] Navarro-Zarza et al. found that among 473 hospitalized patients with SLE with no symptoms or signs of infection at the time of admission, 12.5% developed a nosocomial infection.[9] In this study, length of hospital stay, higher SLE-DAI activity scores, and immunosuppressive medications were significant predictors of nosocomial infection. Other studies have reported higher rates of bacterial sepsis among SLE patients with renal failure.[10] The degree of lymphopenia in patients with SLE has also emerged as an important predictor of significant infections, particularly in the early stages of SLE.[11]

Certain infections may not only act as triggers for SLE exacerbations but may even indirectly contribute to the initial development of autoimmunity in SLE. Pathogens with similar amino acid sequences or antigenic structures that are nearly identical to native molecules have been posited to promote autoantibody production and clinical manifestations of SLE as the result of cross-reactive antibodies or molecular mimicry. For instance, there have been several homologous amino acid sequences noted to exist between Epstein–Barr virus (EBV) nuclear antigens and nuclear autoantigens found among patients with SLE.[12] Serologic evidence of EBV infection has also been shown to be significantly higher in SLE patients compared with healthy matched controls.[12] Other studies have proposed

Systemic Lupus Erythematosus. http://dx.doi.org/10.1016/B978-0-12-801917-7.00045-0

TABLE 1 Infection as Primary Cause of Death in SLE

Author (Reference)	Duration (Years)	Total No. of Patients	Total No. of Deaths	Country	Deaths Caused by Infections (%)
Wallace et al.[54]	30	609	128	United States	21
Rosner et al.[55]	13	1103	222	United States	33
Huicochea Grob et al.[56]	23	65	14	Mexico	29
Kim et al.[57]	4	544	43	Korea	33
Jacobsen et al.[58]	20	513	122	Denmark	21
Mok et al.[59]	24	186	9	China	67
Rodriquez et al.[60]	34	662	161	Puerto Rico	27
Bernatsky et al.[61]	30	9547	1255	United States	5
Wadee et al.[62]	15	226	55	South Africa	44
Nossent et al.[63]	5	2500	91	Europe	57
Al-Arfaj et al.[64]	30	624	25	Saudi Arabia	48
Goldblatt et al.[65]	29	104	67	United Kingdom	25

a relationship between induction of SLE and infection with herpes simplex virus, human herpes virus 8, parvovirus B19, or cytomegalovirus, although additional studies are needed to establish a pathogenic role for these infections.[13–15] Superantigens released from *mycoplasma* species and other common infections have been shown to activate T lymphocytes and B lymphocytes, leading to exacerbations of existing SLE.[16] Gram-negative lipopolysaccharide associated with certain bacterial infections can lead to polyclonal B-cell activation and worsening of disease SLE disease activity.[17]

IMMUNOLOGIC PATHOGENESIS OF INFECTIONS IN SYSTEMIC LUPUS ERYTHEMATOSUS

Long before SLE patients were regularly treated with immunosuppressive drugs, infections represented a major cause of mortality.[18] This fact underscores the native immune dysregulation that renders lupus patients vulnerable to infectious insults. Patients with SLE have numerous immune system defects that increase their propensity for infections (Table 2). However, there is significant heterogeneity between individuals with SLE with respect to quantitative and qualitative immune system defects. These include impairments in phagocyte function, cytokine expression, complement activation, the mannose-binding lectin (MBL) system, and other anomalies of cellular and humoral immunity. Additional susceptibility to infection has been

TABLE 2 Examples of SLE Immune Dysfunction Predisposing to Infection

Humoral immunity
- Hypogammaglobulinemia and Ig subclass deficiencies
- Fc-γ receptor antibodies
- B-cell maturation flaws

Cellular immunity
- Impaired T-cell cytotoxic capability
- Lymphopenia
- NK-cell dysregulation

Phagocyte impairment
- Superoxide deficits
- Defective phagocytosis

Cytokine dysregulation
- Decreased IL-2 production
- Increased TNF-α production
- Increased IL-10

Complement system
- Hypocomplementemia
- Mannose-binding lectin pathway polymorphisms (variant alleles for MBL)
- Complement C1-q deficiency

associated with accrued end-organ tissue damage in SLE and less efficient reticuloendothelial system clearance.

Defects in phagocyte capabilities have been recognized in both neutrophil and macrophage/monocyte cells in lupus sufferers. Untreated patients with SLE have higher rates of phagocyte dysfunction and impaired neutrophil migration than those undergoing active treatment.[19]

One theory attributes the impaired phagocyte function in patients with SLE to their lower levels of macrophage-derived tumor necrosis factor.[19] Lupus patients have also been found to have decreased amounts of superoxide production during phagocytosis; this finding may be linked to certain Fc-γ receptor defects or circulating IgG and IgM anti-Fc-γ receptor antibodies.[20,21] Studies have demonstrated that SLE monocytes have an impaired ability to engulf apoptotic cells and diminished phagocytic activity, which acts to hamper important antigen-presenting functions.[22] Complement-activating anti-neutrophil antibodies and rarer antibodies to myeloid precursors may further diminish neutrophil numbers and function in many patients with SLE.[23] The consumption of complement during SLE-related immune complex formation is yet another mechanism of immune impairment that increases infection risk.

Genetic deficiencies in several constituents of the classical complement pathway are risk factors for the development of SLE as well as infection. Disruption in the classical complement system—especially C1-q—has been linked with impaired clearance of apoptotic cells and the clinical expression of SLE. Patients with C1-q deficiency and/or low levels of MBL have increased vulnerability to both viral and bacterial infections. Such deficiencies have also been recognized as playing a role in SLE pathogenesis via limited recognition and clearance of autoantibodies. Studies have shown that certain MBL alleles associated with MBL deficiency and impaired opsonization are linked with severe infections in patients with SLE.[24,25] A decrease in complement system components C3 and C5–C9 complex in SLE leaves patients less able to fight off encapsulated microorganisms.

CD4[+] T-cell lymphopenia is the most common quantitative immune system impairment in SLE, a finding that increases the risk of infection. CD8[+] T cells in SLE may display dysfunctional cytotoxicity due to low production of interleukin-2 and gamma-interferon levels.[26]

Human and murine studies have demonstrated B- and T-cell-derived cytokine imbalances that may play critical roles in the immune dysregulation and increased infection risk in patients with SLE. Active SLE is associated with increased TNF-α and IL-10 production and reduced levels of IFN-γ. However, the overall impact of these imbalances on immune defense and infection risk remains uncertain.

Although rare, anti-NK cell autoantibodies have been detected in patients with SLE and can hamper the ability to fight infection. However, a decreased number of NK cells is more common.

B-cell anomalies and immunoglobulin deficiency represent additional predispositions of SLE patients to infection. As compared with healthy controls, SLE patients have higher rates of antigen-specific hypogammaglobulinemia and IgG or IgA subclass deficiency, which may be congenital or acquired.[27] Early senescence of hyperactive B cells, B-cell-specific autoantibodies, and other B-cell maturation flaws have been postulated as mechanisms underlying both antibody deficiency and B-cell dysregulation in SLE patients.[28] In fact, there has been much clinical research dedicated to the study of B-cell function in SLE patients, especially with respect to B-cell ablative therapies and therapeutic targets.

Finally, SLE patients may have heightened infection risk due to existing end-organ damage, including impaired splenic and reticuloendothelial system function. Functional hyposplenism is present in up to 5% of SLE patients with a resultant increased risk of infection due to encapsulated microorganisms and bacteria such as *Salmonella*, *Haemophilus* spp., and pneumococci.[29] Inadequate clearance of IgG-sensitized red blood cells from the peripheral circulation by the RES has been shown to correlate with prolonged circulation of immune complexes and higher levels of SLE disease activity.[30] SLE-related end-stage renal disease and pulmonary fibrosis may impair host defense against infectious pathogens. Damage to renal microcirculation and glomerular scarring may contribute to increased rates of urinary tract infections, pyelonephritis, and other kidney infections. Similarly, small vessel gastrointestinal vasculitis may promote the entry of various pathogens into the circulation, leading to sepsis.[31] Lupus skin disease may act to compromise the protective epidermal and deeper skin layers, leading to increased risks of secondary infections from skin microbes.

TREATMENT-ASSOCIATED IMMUNOSUPPRESSION AND INFECTION RISK

While treatments for SLE may control disease and reverse or prevent SLE-associated morbidity, an increased risk of infection is a major concern. Patients with SLE treated with corticosteroids or other immunosuppressives appear to be more susceptible to infections compared with those with other rheumatic disease treated similarly.[32] This highlights the complex and heterogeneous immune defects that place SLE patients at risk for infection independent of their exposure to immunosuppressive medications. Patients with end-organ damage due to active SLE tend to be treated with high doses of both corticosteroids and cytotoxic drugs. Thus, it is not surprising that increased infection rates tallied in many clinical SLE studies may be confounded by more active or advanced SLE. Although minimizing immunosuppression is worthwhile, lower doses of corticosteroids (e.g., <10 mg/day of prednisone) do not necessarily eliminate infection risk.[33]

Patients with SLE receiving active treatment with corticosteroids and/or other immunosuppressive medications may experience clinical improvement as well as improved

TABLE 3 Most Common Opportunistic Pathogens in SLE

Gram-Negative Bacterial	Gram-Positive Bacterial	Viral	Fungal	Parasitic
Escherichia coli	Staphylococcus aureus	Herpes zoster	Candida spp.	Strongyloides
Klebsiella	Streptococcus pneumoniae	Epstein–Barr virus	Cryptococcus neoformans	stercoralis
Enterococcus	Streptococcus pyogenes	Cytomegalovirus	Aspergillus spp.	Toxoplasma
Proteus	Peptococcus	Human papillomavirus	Pneumocystis jirovicii	gondii
Enterobacter Serratia	Listeria monocytogenes		Histoplasmosis	Plasmodium
Bacteroides	Nocardia		Blastomycosis	spp.
Salmonella	Mycobacterium tuberculosis		Coccidioidomycosis	Leishmaniosis
Citrobacter	Non-TB Mycobacterium spp.			Paragonimiasis
Pseudomonas	(M. avium, M. fortuitum,			
Haemophilus influenzae	M. abscessus)			

immune function. For example, treated SLE patients have been shown to have improved neutrophil migration and better overall phagocytic function compared to untreated SLE patients.[19] Hydroxychloroquine and other antimalarial medications have also been found to offer a measure of protection from infection in SLE.[34] Infection risk in SLE may vary depending on the type of immunosuppression administered. In one larger study comparing different maintenance treatments for proliferative nephritis, mycophenolate mofetil and azathioprine were associated with significantly lower risk of severe infection (2%) compared with intravenous cyclophosphamide (25%).[35]

TYPE OF INFECTIONS

The types of infections encountered by people with SLE are quite similar to those affecting the general population: upper respiratory illness, pneumonia, cellulitis, and urinary tract infections are most common. Bacterial infections in SLE include the same common Gram-positive and Gram-negative bacterial pathogens seen in the general population. SLE patients are also more prone to develop a myriad of viral, fungal, and parasitic opportunistic infections (Table 3).

While most viral insults are nonfatal for SLE patients, viral infections can lead to serious morbidity. In addition to the impact of immunosuppressive medications, altered cell-mediated immunity, interferon production defects, CD-4 T-cell lymphopenia, and NK-cell dysfunction have been postulated to play a role in the increased rates of viral infection in SLE populations. Frequent respiratory and gastrointestinal viral insults may be burdensome for patients, although they are usually self-limited. The incidence of herpes zoster virus infection is two- to threefold higher among lupus patients compared to the general population.[36] Aggressive immunosuppressive regimens may also place patients at risk for reactivation of cytomegalovirus or primary cytomegalovirus infection with complications in the CNS, eyes, gastrointestinal tract, or visceral organs. SLE

patients have been shown to have at least a 10-fold increased frequency of EBV-infected peripheral B cells compared to healthy controls. This increase is associated with increased disease activity in SLE patients and is independent of intake of immunosuppressive medication.[37] In addition, an abnormally high EBV viral load in the peripheral blood mononuclear cells (PBMCs) has been demonstrated in SLE patients compared to healthy controls in several studies.[38,39] Kang et al. found a 40-fold increase of EBV load when comparing SLE patients to healthy controls, and Moon et al. found at least a 15-fold increase of EBV load in SLE patients.[38,39] These findings imply that there is more active lytic phase EBV replication in SLE patients. However, whether EBV infection is associated with the development of SLE remains a topic of much debate.

Studies on immunocompetent carriers of EBV demonstrate that they usually show little or no mRNA expression by EBV. However, Gross et al. demonstrated that SLE patients have abnormal expression of several mRNAs, which help facilitate lytic replication in PBMCs, suggesting more active virus in SLE patients. Other research has shown evidence to support abnormal EBV latency states in SLE patients due to overexpression of several latent state mRNAs, which likely act to enhance the lifetime of EBV-infected B cells.[40]

Women with SLE have been shown to have an increased prevalence of human papillomavirus. In one study looking at 173 women with SLE and 217 women without SLE, those with lupus had a threefold increase in HPV infection.[41] The higher rates of HPV infection in this study were associated with immunosuppressive therapy use. These findings not only underscore the importance of early HPV vaccination but speak to the potential need for more frequent cervical cancer screening for women with SLE; this is especially true for those with previously detected HPV.

Among common bacterial infections, pneumonia and respiratory infections are the most frequently encountered.[42] *Staphylococcus aureus*, *Escherichia coli*, and *Streptococcus pyogenes* are common respiratory organisms; the incidence of bacteremic complications appears to be increased.[43] The multifactorial impacts of defects in chemotaxis, poor opsonization, hypocomplementemia, and splenic dysfunction in SLE raise the risk for encapsulated bacterial organisms, particularly streptococcal pneumonia. A recently published study found that the incidence of pneumococcal pneumonia is 13 times higher among SLE patients compared with the general population.[44] In this study, even among those who were *not* taking immunosuppressant medicines, patients with SLE were found to be at a higher risk for pneumococcal disease than the general population. Bacterial urinary tract infections are also seen at higher rates among women with SLE; *E. coli* and *Streptococcus agalactiae* are among those most frequently encountered.[45]

Functional hyposplenism may place SLE patients at increased risk for encapsulated *Haemophilus* and *Salmonella* species. *Salmonella* is more problematic in underdeveloped nations where hygienic food practice is less common. Ingestion of *Salmonella* species may cause gastrointestinal illness with or without complications of bacteremia, osteomyelitis, or septic arthritis.

The most common opportunistic fungal organism causing infection in SLE patients is *Candida*. These infections may present as pharyngitis/esophagitis, skin rash, vaginitis, or bloodstream infections. Another major opportunistic fungal infection encountered by SLE patients is pneumocystis pneumonia (PCP) caused by the yeast-like fungus *Pneumocystis jirovecii*. Lupus patients taking higher doses of oral corticosteroids (at least 40 mg prednisone daily or equivalent) and those with underlying lupus-related alveolitis or other lung conditions are felt to be at increased risk for *P. jirovecii*. Thus, prophylactic antibiotics should be considered in such high risk SLE patients.

Mycobacterial tuberculosis infection is a serious threat to patients with SLE in countries where the infection is endemic, such as India. In that country, rates of active tuberculosis among SLE patients have been cited as high as 16% (while less than 1% in most industrialized countries).[46] Most cases of *Mycobacterium tuberculosis* tend to occur early in the course of SLE due to reactivation of latent infection. However, nontuberculous mycobacterial infections have a tendency to occur as new infections in patients with longer standing SLE.[43]

In underdeveloped areas and more tropical climates, the incidence of parasitic infections rises among SLE patients. One parasite in particular, *Stongyloides stercoralis*, is a soil nematode that causes initial intestinal infection followed by an intricate autoinfection cycle that may lead to blood larvae migration. Suppressed cellular immunity combined with either high-dose corticosteroids and/or immunosuppressive medications may promote a dramatic parasitic burden termed "strongyloides hyperinfection" with dissemination of the organisms that can be fatal. *Toxoplasmosis gondii* represents another opportunistic parasitic threat for lupus patients and can manifest as CNS lesions, overt encephalitis, retinal infection, or a primary pulmonary infection. Recent research examining the origin of increased toxoplasmosis susceptibility in lupus-prone mice revealed a defective antigen-specific IFN-γ response; this may be at least partly to blame for the ineffective clearance and higher parasitic burden in SLE.[47]

Increased malaria risk among patients with SLE has not been commonly reported. In fact, there have been several studies identifying SLE as a protective factor that lowers an individual's risk for malaria. This has been attributed to the existence of several SLE associated autoantibodies that have been discovered to cross-react with *Plasmodium* parasite forms.[48] Other systemic parasitic diseases have also been described in SLE patients, including paragonimiasis and visceral leishmaniasis.[49,50]

Neurologic infections in SLE deserve particular emphasis given their potential to mimic SLE-associated brain disease and the high morbidity and mortality observed with these infections. Bacterial meningitis tends to occur at higher rates in SLE than non-SLE and can prove fatal. The most common CNS bacterial invaders include tuberculosis, followed by *Listeria* monocytogenes.[51] Meningitis due to *Nocardia* species is well-described among patients with SLE. Fungal infections, such as *Cryptococcus neoformans* and various *Aspergillus* species, are also on the list of opportunistic neurological infections.

Clinical Considerations

The most common and concerning complication associated with the treatment of SLE is the increased risk of infection. Despite the judicious use of medications and appropriate monitoring, SLE patients will inevitably face serious morbidity and mortality in the face of infectious diseases. Every clinician caring for patients with SLE faces the challenge of distinguishing manifestations of infection from a flare of SLE. To make patient management even more challenging, infected lupus patients have a tendency to present with active lupus.

Therefore, a thorough history, full physical examination, selected lab testing, and imaging studies are generally necessary to sort out whether a patient has an infection, active SLE, or both. Additional procedures are often necessary as well. For example, while symptoms and signs of pleuritis are common during lupus flares, large pleural effusions or unilateral pleural disease may warrant additional chest imaging, thoracentesis, or even pleural biopsy to definitively rule out underlying infection. Although neuropsychiatric SLE is primarily a clinical diagnosis, extensive imaging and cerebrospinal fluid analysis (and even meningeal biopsy) may be warranted to rule out infectious meningitis.

C-reactive protein (CRP) levels may offer another clue when evaluating the possibility of infection in patients with SLE. CRP levels tend to rise significantly in the midst of an acute infection while normal or only mild elevations are common in SLE disease flares.[52]

PREVENTATIVE STRATEGIES

Efforts to prevent serious infections in patients with SLE should be routine. Judicious use of immunosuppressive drugs (including corticosteroids) and updated vaccinations should be the rule for the care of patients with SLE. A recently published study revealed that the most common reason patients with SLE do not get properly vaccinated is because their health-care provider failed to recommend it.[53] All lupus patients, regardless of treatment regimen, should be strongly encouraged to obtain immunization against influenza, pneumococcus, tetanus, and HPV (females). Many experts recommend that patients on higher doses of corticosteroids (at least 30 mg/day of prednisone or the equivalent) should also be treated with prophylactic therapy to prevent *P. jirovicii* infection. Live vaccinations, including measles/mumps/rubella (MMR), herpes zoster, yellow fever, varicella zoster, and certain live intranasal flu vaccines should be considered in select lupus patients prior to initiating immunosuppressive therapy.

Close monitoring for drug-induced cytopenias and other side effects may also enable physicians to play a more active role in limiting preventable infections in this high-risk group of patients. Blood testing to ascertain immunoglobulin levels in SLE patients may help to further identify lupus patients at even higher risk for infection. There may also be a beneficial role for IVIG to aid certain hypogammaglobulinemic lupus patients when fighting severe infections or following specific exposures.

As a high-risk population, identification and treatment of chronic infections such as tuberculosis, hepatitis B, hepatitis C, and human immunodeficiency virus should be performed prior to the institution of immunosuppression. Select populations should also be screened for other rarer infections, such as toxoplasmosis and strongyloides.

REFERENCES

1. Tektonidou M, Wang Z, Dasgupta A, Ward MM. Burden of serious infections in adults with systemic lupus erythematosus: a national population-based study, 1996–2011. *Arthritis Care Res* 2015;**67**(8): 1078–85. http://dx.doi.org/10.1002/acr.22575.
2. Cervera R, Khamashta MA, Font J, Sebastiani GD, Gil A, Lavilla P, et al. Morbidity and mortality in systemic lupus erythematosus during a 10-year period: a comparison of early and late manifestations in a cohort of 1000 patients. *Medicine* 2003;**82**:299–308.
3. Urowitz MB, Bookman AA, Koehler BE, Gordon DA, Smythe HA, Ogryzlo MA. The bimodal mortality pattern of systemic lupus erythematosus. *Am J Med* 1976;**60**:221–5.
4. Mok CC, Kwok CL, Ho LY, Chan PT, Yip SF. Life expectancy, standardized mortality ratios, and causes of death in six rheumatic diseases in Hong Kong, China. *Arthritis Rheum* 2011;**63**(5):1182–9.
5. Lin H, Wei JC, Tan CY, Liu YY, Li YH, Li FX, et al. Survival analysis of late-onset systemic lupus erythematosus: a cohort study in China. *Clin Rheumatol* 2012;**31**(12):1683–9.
6. Gladman DD, Hussain F, Ibañez D, Urowitz MB. The nature and outcome of infection in systemic lupus erythematosus. *Lupus* 2002;**11**(4):234–9.
7. Barber C, Gold WL, Fortin PR. Infections in the lupus patient: perspectives on prevention. *Curr Opin Rheumatol* 2011;**23**(4):358–65.
8. Ruiz-Irastorza G, Olivares N, Ruiz-Arruza I, Martinez-Berriotxoa A, Egurbide MV, Aguirre C. Predictors of major infections in systemic lupus erythematosus. *Arthritis Res Ther* 2009;**11**(4):R109.
9. Navarro-Zarza JE, Alvarez-Hernandez E, Casasola-Vargas JC, Estrada-Castro E, Burgos-Vargas R. Prevalence of community-acquired and nosocomial infections in hospitalized patients with systemic lupus erythematosus. *Lupus* 2010;**19**(1):43–8.
10. Al-Arfaj AS, Khalil N. Clinical and immunological manifestations in 624 SLE patients in Saudi Arabia. *Lupus* 2009;**18**(5):465–73.
11. Ng WL, Chu CM, Wu AK, Cheng VC, Yuen KY. Lymphopenia at presentation is associated with increased risk of infections in patients with systemic lupus erythematosus. *QJM* 2006;**99**(1):37–47.
12. James JA, Neas BR, Moser KL, Hall T, Bruner GR, Sestak AL, et al. Systemic lupus erythematosus in adults is associated with previous Epstein-Barr virus exposure. *Arthritis Rheum* 2001;**44**(5):1122–6.
13. Sun Y, Sun S, Li W, Li B, Li J. Prevalence of human herpesvirus 8 infection in systemic lupus erythematosus. *Virol J* 2011;**8**:210.
14. Vigeant P, Menard H-A, Boire G. Chronic modulation of the autoimmune response following parvovirus B19 infection. *J Rheumatol* 1994;**21**(6):1165–7.
15. Vasquez V, Barzaga RA, Cunha BA. Cytomegalovirus-induced flare of systemic lupus erythematosus. *Heart Lung* 1992;**21**(4):407–8.
16. Behar SM, Porcelli SA. Mechanisms of autoimmune disease induction: the role of the immune response to microbial pathogens. *Arthritis Rheum* 1995;**38**(4):458–76.
17. Granholm NA, Cavallo T. Autoimmunity, polyclonal B-cell activation and infection. *Lupus* 1992;**1**(2):63–74.
18. Klemperer P, Pollack AD, Baehr G. Pathology of disseminated lupus erythematosus. *Arch Path* 1941;**32**:569.
19. Yu C-L, Chang K-L, Chiu CC, Chiang BN, Han SH. WangSR. Defective phagocytosis, decreased tumor necrosis factor-α production, and lymphocyte hyporesponsiveness predispose patients with systemic lupus erythematosus to infection. *Scand J Rheumatol* 1989;**18**(2):97–105.
20. Gyimesi E, Kavai M, Kiss E, Csipo I, Szucs G, Szegedi G. Triggering of respiratory burst by phagocytosis in monocytes of patients with systemic lupus erythematosus. *Clin Exp Immunol* 1993;**94**(1):140–4.
21. Boros P, Muryoi T, Spiera H, Bona C, Unkeless JC. Autoantibodies directed against different classes of FcgR are found in sera of autoimmune patients. *J Immunol* 1993;**150**(5):2018–24.
22. Robert PJ, Isenberg DA, Segal AW. Defective degradation of bacterial DNA by phagocytes from patients with systemic and discoid lupus erythematosus. *Clin Exp Immunol* 1987;**69**(1):68–78.
23. Rustagi PK, Currie MS, Logue GL. Complement-activating anti-neutrophil antibody in systemic lupus erythematosus. *Am J Med* 1985;**78**(1):971–7.
24. Monticielo OA, Mucenic T, Xavier RM, Brenol JC, Chies JA. The role of mannose-binding lectin in systemic lupus erythematosus. *Clin Rheumatol* 2008;**27**(4):413–9.

25. Mok MY, Ip WK, Lau CS, Lo Y, Wong WH, Lau YL. Mannose-binding lectin and susceptibility to infection in Chinese patients with systemic lupus erythematosus. *J Rheumatol* 2007;**34**(6):1270–6.

26. Tsokos GC. Systemic lupus erythematosus. *N Engl J Med* 2011; **365**(22):2110–21.

27. Kay RA, Wood KJ, Bernstein RM, Holt PJ, Pumphrey RS. An IgG subclass imbalance in connective tissue disease. *Ann Rheum Dis* 1988;**47**(7):536–41.

28. Tarrant TK, Frazer DH, Aya-Ay JP, Patel DD. B cell loss leading to remission in severe systemic lupus erythematosus. *J Rheumatol* 2003;**30**(2):412–4.

29. Alejandro Arce-Salinas C, Villaseñor-Ovies P. Infections and systemic lupus erythematosus. In: Almoallim H, editor. *Systemic lupus erythematosus.* InTech; 2012. ISBN: 978-953-51-0266-3. http://dx.doi.org/10.5772/27509. http://www.intechopen.com.

30. Frank MM, Hamburger MI, Lawley TJ, Kimberly RP, Plotz PH. Defective reticuloendothelial system Fc-receptors function in systemic lupus erythematosus. *N Engl J Med* 1979;**300**(10):518–23.

31. Anand AJ, Glatt AE. Salmonella osteomyelitis and arthritis in sickle cell disease. *Semin Arthritis Rheum* 1994;**24**:211–21.

32. Cohen J, Pinching AJ, Rees AJ, Peters DK. Infection and immunosuppression. *Q J Med* 1982;**51**(201):1–15.

33. Borg TJ, Horst G, Limburg PC, van Rijswijk MH, Kallenberg CG. C-reactive protein levels during disease exacerbations and infections in systemic lupus erythematosus: a prospective longitudinal study. *J Rheumatol* 1990;**17**(12):1642–8.

34. Ruiz-Irastorza G, Olivares N, Ruiz-Arruza I, Martinez-Berriotxoa A, Egurbide MV, Aguirre C. Predictors of major infections in systemic lupus erythematosus. *Arthritis Res Ther* 2009;**11**(4):R109.

35. Contreras G, Tozman E, Nahar N, Metz D. Maintenance therapies for proliferative lupus nephritis: mycophenolate mofetil, azathioprine and intravenous cyclophosphamide. *Lupus* 2005;**14**(Suppl. 1):s33–8.

36. Kang TY, Lee HS, Kim TH, Jun JB, Yoo DH. Clinical and genetic risk factors of herpes zoster in patients with systemic lupus erythematosus. *Rheumatol Int* 2005;**25**(2):97–102.

37. Gross AJ, Hochberg D, Rand WM, Thorley-Lawson DA. EBV and systemic lupus erythematosus: a new perspective. *J Immunol* 2005;**174**(11):6599–607.

38. Kang I, Quan T, Nolasco H, Park SH, Hong MS, Crouch J, et al. Defective control of latent Epstein-Barr virus infection in systemic lupus erythematosus. *J Immunol* 2004;**172**(2):1287–94.

39. Moon UY, Park SJ, Oh ST, Kim WU, Park SH, Lee SH, et al. Patients with systemic lupus erythematosus have abnormally elevated Epstein-Barr virus load in blood. *Arthritis Res Ther* 2004;**6**(4):R295–302.

40. Babcock GJ, Hochberg D, Thorley-Lawson DA. The expression pattern of Epstein-Barr virus latent genes in vivo is dependent upon the differentiation stage of the infected B cell. *Immunity* 2000; **13**(4):497–506.

41. Klumb EM, Pinto AC, Jesus GR, Araujo Jr M, Jascone L, Gayer CR, et al. Are women with lupus at higher risk of HPV infection? *Lupus* 2010;**19**(13):1485–91.

42. Petri M. Infection in systemic lupus erythematosus. *Rheum Dis Clin North Am* 2008;**24**(2):423–56.

43. Cuchacovich R, Gedalia A. Pathophysiology and clinical spectrum of infections in systemic lupus erythematosus. *Rheum Dis Clin North Am* 2009;**35**(1):75–93.

44. Luijten RK, Cuppen BV, Bijlsma JW, Derksen RH. Serious infections in systemic lupus erythematosus with a focus on pneumococcal infections. *Lupus* 2014;**23**(14):1512–6.

45. Duran-Barragan S, Ruvalcaba-Naranjo H, Rodriguez-Gutierrez L, Solano-Moreno H, Hernandez-Rios G, Sanchez-Ortiz A, et al. Recurrent urinary tract infections and bladder dysfunction in systemic lupus erythematosus. *Lupus* 2008;**17**(12):1117–21.

46. Falagas ME, Voidonikola PT, Angelousi AG. Tuberculosis in patients with systemic rheumatic or pulmonary diseases treated with glucocorticosteroids and the preventive role of isoniazid: a review of the available evidence. *Int J Antimicrob Agents* 2007; **30**(6):477–86.

47. Lieberman LA, Tsokos GC. Lupus-prone mice fail to raise antigen-specific T cell responses to intracellular infection. *PLoS One* October 31, 2014;**9**(10):e111382. http://dx.doi.org/10.1371/journal.pone.0111382.

48. Zanini GM, De Moura Carvalho LJ, Brahimi K, De Souza-Passos LF, Guimarães SJ, Da Silva Machado E, et al. Sera of patients with systemic lupus erythematosus react with plasmodial antigens and can inhibit the in vitro growth of *Plasmodium falciparum. Autoimmunity* 2009;**42**(6):545–52.

49. Kraus A, Guerra-Bautista G, Chavarria P. Paragonimiasis: an infrequent but treatable cause of hemoptysis in systemic lupus erythematosus. *J Rheumatol* 1990;**17**:244–6.

50. Ravelli A, Viola S, De Benedetti F. Visceral leishmaniasis as a cause of unexplained fever and cytopenia in systemic lupus erythematosus. *Acta Paediatr* 2002;**91**:246–7.

51. Yang CD, Wang XD, Ye S, Gu YY, Bao CD, Wang Y, et al. Clinical features, prognostic and risk factors of central nervous system infections in patients with systemic lupus erythematosus. *Clin Rheumatol* 2007;**26**(6):895–901.

52. Firooz N, Albert DA, Wallace DJ, Ishimori M, Berel D, Weisman MH. High-sensitivity C-reactive protein and erythrocyte sedimentation rate in systemic lupus erythematosus. *Lupus* 2011;**20**(6):588–97.

53. Lawson EF, Trupin L, Yelin EH, Yazdany J. Reasons for failure to receive pneumococcal and influenza vaccinations among immunosuppressed patients with systemic lupus erythematosus. *Semin Arthritis Rheum* 2015;**44**(6):666–71. http://dx.doi.org/10.1016/j.semarthrit.2015.01.002. pii: S0049–0172(15)00003-7. [epub ahead of print].

54. Wallace DJ, Podell T, Weiner J, Klinenberg JR, Forouzesh S, Dubois EL. Systemic lupus erythematosus- survival patterns: experience with 609 patients. *JAMA* 1981;**245**(9):934–8.

55. Rosner S, Ginzler E, Diamond HS, Weiner M, Schlesinger M, Fries JF, et al. A multicenter study of outcome in systemic lupus erythematosus: causes of death. *Arthritis Rheum* 1982;**25**(6):612–7.

56. Huicochea Grobet ZL, Barron R, Ortega Martell JA, Onuma E. Survival up to 5 and 10 years of Mexican pediatric patients with systemic lupus erythematosus: overhaul of 23 years experience. *Allergol Immunopathol* 1996;**24**:36–8.

57. Kim WU, Min JK, Lee SH, Park SH, Cho CS, Kim HY. Causes of death in Korean patients with systemic lupus erythematosus: a single center retrospective study. *Clin Exp Rheumatol* 1999;**17**(5):539–45.

58. Jacobsen S, Petersen J, Ullman S, Junker P, Voss A, Rasmussen JM, et al. Mortality and causes of death of 513 Danish patients with systemic lupus erythematosus. *Scand J Rheumatol* 1999;**28**(2):75–80.

59. Mok CC, Lee KW, Ho CT, Lau CS, Wang RW. A prospective study of survival and prognostic indicators of systemic lupus erythematosus in a southern Chinese population. *Rheumatology* 2000;**39**(4):399–406.

60. Rodriquez VE, Gonzalez-Pares EN. Mortality study in Puerto Ricans with systemic lupus erythematosus. *P R Health S C J* 2000;**19**(4):335–9.

61. Bernatsky S, Boivin JF, Joseph L, Manzi S, Ginzler E, Gladman DD, et al. Mortality in systemic lupus erythematosus. *Arthritis Rheum* 2006;**54**(8):2550–7.

62. Wadee S, Tikly M, Hopley M. Causes and predictors of death in South Africans with systemic lupus erythematosus. *Rheumatology* 2007;**46**(9):1487–91.

63. Nossent J, Cikes N, Kiss E, Marchesoni A, Nassonova V, Mosca M, et al. Current causes of death in systemic lupus erythematosus in Europe, 2000–2004: relation to disease activity and damage accrual. *Lupus* 2007;**16**(5):309–17.

64. Al Arfaj AS, Khalil N. Clinical and immunological manifestations in 624 SLE patients in Saudi Arabia. *Lupus* 2009;**18**(5):465–73.

65. Goldblatt F, Chambers S, Rahman A, Isenberg DA. Serious infections in British patients with systemic lupus erythematosus: hospitalisations and mortality. *Lupus* 2009;**18**(8):682–9.

Chapter 46

Malignancies in Systemic Lupus Erythematosus

Hiromi Tissera[1], Ann E. Clarke[2], Rosalind Ramsey Goldman[3], Caroline Gordon[4], James E. Hansen[5], Sasha Bernatsky[1]

[1]McGill University Health Centre, Montreal, QC, Canada; [2]Division of Rheumatology, Department of Medicine, University of Calgary, Calgary, AB, Canada; [3]North-western University Feinberg School of Medicine, Chicago, IL, USA; [4]Rheumatology Research Group, College of Medical and Dental Sciences, University of Birmingham, Edgbaston, Birmingham, UK; [5]Department of Therapeutic Radiology, Yale School of Medicine, New Haven, CT, USA

SUMMARY

This chapter focuses on cancer in systemic lupus erythematosus (SLE). While the overall cancer incidence rate in SLE patients compared to the general population is only slightly increased, there is a particularly high risk of lymphoma in SLE. The specific underlying pathophysiology is unclear, but appears to be multifactorial. On the other hand, certain hormone-sensitive cancers appear to be less common in SLE than in the general population. In particular, SLE patients have a reduced risk of breast, ovarian, endometrial, and prostate cancers. Hormonal changes, genetic factors, and drug exposures are discussed as potential reasons for the unique cancer profile in SLE, compared to the general population.

INTRODUCTION

Many studies have shown a link between autoimmune conditions such as rheumatoid arthritis (RA) and systemic lupus erythematosus (SLE) and cancers.[1,2] Although the 5-year survival rate of SLE patients now exceeds 90%, the age and sex adjusted standardized mortality ratios (SMRs) in SLE patients still remain higher compared to the general population. In fact, a recent paper noted a threefold increased risk of death in SLE patients.[1]

Evidence from the past decade ranks cancer as a contributing factor to the increased mortality and morbidity seen in SLE individuals.[3] In this paper, we discuss several cancers that are common in SLE patients. However, not all cancers are increased in SLE patients. In contrast, the incidence of some cancers, such as breast, is observed to be lower in SLE patients. Although much work remains to be done to understand the pathophysiology behind SLE and cancer, possible pathways, including disease activity, medications, and genetics, are discussed below.

HEMATOLOGIC CANCERS

There is an increase in both the incidence and the mortality associated with lymphomas in SLE patients compared to the general population.[2–4] Based on the large multicenter, Systemic Lupus International Collaborating Clinics (SLICC) cohort study, the standardized incidence ratio (SIR) observed for all hematologic cancers was 3.02, 95% CI 2.48–3.63, with an SIR of 4.39, 95% CI 3.46–5.49 observed for non-Hodgkin's lymphoma (NHL) (Table 1).[2] As in the general population, data suggest that lymphoma risk in SLE increases with age.[4]

Myeloid types were found to be the most common non-lymphoma hematological malignancies among SLE patients in contrast to lymphoid types, which are common in the general population.[5] While multiple myeloma (MM) was not found to be increased in SLE cohort studies,[2] an increased risk of MM in patients with a family history of SLE (odds ratio (OR) 2.66, 95% CI 1.12–6.32),[6] as well as an increased risk of monoclonal gammopathy, has been observed.[7]

The cause of the increase in hematological malignancies in SLE remains unclear, but there are several hypotheses. Since chromosomal abnormalities can give rise to certain types of NHL,[8] it is possible that SLE patients with dysregulated lymphocyte proliferation are prone to developing lymphoma through gene translocations, since the chance of translocation is proportional to the rate of proliferation.[9] Increased inflammation present in autoimmune diseases is another hypothesis that may explain the increased incidence of lymphoma.[10] This argument is further strengthened by the fact that diffuse large B-cell lymphomas (DLBCL) arising from activated lymphocytes account for a majority of NHLs in SLE.[2] Another hypothesis is based on a cytokine implicated in SLE and RA, A PRoliferating Inducing Ligand (APRIL). This is known to cause over proliferation by prompting B cells to escape apoptosis.[11] APRIL is strongly expressed in DLBCL in the general population,

TABLE 1 Showing Standardized Incidence Ratio (SIR) or Odds Ratios (OR) of Different Cancers

Cancer Type	Standardized Incidence Ratio (SIR) or Odds Ratio (OR)	References
Hematologic cancers (all lymphomas, leukemias, and multiple myelomas)	SIR: 3.02, 95% CI 2.48–3.63	2
Non-Hodgkin's lymphoma	SIR: 4.39, 95% CI 3.46–5.49	2
Lung	SIR: 1.16, 95% CI 1.12–1.21	16
Cervical	OR: 8.66, 95% CI 3.75–20.00	21
Breast	SIR: 0.76, 95% CI 0.69–0.85	29
Ovarian	SIR: 0.66, 95% CI: 0.49–0.90	29
Endometrial	SIR: 0.71, 95% CI: 0.55–0.91	29
Prostate	SIR: 0.77, 95% CI 0.69–0.87	40
Kidney	SIR: 2.29, 95% CI 1.25–4.18	40
Liver	SIR: 2.44, 95% CI 1.46–4.05	16
Vulva	SIR 3.78, 95% CI 1.52–7.78	2

and was detected at high levels in SLE lymphoma tissues. This may indicate the possibility of APRIL-mediated lymphoma development in this subset of patients.[12] In another study, the role of IL-10 in B-cell lymphomagenesis has been explored. Serum IL-10, which has been correlated with SLE disease activity, was found to be a prognostic factor for NHL based on a study conducted in NHL patients in the general population.[13] Another hypothesis is based on increased serum levels of type 1 IFNs, which are known to be associated with active SLE disease. Studies in mice models have confirmed that IFN-inducible p202 (and its human function homologue IFI16) in B cells is associated with an increased susceptibility to developing B-cell malignancies. However, a complete understanding of the role of p200 proteins in B-cell homeostasis is needed to identify SLE patients with increased B-cell malignancy risk.[12,14,15]

While disease activity has been linked with an increase in lymphoma incidence in rheumatoid arthritis, a recent case–cohort analysis within the multisite SLICC SLE cohort failed to show a link between disease activity and risk of lymphoma.[4] Further, that study suggested an increased risk was with exposure to cyclophosphamide, although the effects were less clear for other immunosuppressive drugs.[4] Data do suggest that the highest risk of lymphoma is observed during the early stages of SLE, suggesting that cumulative exposure to immunosuppressive drugs may not explain all of the lymphoma risk in SLE.[2]

LUNG CANCERS

Studies have consistently reported an augmented risk of lung cancer in persons with certain autoimmune rheumatic

diseases including SLE.[2,16,17] According to a recent meta-analysis, lung cancers observed in SLE patients had an SIR of 1.16 (95% CI 1.12–1.21).[16] Based on the international multisite cohort study, the mortality due to lung cancer is also increased, SMR 2.3 (95% CI 1.6–3.0).[3] Additionally, a study assessing the risk of lung cancer in autoimmune diseases noted that SLE contributed to augmenting the susceptibility to lung cancer, but did not influence the prognosis of the cancer. However, this may be due to the poor prognosis of the lung cancer itself.[17]

The histological distribution of lung cancer observed in SLE patients was overall quite similar to that of the general population,[17] although there remains the possibility that small cell carcinoma may be somewhat overrepresented.[17] Although the exact pathological reason for this remains unclear, few theories have been put forward in the literature. Chronic lung tissue inflammation, occasionally present in autoimmune diseases such as RA and SLE, can contribute to interstitial lung disease and pulmonary fibrosis. Pulmonary fibrosis[18] and increased levels of C-reactive protein (a marker of inflammation)[19] are associated with an increased risk of lung cancer. Studies done specifically in SLE lung cancers have pointed to smoking as an important modifiable risk factor for lung cancer in SLE patients.[2,16] Smoking cessation should be encouraged among SLE patients.

CERVICAL CANCER

Many studies have showed that SLE patients are at risk of developing squamous intraepithelial lesions,[20–23] which precede cervical cancer development. A recent meta-analysis reported an increased risk of high grade squamous intraepithelial lesion (HSIL) in SLE patients (OR, 8.66; 95% CI, 3.75–20.00).[21] Another cohort study looking at patients with systemic inflammatory diseases showed that HSIL and cervical cancers are 1.5 times higher in SLE and RA patients compared to those without systemic inflammatory diseases.[22]

Additionally, studies have consistently shown an increase in human papilloma virus (HPV) infection in SLE patients.[20–22] Interestingly, the use of immunosuppressive drugs has traditionally been linked to a reduced clearance of viruses such as HPV in this population.[24] Most studies have found a link between the prolonged use of immunosuppressants and the risk of abnormal pap results and/or cervical dysplasia.[21,25] However, there are limited data about the specific HPV strains present in SLE patients.[21] Nevertheless, evidence shows that the current HPV vaccines are immunogenic and well tolerated in SLE patients and should be recommended.[23]

In one study, SLE patients received reduced screening for cervical dysplasia in comparison to the general population.[26] Consequently, adherence to screening is highly recommended in women with SLE, particularly those who have been or who currently are exposed to immunosuppressants, or who have any other risk for cervical dysplasia and/or HPV infection (based on their sexual history). Any abnormalities found on screening should of course be closely followed up by the appropriate gynecology team.

BREAST, OVARIAN, AND ENDOMETRIAL CANCERS

Recent multicenter studies and meta-analysis have shown that the incidence of breast cancer in SLE patients is reduced compared to the general population.[27,28] A recent meta-analysis compiling five large SLE cohort studies showed a reduced incidence of breast cancers with an SIR of 0.76 (95% CI 0.69–0.85).[29] Other recent studies have further explored whether certain types of breast cancers are less common among SLE patients. A multicenter study looking at breast cancer histology in SLE reported a slight decrease in ductal carcinoma in SLE patients, which is a subtype that represents 80% of invasive breast cancers in the general population.[27] Another study that looked at older women showed a decrease in estrogen receptor negative carcinoma in SLE patients.[28]

Many factors including genetics, ethnic/racial differences, and medication exposures might contribute to the observed reduced risk of breast cancer. A study exploring the possible relationship between breast cancer and SLE-associated single nucleotide polymorphisms failed to find any link in a population-based genome-wide associated breast cancer study.[30] This invokes the idea that any genetic contribution to reduced breast cancer in SLE is

likely multigenic and influenced by gene–environment interactions.

In addition to breast cancer, ovarian and endometrial cancers are also reported to be decreased in females with SLE.[2,29] Notably, like breast cancer, endometrial and ovarian cancers are also driven by estrogen exposure.[31–33] SLE patients are known to have a higher age at menarche and lower age at menopause compared to the general population;[34] therefore, they are likely to have reduced endogenous estrogen exposure. This may be partially responsible for the reduced incidence of breast and endometrial cancer in SLE, compared to the general population. More recent studies have also attributed antitumor therapeutic effects (especially in breast, ovarian, and prostate cancers) to anti-DNA autoantibodies implicated in lupus. Specifically, these antibodies are involved in DNA repair pathways[35] and can suppress the growth of BRACA2-deficient cells.[36]

Evidence shows that drugs used to treat lupus may also serve to reduce the incidence of cancers in these patients. Specifically, one small cohort study showed a reduced incidence of overall cancer in patients treated with antimalarial drugs.[37] However, specific effects on breast cancer in SLE have never been demonstrated, and the results have not been replicated in larger studies. Similarly, nonsteroidal anti-inflammatory drugs (NSAIDs) used in the general population have been associated with a reduced risk of certain cancers such as estrogen receptor positive breast cancers.[38] To date, there is no clear evidence that NSAIDs drive a decreased risk of breast cancer in SLE. Interestingly, a lower risk of breast cancer has been found in RA, but not scleroderma.[32] In fact, some studies found an increased risk of breast cancer among scleroderma patients. This raises the possibility that some underlying pathologic features of scleroderma, such as increased vascular endothelial growth factor expression in scleroderma, may favor breast cancer development in scleroderma.[39]

Prostate and Other Urological Cancers

Similar to estrogen-driven cancers in females, SLE also appears to have a protective effect on prostate cancers based on recent studies.[16,40–42] In a recent systematic review including nine studies on prostate cancer, an SIR of 0.77 (95% CI 0.69–0.87) was observed.[40] Further, in another literature review of prostate cancer, similar results were observed with an SIR of 0.72 (95% CI 0.57–0.89).[42] While this study compared patients with controls matched for age and geography, a large portion of subjects were Caucasian.[42] Interestingly in another population-based cohort study in Taiwan, SLE patients were found to have a higher risk of developing prostate cancer (HR 3.78, 95% CI 1.30–11.0) compared to the general population. It is possible that the racial and/or lifestyle differences between this study and the other studies contributed to this difference, or that the study suffered from ascertainment bias. Main factors associated with the otherwise consistently reduced prostate cancer rates in SLE might be attributed to hormonal causes. SLE patients are known to have low levels of androgens,[43] which can contribute to the decreased risk of prostate cancer.[16,42]

In contrast to prostate cancer, bladder and kidney cancers have been less extensively studied among SLE patients. A recent systematic review suggested an increase in the incident of kidney cancers (SIR 2.29, 95% CI 1.25–4.18) among SLE patients, but failed to show any clear change in the bladder cancer incidence in SLE compared to the general population.[40]

Risk of Other Cancers in SLE

Other cancers that have been studied in SLE include head and neck malignancies, thyroid, liver, vaginal, and vulva cancers.

In a recent study, the incidence of head and neck malignancies among SLE patients was found to be 2.16-fold higher compared to the general population. Cancers of the oral cavity and nasopharynx were reported to be the sites with the highest incidence risk.[44] Although the cause remains unknown, smoking is a risk factor for oral cancers[41] and the increased susceptibility to viral infections such as Epstein–Barr virus (EBV) in SLE[45] may increase the risk. Increased rates of thyroid cancer have also been reported among SLE patients. One case control study noted an increased prevalence of papillary thyroid cancer and increased thyroid autoimmunity in patients with SLE. Therefore, the authors recommended careful thyroid surveillance using ultrasonography, thyroid stimulating hormone, and thyroid peroxidase antibody during follow-up of SLE patients.[46]

An increased risk of liver cancers has been consistently observed. Based on a meta-analysis, the SIR associated with liver cancers was found to be 2.44, 95% CI 1.46–4.05.[16] However, SIRs vary from 9.9 (with 95% CI 2.5–39.8)[47] to the more conservative estimate in the multicenter study of 1.87 95% CI 0.97–3.27.[2] The authors attribute this increase partly to reduced viral clearance.[2,16] Evidence also suggests an increased reactivation of hepatitis B virus (HBV) in patients with autoimmune diseases,[45,48] possibly due to immunosuppressive therapies.[48] However, this is controversial as some studies have failed to show any increase in hepatitis B and C infection in SLE patients compared to the general population.[49] Nevertheless, a clear increase in incidence has been observed for other viral (HPV, EBV)-associated malignancies such as cervical and oropharyngeal as noted earlier as well as vulva/vaginal, anal cancers, and nonmelanoma skin.[2,47] In the international multicenter study, the incident of cancer of the vulva was reported to be 3.78 times higher in SLE

patients.[2] In one study, the authors suggested that compromised T cells in SLE patients may increase their susceptibility to viral-associated malignancies[47] as has been observed in the HIV population.[50]

CONCLUSIONS

Based on several studies on cancer incidence in SLE patients, it is clear that SLE patients display an altered cancer risk profile. While strong associations are observed in SLE patients for smoking and lung cancer risk, and HPV and cervical cancer risk, further studies are required.

REFERENCES

1. Yurkovich M, Vostretsova K, Chen W, Avina-Zubieta JA. Overall and cause-specific mortality in patients with systemic lupus erythematosus: a meta-analysis of observational studies. *Arthritis Care Res (Hoboken)* 2014;**66**:608–16.
2. Bernatsky S, Ramsey-Goldman R, Labrecque J, Joseph L, Boivin JF, Petri M, et al. Cancer risk in systemic lupus: an updated international multi-centre cohort study. *J Autoimmun* 2013;**42**:130–5.
3. Bernatsky S, Boivin JF, Joseph L, Manzi S, Ginzler E, Gladman DD, et al. Mortality in systemic lupus erythematosus. *Arthritis Rheum* 2006;**54**:2550–7.
4. Bernatsky S, Ramsey-Goldman R, Joseph L, Boivin JF, Costenbader KH, Urowitz MB, et al. Lymphoma risk in systemic lupus: effects of disease activity versus treatment. *Ann Rheum Dis* 2014;**73**:138–42.
5. Lu M, Bernatsky S, Ramsey-Goldman R, Petri M, Manzi S, Urowitz MB, et al. Non-lymphoma hematological malignancies in systemic lupus erythematosus. *Oncology* 2013;**85**:235–40.
6. Landgren O, Linet MS, McMaster ML, Gridley G, Hemminki K, Goldin LR. Familial characteristics of autoimmune and hematologic disorders in 8,406 multiple myeloma patients: a population-based case-control study. *Int J Cancer* 2006;**118**:3095–8.
7. Ali YM, Urowitz MB, Ibanez D, Gladman DD. Monoclonal gammopathy in systemic lupus erythematosus. *Lupus* 2007;**16**:426–9.
8. Ott G, Rosenwald A. Molecular pathogenesis of follicular lymphoma. *Haematologica* 2008;**93**:1773–6.
9. Bernatsky S, Kale M, Ramsey-Goldman R, Gordon C, Clarke AE. Systemic lupus and malignancies. *Curr Opin Rheumatol* 2012;**24**:177–81.
10. Dias C, Isenberg DA. Susceptibility of patients with rheumatic diseases to B-cell non-hodgkin lymphoma. *Nat Rev Rheumatol* 2011;**7**:360–8.
11. He B, Chadburn A, Jou E, Schattner EJ, Knowles DM, Cerutti A. Lymphoma B cells evade apoptosis through the TNF family members BAFF/BLyS and APRIL. *J Immunol* 2004;**172**:3268–79.
12. Tarella C, Gueli A, Ruella M, Cignetti A. Lymphocyte transformation and autoimmune disorders. *Autoimmun Rev* 2013;**12**:802–13.
13. Cortes J, Kurzrock R. Interleukin-10 in non-Hodgkin's lymphoma. *Leuk Lymphoma* 1997;**26**:251–9.
14. Choubey D, Deka R, Ho SM. Interferon-inducible IFI16 protein in human cancers and autoimmune diseases. *Front Biosci* 2008;**13**: 598–608.
15. Veeranki S, Choubey D. Systemic lupus erythematosus and increased risk to develop B cell malignancies: role of the p200-family proteins. *Immunol Lett* 2010;**133**:1–5.
16. Ni J, Qiu LJ, Hu LF, Cen H, Zhang M, Wen PF, et al. Lung, liver, prostate, bladder malignancies risk in systemic lupus erythematosus: evidence from a meta-analysis. *Lupus* 2014;**23**:284–92.

17. Hemminki K, Liu X, Ji J, Sundquist J, Sundquist K. Effect of autoimmune diseases on risk and survival in histology-specific lung cancer. *Eur Respir J* 2012;**40**:1489–95.

18. Franks AL, Slansky JE. Multiple associations between a broad spectrum of autoimmune diseases, chronic inflammatory diseases and cancer. *Anticancer Res* 2012;**32**:1119–36.

19. Siemes C, Visser LE, Coebergh JW, Splinter TA, Witteman JC, Uitterlinden AG, et al. C-reactive protein levels, variation in the C-reactive protein gene, and cancer risk: the rotterdam study. *J Clin Oncol* 2006;**24**: 5216–22.

20. Santana IU, Gomes Ado N, Lyrio LD, Rios Grassi MF, Santiago MB. Systemic lupus erythematosus, human papillomavirus infection, cervical pre-malignant and malignant lesions: a systematic review. *Clin Rheumatol* 2011;**30**:665–72.

21. Zard E, Arnaud L, Mathian A, Chakhtoura Z, Hie M, Touraine P, et al. Increased risk of high grade cervical squamous intraepithelial lesions in systemic lupus erythematosus: a meta-analysis of the literature. *Autoimmun Rev* 2014;**13**:730–5.

22. Kim SC, Glynn RJ, Giovannucci E, Hernandez-Diaz S, Liu J, Feldman S, et al. Risk of high-grade cervical dysplasia and cervical cancer in women with systemic inflammatory diseases: a population-based cohort study. *Ann Rheum Dis* July 2015;**74**(7):1360–7.

23. Soybilgic A, Onel KB, Utset T, Alexander K, Wagner-Weiner L. Safety and immunogenicity of the quadrivalent HPV vaccine in female systemic Lupus Erythematosus patients aged 12 to 26 years. *Pediatr Rheumatol Online J* 2013;**11**:29.

24. Tam LS, Chan PK, Ho SC, Yu MY, Yim SF, Cheung TH, et al. Risk factors for squamous intraepithelial lesions in systemic lupus erythematosus: a prospective cohort study. *Arthritis Care Res (Hoboken)* 2011;**63**:269–76.

25. Rojo-Contreras W, Olivas-Flores EM, Gamez-Nava JI, Montoya-Fuentes H, Trujillo-Hernandez B, Trujillo X, et al. Cervical human papillomavirus infection in Mexican women with systemic lupus erythematosus or rheumatoid arthritis. *Lupus* 2012;**21**:365–72.

26. Bernatsky SR, Cooper GS, Mill C, Ramsey-Goldman R, Clarke AE, Pineau CA. Cancer screening in patients with systemic lupus erythematosus. *J Rheumatol* 2006;**33**:45–9.

27. Tessier Cloutier B, Clarke AE, Ramsey-Goldman R, Wang Y, Foulkes W, Gordon C, et al. Breast cancer in systemic lupus erythematosus. *Oncology* 2013;**85**:117–21.

28. Gadalla SM, Amr S, Langenberg P, Baumgarten M, Davidson WF, Schairer C, et al. Breast cancer risk in elderly women with systemic autoimmune rheumatic diseases: a population-based case-control study. *Br J Cancer* 2009;**100**:817–21.

29. Bernatsky S, Ramsey-Goldman R, Foulkes WD, Gordon C, Clarke AE. Breast, ovarian, and endometrial malignancies in systemic lupus erythematosus: a meta-analysis. *Br J Cancer* 2011;**104**:1478–81.

30. Bernatsky S, Easton DF, Dunning A, Michailidou K, Ramsey-Goldman R, Gordon C, et al. Decreased breast cancer risk in systemic lupus erythematosus: the search for a genetic basis continues. *Lupus* 2012;**21**:896–9.

31. Beral V, Bull D, Green J, Reeves G. Ovarian cancer and hormone replacement therapy in the million women study. *Lancet* 2007;**369**:1703–10.

32. Xu WH, Xiang YB, Ruan ZX, Zheng W, Cheng JR, Dai Q, et al. Menstrual and reproductive factors and endometrial cancer risk: results from a population-based case-control study in urban Shanghai. *Int J Cancer* 2004;**108**:613–9.

33. Pike MC, Peters RK, Cozen W, Probst-Hensch NM, Felix JC, Wan PC, et al. Estrogen-progestin replacement therapy and endometrial cancer. *J Natl Cancer Inst* 1997;**89**:1110–6.

34. Cooper GS, Dooley MA, Treadwell EL, St Clair EW, Gilkeson GS. Hormonal and reproductive risk factors for development of systemic lupus erythematosus: results of a population-based, case-control study. *Arthritis Rheum* 2002;**46**:1830–9.

35. Hansen JE, Chan G, Liu Y, Hegan DC, Dalal S, Dray E, et al. Targeting cancer with a lupus autoantibody. *Sci Transl Med* 2012;**4**:157ra42.

36. Noble PW, Young MR, Bernatsky S, Weisbart RH, Hansen JE. A nucleolytic lupus autoantibody is toxic to BRCA2-deficient cancer cells. *Sci Rep* 2014;**4**.

37. Ruiz-Irastorza G, Ugarte A, Egurbide MV, Garmendia M, Pijoan JI, Martinez-Berriotxoa A, et al. Antimalarials may influence the risk of malignancy in systemic lupus erythematosus. *Ann Rheum Dis* 2007;**66**:815–7.

38. Allott EH, Tse CK, Olshan AF, Carey LA, Moorman PG, Troester MA. Non-steroidal anti-inflammatory drug use, hormone receptor status, and breast cancer-specific mortality in the Carolina Breast Cancer Study. *Breast Cancer Res Treat* 2014;**147**:415–21.

39. Colaci M, Giuggioli D, Vacchi C, Lumetti F, Iachetta F, Marcheselli L, et al. Breast cancer in systemic sclerosis: results of a cross-linkage of an Italian Rheumatologic Center and a population-based Cancer Registry and review of the literature. *Autoimmun Rev* 2014;**13**: 132–7.

40. Huang HB, Jiang SC, Han J, Cheng QS, Dong CB, Pan CM. A systematic review of the epidemiological literature on the risk of urological cancers in systemic lupus erythematosus. *J Cancer Res Clin Oncol* 2014;**140**:1067–73.

41. Petti S, Masood M, Scully C. The magnitude of tobacco smoking-betel quid chewing-alcohol drinking interaction effect on oral cancer in South-East Asia. A meta-analysis of observational studies. *PLoS One* 2013;**8**:e78999.

42. Bernatsky S, Ramsey-Goldman R, Gordon C, Clarke AE. Prostate cancer in systemic lupus erythematosus. *Int J Cancer* 2011;**129**:2966–9.

43. Lavalle C, Loyo E, Paniagua R, Bermudez JA, Herrera J, Graef A, et al. Correlation study between prolactin and androgens in male patients with systemic lupus erythematosus. *J Rheumatol* 1987;**14**:268–72.

44. Chang SL, Hsu HT, Weng SF, Lin YS. Impact of head and neck malignancies on risk factors and survival in systemic lupus erythematosus. *Acta Otolaryngol* 2013;**133**:1088–95.

45. Mohamed DF, Habeeb RA, Hosny SM, Ebrahim SE. Incidence and risk of infection in Egyptian patients with systemic lupus erythematosus. *Clin Med Insights Arthritis Musculoskelet Disord* 2014;**7**:41–8.

46. Antonelli A, Mosca M, Fallahi P, Neri R, Ferrari SM, D'Ascanio A, et al. Thyroid cancer in systemic lupus erythematosus: a case-control study. *J Clin Endocrinol Metab* 2010;**95**:314–8.

47. Dreyer L, Faurschou M, Mogensen M, Jacobsen S. High incidence of potentially virus-induced malignancies in systemic lupus erythematosus: a long-term followup study in a Danish cohort. *Arthritis Rheum* 2011;**63**:3032–7.

48. Watanabe R, Ishii T, Kobayashi H, Asahina I, Takemori H, Izumiyama T, et al. Prevalence of hepatitis B virus infection in patients with rheumatic diseases in Tohoku area: a retrospective multicenter survey. *Tohoku J Exp Med* 2014;**233**:129–33.

49. Abu-Shakra M, El-Sana S, Margalith M, Sikuler E, Neumann L, Buskila D. Hepatitis B and C viruses serology in patients with SLE. *Lupus* 1997;**6**:543–4.

50. Reekie J, Kosa C, Engsig F, Monforte A, Wiercinska-Drapalo A, Domingo P, et al. Relationship between current level of immunodeficiency and non-acquired immunodeficiency syndrome-defining malignancies. *Cancer* 2010;**116**:5306–15.

Chapter 47

The Nervous System in Systemic Lupus Erythematosus

John G. Hanly

Dalhousie University, Halifax, Nova Scotia, Canada; Nova Scotia Health Authority, Halifax, Nova Scotia, Canada

SUMMARY

Approximately one-third of all neuropsychiatric (NP) syndromes in SLE patients are primary manifestations of lupus autoimmunity. Seizure disorders, cerebrovascular disease, acute confusional states, and neuropathies are the most common. Primary NP lupus (NPSLE) events are a consequence of either mircrovasculopathy and thrombosis or autoantibodies and inflammatory mediators. The diagnosis of NPSLE requires the exclusion of other causes and the clinical assessment directs the selection of appropriate investigations. These include measurement of autoantibodies, analysis of cerebrospinal fluid, electrophysiological studies, neuropsychological assessment, and neuroimaging to evaluate brain structure and function. Treatment should include the management of comorbidities contributing to the NP event, use of symptomatic therapies, and more specific interventions with either anticoagulation or immunosuppressive agents, depending on the primary immunopathogenetic mechanism. Although the prognosis is variable, recent studies suggest a more favorable outcome for primary NPSLE manifestations compared to NP events attributed to non-SLE causes.

INTRODUCTION

Although nervous system events are common in SLE patients the majority are not attributable to lupus. Those that are encompass a variety of neurological (N) and psychiatric (P) features. Reports of the prevalence of neuropsychiatric SLE (NPSLE) have been highly variable (21–95%).[1–3] Some of the earlier studies were limited due to: (1) lack of standardized definitions/criteria for NP events including the attribution of NP events to SLE and non-SLE causes; (2) failure to use validated instruments to measure important outcomes such as organ damage and quality of life; (3) retrospective single-center study design.

CLASSIFICATION AND CLINICAL MANIFESTATIONS

In 1999 the American College of Rheumatology (ACR) developed a standard nomenclature and definitions for 19 NP syndromes (Table 1)[4] that can be condensed into central and peripheral,[4] diffuse and focal NP subsets.[5] Guidance on investigations and diagnostic criteria for each of the NP syndromes were also provided. Whether using the ACR classification in a research setting or treating a patient in clinical practice, it is important to determine the attribution of NP events to SLE and non-SLE causes. The ACR classification lists potential causes other than SLE for each of the NP syndromes, responsible in part or entirely for the event. This component of the ACR classification, in combination with other variables, has been used to develop attribution models for NP events in SLE.[6] Depending on the stringency of the attribution decision rules, the proportion of NP events attributed to SLE in newly diagnosed SLE patients varies from 19% to 38% of NP events in 6% to 12% of patients over the first year of the illness. Although headache and mood disorders are the most frequent NP complaints, seizure disorders, cerebrovascular disease, acute confusional states, and neuropathies are the most common NP syndromes attributed to SLE. The cumulative occurrence of NP events increases over time, although the proportion of events attributed to SLE and non-SLE causes remains the same.[7,8] Correctly identifying the attribution of NP events to SLE and non-SLE causes is critical for optimizing treatment and conducting research studies.

Regardless of attribution, most,[6] although not all,[9] NP events in SLE patients are associated with a significant negative impact on health-related quality of life (HRQoL) even when other factors that impact HRQoL such as global SLE disease activity, cumulative organ damage, and medications are taken into account. Clinically meaningful changes in HRQoL concur with physician determination of improvement or deterioration in NP events over time, indicating that HRQoL is a valid patient outcome in clinical studies of NPSLE.

Systemic Lupus Erythematosus. http://dx.doi.org/10.1016/B978-0-12-801917-7.00047-4

TABLE 1 Neuropsychiatric Syndromes in SLE as Defined Using the ACR Nomenclature

Central Nervous System	Peripheral Nervous System
Aseptic meningitis	Guillain Barré syndrome
Cerebrovascular disease	Autonomic neuropathy
Demyelinating syndrome	Mononeuropathy
Headache	Myasthenia gravis
Movement disorder	Cranial neuropathy
Myelopathy	Plexopathy
Seizure disorders	Polyneuropathy
Acute confusional state	
Anxiety disorder	
Cognitive dysfunction	
Mood disorder	
Psychosis	

From Ref. 4 with permission.

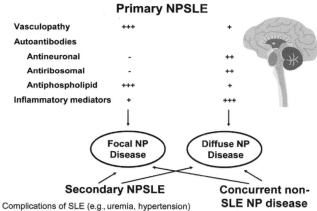

Primary NPSLE

Vasculopathy	+++	+
Autoantibodies		
Antineuronal	-	++
Antiribosomal	-	++
Antiphospholipid	+++	+
Inflammatory mediators	+	+++

Focal NP Disease   Diffuse NP Disease

Secondary NPSLE   **Concurrent non-SLE NP disease**

Complications of SLE (e.g., uremia, hypertension)

Complications of SLE therapy (e.g., steroids, infection)

FIGURE 1 Factors contributing to neuropsychiatric (NP) events in SLE patients. Focal and diffuse nervous system events may result from direct autoimmune/inflammatory mechanisms related to SLE (Primary NPSLE), or a consequence of complications of the disease (e.g., hypertension), or its therapy (e.g., infection) (Secondary NPSLE), or a concurrent non-SLE-related NP event. *Adapted from Hanly JG. Neuropsychiatric lupus. Cur Rheumatol Rep 2001; 3:205–212, with permission.*

ETIOLOGY AND PATHOGENESIS OF NPSLE

Neuropsychiatric SLE (NPSLE) are primary manifestations of the disease, in contrast to complications of the disease (e.g., hypertension), or its therapy (e.g., infection) (Figure 1). Evidence from animal and human studies suggests two autoimmune pathogenic mechanisms for NPSLE (Figure 2): (1) vascular injury involving large and small caliber vessels

Autoimmune Pathogenesis of NPSLE

	Vascular	Inflammatory
Mediators	aPL autoantibodies Immune complexes	Autoantibodies MMPs, Cytokines
Mechanism	Thrombosis Angiopathy (micro)	BBB permeability Immune complexes pDCs activation
Outcome	Focal NP (e.g. stroke) Diffuse NP (e.g. cognitive dysfunction)	Diffuse NP (e.g. psychosis, acute confusion)

FIGURE 2 Autoimmune pathogenic mechanisms for NPSLE: vascular injury involving both large and small caliber vessels mediated by anti-phospholipid antibodies, immune complexes, and leukoagglutination, which results in focal NP events such as stroke and in diffuse NP events such as cognitive dysfunction; injury due to inflammation in which increased permeability of the blood–brain barrier, formation of immune complexes, and production of IFN-α and other inflammatory mediators lead to diffuse NP manifestations such as psychosis and acute confusional states.

mediated by anti-phospholipid antibodies, immune complexes, and leukoagglutination. Clinical sequelae include focal NP events such as stroke and diffuse NP events such as cognitive dysfunction; (2) autoimmune inflammation-mediated injury with increased permeability of the blood–brain barrier, intrathecal formation of immune complexes, production of IFN-α, and other inflammatory mediators. Clinical sequelae include diffuse NP manifestations such as psychosis and acute confusion.

COGNITIVE DYSFUNCTION IN SLE

Cognition is the sum of intellectual functions that include reception of external stimuli, information processing, learning, storage, and expression. Impairment of any of these functions can result in cognitive dysfunction. Cognitive complaints and objectively confirmed cognitive impairment are frequent in SLE and may be considered a distinct subset of NPSLE. Cognitive function is also an indicator of overall brain health that may be affected by a variety of factors including other NP syndromes. Due to the poor correlation between symptoms and objective findings the presence, characteristics, and severity of cognitive impairment should be confirmed by formal neuropsychological assessment. Cognitive dysfunction identified in this way has been reported in up to 80% of SLE patients,[10] though most studies report a prevalence ranging between 17% and 66%.[11,12] Subclinical deficits are common. There in no specific pattern of cognitive dysfunction in SLE but overall cognitive slowing, decreased attention, impaired

TABLE 2 Investigations in NPSLE

- **Autoantibodies:**
  Antineuronal (NR2, Aquaporin-4)
  Antiribosomal P
  Antiphospholipid (aCL, LA)

- **CSF:**
  Exclude infection, assess blood–brain barrier
  Autoantibodies
  Inflammatory mediators, degradation proteins

- **Electrophysiological assessment**

- **Neuropsychological assessment**

- **Neuroimaging:**
  Brain structure (CT, MRI, MTI, DWI, DTI)
  Brain function (PET, SPECT, MRA, MRS, fMRI)

working memory, and executive dysfunction (e.g., difficulty with multitasking, organization, and planning) are the most frequent.

DIAGNOSTIC APPROACH FOR NPSLE

The assessment of an NP event in SLE patients should determine if it is a primary manifestation of the disease, a complication of the disease or its therapy, a coincidental disease process, or combinations thereof. The process is largely one of exclusion based on clinical evaluation and appropriate investigations directed by the clinical circumstances (Table 2).

General Investigations

As emphasized by the EULAR task force recommendations on NPSLE,[13] the diagnostic workup should mimic the approach used in non-SLE patients. For example, patients with a transient ischemic attack or stroke should have an echocardiogram and Doppler ultrasound of the carotids in addition to testing for lupus-specific causes such as antiphospholipid antibodies. Cardiac risk factors such as poorly controlled hypertension and hyperlipidemia should also be considered, given the increased frequency of premature cardiovascular disease in SLE.[14]

Assessment of Global SLE Disease Activity

Some,[14] but not all studies,[15] have found an association between increased global SLE disease activity and NP events attributed to SLE. This association is more robust for diffuse rather than focal NP events.[16]

Autoantibodies in the Circulation and CSF

Peripheral blood anti-phospholipid antibodies should be measured, especially in patients with focal NP events or

cognitive decline. The association between the circulating anti-NR2 antibodies and NPSLE is inconsistent[17–20] but likely to be more informative if measured in the CSF.[21,22] The measurement of CSF cytokines and biomarkers of neurological damage is of academic interest but at this time neither is recommended or even feasible in practice. Neuromyelitis optica (NMO), or Devic's syndrome, is a severe demyelinating disorder of the central nervous system that has been reported in patients with SLE[23] and is associated with NMO autoantibodies whose antigenic target is aquaporin-4.[24]

Electrophysiological Studies

In seizure disorders electroencephalography (EEG) may show asymmetry of the electric cerebral activity, diffuse disorganized background activity, and focal epileptiform discharges.[25] Electrophysiological abnormalities in SLE patients with peripheral neuropathies include axonal neuropathy in 70% and demyelination in 20%.[26]

Neuropsychological Assessment

No simple screening test for cognitive dysfunction in SLE patients is currently available as most lack sensitivity for mild, but clinically significant, dysfunction. Self-report instruments have been validated by some[27] but not others.[28] Computerized testing facilitates efficient screening of SLE patients by nonexperts,[29] but formal testing remains the only definitive way to diagnose cognitive impairment. The ACR battery of neuropsychological tests[4] is comprehensive, but its widespread use remains limited, as such testing is time-consuming, requires specialized training, and is subject to practice effects with repeated use. If abnormalities are detected, repeat testing should be done after a reasonable interval, usually several months, to measure change in cognition following observation or treatment.

Neuroimaging

Standard and more advanced neuroimaging of brain structure and function helps to localize intracranial abnormalities, determine whether the lesions involve white or gray matter, and assess their chronicity and change over time. The assessment of brain structure by CT scanning has largely been replaced by MRI, which is more sensitive, especially T_2 weighted images. Abnormalities occur in white and gray matter in addition to global and regional cerebral atrophy but except for large cerebral infarcts, the correlation between structural changes and clinical NP manifestations of SLE is low.[30] More advanced MRI methodology for detection of structural abnormalities include magnetization transfer imaging (MTI), diffusion weighted imaging (DWI), and diffusion tensor imaging (DTI).[31]

MTI measures magnetization transfer between bound and unbound hydrogen molecules (e.g., between white matter and CSF). The transfer is diminished by either decreased bound molecules (e.g., demyelination) or increased unbound molecules (e.g., edema). Decreased whole brain MTI has been reported in SLE patients even in the absence of other structural MRI changes and tends to be greater in longstanding NPSLE compared to patients with active or acute disease.[31] DWI detects hyperacute brain injury, in particular acute ischemia following stroke when the diffusion of water is highly restricted due to the acute shift of fluid into the intracellular compartment and cytotoxic edema.[30] DTI uses a similar technology to assess the integrity of neural white matter tracts in the brain.[31]

The most objective neuroimaging study of brain function is positron emission tomography (PET) scanning, but practical considerations limit its applicability.[32] Single photon emission computed tomography (SPECT) scanning[32] provides semiquantitative analysis of regional cerebral blood flow and metabolism. It is exquisitely sensitive and has identified both diffuse and focal deficits, which may be fixed or reversible.[33] However, the findings are not specific for SLE and may not correlate with clinical NP manifestations. In fact, up to 50% of SLE patients without clinical manifestations of NP disease may have an abnormal SPECT scan.[34]

Magnetic resonance angiography (MRA) provides noninvasive visualization of cerebral blood flow, although not optimal for small caliber vessels primarily involved in NPSLE. Magnetic resonance spectroscopy (MRS) measures biochemical compounds including *N*-acetylaspartate (NAA), choline, and creatine within predetermined regions of interest. Decreased NAA, believed to reflect neuronal/axonal loss or dysfunction, has been reported in SLE patients, even in the absence of visible damage on structural MRI.[31] fMRI measures changes in local brain deoxyhemoglobin levels that likely reflect neuronal activity. In a study of nine patients with NPSLE,[35] blood-oxygen-level-dependent fMRI showed greater frontoparietal activation in SLE patients than in RA and healthy controls while performing a task that engaged working memory. The findings indicated a compensatory adaptation of neuronal function through recruitment of extracortical pathways, to supplement impaired function of standard pathways.

Despite its limitations, at this time structural MRI remains the neuroimaging method routinely used in clinical practice. More advanced methods such as MTI, DTI, MRS, and fMRI suffer from variability in results between scanners and a lack of normative or standardized guidelines for interpretation. In the future, however, multimodal imaging is likely to become the standard of practice in the diagnosis and monitoring of neurological disorders, including NPSLE.

TREATMENT OF NP EVENTS IN SLE PATIENTS

A thorough clinical assessment and appropriate investigations determine if the NP event is a primary manifestation of SLE, a complication of the disease or prior therapy, or a coincidental disease process. In some cases more than one of these factors may be contributing to the event (Table 3). Identification and treatment of non-SLE-related factors are important in all cases. For example, serious infections and metabolic abnormalities should be addressed in patients presenting with acute confusion and seizures. Patients with vascular NP events should be screened for cardiovascular risk factors. Pharmacological therapies for anxiety and depression, improving poor sleep hygiene, and maintaining normal blood pressure may improve cognitive complaints. Which lupus-specific therapies are used depends on what immunopathogenic mechanism, inflammation-mediated injury, or vascular-mediated injury is predominant.

AUTOIMMUNE INFLAMMATION-MEDIATED INJURY

Serious visceral involvement, such as lupus nephritis, is treated with high-dose corticosteroids and immunosuppressants such as azathioprine, cylclophosphamide, or mycophenolate mofetil. A similar approach is used for NPSLE events due to autoimmune-induced inflammation, despite the relative lack of clinical evidence. An open-label study of 13 patients with lupus psychosis reported a favorable outcome in all patients treated with oral cyclophosphamide for 6 months followed by maintenance therapy with

TABLE 3 Management of NP Events in Patients with SLE

Treatment Strategy	Examples
• Establish diagnosis of NPSLE	CSF examination primarily to exclude infection Autoantibody profile Neuroimaging to assess brain structure and function Neuropsychological assessment
• Identify confounding factors	Hypertension, infection, metabolic abnormalities
• Symptomatic therapy	Anticonvulsants, psychotropics, anxiolytics
• Immunosuppression	Corticosteroids, azathioprine, cyclophosphamide, mycophenolate mofetil, B lymphocyte depletion
• Anticoagulation	ASA, heparin, warfarin

Modified from Hanly JG. Neuropsychiatric lupus. *Cur Rheumatol Rep* 2001, 3:205–212.

azathioprine.[36] A randomized controlled study[37] compared intermittent intravenous cyclophosphamide to intravenous methylprednisone given for up to 2 years in SLE patients with predominantly neurologic disease. There was a significantly better response rate with cyclophosphamide (95%) compared to methylprednisone (54%) (*P*<0.03). More targeted immunosuppressive therapy, such as B-lymphocyte depletion with anti-CD20 used alone or in combination with cyclophosphamide,[38] is promising but requires further study.

VASCULAR-MEDIATED INJURY

Focal NP disease attributed to anti-phospholipid antibodies requires anticoagulation, which is usually lifelong.[10] In the absence of controlled clinical trials for NPSLE due to thrombosis, there is a reliance on studies of prevention of recurrent thrombosis in patients with antiphospholipid syndrome (APS). Two controlled studies of APS found no significant difference between low intensity (target INR: 2.0–3.0) and high intensity (target INR: >3.0) treatment with warfarin in the prevention of recurrent thrombosis.[39,40] However, few patients had arterial thrombosis and the optimal target INR for such cases is unclear.[41] Potential adjunctive therapies in patients with recurrent thrombosis while on warfarin are antiplatelet agents, antimalarials,[42] and statins.[43]

COGNITIVE IMPAIRMENT

Non-SLE causes of cognitive dysfunction should be sought. These include sleep deprivation, mood disorders, fatigue, and medications. Antidepressants, anticonvulsants, and antihypertensive treatments may cause reversible cognitive problems.

Only one placebo-controlled study of pharmacologic therapy for SLE-associated cognitive dysfunction has been performed.[44] Ten SLE patients were enrolled in a double-blind, controlled trial using 0.5 mg/kg prednisone daily. The authors reported improved cognition in five of the eight subjects who completed the trial. A single-center, controlled study of memantine over 12 weeks aimed at "cognitive enhancement" did not demonstrate significant benefit over placebo.[45] Cognitive impairment has been associated with anti-phospholipid antibodies in cross-sectional and longitudinal studies even in the absence of overt thromboembolic disease.[46] Thus, antiplatelet or anticoagulant therapy in such patients is logical, but lacks evidence for efficacy. The use of immunosuppressive therapy in patients with presumed inflammation-mediated brain injury is also logical but again lacks evidence of efficacy from controlled trials, especially in patients with cognitive impairment as the sole manifestation of NPSLE.

Cognitive rehabilitation typically involves intensive retraining of cognitive skills and has been employed in other conditions such as stroke, dementia, traumatic brain injury, multiple sclerosis. One study enrolled 17 women with SLE who reported cognitive difficulties that either interfered with adaptive functioning or caused emotional distress. Treatment involved eight weekly 2-h "psychoeducational group intervention" sessions that focused on cognitive strategy training applied across multiple real-life situations. In addition, there was a psychosocial support component. Patients reported better affect and overall quality of life as well as memory self-efficacy. Although these results are encouraging, controlled and long-term studies are required to confirm these preliminary findings and determine their durability over time.

PROGNOSIS

Clinical trials have been uncontrolled, of short duration, or focused on a single NP manifestation.[36–38,44,47] Longitudinal studies of cognitive function have demonstrated stable cognitive test performance with persistent or progressive cognitive dysfunction in a minority of patients.[48,49] The data from observational cohorts have been inconsistent. For example, increased mortality in patients with NP events has been reported in some studies[50] but not in others.[51] In a follow-up study of 32 patients hospitalized for NPSLE[52] the outcome was generally favorable with either substantial improvement (69%) or stabilization (19%) over 2 years. In SLE patients followed for up to 7 years (mean 3.6 years),[7] there was resolution in approximately 15% of NP events at each annual assessment, although the majority of events were persistent. Of interest, the attribution of NP events to SLE or non-SLE causes did not predict their resolution. Two reports with mean follow-up of 3.7 months[6] and 1.9 years[7] from a large inception cohort study of SLE indicated a more favorable outcome in patients with NP events attributed to SLE. It could be that treatment of NPSLE early in the disease course may have a more favorable outcome and as such may present a therapeutic window of opportunity akin to that seen in other rheumatic diseases.[53,54]

CONCLUSION

The occurrence of NP events in SLE patients poses a diagnostic and therapeutic challenge. The precise characterization and correct attribution of these events to SLE and non-SLE causes are critical. The correct diagnosis relies heavily on careful clinical assessment of the patient and selection of appropriate investigations. Recent studies have provided insight into immunopathogenetic mechanisms for NPSLE, the contribution of non-SLE factors, and the short- and long-term prognosis. Current therapeutic strategies are largely empiric based on knowledge of immunopathogenetic mechanisms and the treatment of other serious organ disease in SLE. Further insights on the immunopathogenetic mechanisms and clinical outcomes of NPSLE are required to inform the design and execution of therapeutic clinical trials.

REFERENCES

1. Ainiala H, Hietaharju A, Loukkola J, Peltola J, Korpela M, Metsanoja R, et al. Validity of the new American college of rheumatology criteria for neuropsychiatric lupus syndromes: a population-based evaluation. *Arthritis Rheum* 2001;**45**(5):419–23.

2. Hanly JG, McCurdy G, Fougere L, Douglas JA, Thompson K. Neuropsychiatric events in systemic lupus erythematosus: attribution and clinical significance. *J Rheumatol* 2004;**31**(11):2156–62.

3. Sibbitt Jr WL, Brandt JR, Johnson CR, Maldonado ME, Patel SR, Ford CC, et al. The incidence and prevalence of neuropsychiatric syndromes in pediatric onset systemic lupus erythematosus. *J Rheumatol* 2002;**29**(7):1536–42.

4. The American college of rheumatology nomenclature and case definitions for neuropsychiatric lupus syndromes. *Arthritis Rheum* 1999;**42**(4):599–608.

5. Hanly JG, Urowitz MB, Sanchez-Guerrero J, Bae SC, Gordon C, Wallace DJ, et al. Neuropsychiatric events at the time of diagnosis of systemic lupus erythematosus: an international inception cohort study. *Arthritis Rheum* 2007;**56**(1):265–73.

6. Hanly JG, Urowitz MB, Su L, Sanchez-Guerrero J, Bae SC, Gordon C, et al. Short-term outcome of neuropsychiatric events in systemic lupus erythematosus upon enrollment into an international inception cohort study. *Arthritis Rheum* 2008;**59**(5):721–9.

7. Hanly JG, Su L, Farewell V, McCurdy G, Fougere L, Thompson K. Prospective study of neuropsychiatric events in systemic lupus erythematosus. *J Rheumatol* 2009;**36**(7):1449–59.

8. Hanly JG, Urowitz MB, Su L, Bae SC, Gordon C, Wallace DJ, et al. Prospective analysis of neuropsychiatric events in an international disease inception cohort of patients with systemic lupus erythematosus. *Ann Rheum Dis* 2010;**69**(3):529–35.

9. Hanly JG, Urowitz MB, Su L, Gordon C, Bae SC, Sanchez-Guerrero J, et al. Seizure disorders in systemic lupus erythematosus results from an international, prospective, inception cohort study. *Ann Rheum Dis* 2012;**71**(9):1502–9.

10. Hanly JG. The nervous system and lupus. In: Lahita RG, editor. *Systemic lupus erythematosus.* 5th ed. Elsevier; 2011. p. 727–46.

11. Denburg SD, Denburg JA. Cognitive dysfunction and antiphospholipid antibodies in systemic lupus erythematosus. *Lupus* 2003;**12**(12):883–90.

12. Hanly JG, Liang MH. Cognitive disorders in systemic lupus erythematosus. Epidemiologic and clinical issues. *Ann NY Acad Sci* 1997;**823**:60–8.

13. Bertsias GK, Ioannidis JP, Aringer M, Bollen E, Bombardieri S, Bruce IN, et al. EULAR recommendations for the management of systemic lupus erythematosus with neuropsychiatric manifestations: report of a task force of the EULAR standing committee for clinical affairs. *Ann Rheum Dis* 2010;**69**(12):2074–82.

14. Govoni M, Bombardieri S, Bortoluzzi A, Caniatti L, Casu C, Conti F, et al. Factors and comorbidities associated with first neuropsychiatric event in systemic lupus erythematosus: does a risk profile exist? A large multicentre retrospective cross-sectional study on 959 Italian patients. *Rheumatol Oxf* 2012;**51**(1):157–68.

15. Jarpa E, Babul M, Calderon J, Gonzalez M, Martinez ME, Bravo-Zehnder M, et al. Common mental disorders and psychological distress in systemic lupus erythematosus are not associated with disease activity. *Lupus* 2011;**20**(1):58–66.

16. Morrison E, Carpentier S, Shaw E, Doucette S, Hanly JG. Neuropsychiatric systemic lupus erythematosus: association with global disease activity. *Lupus* 2014;**23**(4):370–7.

17. Omdal R, Brokstad K, Waterloo K, Koldingsnes W, Jonsson R, Mellgren SI. Neuropsychiatric disturbances in SLE are associated with antibodies against NMDA receptors. *Eur J Neurol* 2005;**12**(5):392–8.

18. Hanly JG, Robichaud J, Fisk JD. Anti-NR2 glutamate receptor antibodies and cognitive function in systemic lupus erythematosus. *J Rheumatol* 2006;**33**(8):1553–8.

19. Harrison MJ, Ravdin LD, Lockshin MD. Relationship between serum NR2a antibodies and cognitive dysfunction in systemic lupus erythematosus. *Arthritis Rheum* 2006;**54**(8):2515–22.

20. Lapteva L, Nowak M, Yarboro CH, Takada K, Roebuck-Spencer T, Weickert T, et al. Anti-N-methyl-D-aspartate receptor antibodies, cognitive dysfunction, and depression in systemic lupus erythematosus. *Arthritis Rheum* 2006;**54**(8):2505–14.

21. Yoshio T, Onda K, Nara H, Minota S. Association of IgG anti-NR2 glutamate receptor antibodies in cerebrospinal fluid with neuropsychiatric systemic lupus erythematosus. *Arthritis Rheum* 2006;**54**(2):675–8.

22. Arinuma Y, Yanagida T, Hirohata S. Association of cerebrospinal fluid anti-NR2 glutamate receptor antibodies with diffuse neuropsychiatric systemic lupus erythematosus. *Arthritis Rheum* 2008;**58**(4):1130–5.

23. Birnbaum J, Kerr D. Devic's syndrome in a woman with systemic lupus erythematosus: diagnostic and therapeutic implications of testing for the neuromyelitis optica IgG autoantibody. *Arthritis Rheum* 2007;**57**(2):347–51.

24. Waters P, Jarius S, Littleton E, Leite MI, Jacob S, Gray B, et al. Aquaporin-4 antibodies in neuromyelitis optica and longitudinally extensive transverse myelitis. *Arch Neurol* 2008;**65**(7):913–9.

25. Vieira-Karuta SC, Silva IC, Liberalesso PB, Bandeira M, Janz Jr L, Lohr Jr A. Epileptic seizures and EEG features in juvenile systemic lupus erythematosus. *Arq Neuropsiquiatr* 2008;**66**(3A):468–70.

26. Florica B, Aghdassi E, Su J, Gladman DD, Urowitz MB, Fortin PR. Peripheral neuropathy in patients with systemic lupus erythematosus. *Semin Arthritis Rheum* 2011;**41**(2):203–11.

27. Julian LJ, Yazdany J, Trupin L, Criswell LA, Yelin E, Katz PP. Validity of brief screening tools for cognitive impairment in rheumatoid arthritis and systemic lupus erythematosus. *Arthritis Care Res Hob* 2012;**64**(3):448–54.

28. Hanly JG, Su L, Omisade A, Farewell VT, Fisk JD. Screening for cognitive impairment in systemic lupus erythematosus. *J Rheumatol* 2012;**39**(7):1371–7.

29. Hanly JG, Omisade A, Su L, Farewell V, Fisk JD. Assessment of cognitive function in systemic lupus erythematosus, rheumatoid arthritis, and multiple sclerosis by computerized neuropsychological tests. *Arthritis Rheum* 2010;**62**(5):1478–86.

30. Peterson PL, Howe FA, Clark CA, Axford JS. Quantitative magnetic resonance imaging in neuropsychiatric systemic lupus erythematosus. *Lupus* 2003;**12**(12):897–902.

31. Appenzeller S, Pike GB, Clarke AE. Magnetic resonance imaging in the evaluation of central nervous system manifestations in systemic lupus erythematosus. *Clin Rev Allergy Immunol* 2008;**34**(3):361–6.

32. Hanly JG. Evaluation of patients with CNS involvement in SLE. *Baillieres Clin Rheumatol* 1998;**12**(3):415–31.

33. Oku K, Atsumi T, Furukawa S, Horita T, Sakai Y, Jodo S, et al. Cerebral imaging by magnetic resonance imaging and single photon emission computed tomography in systemic lupus erythematosus with central nervous system involvement. *Rheumatol Oxf* 2003;**42**(6):773–7.

34. Sibbitt Jr WL, Sibbitt RR, Brooks WM. Neuroimaging in neuropsychiatric systemic lupus erythematosus [see comments]. *Arthritis Rheum* 1999;**42**(10):2026–38.

35. Fitzgibbon BM, Fairhall SL, Kirk IJ, Kalev-Zylinska M, Pui K, Dalbeth N, et al. Functional MRI in NPSLE patients reveals increased parietal and frontal brain activation during a working memory task compared with controls. *Rheumatol Oxf* 2008;**47**(1):50–3.

36. Mok CC, Lau CS, Wong RW. Treatment of lupus psychosis with oral cyclophosphamide followed by azathioprine maintenance: an open-label study. *Am J Med* 2003;**115**(1):59–62.

37. Barile-Fabris L, Ariza-Andraca R, Olguin-Ortega L, Jara LJ, Fraga-Mouret A, Miranda-Limon JM, et al. Controlled clinical trial of IV cyclophosphamide versus IV methylprednisolone in severe neurological manifestations in systemic lupus erythematosus. *Ann Rheum Dis* 2005;**64**(4):620–5.

38. Tokunaga M, Saito K, Kawabata D, Imura Y, Fujii T, Nakayamada S, et al. Efficacy of rituximab (anti-CD20) for refractory systemic lupus erythematosus involving the central nervous system. *Ann Rheum Dis* 2007;**66**(4):470–5.

39. Finazzi G, Marchioli R, Brancaccio V, Schinco P, Wisloff F, Musial J, et al. A randomized clinical trial of high-intensity warfarin versus conventional antithrombotic therapy for the prevention of recurrent thrombosis in patients with the antiphospholipid syndrome (WAPS). *J Thromb Haemost* 2005;**3**(5):848–53.

40. Crowther MA, Ginsberg JS, Julian J, Denburg J, Hirsh J, Douketis J, et al. A comparison of two intensities of warfarin for the prevention of recurrent thrombosis in patients with the antiphospholipid antibody syndrome. *N Engl J Med* 2003;**349**(12):1133–8.

41. Ruiz-Irastorza G, Hunt BJ, Khamashta MA. A systematic review of secondary thromboprophylaxis in patients with antiphospholipid antibodies. *Arthritis Rheum* 2007;**57**(8):1487–95.

42. Jung H, Bobba R, Su J, Shariati-Sarabi Z, Gladman DD, Urowitz M, et al. The protective effect of antimalarial drugs on thrombovascular events in systemic lupus erythematosus. *Arthritis Rheum* 2010;**62**(3):863–8.

43. Meroni PL, Raschi E, Testoni C, Tincani A, Balestrieri G, Molteni R, et al. Statins prevent endothelial cell activation induced by antiphospholipid (anti-beta2-glycoprotein I) antibodies: effect on the proadhesive and proinflammatory phenotype. *Arthritis Rheum* 2001;**44**(12):2870–8.

44. Denburg SD, Carbotte RM, Denburg JA. Corticosteroids and neuropsychological functioning in patients with systemic lupus erythematosus. *Arthritis Rheum* 1994;**37**(9):1311–20.

45. Petri M, Naqibuddin M, Sampedro M, Omdal R, Carson KA. Memantine in systemic lupus erythematosus: a randomized, double-blind placebo-controlled trial. *Semin Arthritis Rheum* 2011;**41**(2):194–202.

46. Hanly JG, Hong C, Smith S, Fisk JD. A prospective analysis of cognitive function and anticardiolipin antibodies in systemic lupus erythematosus. *Arthritis Rheum* 1999;**42**(4):728–34.

47. McCune WJ, Golbus J, Zeldes W, Bohlke P, Dunne R, Fox DA. Clinical and immunologic effects of monthly administration of intravenous cyclophosphamide in severe systemic lupus erythematosus. *N Engl J Med* 1988;**318**(22):1423–31.

48. Hanly JG, Cassell K, Fisk JD. Cognitive function in systemic lupus erythematosus: results of a 5-year prospective study. *Arthritis Rheum* 1997;**40**(8):1542–3.

49. Waterloo K, Omdal R, Husby G, Mellgren SI. Neuropsychological function in systemic lupus erythematosus: a five-year longitudinal study. *Rheumatol Oxf* 2002;**41**(4):411–5.

50. Mody GM, Parag KB, Nathoo BC, Pudifin DJ, Duursma J, Seedat YK. High mortality with systemic lupus erythematosus in hospitalized African blacks. *Br J Rheumatol* 1994;**33**(12):1151–3.

51. Sibley JT, Olszynski WP, Decoteau WE, Sundaram MB. The incidence and prognosis of central nervous system disease in systemic lupus erythematosus. *J Rheumatol* 1992;**19**(1):47–52.

52. Karassa FB, Ioannidis JP, Boki KA, Touloumi G, Argyropoulou MI, Strigaris KA, et al. Predictors of clinical outcome and radiologic progression in patients with neuropsychiatric manifestations of systemic lupus erythematosus [In process citation]. *Am J Med* 2000;**109**(8):628–34.

53. Boers M. Understanding the window of opportunity concept in early rheumatoid arthritis. *Arthritis Rheum* 2003;**48**(7):1771–4.

54. Cush JJ. Early rheumatoid arthritis—is there a window of opportunity? *J Rheumatol Suppl* 2007;**80**:1–7.

Chapter 48

Overlap Syndromes

Eric L. Greidinger

Division of Rheumatology, Miami VAMC, University of Miami Miller School of Medicine, Miami, FL, USA

SUMMARY

Overlap syndromes are inflammatory rheumatic conditions in which patients have clinical manifestations suggestive of multiple distinct immune diseases. The diseases most commonly involved in overlap syndromes include rheumatoid arthritis, lupus, scleroderma, and myositis. The most well-characterized overlap syndrome, mixed connective tissue disease (MCTD), is defined by anti-RNP autoimmunity along with features of at least two of these four conditions, and very often includes sufficient lupus manifestations to fulfill the SLICC lupus classification criteria. Overlap syndromes are generally less common than the conditions they encompass; the prevalence of MCTD, for example, is approximately one-twentieth that of SLE. Some autoantigen systems are particularly linked with overlap syndromes, such as RNP in MCTD. Overlap syndromes provide unique opportunities to understand links between autoimmunity and end organ immune targeting. While insights can be extrapolated from studies of disease processes present in overlap, few treatment trials have focused specifically on overlap syndromes themselves.

INTRODUCTION

Overlap syndromes are inflammatory rheumatic conditions in which patients have simultaneous clinical manifestations suggestive of multiple distinct immune diseases. A well-described and relatively common example of an overlap syndrome is mixed connective tissue disease (or MCTD), a condition characterized by the presence of anti-small nuclear ribonucleoprotein (snRNP, or RNP) autoantibodies in association with clinical manifestations of at least two of the following conditions: lupus, myositis, rheumatoid arthritis, and/or scleroderma.[1] As the example of MCTD illustrates, overlap syndromes can include features of two or more than two conditions. Moreover, patients with overlap syndromes need not meet classification criteria for any or all of the underlying conditions. Thus, a patient with an undefined connective tissue disease (or UCTD), who has evidence of an inflammatory rheumatic syndrome but who does not meet classification criteria for any individual condition, may also have a

rheumatic overlap syndrome.[2] The relationships among the general category of overlap syndromes, the specific overlap syndrome MCTD, and the entity of UCTD are shown in a Venn diagram (Figure 1).

CLINICAL AND LABORATORY MANIFESTATIONS OF OVERLAP SYNDROMES

It is illuminating to contemplate how a patient can be felt to have a condition that is, for example, "lupus-like" (or "scleroderma-like," etc.) without necessarily being lupus itself. Many of the manifestations of inflammatory rheumatic diseases are nonspecific for any particular clinical syndrome. Inflammatory arthritis, for example, is a common manifestation of either lupus or rheumatoid arthritis, and is not uncommon in scleroderma or myositis. Even requiring that the joint involvement be symmetrically distributed in the fingers and wrists excluding the distal interphalangeal joints, while more typical for rheumatoid arthritis, would still be a manifestation seen with at least modest frequency in other inflammatory rheumatic diseases. Rather, to be regarded as "rheumatoid arthritis-like," inflammatory arthritis would typically not only have to involve a typical small joint and symmetrical pattern but also have additional features distinctive to rheumatoid arthritis, such as the presence of typical joint erosions, rheumatoid nodules, and/or autoantibodies that are relatively specific for this condition (such as anti-CCP or other similar anti-citrullinated peptide antibodies).

Distinctions of this sort may be reflective both of differences in underlying disease pathogenesis and of patterns of human perception and cognition: If particular clinical manifestations occur frequently enough in the setting of an otherwise well-defined clinical syndrome, they will likely be regarded as part of the same syndrome rather than as a secondary phenomenon, unless there is a preexisting cognitive schema that conflicts with such a conceptualization. The tendency for disparate clinical manifestations to be lumped together into a unifying diagnosis can be recognized particularly aptly in the case of systemic lupus, where the SLICC classification criteria

Systemic Lupus Erythematosus. http://dx.doi.org/10.1016/B978-0-12-801917-7.00048-6

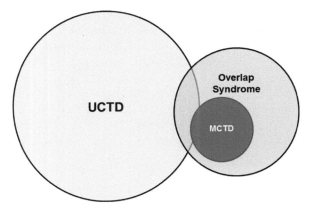

FIGURE 1 Relationship of overlap syndromes to undefined connective tissue disease (UCTD) and to mixed connective tissue disease (MCTD). Some overlap syndromes may have features of multiple rheumatic diseases but not meet classification criteria for any, and thus can be classified as cases of UCTD. MCTD is a subset of overlap syndromes in which anti-RNP antibodies are present. Some MCTD patients may have features of multiple rheumatic diseases but also not meet classification criteria for any of the underlying rheumatic conditions. By virtue of meeting MCTD classification criteria, these cases that would otherwise be considered UCTD no longer meet the definition of UCTD.

could be satisfied by four patients in whom zero clinical or laboratory manifestations were shared.[3] If manifestations that are regarded as aspects of an overlap syndrome occurred more frequently in the setting of an individual disease, those manifestations might either be regarded as additional canonical aspects of that disease or, at least, as nonspecific findings that would not raise the question of whether a "second disease process" was also present.

The point prevalence of MCTD is approximately 3.8 cases per 100,000 adults,[4] roughly 20-fold less prevalent than SLE.[5,6] In analyses of two substantial single center cohorts of patients with anti-RNP autoantibodies, including dozens of patients clinically classified as MCTD, we have found that lupus criteria were satisfied in an overwhelming majority.[7] This difference in the prevalence of "pure" lupus versus the prevalence of this "lupus overlap" syndrome may explain why, at a time when the pathophysiological differences between SLE and MCTD cannot be confidently articulated, MCTD overlap features are not themselves regarded as canonical aspects of lupus. However, it is also worth noting that distinguishing MCTD from SLE has been controversial.[8] This 20-fold difference in prevalence may thus represent an approximate upper limit of the prevalence of an adjunctive syndrome (in the setting of uncertain underlying pathological differences) before it would be considered as a more integral aspect of the more common diagnosis.

Other relatively common clinical manifestations of inflammatory rheumatic diseases that can be associated with multiple individual conditions and are thus difficult to use as evidence for the presence of any particular component of an overlap syndrome include fatigue, serositis, small

vessel vasculitis, and mild Raynaud's phenomenon. Sicca complaints in association with another inflammatory rheumatic disease are generally regarded as secondary Sjogren's syndrome, and are typically also not regarded as a classical overlap syndrome.

Likewise, common laboratory findings in multiple inflammatory rheumatic diseases that thus are not incongruous in the absence of an overlap syndrome include anemia and other cytopenias, elevated acute phase reactants (such as sedimentation rate or C-reactive protein), the presence of anti-nuclear antibodies (ANA), and rheumatoid factor positivity. Additional autoantibodies including Ro/SS-A, La/SS-B, and anti-phospholipid antibodies are also relatively nonspecific for any particular rheumatic condition.

Clinical manifestations that are more suggestive of specific diagnoses that if present concurrently could suggest an overlap syndrome also include the following. Manifestations of a lupus-like overlap syndrome not typically seen in other conditions including typical malar, photosensitive, or discoid rashes (except in dermatomyositis), typical patterns of alopecia, and glomerulonephritis. For scleroderma-like overlap, suggestive findings include cutaneous or visceral fibrosis, gut hypomotility, and severe Raynaud's phenomenon with digital pits or even more prominent ischemic changes. For myositis-like overlap, suggestive findings include clinically significant proximal muscle weakness and classic skin manifestations including heliotrope eyelid rashes, Gottron's papules, and mechanic's hands. While relatively pathognomonic clinical findings exist in additional inflammatory rheumatic syndromes (such as pathergy in Behcet's syndrome, amaurosis fugax in giant cell arteritis, or sausage digits in psoriatic arthritis), the predominance of reports of clinical overlap syndromes are confined to the four cardinal conditions (lupus, rheumatoid arthritis, scleroderma, and/or myositis) seen in overlap in MCTD.

The existence of a clinical overlap syndrome can also be associated with a modulation of the risk or responsiveness to treatment of specific clinical manifestations of the underlying diseases. For example, MCTD has traditionally been regarded as associated with a more benign prognosis than classic lupus,[9] even though the presence of anti-RNP antibodies in classic lupus has been linked to more aggressive disease manifestations.[10] We have recently found that in anti-RNP+ patients meeting classification criteria for systemic lupus erythematosus, the patients who also meet classification criteria for MCTD do have a dramatically lower risk of nephritis compared to those who do not also meet MCTD criteria (odds ratio 4.3 (95% confidence interval 1.3–14.0)).[7] The lung disease in MCTD has likewise been found to be more responsive to immunosuppressive therapy than has typically been observed in scleroderma or myositis.[11]

The modulation of risk associated with an overlap syndrome is not always in a favorable direction, however. In MCTD, the rate of development of lung disease including pulmonary hypertension may be as high as 40%,[7] substantially higher than that reported in unselected cohorts of SLE.[12]

Laboratory studies that may contribute to the suspicion of an individual condition (which could then be a component of an overlap syndrome with other conditions) encompass other relatively specific lab findings, typically specific autoantibodies. Thus, for lupus-like overlap, anti-double-stranded DNA (or anti-native DNA) and anti-Smith antibodies are suggestive, as are classic immunofluorescence and/or electron microscopic patterns on renal biopsy assessment of glomerulonephritis. For scleroderma-like overlap, anti-Scl-70 or other scleroderma-associated anti-nucleolar antibodies may be suggestive. For myositis-like overlap, antibodies including Mi-2 and anti-signal recognition particle may be suggestive. The findings of classic autoantibodies associated with other rheumatic diseases may also lead to consideration of an overlap syndrome, even outside of the four classic rheumatic syndromes described above. This can occur, for example, with anti-neutrophil cytoplasmic antibodies, when confirmed by ELISA for vasculitis-associated specificities and in the clinical context of vasculitic features.

An additional set of autoantibodies has been associated with specific overlap syndromes. These include anti-RNP (with MCTD), anti-PM-Scl (with a scleroderma-myositis overlap syndrome), and anti-Jo-1 or similar anti-tRNA synthetase antibodies (with the antisynthetase syndrome, typically characterized by features including myositis, interstitial lung disease, Raynaud's phenomenon, and erosive polyarthritis). Antisynthetase syndrome is a notable case of overlap syndrome, since anti-Jo-1 antibodies (and aspects of the associated syndrome) are the most common myositis-specific antibody system present in myositis cohorts, potentially contradicting the idea that overlap syndromes are always uncommon manifestations of cardinal rheumatic diseases.[13] This can be explained in part by the fact that the high prevalence of overlap features was identified many years after Jo-1 was linked to myositis, and potentially by the fact that the conditions that occur in overlap with myositis in antisynthetase syndrome are themselves more prevalent. While anti-centromere antibodies are most typical of the CREST syndrome form of scleroderma, these have also been linked to a scleroderma/primary biliary cirrhosis overlap syndrome.[14]

When can a systemic inflammatory rheumatic disease presenting along with second organ-specific autoimmune process be considered an overlap syndrome? There is no clear consensus. Entities such as inflammatory bowel disease-associated arthropathy, for example, in which features of a seronegative spondyloarthropathy and inflammatory enteritis coexist, have not been typically regarded as overlap syndromes. Considering the relatively high prevalence of autoimmune thyroid disease in the general population, there has been a hesitancy to regard thyroid disease plus an inflammatory rheumatic disease as an overlap syndrome, even if highly linked temporally in onset. Multiple sclerosis can be difficult to diagnose as in overlap with lupus, since the clinical and immunological manifestations of neuropsychiatric lupus could be difficult to distinguish from those of MS. On the other hand, the co-occurrence of myositis and myasthenia gravis may be identified clinically, and has recently been found to be associated with a common autoimmune target, cortactin.[15,16] Thus, recognizing the co-occurrence of multiple seemingly distinct immune conditions as potentially due to an overlap syndrome may lead to insight regarding the pathogenesis of each.

IMMUNOLOGY OF OVERLAP SYNDROMES

To the extent that rheumatoid arthritis, lupus, scleroderma, and myositis comprise the most typical elements of rheumatic overlap syndromes, this could be accounted for by similarities in the immune responses that typify each of these conditions when considered in isolation. Each of these conditions have been characterized as associated with type I interferon activation, with largely indistinguishable mediators along this pathway.[17] This type I interferon signature is typical for the response of a sustained cellular response against disease-associated molecular patterns, such as those induced by agonists of Toll-like receptors or other innate immune alarmins. Such signals may be produced by dendritic cells or other antigen-presenting cells with dendritic cell-like properties.

Rheumatoid arthritis, lupus, scleroderma, and myositis are also all conditions in which evidence for the presence of antigen-specific B- and T-cell responses exists, including evidence of isotype switching, affinity maturation, and both intra- and intermolecular epitope spreading. In some cases, as with RNP and dsDNA responses, the antigen-driven disease-specific responses have already been linked with native adjuvant activities that can also drive the dendritic cell-like innate immune responses.[18,19]

Autoantigen targets in each of these conditions have been reported to be susceptible to forms of antigen modification that may facilitate breaking of immune tolerance. Autoantigens associated with each of these conditions have been found to be susceptible to neoepitope creation by granzyme B-mediated enzymatic cleavage.[20] Most of these conditions have also been linked to other forms of autoantigen modification that may be more particular to individual conditions. In rheumatoid arthritis, autoantigen citrullination has been observed as an important phenomenon even in early disease and in extraarticular disease.[21,22] In lupus, recognition of apoptotically modified fragments of autoantigens has been prominently recognized, while in scleroderma, metal-catalyzed oxidative cleavage of disease-associated autoantigens has been observed.[23] While a general scheme of autoantigen modification in forms of myositis has not yet been articulated, there is already some evidence that unique abilities of Jo-1 to conjugate to endogenous adjuvants may be linked to the immunogenicity of this autoantigen in myositis.[24]

While other overlap syndromes have yet to be characterized immunologically at a similar level of detail, there is evidence that MCTD shares immune as well as clinical features with rheumatoid arthritis, lupus, scleroderma, and myositis. MCTD patients show evidence of type I interferon activation (and a pattern of inflammatory cytokine production) that is not distinguishable from that seen in lupus.[7] The snRNP autoantigens, linked clinically to MCTD, U1-RNP, and particularly its 70 kDa protein subunit (U1-70k), is susceptible to antigenic modification by granzyme B cleavage, by apoptotic caspase cleavage (like many lupus autoantigens), and by (scleroderma-like) metal-catalyzed oxidation.[20,23] Additionally, the fact that the U1-RNP complex is part of the primordial spliceosome complex that is largely conserved with organisms without highly developed immune systems may contribute to its tendency to induce autoimmunity, since the U1-RNA subunit is not extensively posttranslationally modified to avoid reactivity with innate immune pattern recognition receptors.

MCTD also has aspects of immunologic distinctiveness from these other conditions. While the hnRNP A2/B1 protein autoantigen targeted in both RA and SLE is also targeted in MCTD, in MCTD the pattern of epitopes targeted is notably different, with a more restricted pattern of epitope targeting.[25] MCTD also has been found to be more strongly associated with pulmonary disease including interstitial lung disease and pulmonary hypertension than rheumatoid arthritis or lupus.[9] In an animal model of anti-RNP autoimmunity, we have found that the interstitial lung disease and plexiform vasculopathy similar to that seen in human MCTD patients developed in an apparently TLR3/TRIF-dependent manner.[26]

The scleroderma/myositis overlap syndrome characterized by anti-PM/Scl antibodies occurs in less than 10% of scleroderma cases, and is associated with a more mild clinical picture regarding lung and gastrointestinal scleroderma manifestations.[27] However, among patients expressing antibodies to both PM/Scl and dsDNA, an overlap syndrome that also meets classification criteria for lupus is seen.[28] As with U1-RNA and the spliceosome, the fact that PM-Scl autoantigens are part of the primordial exosome may likewise increase that potential of these antigens to induce innate immune pattern recognition through diverse pathways.[29]

The relevance of the antigen specificity of the immune responses in rheumatoid arthritis, lupus, scleroderma, myositis, MCTD, and other overlap syndromes is presumably due to the distinctive pathogenic potential of the different antigen/adjuvant specificities. Immune transfer animal models have demonstrated how immunity to particular specificities, even if the antigens/adjuvants targeted may be widely expressed, can induce tissue-specific disease manifestations that are highly correlated with individual aspects of specific inflammatory rheumatic diseases. Examples include the K/BxN serum transfer model of rheumatoid arthritis, and anti-RNP T-cell transfers linked with lupus-like nephritis.[30,31] Within the sphere of anti-RNP overlap syndromes, we have also reported that U1-RNP-stimulated dendritic cells can transfer MCTD-like lung disease, potentially linking this immune phenomenon with other patterns of dendritic cell overactivity that have been linked to scleroderma.[32,33] Meanwhile cases of anti-RNP associated neonatal lupus illustrate that anti-RNP autoantibodies, coupled with sunlight-induced pattern recognition receptor activation, may be sufficient to confer lupus-like photosensitive skin disease.[34,35] Further studies may identify additional tissue targeting determinants of the autoimmune responses seen in rheumatic diseases. These may not only serve to help understand the pathogenesis of these conditions overall, but to assist in the risk assessment and therapeutic planning for individual patients, depending on the immune deviations and associated organ targeting risks identified.

GENETICS

Given the similarities in the immune responses seen among rheumatoid arthritis, lupus, scleroderma, myositis, and MCTD, it is not surprising that to the extent that these conditions have been characterized, many similar patterns of genetic susceptibility have emerged. Even more generally, a series of genetic risk factors for an even more broadly defined risk of autoimmunity, typically also encompassing risk for thyroid disease, type 1 diabetes mellitus, and forms of inflammatory bowel disease have been identified. Many of the risk loci that have been identified to date have functions directly relatable to enhancing immune reactivity, at the B-cell, T-cell, or innate immune levels.[36] When additional loci that are associated with individual diagnoses have been found, these often appear to relate more to factors that predispose toward the recognition of a particular autoantigen and/or self-adjuvant such as Class II HLA polymorphisms, or, for example, in the case of lupus the associations of genes linked with impaired apoptotic debris clearance, or to factors that may be implicated in the organ-specific expression of particular disease manifestations (such as potentially renal toxicity factors linked to lupus nephritis).[37–39]

In each case where features of multiple immune disorders are present, the question may be posed whether the disorders are co-occurring but pathogenically separable, or whether all of the aspects of immune disease relate to a common immunopathology. This is in some ways akin to asking, in a patient with genetic (and/or environmental) cancer risk factors, whether a new tumor appearing in a previously uninvolved organ represents spread of old disease, a "second primary" of the same tissue type, or the development of a pathophysiologically distinct co-occurring lesion. In some cases where multiple autoimmune processes co-occur, as in anti-RNP autoimmunity in MCTD, linking multiple different disease manifestations back to the same autoimmune insult can be reasonably inferred. In other cases, where two autoimmune processes are separable both temporally and antigenically (such as a patient who develops type 1 diabetes mellitus as a child and then develops rheumatoid arthritis in her 40s), it may be intuitive to consider the two autoimmune diseases to be fundamentally separable. However, we have recently found that a shared set of pathogenic T-cell specificities have been recovered predominantly from patients with autoimmune conditions, including diseases as diverse as anti-RNP autoimmunity, rheumatoid arthritis, and type 1 diabetes, suggesting that even in such seemingly disparate cases, the presence of an immunopathological component of overlap cannot be easily dismissed.[31]

ANIMAL MODELS

Some autoimmune-prone animal models have features consistent with multiple cardinal human rheumatic diseases. While primarily considered as a lupus model, for example, the MRL/lpr murine system has also been studied (with the addition of superantigen stimulation) as a model system for rheumatoid arthritis.[40] While Trex1-deficient mice have been studied primarily as a model of myocarditis or of lupus, we have found that these mice also show spontaneous induction of anti-RNP autoantibodies, and can develop MCTD-like lung manifestations similar to those we have previously reported in induced anti-RNP autoimmunity.[19,31] These findings suggest that the Trex1 nuclease may play an important role in the digestion of immunogenic RNAs (such as U1-RNA) in addition to its roles in DNA degradation. Adoptive transfer studies with our induced anti-RNP models have shown how different aspects of the same anti-RNP immune response can potentially mediate distinct disease manifestations including nephritis and lung disease.[32]

TREATMENT

Even for MCTD, the most well-characterized overlap syndrome for which widely adopted formal classification criteria exist, few treatment trials in human subjects have been conducted. Compensating somewhat for this glaring lack of direct experimental data is the fact that patients with clinical overlap syndromes have often not been excluded from clinical trials in other defined rheumatic diseases. Thus, patients meeting classification criteria for MCTD may be found at moderate frequency in lupus clinical trials, for example. To the extent that overlap syndromes represent the coexpression of pathologic manifestations as seen in the underlying cardinal rheumatic diseases, interventions that help the underlying conditions would be expected to have similar efficacy in overlap syndromes. However, the immunopathology present in at least some aspects of overlap

syndromes may be unique to these conditions, making the effects of treatments proven in nonoverlap rheumatic diseases potentially unpredictable in overlap syndromes. As an example of this kind of stratification of drug effects in lupus subsets, it is notable that anti-RNP responses may be relatively resistant to the treatment effects of anti-CD20-mediated B-cell depletion.[41]

REFERENCES

1. Alarcón-Segovia D, Cardiel MH. Comparison between 3 diagnostic criteria for mixed connective tissue disease: study of 593 patients. *J Rheumatol* 1989;**16**(3):328–34.
2. Bodolay E, Csiki Z, Szekanecz Z, Ben T, Kiss E, Zeher M, et al. Five-year follow-up of 665 Hungarian patients with undifferentiated connective tissue disease (UCTD). *Clin Exp Rheumatol* 2003;**21**(3):313–20.
3. Petri M, Orbai AM, Alarcón GS, Gordon C, Merrill JT, Fortin PR, et al. Derivation and validation of the Systemic Lupus International Collaborating Clinics classification criteria for systemic lupus erythematosus. *Arthritis Rheum* 2012;**64**(8):2677–86.
4. Gunnarsson R, Molberg O, Gilboe IM, Gran JT, PAHNOR1 Study Group. The prevalence and incidence of mixed connective tissue disease: a national multicentre survey of Norwegian patients. *Ann Rheum Dis* 2011;**70**(6):1047–51.
5. Somers EC, Marder W, Cagnoli P, Lewis EE, DeGuire P, Gordon C, et al. Population-based incidence and prevalence of systemic lupus erythematosus: the Michigan Lupus Epidemiology and Surveillance program. *Arthritis Rheumatol* 2014;**66**(2):369–78.
6. Lim SS, Bayakly AR, Helmick CG, Gordon C, Easley KA, Drenkard C. The incidence and prevalence of systemic lupus erythematosus, 2002–2004: the Georgia Lupus Registry. *Arthritis Rheumatol* 2014;**66**(2):357–68.
7. Carpintero MF, Martinez L, Fernandez I, Garza Romero AC, Mejia C, Zang Y, et al. Diagnosis and risk stratification in patients with anti-RNP autoimmunity. *Lupus* 2015 Sep;**24**(10):1057–66.
8. Aringer M, Steiner G, Smolen JS. Does mixed connective tissue disease exist? Yes. *Rheum Dis Clin North Am* 2005;**31**(3):411–20. v.
9. Burdt MA1, Hoffman RW, Deutscher SL, Wang GS, Johnson JC, Sharp GC. Long-term outcome in mixed connective tissue disease: longitudinal clinical and serologic findings. *Arthritis Rheum* 1999;**42**(5):899–909.
10. Kirou KA, Lee C, George S, Louca K, Peterson MG, Crow MK. Activation of the interferon-alpha pathway identifies a subgroup of systemic lupus erythematosus patients with distinct serologic features and active disease. *Arthritis Rheum* 2005;**52**(5):1491–503.
11. Jais X, Launay D, Yaici A, Le Pavec J, Tchérakian C, Sitbon O, et al. Immunosuppressive therapy in lupus- and mixed connective tissue disease-associated pulmonary arterial hypertension: a retrospective analysis of twenty-three cases. *Arthritis Rheum* 2008;**58**(2):521–31.
12. Li M, Zhang W, Leng X, Li Z, Ye Z, Li C, et al. Chinese SLE Treatment and Research group (CSTAR) registry: I. Major clinical characteristics of Chinese patients with systemic lupus erythematosus. *Lupus* 2013;**22**(11):1192–9.
13. Hamaguchi Y, Fujimoto M, Matsushita T, Kaji K, Komura K, Hasegawa M, et al. Common and distinct clinical features in adult patients with anti-aminoacyl-tRNA synthetase antibodies: heterogeneity within the syndrome. *PLoS One* 2013;**4**:e60442. http://dx.doi.org/10.1371/journal.pone.0060442. Epub April 3, 2013.

14. Liberal R, Grant CR, Sakkas L, Bizzaro N, Bogdanos DP. Diagnostic and clinical significance of anti-centromere antibodies in primary biliary cirrhosis. *Clin Res Hepatol Gastroenterol* 2013;**37**(6):572–85.

15. Paik JJ, Corse AM, Mammen AL. The co-existence of myasthenia gravis in patients with myositis: a case series. *Semin Arthritis Rheum* 2014;**43**(6):792–6.

16. Berrih-Aknin S. Cortactin: a new target in autoimmune myositis and Myasthenia Gravis. *Autoimmun Rev* 2014;**13**(10):1001–2.

17. Higgs BW, Liu Z, White B, Zhu W, White WI, Morehouse C, et al. Patients with systemic lupus erythematosus, myositis, rheumatoid arthritis and scleroderma share activation of a common type I interferon pathway. *Ann Rheum Dis* 2011;**70**(11):2029–36.

18. Greidinger EL, Zang Y, Martinez L, Jaimes K, Nassiri M, Bejarano P, et al. Differential tissue targeting of autoimmunity manifestations by autoantigen-associated Y RNAs. *Arthritis Rheum* 2007;**56**(5):1589–97.

19. Ahn J, Ruiz P, Barber GN. Intrinsic self-DNA triggers inflammatory disease dependent on STING. *J Immunol* 2014;**193**(9):4634–42.

20. Casciola-Rosen L, Andrade F, Ulanet D, Wong WB, Rosen A. Cleavage by granzyme B is strongly predictive of autoantigen status: implications for initiation of autoimmunity. *J Exp Med* 1999;**190**(6):815–26.

21. Goëb V, Thomas-L'Otellier M, Daveau R, Charlionet R, Fardellone P, Le Loët X, et al. Candidate autoantigens identified by mass spectrometry in early rheumatoid arthritis are chaperones and citrullinated glycolytic enzymes. *Arthritis Res Ther* 2009;**11**(2):R38.

22. Harlow L, Rosas IO, Gochuico BR, Mikuls TR, Dellaripa PF, Oddis CV, et al. Identification of citrullinated hsp90 isoforms as novel autoantigens in rheumatoid arthritis-associated interstitial lung disease. *Arthritis Rheum* 2013;**65**(4):869–79.

23. Greidinger EL, Casciola-Rosen L, Morris SM, Hoffman RW, Rosen A. Autoantibody recognition of distinctly modified forms of the U1-70-kd antigen is associated with different clinical disease manifestations. *Arthritis Rheum* 2000;**43**(4):881–8.

24. Fernandez I1, Harlow L, Zang Y, Liu-Bryan R, Ridgway WM, Clemens PR, et al. Functional redundancy of MyD88-dependent signaling pathways in a murine model of histidyl-transfer RNA synthetase-induced myositis. *J Immunol* 2013;**191**(4):1865–72.

25. Skriner K1, Sommergruber WH, Tremmel V, Fischer I, Barta A, Smolen JS, et al. Anti-A2/RA33 autoantibodies are directed to the RNA binding region of the A2 protein of the heterogeneous nuclear ribonucleoprotein complex. Differential epitope recognition in rheumatoid arthritis, systemic lupus erythematosus, and mixed connective tissue disease. *J Clin Invest* 1997;**100**(1):127–35.

26. Greidinger EL, Zang Y, Jaimes K, Hogenmiller S, Nassiri M, Bejarano P, et al. A murine model of mixed connective tissue disease induced with U1 small nuclear RNP autoantigen. *Arthritis Rheum* 2006;**54**(2):661–9.

27. D'Aoust J, Hudson M, Tatibouet S, Wick J, Canadian Scleroderma Research Group, Mahler M, et al. Clinical and serologic correlates of anti-PM/Scl antibodies in systemic sclerosis: a multicenter study of 763 patients. *Arthritis Rheumatol* 2014;**66**(6):1608–15.

28. Mahler M, Greidinger EL, Szmyrka M, Kromminga A, Fritzler MJ. Serological and clinical characterization of anti-dsDNA and anti-PM/Scl double-positive patients. *Ann NY Acad Sci* August 2007;**1109**:311–21.

29. Staals RH, Pruijn GJ. The human exosome and disease. *Adv Exp Med Biol* 2011;**702**:132–42.

30. Matsumoto I, Lee DM, Goldbach-Mansky R, Sumida T, Hitchon CA, Schur PH, et al. Low prevalence of antibodies to glucose-6-phosphate isomerase in patients with rheumatoid arthritis and a spectrum of other chronic autoimmune disorders. *Arthritis Rheum* 2003;**48**(4):944–54.

31. Zang Y, Martinez L, Fernandez I, Pignac-Kobinger J, Greidinger EL.Conservation of pathogenic TCR homology across class II restrictions in anti-ribonucleoprotein autoimmunity: extended efficacy of T cell vaccine therapy. *J Immunol* 2014;**192**(9):4093–102.

32. Greidinger EL, Zang Y, Fernandez I, Berho M, Nassiri M, Martinez L, et al. Tissue targeting of anti-RNP autoimmunity: effects of T cells and myeloid dendritic cells in a murine model. *Arthritis Rheum* 2009;**60**(2):534–42.

33. van Bon L, Affandi AJ, Broen J, Christmann RB, Marijnissen RJ, Stawski L, et al. Proteome-wide analysis and CXCL4 as a biomarker in systemic sclerosis. *N Engl J Med* 2014;**370**(5):433–43.

34. Heelan K, Watson R, Collins SM. Neonatal lupus syndrome associated with ribonucleoprotein antibodies. *Pediatr Dermatol* 2013;**30**(4):416–23.

35. Bernard JJ, Cowing-Zitron C, Nakatsuji T, Muehleisen B, Muto J, Borkowski AW, et al. Ultraviolet radiation damages self noncoding RNA and is detected by TLR3. *Nat Med* August 2012;**18**(8):1286–90.

36. Baranzini SE. Symposium 2-1 the autoimmunome: similarities and differences among genetic susceptibility to common immune-related diseases. *Nihon Rinsho Meneki Gakkai Kaishi* 2014;**37**(4):261.

37. Morris DL, Fernando MM, Taylor KE, Chung SA, Nititham J, Alarcón-Riquelme ME, et al. MHC associations with clinical and autoantibody manifestations in European SLE. *Genes Immun* 2014;**15**(4):210–7.

38. Galvan MD, Hulsebus H, Heitker T, Zeng E, Bohlson SS. Complement protein C1q and adiponectin stimulate Mer tyrosine kinase-dependent engulfment of apoptotic cells through a shared pathway. *J Innate Immun* 2014;**6**(6):780–92.

39. Zhou XJ, Nath SK, Qi YY, Cheng FJ, Yang HZ, Zhang Y, et al. Brief Report: identification of MTMR3 as a novel susceptibility gene for lupus nephritis in northern Han Chinese by shared-gene analysis with IgA nephropathy. *Arthritis Rheumatol* 2014;**66**(10):2842–8.

40. Edwards 3rd CK, Zhou T, Zhang J, Baker TJ, De M, Long RE, et al. Inhibition of superantigen-induced proinflammatory cytokine production and inflammatory arthritis in MRL-lpr/lpr mice by a transcriptional inhibitor of TNF-alpha. *J Immunol* 1996;**157**(4):1758–72.

41. Cambridge G, Isenberg DA, Edwards JC, Leandro MJ, Migone TS, Teodorescu M, et al. B cell depletion therapy in systemic lupus erythematosus: relationships among serum B lymphocyte stimulator levels, autoantibody profile and clinical response. *Ann Rheum Dis* 2008;**67**(7):1011–6.

Chapter 49

Systemic Lupus Erythematosus and the Eye

Alastair K.O. Denniston[1,2], Erika M. Damato[3], Philip I. Murray[4]

[1]*Department of Ophthalmology, University Hospitals Birmingham NHS Foundation Trust, Birmingham, UK;* [2]*Academic Unit of Ophthalmology, University of Birmingham, Birmingham, UK;* [3]*Birmingham Midland Eye Centre, City Hospital, Birmingham, UK;* [4]*Academic Unit of Ophthalmology, University of Birmingham, City Hospital, Birmingham, UK*

INTRODUCTION

Ocular involvement is common in systemic lupus erythematosus (SLE), with around one-third of patients being affected to some extent. The most common complication is dry eye syndrome, which, though it may cause significant discomfort, is usually responsive to treatment and rarely affects vision. Sight-threatening complications are uncommon but include retinal vaso-occlusive disease, scleritis, and aggressive ocular surface disease (Table 1). Importantly, serious ocular complications may be a warning

TABLE 1 Clinical Presentations in SLE

Causes of "Red Eye"	Cornea	Keratoconjunctivitis Sicca[a]
		Keratitis (Non-KCS Forms)
	Episclera	Episcleritis
	Sclera	Scleritis
	Iris/ciliary body	Anterior uveitis
Causes of loss of vision	Cornea	Keratoconjunctivitis sicca (severe)
	Lens	Cataract[a]
	Vitreous	Vitreous hemorrhage (secondary to proliferative retinopathy)
	Retina	Severe vaso-occlusive retinopathy
		Central retinal vein occlusion (CRVO)
		Branch retinal vein occlusion (BRVO)
		Central retinal artery occlusion (CRAO)
		Branch retinal arteriole occlusion (BRAO)
		Exudative retinal detachment
	Choroid	Choroidopathy
		Choroidal effusion
		Choroidal infarction
	Optic nerve/visual pathway	Optic neuritis
		Anterior ischemic optic neuropathy
		Posterior ischemic optic neuropathy
		Optic chiasmopathy
		Cortical infarcts

[a]*Denotes common causes.*

Systemic Lupus Erythematosus. http://dx.doi.org/10.1016/B978-0-12-801917-7.00049-8

sign of inadequate systemic disease control. The ophthalmologist must therefore treat the ocular manifestations and ensure good liaison with other physicians to ensure that the systemic implications of ophthalmic inflammation are recognized.

THE ROLE OF OPHTHALMIC FEATURES IN THE CRITERIA FOR CLASSIFICATION AND DISEASE ACTIVITY

Despite its high prevalence among patients with SLE, ocular involvement does not form part of the classification criteria, neither as one of the 11 features in the American College of Rheumatologists classification criteria for SLE[1] nor as one of the 17 criteria listed by the SLE International Collaborating Clinics (SLICC) criteria.[2] The recognition of ocular manifestations is important both for the appropriate treatment of ocular disease *per se* and in some cases as an indicator of systemic disease activity, such as the correlation of severe retinopathy to active CNS disease.[3] The "ophthalmic system" is one of the nine categories considered in the updated British Isles Lupus Assessment Group disease activity index (BILAG 2004). The BILAG 2004 Index specifically lists orbital inflammation/myositis/proptosis, severe keratitis, severe scleritis, posterior uveitis, retinal/choroidal vaso-occlusive disease, optic neuritis, and anterior ischemic optic neuropathy as "category A" features (indicating severe disease activity with scoring based on the principle of the physician's intention to treat). In a validation study there was good reliability and physician agreement for the ocular activity index in this single series, which was sufficiently powered for patients with ocular involvement.[4]

CLINICAL PRESENTATION

Anterior Segment

Keratoconjunctivitis Sicca

Keratoconjunctivitis sicca (KCS, "dry eye syndrome") occurs due to secondary Sjögren syndrome and affects around 25% of patients with SLE. It is associated with the autoantibodies, anti-Ro (SSA) and anti-La (SSB). Patients may be asymptomatic, or have symptoms ranging from slight irritation to severe pain and blurred vision. Examination with a biomicroscope ("slit lamp") reveals a reduced tear meniscus with a tear film break-up time of under 10 s. Fluorescein drops and cobalt blue light highlight the corneal changes, which may include punctate epitheliopathy, mucus filaments, strands, or plaques. Additional staining with Lissamine Green eye drops reveals a typical "interpalpebral" pattern in which most staining is nasal and temporal to the corneal limbus.

The Schirmer test can be used to detect reduced tear production. If the test strip is wet by less than 5 mm after 5 min in the unanesthetized eye, this indicates severe tear deficiency. In one series of patients with SLE the median value was 7.5 mm.[5] Symptoms do not correlate well with signs in this context. Many more patients report "dry eyes" than have visible disease.[5] Conversely many asymptomatic patients do have some degree of keratoconjunctivitis sicca on clinical examination.

Other Corneal Disease

Interestingly, superficial punctate keratitis, even in the absence of KCS, may be observed in patients with SLE and DLE, with one series reporting evidence of corneal staining in as many as 21 out of 24 (88%) SLE patients.[6] A response to the immunomodulator quinacrine hydrochloride was noted, suggesting a direct autoimmune phenomenon. Occasionally, deeper corneal involvement may occur, resulting in peripheral ulcerative keratitis, interstitial keratitis, and keratoendotheliitis.[7]

Alterations in the measurement of intraocular pressure have been reported in patients with SLE due to altered biomechanical properties of the cornea. Such mechanical differences may occur from reduced corneal hysteresis and corneal resistance factor, which in turn lead to lower measured intraocular pressures when tested by applanation techniques.[8]

Episcleritis

Episcleritis is reported in up to 2% of SLE patients. Patients present with a red eye with mild (if any) discomfort. Clinically, either sectoral or diffuse injection of the episcleral vasculature, superficial to the sclera, will be seen.

Scleritis

Scleritis is reported in 1% of SLE patients and may indeed be the presenting feature.[9] Scleritis is classified anatomically into "anterior" and "posterior" forms.

Anterior scleritis is the most common type, classically presenting with a severely painful, deeply injected, "beefy red" eye. Involvement of the deeper vascular plexus (cf. episcleritis) is seen with either a "diffuse" or a "nodular" (i.e., focal and associated with a nodule) pattern. It is important to recognize the presence of tissue destruction indicative of "necrotizing scleritis," although this occurs rarely in SLE. Tissue thinning due to scleritis is seen as dark areas on the globe due to the underlying uveal tissue being revealed through the thinned sclera. This may cause high degrees of astigmatism, and in extreme cases globe perforation. Diffuse light (such as from a window) often reveals the degree of inflammation and scleral thinning more easily than the bright focal light of a slit lamp.

The less common "posterior scleritis" may present with ocular pain of variable severity (which may be referred to the brow or jaw), reduced vision, increased long-sightedness, double vision, or photopsia. On examination, features may include shallowing of the anterior chamber, choroidal folds or detachment, exudative retinal detachment, and edema of the macula or optic disc. There may also be lid edema, proptosis, lid retraction, and restricted ocular motility. B-scan ultrasound is the investigation of choice (see "Investigations").

Scleritis is potentially sight threatening and may be an indicator of significant systemic activity. Urgent referral to an ophthalmologist is warranted and systemic therapy is generally indicated.

Other Anterior Segment Complications

Rare anterior segment complications include iris neovascularization (rubeosis iridis, usually indicating severe retinal ischemia) and anterior uveitis, which may be isolated or associated with either scleritis or posterior segment inflammation.[10]

Orbits and Lids

Lid Disease

Both SLE and DLE may affect the eyelids resulting in raised scaly lesions resembling chronic blepharitis.[11] Lid biopsy reveals hyperkeratosis, focal intracellular edema and degeneration of the basal layer, and lymphocytic infiltrates especially around the vessels. The lids may also be involved in the classic malar rash of SLE.

Orbital Disease

Uncommonly SLE may be associated with orbital inflammation or periorbital edema. Orbital inflammation may present with acute proptosis, lid edema, conjunctival injection and chemosis, reduced motility, and raised intraocular pressure. It may mimic orbital cellulitis, thyroid-associated ophthalmopathy, or other forms of orbital inflammation. Orbital inflammation may include myositis or rarely panniculitis (lupus erythematosus profundus); significant orbital involvement may also be associated with DLE.[12] Myositis may be demonstrated by imaging using CT and/or B-scan ultrasound, and confirmed by biopsy. Episodes of orbital myositis may occur concomitantly with a generalized myositis.[13] Orbital inflammation may also be associated with acute ocular ischemia and posterior scleritis.[14] Rare complications include episodic periorbital edema, and septic cavernous sinus thrombosis in the presence of severe immunosuppression.

Posterior Segment

Classic Lupus Retinopathy

Classic lupus retinopathy presents with features including cotton wool spots, retinal hemorrhages, and vascular abnormalities such as arteriolar narrowing, capillary dilation, venous dilation, and tortuosity (see Figures 1–3). Retinal edema, hard exudates, and microaneurysms may also be seen.

The classic "lupus retinopathy" is strongly suggestive of active systemic disease. In one series, retinopathy was associated with active systemic disease in 88% of patients.[15] Although an older series reported the presence of retinopathy in up to 28% of SLE patients, this appears to be declining, presumably due to improved systemic control and earlier diagnosis. More recent studies suggest that its prevalence is nearer 10%, both in adults[16] and in children. Although mild retinopathy is usually asymptomatic, severe disease (and its complications) may be sight threatening, with reduced visual acuity, field defects, distortion, or floaters.

Severe Vaso-occlusive Retinopathy ("Retinal Vasculitis")

Severe vaso-occlusive retinopathy in SLE is rare, but carries a high rate of visual loss with significant visual loss reported in up to 80% of affected patients, and final visual acuity of <20/200 in 50%.[3] Furthermore, this form of retinopathy is strongly associated with the life-threatening complication of CNS lupus.[3] The presence of anti-phospholipid antibodies increases the risk of vaso-occlusive disease (ocular and CNS) by up to four times.[17] A similar retinopathy may also occur in primary antiphospholipid syndrome, although cotton wool spots are less common.

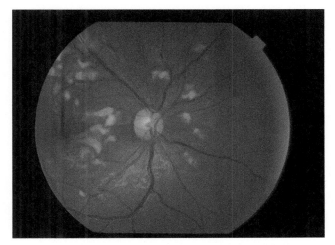

FIGURE 1 Acute lupus retinopathy with cotton wool spots, and narrowing and tortuosity of the retinal arterioles.

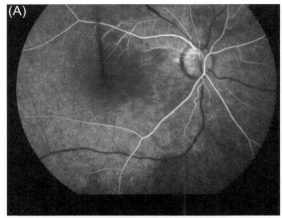

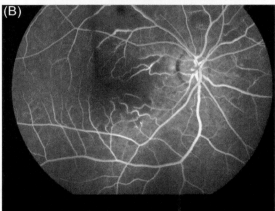

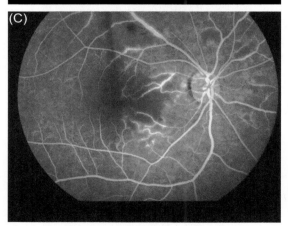

FIGURE 2   Fundus fluorescein angiography of the same patient: (A) early, (B) arteriovenous, and (C) late phases demonstrating capillary "dropout" staining of vessels walls and leakage.

Widespread retinal arteriolar occlusions and capillary nonperfusion are seen (see Figure 4), with subsequent neovascularization of the retina and iris being common (40–72% cases).[3] Proliferative retinopathy may lead to vitreous hemorrhage (up to 63%), retinal traction, and retinal detachment (up to 27%).[3] Fluorescein angiography is extremely valuable in revealing the extent of arterial

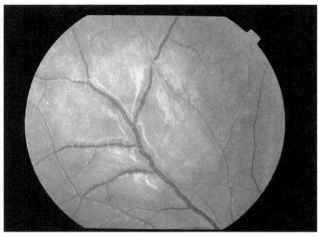

FIGURE 3   Retinal venous beading demonstrated on color fundus photograph of the same patient.

and capillary nonperfusion and leakage from neovascular fronds, and often highlights more extensive disease than is evident clinically.

Severe vaso-occlusive retinopathy is often described as a retinal vasculitis (Table 2); however, true vasculitic changes are not usually present on histologic examination. Microscopy of rare cadaveric specimens reveals hyaline thrombus formation with thickening of the vessel walls and presence of a perivascular infiltrate, in the absence of inflammation of the vessel wall itself.[18] Evidence from such histologic examinations suggests that ophthalmic involvement is perhaps more severe than is clinically apparent. One case study, reporting findings from a patient with lupus, noted degenerative changes of the pericytes and smooth muscle cells of the retinal blood vessels, with partial obliteration of capillary lumen and IgG deposition, despite no ocular disease having been detected clinically.[19]

Arteriole and Venule Occlusions

Occlusion of the larger retinal vessels is a well-recognized complication of SLE and is strongly associated with the presence of anti-phospholipid antibodies, such as anticardiolipin IgG. This may result in central and branch retinal artery occlusions, central and branch retinal vein occlusions, and combined retinal artery and vein occlusions.[3,18] A population-based cohort study from Taiwan published in 2013 found that the incidence of retinal vein occlusion was 3.5 times higher in patients with SLE compared to controls (5.61 vs 1.62 per 10,000 person-years); the risk was significantly higher in the presence of poorly controlled disease.[20] Around two-thirds of retinal vein occlusions in the context of SLE were reported to occur in the first 4 years after diagnosis.[20]

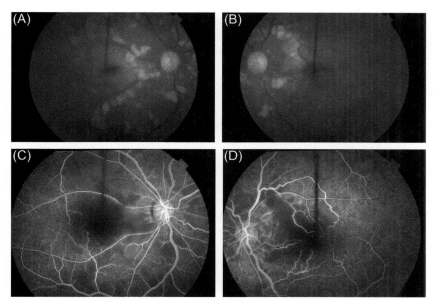

FIGURE 4 Severe vaso-occlusive retinopathy in a different patient. Color fundus photographs demonstrate more severe changes in both eyes including more extensive cotton wool spots in both eyes (A, B), and widespread occlusion of retinal arterioles and capillary "dropout" in both eyes confirmed on fluorescein angiography (C, D).

TABLE 2 Differential Diagnoses of Posterior Segment Disease in SLE

	Noninfectious	Infectious
Conditions that may mimic lupus retinopathy	Behçet's disease	Syphilis
	Granulomatosis with polyangiitis	Lyme disease
	Polyarteritis nodosa	Human immunodeficiency virus (HIV) retinopathy
	Scleroderma	Cytomegalovirus (CMV) retinitis
	Polymyositis	
	Dermatomyositis	
	Sarcoidosis	
	Accelerated hypertension	
	Central retinal vein occlusion (CRVO)	
	Diabetic retinopathy	
Conditions that may mimic lupus choroidopathy	Vogt–Koyanagi–Harada syndrome	
	Central serous chorioretinopathy	
	Sympathetic ophthalmia	
	Sarcoidosis	
	Choroidal metastases	

Other Retinal Manifestations

Rare complications of lupus include a bilateral peripheral pigmentary retinopathy that may mimic retinitis pigmentosa, which is thought to arise due to peripheral vaso-occlusive disease.[21] Hypertensive retinopathy may be seen and may be severe. Infectious complications, associated with the patient's abnormal immune system and/or their immunosuppressant therapy, include varicella zoster virus acute retinal necrosis and CMV retinitis. Exudative retinal detachment may arise due to underlying lupus choroidopathy.[22] As discussed earlier tractional retinal detachment may occur secondary to neovascularization from severe retinal vaso-occlusive disease.

Lupus Choroidopathy

Choroidal involvement is less common than lupus retinopathy but is an important cause of visual morbidity in SLE. Choroidopathy may result in single or multifocal serous detachments of the retina and retinal pigment epithelium (RPE), which mimic typical central serous chorioretinopathy (CSR) (Table 2). Central macular involvement may cause significant visual loss,[23,24] but eccentric lesions often have minimal symptoms. Lesions may progress to extensive exudative retinal detachment,[24] but generally reverse with control of the systemic disease.[24] Fluorescein angiography highlights areas of leakage from the choroid into the subretinal and sub-RPE spaces similar to that seen in typical CSR, but also reveals areas of choroidal ischemia suggestive of the presumed underlying cause.[24] Other choroidal manifestations include choroidal effusions, choroidal infarction, and choroidal neovascular membranes. Indocyanine green (ICG) angiography specifically highlights choroidal perfusion and can be useful in this context.

Neuro-Ophthalmic Complications

Optic Nerve Disease

Optic nerve disease occurs in around 1% of patients with SLE. Clinical presentations include acute optic neuritis and anterior or posterior ischemic optic neuropathy. These may indeed be the presenting feature of SLE. Histological examination reveals either demyelination or axonal necrosis, with ischemia presumed to be the primary cause in either case.[25] In contrast to these acute presentations, chronic retinal or optic nerve disease may result in slowly progressive visual loss and optic atrophy.[25] Bilateral optic disc swelling may indicate papilledema due to idiopathic intracranial hypertension or accelerated hypertension, both of which are more common in SLE.

Ocular Motility Abnormalities

Ocular motility abnormalities are fairly common in SLE, usually due to brain stem or other central disease, although cranial neuropathies, tenosynovitis, and myositis are also seen.[26] Acquired Brown's syndrome, a mechanical problem in which the free movement of the superior oblique muscle/tendon is limited, has been reported and may respond to systemic corticosteroids.[27] Such presentations may predate the diagnosis of SLE, with a case of bilateral sequential trochleitis being recorded 2 years prior to any systemic symptoms that led to the diagnosis of SLE.[28] Severe ophthalmoplegia due to Miller–Fisher syndrome has also been reported in a patient with SLE, which was refractory to conventional immunosuppression but responded to plasmapharesis. Other movement disorders reported include unilateral and rarely bilateral internuclear ophthalmoplegia

(INO),[29] one-and-a-half syndrome,[30] and skew deviations. Transient diplopia may be associated with anti-phospholipid antibodies, possibly due to disturbance of the posterior cerebral circulation. Horizontal and vertical nystagmus are also reported.

Retrochiasmal

CNS disease in SLE can cause a range of visual disorders including visual field defects that may be the first presentation of the disease. Severe occipital involvement may result in cortical blindness.[31] Migraine is common in SLE and both amaurosis fugax and typical fortification spectra are reported. As noted earlier, idiopathic intracranial hypertension is more common in SLE.[32]

INVESTIGATIONS

General

General investigations for suspected SLE are discussed elsewhere but include tests that are diagnostic (e.g., ANA, anti-dsDNA antibodies, anti-Sm antibodies, etc.), tests that assess thrombotic risk (anti-phospholipid antibodies such as anticardiolipin and lupus anticoagulant), and tests that assess disease activity (e.g., complement levels, anti-dsDNA antibody titer). Blood pressure measurement is also imperative.

Ophthalmic

Specific ophthalmic tests are used when clinically indicated.

Anterior Segment

For ocular surface disease: Schirmer's test to measure tear production and direct therapy.

Posterior scleritis: B-scan ultrasonography to detect signs including posterior scleral thickening (usually >1.5 mm) with fluid in Tenon's space (the "T-sign"); CT and MRI may also support the diagnosis.

Orbital disease: CT and/or MRI with contrast enhancement as indicated.

Neuro-ophthalmic disease: MRI with contrast enhancement as indicated; perimetry to document visual field status and monitor change over time.

Posterior Segment

Fundus photography is used to document clinical signs and to help monitor progression reliably. Fundus fluorescein angiography (FFA) is used to assess the retinal circulation, specifically for vaso-occlusion and leakage and to detect new vessels (see Figures 2 and 4). ICG angiography is used to assess the choroidal circulation. Optical coherence tomography (OCT) is used to noninvasively assess the macula.

Although originally limited to the detection of central structural changes in the retina, innovations in OCT hardware and image processing are enabling the adaptation of OCT for use in wide field (i.e., extramacular), enhanced depth (visualizes choroid as well as retina), and OCT angiography (high resolution imaging of the vasculature). This is clearly advantageous compared to the invasive techniques of fluorescein and ICG angiography. The major limitation compared to true angiography is that OCT is a static rather than a dynamic investigation; it shows where the fluid is (and the structural changes arising) rather than using contrast to detect the abnormal movement of fluid from vessels to tissue spaces.

TREATMENT

General

Control of the systemic disease activity is a vital part of controlling ophthalmic disease. Severe ophthalmic complications such as lupus retinopathy are uncommon in well-controlled patients and remission of scleritis, retinopathy, choroidopathy, and CNS lupus usually is usually associated with achieving systemic disease control. Severe ophthalmic disease is an indication for urgent rheumatological assessment and requires systemic treatment. The general principles of systemic treatment for SLE are discussed elsewhere but we would note that immunosuppression should only be managed by those with appropriate experience and facilities for monitoring.

Ophthalmic

Anterior Segment

Keratoconjunctivitis sicca secondary to SLE is primarily controlled with tear replacement therapy adjusted according to the needs of the patient. In very mild cases low viscosity drops (e.g., hypromellose, hydroxyethylcellulose, polyvinyl alcohol) may be sufficient; these have the advantage of causing minimal blurring of vision but only have a short duration of effect. More severe cases usually require combination therapy, e.g., daytime use of a carbomer, which has medium viscosity (and therefore longer duration of effect, but also more blurring of vision) and a paraffin at night, which has high viscosity (even longer-lasting effect but very significant blurring of vision). Preservative-free preparations are preferred when frequent administration is necessary or intolerance develops. Increasingly, sodium hyaluronate-based preparations are being used in addition to, or instead of, other tear replacement therapies. These appear to be effective in reducing dry eye symptoms and improving the health of the ocular surface. In extreme cases autologous serum may be used. These more severe cases should be under the care of an ophthalmologist.

Tear replacement therapy may be supplemented by lacrimal punctal occlusion, initially in the form of punctal plugs, which can be inserted at the slit lamp. Lid margin disease (such as blepharitis) should be looked for and treated. Topical corticosteroid or topical cyclosporin may be appropriate where there is clear evidence of ocular surface inflammation. Environmental modifications that can be trialled include lowering room temperatures, humidifiers, and moist chamber goggles.

Mild anterior segment inflammation, such as most non-KCS forms of keratitis, and anterior uveitis, can be treated with topical corticosteroids (or alternatively topical nonsteroidal anti-inflammatory drugs (NSAIDs) for episcleritis). Even in these milder forms of disease it is usually necessary to improve disease control with systemic therapy in order to maintain remission.

Systemic therapy is even more important in the presence of severe anterior segment inflammation (such as scleritis) or orbital inflammation. For mild, nonnecrotizing scleritis oral NSAIDs are usually used first line, and often sufficient. More severe disease usually requires oral corticosteroids (e.g., prednisone 1 mg/kg/day), but may be preceded by intravenous methylprednisolone (e.g., 500 mg–1 g daily for 3 days). Second-line agents include cyclophosphamide, azathioprine, mycophenolate, cyclosporin, methotrexate, and rituximab.

Posterior Segment

Retinopathy or choroidopathy is an indication for systemic treatment as described above. In unilateral or asymmetric retinal or choroidal disease this is occasionally supplemented by regional corticosteroid injections. Acute presentations of aggressive lupus retinopathy may be florid and can progress rapidly to visual loss. Evidence for the use of additional therapy such as plasmaphoresis or rituxmab is lacking, due to the rarity of such presentations. Despite this, such therapies delivered in a timely fashion could be of use in individual cases.

Retinal vascular occlusions particularly in the context of anti-phospholipid antibodies may be treated with corticosteroids, warfarin, and low-dose acetylsalicylic acid. Retinal neovascularization usually requires treatment with pan-retinal laser photocoagulation, to ablate the ischemic retina. Vitreo-retinal surgery may be required for nonclearing vitreous hemorrhage or tractional retinal detachment.

Neuro-ophthalmic

Neuro-ophthalmic complications reflect active CNS lupus and require systemic therapy as described above. In one small series of SLE-associated optic neuropathy four out of seven patients responded to corticosteroid therapy.[25] Cyclophosphamide may be effective either in conjunction with corticosteroids or in steroid-resistant cases.[33] Although these complications start with inflammation, it is ischemia that causes the permanent loss of function, with only a short window of opportunity to intervene with immunosuppressants to modify the underlying immune process and prevent axonal injury. The presence of anti-phospholipid antibodies in this context may be an indication for anticoagulation to treat and prevent recurrence of optic neuropathy.

Ophthalmic Complications of Systemic Therapy

Although interest tends to focus on chloroquine or hydroxychloroquine therapy, ophthalmic complications associated with corticosteroid treatment are more common. The association between exogenous corticosteroids and posterior subcapsular cataracts is well established. Cataract surgery in patients with SLE is generally very successful, although visual outcomes will be worse if there has been significant posterior segment disease. Exogenous corticosteroids are associated with increased intraocular pressure in up to 30% of the normal population with 5% experiencing an increase of more than 15 mm Hg (normal range 11–21 mm Hg). This steroid-induced ocular hypertension must be monitored (and often treated) to reduce progression to secondary glaucoma. Glaucoma manifests with the cupped optic disc(s) and corresponding visual field loss of glaucomatous optic neuropathy.

The aminoquinolones chloroquine and hydroxychloroquine have been widely used in the treatment of lupus. Both drugs can cause a keratopathy (cornea verticillata), which is visually insignificant and reversible with cessation of treatment. More importantly, both chloroquine and hydroxychloroquine can cause an irreversible sight-threatening maculopathy. Clinically this is seen as a progression from an initial loss of the foveal reflex to a fine granular macular appearance followed by a "bull's eye" maculopathy accompanied by a fall in visual acuity and a central scotoma. In end-stage disease this may be accompanied by generalized atrophy, peripheral pigmentation akin to retinitis pigmentosa, arteriolar attenuation, and optic atrophy.[34] Although both drugs may cause an identical retinopathy, clinically detectable retinopathy is much less common with hydroxychloroquine when used at currently recommended doses (<6.5 mg/kg/day).

Ophthalmic screening is recommended for all patients taking chloroquine.[35,36] For patients taking hydroxychloroquine the revised guidelines of the American Academy of Ophthalmology (AAO) published in 2011 advise a baseline examination comprising subjective tests (visual acuity, dilated fundus examination, and automated 10-2 Humphrey visual field examination) and at least one objective test (Spectral Domain (SD)–OCT, fundus autofluorescence (FAF), and/or multifocal electroretinography (mfERG)).[35] Further screening is then undertaken annually after 5 years of exposure or considered earlier in the presence of additional risk factors. These additional risk factors for HCQ toxicity are defined by the AAO as: (1) duration of use >5 years, (2) cumulative dose >1000 g, (3) daily dose >400 mg/day (>6.5 mg/kg ideal body weight for short individuals) for HCQ and >250 mg/day, (4) renal or hepatic dysfunction, (5) elderly, and (6) preexisting retinal disease or maculopathy. The risk factors for chloroquine are similar but with dosing thresholds set at total dose >460 g and daily dose of >250 mg/day (>3.0 mg/kg/day for short individuals). It is recognized, however, that retinal toxicity is occasionally seen in apparently low-risk individuals.[35,36]

In contrast, the UK recommendations from the Royal College of Ophthalmologists published jointly with the British Society for Rheumatology and the British Association of Dermatologists in 2009 are that low-risk patients do not need screening by an ophthalmologist.[36] They advise the following good practice points for prescribing rheumatologists or dermatologists: (1) maximum dose should not exceed 6.5 mg/kg lean body weight; (2) renal and liver function to be assessed at baseline; (3) ask about visual symptoms at baseline and annual review; (4) record near visual acuity (with reading glasses, if worn) for each eye at baseline and annual review. Patients with visual impairment should then be referred to an optometrist who can refer any significant abnormality not correctable with refraction to the local ophthalmologist in the usual way.[36]

When patients are referred to the ophthalmologist due to an abnormality at baseline or a deterioration in visual function the Royal College of Ophthalmologists guidelines advise that their assessment should include an enquiry about disturbances in their central vision, measurement of distance and near visual acuity, central visual field using either an Amsler chart (for which they recommend red on black) or automated perimetry (e.g., Humphrey 10-2 protocol), and biomicroscopic (slit-lamp) examination of the cornea and retina. The Royal College of Ophthalmologists' guidelines note that additional tests may be indicated, but do not advise that they form a standard part of the assessment.[36] It should be noted that the Royal College of Ophthalmologists' guidelines were published in 2009, and that since then there has been additional evidence to support the potential role of SD-OCT, FAF, and mfERG in detecting early toxicity. Furthermore, although the rate of symptomatic toxicity due to hydroxychloroquine remains low, the use of these newer modalities does indicate that early toxic changes at the macula are much more common than previously thought. Indeed a case–control study of 2361 patients using hydroxychloroquine for more than 5 years in an integrated health organization of 3.4 million members suggested that even at a "safe" daily dose of 4.0–5.0 mg/kg the prevalence of toxicity rose to 20% after 20 years usage; for the first 10 years of usage the prevalence in this group was less than 2%. Interestingly concurrent treatment with tamoxifen was noted to increase the risk of toxicity with an odds ratio of 4.6 (95% confidence intervals 2.1–10.3).[37]

CONCLUSION

Ocular manifestations of SLE, although infrequently severe, are important both in terms of their direct effects (pain, loss of vision, etc.) and in the information they provide as to overall disease activity. Severe retinal vaso-occlusive disease and optic neuropathy are strongly associated with active CNS involvement. As control of systemic disease activity has improved, severe ocular complications have become uncommon. SLE is, however, still a potentially blinding condition. Any visual symptoms require urgent ophthalmic assessment to identify sight-threatening disease requiring systemic therapy.

REFERENCES

1. Tan EM, Cohen AS, Fries JF, et al. The 1982 revised criteria for classification of systemic lupus erythematosus. *Arthritis Rheum* 1982;**25**:1271.
2. Petri M, Orbai AM, Alarcón GS, Gordon C, Merrill JT, et al. Derivation and validation of the Systemic Lupus International Collaborating Clinics classification criteria for systemic lupus erythematosus. *Arthritis Rheum* August 2012;**64**(8):2677–86.
3. Jabs DA, et al. Severe retinal vaso-occlusive disease in systemic lupus erythematous. *Arch Ophthalmol* 1986;**104**(4):558–63.
4. Isenberg DA, et al. BILAG 2004. Development and initial validation of an updated version of the British Isles Lupus Assessment Group's disease activity index for patients with systemic lupus erythematosus. *Rheumatology (Oxford)* 2005;**44**(7):902–6.
5. Jensen JL, et al. Oral and ocular sicca symptoms and findings are prevalent in systemic lupus erythematosus. *J Oral Pathol Med* 1999;**28**(7):317–22.
6. Spaeth GL. Corneal staining in systemic lupus erythematosus. *N Engl J Med* 1967;**276**(21):1168–71.
7. Messmer EM, Foster CS. Vasculitic peripheral ulcerative keratitis. *Surv Ophthalmol* 1999;**43**:379–96.
8. Yazici AT, Kara Yuksel K, Altinkaynak O, et al. The biomechanical properties of the cornea in patients with systemic lupus erythematosus. *Eye* 2011;**28**(8):1005–9.
9. Foster CS. Immunosuppressive therapy for external ocular inflammatory disease. *Ophthalmology* 1980;**87**(2):140–50.
10. Hickman RA, Denniston AK, Yee CS, et al. Bilateral retinal vasculitis in a patient with systemic lupus erythematosus and its remission with rituximab therapy. *Lupus* 2010;**19**(3):327–9.
11. Huey C, et al. Discoid lupus erythematosus of the eyelids. *Ophthalmology* 1983;**90**(12):1389–98.
12. Gupta T, Beaconsfield M, Rose GE, et al. Discoid lupus erythematosus of the periorbita: clinical dilemmas, diagnostic delays. *Eye* 2012;**26**(4):609–12.
13. Grimson BS, Simons KB. Orbital inflammation, myositis, and systemic lupus erythematosus. *Arch Ophthalmol* 1983;**101**(5):736–8.
14. Stavrou P, et al. Acute ocular ischaemia and orbital inflammation associated with systemic lupus erythematosus. *Br J Ophthalmol* 2002;**86**(4):474–5.
15. Stafford-Brady FJ, et al. Lupus retinopathy. Patterns, associations, and prognosis. *Arthritis Rheum* 1988;**31**(9):1105–10.
16. Ushiyama O, et al. Retinal disease in patients with systemic lupus erythematosus. *Ann Rheum Dis* 2000;**59**(9):705–8.
17. Asherson RA, et al. Antiphospholipid antibodies: a risk factor for occlusive ocular vascular disease in systemic lupus erythematosus and the 'primary' antiphospholipid syndrome. *Ann Rheum Dis* 1989;**48**(5):358–61.
18. Graham EM, et al. Cerebral and retinal vascular changes in systemic lupus erythematosus. *Ophthalmology* 1985;**92**(3):444–8.
19. Nag TC, Wadhwa S. Histopathological changes in the eyes in systemic lupus erythematosus: an electron microscope and immunohistochemical study. *Histol Histopathol* 2005;**20**(2):373–82.
20. Yen YC, Weng SF, Chen HA, et al. Risk of retinal vein occlusion in patients with systemic lupus erythematosus: a population-based cohort study. *Br J Ophthalmol* 2013;**97**(9):1192–6.
21. Sekimoto M, et al. Pseudoretinitis pigmentosa in patients with systemic lupus erythematosus. *Ann Ophthalmol* 1993;**25**(7):264–6.
22. Chan WM, et al. Bilateral retinal detachment in a young woman. *Lancet* 2003;**361**(9374):2044.
23. Cunningham Jr ET, Alfred PR, Irvine AR. Central serous chorioretinopathy in patients with systemic lupus erythematosus. *Ophthalmology* 1996;**103**(12):2081–90.
24. Jabs DA, et al. Choroidopathy in systemic lupus erythematosus. *Arch Ophthalmol* 1988;**106**(2):230–4.
25. Jabs DA, et al. Optic neuropathy in systemic lupus erythematosus. *Arch Ophthalmol* 1986;**104**(4):564–8.
26. Keane JR. Eye movement abnormalities in systemic lupus erythematosus. *Arch Neurol* 1995;**52**(12):1145–9.
27. McGalliard J, Bell AL. Acquired Brown's syndrome in systemic lupus erythematosus: another ocular manifestation. *Clin Rheumatol* 1990;**9**(3):399–400.
28. Fonseca P, Manno RLMN. Bilateral sequential trochleitis as the pesenting feature of systemic lupus erythematosus. *J Neuroophthalmol* 2013;**33**(1):74–6.
29. Galindo M, Pablos JL, Gomez-Reino JJ. Internuclear ophthalmoplegia in systemic lupus erythematosus. *Semin Arthritis Rheum* 1998;**28**(3): 179–86.
30. Yigit A, et al. The one-and-a-half syndrome in systemic lupus erythematosus. *J Neuroophthalmol* 1996;**16**(4):274–6.
31. Brandt KD, Lessell S, Cohen AS. Cerebral disorders of vision in systemic lupus erythematosus. *Ann Intern Med* 1975;**83**(2):163–9.
32. Kim JM, Kwok SK, Ju JH, Kim HY, Park SH. Idiopathic intracranial hypertension as a significant cause of intractable headache in patients with systemic lupus erythematosus: a 15-year experience. *Lupus* April 2012;**21**(5):542–7.
33. Rosenbaum JT, Simpson J, Neuwelt CM. Successful treatment of optic neuropathy in association with systemic lupus erythematosus using intravenous cyclophosphamide. *Br J Ophthalmol* 1997;**81**(2):130–2.
34. Hobbs HE, Sorsby A, Freedman A. Retinopathy following chloroquine therapy. *Lancet* 1959;**2**:478–80.
35. Marmor MF, Kellner U, Lai TY, American Academy of Ophthalmology, et al. Revised recommendations on screening for chloroquine and hydroxychloroquine retinopathy. *Ophthalmology* 2011;**118**:415–22. http://dx.doi.org/10.1016/j.ophtha.2010.11.017.
36. The royal college of ophthalmologists. *Hydroxychloroquine and ocular toxicity Recommendations on Screening*. October 2009. http://www.rcophth.ac.uk/core/core_picker/download.asp?id=165&filetitle=Ocular+Toxicity+and+Hydroxychloroquine%3A+Guidelines+for+Screening+2009 (last accessed 01.01.15).
37. Melles RB, Marmor MF. The risk of toxic retinopathy in patients on long-term hydroxychloroquine therapy. *JAMA Ophthalmol* December 1, 2014;**132**(12):1453–60.

Chapter 50

Pregnancy and Fertility in Systemic Lupus Erythematosus

Bonnie L. Bermas[1], Lisa R. Sammaritano[2]

[1]Brigham and Women's Hospital, Boston, MA, USA; [2]Hospital for Special Surgery, New York, NY, USA

SYSTEMIC LUPUS ERYTHEMATOSUS—A MANUAL

Systemic lupus erythematosus (SLE) is a disease of reproductive aged women; as a result, family planning issues such as fertility and pregnancy are an important component of the management of SLE patients. For many years, women who had systemic lupus erythematosus were counseled against becoming pregnant. This directive was founded in the belief that the hormonal and immunologic changes of pregnancy would exacerbate disease activity and contribute to maternal morbidity and poor fetal outcomes. However, with the improved management of SLE, this general prohibition against pregnancy in SLE has become obsolete. While SLE pregnancies are frequently complicated due to higher risk for disease exacerbation in the mother and potential for complications in the fetus, current management that includes careful planning, treatment, and monitoring most often results in successful pregnancy outcomes for these patients.

FERTILITY AND SLE

Fertility in stable SLE patients without identifiable risk factors appears to be comparable to that of the general population.[1] Studies do show a reduction in family size for women with SLE that may relate to effects of disease activity, disease damage, cytotoxic medications, and psychosocial factors.[2]

Etiology of Infertility

Significant causes of decreased fertility in SLE patients include advanced maternal age, active disease or disease-related damage, and medication effects. Onset of SLE is often during the early reproductive years, and given that patients are counseled to avoid pregnancy if disease has not been quiescent, many SLE patients are older when they attempt to conceive and may encounter difficulties related to an age-associated loss of ovarian reserve and oocyte quality.

Premature ovarian failure, defined as persistent amenorrhea with elevated FSH prior to age 40, is sometimes due to autoimmune etiologies but it is rare for these patients to exhibit signs of systemic autoimmune disease.[3] However, SLE patients may have menstrual disturbances or amenorrhea related to active disease.[4] Anti-Mullerian hormone (AMH) serum levels, a marker of ovarian reserve, have been reported to be lower in a group of non-cyclophosphamide-treated SLE patients than in age-matched healthy controls, although use of oral contraceptives and other medications differed between the two groups.[5]

Lupus patients with renal insufficiency or failure may develop hypofertility or infertility through a disruption of the hypothalamic–pituitary axis that can reverse with renal transplantation. While early reports proposed an association among anti-phospholipid antibodies (aPL), infertility, and poor in vitro fertilization (IVF) outcome, recent controlled studies do not support this association and so assessment or treatment for aPL for infertility in the absence of antiphospholipid syndrome with obstetrical complications is not recommended.[6]

Cyclophosphamide (CYC), used for severe lupus manifestations including nephritis and central nervous system disease, accounts for the majority of fertility issues in SLE patients. Patients administered CYC are more likely to maintain fertility if they are younger than 30 years old, the total number of monthly intravenous pulses is six or less, the cumulative dose is less than 7 g, and if there is no amenorrhea before or during administration.[7]

Nonsteroidal anti-inflammatory drugs (NSAIDs) are commonly used for control of mild SLE symptoms and have been suggested as a potential contributor to infertility. Despite experimental and anecdotal data suggesting that these drugs have the potential to interfere with normal follicular rupture and ovulation, systematic clinical data are lacking. High-dose corticosteroids may also affect the menstrual cycle, but it is difficult to distinguish effects of disease activity from those of the corticosteroid itself.

Systemic Lupus Erythematosus. http://dx.doi.org/10.1016/B978-0-12-801917-7.00050-4

Preservation of Fertility

Methods to preserve fertility in female SLE patients include minimizing use of cytotoxic medications, protection of the ovaries, or cryopreservation of ovarian tissue, cells, or embryos. Counseling and frank discussion regarding risk and benefit of both the CYC therapy and any suggested fertility prevention must be done with each individual patient. Every effort should be made to minimize the CYC total dose, especially in older patients. In practice, maximally effective therapy for severe disease to prevent damage and loss of function may dictate dosing. The use of the Euro-Lupus CYC regimen, mycophenolate mofetil, or other non-CYC combination therapies may be helpful in this regard when feasible.[1]

Treatment to provide ovarian protection from CYC effects with gonadotrophic hormone receptor (GnRH) agonists has become common practice, although the benefit of this therapy is still somewhat controversial. In the past, the traditional measure of infertility after CYC has been the development of amenorrhea; newer objective measures such as AMH level may provide a better assessment of ovarian reserve in the future. Administration of the GnRH agonist leuprolide at 10–14 days prior to CYC pulse therapy was shown to be protective against development of persistent amenorrhea in one large series,[8] and a recent meta-analysis calculated a 68% increase in rate of preserved ovarian function in treated versus untreated women.[9] GnRH-agonist therapy should not be administered immediately before CYC: if given in the follicular part of the cycle, it can stimulate the ovaries (potentially worsening ovarian damage) and increase estrogen levels.[10] As a result, patients are rarely treated with GnRH agonists before their first CYC infusion, but can be treated at monthly intervals mid-cycle thereafter.

Long-term preservation of fertility through cryopreservation techniques, while appealing in theory, presents a challenge when administration of CYC is deemed urgent (as is often the case for severe disease). Moreover, patient psychosocial issues and beliefs, the availability and success of advanced reproductive medical therapies, and financial constraints may limit use of these techniques. Cryopreservation of oocytes or embryos requires ovarian hyperstimulation, a procedure that involves a time delay in lupus treatment of at least 2 weeks as well as elevated levels of estrogen, both usually contraindicated in the setting of lupus flare. In contrast, increasing numbers of women in their early to mid-thirties in the general population are pursuing oocyte freezing for fertility preservation, in anticipation of IVF in future years. This fertility-preservation technique can be considered for SLE patients with stable inactive disease who are faced with age-related fertility concerns (discussed below).

Cryopreservation of ovarian tissue is an emerging technique available primarily through research protocols at this time, in which ovarian tissue is removed through laparoscopic oophorectomy, without the need for ovarian stimulation or significant time delay. Oocytes from the retrieved tissue may be matured in vitro and then frozen, or the ovarian tissue itself may be frozen in thin strips for later in vitro oocyte maturation or autotransplantation.[10] At present, when fertility is not or cannot be preserved with available methods, IVF utilizing a donor oocyte and partner's sperm provides an alternative option for pregnancy during a period of quiescent disease.

Assisted Reproductive Techniques

Ovulation induction (OI) and the controlled ovarian hyperstimulation necessary for IVF may increase risk of flare and/or thrombosis in patients with SLE. Risk appears to be related to degree of elevation in 17β-estradiol levels. While individual case reports describe OI- and IVF-related flare and thrombosis in SLE and antiphospholipid syndrome (APS) patients,[3] two large series report overall positive outcomes in a combined total of 177 OI and IVF cycles in patients with SLE and/or APS.[11,12] Flare occurred in 21–42% of SLE patients but was generally mild and responsive to therapy. Risk of both flare and thrombosis was greater if the diagnosis of SLE was not known at the start of the cycle.[11] Flare risk was higher with use of gonadotrophins than with the estrogen antagonist clomiphene, but pregnancy rates for clomiphene were significantly lower. Thrombosis was rare, although almost all patients with positive aPL or APS were treated throughout the cycle with some form of anticoagulation (aspirin and/or heparin). While one group has reported the absence of thrombotic complications in 17 aPL-positive patients undergoing ovulation induction without use of any prophylactic anticoagulation,[13] no controlled studies have been performed. Thrombosis risk is higher with IVF protocols than with OI due to the higher estrogen levels generated, with thrombosis risk most closely associated with the complication of ovarian hyperstimulation syndrome, a capillary-leak syndrome resulting in hemoconcentration.[3]

Options to minimize overall IVF risk for patients with SLE and aPL generally involve modulating the IVF process to avoid very high estrogen levels. Prophylactic aspirin and/or heparin therapy for patients with positive aPL is recommended, given the likely increase in thrombosis risk and the absence of data-derived guidelines. Patients with APS on warfarin are recommended to switch to therapeutic heparin or low molecular weight heparin prior to the start of the cycle and to hold it 12–24 h before oocyte retrieval with resumption 12 h later.[3]

It is not clear that prophylactic low-dose corticosteroid to reduce risk of lupus flare is necessary through IVF cycles; however, patients should be closely observed for evidence of flare and treated promptly with corticosteroid if indicated. Importantly, assisted reproductive techniques should only be performed in lupus patients who have stable inactive disease on pregnancy-compatible medications, i.e., those who would otherwise be considered safe to undertake pregnancy. Occasionally a patient may be considered suitable for IVF but not pregnancy, for example, those with significant renal insufficiency or other severe lupus damage. Such patients may tolerate ovarian stimulation but not the hemodynamic stress of pregnancy; in this situation, IVF followed by embryo transfer to a gestational carrier can result in a biological child. For every patient, and whatever the specific procedure planned, collaboration among the reproductive medicine specialist, high-risk obstetrician, and rheumatologist is critical for maximizing the potential for a successful outcome while minimizing maternal risk.

PREGNANCY IN SLE PATIENTS

During pregnancy, multiple physiologic and immunologic changes occur to maintain the developing fetus. Examples include a 30–50% increase in intravascular volume that results in physiologic anemia; immune system changes of diminished circulating natural killer cells, altered regulatory T-cell sets, and shift to a T-helper 2 type humoral immunity that lead to increased autoantibody production; and increases in prothrombin levels, plasma fibrinogen, and reduced protein S levels that create a prothrombotic state.[14,15] Moreover, common symptoms of pregnancy such as fatigue, joint pain, back aches, headaches, dyspnea, and skin rashes, can easily be confused with symptoms of SLE flare. Standard laboratory assessments of disease activity can be altered by pregnancy as well: sedimentation rate, C-reactive protein, complement components, and white blood cell count all increase during normal pregnancy.[14] These factors contribute to either disease exacerbation or challenges in assessing SLE disease activity in pregnancy.

Pregnancy Impact on SLE Disease Activity

There is no consensus opinion regarding the impact of pregnancy on SLE disease activity. Disparate reports likely reflect the lack of uniformity in flare definition and the compounding effect of pregnancy-specific symptoms on disease activity scales. Recent attempts to rectify this include adjustments to standard disease activity metrics such as the SLEDAI, SLAM, and LAI, to account for the symptoms of pregnancy.

While a few small scale studies have not revealed increased risk of SLE flare during pregnancy,[16] several larger studies suggest that pregnancy flare rates may approach 60%.[17,18] The most common disease manifestations during pregnancy include lupus nephritis, cutaneous disease, arthritis, and thrombocytopenia, and the nature of organ system involvement in the preconception period may predict the type of disease symptoms during pregnancy.[19]

While most flares during pregnancy are mild, about one-fifth of flares will be severe.[20]

Active disease in the 6 months prior to conception increases the risk of flare during pregnancy severalfold.[21] Primagravidas and those patients who have ever had renal disease are likewise vulnerable to flaring during pregnancy.[22,23] Other preconception risk factors for increased disease activity during pregnancy include low complement levels and hematological abnormalities.[24] Patients with active renal disease during the 6 months preceding conception and/or a baseline creatinine value of greater than 1.4 mg/dl are particularly vulnerable to disease flare during pregnancy with the risk of progression to end stage renal disease. They are also at higher risk for preterm delivery, hypertension, preeclampsia, and stroke.[25] Significantly, women with SLE have a 1% maternal mortality rate, 20 times the normal pregnancy mortality risk.[26]

Severe manifestations of disease damage may preclude pregnancy as it puts the mother at too great a risk. These include cardiomyopathy, cardiac valve disease, pulmonary arterial hypertension (PAH), interstitial lung disease, recent cerebral vascular accident, and significant renal insufficiency. PAH in particular is associated with a high risk of pregnancy-related mortality.[27]

Preeclampsia and SLE Flare

Preeclampsia occurs in roughly 25% of women with SLE during pregnancy.[28] Distinguishing a lupus flare from preeclampsia and its variants is challenging, as symptoms largely overlap (Table 1). While hypertension, edema, proteinuria, and low platelets can be found in both disorders, certain features may help distinguish between them. For example, preeclampsia rarely occurs before 20 weeks and most commonly occurs after 34 weeks of gestation, whereas SLE flares can occur throughout pregnancy. Laboratory testing can also be helpful in differentiating a clinical presentation of SLE flare from preeclampsia: low complements, rising anti-dsDNA antibody titers, low white blood cell count, and an active urine sediment suggest a lupus flare, while elevated liver function tests, elevated uric acid, and proteinuria with an acelluar urine sediment are more suggestive of preeclampsia. Management of these disorders differs, as SLE flare is controlled with immunosuppression whereas preeclampsia is treated with immediate delivery. In practice the two entities often coexist and patients may require treatment for both.

SLE Impact on Pregnancy Outcome

Pregnancy outcome for women with lupus has improved; however, SLE pregnancy is still associated with increased rates of pregnancy loss, preterm delivery, and fetal

TABLE 1 Differentiation of SLE Flare from Preeclampsia during Pregnancy

Clinical Finding	SLE Flare	Preeclampsia
Timing	All three trimesters	Rare before 20 weeks, most often after 34 weeks
Hypertension	+/−	+++
Edema	+	+++
Proteinuria	++	+++
Thrombocytopenia	++	+++
LFTs	Unchanged or decreased	++
Uric acid	Normal	Normal or high
Rising dsDNA antibody titer	++	−
Complement levels	Low or falling	Normal or high

growth restriction. In general, most of the risk factors affecting maternal health status in lupus pregnancy, such as disease activity, renal disease, and thrombocytopenia, impact fetal and neonatal outcomes as well. Additionally, the presence of anti-phospholipid antibodies (aPL) anti-SS-A/Ro, and anti-SS-B/La antibodies may negatively affect pregnancy outcome. Clark et al. compared their current cohort to historical data and found the pregnancy loss rate decreased from 40% to 17% over 40 years; rate of preterm delivery, however, did not improve significantly (37% versus 32%, respectively).[29] A large meta-analysis of 2751 lupus pregnancies found overall rates of premature birth to be 39.6% and of intrauterine growth restriction to be 12.7%.[26] These complications are important because severe preterm delivery and growth restriction can have long-term health implications for offspring, including significant neuro-developmental complications.

Pregnancy Loss

Rates of pregnancy loss are clearly increased in patients with SLE and are estimated at 15–30%. Early miscarriage (pregnancy loss at less than 10 weeks gestation) is common in the general population, whereas fetal loss (greater than 10 weeks gestation) and stillbirth (loss after 20 weeks gestation) are infrequent in the general population and are more characteristic of SLE. Factors increasing risk for lupus pregnancy loss include high levels of disease activity before and during pregnancy, presence of aPL, lupus nephritis, renal insufficiency, and hypertension.[20,26,28,30–32] Pregnancy loss rates are threefold higher in patients with active lupus in the first or second trimester of the pregnancy than in patients with quiescent disease.[20]

APL, present in up to 30% of SLE patients, is closely associated with adverse pregnancy outcome: obstetric antiphospholipid syndrome (OB-APS) is defined as recurrent early miscarriage, single fetal loss, or early delivery at less than 34 weeks for preeclampsia or placental insufficiency in the presence of persistent lupus anticoagulant (LAC) or high titer anticardiolipin (aCL) or anti-β2 glycoprotein I (aβ2GPI) IgG or IgM antibodies[33] (Chapters 56–58 and 63). LAC is the most powerful predictor for adverse pregnancy outcome in aPL-positive patients: in the multicenter prospective PROMISSE study (Predictors of pregnancy outcome: biomarker in antiphospholipid antibody syndrome and systemic lupus erythematosus), LAC was associated with a relative risk of 12.33 in a cohort of 144 aPL-positive women with and without SLE. History of thrombosis and concomitant SLE were additional independent risk factors. Overall, adverse outcomes occurred in 39% LAC-positive patients, versus 3% in the LAC-negative group.[34]

Presence of anti-SS-A/Ro and anti-SS-B/La antibodies are associated with a 15–20% risk of neonatal lupus in the offspring, with risk of complete congenital heart block about 2% (see Chapter 51). Complete congenital heart block, especially when associated with other cardiac abnormalities, may result in fetal and/or neonatal death and affected children usually require permanent pacemakers.

Preterm Birth and Intrauterine Growth Restriction

Rates of preterm birth and intrauterine growth restriction are increased in patients with SLE, most commonly for those with high-risk profiles. Intrauterine growth restriction (IUGR) results in infants that are small for gestational age (SGA), defined as being below the 10th percentile of weight for age, and is reported to be more common in SLE pregnancy, especially in the setting of positive aPL and hypertension.[35]

Preterm birth, defined as delivery prior to 37 weeks, may be medically induced for maternal or fetal safety in the setting of complications such as preeclampsia or fetal distress. Spontaneous preterm delivery also occurs, most commonly from preterm labor or preterm premature rupture of membranes (PPROM). Preterm birth rates for SLE patients range from 14 to 50% and rates for Cesarean delivery are also increased.[26,28,30,31] Presence of aPL, lupus disease activity, current or prior nephritis, and hypertension are all associated with earlier delivery. Prednisone use is also significantly associated with PPROM and early delivery.[28]

Even with previous adverse pregnancy outcome, future pregnancies may be successful in patients with SLE. A population-based cohort study recently reported on 177 women with SLE with a previous pregnancy, 69% of whom went on to have a second pregnancy: 89% of second pregnancies resulted in neonates being discharged home. Importantly, 9 of the 10 women with stillbirth or neonatal death in their first pregnancy had a successful second pregnancy.[36]

MANAGEMENT OF SLE DURING PREGNANCY

Disease should be in remission on medications compatible with pregnancy (see below) for 6 months prior to conception. Prepregnancy and early pregnancy evaluation should include assessments for anti-dsDNA and complement levels, anti-SS-A/Ro and anti-SS-B/La antibodies, aPL (including LAC, aCL, and anti-β2GPI), complete blood and platelet count, metabolic panel including renal function and liver function testing, and urinalysis. Patients should be comanaged with a maternal fetal medicine specialist with expertise in SLE. Pregnancy monitoring should be more frequent in SLE pregnancies including nonstress testing and biophysical profiling; in some situations, umbilical artery Doppler testing may be indicated. Complete blood counts with platelets, renal function, liver function testing, complement levels, anti-dsDNA antibody testing, and urinalysis should be performed regularly throughout the pregnancy to monitor for disease flare and preeclampsia.

Medication Management

Medication management of SLE during pregnancy and lactation is challenging, as the potential benefits to the mother of any medication must be weighed against the potential risk to the developing fetus. Information on drug safety is often based on animal studies or case reports and the FDA safety-in-use category designations, A, B, C, D, and X, are often erroneously interpreted to suggest increasing risk with letter progression. The FDA is currently revamping their pregnancy labeling to more accurately reflect drug safety based on current knowledge. Below is a discussion on the safety of commonly used medications for rheumatologic disorders in pregnancy and lactation (Table 2).

Aspirin and NSAIDs are often given to manage joint pain and serositis in SLE patients. Low-dose aspirin is also used to manage antiphospholipid syndrome and in preeclampsia prevention. While these medications are teratogenic in rodents, they are not in humans.[37] There is insufficient data on COX-2 inhibitors to conclude whether these medications can cause congenital anomalies so they are best avoided. Use of NSAIDs can cause premature closure of the ductus arteriosus and these medications should be discontinued after the 30th week of gestation.[38] Both traditional NSAIDs and COX-2-specific inhibitors may interfere with ovulation and implantation; thus these medications should be avoided during a planned conception cycle when possible.[39] There

are conflicting data on whether NSAIDs cause an increased risk of early spontaneous miscarriage; therefore it seems prudent to limit use of these medications during the first trimester.[40,41]

The nonfluorinated glucocorticoids prednisone and prednisolone are mainstays of therapy for SLE symptoms. These steroids cross the placenta in limited amounts and reach the fetus in low concentrations. In contrast, fluorinated glucocorticoids such as betamethasone readily cross the placenta and are used to hasten fetal lung maturity when premature delivery is anticipated.[42] In humans, a 1.5- to 3.4-fold increased risk of cleft palate formation has been reported in offspring of mothers exposed to corticosteroid during the first trimester;[43] however, other congenital anomalies have not been associated. Later in pregnancy, steroid use can contribute to PPROM and SGA infants. Mothers taking glucocorticoids during pregnancy have an increased risk of gestational diabetes, hypertension, and osteoporosis, and so dosage should be minimized when feasible. Prednisone is compatible with nursing,[44] although women taking more than 20 mg per day should discard breast milk produced in the first 4 h after the dose.

The antimalarials hydroxychloroquine and chloroquine are important tools for SLE management. Evidence suggests that continuation of these medications during pregnancy improves pregnancy outcome.[45] While one early case series suggested that antimalarials were ototoxic and retinotoxic,[46] subsequent studies have not shown increased teratogenicity. A 2006 survey of North American rheumatologists revealed that 69% of rheumatologists maintained their patients on hydroxychloroquine during pregnancy.[47] Reassuringly, follow-ups of infants exposed to antimalarials during pregnancy have failed to demonstrate retinal toxicity in offspring.[48]

Large transplant registries including hundreds of pregnancy exposures have not documented increased teratogenicity of azathioprine and cyclosporine. While cyclosporine is considered an FDA category C drug for use during pregnancy and azathioprine is labeled a category D drug, existing data suggest that these medications may be used as immunosuppressive agents during pregnancy.[49] Tacrolimus, another immunosuppressive agent that may be used to manage lupus nephritis, is also considered compatible with pregnancy.[50] Minimal levels of azathioprine and tacrolimus are transferred to breast milk; thus use of these medications in nursing mothers of full-term infants is considered low risk. While low levels of cyclosporine have been found in breast milk, a single breastfed infant was found to have a therapeutic level after nursing,[51] raising concerns about variability in drug transfer to breast milk. Unfortunately, a number of congenital anomalies have been reported after in utero exposure to mycophenolate mofetil so this medication should be discontinued when pregnancy is anticipated and should not be used during breastfeeding.[52]

TABLE 2 Potential Side Effects during Pregnancy and Lactation of Commonly Used Medications in SLE

Drug	Maternal	Fetal	Breastfeeding
Minimal Risk			
Hydroxychloroquine	None	None	Compatible
IVIG	Risk of hepatitis C	Risk of hepatitis C, SGA	Compatible
Some Risk			
Aspirin and NSAIDs	Reduced fertility	Possible increase in miscarriage Premature closure of the ductus arteriosus after 30 weeks	Compatible
Glucocorticoids	Hypertension, glucose intolerance, osteoporosis, PROM	1.5–3.4-fold risk of cleft palate when used in the first trimester, SGA	Compatible >20 mg/day discard first 4 h of breast milk following dose
Azathioprine	None	SGA, prematurity, IUGR	Compatible
Cyclosporine A	Renal insufficiency	SGA, prematurity, IUGR	Equivocal data as some reaches breast milk
Tacrolimus	None	SGA, prematurity, IUGR	Compatible
High Risk			
Methotrexate	None	Embryotoxic, skeletal and facial malformations	Contraindicated
Leflunomide	None	Multiple congenital anomalies	Contraindicated
Mycophenolate mofetil	None	Shortened digits, hypoplastic nails, auditory canal atresia, cleft lip and palate	Contraindicated
Cyclosphosphamide	None	Micrognathia, hypertelorism, SGA, skeletal anomalies, coronary artery agenesis, tumors in offspring	Contraindicated
Unknown Risk			
Rituximab	None		Contraindicated
Abatacept	None		Contraindicated
Belimumab	None		Contraindicated

Methotrexate and leflunomide are both teratogenic and are contraindicated during pregnancy.[53,54] A recent clinical report suggested that preconception and early gestation exposure to leflunomide resulted in few anomalies when patients were treated promptly with a cholestyramine washout.[55] Nonetheless current recommendations are to either stop this medication 2 years prior to conception or to treat with a cholestyramine washout prior to conception to remove active metabolites. Methotrexate and leflunomide should be avoided in lactating women. CYC is extremely teratogenic and is contraindicated during pregnancy with the exception of life-threatening circumstance[56]; it should also be avoided in nursing mothers.

Biological Agents

There is limited information on the safety of biologics during lupus pregnancy. Package inserts for products recommend discontinuation prior to pregnancy ranging from a few months (belimumab, abatacept) to 1 year (rituximab). However, given that IgG does not cross the placenta prior to 12 weeks of gestation, it is unlikely that administration of these medications in the period immediately preceding pregnancy would cause significant exposure to the developing embryo. One large series of 153 pregnancies in which the mother was given rituximab did not demonstrate an increased rate of congenital anomalies.[57] Two pregnancies reported from the belimumab pregnancy registry produced infants without congenital anomalies.[58]

Other Medications

There are limited data on the safety of IVIG during pregnancy, but no cases of congenital anomalies have been reported[59]; it is compatible with pregnancy and lactation and may be a low-risk agent to consider for severe SLE flare or, rarely, for refractory OB-APS.

Anticoagulation is used in women with APS and other thrombotic conditions. Heparin and low molecular weight heparin are compatible with pregnancy while warfarin is not. Angiotensin converting enzyme inhibitors and angiotensin II receptor blockers are contraindicated during pregnancy, although calcium channel blockers and beta blockers may be used to control blood pressure.

Medication Summary

Patients should be kept on their antimalarials during pregnancy. Patients who are aPL positive or who have other risk factors for preeclampsia should be maintained on low-dose aspirin (81–100 mg) throughout pregnancy. Glucocorticoids may be used in low doses for stable disease or in higher doses for flares with the caveat that exposure during the first trimester may increase the risk of cleft lip and palate formation in the offspring. Patients on mycophenolate mofetil, methotrexate, and leflunomide should be taken off of these medications and placed on an immunosuppressive agent compatible with pregnancy such as azathioprine, tacrolimus, or cyclosporine several months prior to conception. Importantly, disease should be stable on these medications for 6 months prior to attempting conception. While CYC is contraindicated during pregnancy, in life-threatening situations this medication has been used in the third trimester with successful pregnancy outcome. The biologics abatacept, belimumab, and rituximab should be discontinued as per the manufacturer's instructions; however, consideration of using these mediations in closer proximity to pregnancy is not unreasonable given that immunoglobulins do not cross the placenta in significant concentrations during the first trimester.

CONCLUSIONS

Fertility and pregnancy for patients with SLE may be affected to varying degrees by both disease and treatment-related factors. Lupus patients with inactive disease who are without renal disease or exposure to CYC can expect fertility comparable to the age-matched population. Lupus itself is unlikely to affect long-term fertility to any significant degree.

Pregnancy evaluation and counseling should include assessment of disease-related damage that might preclude pregnancy, such as PAH or severe renal insufficiency: these patients should not attempt pregnancy due to high risk of maternal morbidity or death. Patients without severe organ damage should be evaluated for current flare or recent disease activity in the preceding 6 months: if recent disease activity is present, they should be counseled to defer pregnancy until disease has been quiescent for at least 6 months on pregnancy-compatible medications, which include hydroxychloroquine, glucocorticoids, azathioprine, cyclosporine, and tacrolimus.

For patients ready to conceive, other risk factors for maternal and fetal complications should be identified including history of renal disease, hypertension, thrombocytopenia, aPL status, and anti-SS-A/Ro and anti-SS-B/La antibodies. Low-dose aspirin is recommended for patients at increased risk for preeclampsia, i.e., those with history of renal disease, hypertension, or aPL. Some experts suggest low-dose aspirin for all patients with SLE. Anticoagulation therapy for patients with OB-APS should be administered according to current guidelines (Chapter 63). With careful evaluation, monitoring, and medical therapy, most SLE patients can have successful pregnancies without long-term adverse effects for mother or child.

REFERENCES

1. Hickman RA, Gordon C. Causes and management of infertility in systemic lupus erythematosus. *Rheumatology* 2011;**50**:1551–8.
2. Vinet E, Pineau C, Cordon C, Clarke AE, Bernatsky S. Systemic lupus erythematosus in women: impact on family size. *Arthritis Care Res* 2008;**59**:1656–60.
3. Bellver J, Pellicer A. Ovarian stimulation for ovulation induction and in vitro fertilization in patients with systemic lupus and antiphospholipid syndrome. *Fertil Steril* 2009;**92**:1803–10.
4. Pasoto SG, Mendonca BB, Bonfa E. Menstrual disturbances in patients with systemic lupus erythematosus without alkylating therapy: clinical hormonal and therapeutic associations. *Lupus* 2002;**11**:175–80.
5. Lawrenze B, Henes JC, Henes M, Neunhoeffler E, Schmalzing M, Fehm T, et al. Impact of systemic lupus erythematosus on ovarian reserve in premenopausal women: evaluation by using anti-Muellerian hormone. *Lupus* 2011;**20**:1193–7.
6. The Practice Committee of the American Society for Reproductive Medicine. Antiphospholipid antibodies do not affect IVF success. *Fertil Steril* 2006;**86**:S224–5.
7. McDermott EM, Powell RJ. Incidence of ovarian failure in systemic lupus erythematosus after treatment with pulse cyclophosphamide. *Ann Rheum Dis* 1996;**55**:224–9.
8. Somers EC, Marder W, Christman GM, Ognenovski V, McCune WJ. Use of a gonadotropin-releasing hormone analog for protection against premature ovarian failure during cyclophosphamide therapy in women with severe lupus. *Arthritis Rheum* 2005;**52**:2761–7.
9. Clowse ME, Behara MA, Anders CK, Copland S, Coffman CJ, Leppert PC, et al. Ovarian preservation by GnRH agonists during chemotherapy: a meta-analysis. *J Womens Health* 2009;**18**(3):311–9.
10. Mersereau J, Dooley MA. Gonadal failure with cyclophosphamide therapy for lupus nephritis: advances in fertility preservation. *Rheum Dis Clin North Am* 2010;**36**:99–108.
11. Guballa N, Sammaritano L, Schwartzman S, Buyon J, Lockshin MD. Ovulation induction and in vitro fertilization in systemic lupus erythematosus and antiphospholipid syndrome. *Arthritis Rheum* 2000;**43**:550–6.
12. Huong DL, Wechsler B, Vauthier-Brouzes D, Duhat P, Costedoat N, Lefebre G, et al. Importance of planning ovulation induction therapy in systemic lupus erythematosus and antiphospholipid syndrome: a single center retrospective study of 21 cases and 114 cycles. *Sem Arthritis Rheum* 2002;**32**:174–88.
13. Balasch J, Cervera R. Reflections on the management of reproductive failure in the antiphospholipid syndrome – the clinician's perspective. *Lupus* 2002;**11**:467–77.

14. Branch DW, Wong LF. Normal pregnancy, pregnancy complications, and obstetric management. In: Sammaritano LR, Bermas BL, editors. *Contraception and pregnancy in patients with rheumatic disease*. New York: Springer; 2014. p. 31–62.

15. Veenstravan Nieuwenhoven AL, Heineman MJ, Faas MM. The immunology of successful pregnancy. *Hum Reprod Update* 2003;9: 347–57.

16. Lockshin MD. Pregnancy does not cause systemic lupus erythematosus to worsen. *Arthritis Rheum* 1989;32:665–70.

17. Petri M, Howard D, Repke J. Frequency of lupus flare in pregnancy. The Hopkins Lupus Pregnancy Center experience. *Arthritis Rheum* 1991;34:1538–45.

18. Cavallasca JA, Laborde HA, Hilda Ruda-Vega H, Nasswetter GG. Maternal and fetal outcomes of 72 pregnancies in Argentine patients with systemic lupus erythematosus (SLE). *Clin Rheumatol* 2008;27:41–6.

19. Tedeschi SK, Massarotti E, Guan H, Fine A, Bermas BL, Costenbader KH. Specific SLE disease manifestations in the six months prior to conception are associated with similar disease manifestations during pregnancy. In: *Oral presentation: American college of rheumatology annual meeting, Boston, MA*. November 2014.

20. Clowse ME, Madger LS, Witter F, Petri M. The impact of increased lupus activity on obstetric outcomes. *Arthritis Rheum* 2005;52:514–21.

21. Clowse ME. Lupus activity in pregnancy. *Rheum Dis Clin North Am* 2007;33:237–52.

22. Saavedra MA, Sanchez A, Morales S, Navarro-Zarza JE, Angeles U, Jara LJ. Primigravida is associated with flare in women with systemic lupus erythematosus. *Lupus* 2015;24(2):180–5.

23. Saavedra MA, Cruz-Reyes C, Vera-Lastra O, Romero GT, Cruz-Cruz P, Arias-Flores R, et al. Impact of previous lupus nephritis on maternal and fetal outcomes during pregnancy. *Clin Rheumatol* 2012;31:813–9.

24. Borilla E, Lojacono A, Gatto M, Andreoli L, Taglietti M, Iaccarino L, et al. Predictors of maternal and fetal complications in SLE patients: a prospective study. *Immunol Rev* 2014;60:170–6.

25. Hou S. Pregnancy in chronic renal insufficiency and end-stage renal disease. *Am J Kidney Dis* 1999;33:235–52.

26. Smyth A, Oliveira GH, Lahr BD, Bailey KR, Norby SM, Garovic VD. A systematic review and meta-analysis of pregnancy outcome in patients with systemic lupus erythematosus and lupus nephritis. *Clin J Am Soc Nephrol* 2010;5:2060–8.

27. Hsu CH, Gomberg-Maitland M, Glassner C, et al. The management of pregnancy and pregnancy-related medical conditions in pulmonary arterial hypertension patients. *Int J Clin Pract Suppl* 2011;172:6–14.

28. Chakravarty EF, Colon I, Langer ES, Nix DA, El-Sayed YY, Genovese MC, et al. Factors that predict prematurity and preeclampsia in pregnancies that are complicated by SLE. *Am J Obstet Gynecol* 2005;192:1897–904.

29. Clark CA, Spitzer KA, Laskin CA. Decrease in pregnancy loss rates in patients with systemic lupus erythematosus over a 40-year period. *J Rheumatol* 2005;32:1709–12.

30. Yasmeen S, Wilkins EE, Field NT, Sheikh RA, Gilbert WM. Pregnancy outcomes in women with systemic lupus. *J Matern Fetal Med* 2001;10:91–6.

31. Johnson MJ, Petrie M, Witter FR, Repke JT. Evaluation of preterm delivery in a systemic lupus erythematosus pregnancy clinic. *Obstet Gynecol* 1995;86:396–9.

32. Clowse ME, Magder LS, Witter F, Petri M. Early risk factors for pregnancy loss in lupus. *Obstet Gynecol* 2006;107:293–9.

33. Miyakis S, Lockshin MD, Atsumi T, Branch DW, Brey RL, Cervera R, et al. International consensus statement on an update of the classification criteria for definite antiphospholipid syndrome (APS). *J Thromb Haemost* 2006;4(2):295–306.

34. Lockshin MD, Kim M, Laskin CA, Guerra M, Branch DW, Merrill J, et al. Lupus anticoagulant, but not anticardiolipin antibody, predicts adverse pregnancy outcome in patients with antiphospholipid antibodies. *Arthritis Rheum* 2012;64(7):2311–8.

35. Cortes-Hernandez J, Ordi-Ros J, Paredes F, Casellas M, Castillo F, Vilardell-Tarres M. Clinical predictors of fetal and maternal outcomes in systemic lupus erythematosus: a prospective study of 103 pregnancies. *Rheumatology* 2002;41(6):643–50.

36. Shand AW, Algert CS, March L, Roberts CL. Second pregnancy outcomes for women with systemic lupus erythematosus. *Ann Rheum Dis* 2013;72:547–51.

37. Van Gelder MM, Roeleveld N, Nordeng H. Exposure to nonsteroidal anti-inflammatory drugs during pregnancy and the risk of selected birth defects: a prospective cohort study. *PloS One* 2011;6:e22174.

38. Koren G, Florescu A, Costei AM, Boskovic R, Moretti ME. Nonsteroidal antiinflammatory drugs during third trimester and the risk of premature closure of the ductus arteriosus: a meta-analysis. *Ann Pharmacother* 2006;40:824–9.

39. Pall M, Friden BE, Brannstrom M. Induction of delayed follicular rupture in the human by the selective COX-2 inhibitor rofecoxib: a randomized double-blind study. *Hum Reprod* 2001;16:1323–8.

40. Nakhai-Pour HR, Broy P, Sheehy O, et al. Use of non-aspirin nonsteroidal anti-inflammatory drugs during pregnancy and the risk of spontaneous abortion. *CMAJ* 2011;183:1713–20.

41. Edwards DR, Aldridge T, Baird DD, et al. Periconceptional over-the-counter nonsteroidal anti-inflammatory drug exposure and risk for spontaneous abortion. *Obstet Gynecol* 2012;120:113–22.

42. Blanford AT, Murphy BE. In vitro metabolism of prednisolone, dexamethasone, betamethasone, and cortisol by the human placenta. *Am J Obstet Gynecol* 1977;127:264–7.

43. Park-Wyllie L, Mazzotta P, Pastuszak A, et al. Birth defects after maternal exposure to corticosteroids: prospective cohort study and meta-analysis of epidemiologic studies. *Teratology* 2000;62: 385–92.

44. Ost L, Wettrell G, Bjorkhem I, Rane A. Prednisolone excretion in human milk. *J Pediatr* 1985;106:1008–11.

45. Clowse ME, Magder L, Witter F, Petri M. Hydroxychloroquine in lupus pregnancy. *Arthritis Rheum* 2006;54:3640–7.

46. Hart CW, Naunton RF. The ototoxicity of chloroquine phosphate. *Arch Otolaryngol* 1964;80:407–12.

47. Al-Herz A, Schulzer M, Esdaile JM. Survey of antimalarial use in lupus pregnancy and lactation. *J Rheumatol* 2002;29:700–8.

48. Osadchy A, Ratnapalan T, Koren G. Ocular toxicity in children exposed in utero to antimalarial drugs: review of the literature. *J Rheumatol* 2011;38:2504–8.

49. Radomski JS, Ahlswede BA, Jarrell BE, et al. Outcomes of 500 pregnancies in 335 female kidney, liver, and heart transplant recipients. *Transplant Proc* 1995;27:1089–90.

50. Kaintz A, Harabacz I, Cowlrick IS, et al. Review of the course and outcome of 100 pregnancies in 84 women treated with tacrolimus. *Transplantation* 2000;70:1718–21.

51. Bermas BL. The medical management of the rheumatology patient during pregnancy. In: Sammaritano LR, Bermas BL, editors. *Contraception and pregnancy in patients with rheumatic disease*. New York: Springer; 2014. p. 273–87.

52. Perez-Aytes A, Ledo A, Boso V, et al. In utero exposure to mycophenolate mofetil: a characteristic phenotype? *Am J Med Genet A* 2008;**146A**:1–7.

53. Feldcamp M, Carey JC. Clinical teratology counseling and consultation case report: low dose methotrexate exposure in the early weeks of pregnancy. *Teratology* 1993;**47**:553–9.

54. Brent RL. Teratogen update: reproductive risks of leflunomide (arava); a pyrimidine synthesis inhibitor: counseling women taking leflunomide before and during pregnancy and men taking leflunomide who are contemplating fathering a child. *Teratology* 2001;**63**:106–12.

55. Cassina M, Johnson DL, Robinson LK, et al. Pregnancy outcome in women exposed to leflunomide before or during pregnancy. *Arthritis Rheum* 2012;**64**:2085–94.

56. Fields CL, Ossorio MA, Roy TM, et al. Wegener's granulomatosus complicated by pregnancy. A case report. *J Reprod Med* 1991;**36**:463–6.

57. Chakravarty EF, Murray ER, Kelman A, et al. Pregnancy outcomes after maternal exposure to rituximab. *Blood* 2011;**117**(5):1499–506.

58. Landy H, Powell M, Hill D, Eudy A, Petri M. Belimumab pregnancy registry: prospective cohort study of pregnancy outcomes. *Obstet Gynecol* 2014;**123**(Suppl.):62S.

59. Parke A. The role of IVIG in the management of patients with antiphospholipid antibodies and recurrent pregnancy losses. *Clin Rev Allergy* 1992;**10**:106–18.

Chapter 51

Neonatal Lupus: Clinical Spectrum, Biomarkers, Pathogenesis, and Approach to Treatment

Jill P. Buyon, Amit Saxena, Peter M. Izmirly

Division of Rheumatology, New York University School of Medicine, New York City, NY, USA

INTRODUCTION

Fetal exposure to maternal autoantibodies transported across the human placenta via FcγRn can result in a spectrum of organ injury: transient if the tissue has regenerative capacity and permanent if this capacity is absent or limited. An important example of passively acquired autoimmunity in a fetus and neonate is that of neonatal lupus (NL) given the concordance between circulating maternal antibody in the fetus and disease manifestations. NL is often referred to as a syndrome since it can comprise one or more manifestations inclusive of cardiac, cutaneous, liver, and hematologic abnormalities. By definition, the maternal autoantibodies associated with NL are directed to antigen targets within the SSA/Ro–SSB/La ribonucleoprotein complex (60 kDa Ro, 52 kDa Ro, 48 kDa La) (reviewed in Ref. 1). NL was coined based on the resemblance of the neonatal rash to the cutaneous lesions seen in SLE.[2,3] Throughout this chapter, cardiac NL refers to the varied spectrum of cardiac disease, inclusive of complete heart block (CHB), cardiomyopathy, and endocardial fibroelastosis (EFE). The transient manifestations of the syndrome mimic the disease characteristics observed in adolescents or adults (rash and cytopenias). However, the permanent manifestation (heart block), with the exception of one published maternal case, is not observed in the adult despite the presence of identical antibodies in the maternal circulation.[4] The term NL is misleading since the neonate does not have SLE and often neither does the mother. In many cases, mothers are clinically asymptomatic and only identified to have serologic abnormalities when gestational surveillance reveals fetal bradycardia.[4,5] Other maternal diseases include an undifferentiated autoimmune syndrome or Sjogren's syndrome.[6]

RISK OF CARDIAC NL AND POPULATION PREVALENCE

The risk of having a child with cardiac NL is approximately 2% for an anti-SSA/Ro-positive woman who has either never been pregnant or has previously had only healthy offspring.[7-10] If an anti-SSA/Ro-positive mother has a previous child affected with cardiac NL or cutaneous NL, the risk of recurrence is 18%[11-16] and 13%,[17] respectively. In general, women with low titers of anti-SSA/Ro antibodies are at less risk than those with high titer antibodies[18]; however, there is considerable overlap in antibody levels between affected and unaffected cases and most women have high titers that remain stable over time. The risk of developing cutaneous manifestations of NL is 7–16%,[8,10] and the recurrence rate of cutaneous NL is estimated to be between 23% and 29%.[17]

The population prevalence of cardiac NL in Finland was reported at 1:17,000 live births[19] with the highest annual estimates at 1:6500. However, this may be an underestimation since only children with pacemakers were included and fetal deaths were not captured. In children born with cardiac NL in the absence of documented structural abnormalities, anti-Ro antibodies are found in over 85%.[20]

The prevalence of anti-SSA/Ro antibodies had been initially reported at 0.20–0.72% in female blood donors,[21] 0.87% in pregnant women,[22] and more recently at 0.86% in healthy females in the general population.[23] The prevalence reported in the latter study may be even higher since only those positive for anti-nuclear antibodies (which may not always detect anti-SSA/Ro) were then tested for anti-SSA/Ro antibodies. For patients with SLE the prevalence of this antibody reactivity is estimated at 40%[24] and in those with Sjogren's syndrome between 60% and 100%.[24]

In aggregate, if the true prevalence of anti-SSA/Ro approaches 0.9% and cardiac NL occurs in 2% and recurrence in 18%, this could yield approximately 600–700 cases per year based on the 2012 National Vital Statistics of 3,952,841 births. Thus, thousands of women in the United States may be faced with the risk of cardiac NL in their offspring, yet prenatal testing does not include an evaluation of anti-SSA/Ro antibodies.

TRANSIENT CLINICAL MANIFESTATIONS OF NL: CUTANEOUS, HEPATIC, HEMATOLOGIC, AND NEUROLOGIC

In contrast to the in utero detection of cardiac NL, cutaneous disease most often appears after birth, with a mean time of detection at 6 weeks and mean duration of 17 weeks.[25] Albeit the specificity of the maternal autoantibodies may be identical, the discordant timing of the cardiac and cutaneous disease supports distinct initiators or amplifiers of injury. The strong association of cutaneous lesions with UV exposure suggests that apoptosis of the keratinocytes and surface translocation of SSA/Ro may result in immune complex formation and tissue injury. All mothers with anti-SSA/Ro antibodies should be counseled regarding UV protection of their infants as both a preventative and therapeutic measure.

The rash is characterized by erythematous annular lesions or arcuate macules with slight central atrophy and raised active margins, which are located primarily on the scalp and face with a characteristic predilection for the upper eyelids. A raccoon-like appearance should immediately raise suspicion for NL. A review of the corporeal distribution of rash among 57 infants with cutaneous NL enrolled in the Research Registry for Neonatal Lupus (RRNL) revealed that 100% had facial involvement. Other affected areas included the scalp, trunk, extremities, neck, intertriginous areas, and rarely the palms or soles, in descending order.[25] The NL rash resembles subacute cutaneous lupus erythematosus, with basal cell damage in the epidermis and a superficial monocyte cell infiltrate in the upper dermis.[26] Immunofluorescence staining of skin biopsies reveals IgG deposition within the epidermis.[26] Of relevance to the pathogenesis of tissue injury mediated by anti-SSA/Ro antibodies, a recent report identified histiocytes consistent with M2 macrophages in the skin lesion of a neonate with cutaneous NL.[27] Although purely speculative, this observation echoes the macrophage infiltrations noted in cardiac NL, suggesting a potential link between these two manifestations: one induced by UV light and the other by apoptosis (see below), both exposing intracellular antigen and inciting an inflammatory infiltrate in response to immune complexes.

The rash is usually self-limiting and almost always resolves by approximately 8 months of age, coincident with the clearance of maternal antibodies from the child's circulation.[26] Residual skin abnormalities are uncommon but can include atrophy, scarring, pitting, hypopigmentation or hyperpigmentation, and telangiectasias.[25,26] On rare occasion, neither anti-SSA/Ro nor SSB/La are detected in the maternal sera of a child with classic NL lesions, but rather antibodies to another ribonucleoprotein, U1-RNP, are present.[28] Thus, evaluation of this latter reactivity should be considered when facing the differential diagnosis of NL in a child with characteristic rash and maternal disease is unsuspected.

In general the self-limiting nature of the rash precludes therapy. Topical steroids (nonfluorinated), have been used. However, data from the RRNL revealed no significant differences in outcome with or without treatment.[25] Systemic therapies are not recommended.

Neonatal liver disease is associated with maternal anti-SSA/Ro but its true prevalence is unknown since routine testing at birth does not include a liver enzyme profile.[29] In one prospective study, 26% of children born to mothers with anti-SSA/Ro had elevated liver enzymes.[8] Laxer described NL associated with significant hepatic involvement in four infants, three living and one who died postnatally.[30] The clinical picture in these neonates was cholestatic. Pathologic changes included giant cell transformation, ductal obstruction, and extramedullary hematopoiesis.[30] Lee and colleagues investigated the incidence of hepatobiliary manifestations among 219 NL patients in the RRNL and noted that recognized hepatobiliary disease occurred in 19 (9%) of 219 infants, usually in conjunction with either cardiac or cutaneous involvement.[29] Three clinical variants were observed: 1, severe liver failure present during gestation or in the neonatal period (least common); 2, conjugated hyperbilirubinemia with mild or no elevations of aminotransferases occurring in the first few weeks of life; and 3, mild elevations of aminotransferases occurring at approximately 2–3 months of life. The prognosis for the children in the last two categories was excellent.[29]

Hematologic manifestations of NL include thrombocytopenia, neutropenia, anemia,[8] and, very rarely, aplastic anemia.[31] Thrombocytopenia was present in 10% of the neonates referred to Lee and her colleagues.[26] While NL thrombocytopenia is presumed to be autoimmune in nature, its exact pathogenesis remains unclear since it is uncertain whether anti-platelet-specific antibodies or anti-SSA/Ro-SSB/La antibodies target the surface of fetal platelets. With regard to the pathogenesis of neutropenia, in vitro exposure of intact neutrophils to anti-SSA/Ro-positive maternal and/or infant serum from affected families results in immunoglobulin deposition, suggesting a possible immune-mediated basis for NL neutropenia.[32] Indeed, the neutrophil/immunoglobulin interactions were neutralized by preincubating the sera with 60 kDa Ro antigen that bound the autoantibody, suggesting that anti-60 kDa SSA/Ro directly drives the pathogenesis of neutropenia.[32] In one prospective study, 25 of 107 infants born to mothers with anti-SSA/Ro or anti-SSB/La antibodies had neutropenia but no cases of neonatal sepsis occurred.[8]

Neurologic dysfunction has been reported in offspring of mothers with anti-SSA/Ro antibodies. In a Canadian cohort of 87 infants exposed to maternal anti-SSA/Ro and/or anti-SSB/La antibodies,[33] 8% (5/47 with and 2/40 without another manifestation of NL) had hydrocephalus, all but one resolving spontaneously. Maternal immunological dysfunction has been associated with reports of developmental language delay, learning difficulties, and left handedness.[34]

In a retrospective study based on detailed questionnaires, telephone interviews, and reviews of medical records of children with NL in the RRNL, their unaffected siblings, and healthy friend controls, it was noted that behavioral problems, either isolated or associated with attention disorder, were present in all groups with no statistical difference.[35] The prevalence of depression, anxiety, developmental delays, learning disability, hearing and speech problems, and use of stimulants were also not significantly different between groups. The authors suggested that parental reporting of neuropsychiatric abnormalities was high in antibody-exposed children; however, it did not meet statistical significance when compared to the controls. More recently, in a study from Sweden, impaired neurodevelopment was reported in 16% of anti-Ro-exposed children (60 siblings with and 54 without CHB [18/114]). Reported problems included speech (9%), motor (8%) and learning (8%) impairment, attention deficit (5%), and behavioral impairment (4%).[36] Impairment in motor skill development was more common in boys ($P < 0.001$) if the child was born preterm ($P < 0.001$). Learning impairment was significantly influenced by maternal SLE ($P < 0.005$), while attention deficits were influenced by both maternal SLE ($P < 0.05$) and cardiac NL in the child ($P < 0.05$).

IMMUTABLE MANIFESTATIONS OF NL: CARDIAC

Cardiac NL covers a broad spectrum of severity. The characteristic clinical presentation is advanced conduction disease (second and third degree heart block, although first degree block is generally considered to be associated with maternal anti-SSA/Ro antibodies but progression is less certain).[37] Other manifestations include cardiomyopathy, endocardial fibrosis (EFE), and valvular abnormalities.[6]

Second degree heart block detected in utero, and first or second degree heart block identified in infants at birth, can progress to complete heart block.[6,11,38] It is unclear whether first degree heart block detected in utero also progresses to more advanced heart block. In part, discordant data on first degree block relate to the specific approaches to measurement and in the cutoffs used for the normal ranges.[39] A recent study based on serial echocardiograms of 165 anti-SSA/Ro-exposed fetuses concluded that fetal AV prolongation does not reliably predict progressive heart block.[37] Third degree block is not reversible but there is evidence for the efficacy of treatment in cases of low-grade heart block.[40]

Other documented arrhythmias and conduction abnormalities seen in cardiac NL include sinus node dysfunction, long QT interval, ventricular and atrial ectopy, ventricular and junctional tachycardia, and atrial flutter, but generally have not been clinically significant in this population.[7,41] Autoantibody-mediated heart block in NL is generally not associated with structural abnormalities, which is logical based on the fact that antibodies are not effectively transported across the placenta until the heart has achieved most of its developmental landmarks (end of first trimester). However, structural abnormalities such as flail mitral valve secondary to chordal disruption from EFE have been reported.[42] Another cardiac abnormality that may be associated with NL is congestive heart failure due to cardiomyopathy, which is often associated with EFE. EFE has been reported both in isolation and in association with conduction defects.[6,43–46] In addition, a few cases of late onset cardiomyopathy have been reported in infants with cardiac NL despite receiving early pacemaker implantation.[44]

FACTORS CONTRIBUTING TO MORTALITY

Case fatality rates and associated risk factors in cardiac NL have been addressed in two large retrospective studies.[6,47] Each confirm and extend findings of previous publications, which included smaller cohorts and in some cases the maternal antibody status was unknown.[11,20,48–51] Data from the Research Registry for Neonatal Lupus (RRNL, a multiethnic/racial US-based registry of anti-SSA/Ro-exposed fetuses with NL), which included 325 cases of cardiac NL, revealed a mortality rate of 17.5%; 30% of whom died in utero.[6] The probability of in utero death was 6%. The cumulative probability of survival at 10 years for a child born alive was 86%. Fetal echocardiographic risk factors associated with increased mortality in a multivariable analysis of all cases included hydrops and EFE. Significant predictors of in utero death were hydrops and earlier diagnosis, and of postnatal death were hydrops, EFE, and lower ventricular rate. The presence of

EFE and dilated cardiomyopathy was associated with an increased case fatality rate of 51.9% and 53.3%, respectively, compared to those who only had isolated advanced block (7.8%). Fetuses born to minorities had a higher case fatality rate, possibly because they were at higher risk for developing hydrops and EFE. Pacing was required in 70% of children and four underwent cardiac transplantation.[6] In a multicenter study including 175 patients with advanced heart block from Europe and Brazil, 75% of whom were exposed to anti-SSA/Ro-SSB/La antibodies, 91% resulted in live births and 93% of those were alive after the neonatal period.[47] Risk factors associated with mortality included gestational age <20 weeks at diagnosis, ventricular rate <50 bpm, fetal hydrops, and impaired left ventricular function at diagnosis. By one year of life, 69% were paced.[47]

SEEKING BIOMARKERS: THE CANDIDATE AUTOANTIBODIES

The association between autoantibodies to the 52 kDa SSA/Ro (Ro52), 60 kDa SSA/Ro (Ro60), and 48 kDa La proteins and NL, inclusive of cutaneous and cardiac manifestations, was reported before 1995.[52] While several studies have attempted to identify epitopes within the SSA/Ro-SSB/La complex that might confer risk of a specific manifestation or increased risk of recurrent disease, no definitive specificities have been reproducibly detected. To date novel reactivities to targets distinct from SSA/Ro–SSB/La have neither increased sensitivity nor appreciably added to specificity. With regard to the detection of anti-Ro60, it is highly relevant that the sensitivity of peptide or recombinant protein ELISAs for anti-Ro60 is low and may result in false negatives.[53–56] Thus, in considering risk of cardiac NL it may be useful to find out what antigen source is being used in the commercial ELISA (at the very least should be native Ro60 or recombinant Ro52).

The titer of maternal autoantibodies has been suggested as a potential biomarker of risk. Jaeggi and colleagues reported that cardiac complications in fetuses are associated with higher titers of maternal anti-SSA/Ro antibodies, although the authors did not distinguish between anti-Ro52 or anti-Ro60 specificities.[18] In this study as in others,[57] titers did not predict recurrent cardiac NL as titers remained high despite a healthy subsequent pregnancy. Of cautionary note, titer is a weak biomarker since anti-SSA/Ro reactivities are generally of high titer. Current commercial ELISAs may not provide final titers since they are often reported as <1 EU being negative, a linear value between 1 and 8 and then >8 but no further titration. One then can only assume that >8 is high titer.

There has been recent excitement in the antibody response against the p200 epitope, spanning Ro52 amino acids (aa) 200–239, as a candidate biomarker conferring an increased maternal risk for the development of cardiac NL in an offspring.[58,59] While several groups have confirmed the high prevalence of the p200 response in women giving birth to a child with cardiac NL, consensus has not been reached as to whether this antibody response is also similarly observed in anti-SSA/Ro-exposed healthy children when all other maternal antibody reactivities to components of the SSA/Ro SSB/La complex, including full-length Ro52, are equivalent.[60]

A limitation of most previous studies is that the prevalence and titer of maternal autoantibodies have not been measured during the time of fetal exposure. To address these limitations and the clinical utility of the p200 response as a diagnostic indicator of cardiac NL, Reed and colleagues evaluated 123 anti-SSA/Ro-exposed umbilical cord blood samples and 115 anti-Ro-positive maternal samples during healthy pregnancies or those complicated by cardiac NL.[57] The frequencies of p200, Ro52, Ro60, and SSB/La autoantibodies were not significantly different between affected and unaffected children. However, neonatal anti-Ro52 and Ro60 titers were highest in cardiac NL and their unaffected siblings compared to unaffected neonates without a cardiac NL sibling. Although both maternal anti-Ro52 and p200 autoantibodies were less than 50% specific for cardiac NL, anti-p200 was the least likely of the SSA/Ro autoantibodies to be false-positive in mothers who have never had an affected child. Titers of anti-Ro52 and p200 did not differ during a cardiac NL or unaffected pregnancy from the same mother.[57] In a very recently reported Italian cohort of 207 pregnant women carrying anti-SSA/Ro antibodies (42 with cardiac NL and 165 unaffected), the risk of disease was significantly decreased in the absence of reactivity to p200 (OR: 0.34; CI: 0.15–0.77), although comparison with the performance of antibody to full-length Ro52 was not evaluated. Of clinical relevance the negative predictive value of anti-Ro60 measured by ELISA was 100%; almost 20% of mothers negative for anti-p200 antibody delivered babies with cardiac NL.[61]

In aggregate, the collective evidence suggests that maternal reactivity to p200 does not confer an added risk to fetal conduction defects over full-length Ro52 or Ro60 autoantibodies. Mothers who may never be at risk for having an affected child have lower anti-Ro60 titers and may require less stringent echocardiographic monitoring compared to women with high-titer autoantibodies.

It has been recently reported that approximately half of sera from 17 anti-SSA/Ro-positive mothers of children with cardiac NL recognize an extracellular epitope of the alpha1G T type calcium channel.[62] Reactivity was mapped to a peptide designated as p305 (corresponding to aa 305–319 of the extracellular loop linking transmembrane segments S5–S6 in a1G repeat I). These results await further confirmation.

LINKING ANTIBODY TO TISSUE DAMAGE AND FIBROSIS: ACCOUNTING FOR ANTIGEN TARGET ACCESSIBILITY

In contrast to autoimmune diseases affecting the blood elements in which the target antigen is normally accessible to the cognate autoantibody by virtue of its surface expression, NL presents a molecular challenge in that the most robust antigen candidates to date are located intracellularly. In considering the cardiac manifestations as a multistep process, two nonmutually exclusive hypotheses have been proposed. One hypothesis is based on molecular mimicry wherein anti-SSA/Ro antibodies cross-react with L-type calcium channels (LTCC) and cause dysregulation of calcium homeostasis.[63] Another posits that intracellular anti-SSA/Ro–SSB/La antigens translocate to the surface of cardiomyocytes undergoing apoptosis during physiological remodeling.[64] Several recent papers have provided advances for both hypotheses.

Based on the prediction that overexpression of LTCC should rescue, whereas knockouts should worsen, the electrocardiographic abnormalities, Karnabi and colleagues reported that transgenic pups with overexpression of LTCC, exposed to anti-SSA/Ro–SSB/La antibodies via passive immunization of the mothers, had significantly less sinus bradycardia and AV block compared to nontransgenic pups.[65] LTCC knockout pups born to immunized mothers had sinus bradycardia, advanced AV block, and decreased fetal parity.

Apoptosis may be particularly relevant in the pathogenesis of cardiac NL since it is a selective process of physiological cell deletion in embryogenesis and normal tissue turnover and plays an important role in shaping morphological and functional maturity. Antibody binding to all three components of the SSA/Ro–SSB/La system, including 48 kDa La, 52 kDa Ro, and 60 kDa Ro, has been demonstrated on the surface membrane of apoptotic cardiocytes and keratinocytes[66,67] and subsequently on apoptotic human fetal cardiomyocytes.[68] Further advancing the mechanism by which anti-SSA/Ro translocates to the cell surface, it has recently been reported that a single point mutation of Ro60 that blocks Y RNA binding and siRNA-mediated knockdown of mY3 RNA attenuates a permissive signal that is required for surface accessibility.[69] Accordingly, the mY3 RNA moiety of the Ro60 ribonucleoprotein may impart a critical role to the pathogenicity of anti-Ro60 antibodies.

The low penetrance of cardiac NL suggests protective fetal factors. Flow cytometry experiments conducted on apoptotic human fetal cardiomyocytes demonstrated dose-dependent binding of β(2)GPI(70). In competitive inhibition experiments, β(2)GPI prevented opsonization of apoptotic cardiomyocytes by maternal anti-Ro60 IgG. However plasmin-mediated cleavage of β2 GPI abrogated this protective effect and promoted the formation of pathogenic anti-Ro60 IgG-apoptotic cardiomyocyte complexes. Based on evaluation of umbilical cord blood from 97 neonates exposed to anti-Ro60 antibodies (53 with cardiac NL and 44 with no cardiac disease), β(2) GPI levels were significantly lower in neonates with cardiac NL. In aggregate these data suggest that intact β(2) GPI in the fetal circulation may be a novel cardioprotective factor in anti-Ro60-exposed pregnancies.[70]

It is generally accepted that apoptotic cells are rapidly removed to obviate inflammatory sequelae. To achieve efficient clearance, human fetal cardiocytes are capable of engulfing apoptotic cardiocytes.[71] This novel physiologic function may account for the nearly complete absence of apoptosis noted on evaluation of healthy hearts from electively terminated fetuses.[72] In contrast, histological studies of hearts from fetuses dying with cardiac NL reveal exaggerated apoptosis, suggesting a potential defect in clearance.[72] The exaggerated apoptosis was accompanied by both intense TGF-β immunoreactivity in the extracellular fibrous matrix and infiltrating macrophages in close proximity to myofibroblasts (transdifferentiated fibroblasts with scarring potential). Notably, multinucleated giant cells were highly characteristic. These histologic findings are supported by in vitro experiments demonstrating that SSA/Ro–SSB/La antibodies inhibit cardiac uptake of apoptotic cardiocytes.[71] Further insights into the mechanism of this impaired efferocytosis were provided by the report that anti-Ro60 surface binding of the apoptotic cardiocyte resulted in a modification of uPAR expression, which served as a "don't eat me" signal and uPA activation.[67] The latter ultimately results in the generation of plasmin and TGF-β activation. The profibrotic consequence of TGF-β activation generated under these conditions was illustrated by myofibroblast transdifferentiation (SMAc staining) of and increased collagen protein expression in the cardiac fibroblasts.[67] A summary of this is shown in Figure 1.

Given the reproducible detection of macrophages and multinucleated giant cells in the region of the conduction tissue in hearts from fetuses dying with cardiac NL, experiments have addressed the potential pathogenic contribution of the macrophage to fibrosis. Dual receptor signaling via uptake of the anti-SSA/Ro immune complex bound apoptotic cardiocytes by FcγR on macrophages, and delivery of associated ssRNA to the endosomal compartment for ligation with TLR7/8 may be critical steps toward conduction damage.[64,73] Since endosomal TLR binds ligand at low pH, pharmacologic approaches to attenuate TLR-dependent readouts have utilized chloroquine, which interferes with acidification.[74,75]

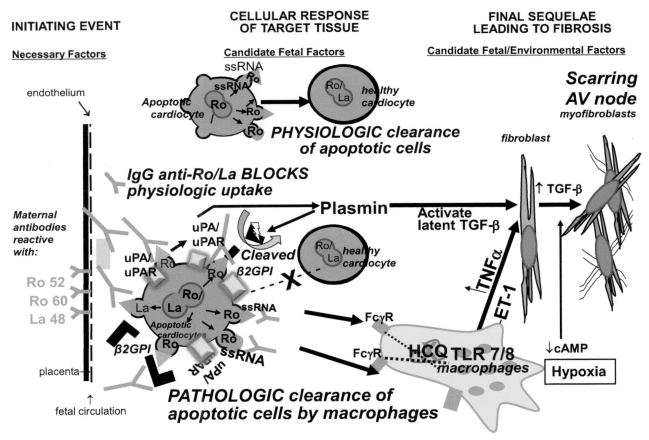

INITIATING EVENT

Necessary Factors

CELLULAR RESPONSE OF TARGET TISSUE

Candidate Fetal Factors

FINAL SEQUELAE LEADING TO FIBROSIS

Candidate Fetal/Environmental Factors

FIGURE 1   Pathologic cascade linking maternal antibody to AV nodal fibrosis and cardiomyopathy.

Macrophage transfection with noncoding ssRNA that bind Ro60 and an immune complex generated by incubation of Ro60 ssRNA with an IgG fraction from a CHB mother or affinity-purified anti-Ro60 significantly increased TNFα secretion, an effect not observed using control RNAs or normal IgG or exploiting apoptotic cells absent Y3 and incapable of Ro60 translocation.[64,73] Dependence on TLR was supported by the significant inhibition of TNFα release by IRS661 (inhibits TLR7) and chloroquine.[64,73] Fibrosis markers were increased in fetal cardiac fibroblasts after incubation with supernatants generated from macrophages transfected with ssRNA or incubated with the immune complex, an effect likewise abrogated by IRS661 or chloroquine.[64,73]

GUIDELINES FOR MONITORING ANTI-SSA/Ro-EXPOSED PREGNANCIES AND APPROACH TO CARDIAC NL

The schema outlined in Figure 2 is a modification of previous published guidelines by the authors. In general mothers known to have anti-SSA/Ro antibodies should undergo weekly fetal echocardiographic surveillance from

16 to 26 weeks. This time frame represents the period during which cardiac NL is most likely to be identified. Weekly surveillance is based on the observation that a fetus can change from normal sinus rhythm to complete block in 1 week. The purpose of monitoring is to identify an abnormality that might be treatable and thus prevent permanent advanced block. While a prolonged PR interval (3 SD above normal is 150 ms, which was used in the U.S. PRIDE study to define first degree block[10]) was considered the most likely marker, spontaneous reversal of first degree block has been reported and clear progression in utero is not robustly documented and extremely rare. There is controversy regarding the efficacy of recommending dexamethasone in this situation.[76] Thus, even the need for serial echocardiograms has been questioned.[37]

However, second degree block may be missed by reliance only on auscultation. Furthermore, extranodal disease would not be identified. These points should provide sufficient rationale for echocardiographic monitoring. Accumulated experience supports the rarity of initial detection of cardiac NL after 26 weeks if serial monitoring has shown no abnormalities; thus earlier recommendations of surveillance until 32 weeks have lost favor.

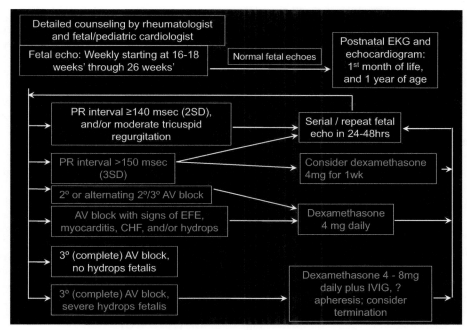

FIGURE 2   Management of the anti-Ro ± anti-La pregnancy.

For established third degree block in which there is no extra nodal disease, the use of dexamethasone (dex) is questionable. While popularized by several groups, its scientific merit is underwhelming, and risks may be substantial.[47,77,78] Since sustained reversal of established block has never been documented, dex might be rationalized only if sufficient evidence suggests that further injury could be forestalled. This remains under intense study and results are anticipated in the near future as large databases are being queried. Prospective studies would be ideal but face challenges of a rare disease and effect size with regard to progression.

TRANSLATING PATHOGENESIS TO PREVENTION

For a mother who has had a child with cardiac NL, the prospect for future pregnancies is one of the most commonly asked questions. This is generally followed by a second question regarding options for preventing another affected child. Despite the attempts of large multicenter studies to forestall disease by careful monitoring, irreversible block and extensive myocardial injury have been documented within 7 days of a normal rhythm and PR interval. Prophylactic and treatment strategies have included maternal steroids, plasmapheresis, sympathomimetics, and in utero cardiac pacing, but unfortunately none have significantly altered mortality.[6]

The initial consideration of IVIG to prevent cardiac NL was based on two presumed mechanisms of efficacy.

The first related to the saturation of FcγRn by IVIG, which would be expected to decrease fetal exposure to anti-SSA/Ro antibodies by accelerating IgG catabolism in the maternal circulation and by decreasing placental transport.[79] The second, a target organ effect, related to the attenuation of anti-inflammatory responses by increasing the macrophage expression of FcγRIIb.[80] Accordingly, a multicenter, prospective, open-label study in the United States was initiated[12] (**P**reventative **IVIG** **T**herapy for **CHB**, PITCH). In parallel with enrollment in U.S. PITCH, a European study followed the same protocol and was terminated after three recurrent cardiac NL cases were identified in 15 mothers.[16] Combining data from both PITCH studies, there were 6 (18%) recurrences in 33 women who had previous pregnancies complicated by cardiac NL. Since each study was designed to conclude inefficacy of IVIG if 6/54 fetuses developed advanced block, the trials were terminated.[12,16]

During the time period of these IVIG trials, basic science exploring the pathogenesis of disease supported the notion that macrophage Toll-like receptor (TLR) signaling following ligation of the ssRNA complexed to the Ro protein contributes to cardiac fibrosis[64,73] as described above. This in vitro observation was initially "translated" to patients by evaluating the use of hydroxychloroquine (HCQ) in an extensive case–control study of anti-Ro antibody-exposed fetuses of SLE mothers (50 cardiac NL and 151 noncardiac NL controls.[81] Seven (14%) cardiac NL children were exposed to HCQ compared with 56 (37%) controls (P = 0.002; OR 0.28).

A multivariable analysis yielded an OR associated with HCQ use of 0.46 (P=0.10). Although HCQ was no longer a statistically significant predictor of cardiac NL, the estimate of the OR remained in the direction of a protective effect, consistent with the results from the overall unadjusted analysis. A subsequent study was performed to evaluate whether HCQ reduces the increased risk of recurrence of cardiac NL, independent of maternal health status.[82] Using an international cohort, 257 pregnancies subsequent to the birth of a child with cardiac NL were evaluated (40 exposed and 217 unexposed to HCQ). The recurrence rate of cardiac NL in fetuses exposed to HCQ was 7.5% (3/40) compared to 21.2% (46/217) in the unexposed group (P=0.05). There were no deaths in the HCQ-exposed group compared to a case fatality rate of 22% in the unexposed group. In both multivariable and propensity score analyses, HCQ use remained significantly associated with a decreased risk of cardiac NL.[82]

In consideration of HCQ it is of note that some physicians remain reluctant to prescribe HCQ during pregnancy given isolated case reports of auditory[83] and retinal toxicity[84] in fetuses exposed to chloroquine, in addition to data from an animal model regarding retinal deposition.[85] Currently, the FDA lists HCQ as pregnancy risk category C (safety in human pregnancy has not been determined). However, recent reviews of the literature suggest that HCQ is safe to use during pregnancy.[86,87] None of the studies (inclusive of over 300 children) found an increased frequency of congenital malformation. A recent prospective study of 114 HCQ-exposed fetuses corroborated those findings, showing no statistical differences in congenital anomalies compared to 455 control pregnancies.[88] In one of the largest studies done to assess for fetal HCQ toxicity, EKGs revealed no differences with regard to duration of the PR or QTC intervals between the 47 unexposed children and the 45 exposed children.[89]

Currently an open label prospective study using the Simon two-stage approach with the hypothesis that HCQ at 400 mg daily significantly reduces the recurrence rate of cardiac NL is enrolling patients. With the completion of 19 patients in the first stage and only one recurrent case,[90] the study is now in the second stage with planned enrollment to at least 54 subjects unless five cases of cardiac NL recur (clinicaltrials.gov).

REFERENCES

1. Buyon J. Neonatal lupus. In: Lahita RG, Tsokos G, Buyon J, Koike T, editors. *Systemic lupus erythematosus.* San Diego: Academic Press; 2011. p. 541–72.
2. Kephart DC, Hood AF, Provost TT. Neonatal lupus erythematosus: new serologic findings. *J Invest Dermatol* 1981;**77**(3):331–3.
3. McCuistion CH, Schoch Jr EP. Possible discoid lupus erythematosus in newborn infant. Report of a case with subsequent development of acute systemic lupus erythematosus in mother. *Arch Dermatol* 1983;**119**(7):615–8.
4. Brucato A, Frassi M, Franceschini F, Cimaz R, Faden D, Pisoni MP, et al. Risk of congenital complete heart block in newborns of mothers with anti-Ro/SSA antibodies detected by counterimmunoelectrophoresis: a prospective study of 100 women. *Arthritis Rheum* 2001;**44**(8):1832–5.
5. Rivera TL, Izmirly PM, Birnbaum BK, Byrne P, Brauth JB, Katholi M, et al. Disease progression in mothers of children enrolled in the Research Registry for Neonatal Lupus. *Ann Rheum Dis* 2009;**68**(6):828–35.
6. Izmirly PM, Saxena A, Kim MY, Wang D, Sahl SK, Llanos C, et al. Maternal and fetal factors associated with mortality and morbidity in a multi-racial/ethnic registry of anti-SSA/Ro-associated cardiac neonatal lupus. *Circulation* 2011;**124**(18):1927–35.
7. Brucato A, Previtali E, Ramoni V, Ghidoni S. Arrhythmias presenting in neonatal lupus. *Scand J Immunol* 2010;**72**(3):198–204.
8. Cimaz R, Spence DL, Hornberger L, Silverman ED. Incidence and spectrum of neonatal lupus erythematosus: a prospective study of infants born to mothers with anti-Ro autoantibodies. *J Pediatr* 2003;**142**(6):678–83.
9. Costedoat-Chalumeau N, Amoura Z, Lupoglazoff JM, Huong DL, Denjoy I, Vauthier D, et al. Outcome of pregnancies in patients with anti-SSA/Ro antibodies: a study of 165 pregnancies, with special focus on electrocardiographic variations in the children and comparison with a control group. *Arthritis Rheum* 2004;**50**(10):3187–94.
10. Friedman DM, Kim MY, Copel JA, Davis C, Phoon CK, Glickstein JS, et al. Utility of cardiac monitoring in fetuses at risk for congenital heart block: the PR Interval and Dexamethasone Evaluation (PRIDE) prospective study. *Circulation* 2008;**117**(4):485–93.
11. Buyon JP, Hiebert R, Copel J, Craft J, Friedman D, Katholi M, et al. Autoimmune-associated congenital heart block: demographics, mortality, morbidity and recurrence rates obtained from a national neonatal lupus registry. *J Am Coll Cardiol* 1998;**31**(7):1658–66.
12. Friedman DM, Llanos C, Izmirly PM, Brock B, Byron J, Copel J, et al. Evaluation of fetuses in a study of intravenous immunoglobulin as preventive therapy for congenital heart block: results of a multicenter, prospective, open-label clinical trial. *Arthritis Rheum* 2010;**62**(4):1138–46.
13. Gladman G, Silverman ED, Yuk L, Luy L, Boutin C, Laskin C, et al. Fetal echocardiographic screening of pregnancies of mothers with anti-Ro and/or anti-La antibodies. *Am J Perinatol* 2002;**19**(2):73–80.
14. Julkunen H, Eronen M. The rate of recurrence of isolated congenital heart block: a population-based study. *Arthritis Rheum* 2001;**44**(2):487–8.
15. Llanos C, Izmirly PM, Katholi M, Clancy RM, Friedman DM, Kim MY, et al. Recurrence rates of cardiac manifestations associated with neonatal lupus and maternal/fetal risk factors. *Arthritis Rheum* 2009;**60**(10):3091–7.
16. Pisoni CN, Brucato A, Ruffatti A, Espinosa G, Cervera R, Belmonte-Serrano M, et al. Failure of intravenous immunoglobulin to prevent congenital heart block: findings of a multicenter, prospective, observational study. *Arthritis Rheum* 2010;**62**(4):1147–52.
17. Izmirly PM, Llanos C, Lee LA, Askanase A, Kim MY, Buyon JP. Cutaneous manifestations of neonatal lupus and risk of subsequent congenital heart block. *Arthritis Rheum* 2010;**62**(4):1153–7.

18. Jaeggi E, Laskin C, Hamilton R, Kingdom J, Silverman E. The importance of the level of maternal anti-Ro/SSA antibodies as a prognostic marker of the development of cardiac neonatal lupus erythematosus a prospective study of 186 antibody-exposed fetuses and infants. *J Am Coll Cardiol* 2010;**55**(24):2778–84.

19. Siren MK, Julkunen H, Kaaja R. The increasing incidence of isolated congenital heart block in Finland. *J Rheumatol* 1998;**25**(9):1862–4.

20. Jaeggi ET, Hornberger LK, Smallhorn JF, Fouron JC. Prenatal diagnosis of complete atrioventricular block associated with structural heart disease: combined experience of two tertiary care centers and review of the literature. *Ultrasound Obstet Gynecol* 2005;**26**(1):16–21.

21. Fritzler MJ, Pauls JD, Kinsella TD, Bowen TJ. Antinuclear, anticytoplasmic, and anti-Sjogren's syndrome antigen A (SS-A/Ro) antibodies in female blood donors. *Clin Immunol Immunopathol* 1985;**36**(1):120–8.

22. Harmon CLL, Huff JC, Norris DA, Weston WL. The frequency of autoantibodies to the SSA/Ro antigen in pregnancy sera [abstract]. *Arthritis Rheum* 1984;**27**(Suppl. 4):S20.

23. Satoh M, Chan EK, Ho LA, Rose KM, Parks CG, Cohn RD, et al. Prevalence and sociodemographic correlates of antinuclear antibodies in the United States. *Arthritis Rheum* 2012;**64**(7):2319–27.

24. Keogan MKG, Jefferies CA. Extractable nuclear antigens and SLE: specificity and role in disease pathogenesis. In: Lahita RG, Tsokos G, Buyon J, Koike T, editors. *Systemic lupus erythematosus*. San Diego: Academic Press; 2011. p. 259–74.

25. Neiman AR, Lee LA, Weston WL, Buyon JP. Cutaneous manifestations of neonatal lupus without heart block: characteristics of mothers and children enrolled in a national registry. *J Pediatr* 2000;**137**(5):674–80.

26. Lee LA. Maternal autoantibodies and pregnancy–II: the neonatal lupus syndrome. *Baillieres Clin Rheumatol* 1990;**4**(1):69–84.

27. Okada N, Okuyama R, Uhara H. Marked histiocytic infiltration in neonatal lupus erythematosus. *J Dermatol* 2014;**41**(2):192–3.

28. Sheth AP, Esterly NB, Ratoosh SL, Smith JP, Hebert AA, Silverman E. U1RNP positive neonatal lupus erythematosus: association with anti-La antibodies? *Br J Dermatol* 1995;**132**(4):520–6.

29. Lee LA, Sokol RJ, Buyon JP. Hepatobiliary disease in neonatal lupus: prevalence and clinical characteristics in cases enrolled in a national registry. *Pediatrics* 2002;**109**(1):E11.

30. Laxer RM, Roberts EA, Gross KR, Britton JR, Cutz E, Dimmick J, et al. Liver disease in neonatal lupus erythematosus. *J Pediatr* 1990;**116**(2):238–42.

31. Wolach B, Choc L, Pomeranz A, Ben Ari Y, Douer D, Metzker A. Aplastic anemia in neonatal lupus erythematosus. *Am J Dis Child* 1993;**147**(9):941–4.

32. Kanagasegar S, Cimaz R, Kurien BT, Brucato A, Scofield RH. Neonatal lupus manifests as isolated neutropenia and mildly abnormal liver functions. *J Rheumatol* 2002;**29**(1):187–91.

33. Boros CA, Spence D, Blaser S, Silverman ED. Hydrocephalus and macrocephaly: new manifestations of neonatal lupus erythematosus. *Arthritis Rheum* 2007;**57**(2):261–6.

34. Gualtieri THR. An immunoreactive theory of selective male affliction. *Behav Brain Sci* 1985;**8**(3):427–41.

35. Askanase AD, Izmirly PM, Katholi M, Mumtaz J, Buyon JP. Frequency of neuro-psychiatric dysfunction in anti-SSA/SSB exposed children with and without neonatal lupus. *Lupus* 2010;**19**(3):300–6.

36. Skog A, Tingstrom J, Salomonsson S, Sonesson SE, Wahren-Herlenius M. Neurodevelopment in children with and without congenital heart block born to anti-Ro/SSA-positive mothers. *Acta Paediatr* 2013;**102**(1):40–6.

37. Jaeggi ET, Silverman ED, Laskin C, Kingdom J, Golding F, Weber R. Prolongation of the atrioventricular conduction in fetuses exposed to maternal anti-Ro/SSA and anti-La/SSB antibodies did not predict progressive heart block. A prospective observational study on the effects of maternal antibodies on 165 fetuses. *J Am Coll Cardiol* 2011;**57**(13):1487–92.

38. Askanase AD, Friedman DM, Copel J, Dische MR, Dubin A, Starc TJ, et al. Spectrum and progression of conduction abnormalities in infants born to mothers with anti-SSA/Ro-SSB/La antibodies. *Lupus* 2002;**11**(3):145–51.

39. Phoon CK, Kim MY, Buyon JP, Friedman DM. Finding the "PR-fect" solution: what is the best tool to measure fetal cardiac PR intervals for the detection and possible treatment of early conduction disease? *Congenit Heart Dis* 2012;**7**(4):349–60.

40. Saleeb S, Copel J, Friedman D, Buyon JP. Comparison of treatment with fluorinated glucocorticoids to the natural history of autoantibody-associated congenital heart block: retrospective review of the research registry for neonatal lupus. *Arthritis Rheum* 1999;**42**(11):2335–45.

41. Hornberger LK, Al Rajaa N. Spectrum of cardiac involvement in neonatal lupus. *Scand J Immunol* 2010;**72**(3):189–97.

42. Cuneo BF, Strasburger JF, Niksch A, Ovadia M, Wakai RT. An expanded phenotype of maternal SSA/SSB antibody-associated fetal cardiac disease. *J Matern Fetal Neonatal Med* 2009;**22**(3):233–8.

43. Guettrot-Imbert G, Cohen L, Fermont L, Villain E, Frances C, Thiebaugeorges O, et al. A new presentation of neonatal lupus: 5 cases of isolated mild endocardial fibroelastosis associated with maternal Anti-SSA/Ro and Anti-SSB/La antibodies. *J Rheumatol* 2011;**38**(2):378–86.

44. Moak JP, Barron KS, Hougen TJ, Wiles HB, Balaji S, Sreeram N, et al. Congenital heart block: development of late-onset cardiomyopathy, a previously underappreciated sequela. *J Am Coll Cardiol* 2001;**37**(1):238–42.

45. Nield LE, Silverman ED, Smallhorn JF, Taylor GP, Mullen JB, Benson LN, et al. Endocardial fibroelastosis associated with maternal anti-Ro and anti-La antibodies in the absence of atrioventricular block. *J Am Coll Cardiol* 2002;**40**(4):796–802.

46. Nield LE, Silverman ED, Taylor GP, Smallhorn JF, Mullen JB, Silverman NH, et al. Maternal anti-Ro and anti-La antibody-associated endocardial fibroelastosis. *Circulation* 2002;**105**(7):843–8.

47. Eliasson H, Sonesson SE, Sharland G, Granath F, Simpson JM, Carvalho JS, et al. Isolated atrioventricular block in the fetus: a retrospective, multinational, multicenter study of 175 patients. *Circulation* 2011;**124**(18):1919–26.

48. Jaeggi ET, Hamilton RM, Silverman ED, Zamora SA, Hornberger LK. Outcome of children with fetal, neonatal or childhood diagnosis of isolated congenital atrioventricular block. A single institution's experience of 30 years. *J Am Coll Cardiol* 2002;**39**(1):130–7.

49. Lopes LM, Tavares GM, Damiano AP, Lopes MA, Aiello VD, Schultz R, et al. Perinatal outcome of fetal atrioventricular block: one-hundred-sixteen cases from a single institution. *Circulation* 2008;**118**(12):1268–75.

50. Waltuck J, Buyon JP. Autoantibody-associated congenital heart block: outcome in mothers and children. *Ann Intern Med* 1994;**120**(7):544–51.

51. Villain E, Coastedoat-Chalumeau N, Marijon E, Boudjemline Y, Piette JC, Bonnet D. Presentation and prognosis of complete atrioventricular block in childhood, according to maternal antibody status. *J Am Coll Cardiol* 2006;**48**(8):1682–7.

52. Buyon JP, Ben-Chetrit E, Karp S, Roubey RA, Pompeo L, Reeves WH, et al. Acquired congenital heart block. Pattern of maternal antibody response to biochemically defined antigens of the SSA/Ro-SSB/La system in neonatal lupus. *J Clin Invest* 1989;**84**(2):627–34.

53. Fritsch C, Hoebeke J, Dali H, Ricchiuti V, Isenberg DA, Meyer O, et al. 52-kDa Ro/SSA epitopes preferentially recognized by antibodies from mothers of children with neonatal lupus and congenital heart block. *Arthritis Res Ther* 2006;**8**(1):R4.

54. Gordon P, Khamashta MA, Rosenthal E, Simpson JM, Sharland G, Brucato A, et al. Anti-52 kDa Ro, anti-60 kDa Ro, and anti-La antibody profiles in neonatal lupus. *J Rheumatol* 2004;**31**(12):2480–7.

55. Reed JH, Jackson MW, Gordon TP. A B cell apotope of Ro 60 in systemic lupus erythematosus. *Arthritis Rheum* 2008;**58**(4):1125–9.

56. Ricchiuti V, Briand JP, Meyer O, Isenberg DA, Pruijn G, Muller S. Epitope mapping with synthetic peptides of 52-kD SSA/Ro protein reveals heterogeneous antibody profiles in human autoimmune sera. *Clin Exp Immunol* 1994;**95**(3):397–407.

57. Reed JH, Clancy RM, Lee KH, Saxena A, Izmirly PM, Buyon JP. Umbilical cord blood levels of maternal antibodies reactive with p200 and full-length Ro 52 in the assessment of risk for cardiac manifestations of neonatal lupus. *Arthritis Care Res* 2012;**64**(9):1373–81.

58. Salomonsson S, Dorner T, Theander E, Bremme K, Larsson P, Wahren-Herlenius M. A serologic marker for fetal risk of congenital heart block. *Arthritis Rheum* 2002;**46**(5):1233–41.

59. Strandberg L, Winqvist O, Sonesson SE, Mohseni S, Salomonsson S, Bremme K, et al. Antibodies to amino acid 200-239 (p200) of Ro52 as serological markers for the risk of developing congenital heart block. *Clin Exp Immunol* 2008;**154**(1):30–7.

60. Clancy RM, Buyon JP, Ikeda K, Nozawa K, Argyle DA, Friedman DM, et al. Maternal antibody responses to the 52-kd SSA/RO p200 peptide and the development of fetal conduction defects. *Arthritis Rheum* 2005;**52**(10):3079–86.

61. Scarsi M, Radice A, Pregnolato F, Ramoni V, Grava C, Bianchi L, et al. Anti-Ro/SSA-p200 antibodies in the prediction of congenital heart block. An Italian multicentre cross-sectional study on behalf of the 'Forum Interdisciplinare per la Ricerca nelle Malattie Autoimmuni (FIRMA) Group'. *Clin Exp Rheumatol* 2014;**32**(6):848–54.

62. Strandberg LS, Cui X, Rath A, Liu J, Silverman ED, Liu X, et al. Congenital heart block maternal sera autoantibodies target an extracellular epitope on the alpha1G T-type calcium channel in human fetal hearts. *PloS One* 2013;**8**(9):e72668.

63. Karnabi E, Boutjdir M. Role of calcium channels in congenital heart block. *Scand J Immunol* 2010;**72**(3):226–34.

64. Clancy RM, Alvarez D, Komissarova E, Barrat FJ, Swartz J, Buyon JP. Ro60-associated single-stranded RNA links inflammation with fetal cardiac fibrosis via ligation of TLRs: a novel pathway to autoimmune-associated heart block. *J Immunol* 2010;**184**(4):2148–55.

65. Karnabi E, Qu Y, Mancarella S, Boutjdir M. Rescue and worsening of congenital heart block-associated electrocardiographic abnormalities in two transgenic mice. *J Cardiovasc Electrophysiol* 2011;**22**(8):922–30.

66. Ambrosi A, Dzikaite V, Park J, Strandberg L, Kuchroo VK, Herlenius E, et al. Anti-Ro52 monoclonal antibodies specific for amino acid 200-239, but not other Ro52 epitopes, induce congenital heart block in a rat model. *Ann Rheum Dis* 2012;**71**(3):448–54.

67. Briassouli P, Komissarova EV, Clancy RM, Buyon JP. Role of the urokinase plasminogen activator receptor in mediating impaired efferocytosis of anti-SSA/Ro-bound apoptotic cardiocytes: implications in the pathogenesis of congenital heart block. *Circ Res* 2010;**107**(3):374–87.

68. Miranda-Carus ME, Askanase AD, Clancy RM, Di Donato F, Chou TM, Libera MR, et al. Anti-SSA/Ro and anti-SSB/La autoantibodies bind the surface of apoptotic fetal cardiocytes and promote secretion of TNF-alpha by macrophages. *J Immunol* 2000;**165**(9):5345–51.

69. Reed JH, Sim S, Wolin SL, Clancy RM, Buyon JP. Ro60 requires Y3 RNA for cell surface exposure and inflammation associated with cardiac manifestations of neonatal lupus. *J Immunol* 2013;**191**(1):110–6.

70. Reed JH, Clancy RM, Purcell AW, Kim MY, Gordon TP, Buyon JP. beta2-glycoprotein I and protection from anti-SSA/Ro60-associated cardiac manifestations of neonatal lupus. *J Immunol* 2011;**187**(1):520–6.

71. Clancy RM, Neufing PJ, Zheng P, O'Mahony M, Nimmerjahn F, Gordon TP, et al. Impaired clearance of apoptotic cardiocytes is linked to anti-SSA/Ro and -SSB/La antibodies in the pathogenesis of congenital heart block. *J Clin Invest* 2006;**116**(9):2413–22.

72. Clancy RM, Kapur RP, Molad Y, Askanase AD, Buyon JP. Immunohistologic evidence supports apoptosis, IgG deposition, and novel macrophage/fibroblast crosstalk in the pathologic cascade leading to congenital heart block. *Arthritis Rheum* 2004;**50**(1):173–82.

73. Reed JH, Sim S, Wolin SL, Clancy RM, Buyon JP. Ro60 requires Y3 RNA for cell surface exposure and inflammation associated with cardiac manifestations of neonatal lupus. *J Immunol* July 1 2013;**191**(1):110–6.

74. Lovgren T, Eloranta ML, Bave U, Alm GV, Ronnblom L. Induction of interferon-alpha production in plasmacytoid dendritic cells by immune complexes containing nucleic acid released by necrotic or late apoptotic cells and lupus IgG. *Arthritis Rheum* 2004;**50**(6):1861–72.

75. Kelly KM, Zhuang H, Nacionales DC, Scumpia PO, Lyons R, Akaogi J, et al. "Endogenous adjuvant" activity of the RNA components of lupus autoantigens Sm/RNP and Ro 60. *Arthritis Rheum* 2006;**54**(5):1557–67.

76. Pike JI, Donofrio MT, Berul CI. Ineffective therapy, underpowered studies, or merely too little, too late? Risk factors and impact of maternal corticosteroid treatment on outcome in antibody-associated fetal heart block. *Circulation* 2011;**124**(18):1905–7.

77. Costedoat-Chalumeau N, Amoura Z, Le Thi Hong D, Wechsler B, Vauthier D, Ghillani P, et al. Questions about dexamethasone use for the prevention of anti-SSA related congenital heart block. *Ann Rheum Dis* 2003;**62**(10):1010–2.

78. Jaeggi ET, Fouron JC, Silverman ED, Ryan G, Smallhorn J, Hornberger LK. Transplacental fetal treatment improves the outcome of prenatally diagnosed complete atrioventricular block without structural heart disease. *Circulation* 2004;**110**(12):1542–8.

79. Li N, Zhao M, Hilario-Vargas J, Prisayanh P, Warren S, Diaz LA, et al. Complete FcRn dependence for intravenous Ig therapy in autoimmune skin blistering diseases. *J Clin Invest* 2005;**115**(12):3440–50.

80. Samuelsson A, Towers TL, Ravetch JV. Anti-inflammatory activity of IVIG mediated through the inhibitory Fc receptor. *Science* 2001;**291**(5503):484–6.

81. Izmirly PM, Kim MY, Llanos C, Le PU, Guerra MM, Askanase AD, et al. Evaluation of the risk of anti-SSA/Ro-SSB/La antibody-associated cardiac manifestations of neonatal lupus in fetuses of mothers with systemic lupus erythematosus exposed to hydroxychloroquine. *Ann Rheum Dis* 2010;**69**(10):1827–30.

82. Izmirly PM, Costedoat-Chalumeau N, Pisoni CN, Khamashta MA, Kim MY, Saxena A, et al. Maternal use of hydroxychloroquine is associated with a reduced risk of recurrent anti-SSA/Ro-antibody-associated cardiac manifestations of neonatal lupus. *Circulation* 2012;**126**(1):76–82.

83. Matz GJ, Naunton RF. Ototoxicity of chloroquine. *Arch Otolaryngol* 1969;**88**:370–2.

84. Paufique L, Magnard P. Retinal degeneration in 2 children following preventive antimalarial treatment of the mother during pregnancy. *Bull Soc Ophtalmol Fr* 1969;**69**(4):466–7.

85. Ullberg S, Lindquist NG, Sjostrand SE. Accumulation of chorioretinotoxic drugs in the foetal eye. *Nature* 1970;**227**(5264):1257–8.

86. Costedoat-Chalumeau N, Amoura Z, Huong DL, Lechat P, Piette JC. Safety of hydroxychloroquine in pregnant patients with connective tissue diseases. Review of the literature. *Autoimmun Rev* 2005;**4**(2):111–5.

87. Ruiz-Irastorza G, Ramos-Casals M, Brito-Zeron P, Khamashta MA. Clinical efficacy and side effects of antimalarials in systemic lupus erythematosus: a systematic review. *Ann Rheumatic Dis* 2010;**69**(1):20–8.

88. Diav-Citrin O, Blyakhman S, Shechtman S, Ornoy A. Pregnancy outcome following in utero exposure to hydroxychloroquine: a prospective comparative observational study. *Reprod Toxicol* 2013;**39**:58–62.

89. Costedoat-Chalumeau N, Amoura Z, Duhaut P, Huong DL, Sebbough D, Wechsler B, et al. Safety of hydroxychloroquine in pregnant patients with connective tissue diseases: a study of one hundred thirty-three cases compared with a control group. *Arthritis Rheum* 2003;**48**(11):3207–11.

90. Izmirly PM, Costedoat-Chalumeau N, Saxena A, Zink A, Smith Z, Friedman D, et al. First stage of a Simon's two-stage optimal approach supports placental transfer of hydroxychloroquine and a reduced recurrence rate of the cardiac manifestations of neonatal lupus. *Arthritis Rhuem* 2013;**66**(Suppl. 10):S1212.

Chapter 52

Incomplete Lupus

George Stojan
Harvard Medical School, Division of Rheumatology, Beth Israel Deaconess Medical Center, Boston, MA, USA

SUMMARY

Patients who meet less than four American College of Rheumatology (ACR) criteria or have other representative, noncriteria systemic lupus erythematosus (SLE) manifestations have incomplete lupus erythematosus. The most common clinical manifestations in patients with incomplete lupus include rashes, arthritis, Raynaud's phenomenon, and cytopenias. ANA (anti-nuclear antibodies) is the most commonly detected serological finding, but the presence of anti-dsDNA, anti-phospholipid antibodies, and low complements is associated with higher risk of progression to SLE. Despite a generally mild clinical course without nephritis, vasculitis, or CNS involvement, the disease-related mortality and cardiovascular morbidity are indistinguishable from the one in SLE, indicating a need for continued monitoring, vigilance in recognizing this entity, and consideration of early start of treatment.

DEFINITION

The introduction of systemic lupus erythematosus (SLE) classification criteria was a major step forward in the study of SLE and revolutionized both basic and clinical research in the field. The purpose of the classification criteria was to facilitate enrollment into clinical trials; thus they needed to be unambiguous, easy to apply, and highly specific. When the American College of Rheumatology (ACR) classification criteria for SLE were adopted, the authors did not propose their use as diagnostic criteria,[1,2] but their adoption in clinical practice as the sine qua non of systemic lupus diagnosis has created major obstacles in the clinical approach to patients who do not fulfill the required four criteria.

When patients present with signs and symptoms of an autoimmune diathesis within the realm of systemic lupus erythematosus yet do not fulfill four of the ACR classification criteria, they are said to have "incomplete lupus." It should be noted that there is no universally accepted definition of incomplete lupus with proposals ranging from anti-nuclear antibodies (ANA) with a single organ manifestation of SLE to three separate ACR criteria for SLE. Adding to the difficulty of performing a comprehensive literature search is the differing nomenclature for the entity itself, which is also being referred to as subclinical lupus, variant lupus, or latent lupus.[3–5]

INCOMPLETE LUPUS VERSUS UNDIFFERENTIATED CONNECTIVE TISSUE DISEASE (UCTD)

It is estimated that approximately 50% of patients with an autoimmune diathesis have an unclassifiable profile at the time of disease onset.[6] This inevitably leads to another controversy in the field, which is distinguishing between incomplete lupus and UCTD.

UCTD refers to unclassifiable systemic autoimmune diseases that share clinical and serological manifestations with definite connective tissue diseases such as systemic lupus, systemic sclerosis, and rheumatoid arthritis, but do not fulfill any of the existing classification criteria.[7] SLE is the most frequently reported diagnosis (20–60% of cases) among patients with UCTD who develop a defined CTD.[8] The evolution is likely to occur during the first 1–5 years after the appearance of symptoms but some late evolutions are also described.[8]

How does one then distinguish between UCTD and incomplete lupus? The distinction between the two conditions is not well defined, but it would be reasonable to regard incomplete lupus as a subset of UCTD, where presenting features are compatible with the potential for SLE development.[9]

EPIDEMIOLOGY

There is a paucity of data in regard to the incidence and/or prevalence of incomplete lupus. In an 8 year prospective study in Denmark, the median annual incidence of definite SLE was 1.04 per 100,000 and of incomplete SLE was 0.36 per 100,000. The point prevalence of incomplete lupus in 1994 was 6.59 per 100,000 and it increased to 7.53 per 100,000 in 2002. Over the 8 years of follow-up, seven patients with incomplete lupus transformed into definite SLE at a progression rate of 3.64 per 100 person-years at risk.[10,11]

Systemic Lupus Erythematosus. http://dx.doi.org/10.1016/B978-0-12-801917-7.00052-8

TABLE 1 Summary of Incomplete Lupus Studies

	Ganczarczyk et al.[4]	Greer and Panush[5]	Vila et al.[12]	Swaak et al.[13]	Stahl et al.[14-16]	Al Attia[17]	Laustrup et al.[10]	Olsen et al.[18]
Design	Single center	Single center	Single center	Multicenter	Population	Single center	Population	Single center
Inclusion	>1 ACR ≤2 + one other symptom	>2 ACR <4	>1 ACR <4	ANA and at least one ACR clinical criterion	ANA and at least one ACR clinical criterion	>1 ACR <4	>1 ACR <4	>1 ACR <4
Number of patients	22	38	87	122	28	12	37	22
Observation	8	1.6 years	2.2 years	3 years	5.3 years	1.8 years	8 years	2.4 years
Transition to SLE	7 (32%)	2 (5.3%)	8 (9%)	25	16 (57%)	0	7 (26.9%)	3 (14%)
Predictors of transition	None	None	Photosensitivity, malar rash, oral ulcers, low C3 levels, and anti-dsDNA	None	Malar rash and anticardiolipin	N/A	Mild disease, absence of renal and CNS involvement	Young females, increased IgG specificities to proliferating cell nuclear antigen (PCNA), beta 2 microglobulin, C1q, and hemocyanin

TRANSITION FROM INCOMPLETE LUPUS ERYTHEMATOSUS (ILE) TO SLE

In Table 1, the most important studies in the field of incomplete lupus are summarized. The most common clinical manifestations in patients with incomplete lupus include rashes, arthritis, Raynaud's phenomenon, and cytopenias. The disease course tends to be mild, without nephritis, vasculitis, or CNS involvement. The most commonly identified serological findings include ANA, while anti-Ro/La antibodies are more frequently detected than anti-Sm or anti-dsDNA.

When faced with a patient who has incomplete lupus, there is no question more important than whether an imminent progression to systemic lupus will occur. As evident from Table 1, the studies to date have been heterogeneous with varying inclusion criteria and length of observation. The range of progression to SLE varied from 5.3% to 57%. The predictors of transition have included female sex and young age as demographic factors, malar rash, photosensitivity and oral ulcers as clinical factors, and, ultimately, low complements, anti-dsDNA, and anticardiolipins as laboratory markers but there is no factor that was uniformly associated with progression across the studies. Incomplete lupus may continue to evolve to SLE over time as evidenced by the highest progression rates seen in the studies with the longest follow-up. The first 4 years from the time of diagnosis carry the highest risk of progression.[19,20]

Data from the RELESSER registry[21] deserve a special mention and were purposefully not included in the table above. RELESSER-T was a cross-sectional multicenter study, the largest one to date, that focused on the difference between patients who fulfilled the 1997 ACR SLE criteria and those with less than four criteria.

Malar rash, oral ulcers, lupus nephritis, and antiphospholipid syndrome were the features that were most strongly associated with SLE. Renal and CNS involvement was rare in patients with incomplete lupus (4% and 1.2%, respectively). Patients with SLE had higher disease activity, more damage, and a higher mortality rate compared to patients with incomplete lupus.

Although disease activity scores were low, one of every four deaths documented in RELESSER was due to SLE activity. There were no differences between patients with SLE and incomplete SLE when it comes to disease activity-related death. The authors brought up several potential confounding factors like underestimating disease activity in incomplete lupus, which may have led to poor follow-up, less immunosuppressive use, and finally infrequent use of antimalarials since one-third of incomplete SLE patients were never prescribed antimalarials.

In regard to comorbidities, the rates of cardiovascular events were numerically higher in patients with incomplete SLE, although without reaching statistical significance. Patients with incomplete lupus were older and had higher rates of certain risk factors for coronary disease such as smoking and diabetes, although this was once again not statistically different compared to the SLE group.

TREATMENT

The new findings from the RELESSER registry add new insight into the morbidity and mortality of patients with incomplete lupus. Despite a uniform agreement that incomplete lupus tends to be a less aggressive form of disease, with lower disease activity scores and less renal and CNS involvement, the cardiovascular morbidity and long-term mortality seem to be similar to those in patients with SLE. How different treatment regimens influence clinical expression, progression to SLE, and long-term mortality and morbidity is not known. In a retrospective study involving sera from 130 United States military personnel who later developed SLE, hydroxychloroquine was associated with a longer time between the onset of the first clinical symptom and the SLE diagnosis, a lower rate of autoantibody accumulation, and a decreased number of autoantibody specificities at and after diagnosis.[22] No such effect was seen for NSAID treatment. These important preliminary findings provide limited support for the early use of immunosuppressive therapies in incomplete lupus, although prospective studies are needed to clearly elucidate the role of pharmacologic interventions in halting the progression to SLE in high risk patients.

REFERENCES

1. Hochberg MC. Updating the American college of rheumatology revised criteria for the classification of systemic lupus erythematosus. *Arthritis Rheum* September 1997;**40**(9):1725.
2. Tan EM, Cohen AS, Fries JF, Masi AT, McShane DJ, Rothfield NF, et al. The 1982 revised criteria for the classification of systemic lupus erythematosus. *Arthritis Rheum* November 1982;**25**(11):1271–7.
3. Asherson RA, Cervera R, Lahita RG. Latent, incomplete or lupus at all? *J Rheumatol* December 1991;**18**(12):1783–6.
4. Ganczarczyk L, Urowitz MB, Gladman DD. Latent lupus. *J Rheumatol* April 1989;**16**(4):475–8.
5. Greer JM, Panush RS. Incomplete lupus erythematosus. *Arch Intern Med* November 1989;**149**(11):2473–6.
6. Alarcón GS, Williams GV, Singer JZ, Steen VD, Clegg DO, Paulus HE, et al. Early undifferentiated connective tissue disease. I. Early clinical manifestation in a large cohort of patients with undifferentiated connective tissue diseases compared with cohorts of well established connective tissue disease. *J Rheumatol* September 1991;**18**(9):1332–9.
7. Mosca M, Neri R, Bombardieri S. Undifferentiated connective tissue diseases (UCTD): a review of the literature and a proposal for preliminary classification criteria. *Clin Exp Rheumatol* October 1999;**17**(5):615–20.
8. Mosca M, Tani C, Vagnani S, Carli L, Bombardieri S. The diagnosis and classification of undifferentiated connective tissue diseases. *J Autoimmun* March 2014;**48–49**:50–2.
9. Nossent J, Swaak T. *Incomplete lupus erythematosus. Systemic lupus erythematosus.* 5th ed. Elsevier; 2011. p. 707–17.

10. Laustrup H, Voss A, Green A, Junker P. Occurrence of systemic lupus erythematosus in a Danish community: an 8-year prospective study. *Scand J Rheumatol* April 2009;**38**(2):128–32.

11. Voss AB, Green A, Junker P. Systemic lupus erythematosus in the county of Fynen. An epidemiologic study. *Ugeskr Laeger* June 21, 1999;**161**(25):3837–40.

12. Vilá LM, Mayor AM, Valentín AH, García-Soberal M, Vilá S. Clinical outcome and predictors of disease evolution in patients with incomplete lupus erythematosus. *Lupus* 2000;**9**(2):110–5.

13. Swaak AJ, van de Brink H, Smeenk RJ, Manger K, Kalden JR, Tosi S, et al. Incomplete lupus erythematosus: results of a multicentre study under the supervision of the EULAR Standing Committee on International Clinical Studies Including Therapeutic Trials (ESCISIT). *Rheumatol Oxf Engl* January 2001;**40**(1):89–94.

14. Alarcón GS, McGwin G, Roseman JM, Uribe A, Fessler BJ, Bastian HM, et al. Systemic lupus erythematosus in three ethnic groups. XIX. Natural history of the accrual of the American college of rheumatology criteria prior to the occurrence of criteria diagnosis. *Arthritis Rheum* August 15, 2004;**51**(4):609–15.

15. Danieli MG, Fraticelli P, Franceschini F, Cattaneo R, Farsi A, Passaleva A, et al. Five-year follow-up of 165 Italian patients with undifferentiated connective tissue diseases. *Clin Exp Rheumatol* October 1999;**17**(5):585–91.

16. Ståhl Hallengren C, Nived O, Sturfelt G. Outcome of incomplete systemic lupus erythematosus after 10 years. *Lupus* 2004;**13**(2):85–8.

17. Al Attia HM. Borderline systemic lupus erythematosus (SLE): a separate entity or a forerunner to SLE? *Int J Dermatol* April 2006;**45**(4):366–9.

18. Olsen NJ, Li Q-Z, Quan J, Wang L, Mutwally A, Karp DR. Autoantibody profiling to follow evolution of lupus syndromes. *Arthritis Res Ther* 2012;**14**(4):R174.

19. Dijkstra S, Nieuwenhuys EJ, Swaak AJ. The prognosis and outcome of patients referred to an outpatient clinic for rheumatic diseases characterized by the presence of antinuclear antibodies (ANA). *Scand J Rheumatol* 1999;**28**(1):33–7.

20. Vlachoyiannopoulos PG, Tzavara V, Dafni U, Spanos E, Moutsopoulos HM. Clinical features and evolution of antinuclear antibody positive individuals in a rheumatology outpatient clinic. *J Rheumatol* May 1998;**25**(5):886–91.

21. Rúa-Figueroa Í, Richi P, López-Longo FJ, Galindo M, Calvo-Alén J, Olivé-Marqués A, et al. Comprehensive description of clinical characteristics of a large systemic lupus erythematosus cohort from the Spanish Rheumatology Society Lupus Registry (RELESSER) with emphasis on complete versus incomplete lupus differences. *Medicine (Baltimore)* January 2015;**94**(1):e267.

22. James JA, Kim-Howard XR, Bruner BF, Jonsson MK, McClain MT, Arbuckle MR, et al. Hydroxychloroquine sulfate treatment is associated with later onset of systemic lupus erythematosus. *Lupus* 2007;**16**(6):401–9.

Chapter 53

Childhood-Onset Systemic Lupus Erythematosus

Mindy S. Lo

Boston Children's Hospital, Harvard Medical School, Boston, MA, USA

SUMMARY

Childhood-onset disease represents 10–20% of systemic lupus erythematosus (SLE) cases. The demographic characteristics largely parallel those seen in adult-onset disease, although the female:male ratio is less skewed in children, and may approach equal in very early onset SLE. The genetic contribution is thought to be stronger in childhood-onset disease, and this is supported by younger onset of disease in cases of familial lupus.

The clinical manifestations of pediatric lupus are similar to those seen in adults. However, children generally present with more severe disease and higher prevalence of lupus nephritis. This, together with their longer lifetime burden of disease, means that patients with childhood-onset SLE have higher morbidity and mortality overall. They may experience greater effects of medication toxicity due to higher cumulative exposure and exposure during their critical period of growth.

EPIDEMIOLOGY

Among all patients with SLE, it is estimated that 10–20% have onset in childhood. Definition of childhood-onset, or pediatric SLE (pSLE), however, varies by study as the age thresholds used can be quite variable. In general, the majority of pSLE cases develop in adolescents, while prepubertal onset is relatively rarer.

Limited data are available on incidence and prevalence of lupus in children. A recent review of the Medicaid database estimated an overall SLE prevalence of 9.73 per 100,000 children in the United States.[1] Incidence rate was calculated at 2.22 cases/100,000/year, substantially higher than a prior estimation of 0.28 based on data gathered by a Canadian disease registry.[2] This difference may be explained by differences in racial composition, or possibly increasing frequency of pSLE over time, as has been suggested in studies of SLE in adults.[3,4]

In the Medicaid study, non-White children were disproportionately affected at higher rates, consistent with what has been reported in adults with SLE.[1,5,6] Among the racial groups, Asian children had the highest prevalence of both SLE and lupus nephritis at 23.79 and 11.21, respectively, followed by African–American, Native American, and Hispanic children.[1] Non-Caucasian children with SLE also have younger age of onset and higher prevalence of renal disease.[7] In a large study of hospital admissions for pSLE, African–American and Hispanic children had higher rates of end-stage renal disease (ESRD) and death; Hispanic patients also had longer lengths of stay and more readmissions.[8] Socioeconomic status may play a role in some of the observed racial and ethnic differences, but these factors remain inadequately studied at this point.

Females are also disproportionately affected by pSLE, as is the case in adult-onset SLE. However, the female-to-male ratio is lower in children than in adults, with estimates ranging from 3.6–5.3 to 1.[1,9,10] Most studies have suggested a trend toward less skewed sex ratios in children with prepubertal disease, and the sex ratio is nearly even in infantile-onset SLE.[11]

In contrast to SLE, subacute cutaneous lupus erythematosus and other cutaneous-limited forms of lupus are extremely rare in children, with literature limited to case reports only.[12]

CLINICAL MANIFESTATIONS

Clinical manifestations of pSLE generally parallel those seen in adult onset disease. Hematologic, musculoskeletal, and cutaneous manifestations are the most common presenting features in pSLE, each observed in 55–70% of cases.[9,13] Initial presentations of SLE in children are often severe, with severe organ involvement in 40% of children at onset. In one cohort of 256 patients followed for a mean of 3.5 years, three of six deaths occurred at first presentation.[13]

Initial presenting features also often include constitutional symptoms, such as fever and fatigue.[9,13] Raynaud phenomenon is noted at presentation in 10–14% of children with SLE.[9,13]

Systemic Lupus Erythematosus. http://dx.doi.org/10.1016/B978-0-12-801917-7.00053-X

Hematologic manifestations most typically include Coombs-positive hemolytic anemia, thrombocytopenia, and leukopenia. Hemolytic anemia is more common in children with SLE compared to adults.[14,15] Antiphospholipid antibodies are found in 30–50% of pSLE cases.

In contrast to adult SLE, anti-dsDNA antibodies are found in high frequency (61–93%) in pSLE.[9,13,15,16] The strength of association between anti-DNA antibodies and renal disease may also be stronger in children than in adults.[15] Rheumatoid factor is comparatively rare in pSLE.[16] Anti-histone and anti-ribosomal P antibodies are also more common in children with SLE, while other autoantibody profiles are generally similar between children and adults.[15] Although the frequencies of Ro/SSA and La/SSB antibodies are not significantly different in pediatric and adult SLE, sicca symptoms are relatively uncommon in children.[9,15]

Hypocomplementemia is noted in >70% of children with SLE. Inherited complement deficiencies are more commonly seen in pSLE, as typically complement deficiency is associated with early onset of autoimmune manifestations.[17] Other laboratory manifestations are generally similar to those seen in adults; both hyper- and hypogammaglobulinemia are reported.[18]

Arthritis in pSLE is usually nonerosive, most commonly symmetric and affecting knees, fingers, wrists, and ankles. In most patients with joint involvement, the arthritis is present at initial diagnosis. Thus, joint symptoms that develop more than 1 year after disease onset should prompt consideration of other causes, especially avascular necrosis. Children may be relatively protected from osteonecrosis, however; one prospective study found significantly lower rates of osteonecrosis in pediatric patients (defined as <15 years of age) compared to adolescent and adult patients, despite receiving higher daily corticosteroid doses.[19]

Cutaneous manifestations are similar to those seen in adults; malar rash, vasculitis, photosensitivity, and oral ulcers are most common. Alopecia is also seen in 10–29% of children with SLE.[9,13]

Renal involvement occurs at significantly higher rates in children and adolescents with SLE compared to adults.[14,15] Prevalence of nephritis in pSLE is estimated between 37% and 55%, and, if present, is found at initial diagnosis or within 2 years of disease onset in 90% of patients.[1,9,13] The distribution of nephritis histological class mirrors that seen in adults; more than half of these children will have proliferative (WHO class III–IV) disease.[14] Renal disease in children is more severe than that in adults, and is a major cause of morbidity.[20,21]

Neuropsychiatric disease is a concerning feature that affects 15–30% of children with SLE.[9,13] As with other severe organ involvement in pSLE, onset typically occurs early in the course.[22] Headaches, seizures, and psychosis

are the most commonly reported symptoms. Chorea is rare but seen more often in children than adults.[23] Overt lupus cerebritis presenting with these features is easily recognized; however, cognitive impairment and depression/mood disorders due to SLE are often overlooked. In adolescents in particular, a decline in school performance and depressive symptoms can also be attributed to a number of noninflammatory causes that must be considered. These include difficulty adjusting to chronic illness, missed school days due to medical appointments, and corticosteroid side effects.

Macrophage activation syndrome (MAS) is a serious complication of SLE that may be underrecognized. MAS is more commonly associated with juvenile idiopathic arthritis (JIA); while the true prevalence of MAS development in pSLE is not known, the severity of illness may be greater in SLE than in JIA, with higher rates of ICU admission, need for mechanical ventilation, and longer hospital stays.[24] The mortality of MAS development in pSLE may be as high as 11%.[24,25]

FAMILIAL SLE

Though typically thought to be of multigenic or oligogenic origin, familial cases of SLE demonstrate the potentially strong contribution of single genevariants to lupus pathogenesis. In many instances of familial lupus, the autoimmune phenotype develops early in life. Inherited deficiencies of complement are the best known examples of this. Patients with deficiency of C1q have >90% lifetime risk of developing SLE; in these cases, onset of SLE features occurs at a median age of 6 years.[26]

Detailed examination of families with multiple affected members has yielded new insights into the pathogenesis of SLE. In addition to complement factors, other contributory genes identified through analysis of families with SLE or lupus-like diseases include TREX1, DNASE1L3, and PRKCD, among others.[27,28] The implicated pathways include those involved in sensing DNA damage, clearance of DNA in apoptosis, and B-cell signaling. As most cases of familial SLE do not have an identified genetic mutation, it can be expected that more gene variants important for lupus pathogenesis will be discovered in future studies of these families.

The genetic basis of SLE is discussed in greater depth elsewhere (Chapter 10).

MORBIDITY AND MORTALITY

Multiple studies over the years have demonstrated the higher severity of disease when SLE presents in childhood versus adulthood. Childhood onset conveys a mortality risk 3.1-fold higher than adult-onset disease.[29] Mortality rates have been improving over the years with advances in both diagnosis and management. The 5-year survival estimate for childhood-onset SLE has improved from 59% to 93% in the 1980s to near 100% currently.[30] Ten year survival is less favorable at only 86%.[31] Improved survival rates also mean, however, that more patients are living with long-term morbidity. In one study of pSLE hospitalizations over a 10 year period, mortality declined significantly from 1% to 0.6%, while the rate of dialysis, blood transfusions, and vascular catheterization procedures increased with time.[32] Most children do not achieve durable remission, and thus organ damage continues to accrue with time. In addition, even accounting for disease duration, patients with childhood-onset SLE accrue damage faster than patients with adult-onset disease.[33]

Causes of death in children, as with adults, have historically been related mostly to renal disease and infection. As renal outcomes have improved over the years, causes of death in pSLE have shifted. In one retrospective, multi-center study of 12 children and adolescents with SLE, none were related to renal disease.[34] Infection was responsible for three deaths; SLE pancreatitis for three deaths; pulmonary thromboembolism in two patients; pulmonary hemorrhage in one patient; encephalitis in one patient; myocardial infarction in one patient; and one child committed suicide.[34]

Among children with renal involvement, outcome is predicted by histological class. As in adults, proliferative disease conveys the worst prognosis.[35] In a large Asian cohort of pediatric lupus nephritis, most of whom had class IV disease, rates of ESRD were overall low; the 5-, 10-, and 15-year ESRD-free survival rates were 95%, 94%, and 90%, respectively.[36] Infection was the leading cause of death in this cohort.

THERAPEUTIC CONSIDERATIONS IN CHILDREN

Although pathogenesis and diagnosis of SLE are generally similar among children and adults, there are many unique considerations that must be made in the care of pediatric patients.

Medication Toxicity

First, medication toxicity profiles must take into account differences in the physiology of a child versus an adult. In addition, the longer duration of disease that these children face also means that their cumulative exposure to medications will be greater. The first example of this is corticosteroid use. Multiple studies have demonstrated that significantly higher rates of steroid medications, both intravenous and oral, are prescribed for children with SLE compared to adults.[20,30,37] This most likely reflects the increased disease severity in pediatric patients. Complications of chronic steroid use are well known; in children, growth suppression is a major concern that is not typically relevant for adults. The effect of steroids on growth is

difficult to distinguish from that of chronic disease activity. An estimated 15–16% of pediatric SLE patients experience growth failure during the course of their disease.[38] However, the effect of this growth failure on final height has not yet been studied.

Steroid use also contributes to the early atherosclerosis and osteopenia reported in patients with childhood-onset SLE.[39] Although the exact prevalence of atherosclerosis in pSLE is not known, carotid intima–media thickening (CIMT) has been used as a proxy measure. The use of statins to prevent atherosclerosis in adults with SLE has previously been proposed as a preventive health measure, although the effectiveness of this approach is unclear. A study of pSLE patients randomized to therapy with atorvastatin or placebo for 3 years did not show a difference in outcome as measured by CIMT. However, the group treated with atorvastatin did show lower C-reactive protein and cholesterol levels.[40] Further subgroup analysis of this cohort has suggested that patient characteristics such as older age and normal vitamin D levels may correlate with better response to therapy.[41,42]

There are multiple mechanisms which contribute to the effect of chronic steroid use on bone mineral density. These include inhibition of intestinal calcium absorption, increased urinary calcium excretion, inhibition of osteoblast activity, and accelerated bone resorption.[43] The risk of fragility fractures in glucocorticoid-induced osteopenia is not well defined in children. Similarly, there are no standardized guidelines for the prevention or treatment of glucocorticoid-induced osteopenia. Based on adult data, calcium and vitamin D supplementation are recommended for all children receiving long-term therapy with glucocorticoids. Bisphosphonate use is typically reserved for patients with osteopenic fractures, as these medications are incorporated into bone for years and long-term effects on growth are not known.

Other Cushingoid effects of chronic steroid use are also of particular concern in children and adolescents, as they contribute to nonadherence. In one study, 15% of adolescent patients gained ≥20 kg over the course of corticosteroid therapy, and 10% met criteria for obesity at the end of the study.[44] Additional cosmetic side effects of steroid use such as hirsutism and acne have also been reported as factors affecting adherence to therapy.

Effects of therapy on future fertility are a major concern in the care of pediatric and adolescent patients, both male and female. Cyclophosphamide, in particular, is associated with gonadal toxicity in both males and females. Suppression of spermatogenesis by cyclophosphamide disproportionately affects postpubertal, as opposed to prepubertal, males, and this effect may be temporary or permanent.[45] In one study of 35 males with SLE, ages 15–45, all patients had abnormal semen analyses. Cryopreservation of sperm should be discussed with patients for whom cyclophosphamide therapy is being considered. In females, prepubertal patients are again less susceptible to the gonadal toxicity of cyclophosphamide as compared to postpubertal adolescents. Multiple studies have shown that while the risk of premature ovarian failure in pediatric/adolescent SLE is significant (0–36%), it is substantially less than that observed in older patients.[45] However, even in the absence of overt ovarian failure, ovarian reserve may still be diminished in adolescents exposed to cyclophosphamide.[46,47] Suppression of ovulation may be a feasible method of ovarian protection, and should be a consideration for all postpubertal patients receiving alkylating agents.

Malignancy Risk

Lifetime risk for malignancy, especially lymphoma, has been reported in multiple studies to be higher in adult patients with SLE.[48] The risk for children, who have longer disease burden, has not been as well characterized. In one multicenter study of 1020 patients observed for a total of 7986 patient-years, 14 cancers were reported.[49] As only three were expected from matched cancer registry data, this was estimated to represent a standardized incidence ratio of 4.7 (95% CI, 2.6–7.8). Three of the 14 were hematologic malignancies. Mean SLE duration at the time of cancer diagnosis was 12.3 years.

A major question for both pediatric and adult patients is whether this increased malignancy risk is related to the specific disease pathophysiology or the effects of immunosuppressive medication. One study suggests that cyclophosphamide exposure, more so than disease activity, contributes to the increased risk for lymphoma.[50] Another speculation has been the role of Epstein–Barr virus (EBV), which may be more important for pathophysiology in childhood-onset lupus.[51] It has not, however, been studied whether EBV-associated malignancies specifically are overrepresented in SLE.

Psychosocial Issues

Adolescent SLE patients commonly struggle with adherence to therapy. In one study, fewer than a third of adolescent patients who were adherent to clinic visits were also adherent to hydroxychloroquine treatment.[52] Poor medication adherence is multifactorial; cited factors include mood disorders, medication side effects, changes in physical appearance, and fear of being viewed differently from peers. Guidelines restricting sun exposure, smoking, and oral contraceptives may negatively impact social behavior, or at least be perceived as such by the patient.[53] Adolescents who feel generally well may also fail to understand the importance of continuing treatment.

Transition from pediatric to adult care providers is also a vulnerable time for young patients. Patients at this stage are struggling to achieve emotional and physical independence

from parents/caregivers while establishing their own careers and identities.[54] The self-management skills adolescents require for successful transition are many, and may not be immediately obvious to adult providers. They include maintaining a medical file, filling prescriptions and taking medications appropriately, scheduling medical appointments, navigating the insurance system, and arranging transportation to appointments.[55] Patients also need to have adequate understanding of the disease and its symptoms in order to communicate effectively with their providers and participate in medical decision making. The parent's ability to relinquish control is also necessary for the transition to independence. Transition planning and/or specialized transition clinics are thus recommended for all adolescent patients.

REFERENCES

1. Hiraki LT, Feldman CH, Liu J, Alarcon GS, Fischer MA, Winkelmayer WC, et al. Prevalence, incidence, and demographics of systemic lupus erythematosus and lupus nephritis from 2000 to 2004 among children in the US Medicaid beneficiary population. *Arthritis Rheum* 2012;**64**:2669–76.
2. Malleson PN, Fung MY, Rosenberg AM. The incidence of pediatric rheumatic diseases: results from the Canadian Pediatric Rheumatology Association Disease Registry. *J Rheumatol* 1996;**23**:1981–7.
3. Danchenko N, Satia JA, Anthony MS. Epidemiology of systemic lupus erythematosus: a comparison of worldwide disease burden. *Lupus* 2006;**15**:308–18.
4. Uramoto KM, Michet Jr CJ, Thumboo J, Sunku J, O'Fallon WM, Gabriel SE. Trends in the incidence and mortality of systemic lupus erythematosus, 1950–1992. *Arthritis Rheum* 1999;**42**:46–50.
5. Hopkinson ND, Doherty M, Powell RJ. Clinical features and race-specific incidence/prevalence rates of systemic lupus erythematosus in a geographically complete cohort of patients. *Ann Rheum Dis* 1994;**53**:675–80.
6. Hart HH, Grigor RR, Caughey DE. Ethnic difference in the prevalence of systemic lupus erythematosus. *Ann Rheum Dis* 1983;**42**:529–32.
7. Hiraki LT, Benseler SM, Tyrrell PN, Harvey E, Hebert D, Silverman ED. Ethnic differences in pediatric systemic lupus erythematosus. *J Rheumatol* 2009;**36**:2539–46.
8. Son MB, Johnson VM, Hersh AO, Lo MS, Costenbader KH. Outcomes in hospitalized pediatric patients with systemic lupus erythematosus. *Pediatrics* 2014;**133**:e106–13.
9. Bader-Meunier B, Armengaud JB, Haddad E, Salomon R, Deschenes G, Kone-Paut I, et al. Initial presentation of childhood-onset systemic lupus erythematosus: a French multicenter study. *J Pediatr* 2005;**146**:648–53.
10. Zhu J, Wu F, Huang X. Age-related differences in the clinical characteristics of systemic lupus erythematosus in children. *Rheumatol Int* 2013;**33**:111–5.
11. Pluchinotta FR, Schiavo B, Vittadello F, Martini G, Perilongo G, Zulian F. Distinctive clinical features of pediatric systemic lupus erythematosus in three different age classes. *Lupus* 2007;**16**:550–5.
12. Schoch JJ, Peters MS, Reed AM, Tollefson MM. Pediatric subacute cutaneous lupus erythematosus: report of three cases. *Int J Dermatol* 2014. http://dx.doi.org/10.1111/ijd.12661.

13. Hiraki LT, Benseler SM, Tyrrell PN, Hebert D, Harvey E, Silverman ED. Clinical and laboratory characteristics and long-term outcome of pediatric systemic lupus erythematosus: a longitudinal study. *J Pediatr* 2008;**152**:550–6.

14. Amaral B, Murphy G, Ioannou Y, Isenberg DA. A comparison of the outcome of adolescent and adult-onset systemic lupus erythematosus. *Rheumatology (Oxford)* 2014;**53**:1130–5.

15. Hoffman IE, Lauwerys BR, De Keyser F, Huizinga TW, Isenberg D, Cebecauer L, et al. Juvenile-onset systemic lupus erythematosus: different clinical and serological pattern than adult-onset systemic lupus erythematosus. *Ann Rheum Dis* 2009;**68**:412–5.

16. Livingston B, Bonner A, Pope J. Differences in autoantibody profiles and disease activity and damage scores between childhood- and adult-onset systemic lupus erythematosus: a meta-analysis. *Semin Arthritis Rheum* 2012;**42**:271–80.

17. Bryan AR, Wu EY. Complement deficiencies in systemic lupus erythematosus. *Curr Allergy Asthma Rep* 2014;**14**:448.

18. Lim E, Tao Y, White AJ, French AR, Cooper MA. Hypogammaglobulinemia in pediatric systemic lupus erythematosus. *Lupus* 2013;**22**:1382–7.

19. Nakamura J, Saisu T, Yamashita K, Suzuki C, Kamegaya M, Takahashi K. Age at time of corticosteroid administration is a risk factor for osteonecrosis in pediatric patients with systemic lupus erythematosus: a prospective magnetic resonance imaging study. *Arthritis Rheum* 2010;**62**:609–15.

20. Brunner HI, Gladman DD, Ibanez D, Urowitz MD, Silverman ED. Difference in disease features between childhood-onset and adult-onset systemic lupus erythematosus. *Arthritis Rheum* 2008;**58**:556–62.

21. Pereira T, Abitbol CL, Seeherunvong W, Katsoufis C, Chandar J, Freundlich M, et al. Three decades of progress in treating childhood-onset lupus nephritis. *Clin J Am Soc Nephrol* 2011;**6**:2192–9.

22. Benseler SM, Silverman ED. Neuropsychiatric involvement in pediatric systemic lupus erythematosus. *Lupus* 2007;**16**:564–71.

23. Klein-Gitelman M, Reiff A, Silverman ED. Systemic lupus erythematosus in childhood. *Rheum Dis Clin North Am* 2002;**28**:561–77. vi–vii.

24. Bennett TD, Fluchel M, Hersh AO, Hayward KN, Hersh AL, Brogan TV, et al. Macrophage activation syndrome in children with systemic lupus erythematosus and children with juvenile idiopathic arthritis. *Arthritis Rheum* 2012;**64**:4135–42.

25. Parodi A, Davi S, Pringe AB, Pistorio A, Ruperto N, Magni-Manzoni S, et al. Macrophage activation syndrome in juvenile systemic lupus erythematosus: a multinational multicenter study of thirty-eight patients. *Arthritis Rheum* 2009;**60**:3388–99.

26. Kallel-Sellami M, Baili-Klila L, Zerzeri Y, Laadhar L, Blouin J, Abdelmoula MS, et al. Pediatric systemic lupus erythematosus with C1q deficiency. *Ann N Y Acad Sci* 2007;**1108**:193–6.

27. Belot A, Cimaz R. Monogenic forms of systemic lupus erythematosus: new insights into SLE pathogenesis. *Pediatr Rheumatol Online J* 2012;**10**:21.

28. Belot A, Kasher PR, Trotter EW, Foray AP, Debaud AL, Rice GI, et al. Protein kinase cdelta deficiency causes mendelian systemic lupus erythematosus with B cell-defective apoptosis and hyperproliferation. *Arthritis Rheum* 2013;**65**:2161–71.

29. Hersh AO, Trupin L, Yazdany J, Panopalis P, Julian L, Katz P, et al. Childhood-onset disease as a predictor of mortality in an adult cohort of patients with systemic lupus erythematosus. *Arthritis Care Res (Hoboken)* 2010;**62**:1152–9.

30. Hersh AO, von Scheven E, Yazdany J, Panopalis P, Trupin L, Julian L, et al. Differences in long-term disease activity and treatment of adult patients with childhood- and adult-onset systemic lupus erythematosus. *Arthritis Rheum* 2009;**61**:13–20.

31. Miettunen PM, Ortiz-Alvarez O, Petty RE, Cimaz R, Malleson PN, Cabral DA, et al. Gender and ethnic origin have no effect on longterm outcome of childhood-onset systemic lupus erythematosus. *J Rheumatol* 2004;**31**:1650–4.

32. Knight AM, Weiss PF, Morales KH, Keren R. National trends in pediatric systemic lupus erythematosus hospitalization in the United States: 2000–2009. *J Rheumatol* 2014;**41**:539–46.

33. Kamphuis S, Silverman ED. Prevalence and burden of pediatric-onset systemic lupus erythematosus. *Nat Rev Rheumatol* 2010;**6**:538–46.

34. Klein A, Cimaz R, Quartier P, Decramer S, Niaudet P, Baudouin V, et al. Causes of death in pediatric systemic lupus erythematosus. *Clin Exp Rheumatol* 2009;**27**:538–9.

35. Bogdanovic R, Nikolic V, Pasic S, Dimitrijevic J, Lipkovska-Markovic J, Eric-Marinkovic J, et al. Lupus nephritis in childhood: a review of 53 patients followed at a single center. *Pediatr Nephrol* 2004; **19**:36–44.

36. Lee PY, Yeh KW, Yao TC, Lee WI, Lin YJ, Huang JL. The outcome of patients with renal involvement in pediatric-onset systemic lupus erythematosus–a 20-year experience in Asia. *Lupus* 2013; **22**:1534–40.

37. Brunner HI, Klein-Gitelman MS, Ying J, Tucker LB, Silverman ED. Corticosteroid use in childhood-onset systemic lupus erythematosus-practice patterns at four pediatric rheumatology centers. *Clin Exp Rheumatol* 2009;**27**:155–62.

38. Hiraki LT, Hamilton J, Silverman ED. Measuring permanent damage in pediatric systemic lupus erythematosus. *Lupus* 2007;**16**:657–62.

39. Ilowite NT, Samuel P, Ginzler E, Jacobson MS. Dyslipoproteinemia in pediatric systemic lupus erythematosus. *Arthritis Rheum* 1988;**31**:859–63.

40. Schanberg LE, Sandborg C, Barnhart HX, Ardoin SP, Yow E, Evans GW, et al. Use of atorvastatin in systemic lupus erythematosus in children and adolescents. *Arthritis Rheum* 2012;**64**:285–96.

41. Ardoin SP, Schanberg LE, Sandborg CI, Barnhart HX, Evans GW, Yow E, et al. Secondary analysis of APPLE study suggests atorvastatin may reduce atherosclerosis progression in pubertal lupus patients with higher C reactive protein. *Ann Rheum Dis* 2014;**73**:557–66.

42. Robinson AB, Tangpricha V, Yow E, Gurion R, Schanberg LE, McComsey GA. Vitamin D status is a determinant of atorvastatin effect on carotid intima medial thickening progression rate in children with lupus: an Atherosclerosis Prevention in Pediatric Lupus Erythematosus (APPLE) substudy. *Lupus Sci Med* 2014;**1**:e000037.

43. Buehring B, Viswanathan R, Binkley N, Busse W. Glucocorticoid-induced osteoporosis: an update on effects and management. *J Allergy Clin Immunol* 2013;**132**:1019–30.

44. Manaboriboon B, Silverman ED, Homsanit M, Chui H, Kaufman M. Weight change associated with corticosteroid therapy in adolescents with systemic lupus erythematosus. *Lupus* 2013;**22**:164–70.

45. Silva CA, Brunner HI. Gonadal functioning and preservation of reproductive fitness with juvenile systemic lupus erythematosus. *Lupus* 2007;**16**:593–9.

46. Aikawa NE, Sallum AM, Pereira RM, Suzuki L, Viana VS, Bonfa E, et al. Subclinical impairment of ovarian reserve in juvenile systemic lupus erythematosus after cyclophosphamide therapy. *Clin Exp Rheumatol* 2012;**30**:445–9.

47. Brunner HI, Bishnoi A, Barron AC, Houk LJ, Ware A, Farhey Y, et al. Disease outcomes and ovarian function of childhood-onset systemic lupus erythematosus. *Lupus* 2006;**15**:198–206.

48. Cloutier BT, Clarke AE, Ramsey-Goldman R, Gordon C, Hansen JE, Bernatsky S. Systemic lupus erythematosus and malignancies: a review article. *Rheum Dis Clin North Am* 2014;**40**:497–506. viii.

49. Bernatsky S, Clarke AE, Labrecque J, von Scheven E, Schanberg LE, Silverman ED, et al. Cancer risk in childhood-onset systemic lupus. *Arthritis Res Ther* 2013;**15**:R198.

50. Bernatsky S, Ramsey-Goldman R, Joseph L, Boivin JF, Costenbader KH, Urowitz MB, et al. Lymphoma risk in systemic lupus: effects of disease activity versus treatment. *Ann Rheum Dis* 2014;**73**:138–42.

51. McClain MT, Poole BD, Bruner BF, Kaufman KM, Harley JB, James JA. An altered immune response to Epstein-Barr nuclear antigen 1 in pediatric systemic lupus erythematosus. *Arthritis Rheum* 2006;**54**:360–8.

52. Ting TV, Kudalkar D, Nelson S, Cortina S, Pendl J, Budhani S, et al. Usefulness of cellular text messaging for improving adherence among adolescents and young adults with systemic lupus erythematosus. *J Rheumatol* 2012;**39**:174–9.

53. Kone-Paut I, Piram M, Guillaume S, Tran TA. Lupus in adolescence. *Lupus* 2007;**16**:606–12.

54. Falcini F, Nacci F. Systemic lupus erythematosus in the young: the importance of a transition clinic. *Lupus* 2007;**16**:613–7.

55. Lawson EF, Hersh AO, Applebaum MA, Yelin EH, Okumura MJ, von Scheven E. Self-management skills in adolescents with chronic rheumatic disease: a cross-sectional survey. *Pediatr Rheumatol Online J* 2011;**9**:35.

Chapter 54

Drug-Induced Lupus

Mary Anne Dooley

Dooley Rheumatology, Chapel Hill, NC, USA

SUMMARY

Drug-induced lupus (DIL) is a disorder with clinical, histological, and immunological features similar to idiopathic systemic lupus erythematosus, but that occurs when certain drugs are taken and resolves after discontinuation of the offending agent. No uniform diagnostic criteria exist for the disorder. The list of drugs that are associated with this disorder exceeds 100, including newer biologic agents, and the list continues to expand. Despite recognition of this entity over 70 years ago, data regarding the causality of drugs in inducing lupus are mostly limited to case series and reports. Positive/antinuclear antibodies and anti-histone antibodies are usually present. Various mechanisms proposed for DIL include genetic predisposition, reduced DNA methylation by direct inhibition of DNA methyltransferases or indirectly by ERK pathway signaling, and haptenization—a drug binding to plasma or tissue proteins inducing an immune response. Additionally, local drug metabolism within leukocytes or hepatocytes may convert drugs to cytotoxic reactive compounds, increasing necrotic cell debris and activating macrophages; alternatively drugs may impair or increase apoptosis. Diagnosis of DIL requires careful patient examination, medication and history review, and diligent assessment of disease symptoms and time course following drug exposure, removal, and potential rechallenge.

INTRODUCTION

There are no uniformly accepted definitions of drug-induced lupus (DIL). The primary features are an immunologically mediated drug reaction with clinical features similar to systemic lupus erythematosus that is temporally associated with a drug exposure and that resolves after removal of the culprit drug. DIL is a "type B" drug reaction: unpredictable and influenced by many individual factors including genetic susceptibility, sex, race, concomitant drug interactions, overall health, and environmental and dietary factors.[1] In 1954 hydralazine was reported to induce DIL. Since these initial reports, over 100 drugs have been associated with DIL.[1–4] Hydralazine and procainamide remain the

only high-risk drugs for developing DIL with 20% of procainamide-treated patients and 5–8% of hydralazine-treated patients developing the syndrome within the first year of therapy. Quinidine is recognized as "intermediate" risk with an incidence of <1%. Most other drugs are classified as "low risk" or "very low risk" based on case series or single case reports. Fewer cases of DIL are attributed to these high-risk drugs as their use has declined. However, the new age of biologic modulators for treating cancer and autoimmune diseases has been associated with increasing reports of DIL associated with tumor necrosis factor (TNF)-α inhibitors, cytokines, and interferons (IFNs).

In 2007, Borchers et al. proposed diagnostic criteria for DIL.[6] These include: (1) sufficient and continuous exposure to the drug prior to development of the disorder, (2) at least one characteristic of systemic lupus, (3) absence of prior features of lupus or any other autoimmune disorder, and (4) resolution of the disorder within weeks to months of drug discontinuation, though serologies may take much longer. These criteria have been criticized.[4] A threshold dose for a drug to induce DIL has not been defined as individual factors such as genetic susceptibility and health status including renal and hepatic function confound this relationship. Additionally, concomitant drug interactions may promote DIL. Adhering to the third criterion is difficult as the indication for treatment with some of the biologics recognized to induce DIL may be an underlying autoimmune disease such as rheumatoid arthritis or inflammatory bowel disease for which the drugs are used.

EPIDEMIOLOGY

Drug-induced lupus remains an underappreciated entity that has not been evaluated in prospectively designed studies. The incidence of DIL in the United States has been estimated to be 15,000–30,000 new cases per year.[1–3,6] The frequency of DIL is probably underreported. As many cases are mild and resolve once the offending drug is removed, laboratory and other diagnostic assessments are often not performed. Autoantibodies develop in a significant number of patients prescribed certain medications; most of these patients do not develop signs of an autoantibody-associated

Systemic Lupus Erythematosus. http://dx.doi.org/10.1016/B978-0-12-801917-7.00054-1

disease. Recent studies have used large patient databases to quantify the risk of DIL. Schoonen et al. used a matched nested case–control study using primary care data from the UK General Practice Research Database to evaluate the incidence of lupus and the proportion of patients exposed to drugs selected as known risks for DIL.[7] This study confirmed the risks associated with hydralazine, minocycline, and carbamazepine and noted that 12% of incident lupus cases occurred in patients exposed to suspect drugs. A population-based matched case–control study in Sweden confirmed the association of subacute cutaneous lupus with TNF-α inhibitors with an eightfold odds ratio.[8] Moulis et al. compared the frequency of reported DIL in the French pharmacovigilance database.[9] The association of TNF inhibitors with DIL was confirmed with differential risks of the drugs observed. The reported odds ratio was decreased twofold for etanercept compared to the monoclonal antibody drugs adalimumab and infliximab. Case reports of patients with DIL on monoclonal anti-TNF-α inhibitor able to switch to a nonmonoclonal agent have reported recurrence in some though not all patients.[10,11]

The association of particular drugs with DIL may reflect the length of time the drug has been available, the frequency it is prescribed, and the population exposed. For example, women are two to four times more likely than males to develop DIL on procainamide or hydralazine, but males are more frequently reported due to their increased risk of cardiovascular disease and exposure to the drugs.[2,3] Estrogen-associated DIL has been associated with women due to the rarity of men receiving estrogen-containing drugs.[12] Minocycline-induced DIL is more frequently observed in young females being treated for acne, in whom use of this agent is more common.[13] Little is known about racial susceptibility to DIL. Caucasians have been reported to be affected up to six times more frequently than African-Americans and to exhibit a more severe disease.[1–3] However, this may simply represent bias in the populations studied or socioeconomic issues associated with costly medications. A recent publication of DIL associated with rifabutin therapy in a 55-year-old African-American woman counters the view that DIL is not seen in patients with African ancestry.[14]

Medications Associated with DIL

A variety of drugs have been identified as being definite, probable, or possible causes of DIL (Table 1). Those drugs currently associated with the highest risk of inducing lupus in an individual patient are procainamide, hydralazine, and minocycline. The expansion in use of biologic therapies suggests that these agents will increasingly account for future cases of DIL.

- **Procainamide**—Procainamide-induced DIL may be mediated by the reactive metabolite procainamide

hydroxylamine. A positive ANA occurs in almost all patients given the drug for more than 2 years; one-third of those who have taken procainamide for more than 1 year develop symptoms. Clinical symptoms are more likely to develop in slow acetylators. Risk factors include HLA-DR6Y, but not DR4 or DR3. In contrast, there is little ANA formation or symptoms following the administration of *N*-acetylprocainamide (NAPA), the major active metabolite of procainamide; remission of procainamide-induced lupus can be achieved by switching to NAPA.

- **Hydralazine**—The incidence of clinical disease averages 5–10% of patients exposed to hydralazine. A number of risk factors have been identified including drug dose (more than 200 mg/day and/or cumulative dose of more than 100 g), female sex, slow hepatic acetylation, the HLA-DR4 genotype, and the C4 null gene. In one study, lupus developed in 19% of women taking 200 mg of hydralazine per day as compared to 13 of 13 who also had the HLA-DR4 genotype. Even low doses may not be safe as clinical disease can develop in up to 5% of slow acetylators taking 100 mg per day.[16]

- **Minocycline**—Minocycline, in contrast to other tetracyclines, is associated with DIL, particularly in young women given the drug to treat acne. The average age of patients with minocycline-induced lupus (22 years) is younger than

TABLE 1 Differentiating Drug-Induced Lupus from Idiopathic Systemic Lupus

	Drug-Induced Lupus	Systemic Lupus
Gender predisposition	N/A	+++
Age predisposition	N/A	+++
Arthralgias	+++	+++
Myalgias	++	+++
Fever/pleurisy/pericarditis	+	+++
Malar rash/alopecia/discoid lesions	+	+++
Purpura, erythematous papules	+++	+
Mucosal ulcers/lymphadenopathy	+	+++
CNS/renal manifestations	+	+++
ANA	+++	+++
Anti-histone antibodies	+++	+
Anti-ssDNA antibodies	+++	+
Anti-dsDNA antibodies	+	+++
Reduced complement	+	+++

those with procainamide- or hydralazine-induced lupus. The majority of patients received the drug for over a year prior to the onset of their lupus symptoms. About half the affected patients have laboratory evidence of liver involvement and 20% have skin rashes. Hepatic damage associated with minocycline may be the result of reactive metabolites being produced by the liver. Symptoms include arthralgia (73–100%), arthritis (12–45%), fever (38%), and rash (29%). A positive ANA and P-ANCA have been found in 92% and 83% of tested sera; however, anti-histone antibodies are uncommon (0%–13%). Although most cases of minocycline-induced lupus resolve within a relatively short time after drug discontinuation, young children may be at increased risk for prolonged disease following minocycline exposure.[17]

- **Anti-TNF agents**—Tumor necrosis factor α antagonist-induced lupus-like syndrome (TAILS) has been reported for infliximab, adalimumab, certolizumab pegol, golimumab, and etanercept; and has been associated with the development of positive ANA (13–83%), anti-DNA (3–32%), and/or anti-histone antibodies. Several cases of anti-TNF-α DIL with renal disease have been reported. Low serum complement levels, anti-extractable nuclear antigen antibodies, and anti-dsDNA antibodies are reported in half the cases of anti-TNF-α DIL; anti-histone antibodies are less common than in classic DIL.[18] Recognition of DIL in patients receiving anti-TNF-α therapy can be difficult due to the symptoms of their underlying disease. A temporal association (months to years) of the offending drug with characteristic or suggestive symptoms, and resolution of symptoms on drug withdrawal, is the best evidence for diagnosis of DIL.

- **Interferons**—IFNs are a family of cytokines widely used in the treatment of various conditions such as melanoma, Kaposi's sarcoma, viral hepatitis, chronic myeloid leukemia, renal-cell and carcinoid tumors, and multiple sclerosis. The use of α-, β-, and γ-IFN have been linked to the development of DIL.[19,20] Studies have reported a 1–14% frequency of IFN-induced lupus, with up to 8% of patients receiving long-term IFN therapy developing anti-dsDNA antibodies. Type 1 IFN levels correlate with cutaneous features in SLE and have been found to be involved in the development of UVB-induced photosensitivity in patients with lupus. In some lupus patients, IFN levels correlate with ANA and anti-DNA antibody titers and degree of clinical disease activity.

Clinical Features

There is no clear distinction in clinical or serologic findings between patients with DIL or idiopathic systemic lupus erythematosus. In general, DIL has been described as being milder than systemic lupus. Table 2 summarizes these differences. DIL patients more frequently develop rashes characteristic of a drug-induced process (purpuric, erythematous, and/or papular) versus the classic lupus malar rash or discoid lesions. Qualitative laboratory differences can also differentiate DIL from systemic lupus. The ANA in DIL is typically a homogeneous pattern as anti-histone antibodies are found in up to 75% of DIL cases.[1–3] Distinguishing idiopathic lupus and DIL has become less clear with symptomatology and laboratory reports of DIL associated with increasing clinical use of biologic agents (such as anti-TNF-α inhibitors and IFN therapies), which may induce anti-dsDNA antibodies.[5,15] Though DIL is generally less severe than idiopathic lupus, life-threatening cases of pericardial tamponade,[21] fatal statin-induced DIL,[22,23] and transient inability to determine blood group delaying transfusion in a case of dabigatran-induced DIL are reported.[24]

Similar to idiopathic lupus, DIL can be divided into systemic, subacute cutaneous, and chronic cutaneous lupus. Systemic DIL is characterized by lupus-like symptoms including fever, rash, and joint pain with positive antinuclear and anti-histone antibodies, while anti-double-strand DNA and anti-extractable nuclear antigen antibodies are rare. The frequency of lupus manifestations may vary with the drug. For example, pleuritis occurs in approximately half of the procainamide-induced lupus patients, 22% of those with quinidine-induced disease, and less than 1% of those with minocycline.[25] Minocycline-induced DIL more frequently affects the liver (32–54%), and increased CRP levels are seen in nearly 90% of patients.[26] Quinidine-induced DIL frequently includes neurologic involvement (30%) though this feature is rare with other drugs causing DIL.[2,5,6] Thrombocytopenia and hypocomplementemia are reported in nearly half of quinidine-induced cases and frequently in TNF-α inhibitor DIL.[5] Anti-dsDNA antibodies are unusual, with the exceptions of IFN-α and anti-TNF-α-induced disease.[5,27]

The causative drugs and serologic findings for cutaneous DIL differ from systemic DIL. Drug-induced SCLE is similar to idiopathic SCLE in clinical features and serologic characteristics including anti-Ro SSA antibody positivity, and is more common than the systemic form of DIL.[28] Drug-induced subacute cutaneous lupus was first described in 1985 by Reed et al.[29] This cutaneous form is more frequently seen in older women with a mean age of 58 years. The most common features are erythema on sun-exposed skin and characteristic annular polycyclic or papulosquamous lesions. Patients commonly have not only ANA but also anti-Ro/SSA and anti-La/SSB autoantibodies. Anti-histone antibodies are seen in fewer than half of these patients and anti-DNA antibodies are rare. Drugs associated with this form include antihypertensives (calcium channel blockers, ACE inhibitors, beta blockers); other drugs implicated include IFN, the antifungal terbinafine, ticlodipine, and leflunomide.[28,29] The chronic cutaneous form is rare, usually seen with fluorouracil exposure.[30] Discoid skin

TABLE 2 Medications Associated with Drug-Induced Lupus

Drug	High Risk >5%	Low Risk <1%	Very Low Risk < 0.1%
Nonbiologics			
Antiarrythmics	Procainamide (15–20%)	Quinidine <1%	Disopyramide, propafenone
Antihypertensives	Hydralazine (5–8%)	Methyldopa, captopril, acebutol	Clonidine, enalapril, labetalol, minoxidil, pindolol, prazosin chlorthalidone, hydrochlorothiazide diltiazem, verapamil, nifedipine, reserpine
Antipsychotics		Chlorpromazine	Clozapine, perphenazine, phenelzine, chloprothixine, lithium carbonate, buproprion
Antibiotics		Minocycline isonioazid	Nitrofurantoin, *para*-aminosalicylic acid, sulfonamides, penicillins, rifabutin
Antifungals			Terbinafine, griseofulvin
Anticonvulsants		Carbamazepine	Ethosuximide, phenytoin, primidone, trimethadione, valproic acid, clobazam
Antithyroidals			Propylthiouracil, methylthiouracil
Anti-inflammatories		Sulfasalazine, ᴅ-penicillamine	Leflenamide Piroxicam, Naproxene Phenylbutazone
Anticholesterolemics			Atorvastatin, fluvastatin, lovastatin, pravastatin, simvastatin
Diuretics			Clorthalidone, hydrochlorothiazine
Biologicals			
TNFα inhibitors			Etanercept, infliximab adalimumab; golimumab, certolizumab pegol
Interferons			IFN-α, β, and γ
Cytokines			IL-2, toclizumab (anti-IL6)
Others			Fluorouracile agents, timolol eye drops, ticlodipine, levodopa, abatacept (CTLA4-Ig)

lesions, rare in other types of DIL, frequently occur. Nearly 70% have detectable ANA but anti-histone, anti-Ro/SSA, anti La/SSB, and anti-dsDNA are usually not seen.

Autoantibodies

Many of the autoantibodies developed during therapy with the agents above react with histone or histone–DNA complexes. However, anti-histone antibodies lack specificity for DIL as they are also found in systemic lupus (up to 80% of patients), adult and juvenile rheumatoid arthritis, Felty's syndrome, undifferentiated connective tissue disease, and other disease states. In those taking procainamide, hydralazine, chlorpromazine, and quinidine, anti-histone antibodies are present in 95% of cases; other autoantibodies are uncommon in this disorder.[2,3] The development of IgG antibodies to the complex of H2A–H2B and DNA soon after starting procainamide is associated with a high risk of developing drug-induced lupus[31]; autoantibodies to

single-stranded DNA or histones alone do not distinguish between symptomatic or asymptomatic patients. Although studies of anti-histone antibodies may provide important insights into the mechanisms behind DIL, their diagnostic value for individual patients is limited.

- Anti-double-stranded DNA antibodies—Anti-double-stranded DNA antibodies are typically present in DIL due to with IFN-α and anti-TNF-α agents. Although patients develop autoantibodies, relatively few patients, including those with anti-DNA antibodies, develop clinical DIL.
- Anti-phospholipid antibodies. Anti-phospholipid antibodies including the lupus anti-coagulant and anti-cardiolipin antibodies have been reported to be associated with a number of drugs, including chlorpromazine, procainamide, hydralazine, perphenazine, quinine, and sulfasalazine. The autoantibodies are frequently IgM, and generally not associated with thrombotic events.[32]
- Anti-neutrophil cytoplasmic antibodies—Although an immune complex-mediated glomerulonephritis can

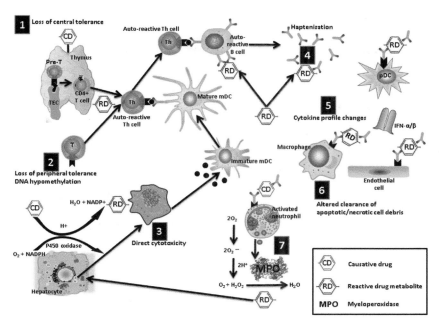

FIGURE 1 **Proposed mechanisms of drug-induced lupus.** 1. Reactive drug and/or metabolites disrupt central tolerance in the thymus leading to increased survival of autoreactive Th cells. 2. Causative drug and/or metabolites inhibit DNA methylation leading to increased LFA-1 and B-cell stimulators resulting in enhanced lymphocyte responsiveness. 3. Causative drugs and/or their metabolites may be directly cytotoxic producing cellular debris. Immature dendritic cells activate and process peptides, maturing to antigen-presenting cells interacting with autoreactive Th cells. This triggers lymphocyte interaction and the production of autoantibodies. 4. The drug or metabolites bind plasma or tissue antigens and become immunologically active leading to immune complex formation—a process called haptenization. 5. Immune complexes are endocytosed by plasmacytoid dendritic cells and trigger release of type 1 IFNs, changing the cytokine profile. 6. Haptenized reactive drug metabolites may bind directly to macrophages altering clearance of apoptotic/necrotic cell debris. 7. Causative drugs may trigger neutrophil activation and the production of reactive oxygen species.

occur, renal disease in DIL is most often due to a necrotizing glomerulonephritis with little or no immune complex deposition. These patients usually show a P-ANCA pattern on immunofluorescence microscopy with anti-MPO plus either anti-lactoferrin or anti-elastase (the latter antibodies are called atypical P-ANCA). This combination of ANCAs appears to be relatively specific for this form of hydralazine-induced vasculitis.[33–35] These patients may also have anti-double-stranded DNA antibodies.

Pathophysiology

A single mechanism for DIL is unlikely given the diverse drugs implicated from many drug categories. Several mechanisms have been proposed, including genetic risk factors, loss of central tolerance, DNA demethylation, direct cytotoxicity, biotransformation of drugs by neutrophils to active metabolites capable of stimulating immune cells, drugs or their metabolites acting as haptens, and interference with apoptosis or the clearance of apoptotic or necrotic cell debris.[36] Figure 1 summarizes mechanisms proposed for induction of DIL.

- **Genetic risk factors**—Acetylator status: For drugs metabolized by acetylation such as procainamide and

hydralazine, DIL is more likely to develop and more rapid in onset in patients who are slow acetylators because of a genetically mediated decrease in the hepatic synthesis of *N*-acetyltransferase.[37,38] In comparison, acetylation rate is not a risk factor for spontaneous lupus or DIL related to other agents such as minocycline and TNF-α inhibitors. Other genetic risk factors include HLA-DR4, HLA-DR0301, and the complement C4 null allele.[1–3]

- **Loss of central tolerance**—Antibodies to the histone (H2A–H2B)–DNA complex can be induced in mice by the intrathymic injection of PAHA.[39] In another study by Rubin and colleagues, the incubation of PAHA with T-cell clones resulted in resistance to anergy induction.[40] Taken together, these observations suggest that PAHA induces autoimmunity via the emergence of autoreactive T cells followed by the production of anti-histone antibodies.

- **DNA demethylation**—Notably, the two most commonly implicated drugs in DIL (procainamide and hydralazine) inhibit DNA methylation.[1–3] Procainamide is a competitive DNA methyltransferase inhibitor. Hydralazine is a selective ERK pathway inhibitor, preventing induction of DNA methyltransferase in stimulated T cells. DNA hypomethylation can lead to increased LFA-1 and B-cell stimulators, resulting in enhanced lymphocyte responsiveness and production of autoantibodies.

- **Drug biotransformation** to reactive metabolites is another metabolism-mediated mechanism for DIL. Drug metabolism by NADPH oxidase, myeloperoxidase, nitric oxide, cytochrome P450, and prostaglandin synthetase can occur in activated leukocytes.[41–43] This interaction results in the formation of reactive drug metabolites, which may directly affect lymphocyte function. These reactions can lead directly to cytotoxic compounds that can then covalently bond to and alter DNA.
- **Haptenization**—Alternatively, these reactive metabolites can bond to proteins, a process called haptenization and induce an immune response.
- **Direct cytotoxicity/immunogenicity**—Other cells in the immune system also contribute; D-penicillamine has been shown to directly bind to macrophages and alter their function.[44,45] In the case of biologic agents, the drug may be the target.[46–48]

DIAGNOSIS

The presence of drug-induced lupus should be suspected when a patient taking one or more suspect drugs for at least 1 month, and usually much longer, presents with some combination of arthralgia, myalgia, malaise, fever, rash, and/or serositis. Confirming the diagnosis is difficult, however, because of the clinical overlap with the more common idiopathic disease. If available, the finding of anti-histone antibodies in the absence of other autoantibodies strongly suggests that a drug is responsible. The "gold standard" is spontaneous resolution of the disease within 1 to 7 months after the offending drug has been discontinued.

TREATMENT OF DRUG-INDUCED LUPUS

The most important aspect of DIL management involves recognizing that a drug is responsible for the illness. As a rule, symptoms of DIL are self-limiting once the offending drug is stopped. The development of a positive ANA while receiving a drug is not sufficient to diagnose DIL or to discontinue the drug, although careful monitoring for subsequent clinical features is important. Treatment will vary among patients, depending on the severity and manifestation(s) of the increased disease activity. Constitutional and musculoskeletal symptoms are usually adequately controlled with aspirin or NSAIDs. Low-dose prednisone may be necessary for refractory symptoms, and higher doses may be used for resistant features or symptomatic pericardial effusion. In contrast, patients with hydralazine-induced vasculitis often require cytotoxic therapy as in other ANCA-positive vasculitides. The rare case of biopsy-proven renal disease or vasculitis should be treated similarly to systemic lupus with corticosteroids and immunosuppressive agents. Although most symptoms of DIL resolve within a few weeks of

discontinuing the offending drug, occasionally patients may take up to 1 year to recover completely. Anti-nuclear antibody expression may also be prolonged or fail to resolve over time even as clinical symptoms disappear.

CONCLUSION

As the frequency of use of biologic agents associated with DIL increases, the practicing clinician must have heightened awareness of the potential problem of DIL. Prompt recognition and discontinuation of the suspected drug are associated with excellent outcomes in most cases. The number of reported associations is expected to increase as new drugs are developed. Because some of these case reports may represent idiosyncratic reactions or the coincidental development of systemic lupus, rigorous epidemiological, clinical, and laboratory testing should be done to confirm the association. Finally, physicians need to be aware that many patients with chronic diseases ingest over-the-counter and alternative medicines that could potentially induce the development of autoimmune diseases, including lupus.

REFERENCES

1. Rubin RL. Drug-induced lupus. *Expert Opin Drug Saf* 2015;**2**:1–18.
2. Chang C, Gershwin ME. Drug-induced lupus erythematosus. Incidence, management and prevention. *Drug Saf* 2011;**34**:357–74.
3. Patel D, Richardson B. Drug-induced lupus. In: Wallace D, Hahn B, editors. *Dubois' lupus erythematosus and related syndromes*. 2013. p. 484–94.
4. Xiao X, Chang C. Diagnosis and classification of drug-induced autoimmunity (DIA). *J Autoimmun* 2014;**48-49**:66–72.
5. Araujo-Fernandez S, Ahijon-Lana M, Isenberg DA. Drug-induced lupus: Including anti-tumour necrosis factor and interferon induced. *Lupus* 2014;**23**:545–53.
6. Borchers AT, Keen CL, Gershwin ME. Drug-induced lupus. *Ann N Y Acad Sci* 2007;**1108**:166–82.
7. Schoonen WM, Thomas SL, Somers EC, Smeeth L, Kim J, Evans S, et al. Do selected drugs increase the risk of lupus? A matched case-control study. *Br J Clin Pharmacol* 2010;**70**:588–96.
8. Gronhagen CM, Fored CM, Linder M, Granath F, Nyberg F. Subacute cutaneous lupus erythematosus and its association with drugs: a population-based case-control study of 234 patients in Sweden. *Br J Dermatol* 2012;**167**:296–305.
9. Moulis G, Sommet A, Lapeyre-Mestre M, Montastruc J-L. Is the risk of tumour necrosis factor inhibitor-induced lupus or lupus-like syndrome the same with monoclonal antibodies and soluble receptor? A case/non-case study a nationwide pharmacovigilance database. *Rheumatology (Oxford)* 2014;**53**:1864–71.
10. Subramanian S, Yajnik V, Sands BE, Cullen G, Korzenik JR. Characterization of patients with infliximab-induced lupus erythematosus and outcomes after retreatment with a second anti-TNF agent. *Inflamm Bowel Dis* 2011;**17**:99–104.
11. Williams VL, Cohen PR. TNF alpha antagonist-induced lupus-like syndrome:report and review of the literature with implications for treatment with alternative TNF α antagonists. *Int J Dermatol* 2011;**50**:619–25.

12. Vasoo S. Drug-induced lupus: an update. *Lupus* 2006;**15**:757–61.
13. Lawson TM, Amos N, Bulgen D, Williams BD. Minocycline-induced lupus: clinical features and response to rechallenge. *Rheumatology (Oxford)* 2001;**40**:329.
14. Anyimadu H, Saadia N, Mannheimer S. Drug-induced lupus associated with rifabutin: a literature review. *J Int Assoc Provid AIDS Care* 2013;**12**:166–8.
15. De Rycke L, Baeten D, Kruithof E, et al. The effect of TNF alpha blockade on the antinuclear antibody profile in patients with chronic arthritis: biological and clinical implications. *Lupus* 2005;**14**:931.
16. Cameron HA, Ramsey LE. The lupus syndrome induced by hydralazine: a common complication with low dose treatment. *Br Med J (Clin Res Ed)* 1984;**289**:410–2.
17. El-Hallak M, Giani T, Yeniay BS, et al. Chronic minocycline-induced autoimmunity in children. *J Pediatr* 2008;**153**:314–9.
18. Pretel M, Marques L, Espana A. Drug-induced lupus erythematosus. *Actas Dermosifiliorgr* 2014;**105**:18–30.
19. Mistry N, Shapero J, Crawford RI. A review of adverse cutaneous drug reactions resulting from the use of interferon and ribavirin. *Can J Gastroenterol* 2009;**23**:677.
20. Lee HY, Pang SM. Subacute cutaneous lupus erythematosus after immunotherapy for renal-cell carcinoma: the case for interferon-alpha. *Clin Exp Dermatol* 2010;**35**:491–2.
21. Siddique MA, Khan IA. Isoniazide-induced lupus erythematosus presenting with cardiac tamponade. *Am J Ther* 2002;**9**:163–5.
22. Noel B. Lupus erythematosus and other autoimmune diseases related to statin therapy: a systematic review. *J Eur Acad Dermatol Venereol* 2007;**21**:17.
23. Sridhar MK, Abdulla A. Fatal lupus-like syndrome and ARDS induced by fluvastatin. *Lancet* 1998;**352**:114.
24. Stollberger C, Krutisch G, Finsterer J, Wolf HM. Dabigatran-induced lupus temporarily preventing blood group determination. *Blood Coagul Fibrinolysis* 2014;**25**:625–7.
25. Sarzi-Puttini P, Atzeni F, Capsoni F, et al. Drug-induced lupus erythematosus. *Autoimmunity* 2005;**38**:507.
26. Vedove CD, Del Giglio M, Schena D, et al. Drug-induced lupus. *Arch Dermatol Res* 2009;**301**:99–105.
27. Ioannou Y, Isenberg DA. Current evidence for the induction of autoimmune rheumatic manifestations by cytokine therapy. *Arthritis Rheum* 2000;**43**:1431–42.
28. Lowe G, Henderson CL, Grau RH, Sontheimer RD. A systematic review of drug-induced subacute cutaneous lupus erythematosus. *Br J Dermatol* 2010;**164**:465–72.
29. Reed BR, Huff JC, Jones SK, Orton PW, Lee LA, Norris DA. Subacute cutaneous lupus associated with hydrochlorothiazide therapy. *Ann Intern Med* 1985;**103**:49–51.
30. Funke AA, Kulp-Shorten CL, Callen JP. Subacute cutaneous lupus erythematosus exacerbated or induced by chemotherapy. *Arch Dermatol* 2010;**146**:1113–6.
31. Totoritis MC, Tan EM, McNally EM, Rubin RL. Association of antibody to histone complex H2A-H2B with symptomatic procainamide-induced lupus. *N Engl J Med* 1988;**318**:1431.
32. Dlott JS, Roubey RAS. Drug-induced lupus anticoagulants and antiphospholipid antibodies. *Curr Rheumatol Rep* 2012;**14**:71–8.
33. Nässberger L, Johansson AC, Björck S, Sjöholm AG. Antibodies to neutrophil granulocyte myeloperoxidase and elastase: autoimmune responses in glomerulonephritis due to hydralazine treatment. *J Intern Med* 1991;**229**:261.
34. Short AK, Lockwood CM. Antigen specificity in hydralazine associated ANCA positive systemic vasculitis. *QJM* 1995;**88**:775.
35. Cambridge G, Wallace H, Bernstein RM, Leaker B. Autoantibodies to myeloperoxidase in idiopathic and drug-induced systemic lupus erythematosus and vasculitis. *Br J Rheumatol* 1994;**33**:109.
36. Chang C, Gershwin ME. Drugs and autoimmunity- A contemporary review and mechanistic approach. *J Autoimmun* 2010;**34**:266–75.
37. Sim E, Lack N, Wang CJ, et al. Arylamine N-acetyltransferases: structural and functional implications of polymorphisms. *Toxicology* 2008;**254**:170.
38. Grant DM, Mörike K, Eichelbaum M, Meyer UA. Acetylation pharmacogenetics. The slow acetylator phenotype is caused by decreased or absent arylamine N-acetyltransferase in human liver. *J Clin Invest* 1990;**85**:968.
39. Kretz-Rommel A, Duncan SR, Rubin RL. Autoimmunity caused by disruption of central T cell tolerance. A murine model of drug-induced lupus. *J Clin Invest* 1997;**99**:1888.
40. Kretz-Rommel A, Rubin RL. A metabolite of the lupus-inducing drug procainamide prevents anergy induction in T cell clones. *J Immunol* 1997;**158**:4465.
41. Mannargudi B, McNally D, Reynolds W, Uetrecht J. Bioactivation of minocycline to reactive intermediates by myeloperoxidase, horseradish peroxidase, and hepatic microsomes: implications for minocycline-induced lupus and hepatitis. *Drug Metab Dispos* 2009;**37**:1806–18.
42. McKinnon RA, Nebert DW. Possible role of cytochromes P450 in lupus erythematosus and related disorders. *Lupus* 1994;**3**:473.
43. Lu W, Uetrecht JP. Peroxidase-mediated bioactivation of hydroxylated metabolites of carbamazepine and phenytoin. *Drug Metab Dispos* 2008;**36**:1624.
44. Masson MJ, Teranishi M, Shenton JM, Uetrecht JP. Investigation of the involvement of macrophages and T cells in D-penicillamine-induced autoimmunity in the Brown Norway rat. *J Immunotoxicol* 2004;**1**:79.
45. Li J, Mannargudi B, Uetrecht JP. Covalent binding of penicillamine to macrophages: implications for penicillamine-induced autoimmunity. *Chem Res Toxicol* 2009;**22**:1277.
46. Fadel F, El Karoui K. Knebelmann B Anti-CTLA4 antibody-induced lupus nephritis. *N Engl J Med* 2009;**361**:211–2.
47. Neradová A, Stam F, van den Berg JG, Bax WA. Etanercept-associated SLE with lupus nephritis. *Lupus* 2009;**18**:667.
48. Brunasso AM, Aberer W, Massone C. Subacute lupus erythematosus during treatment with golimumab for seronegative rheumatoid arthritis. *Lupus* 2014;**23**:201–3.

Chapter 55

Vasculitis in Lupus

Anisur Rahman
Division of Medicine, University College London, London, UK

SUMMARY

Although vasculopathy and endothelial activation may be important in the pathogenesis of lupus, true vasculitis demonstrated by histology, arteriography, or classical clinical presentation is less common. Estimates of the prevalence of vasculitis in patients with lupus range from 11% to 36% and the vast majority of cases are cutaneous and respond to antimalarials or oral corticosteroids.

Visceral vasculitis is less common but more serious. Vasculitis of the large vessels is rare and has mainly been described in case reports. Lupus mesenteric vasculitis typically presents with abdominal pain and should be considered in any lupus patient presenting with an acute abdomen. Although earlier reports recommended early laparotomy in these patients, diagnosis using computed tomography (CT) scanning followed by intravenous corticosteroids (and sometimes immunosuppressants) is now recommended.

PREVALENCE AND ASSOCIATED FEATURES OF VASCULITIS IN LUPUS

It is difficult to obtain exact figures for the prevalence of vasculitis in lupus, as the definition of what constitutes vasculitis differs between different authors. A recent review[1] cites a prevalence of 11% to 36% Most of the evidence comes from large retrospective studies in single centers. Drenkard et al. in 1997 reported on a cohort of 540 Mexican patients followed for a mean of 7.2 years to 1990.[2] Of these patients, 194 (36%) were reported to have suffered at least one episode of vasculitis, though this was only proved by histology or imaging in 54 cases (28%). The majority of cases (174) had cutaneous vasculitis, which occurred with no visceral involvement in 164 patients, and over 90% of biopsies were of the skin. Among 29 patients with visceral vasculitis, most (19) had mononeuritis multiplex. There was only one case of mesenteric vasculitis. Perhaps because of the predominance of cutaneous disease there was no difference in mortality between the 194 SLE patients with vasculitis and the 346 without vasculitis, but patients with visceral involvement were more likely to die than those with cutaneous vasculitis

(p = 0.006). In a more recent retrospective study from Barcelona,[3] Ramos-Casals et al. reported on 670 patients with SLE seen between 1980 and 2004. Their figure for prevalence of vasculitis was much lower than that of the earlier Mexican study[2] at 11%, but they also found that the majority of cases (89%) were cutaneous vasculitis. Their lower prevalence may have been due to a stricter definition of vasculitis; 45/76 patients (59%) with vasculitis in the Spanish study had histological and/or imaging evidence and the others had typical vasculitic skin lesions assessed by a dermatologist. Of 14 patients with visceral vasculitis, 7 had mononeuritis (proved by biopsy).

In Drenkard's study,[2] patients with vasculitis had longer SLE disease duration (p = 0.05) and younger age of onset (p = 0.006) than those with no vasculitis. In the study of Ramos-Casals,[3] the patients with vasculitis had higher mean activity scores measured by the European Consensus Lupus Activity Measure (ECLAM) (p < 0.001). Regarding serological markers, Ramos-Casals et al. found that vasculitis was associated with anemia (p < 0.001), ESR over 50 (p < 0.001), and anti-La/SSB antibodies (p = 0.014, though only 19% of patients with vasculitis were actually anti-La-positive) in multivariate analysis. Positivity for anti-phospholipid antibodies (aPL) was significantly associated with vasculitis in univariate but not multivariate analysis with 52% of patients with lupus vasculitis being aPL-positive.

Ramos-Casals et al. reported that 65/76 patients had small vessel vasculitis while the other 11 had medium vessel vasculitis.[3] Histologically, 29 of 45 patients who had a biopsy had leukocytoclastic vasculitis and 10 had necrotizing vasculitis. All patients with medium vessel vasculitis, but only 5% of those with small vessel vasculitis, had visceral involvement.

CUTANEOUS VASCULITIS

In a study of cutaneous manifestations in 73 patients with SLE, 11% were found to have cutaneous vasculitis.[4] Many different types of rash have been described, but the most common presentations are punctate vasculitic lesions and

Systemic Lupus Erythematosus. http://dx.doi.org/10.1016/B978-0-12-801917-7.00055-3

palpable purpura. These two types accounted for 143/160 cases of cutaneous lupus vasculitis described by Drenkard et al.[2] and 46 of 68 described by Ramos-Casals et al.[3] The latter group described a subset of 20 patients with cryoglobulinemia and a small vessel cutaneous vasculitis affecting particularly the legs. One-quarter of these patients had serology suggestive of hepatitis C infection.[3] It may be helpful to test for cryoglobulins and hepatitis C in patients with lupus and palpable purpura of the legs. There are no published clinical trials investigating treatment of cutaneous vasculitis specifically but most patients respond well to antimalarials, with oral steroids added in more severe cases.[1] Dapsone and thalidomide may be considered in rare cases.[1]

LUPUS MESENTERIC VASCULITIS

Visceral vasculitis is rare, typically composing about 10% of all cases of lupus vasculitis.[3] Lupus mesenteric vasculitis (LMV) has been the most frequently studied form of visceral vasculitis in lupus. Prevalence of LMV in patients with lupus varies geographically: 0.2–6.4% in European and American studies but higher (5.8–9.7%) in Korea.[5] Abdominal pain itself is a common symptom in patients with lupus.[6,7] Most of those patients do not have LMV,[7] but those who do are at risk of serious outcomes including death.[8] Thus many papers have concentrated on how to diagnose the minority of patients with lupus and abdominal pain who have true LMV and how to manage those cases.

Medina et al. advocated early laparotomy in patients with lupus admitted with acute abdomen.[9] They described 51 such patients admitted over an 8-year period, 19 of whom had LMV, and they found that a delay in laparotomy adversely influenced outcome. However, most publications since then have stressed that assessing disease activity and use of computed tomography (CT) imaging can reliably diagnose LMV without the need for surgery and that this should be followed by treatment with corticosteroids and sometimes immunosuppression.[5,8,10,11] Characteristic findings on abdominal CT include prominent mesenteric vessels, diffuse dilated loops of bowel, and the "comb" sign—mesenteric vessels arranged in a palisade or comb-like pattern.[12] These changes are reversible on treating LMV.[12] CT is more helpful than endoscopic biopsy, which can miss the vasculitic lesions as they are too deep beneath the mucosa.[10]

In a review from New Orleans, Buck et al. found that 56 of a total cohort of 319 patients with lupus were admitted with abdominal pain between 1980 and 1999.[8] Only five presented with an acute abdomen and underwent laparotomy. None of them were found to have vasculitis. Of the remaining 51 with subacute abdominal pain, three had LMV and the two factors most helpful in identifying these cases were Systemic Lupus Disease Activity Index (SLEDAI)

score > 8 and characteristic CT changes. These patients were successfully treated with corticosteroids. In a larger Korean study,[11] Kwok et al. reported that 87 of 706 patients with lupus followed between 1990 and 2006 were admitted with abdominal pain, 41 of whom had a diagnosis of LMV on clinical assessment and CT scanning. There was only one laparotomy and patients were treated with high-dose intravenous corticosteroids (1–2 mg/kg methylprednisolone per day for 3 days) and bowel rest with good response and no deaths from LMV. Only one patient received intravenous cyclophosphamide.

In contrast, a very large Chinese study of 3823 patients with SLE followed between 2002 and 2011 described 97 patients with LMV, 47 of whom presented with acute abdomen.[10] In fact, cases of LMV constituted 2.5% of hospital admissions of patients with lupus but 49.5% of those admitted with acute abdomen. This cohort of 97 patients with LMV was different than those presented in other studies as many patients had a short history of lupus and LMV was the presenting symptom in almost half the cases. Treatment was with high-dose oral (not intravenous) corticosteroids, but most patients also received immunosuppression, including intravenous cyclophosphamide in 67 cases. Of the 97 patients, 82 achieved remission with medical therapy alone and only two required surgery. The 13 patients who died included 8 with pneumonia and 5 with multiorgan failure. Factors statistically associated with mortality were low white count, low albumin, elevated amylase, and not being treated with cyclophosphamide. Use of cyclophosphamide was also associated with lower relapse rate in this study,[10] but the same has not been reported by others.[8,11]

Overall, these results suggest that LMV should be considered seriously in patients with lupus who present with an acute abdomen, especially in the context of a flare of disease and high SLEDAI score. Abdominal CT is valuable in making the diagnosis after which high-dose intravenous steroids should be used, with cyclophosphamide added for severe or refractory cases. Surgery is not often necessary.

LARGE VESSEL VASCULITIS

Large vessel vasculitis is very rare in lupus. Among the 670 patients followed for 24 years by Ramos-Casals et al.[3] there were no cases of large vessel vasculitis. There have been case reports of giant cell arteritis,[13,14] Takayasu's arteritis,[15] cerebral vasculitis,[16] and fulminant rapidly fatal systemic vasculitis,[17] but many reports are old and have not been followed by further similar reports and in some cases the diagnosis of SLE was doubtful. For example, over half the cases of Takayasu's arteritis reviewed by Sachetto et al. did not fulfill American College of Rheumatology classification criteria for SLE.[15]

OTHER FORMS OF VASCULITIS

A recent review[1] summarizes the evidence for hepatic, pancreatic, pulmonary, and coronary vasculitis in SLE, all of which are so rare clinically that the literature consists primarily of case reports and autopsy studies.

REFERENCES

1. Barile-Fabris L, Hernandez-Cabrera MF, Barragan-Garfias JA. Vasculitis in systemic lupus erythematosus. *Curr Rheumatol Rep* 2014;**16**(9):440.
2. Drenkard C, Villa AR, Reyes E, Abello M, Alarcon-Segovia D. Vasculitis in systemic lupus erythematosus. *Lupus* 1997;**6**(3):235–42.
3. Ramos-Casals M, Nardi N, Lagrutta M, Brito-Zeron P, Bove A, Delgado G, et al. Vasculitis in systemic lupus erythematosus: prevalence and clinical characteristics in 670 patients. *Medicine (Baltimore)* 2006;**85**(2):95–104.
4. Yell JA, Mbuagbaw J, Burge SM. Cutaneous manifestations of systemic lupus erythematosus. *Br J Dermatol* 1996;**135**(3):355–62.
5. Ju JH, Min JK, Jung CK, Oh SN, Kwok SK, Kang KY, et al. Lupus mesenteric vasculitis can cause acute abdominal pain in patients with SLE. *Nat Rev* 2009;**5**(5):273–81.
6. Shapeero LG, Myers A, Oberkircher PE, Miller WT. Acute reversible lupus vasculitis of the gastrointestinal tract. *Radiology* 1974;**112**(3):569–74.
7. al-Hakeem MS, McMillen MA. Evaluation of abdominal pain in systemic lupus erythematosus. *Am J Surg* 1998;**176**(3):291–4.
8. Buck AC, Serebro LH, Quinet RJ. Subacute abdominal pain requiring hospitalization in a systemic lupus erythematosus patient: a retrospective analysis and review of the literature. *Lupus* 2001;**10**(7):491–5.
9. Medina F, Ayala A, Jara LJ, Becerra M, Miranda JM, Fraga A. Acute abdomen in systemic lupus erythematosus: the importance of early laparotomy. *Am J Med* 1997;**103**(2):100–5.
10. Yuan S, Ye Y, Chen D, Qiu Q, Zhan Z, Lian F, et al. Lupus mesenteric vasculitis: clinical features and associated factors for the recurrence and prognosis of disease. *Semin Arthritis Rheum* 2014;**43**(6):759–66.
11. Kwok SK, Seo SH, Ju JH, Park KS, Yoon CH, Kim WU, et al. Lupus enteritis: clinical characteristics, risk factor for relapse and association with anti-endothelial cell antibody. *Lupus* 2007;**16**(10):803–9.
12. Ko SF, Lee TY, Cheng TT, Ng SH, Lai HM, Cheng YF, et al. CT findings at lupus mesenteric vasculitis. *Acta Radiol* 1997;**38**(1):115–20.
13. Bunker CB, Dowd PM. Giant cell arteritis and systemic lupus erythematosus. *Br J Dermatol* 1988;**119**(1):115–20.
14. Scharre D, Petri M, Engman E, DeArmond S. Large intracranial arteritis with giant cells in systemic lupus erythematosus. *Ann Intern Med* 1986;**104**(5):661–2.
15. Sachetto Z, Fernandes SR, Del Rio AP, Coimbra IB, Bertolo MB, Costallat LT. Systemic lupus erythematosus associated with vasculitic syndrome (Takayasu's arteritis). *Rheumatol Int* 2010;**30**(12):1669–72.
16. Rowshani AT, Remans P, Rozemuller A, Tak PP. Cerebral vasculitis as a primary manifestation of systemic lupus erythematosus. *Ann Rheum Dis* 2005;**64**(5):784–6.
17. Medina G, Gonzalez-Perez D, Vazquez-Juarez C, Sanchez-Uribe M, Saavedra MA, Jara LJ. Fulminant systemic vasculitis in systemic lupus erythematosus. Case report and review of the literature. *Lupus* 2014;**23**(13):1426–9.

Part V

Antiphospholipid Syndrome

Pathogenesis of Antiphospholipid Syndrome

Olga Amengual, Tatsuya Atsumi

Division of Rheumatology, Endocrinology and Nephrology, Hokkaido University Graduate School of Medicine, Sapporo, Japan

INTRODUCTION

The presence of antiphospholipid antibodies (aPL) is the defining feature of antiphospholipid syndrome (APS). It is now well accepted that, despite their name, the majority of aPL associated with APS are directed against phospholipid-binding proteins, among them β2-glycoprotein I (β2GPI) and prothrombin are regarded as the most relevant antigenic targets.[1,2]

In the laboratory, aPL can be broadly categorized into those antibodies that are detected using enzyme-linked immunosorbent assay (ELISA) such as anticardiolipin antibodies (aCL) or anti-β2GPI antibodies, and those antibodies detected by their ability to prolong phospholipid-dependent coagulation tests, known as lupus anticoagulant (LA).

The majority of aCL detected in APS are directed against epitopes expressed on β2GPI, which are exposed when β2GPI interacts with negatively charged phospholipids or when β2GPI is adsorbed on a polyoxygenated polystyrene plate treated with γ-irradiation. Prolongation of phospholipid-dependent coagulation tests (prothrombin time, activated partial thromboplastin time, kaolin clotting time, dilute Russell's viper venom time) is caused by antibodies with different specificities against phospholipid-binding proteins.

Several other "cofactors," including prothrombin, annexin V, protein S, protein C, and high- and/or low-molecular-weight kininogen, have been described to relate to the clinical manifestations of APS. In particular, prothrombin has been recognized as the "second" major antigenic target of autoimmune aPL. ELISAs for the detection of antiprothrombin antibodies identify two populations of antibodies: those binding to prothrombin alone, aPT-A, and those that bind to phosphatidylserine–prothrombin complexes, phosphatidylserine-dependent antiprothrombin antibodies (aPS/PT).[3,4]

Thrombotic complications in APS can occur in most vessels and numerous pathogenic mechanisms have been implicated. aPL promote thrombosis through inhibition of the natural anticoagulation pathways, impairment of the fibrinolytic system, activation of the complement system, and activation of procoagulant cells (Table 1). In this chapter, we detail the suggested pathogenic mechanisms related to the aPL-mediated induction of a hypercoagulable state in APS.

PATHOGENESIS OF aPL

aPL are thought to be pathogenic antibodies due to their strong relationship with the clinical manifestations of APS. The action of aPL on prothrombotic cells via phospholipid-binding proteins, β2GPI and prothrombin, was shown to be more important than the modifications of the function of the proteins by aPL.

aPL and the Coagulation System

The coagulation system is an amplification cascade of enzymatic reactions resulting in thrombin formation. Protein C is a major constituent of the anticoagulant system. Thrombin binds to thrombomodulin and activates protein C; activated protein C complexes with protein S. These complexes function as an anticoagulant by proteolytically catalyzing the inactivation of activated factors V and VIII. Both protein C and protein S are phospholipid-binding plasma proteins.

Resistance, related to aPL, against activated protein C is one of the classical mechanisms responsible for thrombosis.[5] The protein C system may be interfered by aPL in different ways. aPL inhibit both the activation of protein C by the thrombin/thrombomodulin complex and the proteolytic effect of activated protein C on inactivation of activated factors. Rabbit polyclonal antibodies[6] and a human monoclonal anti-β2GPI antibody inhibit activated protein C function.[7,8] Most prothrombin–antiprothrombin antibodies immune complexes may predispose to thrombosis by interfering with the inactivation of activated factor V by activated protein C in the presence and absence of protein S.[9] aPL may alter the effect of protein S in the protein C pathway. Decreased levels of protein S were found in plasma from APS patients. Some of the immunoglobulin (Ig) G that inhibit activated factor V degradation were directed not only to

TABLE 1 Mechanisms of Antiphospholipid Antibodies (aPL)-Mediated Pathogenicity

Effects of aPL on coagulation system

  Protein C pathway

  Contact activation pathway

  β2-glycoprotein I/thrombin interaction

  Decreased tissue factor pathway inhibitor activity

  Protein Z

Effect of aPL on fibrinolysis

  Upregulation of plasminogen activator inhibitor 1

  Interference with activated factor XII

  Effects of lipoprotein(a)

Effect of aPL on cells

  Induction of procoagulant activity (*endothelial cells and monocytes*)

  Induction of proinflammatory activity (*endothelial cells and monocytes*)

  Release of membrane-bound microparticles (*endothelial cells and platelets*)

  Stimulation of platelet activation and aggregation

  Disruption of the annexin A5 shield

  T cell interaction

  Placenta damage

  Trophoblast perturbation

  Neutrophil activation

  Endometrial angiogenesis

aPL and atherothrombosis

Complement activation

phospholipid-bound protein C but also to phospholipid-bound protein S.

The interference of aPL with the contact pathway of coagulation is another proposed thrombotic mechanism in APS. The contact activation pathway is initiated with activation of factor XII by negatively charged surfaces. Activated factor XII cleaves factor XI to activated factor XI in the presence of high-molecular-weight kininogen and prekalikrein. β2GPI inhibited the phospholipid-mediated autoactivation of factor XII and the contact activation pathway of coagulation. Moreover, β2GPI binds to factor XI and inhibits activation of factor XI by thrombin and activated factor XII; this inhibition attenuates thrombin generation. Monoclonal anti-β2GPI antibodies enhanced the inhibition of factor XI activation by β2GPI and thrombin complexes.[10]

Thrombin is one of the more potent enzymes involved in the regulation of many biological functions in vivo including inflammation, angiogenesis, arteriosclerosis, neoplastic transformation, and tissue repair. Thrombin is generated, on the surface of activated cells, from its inactive precursor prothrombin by activated factor X, as part of the prothrombinase complex. Thrombin acts as procoagulant by cleaving fibrinogen to fibrin and interacts with protease-activated receptors to activate various procoagulant cells. Thrombin binds glycoprotein (GP) Ib–IX–V complexes on the surface of platelets to promote platelet aggregation and activation. On the other hand, thrombin behaves as anticoagulant on binding to thrombomodulin to favor activation of protein C. The participation of β2GPI in thrombin generation has been demonstrated by the significant reduction of in vitro ability to generate thrombin observed in plasma from β2GPI-null mice. β2GPI directly binds to thrombin and β2GPI/thrombin interaction may interfere not only with the coagulation system but also with many of the biological functions in which thrombin participates.[10]

The tissue factor pathway inhibitor (TFPI) is a natural anticoagulant that regulates tissue factor (TF)-induced blood coagulation. Anti-TFPI activity identified in the IgG fraction of patients with APS was associated with increased in vitro TF-induced thrombin generation.[11] Inhibitors of TFPI or interference to TFPI activity could upregulate the TF pathway and contribute to the hypercoagulability in APS.

The inhibition of protein Z by aPL is another thrombotic mechanism in APS. Protein Z functions as a natural anticoagulant serving as cofactor for the inactivation of activated factor X by the protein Z-dependent protease inhibitor. Reduced plasma levels of protein Z detected in patients with aPL were associated with thrombosis. In the presence of β2GPI, aPL greatly impair the inhibition of activated factor X by protein Z/protein Z-dependent protease inhibitor.[12]

aPL and the Fibrinolytic System

Fibrinolysis is a tightly regulated process by which fibrin-rich thrombus is remodeled and degraded. The fibrinolytic system involves the conversion of plasminogen to plasmin from plasminogen by the tissue-type plasminogen activator (tPA) or urokinase-type plasminogen activator and the hydrolytic cleavage of fibrin to fibrin degradation products by plasmin.

The regulation of plasmin generation and activity is highly important for maintaining the homeostatic balance in vivo. Inhibition of the fibrinolytic system may occur at the level of plasminogen activator by specific plasminogen activator inhibitors (PAI-1 and PAI-2) or at the level of plasmin by α2-macroglobulin and α2-plasmin inhibitors.

Impairment of fibrinolysis due to aPL may contribute to the development of thrombosis. Upregulation of PAI-I levels and decreased tPA release were reported in patients with primary APS and venous thrombosis, suggesting that tPA/PAI-1 balance is crucial for developing thrombosis.[13]

Several studies demonstrated that β2GPI and anti-β2GPI antibodies interact with components of the fibrinolytic system. aPL may inhibit both the intrinsic and the extrinsic fibrinolysis pathways. β2GPI blocks the neutralization of tPA by PA-1 in a concentration-dependent manner. The addition of monoclonal aCL blocked this activity, inhibiting the fibrinolysis by an elevation in PAI-1 activity.[14] Monoclonal anti-β2GPI antibodies significantly suppressed the intrinsic fibrinolytic activity in vitro; this inhibition was attributed to a reduced contact activation reaction initiated by activated factor XII.[15] Impaired activated factor XII-dependent activation of fibrinolysis was observed in pregnant women with APS women who developed late-pregnancy complications.[16] Antibodies interacting with the catalytic domain of tPA have been detected in APS patients and could represent a cause of hypofibrinolysis.

β2GPI could regulate the fibrinolysis by direct interaction with plasminogen. The fifth domain in β2GPI can be proteolytically cleaved by plasmin to create "nicked" β2GPI, which is unable to bind to phospholipids. Nicked β2GPI binds to plasminogen and blocks the formation of plasmin by tPA controlling the extrinsic fibrinolysis through a negative feedback mechanism.[17] On the other, in the presence of plasminogen and tPA, intact β2GPI may promote plasmin generation. Therefore, intact β2GPI may stimulate fibrinolysis, but following plasminogen activation and cleavage, nicked β2GPI could inhibit further plasmin generation.

β2GPI interacts with tPA and stimulates fibrinolysis in plasma. Monoclonal aCL with anti-β2GPI activity, obtained from APS patients, could impair activated factor XII-dependent activation of fibrinolysis during pregnancy.[18]

Finally, patients with APS had elevated levels of lipoprotein (a) (Lp(a)). Patients with maximal elevation of Lp(a) showed a reduced fibrinolytic activity, estimated by low D-dimer and PAI-1.[19] Lp(a) competes with plasminogen for binding sites, leading to reduced fibrinolysis. Lp(a) also increases PAI-1 expression by endothelial cells and could interact with cellular plasminogen receptors. This behavior confers Lp(a) a prothrombotic potential.

Annexin 2, an endothelial cell receptor for β2GPI, stimulates fibrinolysis through binding to tPA and plasminogen. Antibodies against annexin 2 found in patients with APS correlated with a history of thrombosis. These antibodies could inhibit cell surface fibrinolysis through direct interaction with endothelial cell annexin 2.[20]

INTERACTION OF aPL WITH CELLS

Activated or damaged endothelial cells, monocytes, and platelets are predominant targets of aPL. aPL induce TF in endothelial cells and monocytes and cause increased release by endothelial cells of leukocyte adhesion molecules, endothelin-1, inflammatory cytokines, and the fibrinolysis inhibitor PAI-1.[21–23] These effects are mediated by β2GPI and cell surface receptors promoting thrombosis and inflammation. Prothrombin also binds to endothelial cells; this binding is enhanced by a human monoclonal IgG antiprothrombin antibody (IS6), which upregulates the expression of TF and E-selectin on endothelial cells.[24]

Platelets are prone to agglutinate and aggregate after exposure to aPL.[25] β2GPI binds to surface membranes of activated platelets and inhibits the generation of activated factor X. Anti-β2GPI antibodies interfered with this inhibition.

Disruption of the annexin A5 anticoagulant shield is another thrombogenic mechanism in APS. Annexin A5 is a potent anticoagulant protein found in a variety of tissues including the placenta and the vascular endothelium. Annexin A5 binds anionic phospholipids with high affinity and crystallizes over phospholipid bilayers, blocking their availability for coagulation reactions forming a protective anticoagulant shield on vascular cells. aPL interfere with annexin A5 binding and crystallization, resulting in acceleration of coagulation reactions. Levels of annexin A5 were markedly reduced on placental villi in patients with APS and on apical membranes of placental villi when cultured with aPL IgG fractions from APS patients. The aPL reduction of annexin A5, also demonstrated on endothelial cells and platelets, occurs via its displacement by aPL in the presence of β2GPI.[26]

aPL interact with T cells. The binding of β2GPI to anionic phospholipid facilitates the processing and presentation of a cryptic epitope that activate pathogenic autoreactive CD4+ T cells. β2GPI-reactive CD4+ T cell proliferation depends on monocytes as antigen-presenting cells.[27] This reaction was observed only in the presence of anti-β2GPI antibodies and was mediated by Fcγ receptor I. These findings suggested that the opsonization of the β2GPI/phosphatidylserine complex by the IgG anti-β2GPI antibody is essential for efficient antigen presentation from monocytes to T cells and eventually for maintaining the pathogenic anti-β2GPI antibody response in APS.

Direct placenta damage and trophoblast perturbation are thought to be involved in aPL-mediated fetal loss. Sera from patients with APS reduce placental growth and increase trophoblastic apoptosis in vitro. Perturbation of trophoblast by aPL includes the promotion of nonapoptotic trophoblasts shed from the placenta causing endothelial cell activation. Anti-β2GPI antibodies modulated human first trimester trophoblast cytokine/chemokine production, triggering placental inflammation and cell death.[28] Furthermore, aPL suppress placenta growth factor production, leading to the failure of placenta formation and function, and alter the trophoblast secretion of angiogenic factors. Finally, neutrophil activation and inhibition of endometrial angiogenesis by aPL have been related to aPL-mediated pregnancy failure.[29]

Cell Receptors for aPL Interactions

The cell activation mediated by aPL requires the interaction between the phospholipid-binding plasma proteins and a specific cell receptor(s). Several candidate receptors for the binding of β2GP to cellular membranes have been identified including annexin A2 apolipoprotein E receptor 2, low-density lipoprotein receptor (LDL-R)-related protein, megalin, Toll-like receptor (TLR) 2, TLR 4, TLR 8, CD14, the very-LDL-R, P-selectin GP ligand-1, GP Ibα, integrin α5β1, platelet factor 4, and several complement factors. Most of these receptors are expressed on various cell types and whether many different receptors are involved in the pathophysiology of thrombosis is still a matter of controversy.[30]

The role of members of the TLR family in aPL-mediated cell activation has been widely evaluated. Some reports underlined the essential role of TLR2 for the pathogenic effects of aPL whereas others showed the involvement of TLR4 in the activation of the cell by aPL. β2GPI binds to TLR2 on the endothelial cell surface, and it was reported that TLR2 but not TLR4 mediates the activation of human monocytes and endothelial cells by aPL.[31] This effect was enhanced in the presence of CD14, a coreceptor for TLR2 and TLR4. On the other hand, TLR4-like signaling was shown in monocytes after incubation with anti-β2GPI antibodies,[32] and a mutation in murine TLR4 attenuated the increased prothrombotic state observed in wild-type mice injected with aPL. A direct interaction between TLR4 and β2GPI immune complexes, however, remains to be confirmed. Recent findings show that the response of aPL-activated monocytes could depend on activation of TLR7 and TLR8.[33]

β2GPI directly binds to the GPIbα subunit of the platelet adhesive receptor GPIb/IX/V, leading to increased thrombus formation in vitro.[34] Binding of β2GPI to GPIbα enables anti-β2GPI antibodies, directed against domain I, to activate platelets, resulting in thromboxane production, and also to activate the phosphoinositol-3 kinase (PI3-kinase)/Akt pathway contributing to platelet adhesion and aggregation.

Platelet factor 4 is a member of the C-X-C chemokine family secreted by activated platelets, and also has the ability to bind to the platelet surface. The direct binding of β2GPI to platelet factor 4 has been reported. β2GPI forms stable complexes with platelet factor 4, leading to the stabilization of the β2GPI dimeric structure, facilitating antibody recognition.[35] The β2GPI/platelet factor 4 complex is strongly recognized by APS patients' sera. Moreover, platelets may be activated by β2GPI/anti-β2GPI antibody/platelet factor 4 or β2GPI/ platelet factor 4 complexes.

CD36 is a member of the class B scavenger receptors expressed on monocytes, macrophages, platelets, and capillary endothelial cells. CD36 resides in lipid rafts and interacts with a variety of membrane receptors, mediating multiple functions including inflammation, atherogenesis, and thrombosis. Procoagulant cell activation mediated by aPL could involve the recruitment of cell surface receptors on lipid rafts; therefore, CD36 could interact with other β2GPI or prothrombin receptors involved in the pathogenesis of APS.[36]

Numerous receptors have been proposed to be involved in the aPL-mediated cell activation in APS. To date there is no consensus on which receptor or coreceptor is mainly responsible for cell activation mediated by aPL. Additional studies are needed to clarify the biological and pathological roles of the identified receptors in APS.

Signaling Transduction Pathways of Cell Activation

Different signaling transduction pathways have been involved in the cell activation mediated by aPL. Among the important signaling intermediates that play a central role in this processes are the nuclear factor kappa B (NFκB), p38 mitogen-activated protein kinase (MAPK), extracellular signal-regulated kinases (ERK), interleukin (IL)-1 receptor-associated kinase (IRAK), and myeloid differentiation protein 88 (MyD88).

Incubation of endothelial cells or monocytes with anti-β2GPI antibodies resulted in a redistribution of NFκB from the cytoplasm to the nucleus, promoting an increased expression of TF, leukocyte adhesion molecules and inflammatory cytokines, IL-6, IL8, and tumor necrosis factor (TNF)α.[37,38]

The p38 MAPK pathway is an important component of intracellular signaling cascades and has a crucial role in mediating the effect of aPL in different cell types.[39–41] Stimulation of monocytes by monoclonal anti-β2GPI antibodies from APS patients leads to p38 MAPK phosphorylation, a locational shift of NFκB into the nucleus, and upregulation of TF expression. Such activation was not seen in the absence of β2GPI, indicating that the disturbance of monocyte by anti-β2GPI antibodies is started by interaction between the cell and the autoantibody-bound β2GPI. Activation of the p38 MAPK pathway also increases activities of TNFα, IL-1β, and macrophage inflammatory cytokine 3β.

The induction of TF expression was also reported through the simultaneous activation of NFκB via the p38 MAPK pathway, and of the mitogen extracellular signal-regulated kinase (MEK)-1/ERK pathway.[42] However, the expression of TF could not be suppressed by an inhibitor of the MEK-1/ERK pathway, suggesting that the p38 MAPK system plays the main role in these reactions.

IgG purified from APS patients induced phosphorylation of ERK. Furthermore, affinity-purified anti-β2GPI antibodies obtained from patients with APS react with β2GPI in lipid rafts in the monocyte plasma membrane. Anti-β2GPI antibody binding triggers IRAK phosphorylation and NFκB translocation, leading to a proinflammatory and procoagulant monocyte phenotype characterized by the release of TNFα and TF, respectively.[43] The adapter molecule MyD88-dependent signaling pathway and the TNF receptor-associated factor (TRAF6) have also been implicated in the aPL-mediated cell activation. Krüppel-like factors (KLFs) are essential in regulating the endothelial response to inflammatory stimuli and have been implicated in the endothelial proinflammatory response to anti-β2GPI antibodies. Incubation of endothelial cells with anti-β2GPI antibodies leads to a decreased expression of KLFs, which in turn could facilitate cellular activation mediated through NFκB. These results provide new evidence for novel protein–protein interactions on endothelial cells that may contribute to endothelial cell activation and the pathogenesis APS.[30] Finally, the PI3-kinase/Akt pathway seems to play a specific role in platelet activation by aPL.[44] Figure 1 shows some of the proposed mechanisms of procoagulant cell activation mediated by aPL.

aPL and Atherothrombosis

aPL have been related to atherosclerotic diseases such as myocardial infarction and stroke. Oxidized LDL (oxLDL) is the principal lipoprotein found in atherosclerotic lesions. OxLDL colocalizes with β2GPI, immunoreactive CD4+ lymphocytes, and Igs, indicating that aPL could contribute to the development of atherosclerosis. OxLDL binds to β2GPI to form oxLDL/β2GPI complexes, and circulating oxLDL/β2GPI complexes are the antigen targets for anti-β2GPI antibodies in patients with APS. IgG anti-β2GPI immune complexes containing oxLDL facilitate the accumulation of oxLD in macrophages and allowed the presentation of β2GPI epitopes to pathogenic autoreactive T cells. Both mechanisms required Fcγ type I receptor-mediated uptake by macrophages/monocytes.[45] Thus, oxLDL/β2GPI complexes are a major atherogenic autoantigen and IgG anti-β2GPI antibodies may facilitate antigen presentation and foam cell formation in APS.

aPL and Complement Activation

The complement system has been identified as essential for the pathogenicity of aPL. Complement activation by aPL is one of the mechanisms implicated in the pregnancy morbidity in APS[46] and may also be a contributor to the thrombophilia characteristic of APS. Further, there is a close relationship between complement and coagulation pathways.

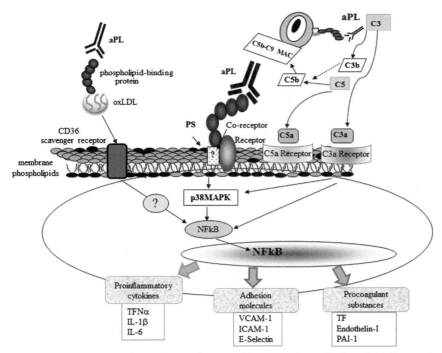

FIGURE 1 **Mechanisms of cell activation mediated by aPL.** aPL interact with procoagulant cells through binding to phospholipid-binding plasma proteins (β2GPI or prothrombin) on cell surfaces. This interaction requires specific cell receptors and provokes the phosphorylation of p38 MAPK and the nuclear translocation of NFκB. The activation of signaling cascade mediates upregulation of procoagulant substances, adhesion molecules, and proinflammatory cytokines resulting in thrombus formation and the establishment of a proinflammatory state. Circulating oxLDL molecules bind to β2GPI to form oxLDL/β2GPI complexes that become antigenic targets for anti-β2GPI antibodies. Immunocomplexes containing anti-β2GPI antibodies and oxLDL/β2GPI are uptaken by CD36 scavenger receptors, which triggers signaling cascades for inflammatory responses. Finally, aPL activate complement through the classical pathway. C3a, C5a, and C5b-9 MAC may bind to specific receptors on the cell surface and enhance the effects of aPL in cells. aPL, anti-phospholipid antibodies; p38 MAPK, p38 mitogen-activated protein kinase; NFκB, nuclear factor kappa B; ox/LDL, oxidized low-density lipoprotein; β2GPI, β2-glycoprotein I; PS, phosphatidylserine; TNFα, tumor necrosis factor α; IL, interleukin; VCAM; vascular cell adhesion molecule 1; ICAM-1, intercellular adhesion molecule 1; TF, tissue factor; PAI-1, plasminogen activator inhibitor 1; MAC, membrane attack complex.

Human and mouse studies showed that aPL are specifically targeted to trophoblasts. Complement deposition was found in the placental tissues of women with aPL.[47] Placenta trophoblast cells are targeted by phospholipid-binding protein–aPL complexes, which can activate complement via the classical pathway. C3 and subsequently C5 are activated. Generated C5a recruits and activates polymorphonuclear leukocytes and monocytes and stimulates the release of mediators of inflammation, ultimately resulting in placenta injury and fetal death.

The essential role of complement activation in pregnancy loss and fetal growth restriction was reported in a murine model of APS. Inhibition of the complement cascade in vivo, using the C3 convertase inhibitor complement receptor 1-related gene/protein y (Crry)-Ig, blocks aPL-mediated fetal loss.[48] In addition, deficiency of complement C3 prevented fetal loss and growth restriction in these mice and antibodies that block C5a–C5a receptor interactions prevent pregnancy complications. Furthermore, mice deficient in alternative and classical pathway complements were resistant to fetal injury induced by aPL, indicating that both classical and alternative complement pathway activation contributes to damage. Finally, treatment with heparin prevented aPL-induced complement activation in vivo and in vitro and protected mice from aPL-related pregnancy complications.[46]

TNFα is a mediator that links complement activation and aPL to fetal death. Miscarriages induced by aPL are less frequent in mice deficient in TNFα or treated with TNFα blockade.[49] Complement activation triggers also the induction of TF in decidual tissues, which leads to trophoblast injury and pregnancy loss.

Complement activation takes part in the thrombotic manifestations in APS. Higher levels of complement activation products were detected in the plasma of APS patients with cerebral ischemic events compared with patients with non-APS-related cerebral ischemia. Mice deficient in component complement C3, C5, or C5a receptors were resistant to aPL-induced enhanced thrombophilia and endothelial cell activation, and anti-C5 monoclonal antibody prevented these effects.[50]

Low serum complement levels of C3, C4, and CH50 were observed in patients with primary APS and related to consumption of complement as a result of complement activation. Serum complement levels correlated with LA activity and plasma levels of TNFα, implying that complement activation may be a contributor to thrombophilia in APS.[51] The IgG isotype of aPL is the most frequently found in patients, with APS and IgG2 subclass the most prevalent. IgG2 and IgG4 subclasses have a relatively weak ability to fix complement via the classical pathways, thus other additional mechanisms may be involved in the enhancement of complement activation in patients with aPL. The inflammatory process accompanied by complement activation is an important phenomenon that mediates the crossroads between the immune response and the thrombosis.

CONCLUSION

The pathogenesis of APS is multifactorial. The recognition of candidate cell receptors for aPL binding and the elucidation of the intracellular signaling pathways of the cell activation mediated by aPL have greatly increased our understanding of the singular thrombophilia state in patients with APS. There are various pathways by which aPL lead to a prothrombotic state, and whether the generalized thrombotic manifestations in APS indicate the multiple effects of aPL or are related to a still unidentified mechanism remains unclear.

ACKNOWLEDGMENTS

The authors are supported by grants from the Japanese Ministry of Health, Labor, and Welfare, and the Japanese Ministry of Education, Culture, Sports, Science, and Technology.

REFERENCES

1. McNeil HP, Simpson RJ, Chesterman CN, Krilis SA. Anti-phospholipid antibodies are directed against a complex antigen that induces a lipid-binding inhibitor of coagulation: b2-glycoprotein I (apolipoprotein H). *Proc Natl Acad Sci USA* 1990;**87**:4120–4.
2. Bevers EM, Galli M, Barbui T, Comfurius P, Zwaal RF. Lupus anticoagulant IgG's (LA) are not directed to phospholipids only, but to a complex of lipid-bound human prothrombin. *Thromb Haemost* 1991;**66**:629–32.
3. Galli M, Beretta G, Daldossi M, Bevers EM, Barbui T. Different anticoagulant and immunological properties of anti-prothrombin antibodies in patients with antiphospholipid antibodies. *Thromb Haemost* 1997;**77**:486–91.
4. Atsumi T, Ieko M, Bertolaccini ML, Ichikawa K, Tsutsumi A, Matsuura E, et al. Association of autoantibodies against the phosphatidylserine-prothrombin complex with manifestations of the antiphospholipid syndrome and with the presence of lupus anticoagulant. *Arthritis Rheum* 2000;**43**:1982–93.
5. de Laat B, Eckmann CM, van Schagen M, Meijer AB, Mertens K, van Mourik JA. Correlation between the potency of a beta2-glycoprotein I-dependent lupus anticoagulant and the level of resistance to activated protein C. *Blood Coagul Fibrinolysis* 2008;**19**:757–64.
6. Matsuda J, Gotoh M, Gohchi K, Kawasugi K, Tsukamoto M, Saitoh N. Resistance to activated protein C activity of an anti-beta 2-glycoprotein I antibody in the presence of beta 2-glycoprotein I. *Br J Haematol* 1995;**90**:204–6.
7. Ieko M, Ichikawa K, Triplett DA, Matsuura E, Atsumi T, Sawada K, et al. Beta2-glycoprotein I is necessary to inhibit protein C activity by monoclonal anticardiolipin antibodies. *Arthritis Rheum* 1999;**42**:167–74.
8. Atsumi T, Khamashta MA, Amengual O, Donohoe S, Mackie I, Ichikawa K, et al. Binding of anticardiolipin antibodies to protein C via b2-glycoprotein I (b2-GPI): a possible mechanism in the inhibitory effect of antiphospholipid antibodies on the protein C system. *Clin Exp Immunol* 1998;**112**:325–33.

9. Galli M, Willems GM, Rosing J, Janssen RM, Govers-Riemslag JW, Comfurius P, et al. Anti-prothrombin IgG from patients with antiphospholipid antibodies inhibits the inactivation of factor Va by activated protein C. *Br J Haematol* 2005;**129**:240–7.

10. Rahgozar S, Yang Q, Giannakopoulos B, Yan X, Miyakis S, Krilis SA. Beta2-glycoprotein I binds thrombin via exosite I and exosite II: anti-beta2-glycoprotein I antibodies potentiate the inhibitory effect of beta2-glycoprotein I on thrombin-mediated factor XIa generation. *Arthritis Rheum* 2007;**56**:605–13.

11. Adams MJ, Donohoe S, Mackie IJ, Machin SJ. Anti-tissue factor pathway inhibitor activity in patients with primary antiphospholipid syndrome. *Br J Haematol* 2001;**114**:375–9.

12. Forastiero RR, Martinuzzo ME, Lu L Broze GJ. Autoimmune antiphospholipid antibodies impair the inhibition of activated factor X by protein Z/protein Z-dependent protease inhibitor. *J Thromb Haemost* 2003;**1**:1764–70.

13. Ames PR, Tommasino C, Iannaccone L, Brillante M, Cimino R, Brancaccio V. Coagulation activation and fibrinolytic imbalance in subjects with idopathic antiphospholipid antibodies - a crucial role for acquired free protein S deficiency. *Thromb Haemost* 1996;**76**:190–4.

14. Ieko M, Ichikawa K, Atsumi T, Takeuchi R, Sawada KI, Yasukouchi T, et al. Effects of beta2-glycoprotein I and monoclonal anticardiolipin antibodies on extrinsic fibrinolysis. *Semin Thromb Hemost* 2000;**26**:85–90.

15. Takeuchi R, Atsumi T, Ieko M, Amasaki Y, Ichikawa K, Koike T. Suppressed intrinsic fibrinolytic activity by monoclonal anti-beta-2 glycoprotein I autoantibodies: possible mechanism for thrombosis in patients with antiphospholipid syndrome. *Br J Haematol* 2002;**119**:781–8.

16. Carmona F, Lazaro I, Reverter JC, Tassies D, Font J, Cervera R, et al. Impaired factor XIIa-dependent activation of fibrinolysis in treated antiphospholipid syndrome gestations developing late-pregnancy complications. *Am J Obstet Gynecol* 2006;**194**:457–65.

17. Yasuda S, Atsumi T, Ieko M, Matsuura E, Kobayashi K, Inagaki J, et al. Nicked beta2-glycoprotein I: a marker of cerebral infarct and a novel role in the negative feedback pathway of extrinsic fibrinolysis. *Blood* 2004;**103**:3766–72.

18. Lazaro I, Carmona F, Reverter JC, Cervera R, Tassies D, Balasch J. Antiphospholipid antibodies may impair factor XIIa-dependent activation of fibrinolysis in pregnancy: in vitro evidence with human endothelial cells in culture and monoclonal anticardiolipin antibodies. *Am J Obstet Gynecol* 2009;**201**(87):e1–6.

19. Atsumi T, Khamashta MA, Andujar C, Leandro MJ, Amengual O, Ames PR, et al. Elevated plasma lipoprotein(a) level and its association with impaired fibrinolysis in patients with antiphospholipid syndrome. *J Rheumatol* 1998;**25**:69–73.

20. Cesarman-Maus G, Rios-Luna NP, Deora AB, Huang B, Villa R, Cravioto Mdel C, et al. Autoantibodies against the fibrinolytic receptor, annexin 2, in antiphospholipid syndrome. *Blood* 2006;**107**:4375–82.

21. Amengual O, Atsumi T, Khamashta MA, Hughes GRV. The role of the tissue factor pathway in the hypercoagulable state in patients with the antiphospholipid syndrome. *Thromb Haemost* 1998;**79**:276–81.

22. Pierangeli SS, Espinola RG, Liu X, Harris EN. Thrombogenic effects of antiphospholipid antibodies are mediated by intercellular cell adhesion molecule-1, vascular cell adhesion molecule-1, and P-selectin. *Circ Res* 2001;**88**:245–50.

23. Atsumi T, Khamashta MA, Haworth RS, Brooks G, Amengual O, Ichikawa K, et al. Arterial disease and thrombosis in the antiphospholipid syndrome: a pathogenic role for endothelin 1. *Arthritis Rheum* 1998;**41**:800–7.

24. Vega-Ostertag M, Liu X, Kwan-Ki H, Chen P, Pierangeli S. A human monoclonal antiprothrombin antibody is thrombogenic in vivo and upregulates expression of tissue factor and E-selectin on endothelial cells. *Br J Haematol* 2006;**135**:214–9.

25. Wiener MH, Burke M, Fried M, Yust I. Thromboagglutination by anticardiolipin antibody complex in the antiphospholipid syndrome: a possible mechanism of immune-mediated thrombosis. *Thromb Res* 2001;**103**:193–9.

26. de Laat B, Wu XX, van Lummel M, Derksen RH, de Groot PG, Rand JH. Correlation between antiphospholipid antibodies that recognize domain I of beta2-glycoprotein I and a reduction in the anticoagulant activity of annexin A5. *Blood* 2007;**109**:1490–4.

27. Yamaguchi Y, Seta N, Kaburaki J, Kobayashi K, Matsuura E, Kuwana M. Excessive exposure to anionic surfaces maintains autoantibody response to beta(2)-glycoprotein I in patients with antiphospholipid syndrome. *Blood* 2007;**110**:4312–8.

28. Mulla MJ, Brosens JJ, Chamley LW, Giles I, Pericleous C, Rahman A, et al. Antiphospholipid antibodies induce a pro-inflammatory response in first trimester trophoblast via the TLR4/MyD88 pathway. *Am J Reprod Immunol* 2009;**62**:96–111.

29. Redecha P, Franzke CW, Ruf W, Mackman N, Girardi G. Neutrophil activation by the tissue factor/Factor VIIa/PAR2 axis mediates fetal death in a mouse model of antiphospholipid syndrome. *J Clin Invest* 2008;**118**:3453–61.

30. Brandt KJ, Kruithof EK, de Moerloose P. Receptors involved in cell activation by antiphospholipid antibodies. *Thromb Res* 2013;**132**:408–13.

31. Satta N, Kruithof EK, Fickentscher C, Dunoyer-Geindre S, Boehlen F, Reber G, et al. Toll-like receptor 2 mediates the activation of human monocytes and endothelial cells by antiphospholipid antibodies. *Blood* 2011;**117**:5523–31.

32. Zhou H, Yan Y, Xu G, Zhou B, Wen H, Guo D, et al. Toll-like receptor (TLR)-4 mediates anti-beta2GPI/beta2GPI-induced tissue factor expression in THP-1 cells. *Clin Exp Immunol* 2011;**163**:189–98.

33. Prinz N, Clemens N, Strand D, Putz I, Lorenz M, Daiber A, et al. Antiphospholipid antibodies induce translocation of TLR7 and TLR8 to the endosome in human monocytes and plasmacytoid dendritic cells. *Blood* 2011;**118**:2322–32.

34. Pennings MT, Derksen RH, van Lummel M, Adelmeijer J, VanHoorelbeke K, Urbanus RT, et al. Platelet adhesion to dimeric beta-glycoprotein I under conditions of flow is mediated by at least two receptors: glycoprotein Ibalpha and apolipoprotein E receptor 2'. *J Thromb Haemost* 2007;**5**:369–77.

35. Sikara MP, Routsias JG, Samiotaki M, Panayotou G, Moutsopoulos HM, Vlachoyiannopoulos PG. {beta}2 Glycoprotein I ({beta}2GPI) binds platelet factor 4 (PF4): implications for the pathogenesis of antiphospholipid syndrome. *Blood* 2010;**115**:713–23.

36. Kato M, Atsumi T, Oku K, Amengual O, Nakagawa H, Fujieda Y, et al. The involvement of CD36 in monocyte activation by antiphospholipid antibodies. *Lupus* 2013;**22**:761–71.

37. Dunoyer-Geindre S, De Moerloose P, Galve-De Rochemonteix B, Reber G, Kruithof E. NFkappaB is an essential intermediate in the activation of endothelial cells by anti-beta(2) glycoprotein 1 antibodies. *Thromb Haemost* 2002;**88**:851–7.

38. Zhou H, Sheng L, Wang H, Xie H, Mu Y, Wang T, et al. Anti-beta2GPI/beta2GPI stimulates activation of THP-1 cells through TLR4/MD-2/MyD88 and NF-kappaB signaling pathways. *Thromb Res* 2013;**132**:742–9.

39. Bohgaki M, Atsumi T, Yamashita Y, Yasuda S, Sakai Y, Furusaki A, et al. The p38 mitogen-activated protein kinase (MAPK) pathway mediates induction of the tissue factor gene in monocytes stimulated with human monoclonal anti-beta2Glycoprotein I antibodies. *Int Immunol* 2004;**16**:1633–41.

40. Vega-Ostertag M, Harris EN, Pierangeli SS. Intracellular events in platelet activation induced by antiphospholipid antibodies in the presence of low doses of thrombin. *Arthritis Rheum* 2004;**50**:2911–9.

41. Vega-Ostertag M, Casper K, Swerlick R, Ferrara D, Harris EN, Pierangeli SS. Involvement of p38 MAPK in the up-regulation of tissue factor on endothelial cells by antiphospholipid antibodies. *Arthritis Rheum* 2005;**52**:1545–54.

42. Lopez-Pedrera C, Buendia P, Cuadrado MJ, Siendones E, Aguirre MA, Barbarroja N, et al. Antiphospholipid antibodies from patients with the antiphospholipid syndrome induce monocyte tissue factor expression through the simultaneous activation of NF-kappaB/Rel proteins via the p38 mitogen-activated protein kinase pathway, and of the MEK-1/ERK pathway. *Arthritis Rheum* 2006;**54**:301–11.

43. Sorice M, Longo A, Capozzi A, Garofalo T, Misasi R, Alessandri C, et al. Anti-beta2-glycoprotein I antibodies induce monocyte release of tumor necrosis factor alpha and tissue factor by signal transduction pathways involving lipid rafts. *Arthritis Rheum* 2007;**56**:2687–97.

44. Shi T, Giannakopoulos B, Yan X, Yu P, Berndt MC, Andrews RK, et al. Anti-beta2-glycoprotein I antibodies in complex with beta2-glycoprotein I can activate platelets in a dysregulated manner via glycoprotein Ib-IX-V. *Arthritis Rheum* 2006;**54**:2558–67.

45. Kajiwara T, Yasuda T, Matsuura E. Intracellular trafficking of beta2-glycoprotein I complexes with lipid vesicles in macrophages: implications on the development of antiphospholipid syndrome. *J Autoimmun* 2007;**29**:164–73.

46. Girardi G, Redecha P, Salmon JE. Heparin prevents antiphospholipid antibody-induced fetal loss by inhibiting complement activation. *Nat Med* 2004;**10**:1222–6.

47. Shamonki JM, Salmon JE, Hyjek E, Baergen RN. Excessive complement activation is associated with placental injury in patients with antiphospholipid antibodies. *Am J Obstet Gynecol* 2007;**196**(167):e1–5.

48. Girardi G, Berman J, Redecha P, Spruce L, Thurman JM, Kraus D, et al. Complement C5a receptors and neutrophils mediate fetal injury in the antiphospholipid syndrome. *J Clin Invest* 2003;**112**:1644–54.

49. Berman J, Girardi G, Salmon JE. TNF-alpha is a critical effector and a target for therapy in antiphospholipid antibody-induced pregnancy loss. *J Immunol* 2005;**174**:485–90.

50. Pierangeli SS, Girardi G, Vega-Ostertag M, Liu X, Espinola RG, Salmon J. Requirement of activation of complement C3 and C5 for antiphospholipid antibody-mediated thrombophilia. *Arthritis Rheum* 2005;**52**:2120–4.

51. Oku K, Atsumi T, Bohgaki M, Amengual O, Kataoka H, Horita T, et al. Complement activation in patients with primary antiphospholipid syndrome. *Ann Rheum Dis* 2009;**68**:1030–5.

Chapter 57

Antibodies and Diagnostic Tests in Antiphospholipid Syndrome

Cecilia Beatrice Chighizola[1,2], Maria Orietta Borghi[1,2], Pier Luigi Meroni[1,2,3]

[1]Immunology Research Laboratory, IRCCS Istituto Auxologico Italiano, Milan, Italy; [2]Department of Clinical Sciences and Community Health, University of Milan, Milan, Italy; [3]Division of Rheumatology, Istituto Ortopedico Gaetano Pini, Milan, Italy

SUMMARY

The current classification criteria for antiphospholipid syndrome (APS) recommend testing for three assays, namely antibodies against cardiolipin (aCL) and β2-glycoprotein I (anti-β2GPI) plus lupus anticoagulant (LA). β2GPI-dependent antibodies are those mainly responsible for the positivity in the APS laboratory assays and for most of the pathogenic mechanisms involved in the syndrome. To overcome the technical limitations of APS assays and to identify a broader spectrum of patients, several tests have been assessed as additional laboratory tools: antibodies against domain I of β2GPI, aCL, anti-β2GPI IgA and antibodies against PT are among the most promising but still under evaluation. Other nonclassification/diagnostic autoantibodies have been described in APS, some directly contributing to the clinical manifestations (antibodies against proteins involved in hemostasis, anti-platelet and anti-endothelial cell antibodies) and some others reflecting the ongoing systemic autoimmunity characteristic of the syndrome (anti-nuclear, anti-mitochondrial, anti-red cell, anti-thyroid antibodies, and antibodies against plasma lipoproteins).

ANTIPHOSPHOLIPID SYNDROME AS AN AUTOANTIBODY-MEDIATED DISEASE

Antiphospholipid syndrome (APS) is the most recent example of an autoantibody-mediated disease. Indeed, antibodies directed against phospholipid (PL)-binding proteins—the anti-phospholipid antibodies (aPL)—not only are significantly associated with both vascular and obstetric manifestations of the syndrome but also mediate pathogenic pathways.[1,2] aPL trigger thrombotic events only occasionally and in association with additional thrombophilic factors, suggesting that a "second hit" is required to unveil an aPL thrombogenic effect. aPL still represent a strong risk factor for miscarriages but the potential "second hits" are less known.[2]

aPL specifically recognize two antigens: beta2-glycoprotein-I (β2GPI) and prothrombin (PT), which provide the main targets of the classification/diagnostic laboratory tests for APS[3] (Table 1). The same autoantibodies mediate most of the pathogenic mechanisms involved in the syndrome: the bulk of evidence—in in vitro as well as in animal models—supports a major role for anti-β2GPI antibodies[4] (Table 2).

Additional autoantibodies have been described in APS, some directly contributing to the clinical manifestations and some others reflecting the ongoing systemic autoimmunity[5] (Table 3).

CLASSIFICATION LABORATORY ASSAYS

Current criteria for APS classification recommend testing for three assays: IgG/IgM antibodies against cardiolipin (aCL) and β2GPI and lupus anticoagulant (LA). A medium/high-titer positivity in at least one test, confirmed 12 weeks apart, is required to diagnose APS.[3]

Result comparability and data extrapolation among the criteria tests still provide a major issue and are the target of many efforts toward harmonization; guidelines for correct assaying have been published, leading to amelioration of result reproducibility. The recent introduction of automated platforms and the use of reference materials might help in improving harmonization.[6]

Lupus Anticoagulant

LA is a functional test that detects immunoglobulins inducing an in vitro elongation of PL-dependent clotting time. LA phenomenon is mediated by high-titer antibodies, usually IgG, targeting β2GPI (most commonly, domain (D) I of the molecule) or PT.[7]

According to updated guidelines, LA should be assessed by a three-step strategy envisaging: (1) a screening test (to demonstrate the prolongation of clotting time); (2) a mixing test (to exclude a deficiency in coagulation factor); and (3) a confirming test (to identify the inhibitor

Systemic Lupus Erythematosus. http://dx.doi.org/10.1016/B978-0-12-801917-7.00057-7

TABLE 1 Target Antigens and Type of Antibodies in aPL Laboratory Assays

Target Antigen	Assay Characteristics	Coating	Detectable Antibodies
Bovine/human β2GPI	aCL solid-phase assay	CL	Mainly β2GPI-dependent aPL
Human β2GPI	Anti-β2GPI solid-phase assay	Human β2GPI	β2GPI-specific aPL
Human β2GPI–whole DI or conformational DI epitope	Anti-DI solid-phase assay	β2GPI–whole DI or conformational epitope	DI-β2GPI-dependent aPL
Human PT	aPS/PT ELISA	PS/PT	aPS/PT complex
Protein C, protein S, and C4b-binding protein, activated protein C, thrombomodulin	aCL solid-phase assay	CL	Mainly β2GPI-dependent aPL and antibodies to coagulation factors
High molecular weight kininogen	aPE ELISA	Neutral PL (PE)	Anti-high molecular weight kininogen antibodies
Human β2GPI/PT (main antigens)	LA: Functional PL-dependent coagulation assay	Not applicable	β2GPI-dependent aPL and aPT and others (?)

aCL, Anti-cardiolipin; β2GPI, anti-beta2-glycoprotein-I; LA, lupus anticoagulant are the APS classification laboratory assays. β2GPI-dependent antibodies are detectable specifically by the anti-β2GPI assay and are the main antibodies identified by the aCL assay. Antibodies for domain (D) I (anti-DI) require a specific coating. Antibodies against a conformational phosphatidylserine (PS)–prothrombin (PT) complex (aPS/PT) can be detected by a specific ELISA. aCL assay may also detect antibodies against other phospholipid (PL)-binding proteins (protein C, protein S, C4b-binding protein, activated protein C, thrombomodulin). Plates coated with phosphatidylethanolamine (PE) are used to detect anti-high molecular weight kininogen antibodies. LA phenomenon is mainly mediated by anti-β2GPI and anti-PT antibodies (aPT), but additional antibodies may be involved.

TABLE 2 Role of Anti-β2GPI Antibodies in the Main APS Pathogenic Mechanisms

aPL-Mediated Mechanisms of Thrombosis	aPL-Mediated Mechanisms of Fetal Loss
✓ Disruption of fluid phase coagulation Interference with coagulation soluble factors[a] Interference with activation of anticoagulant protein C[a] Interference with annexin A5[a] Inhibition of fibrinolysis[b] ✓ Disruption of coagulation cascade cell function Endothelial cell perturbation[a] Induction of TF expression on circulating monocytes[a] Platelet activation[a] ✓ Complement activation[a]	✓ Placental tissue thrombosis[a] ✓ Acute inflammation[a] ✓ Inhibition of syncytium/trophoblast differentiation[a] ✓ Complement activation[a] ✓ Embryo and/or placental apoptosis[b]

[a]β2GPI-dependent mechanism.
[b]Partially β2GPI-dependent mechanism.

TABLE 3 Additional Autoantibodies in APS

Antibodies Potentially Involved in Thrombus Formation	Autoantibodies Not Related to Thrombus Formation
✓ Antibodies against coagulation factors ✓ Antibodies against platelets ✓ Anti-endothelial antibodies	✓ Anti-nuclear antibodies ✓ Anti-mitochondrial antibodies ✓ Antibodies to red blood cells ✓ Anti-thyroid antibodies ✓ Anti-plasma lipoprotein antibodies

of coagulation as PL dependent).[8] Besides the several standardization issues affecting LA reproducibility, its interpretation is affected by the interference of concomitant oral anticoagulation, with obvious clinical implications in APS. Nevertheless, LA has consistently been identified as the strongest thrombotic risk factor among the three aPL assays. In a systematic literature review, LA emerged as an independent predictor of thrombosis; noteworthy, this association held significance irrespectively of thrombotic site and of an associated diagnosis of systemic lupus erythematosus (SLE).[9] Similarly, LA was the strongest predictor of recurrent pregnancy loss (RPL)[10] and placenta-mediated pregnancy complications.[11]

A recent study has addressed the clinical significance of isolated, β2GPI-independent LA: patients with a mere LA positivity presented a thrombotic risk similar to that of the general population.[12] Therefore, an isolated LA conveys a very different clinical risk compared to LA associated with aCL/anti-β2GPI antibody positivity.

Anti-cardiolipin Antibodies

aCL are usually detected by solid-phase assays employing cardiolipin (CL)-coated matrix in the presence of bovine serum, thus detecting antibodies binding to CL alone (β2GPI-independent aCL) and those that bind to CL bound to bovine β2GPI (β2GPI-dependent aCL). Some assays employ human β2GPI, to avoid missing aCL that recognize CL when bound to human—but not bovine—β2GPI. IgG and IgM aCL are expressed in IgG (GPL) and IgM antiphospholipid (MPL) units, established using calibrators (affinity-purified polyclonal IgG and IgM aCL).[1,6] Medium/high titers, required to diagnose APS, are defined as above 40 GPL/MPL or the 99th percentile.[3]

In a systematic literature review, aCL IgG were associated with thrombosis, either venous or arterial; on further analysis, aCL correlated with cerebral stroke and myocardial infarction, but not deep vein thrombosis.[9] With regard to pregnancy morbidity, aCL IgG have been related to early and late fetal losses, while aCL IgM were associated with late losses only.[10] When considering placenta-mediated adverse outcomes, an association of aCL was reported with preeclampsia[11]; the association was stronger for severe preeclampsia.[13] Unfortunately, data interpretation is affected by the wide heterogeneity in aCL testing, which partially prevents result comparability.

Anti-β2 Glycoprotein I Antibodies

Anti-β2GPI antibodies are usually detected by solid-phase assays using matrix coated with purified human β2GPI; current classification criteria consider an antibody titer greater than the 99th percentile.[3] Even though interlaboratory agreement in anti-β2GPI assays appeared to be higher than aCL ELISA, the lack of accepted calibrators raises harmonization issues. International efforts have been recently focused to identify a suitable reference material: monoclonal and affinity-purified polyclonal anti-β2GPI IgG have been evaluated. The latter has been found to produce stable and reproducible results, a start for establishing international units.[6]

In a 2003 meta-analysis, anti-β2GPI antibodies were associated with thrombosis in 57% of evaluated studies; the rate increased to 61% when considering IgG isotypes and decreased to 47% for IgM.[14] With regard to pregnancy morbidity, anti-β2GPI antibody positivity was not related to RPL[10] but with placenta-mediated complications.[11] Unfortunately, anti-β2GPI antibodies to date have been assessed in few studies; such paucity of data prevents the drawing of definite conclusions about their clinical significance, despite their widely accepted pivotal pathogenic role in experimental models.[2]

Every aPL test conveys a different clinical significance, implying that each aPL profile carries a characteristic hazard for related events. On one hand of the spectrum, there are patients with double/triple aPL positivity, likely driven by reactivity against β2GPI. On the other hand, there are subjects with single aPL positivity, whose clinical significance is still under investigation.[15] Another critical issue concerns low-titer antibody positivity: aPL are widely accepted to confer prothrombotic susceptibility only at medium/high titers (in solid-phase assays), while it is increasingly recognized that low-titer aPL might be implicated in pregnancy morbidity.[16] Attempts to better characterize the clinical risk of an aPL profile culminated in the development of two independent scoring systems, aPL-S (aPL score, comprising five clotting assays and six ELISA) and GAPSS (Global APS score, which includes also independent risk factors for thrombosis and pregnancy morbidity), whose utility in clinical practice is currently being evaluated.[17]

NONCLASSIFICATION LABORATORY ASSAYS

Several tests have been assessed as additional laboratory assays to detect circulating aPL, to: (1) identify a broader spectrum of patients, comprising subjects with so-called "seronegative APS" (a clinical picture highly suggestive of APS with no detectable aPL); (2) improve assay specificity to overcome false aPL (particularly aCL) positivity, which is a rather common finding in subjects with infectious or malignant diseases; (3) overcome technical limitations in aPL testing, and (4) increase the predictivity of clinical events, with a more accurate risk stratification.[17]

Anti-β2-Glycoprotein I Domain I Antibodies

A positively charged discontinuous epitope in DI of β2GPI has been identified as the most relevant antigenic target involved in β2GPI/anti-β2GPI antibody binding.[4] The pathogenicity of anti-DI antibodies has been progressively characterized: passive infusion of a synthetic peptide targeting DI partially protected naïve mice from thrombogenic effects of human polyclonal aPL IgG fractions; more recently, a human monoclonal anti-DI IgG induced clotting and fetal loss in animals.[18] Several methodologies can be employed to detect anti-DI antibodies: a two-step solid-phase assay using hydrophilic–hydrophobic plates, several one-step solid-phase assays, and counterimmunoelectrophoresis employing different DI sources.[4] Antibodies against DI are more specific for APS compared to antibodies targeting the whole molecule; they are detectable in most APS patients, providing the prevalent β2GPI antibody specificity not only in primary APS but also among aPL-positive patients with associated autoimmune conditions. Furthermore, anti-β2GPI-DI IgG antibodies have been found to be associated with LA, vascular thrombosis, and, to a lesser extent, with pregnancy complications.[17] Interestingly, patients at higher clinical risk, namely those with double/triple aPL positivity, display greater prevalence and titers of anti-DI antibodies. It is still not clear whether anti-DI antibodies offer additional prognostic value over double/triple positivity, or simply reflect the fact that APS patients with two to three positive tests are more likely to carry anti-DI antibodies.[15] A small but consistent proportion of full-blown APS patients display autoantibodies reacting with β2GPI epitopes other than DI, implying that the assay for the whole molecule cannot yet be replaced.[15]

IgA Anti-cardiolipin and Anti-β2-Glycoprotein I Antibodies

In vivo findings are supportive for a pathogenic role of IgA aCL[19,20]; however, their association with clinical events is inconsistent.[20-22] IgA anti-β2GPI antibodies are more promising, particularly in SLE, where few studies have reported isolated anti-β2GPI IgA positivity associated with vascular events[20] or RPL.[21] Based on these data, IgA aPL were included in the recent SLICC classification, prompting some investigators to advocate the incorporation of IgA antibodies among APS criteria. Currently, IgA testing might be reasonable when APS is clinically suspected but conventional markers are negative.[22]

Anti-prothrombin Antibodies

Antibodies against PT (aPT) exert in vitro thrombogenic effects interfering with fluid-phase coagulation components and activating endothelial cells (EC). Owing to this finding, aPT were thought to represent promising diagnostic/prognostic aPL. However because of the lack of cross-reactivity of human aPT with animal PT, in vivo evidence for their pathogenic effect is still lacking. ELISA detecting antibodies against PT employs as antigenic target the mere PT or the PS/PT complex; the latter identifies antibodies against PS/PT (aPS/PT), a separate autoantibody population recognizing a conformational epitope(s) different from those present on plain PT.[15] The clinical significance of aPT positivity in APS is still debated: conflicting results emerged about the association with thrombosis. Conversely, most studies highlighted a significant association of aPS/PT with aPL-associated manifestations, particularly venous thrombosis. Consistently, a systematic review found that both aPT and aPS/PT increase the thrombotic hazard, with aPS/PT representing a stronger risk factor for thrombosis than aPT.[23] Noteworthy, aPS/PT, together with anti-β2GPI antibodies and LA, displayed the best diagnostic accuracy for both vascular and obstetric APS among several combinations of six aPL assays. Testing for anti-PS/PT has been suggested to be useful to: (1) better stratify the clinical risk; (2) characterize an isolated LA positivity (i.e., anti-β2GPI negative); and (3) assess patients on anticoagulation, as surrogate test for an isolated LA when the functional assay cannot be performed. However, current evidence is not solid enough to recommend routine testing, even though the aPS/PT assay deserves attention.[15,17]

Antibodies against Phosphatidylethanolamine

Phosphatidylethanolamine (PE) is a zwitterionic PL that promotes thrombosis by activating factor (F)X and PT and works as anticoagulant potentiating activated protein C (APC) activity. Subsets of antibodies against PE (aPE) bind to high molecular weight kininogen, leading to the formation of antibody–PE–kininogen trimolecular complexes that enhance platelet aggregation.[15] An in vivo demonstration of aPE pathogenicity in mediating vascular events is lacking; conversely, aPE infusion to pregnant mice triggered placental thrombosis and hemorrhage, with increased apoptosis.[24] aPE, currently detected by a poorly standardized ELISA, seem to hold some clinical significance among women experiencing RPL, who displayed a higher aPE prevalence than healthy controls (between 23% and 31.7%). Most studies confirmed the association of aPE with RPL, but not those considering merely SLE patients. Conversely, the majority of authors failed to find any association between aPE and thrombosis.[15] Having been reported as the sole aPL among some patients with vascular or obstetric manifestations, aPE were proposed as serological markers of seronegative APS. However, overall evidence is inconsistent and comes from few small studies[25]; aPE testing is thus not recommended.[17]

Antibodies against Anionic Phospholipids Other than Cardiolipin

Autoantibodies targeting negatively charged PL other than CL have been evaluated as diagnostic and prognostic APS markers: PS, phosphatidylinositol (PI) and phosphatidic acid (PA) are the best-characterized antigens. Noteworthy, aCL and anti-β2GPI antibodies broadly cross-react with both PS and PI, a cross-reactivity mostly mediated by the recognition of β2GPI complexed with PL. Therefore, antibodies against negatively charged PL are reported in subjects with at least one criteria assay: testing for antibodies against PS, PI, and PA does not improve the likelihood of diagnosing APS.[26]

A novel ELISA kit detecting antibodies against a mixture of negatively charged PL comprising PS, PA, and β2GPI (APhL) has been recently developed. The APhL assay displays higher positive and negative predictive values for APS diagnosis compared to LA and commercially available aCL/anti-β2GPI antibody assays, particularly in SLE patients.[15,17] These preliminary data need further confirmation.

Annexin A5 Resistance Assay

Annexin (Ann)A5 is a potent anticoagulant protein which, on PL binding, undergoes oligomerization, providing a shield against coagulation enzymes. The AnnA5-mediated endothelial protection is prevented by β2GPI-dependent aPL, thus favoring thrombosis. AnnA5 resistance is assessed by a novel two-stage coagulation assay; more than half of APS patients were AnnA5 resistant, compared to 2–5% of controls. Resistance to AnnA5 inversely correlated with anti-DI antibody titers, suggesting its potential utility in identifying pathogenic anti-β2GPI antibodies.[15]

OTHER AUTOANTIBODIES IN ANTIPHOSPHOLIPID SYNDROME

Antibodies Possibly Involved in Thrombosis

Antibodies against Proteins Involved in Hemostasis

Autoantibodies specific for several coagulation factors as well as for proteins involved in the feedback regulatory mechanisms have been described in APS. At least some of these antibodies, as evinced from studies using monoclonal antibodies, bind to β2GPI conformational epitope(s) shared by several serine proteases involved in hemostasis (thrombin, protein C (pC), APC, tissue type plasminogen activator (tPA), and FIXa[27]); conversely, other autoantibodies seem to be unrelated to aPL.

Antibodies against Protein C and S

The anticoagulant pC pathway plays a central role in the regulation of coagulation due to the proteolytic inactivation of FVa and FVIIIa, which is catalyzed by cofactors (protein S [pS] and FV). aPL might initiate thrombosis interfering with APC anticoagulant activity, resulting in acquired APC resistance (APCr). Accordingly, some clinical studies reported an association of APCr with aPL positivity, mainly LA, and thrombosis, especially venous. APCr in aPL carriers may be due to different mechanisms: (1) antibodies unrelated to aPL specifically reacting with pC or pS, (2) aPL cross-reacting with pC system components, (3) aPL targeting β2GPI bound to pC, with the in situ formation of immune complexes affecting pC function, and (4) aPL immune complexes competing with pC for PL binding.[28]

The positivity rates of anti-pC and anti-pS antibodies in APS populations vary widely across reports: some early studies reported anti-pS to be more prevalent than those targeting pC, which were associated with thrombosis and APCr.[28] Conversely, in a recent study anti-pC were much more frequent than anti-pS; to note, anti-pC were specific for APS, being associated, when at higher avidity, with greater APCr and severe thrombotic phenotype.[29]

Antibodies against Coagulation Factors

Autoantibodies against coagulation factors are detectable in many autoimmune diseases, including APS. They neutralize, partially or completely, the activation or function of a given clotting factor, or promote its clearance.[30] *Antibodies*

targeting thrombin have been shown to be elevated in APS patients, significantly interfering with the inactivation of thrombin, FIXa, and FXa by antithrombin, thus contributing to prothrombotic effects.[30] *Antibodies to FVII/VIIa and FXa* have been reported in small APS series, without sound evidence for a diagnostic/predictive value.[31] *Antibodies against FVIII* can rarely be found associated with LA and an abnormal activated partial thromboplastin time, with bleeding as the most frequent manifestation.[30] *Antibodies against FXII* were originally described in LA-positive subjects, associated with lower levels of FXII. Among SLE subjects, their positivity was described in up to 40% of cases, being associated with both thrombosis and adverse pregnancy outcome.[30] In small cohorts, *anti-tissue factor (TF) pathway inhibitor (TFPI) IgG antibodies* were reported in 65% of aPL carriers with a variable interference on TFPI function and TF-induced thrombin generation.[32]

Antibodies against Tissue Type Plasminogen Activator

Hypofibrinolysis has been suggested as an additional mechanism for the APS thrombophilic state; lesser permeable fibrin clot and prolonged fibrinolysis time were recently reported in APS subjects, particularly among those with arterial thrombosis.[33] Antibodies specifically interacting with the tPA catalytic domain can be found in APS patients, potentially leading to hypofibrinolysis.[34]

Antibodies against Annexin A2

AnnA2 is a cofactor for plasmin generation and cell-surface localization of fibrinolytic activity, acting as a β2GPI receptor on EC. Autoantibodies against AnnA2 were demonstrated to exert in vitro prothrombotic activity by activating EC, inducing TF expression and blocking tPA-induced plasminogen activation. A high prevalence of AnnA2 antibodies has been described not only in APS but also in other autoimmune conditions, thus lowering the specificity of this biomarker.[15]

Anti-platelet Antibodies

Thrombocytopenia is one of the most common noncriteria manifestations of the syndrome, but its etiopathogenesis has not yet been unraveled. Experimental studies failed to demonstrate a direct cross-reactivity of aPL with resting platelets; however, on activation, β2GPI might complex with either PS or cell membrane receptor(s), thus targetable by β2GPI-dependent aPL. Consistently, there is sound evidence that β2GPI-dependent aPL enhance platelet activation after agonist stimulation.[2] Antibodies directed against platelet glycoproteins (GP) IIb–IIIa and/or GPIb–IX can be detected in 40% of aPL carriers, which are significantly more frequent among APS patients with thrombocytopenia compared to those with a normal platelet count. Anti-heparin platelet factor 4 antibodies have been also reported in aPL carriers, even in those heparin-naïve, without any association with laboratory or clinical findings.[35]

Anti-endothelial Cell Antibodies

Because of its active role in hemostasis and the large body distribution, endothelium provides the main aPL target. aPL have been shown to activate EC both in vitro and in vivo, inducing a procoagulant and inflammatory phenotype. Not surprisingly, a high rate of APS sera (up to 86%) display endothelial binding activity as assessed by cell ELISA. Most of this reactivity against the endothelium was shown to be mediated by anti-β2GPI antibodies targeting the antigen on the EC surface. However, immunoprecipitation studies showed that APS sera can react against other constitutive EC membrane proteins; the potential pathogenicity of this subset, at variance of anti-β2GPI antibodies, is still debated.[36]

Autoantibodies Not Involved in Thrombosis

The detection of *anti-nuclear antibodies* (ANA) at titers higher then 1:320 as well as of antibodies against double-stranded DNA (anti-dsDNA) or extractable nuclear antigens (ENA) was initially regarded as exclusion criteria for primary APS. However, even in a large international cohort, ANA were reported in 22% of patients with primary APS[37] and higher frequencies were described in smaller series.[38] ANA with specificity for lamins B1 (constituent of the nuclear lamin) and for nucleosomes have been found to be responsible for the high ANA prevalence, although at variable frequencies among the studies.[39–41] Although ANA can be detected at higher frequency in APS patients with lupus-like systemic manifestations, still open is the question of their predictivity for the evolution to a full-blown lupus.[39,41]

Anti-mitochondrial antibodies (AMA) producing an M5 pattern (a cytoplasmic fluorescence brighter on proximal than distal renal tubules, without gastric parietal cell reactivity) by indirect immunofluorescence on rodent tissues have been frequently identified in APS sera, with a positivity rate of 28% in the largest published study.[42] The AMA-M5 pattern is rarely seen in different clinical settings but detectable in primary as well as secondary APS, correlating with thrombocytopenia and RPL but not thrombotic events.[42,43]

The prevalence of *antibodies against thyroid antigens* was reported similar in unselected APS patients and healthy controls.[44] Conversely, they have been detected in 27% of women with obstetric APS, suggesting an addictive effect with aPL for a negative pregnancy outcome.[45]

Positive direct Coomb's test and autoimmune hemolytic anemia have been reported in APS.[35] Although there are anecdotal cases showing cross-reactivity between aPL and erythrocyte antigens, *anti-red blood cell antibodies* are in general unrelated to aPL.[35]

Similarly both ANA and AMA-M5 are not apparently due to aPL cross-reacting with nuclear or mitochondrial constituents and all these autoantibodies are thought to represent an aspect of the "systemic autoimmunity" of the syndrome.[39]

Anti-oxidized low-density lipoprotein antibodies (anti-oxLDL), which have been described in patients with primary or secondary APS, may play a role in atherosclerotic plaque formation; however, they were found to be mainly related to β2GPI-dependent aPL recognition of β2GPI complexed with oxLDL molecules.[46]

REFERENCES

1. Giannakopoulos B, Passam F, Ioannou Y, Krilis SA. How we diagnose the antiphospholipid syndrome. *Blood* 2008;**113**:985–94.
2. Meroni PL, Borghi MO, Raschi E, Tedesco F. Pathogenesis of antiphospholipid syndrome: understanding the antibodies. *Nat Rev Rheumatol* 2011;**7**:330–9.
3. Miyakis S, Lockshin MD, Atsumi T, Branch DW, Brey RL, Cervera R, et al. International consensus statement on an update of the classification criteria for definite antiphospholipid syndrome (APS). *J Thromb Haemost* 2006;**4**:295–306.
4. Chighizola CB, Gerosa M, Meroni PL. New tests to detect antiphospholipid antibodies: anti-domain I beta-2-glycoprotein-I antibodies. *Curr Rheumatol Rep* 2014;**16**:402–9.
5. Shoenfeld Y, Twig G, Katz U, Sherer Y. Autoantibody explosion in antiphospholipid syndrome. *J Autoimmun* 2008;**30**:74–83.
6. Meroni PL, Biggioggero M, Pierangeli SS, Sheldon J, Zegers I, Borghi MO. Standardization of autoantibody testing: a paradigm for serology in rheumatic diseases. *Nat Rev Rheumatol* 2014;**10**:35–43.
7. Pengo V, Banzato A, Denas G, Jose SP, Bison E, Hoxha A, et al. Correct laboratory approach to APS diagnosis and monitoring. *Autoimmun Rev* 2013;**12**:832–4.
8. Pengo V. ISTH guidelines on lupus anticoagulant testing. *Thromb Res* 2012;**130**:S76–7.
9. Galli M, Luciani D, Bertolini G, Barbui T. Lupus anticoagulants are stronger risk factors for thrombosis than anticardiolipin antibodies in the antiphospholipid syndrome: a systematic review of the literature. *Blood* 2003;**101**:1827–32.
10. Opatrny L, David M, Kahn SR, Shrier I, Rey E. Association between antiphospholipid antibodies and recurrent fetal loss in women without autoimmune disease: a metaanalysis. *J Rheumatol* 2006;**33**:2214–21.
11. Abou-Nassar K, Carrier M, Ramsay T, Rodger MA. The association between antiphospholipid antibodies and placenta mediated complications: a systematic review and meta-analysis. *Thromb Res* 2011;**128**:77–85.
12. Pengo V, Testa S, Martinelli I, Ghirarduzzi A, Legnani C, Gresele P, et al. Incidence of a first thromboembolic event in carriers of isolated lupus anticoagulant. *Thromb Res* 2015;**135**:46–9.
13. do Prado AD, Piovesan DM, Staub HL, Horta BL. Association of anticardiolipin antibodies with preeclampsia: a systematic review and meta-analysis. *Obstet Gynecol* 2010;**116**:1433–43.
14. Galli M, Luciani D, Bertolini G, Barbui T. Anti-β2-glycoprotein I, antiprothrombin antibodies, and the risk of thrombosis in the antiphospholipid syndrome. *Blood* 2003;**102**:2717–23.

15. Meroni PL, Chighizola CB, Rovelli F, Gerosa M. Antiphospholipid syndrome in 2014: more clinical manifestations, novel pathogenic players and emerging biomarkers. *Arthritis Res Ther* 2014;**16**:209.

16. Meroni PL, Chighizola CB, Gerosa M, Trespidi L, Acaia B. Obstetric antiphospholipid syndrome: lobsters only? Or should we also look for selected red herrings? *J Rheumatol* 2015;**42**:158–60.

17. Bertolaccini ML, Amengual O, Andreoli L, Atsumi T, Chighizola CB, Forastiero R, et al. 14th International Congress on Antiphospholipid Antibodies Task Force. Report on antiphospholipid syndrome laboratory diagnostics and trends. *Autoimmun Rev* 2014;**13**:917–30.

18. Agostinis C, Durigutto P, Sblattero D, Borghi MO, Grossi C, Guida F, et al. A non-complement-fixing antibody to β2 glycoprotein I as a novel therapy for antiphospholipid syndrome. *Blood* 2014;**123**:3478–87.

19. Pierangeli SS, Liu XW, Barker JH, Anderson G, Harris EN. Induction of thrombosis in a mouse model by IgG, IgM and IgA immunoglobulins from patients with the antiphospholipid syndrome. *Thromb Haemost* 1995;**74**:1361–7.

20. Murthy V, Willis R, Romay-Penabad Z, Ruiz-Limón P, Martínez-Martínez LA, Jatwani S, et al. Value of isolated IgA anti-β2-glycoprotein I positivity in the diagnosis of the antiphospholipid syndrome. *Arthritis Rheum* 2013;**65**:3186–93.

21. Meijide H, Sciascia S, Sanna G, Khamashta MA, Bertolaccini ML. The clinical relevance of IgA anticardiolipin and IgA anti-β2 glycoprotein I antiphospholipid antibodies: a systematic review. *Autoimmun Rev* 2013;**12**:421–5.

22. Andreoli L, Fredi M, Nalli C, Piantoni S, Reggia R, Dall'Ara F, et al. Clinical significance of IgA anti-cardiolipin and IgA anti-β2 glycoprotein I antibodies. *Curr Rheumatol Rep* 2013;**15**:343.

23. Sciascia S, Sanna G, Murru V, Roccatello D, Khamashta MA, Bertolaccini ML. Anti-prothrombin (aPT) and anti-phosphatidylserine/prothrombin (aPS/PT) antibodies and the risk of thrombosis in the antiphospholipid syndrome. *Thromb Haemost* 2014;**111**:354–64.

24. Velayuthaprabhu S, Matsubayashi H, Sugi T, Nakamura M, Ohnishi Y, Ogura T, et al. A unique preliminary study on placental apoptosis in mice with passive immunization of anti-phosphatidylethanolamine antibodies and anti-factor XII antibodies. *Am J Reprod Immunol* 2011;**66**:373–84.

25. Bertolaccini M, Amengual O, Atsumi T, Binder W, Laat BD, Forastiero R, et al. "Non-criteria" aPL tests: report of a task force and preconference workshop at the 13th International Congress on Antiphospholipid Antibodies, Galveston, TX, USA, April 2010. *Lupus* 2011;**20**:191–205.

26. Tebo AE. Antiphospholipid syndrome and the relevance of antibodies to negatively charged phospholipids in diagnostic evaluation. *Lupus* 2014;**23**:1313–6.

27. Chen PP, Giles I. Antibodies to serine proteases in the antiphospholipid syndrome. *Curr Rheumatol Rep* 2010;**12**:45–52.

28. Wahl D, Membre A, Perret-Guillaume C, Regnault V, Lecompte T. Mechanisms of antiphospholipid-induced thrombosis: effects on the protein C system. *Curr Rheumatol Rep* 2009;**11**:77–81.

29. Arachchillage DRJ, Efthymiou M, Mackie IJ, Lawrie AS, Machin SJ, Cohen H. Anti-protein C antibodies are associated with resistance to endogenous protein C activation and a severe thrombotic phenotype in antiphospholipid syndrome. *J Thromb Haemost* 2014;**12**:1801–9.

30. Cugno M, Gualtierotti R, Tedeschi A, Meroni PL. Autoantibodies to coagulation factors: from pathophysiology to diagnosis and therapy. *Autoimmun Rev* 2014;**13**:40–8.

31. Yang Y-H, Hwang K-K, FitzGerald J, Grossman JM, Taylor M, Hahn BH, et al. Antibodies against the activated coagulation factor X (FXa) in the antiphospholipid syndrome that interfere with the FXa inactivation by antithrombin. *J Immunol* 2006;**177**:8219–25.

32. Adams M, Breckler L, Stevens P, Thom J, Baker R, Oostryck R. Anti-tissue factor pathway inhibitor activity in subjects with antiphospholipid syndrome is associated with increased thrombin generation. *Haematologica* 2004;**89**:985–90.

33. Vikerfors A, Svenungsson E, Ågren A, Mobarrez F, Bremme K, Holmström M, et al. Studies of fibrin formation and fibrinolytic function in patients with the antiphospholipid syndrome. *Thromb Res* 2014;**133**:936–44.

34. Cugno M, Cabibbe M, Galli M, Meroni PL, Caccia S, Russo R, et al. Antibodies to tissue-type plasminogen activator (tPA) in patients with antiphospholipid syndrome: evidence of interaction between the antibodies and the catalytic domain of tPA in 2 patients. *Blood* 2004;**103**:2121–6.

35. Barcellini W, Artusi C. Non-thrombotic hematologic manifestations in APS. In: Meroni PL, editor. *Antiphospholipid antibody syndrome - from bench to bedside*. Milan: Springer International Publishing; 2014. p. 113–26.

36. Ronda N, Raschi E, Borghi MO, Meroni PL. Anti-endothelial cell autoantibodies. In: Shoenfeld Y, Meroni PL, Gershwin E, editors. *Autoantibodies*. Oxford: Elsevier; 2013. p. 723–30.

37. Cervera R, Piette J-C, Font J, Khamashta MA, Shoenfeld Y, Camps M'T, et al. Antiphospholipid syndrome: clinical and immunologic manifestations and patterns of disease expression in a cohort of 1000 patients. *Arthritis Rheum* 2002;**46**:1019–27.

38. de Carvalho JF, Caleiro MTC, Vendramini M, Bonfá E. Clinical and laboratory evaluation of patients with primary antiphospholipid syndrome according to the frequency of antinuclear antibodies (ANA Hep-2). *Rev Bras Reumatol* 2010;**50**:262–72.

39. Tincani A, Franceschini F, Spunghi M, Panzeri P, Balestrieri G, Meroni PL. Immunological abnormalities in the antiphospholipid syndrome. In: Asherson RA, Cervera R, Piette JC, Shoenfeld Y, editors. *The antiphospholipid syndrome II*. Amsterdam: Elsevier; 2002. p. 271–83.

40. Gómez-Puerta JA, Burlingame RW, Cervera R. Anti-chromatin (antinucleosome) antibodies: diagnostic and clinical value. *Autoimmun Rev* 2008;**7**:606–11.

41. Andreoli L, Pregnolato F, Burlingame RW, Allegri F, Rizzini S, Fanelli V, et al. Antinucleosome antibodies in primary antiphospholipid syndrome: a hint at systemic autoimmunity? *J Autoimmun* 2008;**30**:51–7.

42. La Rosa L, Covini G, Galperin C, Catelli L, Del Papa N, Reina G, et al. Anti-mitochondrial M5 type antibody represents one of the serological markers for anti-phospholipid syndrome distinct from anti-cardiolipin and anti-beta2-glycoprotein I antibodies. *Clin Exp Immunol* 1998;**112**:144–51.

43. Andrejevic S, Bonaci-Nikolic B, Sefik-Bukilica M, Petrovic R. Clinical and serological follow-up of 71 patients with anti-mitochondrial type 5 antibodies. *Lupus* 2007;**16**:788–93.

44. Mavragani CP, Danielides S, Zintzaras E, Vlachoyiannopoulos PG, Moutsopoulos HM. Antithyroid antibodies in antiphospholipid syndrome: prevalence and clinical associations. *Lupus* 2009;**18**:1096–9.

45. De Carolis C, Greco E, Guarino MD, Perricone C, Dal Lago A, Giacomelli R, et al. Anti-thyroid antibodies and antiphospholipid syndrome: evidence of reduced fecundity and of poor pregnancy outcome in recurrent spontaneous aborters. *Am J Reprod Immunol* 2004;**52**:263–6.

46. Matsuura E, Lopez LR, Shoenfeld Y, Ames PRJ. β2-glycoprotein I and oxidative inflammation in early atherogenesis: a progression from innate to adaptive immunity? *Autoimmun Rev* 2012;**12**:241–9.

Chapter 58

Clinical Manifestations

Miyuki Bohgaki[1], Takao Koike[1,2]

[1]NTT Sapporo Medical Center, Sapporo Hokkaido, Japan; [2]Department of Medicine II, Hokkaido University Graduate School of Medicine, Sapporo Hokkaido, Japan

SUMMARY

The most common state of antiphospholipid syndrome (APS) is thrombophilic prone. However, the clinical manifestations of APS are not exclusive to vascular thrombosis or obstetric complications. Antiphospholipid antibody-associated features are not included in classification criteria but are recognized, such as heart valve diseases, livedo reticularis, thrombocytopenia, nephropathy, and neurological disorders. Because several other nonthrombotic manifestations are also reported to be associated with antiphospholipid antibodies, they are perceived to be unique disease-causing pathogenic antibodies in a systemic autoimmune disorder. Common clinical manifestations include deep vein thrombosis, thrombocytopenia, livedo reticularis, cerebrovascular accident, superficial thrombophlebitis, pulmonary embolism, and fetal loss. Hemolytic anemia, skin ulcers, epilepsy, myocardial infarction, amaurosis fugax, and digital necrosis are also found, although rarely.

INTRODUCTION

Antiphospholipid syndrome (APS) is a systemic autoimmune disease, and its most critical manifestation is acquired thrombogenicity.[1,2] It is classified by at least one clinical and one laboratory criterion (Table 1). Vascular thrombosis and pregnancy morbidity are the manifestations for the clinical criteria. The presence of at least one antiphospholipid antibody (aPL)—lupus anticoagulant (LA), anticardiolipin (aCL), and/or anti-β2 glycoprotein I antibodies (aβ2GPI)[3]—on two separate occasions 12 weeks apart is required to meet the laboratory criteria.

VASCULAR THROMBOSIS

Thrombosis lies at the core in symptoms of APS. The most significant and exclusive characteristic of thrombosis in APS is that patients present arterial as well as venous thrombosis.[4] Any tissue and organ can be involved, but common thromboses are deep venous thrombosis (DVT) of lower limbs, pulmonary embolism, and cerebral ischemic attack.

The prevalence of thrombosis varies among racial backgrounds, and arterial thrombotic events have been shown more in Japanese patients with APS compared to white patients.[5]

Cerebral vessels are the site of predilection for arterial thrombosis, accounting for more than 90%, while ischemic cardiac events occur relatively infrequently. APS is recognized as a most important causative disease of early-onset cerebrovascular thrombosis, such as strokes and transient ischemic attacks (TIAs).[6,7] Other affected organs include the eyes (retinal arteries), abdomen (mesenteric arteries), and digits and limbs (peripheral arteries). Thrombosis usually remains local, with the exception of catastrophic antiphospholipid syndrome (CAPS), but it is often recurrent.

The DVT of lower limbs occurs most frequently (~40%), and superficial leg vein thrombosis also occurs (~12%).[6] Pulmonary thromboembolism accompanying DVT or even solely has been often presented. While rare, other venous thromboses related to APS are axillary venous thrombosis, retinal vein thrombosis, renal vein thrombosis, Budd-Chiari syndrome (hepatic veno-occlusive disease), cerebral venous thrombosis (sagittal sinus thrombosis) or adrenal vein thrombosis.[8] Budd-Chari syndrome may be the first clinical manifestation of APS.

PREGNANCY MORBIDITY

Obstetric manifestations are the defining characteristics of APS. Recurrent pregnancy loss, occasionally in the second trimester, is a classic and characteristic feature of APS.[4] Recently, obstetric APS have been recognized as different from thrombotic APS.[9] Current evidence demonstrates that fetal loss and severe preeclampsia or placental insufficiency are associated with APS.[10] However, the association between recurrent early pregnancy loss (prior to 10 weeks of gestation) and aPL remains inconclusive.[10]

The most frequent fetal complication in APS is recurrent pregnancy loss. Between 7% and 25% of recurrent pregnancy loss is owed to the presence of aPLs.[9] Secondary APS, history of both thrombosis and pregnancy morbidity,

TABLE 1 Criteria for Defining Antiphospholipid Syndrome

Antiphospholipid Antibody Syndrome (APS) Is Present if At Least One of the Clinical Criteria and One of the Laboratory Criteria That Follow Are Met

Clinical Criteria

1. Vascular thrombosis
One or more clinical episodes of arterial, venous, or small vessel thrombosis, in any tissue or organ. Thrombosis must be confirmed by objective validated criteria. For histopathologic confirmation, thrombosis should be present without significant evidence of inflammation in the vessel wall.
2. Pregnancy morbidity
    a. One or more unexplained deaths of a morphologically normal fetus at or beyond the 10th week of gestation, with normal fetal morphology documented by ultrasound or by direct examination of the fetus, or
    b. One or more premature births of a morphologically normal neonate before the 34th week of gestation because of: (1) eclampsia or severe preeclampsia defined according to standard definitions, or (2) recognized features of placental insufficiency, or
    c. Three or more unexplained consecutive spontaneous abortions before the 10th week of gestation, with maternal anatomic or hormonal abnormalities and paternal and maternal chromosomal causes excluded.
In studies of populations of patients who have more than one type of pregnancy morbidity, investigators are strongly encouraged to stratify groups of subjects according to a, b, or c above.

Laboratory Criteria

1. Lupus Anticoagulant (LA) present in plasma, on two or more occasions at least 12 weeks apart, detected according to the guidelines of the International Society on Thrombosis and Haemostasis (Scientific Subcommittee on LAs/phospholipid-dependent antibodies).
2. Anticardiolipin (aCL) antibody of IgG and/or IgM isotype in serum or plasma, present in medium or high titer (i.e., >40 GPL or MPL, or >the 99th percentile), on two or more occasions, at least 12 weeks apart, measured by a standardized ELISA.
3. Anti-β2 glycoprotein-I antibody of IgG and/or IgM isotype in serum or plasma (in titer >the 99th percentile), present on two or more occasions, at least 12 weeks apart, measured by a standardized ELISA, according to recommended procedures.

ELISA, enzyme-linked immunosorbent assay; GPL units, IgG antiphospholipid units; MPL units, IgM antiphospholipid units.
Modified from Miyakis et al.[3]

and triple aPL positivity are reportedly associated with pregnancy failure in patients with APS.[11] Treatment of APS patients with anticoagulant or antiplatelet agents shows remarkable improvement in live birth rates. Expecting women with APS have the likelihood of live birth of almost 80% with proper management, compared with only 15% of patients without treatment.[12]

On the other hand, even with anticoagulant or antiplatelet treatment, the risk of other obstetric morbidities, such as preeclampsia, intrauterine growth restriction (IUGR), and prematurity remains high. Premature birth occurs as the common neonatal complication of APS, as a consequence of preeclampsia, IUGR and hemolysis, elevated liver enzyme levels, and low platelet levels (HELLP) syndrome.[10] As for fertility, available evidence suggests that aPL is not a mediator of infertility, and aPL positivity does not seem to influence in vitro fertilization outcomes.[10]

Multiple mechanisms likely contribute to obstetric manifestation in APS. Initially, thrombotic predisposition has been simply sought to induce placental events in APS, although evidence of thrombosis of the uteroplacental vasculature was invalid.[13] APLs might disrupt trophoblast invasion and endometrial angiogenesis and, consequently, lead to placental dysfunction. Studies have demonstrated that complement activation by aPL has a responsible role.[10,14,15] The activation of complement by aPL, both classical and alternative pathways, may cause fetal loss, IUGR, and preeclampsia.

CATASTROPHIC APS

As a particular state of APS, CAPS manifests rapidly progressing simultaneous systemic thromboses driving to fatal multiple organ failure (Table 2).[16] The principle of CAPS is acute thrombotic microangiopathy associated with aPL. Thrombotic storm, extensive microvascular thrombosis, may bring chaos to whole body of host. CAPS is low frequency but high consequence, characterized by the evolvement of at least three organs over several days or weeks with multiple occlusion of medium or small vessels and the presence of aPLs, generally high titer.[17] More than half of the patients presented with primary APS (59%), 26.9% presented with SLE,[16] and almost half of patients developed CAPS as the first manifestation of APS.[16]

Most CAPS events (65.4%) are thought to be triggered by a particular condition.[16] Infection is the most common precipitating cause of CAPS. Malignancies, surgical procedures, withdrawal or poor control of anticoagulant therapy, obstetric complications, and SLE flares also trigger CAPS. CAPS is occasionally accompanied by systemic inflammatory response syndrome.[18]

Various organs are involved and the clinical manifestations depend on the affected region and extent of the occlusion. The most commonly affected organs are kidneys (73.0%), followed by lungs (58.9%), brain (55.9%), heart (49.7%), and skin (45.5%). The intestine, spleen, adrenal glands, pancreas, retina, bone marrow, and, rarely, testis or ovary, prostate, and gallbladder are affected. Small-vessel involvement causes thrombotic microangiopathy that results in hemolytic anemia or failure of the affected organs. Patients with thrombocytopenia are more predisposed to develop hemolysis, schistocytes, disseminated intravascular coagulation (DIC), and high-fibrin degradation products.[19] CAPS

TABLE 2 Diagnostic Criteria for CAPS

1. Evidence of involvement of three organs, systems, and/or tissues.
2. Development of manifestations simultaneously or in less than 1 week.
3. Laboratory confirmation of the presence of aPL (LAC and/or aCL and/or anti-β2GPI antibodies) in titers higher than 40 UI/l.
4. Exclude other diagnosis.

Definite CAPS:
  All 4 criteria.
Probable CAPS:
  All 4 criteria, except for involvement of only 2 organs, system, and/or tissues.
  All 4 criteria, except for the absence of laboratory confirmation at least 6 weeks apart associable to the early death of a patient never tested for aPL before onset of CAPS.
  1, 2, and 4.
  1, 3, and 4, and the development of a third event in >1 week but <1 month, despite anticoagulation treatment.

Cervera et al.[16,17]

patients with severe thrombocytopenia and/or schistocytosis sometimes present overlap with other thrombotic microangiopathies (TMAs), thrombotic thrombocytopenic purpura (TTP), hemolytic-uremic syndrome (HUS), HELLP syndrome, and heparin-induced thrombocytopenia (HIT).

Renal, pulmonary, and cerebral involvement can cause a crisis of life. Patients with affected kidneys may present with acute renal failure, malignant hypertension, proteinuria, and hematuria. Lung manifestations include acute respiratory distress syndrome, pulmonary embolism (frequent), and pulmonary hemorrhage (occasional). In descending order of frequency, encephalopathy, stroke, seizures, headache, and coma are cerebral manifestations. Heart failure, myocardial infarction, and mitral or aortic valvular defects have been also reported. Skin problems arise in the form of livedo reticularis, skin necrosis, ulcers, and digital ischemia. In one study, more patients presented with peripheral vessel involvement (69.2%) versus arterial (47.8%).[16]

CAPS is life-threatening with an almost 50% mortality rate.[20] However, 66% of recovered patients have maintained remission during 5 years of follow-up.[21] Further APS-related events were found in 19% of patients, but no patients demonstrated further CAPS.[21] Older age (over 36 years old), SLE, pulmonary and renal involvement, and positive antinuclear antibody titers are associated with higher mortality in patients with catastrophic APS.[20]

FEATURES ASSOCIATED WITH aPL

Cardiac Manifestations

APS exhibits diverse cardiac manifestations. Heart valvulopathy, the presence of thickening or vegetation of the valves

(mainly mitral and aortic), is the most frequent cardiac manifestation of APS. Valvulopathy-associated aPL is defined by the presence of valve lesions (global thickening >3 mm, localized thickening involving the leaflet proximal or middle portion, or irregular nodules and/or vegetations of the edge of the valve known as Libman–Sacks endocarditis) and/or moderate to severe valve dysfunction (regurgitation, stenosis) in the absence of a history of rheumatic fever and infective endocarditis.[3] Among SLE patients with aPLs compared with patients negative for these antibodies, the risk of heart valve disease (HVD) is increased threefold.[22] Despite anticoagulant and/or antiplatelet therapies, one-third of the patients presented with worsening of the valve lesion.[23] Patients with HVD are more likely to develop arterial thrombotic events, livedo, migraine, and convulsion.[24] Although around 4–6% of the APS patients with HVD will require valve replacement surgery, the surgery may put the patients in a tough situation. Surgical death in APS patients has been reported more than twice as often than in non-APS patients, and only half of the patients resolve without complications.[25]

Coronary artery disease bears the thrombosis criteria for APS.[3] The prevalence of myocardial infarction (MI) was noted 5.5%, and APS patients have seven times the risk for MI compared to the general population.[7]

Hematological Manifestations

Almost 20–40% patients with APS present with thrombocytopenia,[6] which is generally mild (platelet counts are more than $50\times10^9\,L^{-1}$) and rarely causes hemorrhage.[26] Thrombocytopenia is more common in patients with APS and SLE than primary APS, and aPL is associated with thrombocytopenia in patients of other autoimmune diseases with APS.[27,28] One-third of patients newly diagnosed with idiopathic thrombocytopenic purpura were positive for aPL.[27] Furthermore, patients with aPL-positive thrombocytopenia tend to experience thrombosis or pregnancy loss.[28]

Approximately 10–20% of patients with APS may present with Coombs-positive hemolytic anemia.[6] Although the IgM isotype aCL or LA are suggested to cause autoimmune hemolytic anemia in APS patients, the exact roles and clinical importance of aPLs in autoimmune hemolytic anemia are not still clear.[29]

Bone marrow necrosis (BMN) is defined morphologically by the destruction of hematopoietic tissue, including stroma with preservation of the bone, and is regarded as a potentially rare and fatal syndrome.[29] The best-accepted mechanism of BMN is microvascular obstruction of the bone marrow. Several cases of BMN associated with aPL have been reported; the majority occurred in CAPS patients. Pregnancy and puerperium were possible precipitating factors in 50% of the cases, and mortality was fairly high (37.5%) due to multiorgan failure.[29]

Renal Manifestations

Renal involvement is also remarkable in APS.[30] APS nephropathy is characterized by clinical and histological manifestations.[31] Vascular nephropathy, relating hypertension, renal insufficiency, and proteinurea, is observed as clinical manifestations. Systemic hypertension is observed frequently as more than 40% of patients with APS nephropathy. Proteinuria may range from low grade to nephrotic grade. Histological findings are TMA (acute thrombi), arterial fibrous intimal hyperplasia (chronic lesions), organized thrombi with recanalization, fibrous arterial occlusion, and focal cortical atrophy.[31] Renal TMA causes proteinuria without cells in the urine or hypocomplementemia. Aside from microvessel or capillary arteries, all levels within the renal vasculature are involved, such as trunk of renal artery or veins.[32] The range of renal manifestations associated with APS is broadening and, therefore, aPLs have increasing relevance in end-stage renal disease, transplantation, and pregnancy. APS nephropathy is an independent risk factor of lupus nephritis by hypertension, elevated creatinine, and increased interstitial fibrosis. The outcome of renal transplantation is worse in patients with SLE in the presence of aPLs than absence of aPLs, due to early graft loss from arterial or venous thrombosis, or TMA.[33]

Neurological Manifestations

Neurological symptoms are significant manifestations of APS. APS often affects the central nervous system (CNS) and causes cerebral infarction, epilepsy, consciousness disorder, migraine, or limb dysfunction.[34] In 1983, in the original description of the syndrome, Hughes emphasized the importance of cerebral involvement in patients with APS, including cerebrovascular accidents (TIAs or visual field defects or progressive cerebral ischemia) and myelitis.[4] The underlying mechanism can be related to ischemic damage to brain tissue due to thrombophilicity or to direct damage to brain tissue distinct from hypercoagulability.[35]

Almost half of arterial thrombosis in APS patients is stroke or TIA.[36] In young and female stroke patients, the presence of aPL is an important element to consider.[7] More than 20% of strokes in patients younger than 45 years are related to aPL positivity.[37] The strokes often recur at wide intervals and different regions, and sometimes cause convulsions or dementia with multifocal infarction.[37] Sneddon's syndrome demonstrates progressive cerebrovascular disease, including stroke and severe TIA and early onset dementia, and livedo reticularis.[37] More than 40% patients suffering from Sneddon's syndrome are positive for aPL.

Chronic and recurrent stroke in APS affect small vessels and lead to multifocal damage to the brain and cause early-onset, multi-infarct dementia.[38] Findings from magnetic resonance imaging (MRI) for infarct features of APS adhered to vascular dementia include bilaterality, multiplicity, location in the dominant hemisphere, and location in the frontal or medial limbic structures.[37] Mild cognitive dysfunctions in APS are attention and memory deficit and difficulty in concentration, and some of these patients had no history of stroke and no ischemic lesions of the brain.[36] In SLE patients, verbal memory loss, reduced psychomotor speed, and executive dysfunctions have been significantly correlated with the presence of aPL and its levels.[36]

In movement disorders, chorea, tics, hemidystonia, paroxysmal nonkinesigenic dyskinesias, parkinsonism, cerebellar ataxia, and complex mixed presentations have been presented.[36] The highest incidence of aPL-related chorea is detected in children and females, and the prevalence of aPL is almost 60–90% patients with lupus chorea.[39]

Multiple sclerosis (MS)-like symptoms can also occur.[40] Some features exhibited in APS, such as optic neuritis, Devic's syndrome, brainstem/cerebellar syndromes, and diplopia, are often identified as the first manifestations of MS. While the prevalence of aPL in MS patients has been reported to be between 2% and 88%, the implications of aPLs on the clinical presentation of MS are still unclear.[40]

Transverse myelitis (TM) is a rare symptom of APS, although there is a strong association between aPL positivity and the occurrence of TM in SLE patients.[38] Convulsions in APS are almost 7–10%, and epilepsy is more frequent in secondary APS than primary.[6,37] The remarkable neurological symptom in APS is the headache, with almost 20% of patients presenting with chronic and untreatable migraine.[6]

Ophthalmological or otological manifestations are also major feature of APS.[38] Retinal and choroidal vessel involvement causes acute ischemia of eyes. Patients complain of amaurosis fugax, transient blurring of eyes, diplopia, decreased vision, or transient field defects resulting from venous stasis retinopathy or opthalmo-neuropathy. Sudden sensorineural hearing loss has also been reported as a manifestation of APS.[41]

Skin Manifestations

Almost 40–50% of the patients present with cutaneous symptoms.[42] Histologically, noninflammatory thrombosis in small vessels throughout the dermis and the subcutaneous fat tissue are characteristic, observed in circumscribed skin ulcerations, widespread cutaneous necrosis, and pseudo-vasculitis lesions. In contrast, thrombosis is rarely observed from biopsies in livedo reticularis.[42]

Livedo reticularis is the most common cutaneous symptom in APS. A significant association between livedo and arterial thrombosis, heart valve abnormalities, and hypertension has been indicated. Conversely, livedo reticularis was observed less frequently in patients with only venous thrombosis.[42] Skin ulcers are also observed in APS patients. Postphlebitic ulcers resulting from chronic venous insufficiency due to DVT and/or venous reflux are observed in almost 4% of patients with APS. Large ulcers resembling pyoderma gangrenosum are also observed. Digital gangrene has been found following distal ischemic symptoms. Pseudo vasculitis, including purpura, ecchymoses, red macules, small erythematous, painful papules, or nodules has been also found.

Pulmonary Manifestations

Pulmonary embolism and infarction are most common pulmonary complication, occurring in almost 40% of patients with APS.[43] Pulmonary microthrombosis, recurrent pulmonary embolisms resulting from DVT, and heart valvulopathy are thought to contribute to the development of pulmonary hypertension in APS. Activated platelets or altered endothelial cells on the lung vessels or the implication of endothelin-1 are also assumed to be related.[43–45] Primary thrombosis of lung vessels and large, small, or pulmonary capillaries may also occur.[43] Although pulmonary endarterectomy is one of the options to treat chronic thromboembolic pulmonary hypertension, stroke and severe thrombocytopenia are more frequent as postoperative complications in patients with APS than without APS.[46] Diffuse alveolar hemorrhage is a rare manifestation due to capillaritis.[47] Patients are usually middle-aged men with cough and dyspnea progressing to acute respiratory failure.[48]

APS manifests diverse symptoms (Table 3), and it is seemingly impossible to confine to one entity. However, from the perspective of APS as a systemic autoimmune disease, every manifestation may make a great deal of sense.

TABLE 3 Clinical Manifestations of Antiphospholipid Syndrome

Frequent (>20% of cases)	Venous thromboembolism Miscarriage or fetal loss Stroke or transient ischemic attack Migraine Livedo reticularis
Less common (10–20% of cases)	Heart valve disease Preeclampsia or eclampsia Premature birth Hemolytic anemia Coronary artery disease
Unusual (<10% of cases)	Epilepsy Vascular dementia Chorea Retinal artery or vein thrombosis Amaurosis fugax Pulmonary hypertension Leg ulcers Digital gangrene Osteonecrosis Antiphospholipid syndrome nephropathy Mesenteric ischemia
Rare (<1% of cases)	Adrenal hemorrhage Transverse myelitis Budd-Chiari syndrome

Ruiz-Irastorza et al.[49]

REFERENCES

1. Hughes GR. Hughes syndrome/APS. 30 years on, what have we learnt? Opening talk at the 14th International Congress on Antiphospholipid Antibodies Rio de Janiero, October 2013. *Lupus* 2014;**23**(4): 400–6.
2. Koike T, Bohgaki M, Amengual O, Atsumi T. Antiphospholipid antibodies: lessons from the bench. *J Autoimmun* 2007;**28**(2–3):129–33.
3. Miyakis S, Lockshin MD, Atsumi T, et al. International consensus statement on an update of the classification criteria for definite antiphospholipid syndrome (APS). *J Thromb Haemost* 2006;**4**(2):295–306.
4. Hughes GR. Thrombosis, abortion, cerebral disease, and the lupus anticoagulant. *Br Med J* 1983;**287**(6399):1088–9.
5. Fujieda Y, Atsumi T, Amengual O, et al. Predominant prevalence of arterial thrombosis in Japanese patients with antiphospholipid syndrome. *Lupus* 2012;**21**(14):1506–14.
6. Cervera R, Boffa MC, Khamashta MA, Hughes GR. The Euro-Phospholipid project: epidemiology of the antiphospholipid syndrome in Europe. *Lupus* 2009;**18**(10):889–93.
7. Urbanus RT, Siegerink B, Roest M, Rosendaal FR, de Groot PG, Algra A. Antiphospholipid antibodies and risk of myocardial infarction and ischaemic stroke in young women in the RATIO study: a case-control study. *Lancet Neurol* 2009;**8**(11):998–1005.
8. Hughes GR. Hughes syndrome (the antiphospholipid syndrome): a disease of our time. *Inflammopharmacology* 2011;**19**(2):69–73.
9. D'Ippolito S, Meroni PL, Koike T, Veglia M, Scambia G, Di Simone N. Obstetric antiphospholipid syndrome: a recent classification for an old defined disorder. *Autoimmun Rev* 2014;**13**(9):901–8.
10. de Jesus GR, Agmon-Levin N, Andrade CA, et al. 14th International Congress on Antiphospholipid Antibodies Task Force report on obstetric antiphospholipid syndrome. *Autoimmun Rev* 2014;**13**(8):795–813.
11. Ruffatti A, Del Ross T, Ciprian M, et al. Risk factors for a first thrombotic event in antiphospholipid antibody carriers: a prospective multicentre follow-up study. *Ann Rheum Dis* 2011;**70**(6):1083–6.
12. de Jesus GR, dos Santos FC, Oliveira CS, Mendes-Silva W, de Jesus NR, Levy RA. Management of obstetric antiphospholipid syndrome. *Curr Rheumatol Rep* 2012;**14**(1):79–86.
13. Meroni PL, Borghi MO, Raschi E, Tedesco F. Pathogenesis of antiphospholipid syndrome: understanding the antibodies. *Nat Rev Rheumatol* 2011;**7**(6):330–9.
14. Oku K, Atsumi T, Bohgaki M, et al. Complement activation in patients with primary antiphospholipid syndrome. *Ann Rheumatic Dis* 2009;**68**(6):1030–5.
15. Shamonki JM, Salmon JE, Hyjek E, Baergen RN. Excessive complement activation is associated with placental injury in patients with antiphospholipid antibodies. *Am J Obstet Gynecol* 2007;**196**(2):167 e1–5.
16. Cervera R, Rodriguez-Pinto I, Colafrancesco S, et al. 14th International Congress on Antiphospholipid Antibodies Task Force report on catastrophic antiphospholipid syndrome. *Autoimmun Rev* 2014;**13**(7): 699–707.
17. Asherson RA, Cervera R, de Groot PG, et al. Catastrophic antiphospholipid syndrome: international consensus statement on classification criteria and treatment guidelines. *Lupus* 2003;**12**(7):530–4.
18. Bucciarelli S, Espinosa G, Cervera R. The CAPS Registry: morbidity and mortality of the catastrophic antiphospholipid syndrome. *Lupus* 2009;**18**(10):905–12.
19. Bayraktar UD, Erkan D, Bucciarelli S, Espinosa G, Asherson R. Catastrophic Antiphospholipid Syndrome Project G. The clinical spectrum of catastrophic antiphospholipid syndrome in the absence and presence of lupus. *J Rheumatol* 2007;**34**(2):346–52.

20. Bucciarelli S, Erkan D, Espinosa G, Cervera R. Catastrophic antiphospholipid syndrome: treatment, prognosis, and the risk of relapse. *Clin Rev Allergy Immunol* 2009;**36**(2–3):80–4.

21. Erkan D, Asherson RA, Espinosa G, et al. Long term outcome of catastrophic antiphospholipid syndrome survivors. *Ann Rheum Dis* 2003;**62**(6):530–3.

22. Zuily S, Regnault V, Selton-Suty C, et al. Increased risk for heart valve disease associated with antiphospholipid antibodies in patients with systemic lupus erythematosus: meta-analysis of echocardiographic studies. *Circulation* 2011;**124**(2):215–24.

23. Kampolis C, Tektonidou M, Moyssakis I, Tzelepis GE, Moutsopoulos H, Vlachoyiannopoulos PG. Evolution of cardiac dysfunction in patients with antiphospholipid antibodies and/or antiphospholipid syndrome: a 10-year follow-up study. *Semin Arthritis Rheum* 2014;**43**(4):558–65.

24. Shoenfeld Y, Lev S, Blatt I, et al. Features associated with epilepsy in the antiphospholipid syndrome. *J Rheumatol* 2004;**31**(7):1344–8.

25. Erdozain JG, Ruiz-Irastorza G, Segura MI, et al. Cardiac valve replacement in patients with antiphospholipid syndrome. *Arthritis Care Res* 2012;**64**(8):1256–60.

26. (IR-APA) IRoAA. Thrombosis and thrombocytopenia in antiphospholipid syndrome (idiopathic and secondary to SLE): first report from the Italian Registry. Italian Registry of Antiphospholipid Antibodies (IR-APA). *Haematologica* 1993;**78**(5):313–8.

27. Diz-Kucukkaya R, Hacihanefioglu A, Yenerel M, et al. Antiphospholipid antibodies and antiphospholipid syndrome in patients presenting with immune thrombocytopenic purpura: a prospective cohort study. *Blood* 2001;**98**(6):1760–4.

28. Atsumi T, Furukawa S, Amengual O, Koike T. Antiphospholipid antibody associated thrombocytopenia and the paradoxical risk of thrombosis. *Lupus* 2005;**14**(7):499–504.

29. Uthman I, Godeau B, Taher A, Khamashta M. The hematologic manifestations of the antiphospholipid syndrome. *Blood Rev* 2008;**22**(4):187–94.

30. Tektonidou MG. Identification and treatment of APS renal involvement. *Lupus* 2014;**23**(12):1276–8.

31. Daugas E, Nochy D, Huong DL, et al. Antiphospholipid syndrome nephropathy in systemic lupus erythematosus. *J Am Soc Nephrol* 2002;**13**(1):42–52.

32. Uthman I, Khamashta M. Antiphospholipid syndrome and the kidneys. *Semin Arthritis Rheum* 2006;**35**(6):360–7.

33. Barbour TD, Crosthwaite A, Chow K, et al. Antiphospholipid syndrome in renal transplantation. *Nephrology* 2014;**19**(4):177–85.

34. Zhu DS, Fu J, Zhang Y, et al. Neurological antiphospholipid syndrome: clinical, neuroimaging, and pathological characteristics. *J Neurol Sci* 2014;**346**(1–2):138–44.

35. Arnson Y, Shoenfeld Y, Alon E, Amital H. The antiphospholipid syndrome as a neurological disease. *Semin Arthritis Rheum* 2010;**40**(2):97–108.

36. Carecchio M, Cantello R, Comi C. Revisiting the molecular mechanism of neurological manifestations in antiphospholipid syndrome: beyond vascular damage. *J Immunol Res* 2014;**2014**:239398.

37. Rodrigues CE, Carvalho JF, Shoenfeld Y. Neurological manifestations of antiphospholipid syndrome. *Eur J Clin Invest* 2010;**40**(4):350–9.

38. Sanna G, D'Cruz D, Cuadrado MJ. Cerebral manifestations in the antiphospholipid (Hughes) syndrome. *Rheum Dis Clin N Am* 2006;**32**(3):465–90.

39. Avcin T, Cimaz R, Silverman ED, et al. Pediatric antiphospholipid syndrome: clinical and immunologic features of 121 patients in an international registry. *Pediatrics* 2008;**122**(5):e1100–7.

40. Uthman I, Noureldine MH, Berjawi A, et al. Hughes syndrome and multiple sclerosis. *Lupus* 2015;**24**(2):115–21.

41. Wiles NM, Hunt BJ, Callanan V, Chevretton EB. Sudden sensorineural hearing loss and antiphospholipid syndrome. *Haematologica* 2006;**91**(Suppl. 12):ECR46.

42. Asherson RA, Frances C, Iaccarino L, et al. The antiphospholipid antibody syndrome: diagnosis, skin manifestations and current therapy. *Clin Exp Rheumatol* 2006;**24**(1 Suppl. 40):S46–51.

43. Espinosa G, Cervera R, Font J, Asherson RA. The lung in the antiphospholipid syndrome. *Ann Rheum Dis* 2002;**61**(3):195–8.

44. Wilson WA, Gharavi AE, Koike T, et al. International consensus statement on preliminary classification criteria for definite antiphospholipid syndrome: report of an international workshop. *Arthritis Rheum* 1999;**42**(7):1309–11.

45. Stojanovich L. Pulmonary manifestations in antiphospholipid syndrome. *Autoimmun Rev* 2006;**5**(5):344–8.

46. Camous J, Decrombecque T, Louvain-Quintard V, Doubine S, Dartevelle P, Stephan F. Outcomes of patients with antiphospholipid syndrome after pulmonary endarterectomy. *Eur J Cardiothoracic Surg* 2014;**46**(1):116–20.

47. Cartin-Ceba R, Peikert T, Ashrani A, et al. Primary antiphospholipid syndrome-associated diffuse alveolar hemorrhage. *Arthritis Care Res* 2014;**66**(2):301–10.

48. Asherson RA, Greenblatt MA. Recurrent alveolar hemorrhage and pulmonary capillaritis in the "primary" antiphospholipid syndrome. *J Clin Rheumatol* 2001;**7**(1):30–3.

49. Ruiz-Irastorza G, Crowther M, Branch W, Khamashta MA. Antiphospholipid syndrome. *Lancet* 2010;**376**(9751):1498–509.

Part VI

Treatment of the Disease

Chapter 59

Nonsteroidal Anti-inflammatory Drugs in Systemic Lupus Erythematosus

Robert G. Lahita[1,2], Chengqun Shao[1]

[1]Newark Beth Israel Medical Center, Newark, NJ, USA; [2]Rutgers New Jersey Medical School, Newark, NJ, USA

INTRODUCTION

Nonsteroidal anti-inflammatory drug (NSAID) use in systemic lupus erythematosus (SLE) dates back to the early 1950s, when phenylbutazone, the first nonsalicylate NSAID, was used to treat "subacute" lupus in 1953. Despite their common use, NSAIDs are still not approved by the U.S. Food and Drug Administration (FDA) for the management of SLE. To date, there are no controlled studies that document the efficacy or side effects of NSAIDs in systemic lupus erythematosus patients, but use among rheumatologists is popular. A survey among private rheumatologists at Cedars-Sinai Medical Center showed that 84% of 925 SLE patients were prescribed NSAIDs. NSAIDs are thought to help with fever, synovitis, serositis, fatigue, arthritis, and headache.[1,2] The most commonly prescribed NSAIDs were naproxen (46%), sulindac (29%), indomethacin (13%). and ibuprofen (12%).

Although NSAIDs are commonly used in SLE and non-SLE patients, the data on NSAID-induced adverse events in SLE patients is limited; however, their adverse effects have major health implications given the large number of users. This chapter discusses some of the major side effects associated with NSAID use in SLE patients.

INHIBITORY ROLE OF NSAIDs

NSAIDs collectively inhibit the synthesis of prostaglandins, a group of active lipid compounds that have diverse effects in various organ systems. The cellular membrane contains phospholipids for the synthesis of prostaglandins and thromboxane. Phospholipids are metabolized by phospholipase A into arachidonic acid; arachidonic acid is then further metabolized by cyclooxygenase to form prostaglandins. NSAIDs inhibit cyclooxygenase and inhibit the rate-limiting step of prostaglandin synthesis.[3] Two isoforms of the cyclooxygenase enzyme have been identified—COX-1 and COX-2. The expression of COX-1 is more constitutive compared to COX-2 but the latter is more inducible, with a 20-fold increase compared to a two- to threefold increase in COX-1 enzyme. COX-1 is thought to be ubiquitous throughout the body, whereas COX-2 expression is more selective, mainly in the brain, kidneys, and reproductive system.[4] COX-1 and COX-2 inhibitors have been shown to be equally effective for pain control in rheumatoid arthritis and osteoarthritis patients, but the extent of serious gastrointestinal injury is less with COX-2 inhibitors.[5]

EFFECTS ON THE KIDNEYS

Significant proteinuria is long recognized as a poor prognostic indicator in patients with nephrotic syndrome. Starting in the early 1950s, physicians have reported successful reduction in proteinuria in nephrotic patients who were treated with NSAIDs, particularly indomethacin.[6,7] Since then, there have been case reports detailing the same successful outcome in lupus nephritis patients. Espinoza et al.[8] reported six SLE patients with lupus nephritis and persistent nephrotic syndrome. The average age of the patients was 40.5 years, and a significant reduction in urinary protein excretion was demonstrated after treatment with indomethacin. The mechanism of this reduction is not clear, but some have hypothesized a reduction in renal blood flow and glomerular filtration rate, which might account for this phenomenon. Although this beneficial effect seems attractive for long-term nephroprotection, it should be noted that the kidney depends on intact prostaglandin synthesis to counteract acute hemodynamic insults.[9] Thus, if the goal of NSAID use is nephroprotection, close monitoring of clinical and laboratory data is required in cases of SLE renal disease.

Just as there are reports on the beneficial role of NSAIDs in proteinuria, the first report on NSAID-induced acute interstitial nephritis with nephrotic syndrome in SLE patients was published in 1990.[10] NSAID-induced acute renal insufficiency is one of the most common and well-recognized side effects from this class of drug. In addition to interstitial nephritis, minimal change disease, papillary necrosis, and nephrotic syndrome are other rare reactions to NSAIDs.[9,11] The pathophysiology behind most forms of NSAID-induced renal pathology is attributed to decreased synthesis of prostaglandins. The effect of prostaglandins on renal vasculature is well validated by in vivo studies[12,13]; after infusion of prostaglandin in dog kidneys, a vasodilation effect on the renal vascular bed was observed. This would lead one to hypothesize that NSAID-induced inhibition of prostaglandins would decrease renal blood flow via the afferent glomerular circulation and increase serum creatinine. However, animal and human models suggest that the loss of autoregulation occurs only when it is superimposed on an underlying hemodynamic insult.[14,15] In general, SLE-specific data on NSAIDs is limited, but it appears that active lupus nephritis increases the serum creatinine level and decreases creatinine clearance, and the addition of NSAIDS further decreases the afferent glomerular circulation. Kimberly and Plotz noted a 58% reduction in creatinine clearance as well as a 163% increase in serum creatinine in 13 of 23 lupus patients after a minimum of 7 days of aspirin therapy.[16] Patients with active lupus nephritis in this study were more likely to have NSAID-related renal dysfunction as compared to those without active lupus nephritis; additional studies also corroborated this theory.[10]

GASTROINTESTINAL SIDE EFFECTS

The relationship between nonselective NSAIDs and the risk of serious gastrointestinal (GI) injury in the form of gastritis, ulceration, bleed, and perforation is well established.[17] The mechanism of adverse GI events is linked to blockade of COX-1 mediated synthesis of prostaglandin E2, which is known to confer a cytoprotective role in the gastrointestinal epithelium.[5] Thus, the introduction of selective cyclooxygenase (COX)-2 inhibitors to the market in 1999 was welcomed in anticipation of a better gastrointestinal side effect profile.

The Vioxx Gastrointestinal Outcomes Research (VIGOR) study randomized 8076 patients with rheumatoid arthritis to receive either oral rofecoxib (50 mg) or naproxen (500 mg twice daily) for 9 months.[18] The results demonstrated 54% relative risk reduction in upper GI events, including symptomatic ulcer, upper GI bleed, and perforation in the Rofecoxib group.[19] However, another large randomized controlled study, the Celecoxib Long-Term Arthritis Safety Study Trial (CLASS) trial, demonstrated no difference in GI toxicity between selective and nonselective COX-2 inhibitors.[20] Despite this, the outcome of the VIGOR study affords the most definitive support that selective COX-2 inhibitors reduce gastrointestinal adverse events compared with nonselective NSAIDS.

Given these studies, it would be reasonable to question the risk of adverse GI events (i.e., mouth ulcers, dysphagia, anorexia, nausea, vomiting, hemorrhage, and abdominal pain) in SLE patients treated with nonselective and selective

NSAIDs. To date, there are no published studies assessing GI side effects in SLE patients who are treated with NSAIDS. We assume a reduced risk of gastrointestinal toxicity with COX-2 inhibitors in lupus patients from data gathered from rheumatoid arthritis and osteoarthritis population. A large-scale study involving SLE patients on NSAID treatment, with and without the use of gastroprotective agents, should illuminate the true incidence of NSAID-induced GI side effects.

INCREASED CARDIOVASCULAR RISK: WHAT IS THE VERDICT?

The cardiovascular side effects of NSAIDS are an ongoing concern after rofecoxib was withdrawn from the market in September 2004. Rofecoxib (Vioxx) was associated with an increased risk of cardiovascular events (e.g., myocardial infarction, angina, cerebral vascular accident) in the VIGOR study.[18] In 2005, this prompted the FDA to require that all NSAID products carry a warning for cardiovascular risk, but the evidence is controversial. The increased risk of cardiovascular events is possibly due to an imbalance between prostacyclin and platelet thromboxane levels. COX-2 inhibitors decrease prostacyclin and increase platelet thromboxane, which promote atherogenesis and destabilize atherosclerotic plaques.[21]

Although there are randomized controlled and observational studies that support an increase in cardiovascular risk with COX-2 inhibitors,[22–25] the data, thus far, have been inconclusive. The data are also criticized because their accrual is limited by short-term follow-up, the difference in baseline cardiovascular risk, and variable dosage use. Furthermore, the CLASS trial did not demonstrate a significant difference in cardiovascular events among NSAID takers.[20]

Due to such controversy, the Prospective Randomized Evolution of Celecoxib Integrated Safety (PRECISION) trial was conducted to answer the safety profile of NSAIDs. The PRECISION trial, expected to be completed toward the end of 2015, will help better define the relative cardiovascular safety profile of celecoxib, ibuprofen, and naproxen specifically. The number of randomized clinical trials monitoring cardiovascular side effects of NSAIDs in SLE patients is extremely small. Therefore, current clinical use and the side effect profile of NSAIDS in SLE is based on case reports and randomized controlled trials in non-SLE patients.

CENTRAL NERVOUS SYSTEM (ASEPTIC MENINGITIS) SIDE EFFECTS

NSAID-induced aseptic meningitis is an uncommon adverse effect of NSAIDS, but it is known to occur in patients with immune diseases like SLE.[26] Multiple case reports have linked this complication with tolmetin, sulindac, naproxen, diclofenac, and ibuprofen use.[27–30] The pathogenesis of NSAID-induced aseptic meningitis is not clear, but it seems that the inhibition of the cyclooxygenase pathway does not play a role because patients seem to tolerate other NSAIDs prior to and after the meningitis episode.[31] Most agree with a hypersensitivity reaction hypothesis given the rapid onset of meningitis symptoms, quick resolution of symptoms after stopping the offending drug, and the presence of allergic signs.

The vast majority of patients present with complaints of headache, fever, meningeal signs, and changes in mental status.[26] Interpretation of these ubiquitous symptoms and signs is challenging in the setting of SLE because NSAID-induced aseptic meningitis must be differentiated from lupus cerebritis since treatment differs significantly. Unlike NSAID-induced aseptic meningitis, the cerebral spinal fluid in lupus cerebritis is lymphocytic (<50 cells) and accompanied by clinical and laboratory data consistent with a lupus flare.[32,33] Therefore, careful interpretation of laboratory data and drug history in SLE patients presenting with meningitis may help avoid unnecessary antimicrobial therapy.

EFFECTS ON REPRODUCTION

NSAIDs are widely used in pregnant women; therefore, even a small increase in the risk of adverse events can lead to major public health consequences. Aspirin and indomethacin are the two most commonly studied NSAIDs in pregnancy. Indomethacin was linked to a higher risk of fetal congenital abnormalities such as oligohydramnios, premature closure of the fetal ductus arteriosus, nephrotoxicity, periventricular hemorrhage, and low birth weight.[4,34] Other investigators have failed to corroborate this finding.[35,36] NSAIDs, like ibuprofen, are not studied in pregnant women, but a postmarketing voluntary study by Barry et al.[37] reported 50 cases of in utero ibuprofen overdose with no evidence of fetal abnormalities.

Several population-based studies correlated NSAID use with an increased risk of miscarriage.[38,39] The highest risk of miscarriage occurred with NSAID use around the time of conception, which is likely linked to altered implantation from decreased synthesis of prostaglandins. There has been considerable evidence accumulated from animal studies involving rats and hamsters exposed to prostaglandin inhibitors indicating that prostaglandins play an important role in the early events of implantation.[40-42] However, the prostaglandins involved are controversial; it is believed that different prostaglandins could be involved at different stages of implantation. Furthermore, retrospective and prospective studies on pregnant SLE patients showed more frequent premature births and spontaneous abortions compared to non-SLE patients.[43] Although there are no trials assessing the true combined risk of miscarriage in pregnant SLE patients taking NSAID, given the preponderance of studies detailing pregnancy related complications in SLE and NSAIDS separately, it is wise to avoid NSAIDs in this high-risk group.

CONCLUSION

NSAIDs are an integral part of lupus treatment particularly for headache, fever, arthritis, and serositis. Given the available data, caution is advised when prescribing NSAIDs to patients with lupus nephritis and those at high risk for cardiovascular events at baseline. Some side effects of NSAIDs are increased in SLE patients, such as aseptic meningitis and heightened risk of miscarriage. Monitoring of NSAIDs toxicity in SLE patients should be vigilant and include periodic surveillance of liver function, blood count, and renal function, particularly those with lupus nephritis. In summary, current lupus-specific data on NSAID toxicity is rather limited; more randomized controlled and large population studies are needed to clarify if absolute contraindications of NSAIDs use in SLE exist.

REFERENCES

1. Wallace DJ, Metzger AL, Klinenberg JR. NSAID usage patterns by rheumatologists in the treatment of SLE. *J Rheumatol* 1989;**16**(4):557–60.
2. Dubois EL. Letter: ibuprofen for systemic lupus erythematosus. *N Engl J Med* 1975;**293**(15):779.
3. Ostensen M, Villiger PM. Nonsteroidal anti-inflammatory drugs in systemic lupus erythematosus. *Lupus* 2000;**9**(8):566–72.
4. Horizon AA, Wallace DJ. Risk: benefit ratio of nonsteroidal anti-inflammatory drugs in systemic lupus erythematosus. *Expert Opin Drug Saf* 2004;**3**(4):273–8.
5. Meagher EA. Balancing gastroprotection and cardioprotection with selective cyclo-oxygenase-2 inhibitors: clinical implications. *Drug Saf* 2003;**26**(13):913–24.
6. Arisz L, Donker AJ, Brentjens JR, van der Hem GK. The effect of indomethacin on proteinuria and kidney function in the nephrotic syndrome. *Acta Medica Scand* 1976;**199**(1–2):121–5.
7. Shehadeh IH, Demers LM, Abt AB, Schoolwerth AC. Indomethacin and the nephrotic syndrome. *JAMA* 1979;**241**(12):1264–6.
8. Espinoza LR, Jara LJ, Martinez-Osuna P, Silveira LH, Cuellar ML, Seleznick M. Refractory nephrotic syndrome in lupus nephritis: favorable response to indomethacin therapy. *Lupus* 1993;**2**(1):9–14.
9. Clive DM, Stoff JS. Renal syndromes associated with nonsteroidal antiinflammatory drugs. *N Engl J Med* 1984;**310**(9):563–72.
10. Ling BN, Bourke E, Campbell Jr WG, Delaney VB. Naproxen-induced nephropathy in systemic lupus erythematosus. *Nephron* 1990;**54**(3):249–55.
11. Warren GV, Korbet SM, Schwartz MM, Lewis EJ. Minimal change glomerulopathy associated with nonsteroidal antiinflammatory drugs. *Am J Kidney Dis Off J Natl Kidney Found* 1989;**13**(2):127–30.
12. Lifschitz MD. Prostaglandins and renal blood flow: in vivo studies. *Kidney Int* 1981;**19**(6):781–5.
13. Swain JA, Heyndrickx GR, Boettcher DH, Vatner SF. Prostaglandin control of renal circulation in the unanesthetized dog and baboon. *Am J Physiol* 1975;**229**(3):826–30.
14. Blasingham MC, Nasjletti A. Differential renal effects of cyclooxygenase inhibition in sodium-replete and sodium-deprived dog. *Am J Physiol* 1980;**239**(4):F360–5.
15. Donker AJ, Arisz L, Brentjens JR, van der Hem GK, Hollemans HJ. The effect of indomethacin on kidney function and plasma renin activity in man. *Nephron* 1976;**17**(4):288–96.

16. Kimberly RP, Plotz PH. Aspirin-induced depression of renal function. *N Engl J Med* 1977;**296**(8):418–24.

17. Singh G, Ramey DR, Morfeld D, Shi H, Hatoum HT, Fries JF. Gastrointestinal tract complications of nonsteroidal anti-inflammatory drug treatment in rheumatoid arthritis. A prospective observational cohort study. *Arch Intern Med* 1996;**156**(14):1530–6.

18. Bombardier C, Laine L, Reicin A, Shapiro D, Burgos-Vargas R, Davis B, et al. Comparison of upper gastrointestinal toxicity of rofecoxib and naproxen in patients with rheumatoid arthritis. VIGOR Study Group. *N Engl J Med* 2000;**343**(21):1520–8. 2 p following 1528.

19. Bjarnason I, Macpherson A, Rotman H, Schupp J, Hayllar J. A randomized, double-blind, crossover comparative endoscopy study on the gastroduodenal tolerability of a highly specific cyclooxygenase-2 inhibitor, flosulide, and naproxen. *Scand J Gastroenterol* 1997;**32**(2):126–30.

20. Silverstein FE, Faich G, Goldstein JL, Simon LS, Pincus T, Whelton A, et al. Gastrointestinal toxicity with celecoxib vs nonsteroidal anti-inflammatory drugs for osteoarthritis and rheumatoid arthritis: the CLASS study: a randomized controlled trial. Celecoxib Long-term Arthritis Safety Study. *JAMA* 2000;**284**(10):1247–55.

21. Grosser T, Fries S, FitzGerald GA. Biological basis for the cardiovascular consequences of COX-2 inhibition: therapeutic challenges and opportunities. *J Clin Invest* 2006;**116**(1):4–15.

22. Cannon CP, Curtis SP, FitzGerald GA, Krum H, Kaur A, Bolognese JA, et al. Cardiovascular outcomes with etoricoxib and diclofenac in patients with osteoarthritis and rheumatoid arthritis in the Multinational Etoricoxib and Diclofenac Arthritis Long-term (MEDAL) programme: a randomised comparison. *Lancet* 2006;**368**(9549):1771–81.

23. Mukherjee D, Nissen SE, Topol EJ. Risk of cardiovascular events associated with selective COX-2 inhibitors. *JAMA* 2001;**286**(8):954–9.

24. McGettigan P, Henry D. Cardiovascular risk and inhibition of cyclooxygenase: a systematic review of the observational studies of selective and nonselective inhibitors of cyclooxygenase 2. *JAMA* 2006;**296**(13):1633–44.

25. Antman EM, DeMets D, Loscalzo J. Cyclooxygenase inhibition and cardiovascular risk. *Circulation* 2005;**112**(5):759–70.

26. Moris G, Garcia-Monco JC. The challenge of drug-induced aseptic meningitis. *Arch Intern Med* 1999;**159**(11):1185–94.

27. Gilbert GJ, Eichenbaum HW. Ibuprofen-induced meningitis in an elderly patient with systemic lupus erythematosus. *South Med J* 1989;**82**(4):514–5.

28. Widener HL, Littman BH. Ibuprofen-induced meningitis in systemic lupus erythematosus. *JAMA* 1978;**239**(11):1062–4.

29. Ballas ZK, Donta ST. Sulindac-induced aseptic meningitis. *Arch Intern Med* 1982;**142**(1):165–6.

30. Ruppert GB, Barth WF. Ibuprofen hypersensitivity in systemic lupus erythematosus. *South Med J* 1981;**74**(2):241–3.

31. Bernstein RF. Ibuprofen-related meningitis in mixed connective tissue disease. *Ann Intern Med* 1980;**92**(2 Pt 1):206–7.

32. Gibson T, Myers AR. Nervous system involvement in systemic lupus erythematosus. *Ann Rheum Dis* 1975;**35**(5):398–406.

33. Canoso JJ, Cohen AS. Aseptic meningitis in systemic lupus erythematosus. Report of three cases. *Arthritis Rheum* 1975;**18**(4):369–74.

34. Turner G, Collins E. Fetal effects of regular salicylate ingestion in pregnancy. *Lancet* 1975;**2**(7930):338–9.

35. Shapiro S, Siskind V, Monson RR, Heinonen OP, Kaufman DW, Slone D. Perinatal mortality and birth-weight in relation to aspirin taken during pregnancy. *Lancet* 1976;**1**(7974):1375–6.

36. Werler MM, Mitchell AA, Shapiro S. The relation of aspirin use during the first trimester of pregnancy to congenital cardiac defects. *N Engl J Med* 1989;**321**(24):1639–42.

37. Barry WS, Meinzinger MM, Howse CR. Ibuprofen overdose and exposure in utero: results from a postmarketing voluntary reporting system. *Am J Med* 1984;**77**(1A):35–9.

38. Li DK, Liu L, Odouli R. Exposure to non-steroidal anti-inflammatory drugs during pregnancy and risk of miscarriage: population based cohort study. *BMJ* 2003;**327**(7411):368.

39. Nielsen GL, Sorensen HT, Larsen H, Pedersen L. Risk of adverse birth outcome and miscarriage in pregnant users of non-steroidal anti-inflammatory drugs: population based observational study and case-control study. *BMJ* 2001;**322**(7281):266–70.

40. Kennedy TG, Gillio-Meina C, Phang SH. Prostaglandins and the initiation of blastocyst implantation and decidualization. *Reproduction* 2007;**134**(5):635–43.

41. Evans CA, Kennedy TG. The importance of prostaglandin synthesis for the initiation of blastocyst implantation in the hamster. *J Reprod Fertil* 1978;**54**(2):255–61.

42. Kennedy TG. Evidence for a role for prosaglandins in the initiation of blastocyst implantation in the rat. *Biol Reprod* 1977;**16**(3):286–91.

43. Devoe LD, Taylor RL. Systemic lupus erythematosus in pregnancy. *Am J Obstet Gynecol* 1979;**135**(4):473–9.

Chapter 60

Value of Antimalarial Drugs in the Treatment of Lupus

Ziv Paz

Division of Rheumatology & Lupus Center, BIDMC, Harvard Medical School, Boston, MA, USA

INTRODUCTION

Antimalarial agents are now used as the standard of care for the treatment of systemic lupus erythematosus (SLE). The first documented use of antimalarial medications dates back to the sixteenth century, when powder from the cinchona bark tree, which grows in the Andes, was used successfully to treat malaria and was distributed through Europe by the Jesuits.[1] In the nineteenth century, chemical analysis showed that Cinchona bark contained 25 different alkaloids. Payne reported the first evidence-based successful use of quinine for cutaneous lupus in 1894.[2] However, quinacrine (atabrine) was patented only 35 years after.

Quinacrine was used as antimalarial prophylactic drug by millions of US soldiers during World War II—the biggest unplanned safety trial for a single medication in history. During these years, the beneficial effects of quinacrine on inflammatory arthritis and skin rash were recognized. These observations led to the development of new drugs, looking for more favorable safety profile and better effectivity against inflammatory conditions. There were early European reports on the use of antimalarial agents for the treatment of SLE.[3–6] However, it was not until 1951 when Page, extrapolating from the observations he made during World War II, demonstrated a clear success in treating 18 patients with cutaneous lupus.[7] This was the beginning of a new era. Hydroxychloroquine (HCQ) came on the market in 1955 and, over the course of a few decades, became the cornerstone of SLE treatment.

PHARMACOKINETICS AND PHARMACODYNAMICS OF ANTIMALARIALS

The most commonly used antimalarial in the United States for the treatment of SLE is HCQ. HCQ's bioavailability in healthy volunteers ranges between 0.67 and 0.74.[8] HCQ and chloroquine have a very large volume of distribution and distribute extensively in tissues (particularly those containing melanin).[9] Plasma protein binding of chloroquine ranges between 50% and 67%.[10] Chloroquine apparently binds more avidly to corneal tissue than HCQ.[11] Based on eye examinations, 95% of patients on chloroquine had corneal deposits, while this was seen only in 10% of the patients who were using HCQ. Transplacental distribution is slow and the relative peak concentration in the fetus was only 1% of that in the mother.[12]

In 16 rheumatoid arthritis (RA) patients, chloroquine remained in the skin for 6–7 months after cessation of therapy.[13] Chloroquine appears to concentrate in muscles.[14] This observation led to a study that was designed to assess the effects of chloroquine on the heart, which were described only on rare occasions before. Chloroquine and its main metabolite were investigated in 12 volunteers that were given 3 mg/kg of intravenous chloroquine. The systolic blood pressure fell by 10 mm Hg, with an increase in the heart rate and a prolongation of the QR interval (from 81 to 92 ms) but without change in the QTc interval.[15]

The half-life of HCQ in the blood is 50 ± 16 days.[8] The renal clearance of unchanged HCQ accounted for only 21% of the dose.[16] In contrast to HCQ, between 28% and 47% of a chloroquine dose is excreted unchanged in the urine.[17] Although hepatic metabolism is the principal route by which chloroquine is excreted, small amounts (between 0.7% and 4.2%) are excreted through breast milk.[18]

There is a linear relationship between the dose used and the clinical response and toxicity. In one study, a group of 34 RA patients had decreased morning stiffness and a better overall response with higher HCQ concentrations (697 ng/ml compared to 248 ng/ml).[19] When the blood concentrations of HCQ were above 800 ng/ml, 80% of patients reported side effects, whereas no patients had side effects with blood concentrations below 400 ng/ml.[20] Important drug–drug interactions were described with D-penicillamine and cimetidine but not with other medications used in combination with antimalarials.

MECHANISMS OF ACTION

Modification of the Lysosome pH

HCQ and chloroquine are weak diprotic bases that can pass through the lipid cell membrane and preferentially concentrate in the acidic cytoplasmic vesicles. It was demonstrated that the interaction between macrophages and T cells is inhibited by chloroquine.[21] It was hypothesized that the changes in the acidic environment of the lysosomes lead to defects in internalization, proteolytic cleavage, and assembly of the antigenic peptide with class II major histocompatibility complex (MHC) molecules. These, in turn, lead to the observed malfunction of macrophages or other antigen-presenting cells and modification of the effector immune response with decrease in the levels of the proinflammatory cytokines IL-1, IL-6, and tumor necrosis factor.[22]

Blockade of Toll-like Receptors

Toll-like receptors (TLRs) are type I transmembrane receptors that form the early defense mechanism against foreign organisms. These receptors recognize specific molecular patterns associated with pathogenic species. Several TLRs can sense nucleic acid sequences. The nucleic acid sensing TLRs are located mainly in the intracellular compartments. When activated in plasmacytoid dendritic cells (pDCs), the TLRs stimulate the production of type I interferons and proinflammatory cytokines. The presence of antinuclear antibodies is a hallmark of SLE. It is hypothesized that in SLE there is defected clearance of apoptotic material. The persistent exposure of potent neoantigens (e.g., nucleic acids) activates the pDCs' TLRs and leads to excessive production of type I interferons and proinflammatory cytokines.

Interferon (IFN)-α was shown to be significant in the pathogenesis of SLE to the extent that the term *interferon signature* became the hallmark of SLE pathophysiology.[23] Antimalarials block this TLR-mediated immune response by pH alteration of the TLRs' intracellular compartments and by direct competitive binding to the TLRs.[24] The blockade of this response leads to decrease in production of type I interferons and other proinflammatory cytokines.

Nonimmunological Effects of Antimalarials

The immune-modulatory effects of antimalarials are well studied, as briefly outlined above. Over the many years of clinical use of antimalarials in SLE, many additional benefits were observed and described. The lipid-lowering effects of antimalarials were demonstrated in 1990.[25] These effects are mediated via upregulation of the low-density lipoprotein receptor and interaction with the TLRs, which also play a role in lipid metabolism.[26,27]

Thrombotic events are devastating manifestations of SLE. These events are associated with the presence of antiphospholipid antibodies. It is thought that these antibodies disrupt the phospholipid bilayer of the cell membrane and expose the phospholipids. The exposed phospholipids are thrombogenic and lead to activation of the coagulation system and thrombus formation. In vitro studies demonstrated that HCQ blocks these effects of antiphospholipid antibodies on platelet aggregation and thrombus formation.[28]

Finally, one of the most established observations is the beneficial effect of antimalarials in cutaneous lupus. Exposure to ultraviolet light can lead to flare of SLE and especially its cutaneous manifestations.[29] Antimalarial agents accumulate in the skin and block the ultraviolet-associated inflammation.[30]

THE BENEFICIAL EFFECTS OF ANTIMALARIALS IN SLE

HCQ is used as first line treatment in SLE. Its in vitro beneficial effects were outlined previously. Most of the data on its in vivo clinical effects are based on observational studies. The only randomized double-blinded placebo-controlled trial has been the Canadian Hydroxychloroquine Study Group trial.[31] In this study, a group of 47 SLE patients were divided to treatment with HCQ (n=25) or placebo (n=22). Discontinuation of HCQ increased the relative risk of a clinical flare by 2.5 times over a 6-month period with 6.1 times higher risk for severe disease exacerbation.

Several interesting publications came out from the LUMINA cohort over the years, signifying the variety of the clinical effects associated with the use of HCQ. HCQ use was associated with reduced accrual of new damage, improved survival (5% of deaths occurred in patients using HCQ compared with 17% in patients not receiving HCQ), decreased rates of thrombotic events (OR 0.536), lower frequency of World Health Organization class IV glomerulonephritis, lower disease activity, lower steroid requirements, and longer time to skin damage (HR 0.23).[32–36] Finally, it was shown retrospectively in military personnel that early initiation of HCQ can delay the onset of clinical SLE by median time of 1 year and is associated with less severe disease.[37] Wallace et al. summarized the results of many other trials in his excellent *Nature* review.[38]

PRACTICAL ASPECTS RELATED TO THE USE OF ANTIMALARIALS

Antimalarials are safe drugs with favorable profiles, especially with appropriate dosing and monitoring (Table 1). There are several aspects that need to be considered before and during treatment, as discussed in the following sections.

TABLE 1 Recommended Use for Antimalarials in the United States

	Brand Names in US	Dosage Forms in US	Administration	Dosing: Renal Impairment	Dosing: Hepatic Impairment	Monitoring
Hydroxychloroquine	Plaquenil	200 mg	6.5 mg/kg of IBW/day	Use with caution.	Use with caution.	CBC, kidney function, and LFTs every 3 months. Eye exam as per AAO guidelines
Chloroquine	Aralen	250 and 500 mg	250 mg once daily. In severe cases can use 500 mg daily for up to two months and then taper.	CrCl <10 ml/min: Administer 50% of dose.	Use with caution.	CBC, kidney function and LFTs every 3 months. Eye exam as per AAO guidelines
Quinacrine	Not commercially manufactured in the USA but can be ordered from pharmacies that compound it					

Hydroxychloroquine sulfate 200 mg is equivalent to 155 mg hydroxychloroquine base and 250 mg chloroquine phosphate.
Abbreviations: IBW, ideal body weight; CBC, complete blood counts; LFTs, liver function tests; AAO, American Academy of Ophthalmology.

SCREENING FOR GLUCOSE-6-PHOSPHATE DEHYDROGENASE DEFICIENCY

Glucose-6-phosphate deficiency is the most prevalent enzyme deficiency, with 400 million people affected worldwide. This condition is especially prevalent among the African population. This population is also the most vulnerable with regard to SLE. One of the specific and relevant concerns is the development of hemolytic anemia in response to the administration of the antimalarial drugs in patients with glucose-6-phosphate dehydrogenase (G6PD) deficiency.

In the 1950s, a series of investigations by United States Army researchers identified G6PD deficiency as the cause of hemolysis after administration of the primaquine. For decades, there was a concern that other antimalarials like HCQ and cholorquine can lead to hemolytic anemia in G6PD-deficient patients. As a result, many practitioners were screening their patients for the presence of G6PD deficiency. However, it seems that with the current doses of HCQ, even in the presence of G6PD deficiency, the chances for hemolytic anemia are low. Currently, there are no clear guidelines and no recommendations to screen patients for the presence of G6PD deficiency prior to initiation of treatment with HCQ. One of the remaining controversial issues is the use of HCQ in patients with known G6PD deficiency. The U.S. Federal Drug Administration currently recommends against the use of HCQ in this population.

NONOPHTHALMOLOGIC ADVERSE EFFECTS OF ANTIMALARIAL AGENTS

Antimalarial agents are considered to be safe and are well tolerated. Most of the documented adverse effects were more commonly seen with the use of chloroquine and less with HCQ. The most common nonophthalmologic adverse effects are nausea, vomiting, pruritus, maculopapular rash, skin and mucosal pigmentation, insomnia, nightmares, and nervousness. Rarely, patients present with tinnitus, neuropathy, seizures, leukopenia, anemia, depigmentation of hair, hair loss, and elevated liver function tests.

OPHTHALMOLOGIC ADVERSE EFFECTS OF ANTIMALARIAL AGENTS

The ophthalmologic adverse effects of antimalarials are the most concerning. The most common manifestations are keratopathy due to corneal deposits and retinal toxicity ("bull's eye maculopathy"). There is no consensus on the incidence of retinal toxicity, the best technique for screening, or the frequency of screening. HCQ and chloroquine bind to the melanin pigment in the retinal pigmented epithelium (RPE) and accumulate over time. The risk of toxicity depends on the presence of pre-existing risk factors (Table 2).[39]

Retinal toxicity was considered to be rare, with a reported prevalence of 0.5–2%.[40] However, these numbers were based mainly on studies reviewing cases with reported visual loss, which represent already advanced stages. The use of modern techniques can lead to early detection of retinopathy. Central visual field 10-2 testing and spectral-domain optical coherence tomography (SD-OCT) are very sensitive to early changes.[41]

In a retrospective case–control study, the prevalence and risk factors for retinal toxicity were assessed in 2361 patients who had used HCQ continuously for at least 5 years.[42] In this seminal work, the authors found that 7.5% of long-term HCQ users screened with modern techniques had evidence of retinal toxicity. This prevalence is approximately 3 times higher than previously reported.[40] In this study, most of the patients who were diagnosed with retinal toxicity were detected before bull's eye maculopathy was visible. Moreover, the risk rises markedly with concurrent kidney disease, with prevalence of above 50% with use of doses above 5.0 mg/kg and with duration of use beyond 20 years. Finally, even though the common practice was to use ideal or lean body weight for dosing, they showed that real body weight correlates better with retinal toxicity. The importance of early detection is further emphasized by the fact that the retinal disease progresses even 3 years after the discontinuation of HCQ if RPE damage was already present at the time of discontinuation.[43]

The American Academy of Ophthalmology currently recommends using objective measures, such as SD-OCT and multifocal electroretinography (mfERG) along with visual fields for screening for HCQ retinopathy[44] (Table 3). More than one technique is required, as 10% of patients with early HCQ toxicity will demonstrate prominent ring scotomas on visual field testing without obvious SD-OCT abnormality.[45] Unfortunately, not all the RA and SLE patients treated with HCQ are adequately screened. It has been shown that among 6339 RA and SLE patients using HCQ or chloroquine, 1409 (7.8%) had used chloroquine or HCQ for at least 4 years. Among those, 27.9% lacked regular eye care visits, 6.1% had no visits to eye care providers, and 34.5% had no diagnostic testing for maculopathy during the 5-year period.[46]

USE OF ANTIMALARIALS IN PREGNANCY AND LACTATION

HCQ is safe during both pregnancy and lactation. Several retrospective studies and cohort registries of pregnant SLE patients showed no teratogenic effects or poor outcomes associated with the use of HCQ.[47,48] The use of HCQ in pregnancy is associated with decreased disease activity and decreased rates of neonatal lupus.[49] HCQ is secreted in breastmilk in a very low concentration that is unlikely to lead to any harm.

TABLE 2 Risk Factors for Retinal Toxicity Associated with the Use of Antimalarials

1. Daily dosage exceeding 6.5 mg/kg
2. Obesity
3. Duration longer than 5 years
4. Renal or liver impairment
5. Age greater than 60 years
6. Pre-existing retinal disease
7. Concurrent tamoxifen citrate therapy

TABLE 3 American Academy of Ophthalmology Recommendations on Screening for Chloroquine and Hydroxychloroquine Retinopathy

Dose of 400 mg of HCQ daily (or 250 mg CQ). For individuals of short stature, the dose should be determined on the basis of ideal body weight.

A baseline examination. Annual screening should begin after 5 years (or annually if any risk factors; Table 2).

Along with 10-2 automated fields, at least one advanced procedure[a] should be used for routine screening.

mfERG testing may be used in place of visual fields.

Amsler grid testing is no longer recommended.

Fundus examinations are advised for documentation, but visible bull's eye maculopathy is a late change, and the goal of screening is to recognize toxicity at an earlier stage.

The drugs should be stopped if possible when toxicity is recognized or strongly suspected.

HCQ, Hydroxychloroquine; CQ, Chloroquine.
[a]Multifocal electroretinogram (mfERG), spectral domain optical coherence tomography (SD-OCT), and fundus autofluorescence (FAF).

REFERENCES

1. Wallace DJ. The history of antimalarials. *Lupus* 1996;**5**(Suppl. 1):S2–3.

2. Payne JF. A postgraduate lecture on lupus erythematosus. *Clin J* 1894;**4**:223–39.

3. Martenstein H. Subacute lupus erythematosus and tubercular cervical adenopathy. Treatment with plasmochin. *Z Haut Geschlechtskr* 1928;**27**:239–48.

4. Davidson AM, Birt AR. Quinine bisulfate as a desensitizing agent in the treatment of lupus erythematosus. *Arch Dermatol* 1938;**37**:247–53.

5. Prokoptchouk AJ. Traitment du loup erythemateux par l'ariquine. *Z Haut Geschlechskr* 1940;**66**:112. Translated into English in Arch Dermatol Syph 1955;**71**:250.

6. Sorinson NS. Acrichin in therapy of lupus erythematosus. *Vrach Delu* 1941;**23**:441–6.

7. Page F. Treatment of lupus erythematosus with mepacrine. *Lancet* 1951;**2**:755–8.

8. Tett SE, Cutler DJ, Day RO, Brown KF. Bioavailability of hydroxychloroquine tablets in healthy volunteers. *Br J Clin Pharmacol* 1989;**27**:771–9.

9. Tett SE, Cutler DJ, Day RO, Brown KF. A dose-ranging study of the pharmacokinetics of hydroxychloroquine following intravenous administration to healthy volunteers. *Br J Clin Pharmacol* 1988;**26**:303–13.

10. Augustijns P, Verbeke N. Stereoselective pharmacokinetic properties of chloroquine and desthylchloroquine (sie) in humans. *Clin Pharmacokinet* 1993;**24**:259–69.

11. Easterbrook M. Is corneal deposition of anti-malarial any indication of retinal toxicity? *Can J Ophthalmol* 1990;**25**:249–51.

12. Augustijns P, Jongsma HW, Verbeke N. Transplacental distribution of chloroquine in sheep. *Dev Pharmacol Ther* 1991;**17**:191–9.

13. Sjolin-Forsberg G, et al. Chloroquine phosphate: a long-term follow-up of drug concentrations in skin suction blister fluid and plasma. *Acta Derm Venereol* 1993;**73**:426–9.

14. MacIntyre AC, Cutler DJ. In vitro binding of chloroquine to rat muscle preparations. *J Pharm Sci* 1986;**75**:1068–70.

15. Looareesuwan S, et al. Cardiovascular toxicity and distribution kinetics of intravenous chloroquine. *Br J Clin Pharmacol* 1986;**6**:12312–3.

16. Cutler DJ, MacIntyre AC, Tett SE. Pharmacokinetics and cellular uptake of 4-aminoquinolone antimalarials. *AAS* 1988;**24**:142–57.

17. White NJ. Clinical pharmacokinetics of antimalarial drugs. *Clin Pharmacokinet* 1985;**10**:187–215.

18. Ogunbona FA, Onyeji CO, Bolaji OO, Torimori SE. Excretion of chloroquine and desethylchloroquine in human milk. *Br J Clin Pharmacol* 1987;**23**:473–6.

19. Tett SE, McLachlan A, Day RO, Cutler D. Insights from pharmacokinetic and pharmacodynamic studies of hydroxychloroquine. *Agents Actions* 1993;**4**(Suppl.):145–90.

20. Frisk-Holmberg M, et al. Chloroquine serum concentration and side-effects: evidence for dose-dependent kinetics. *Clin Pharmacol Ther* 1979;**25**:345–50.

21. Unanue E. Antigen-presenting function of the macrophage. *Annu Rev Immunol* 1984;**2**:395.

22. Wallace DJ, Linker-Israeli M, Hyun S, Klinenberg JR, Stecher V. The effect of hydroxychloroquine therapy on serum levels of immunoregulatory molecules in patients with systemic lupus erythematosus. *J Rheumatol* 1994;**21**:375–6.

23. Vallin H, Blomberg S, Alm GV, Cederblad B, Ronnblom L. Patients with systemic lupus erythematosus (SLE) have a circulating inducer of interferon-α (IFN-α) production acting on leucocytes resembling immature dendritic cells. *Clin Exp Immunol* 1999;**115**:196–202.

24. Kuznik A, et al. Mechanism of endosomal TLR inhibition by antimalarial drugs and imidazoquinolines. *J Immunol* 2011;**186**:4794–804.

25. Wallace DJ, Metzger AL, Stecher VJ, Turnbull BA, Kern PA. Cholesterol-lowering effect of hydroxychloroquine in patients with rheumatic disease: reversal of deleterious effects of steroids on lipids. *Am J Med* 1990;**89**:322–6.

26. Lange Y, Duan H, Mazzone T. CKholesterol homeostasis is modulated by amphiphiles at transcriptional and post-transcriptional loci. *J Lipid Res* 1996;**37**:534–9.

27. Gu JQ, et al. A Toll-like receptor 9-mediated pathway stimulates perilipin 3 (TIP47) expression and induces lipid accumulation in macrophages. *Am J Physiol Endocrinol Metab* 2010;**299**:E593–600.

28. Espinola RG, Pierangeli SS, Gharavi AE, Harris EN. Hydroxychloroquine reverses platelet activation induced by human IgG antiphospholipid antibodies. *Thromb Haemost* 2002;**87**:518–22.

29. Furukawa F, Kashihara-Sawami M, Lyons MB, Norris DA. Binding of antibodies to the extractable nuclear antigens SS-A/Ro and SS-B/La is induced on the surface of human keratinocytes by ultraviolet light (UVL): implications for the pathogenesis of photosensitive cutaneous lupus. *J Invest Dermatol* 1990;**94**:77–85.

30. Nguyen TQ, Capra JD, Sontheimer RD. 4-aminoquinoline antimalarials enhance UV-B induced c-jun transcriptional activation. *Lupus* 1998;**7**:148–53.

31. The Canadian Hydroxychloroquine Study Group. A randomized study of the effect of withdrawing hydroxychloroquine sulfate in systemic lupus erythematosus. *N Engl J Med* 1991;**324**:150–4.

32. Fessler BJ, et al. Systemic lupus erythematosus in three ethnic groups: XVI. Association of hydroxychloroquine use with reduced risk of damage accrual. *Arthritis Rheum* 2005;**52**:1473–80.

33. Alarcon GS, et al. Effect of hydroxychloroquine on the survival of patients with systemic lupus erythematosus: data from LUMINA, a multiethnic US cohort (LUMINA L). *Ann Rheum Dis* 2007;**66**:1168–72.

34. Pons-Estel GJ, et al. Possible protective effect of hydroxychloroquine on delaying the occurrence of integument damage in lupus: LXXI, data from a multiethnic cohort. *Arthritis Care Res (Hoboken)* 2010;**62**:393–400.

35. Ho KT, et al. Systemic lupus erythematosus in a multiethnic cohort (LUMINA): XXVIII. Factors predictive of thrombotic events. *Rheumatology (Oxford)* 2005;**44**:1303–7.

36. Pons-Estel GJ, et al. Protective effect of hydroxychloroquine on renal damage in patients with lupus nephritis: LXV, data from a multiethnic US cohort. *Arthritis Rheum* 2009;**61**:830–9.

37. James JA, et al. Hydroxychloroquine sulfate treatment is associated with later onset of systemic lupus erythematosus. *Lupus* 2007;**16**:401–9.

38. Wallace DJ, Gudsoorkar VS, Weisman MH, Venuturupalli SR. New insights into mechanisms of therapeutic effects of antimalarial agents in SLE. *Nat Rev Rheumatol* 2012;**8**:522–33.

39. Marmor MF, Carr RE, Easterbrook M, Farjo AA, Mieler WF, American Academy of Ophthalmology. Recommendations on screening for chloroquine and hydroxychloroquine retinopathy: a report by the American Academy of Ophthalmology. *Ophthalmology* 2002:1377–82.

40. Mavrikakis I, Sfikakis PP, Mavrikakis E, et al. The incidence of irreversible retinal toxicity in patients treated with hydroxychloroquine: a reappraisal. *Ophthalmology* 2003;**110**:1321–6.

41. Marmor MF. Comparison of screening procedures in hydroxychloroquine toxicity. *Arch Ophthalmol* 2012;**130**:461–9.

42. Melles RB, Marmor MF. The risk of toxic retinopathy in patients on long-term hydroxychloroquine therapy. *JAMA Ophthalmol* 2014;**132**:1453–60.

43. Marmor MF, Hu J. Effect of disease stage on progression of hydroxychloroquine retinopathy. *JAMA Ophthalmol* 2014;**132**:1105–12.

44. Marmor MF, Kellner U, Lai TY, et al. American Academy of Ophthalmology. Revised recommendations on screening for chloroquine and hydroxychloroquine retinopathy. *Ophthalmology* 2011;**118**: 415–22.

45. Marmor MF, Melles RB. Disparity between visual fields and optical coherence tomography in hydroxychloroquine retinopathy. *Ophthalmology* 2014;**121**:1257–62.

46. Nika M, Blachley TS, Edwards P, Lee PP, Stein JD. Regular examinations for toxic maculopathy in long-term chloroquine or hydroxychloroquine users. *JAMA Ophthalmol* 2014;**132**:1199–208.

47. Clowse ME, Magder L, Witter F, Petri M. Hydroxychloroquine in lupus pregnancy. *Arthritis Rheum* 2006;**54**:3640–7.

48. Levy RA, et al. Hydroxychloroquine (HCQ) in lupus pregnancy: double-blind and placebo-controlled study. *Lupus* 2001;**10**:401–4.

49. Izmirly PM, et al. Evaluation of the risk of anti-SSA/Ro-SSB/La antibody-associated cardiac manifestations of neonatal lupus in fetuses of mothers with systemic lupus erythematosus exposed to hydroxychloroquine. *Ann Rheum Dis* 2010;**69**:1827–30.

Chapter 61

Systemic Glucocorticoids

Zahi Touma[1,2], Murray B. Urowitz[1,2,3]

[1]University of Toronto Lupus Clinic, Toronto Western Hospital, Centre for Prognosis Studies in the Rheumatic Diseases, Toronto, ON, Canada; [2]Department of Internal Medicine, Division of Rheumatology, University of Toronto, Toronto, ON, Canada; [3]Toronto Western Research Institute, Toronto, ON, Canada

INTRODUCTION

Since their discovery in 1949 by Philip S. Hench and colleagues, glucocorticoids continue to be the cornerstone of the treatment of several rheumatic diseases, including systemic lupus erythematosus (SLE).[1] In the initial trial of synthetic cortisone in 1949 on patients with rheumatoid arthritis, Hench et al. found that some clinical and laboratory features of rheumatoid arthritis benefited from the daily intramuscular injection with either the adrenal cortical hormone, 17-hydroxy-11-dehydrocorticosterone, or the pituitary adrenocorticotropic hormone (ACTH).[1] In 1950, Edward Kendall, Tadeus Reichstein, and Philip Hench won the Nobel Prize in Physiology or Medicine for the discovery of cortisone.

As a result of their potent anti-inflammatory effects, glucocorticoids were extensively used to treat different rheumatic diseases, including SLE. Pollak and colleagues in 1961 and Smith and colleagues in 1965 reported on the effect of a large glucocorticoids dose in the management of renal function in adult lupus nephritis patients as well as in children with lupus nephritis.[2,3] Pollak et al. followed 16 patients for 6 months and reported that histological signs of activity either disappeared or decreased in 10 of the 16 patients on glucocorticoids.[2] Soon thereafter, oral glucocorticoids gained acceptance in the treatment of SLE. In 1976, Cathcart et al. treated seven patients with diffuse proliferative lupus nephritis with high-dose intravenous methylprednisolone (pulse) therapy. Following the pulse therapy, five patients with rapidly deteriorating renal function demonstrated a remarkable improvement in their renal function and all patients showed serological amelioration.[4] Unfortunately, along with their potent anti-inflammatory effects, the use of glucocorticoids was associated with several serious side effects.

In this chapter, we review the properties of glucocorticoids (anti-inflammatory and immunosuppressive effects), their role in the management of SLE, their adverse events, and future directions regarding their use. We also reflect on the experience with glucocorticoids of the University of Toronto Lupus Clinic, a prospective observational cohort study of 42 years duration.[5]

NOMENCLATURE

In the literature, there is confusion between the use of the term *glucocorticoids* and *corticosteroids*, which are often used as synonyms. The term *corticosteroids* covers both mineralocorticoids and glucocorticoids hormones. Buttgereit et al. proposed the use of the term *glucocorticoids* to describe the class of drug steroids otherwise referred to as corticosteroids, corticoids, glucocorticosteroids, and glucocorticoids.[6] The use of the term *steroids* is too broad and can be misleading, especially because steroids encompass chemical compounds characterized by a common multiple ring structure (sterol skeleton formed by six-carbon hexane rings and one-five carbon pentane ring) that include molecules such as cholesterol, sex hormones, and corticosteroids.[6] The adrenal cortex produces two major classes of steroids: the corticosteroids and androgens. Based on their activity, the adrenal corticosteroids are further subgrouped into glucocorticoids (carbohydrate metabolism regulating) and mineralocorticoids (electrolyte balance regulating).[6]

RATIONALE AND MECHANISM OF ACTION OF GLUCOCORTICOIDS IN SLE

Glucocorticoids exhibit very potent anti-inflammatory and immunosuppressive effects, which constitute the rationale for their use in SLE and other autoimmune diseases. Both glucocorticoids, which are primarily regulated by corticotropin (ACTH) and the hypothalamic-pituitary-adrenal axis, participate in controlling the inflammatory process in the short term.[7] The hypothalamic-pituitary-adrenal axis role is mediated via the glucocorticoid receptors expressed in almost all cells.[8] It is also known that the glucocorticoids' anti-inflammatory role is mediated by their ability to inhibit antibody synthesis in the long term.[9]

Mechanism of Action of Glucocorticoids

The effects of glucocorticoids are mediated via genomic and nongenomic mechanisms. In general, with the use of oral therapeutic glucocorticoids, the effect of glucocorticoids

Systemic Lupus Erythematosus. http://dx.doi.org/10.1016/B978-0-12-801917-7.00061-9

is mediated via genomic mechanisms. The human gluco-corticoid receptor (GR) gene is one locus on chromosome 5_q31-32, and the human GR messenger RNA has alternative splice variants that produce the target proteins.[10] The GR binds to cortisone and initiates the dissociation of molecular chaperones, such as heat-shock proteins, from the receptor.

Within the cell, glucocorticoids act through genomic and nongenomic paths in three ways.[8] First, the glucocorticoid-GR complex penetrates the nucleus and binds to the DNA sequences called glucocorticoid-responsive elements, which initiate the transcription process mediated by RNA polymerase II. In the second way, interactions between the cortisol-glucocorticoid-receptor complex and other transcription factors (such as nuclear factor-kB [NF-kB]) are involved in the regulation of other glucocorticoid-responsive genes. Most anti-inflammatory effects are thought to occur due to inhibited gene transcription via NF-kB and the adverse effects of glucocorticoids are mediated via activation of transcription of certain genes (transactivation).[11] The third way involves nongenomic mechanisms and consists of glucocorticoids signaling through membrane-associated receptors and secondary messengers.[8]

At dosages of more than 100 mg/day of prednisolone, glucocorticoid receptors become saturated, and this involves the emergence of nongenomic mechanisms.[12] When acting through genomic mechanisms, glucocorticoids take at least 30 min to several hours to show an effect and glucocorticoids can have also a rapid onset (seconds to minutes). In pulse therapy, glucocorticoids act faster (within minutes) via nongenomic mechanisms.[12,13] The response to pulse therapy might be biphasic, involving an early rapid nongenomic effect and a delayed and more sustained genomic effect.[14]

Anti-inflammatory and Immunosuppressive Effects of Glucocorticoids

Glucocorticoids exert their anti-inflammatory and immunosuppressive effects by acting on different cellular pathways, which are considered complex.[15] Glucocorticoids act first via their anti-inflammatory effects and promote immunosuppressive effects at a later stage through the inhibition of antibody synthesis and its effects on humoral immune response.[15] Anti-inflammatory effects of glucocorticoids are mediated by their ability to:

1. Increase the blood count of neutrophils and decrease their trafficking
2. Decrease the blood count of macrophages and monocytes, trafficking, and their phagocytosis and bactericidal effects, and inhibit antigen presentation, which may increase susceptibility to infection
3. Decrease lymphocytes' blood count, trafficking, and cytokine production

4. Decrease the blood count of eosinophils and increase apoptosis
5. Decrease the blood count of basophils and the release of mediators of inflammation[16]

Glucocorticoids also suppress fibroblast proliferation IL-1 and tumor necrosis factor-induced metalloproteinase synthesis.[17] Glucocorticoids inhibit the activity of several T-helper type 1 cytokines, including IL-1β, IL-2, IL-3, and IL-6. Glucocorticoids also have the ability to inhibit the production of cylcoxygenase-2 and the formation of arachidonic acid metabolites through the induction of expression of lipocortin-1 (an inhibitor of phospholipase A2).

Glucocorticoids have the ability to block antibody production via different mechanisms:

1. Lymphopenia (T cells are affected more than B cells), which is secondary to lymphocyte redistribution, mainly to the bone marrow and spleen, or apoptosis[18]
2. Inhibition of IL-2 synthesis and signaling
3. Inhibition of signal transduction events critical for T-cell activation
4. Inhibition of antigen-presenting cell function
5. B-cell suppression via inhibition of BLys (by high dose dexamethasone)[19]

FORMS AND MODE OF ADMINISTRATION OF SYSTEMIC CORTICOSTEROIDS

Forms of Synthetic Steroids

Synthetic steroids are more potent than natural steroid hormones. Glucocorticoids with an 11-keto such as cortisone and prednisone are biologically inactive. Cortisone and prednisone activation is processed in the liver via the hepatic enzymes, where 11-keto is reduced to 11-hydroxy configuration to become active. This phenomenon results in the conversion of cortisone to cortisol and prednisone to prednisolone. The use of prednisolone might be more efficacious in patients with liver disease.[16] Tissue concentration of biologically active glucocorticoids is controlled by two intracellular enzymes: 11 β-hydroxysteroid dehydrogenase type 1, which promotes the activation of inactive forms of glucocorticoids; and 11 β-hydroxysteroid dehydrogenase type 2, which promotes the conversion of active glucocorticoids to inactive forms.[20] The potency of glucocorticoids is related to the structural differences in the steroid configuration, where the introduction of a double bond between the 1 and 2 positions of cortisol results in prednisolone and the addition of the 6-methyl group to the last produces methylprednisolone.

It is known that prednisolone is four times more potent than cortisol and methylprednisolone is five times more potent than cortisol. Glucocorticoids' biologic half-lives (8–48 h) are longer than their plasma half-lives (0.5–4 h) (Table 1).[16]

TABLE 1 Forms of Glucocorticoids

Glucocorticoid	Equivalent Commercial Tablet (mg)	Plasma Half-life (min)	Biologic Half-life (h)	Relative Anti-inflammatory Effect	Relative Mineralocorticoid Effect	Protein Binding
Short Acting						
Cortisone	25	30	8–12	0.8	0.8	None
Cortisol	20	90–120	8–12	1	1	Very high
Intermediate Acting						
Methylpredniso-lone	4	>180	12–36	5	0.5	None
Prednisolone	5	200	12–36	4	0.6	High
Prednisone	5	200	12–36	4	0.6	Very high
Triamcinolone	4	200	12–36	5	0	High
Long Acting						
Dexamethasone	0.75	180–270	48	25	0	High
Betamethasone	0.65	180–300	48	25	0	High

The metabolism of synthetic steroids is in the liver and inactive metabolites are eliminated by the kidneys. Synthetic steroids bounded to transport protein cannot pass the placenta. The placenta contains 11 β-hydroxysteroid dehydrogenase type 2, which catalyzes the active glucocorticoids received from the blood of the mother to inactive forms. Dexamethasone and betamethasone have almost no affinity for transport proteins and are usually not metabolized by 11 β-hydroxysteroid dehydrogenase type 2 in the placenta, thus reaching the fetal blood without alteration.[16] Prednisone is the most frequently prescribed synthetic steroid in lupus and other rheumatic diseases due to its short plasma half-life and the availability of tablets in different doses.[9,21] Both prednisone and prednisolone are excreted in breast milk but in small quantities; it is recommended to avoid breastfeeding 4 h after the intake of prednisone and prednisolone.[22]

Mode of Administration of Local Glucocorticoids

Glucocorticoids in the management of SLE can be administered locally in the form of topical, intrasynovial, or intralesional. Topical preparations are mainly used in the treatment of localized lupus skin rash without evidence of vasculitis. Formulations include short-acting hydrocortisone (0.125–1.0%), intermediate-acting products with triamcinolone (0.025–0.5%), and long-acting products with betamethasone (0.01–0.1%). The intrasynovial mode of administration is used in the treatment of limited soft tissue and joint inflammations from SLE (e.g., methylprednisolone

acetate). Intralesional delivery is used to treat patchy alopecia and discoid lupus (e.g., triamcinlone cetonide).

Oral Glucocorticoids

Oral glucocorticoids is the most frequent route of administration used by clinicians in the management of SLE. The absorption of glucocorticoids is excellent on either an empty or full stomach. The most commonly prescribed forms are prednisone in North America and prednisolone in Europe. Glucocorticoids may be prescribed as a single morning dose or in a divided dose regimen (two to four times a day). For patients with more severe lupus disease activity, a divided dose regimen might be a preferable approach over the single daily dose, which is used more often in patients with less active disease.

Glucocorticoid resistance could be related to decreased absorption (e.g., by cholestyramine), interaction with drugs that induce hepatic microsomal enzymes (especially CYP3A4), or increased metabolism by drugs such as barbiturates and rifampin. Other medications such as ketoconazole and clarithromycin increase glucocorticoid activity through the inhibition of CYP3A4. Patients with liver disease are unable to metabolize prednisone and may be given prednisolone (in the same dose as prednisone). Patients suffering from mineralocorticoid side effects such as fluid retention can be switched to methylprednisolone (medrol) at a 20% lower dose. In addition, medrol binds exclusively to high-capacity albumin and has a concentration-independent protein-bound fraction (60–70%). Only the free fraction of glucocorticoids is biologically active. The protein binding for prednisolone and prednisone is concentration dependent and varies from 90% (with standard oral doses) to 60% (at higher doses).

The therapeutic dose of glucocorticoids in the management of SLE patients is determined based on the approach of body weight, 1 mg/kg/day, which has no scientific basis. The dosages of prednisone that have been suggested include low or maintenance dosage (0.1–0.25 mg/kg/day), moderate dosage (0.5 mg/kg/day), high dosage (1–3 mg/kg/day), and massive dosage (15–30 mg/kg/day).[23] Clinical experience has shown that the responsiveness to glucocorticoids is individual and varies between patients. Three major factors determine the responsiveness to glucocorticoids: disease factors, organ-specific factors, and host factors. It is well known that rheumatoid arthritis and polymyalgia rheumatica are more sensitive as a disease to glucocorticoids than is SLE.

The dosage of glucocorticoids used in the treatment of mucocutaneous SLE manifestations is different from the treatment of central nervous system or renal involvement. Some organs, such as mucocutaneous, are more sensitive to glucocorticoids compared to the central nervous system or renal system. Furthermore, some patients may develop comorbidities such as osteonecrosis or cataracts on 20 mg/day of prednisone for 6 months, whereas other patients never develop osteonecrosis or cataracts on a much higher dose. It is not unusual to have variation in the responsiveness to the same organ between patients, where 10 mg/day of prednisone for mucocutaneous manifestations might be successful in one patient while a higher dose is required in another patient.

Each of these factors (disease, organ, and host) need to be considered when deciding the dosage of glucocorticoids. Another factor to consider in determining the dosage of glucocorticoids is the phase of treatment: induction, maintenance, and withdrawal of glucocorticoids. In general clinical practice, clinicians induce with the highest dose of glucocorticoids for the corresponding organ (e.g., 10–15 for mucocutaneous). If improvement is achieved in 2–6 weeks, the dose of glucocorticoids is tapered progressively, and it is not unusual to maintain the same level for a period of time to ensure the consolidation of the improvement. In a select group of patients in remission, further tapering and stopping the prednisone is considered. It is very important to remember that in clinical practice the aim is to stop glucocorticoids if possible.

At the Toronto Lupus Clinic, we use a different approach regarding the dosage of glucocorticoids and we recommend this approach to induce adult lupus patients. In adults, the induction dose can be defined using four levels: low (up to 20 mg/day), moderate (20–40 mg/day), high (40–80 mg/day), and very high (>80 mg/day) doses of prednisone. The very high dose includes oral and intravenous "pulse

therapy"/intermittent infusion. These doses are not based on the body weight of the patient. This approach is derived based on the factors described above (disease, organ, and host). The treating physician could choose a low, moderate, high, or very high dose as induction therapy. Therapeutic dilemmas occur when a patient does not respond to a high dose of prednisone. In this case, clinicians tend to consider pulse therapy in massive doses rather than a stepwise increase in the dose. It is not unusual to find in published literature patients receiving 0.5 or 1 g/day of methylprednisolone for 3–5 consecutive days to induce a response in lupus nephritis and central nervous system manifestations, although good studies to confirm this approach are lacking.

Intravenous Glucocorticoids

Pulse therapy is often linked to 1 g/day for 3–5 consecutive days of methylprednisolone (Medrol, Depo-Medrol, Solu-Medrol), which is a water-soluble glucocorticoid. Methylprednisolone was first used to treat lupus nephritis using the same protocol as for renal transplant.[24] This protocol continues to be used in the management of life or organ-threatening complications of SLE (lupus nephritis, myelopathy, alveolar hemorrhage, optic neuritis, and others). Others believe that the use of glucocorticoids intravenously ensures that the drug works faster compared to oral administration.[25,26] An advantage of intravenous glucocorticoids is that they can be given intermittently to control disease activity rather than keeping the patient on a very high dose of prednisone for a long period. Studies on rheumatoid arthritis confirmed that low and moderate doses of methylprednisolone are efficacious when compared to high doses of glucocorticoids.[27,28]

Based on our experience at the Toronto Lupus Clinic, if intravenous glucocorticoids pulse therapy is considered as induction, we advocate a stepwise increase of the pulse doses depending on the response of the patients rather than starting with megadoses like 0.5–1 g/day of methylprednisolone. There is little evidence as yet to support the use of megadoses in SLE. There is a need for randomized controlled trials comparing moderate doses of pulse methylprednisolone and megadoses of this agent in SLE. In addition, evidence from the literature in several studies confirmed that high doses do not show any superiority over moderate doses. This approach will minimize the comorbidities linked to glucocorticoids in particular infections.[29–31]

The duration of the pulse therapy is also not well defined, and it varies from 3–5 consecutive days.[32] There is no evidence for this approach; in general, because patients are continued on a high dose of prednisone after the pulse, there is no rationale to extend the pulse to 5 days. Intravenous pulse therapy can be considered in situations where other treatment approaches have failed or in cases of refractory disease that does not respond to high doses of oral prednisone. Other indications for intravenous pulse therapy can be cases of severe lupus nephritis with acute renal failure or refractory rapid progressive glomerulonephritis, severe thrombocytopenia or hemolytic anemia, or vasculitis. Another instance where intravenous pulse glucocorticoids might be considered is in a noncompliant patient with active disease in the context of life-threatening and organ-threatening lupus.

Intramuscular Therapy

Intramuscular (IM) administration of glucocorticoids is reserved for patients who are not able to receive oral or intravenous glucocorticoids, such as patients with difficult intravenous access or situations related to inadequate absorption of oral glucocorticoids. Long-acting glucocorticoids (e.g., triamcinolone acetonide) can be administered IM and can be used for induction of mild to severe flares of SLE. The Flares in Lupus Outcome Assessment Trial (FLOAT) compared oral methylprednisolone and IM intramuscular triamcinolone use.[33] In this clinical trial, 50 patients with SLE with a mild or moderate flare were randomized to receive oral methylprednisolone with rapid tapering (Medrol) or triamcinolone 100 mg IM. Both groups did equally well, but IM triamcinolone resulted in a more rapid response than the oral methylprednisolone at days 1 and 2.[33]

APPROACH TO THE USE OF GLUCOCORTICOIDS BASED ON ORGAN SYSTEM INVOLVEMENT

Glucocorticoids are often initiated in the setting of lupus flare, worsening of disease activity, or sometimes for persistently active disease.[34] The goal for the use of glucocorticoids is to suppress the inflammatory and autoimmune processes related to SLE and clinically to induce remission or improvement in disease activity. In this section, we provide an approach based on organ system involvement (Table 2).

Mucocutaneous

While the majority of mucocutaneous manifestations of SLE are treated with antimalarial medications (e.g., hydroxychloroquine) with or without topical glucocorticoids or immunosuppressants, occasionally glucocorticoids are required. Glucocorticoids are prescribed in particular when the skin rash involves a large part of the body's surface area where it becomes difficult to target with local glucocorticoids. Glucocorticoids are also prescribed as a bridge therapy until antimalarial or immunosuppressants start to take effect. It is very important to note that a low to moderate dose of glucocorticoids (oral prednisone) is usually enough to control the majority of mucocutaneous manifestations.[35,36]

Musculoskeletal

Arthritis, myositis, and tendonitis are the major manifestations in this system. Arthritis is very common in SLE and the mainstay treatment is nonsteroidal anti-inflammatory drugs (NSAIDs) and hydroxychloroquine. While mild arthritis can be treated with NSAIDs, more severe forms require the use of low (up to 20 mg/day) doses of prednisone and often immunosuppressants if patients exhibit signs of flare while tapering the prednisone dose below 7.5 mg/day. Methotrexate, azathioprine, and mycophenolate mofetil can be added to the treatment of arthritis. Myositis is uncommon in SLE and often occurs in the context of other manifestations of SLE. In general, mild myositis requires a low dose of prednisone and more severe cases might need moderate to high doses of prednisone along with immunosuppressants.

Cardiopulmonary

Serositis (pleuritis and pericarditis) with or without small effusions requires a low to moderate prednisone dose. NSAIDs are often used in the management of mild serositis, especially if it is occurring without other SLE manifestations. Myocarditis is usually associated with significant comorbidities for SLE patients and requires moderate to high dose of prednisone. Acute lupus pneumonitis can be a very serious manifestation of SLE requiring the use of high to very high doses of glucocorticoids.[37]

Renal

Lupus nephritis occurs in 50–75% of adults with SLE. It is a major cause of morbidity and predicts poor survival. In general, the manifestation of lupus nephritis emerges within the first 36 months from diagnosis, although some patients developed it later.[38] The cornerstone of treatment of lupus nephritis continues to be glucocorticoids.[25,26,39] Proliferative lupus nephritis will usually require high doses of corticosteroids as part of the induction treatment along with immunosuppressive agents.[40–42] Pulse therapy might be justified in selected patients with disease resistant to high doses of prednisone after 4–6 weeks. Patients with pure mesangial or membranous lupus nephritis are in general also treated with glucocorticoids. The effects of cyclosporine or pulse cyclophosphamide in patients with membranous disease was evaluated in 41 patients in a randomized trials. Austin et al. showed that the rate of complete remission (proteinuria <0.3 g/day) was higher in the group who received immunosuppressive agents compared to glucocorticoids alone (46% vs 13% respectively at 1 year).[43] Clinical trials in lupus nephritis focus mainly on patients with

TABLE 2 Regimen of Glucocorticoids for Systemic Lupus Erythematosus Manifestations

Manifestations	Low (e.g., Prednisone up to 20 mg/day)	Moderate (e.g., Prednisone 20–40 mg/day)	High (e.g., Prednisone 40–80 mg/day)	Intravenous (e.g., Pulses x 1–3)
Mucocutaneous	Initial or bridging until hydroxychloroquine in full effect	If unresponsive to low of bridging until hydroxy-chloroquine in full effect	Severe discoid	No
Vasculitic skin lesions ONLY	Yes	Yes, if unresponsive to lower doses	No	No
Arthralgia and/or arthritis myositis	Moderate to severe polyarthritis	No	No	No
	Mainly increased creatine Kinase with little weakness	With significant muscle weakness	No	No
Constitutional	Usually dramatic response	No	No	No
Acute lupus pneumonitis	No	May respond	If unresponsive to moderate	No
Myocarditis	No	May respond	If unresponsive to moderate	If unresponsive to moderate
Serositis	If unresponsive to NSAIDs	If unresponsive to low	If unresponsive to moderate	No
Lupus nephritis (WHO I, II)	May respond	If unresponsive to low	No	No
Lupus nephritis (WHO III, IV, V)	No	No	Induction dose	Unresponsive to high dose
Thrombocytopenia	For moderate thrombocytopenia (50–120,000)	No	For refractory thrombo-cytopenia or very low initial levels (<50,000)	Severe, life-threat-ening, refractory
Vasculitic skin lesions with major organ involvement	No	No	Yes	Unresponsive to high dose
Neuropsychiatric lupus	No	Lupus headache	Yes	Unresponsive to high dose

proliferative or proliferative and membranous nephritis.[40,44] There is a lack of clinical trials to determine the role of immunosuppressive therapy in pure mesangial or membranous nephritis where glucocorticoids alone might be beneficial.[32] Patients with more severe mesangial or membranous disease may respond to moderate (20–40 mg/day) doses of glucocorticoids in the induction phase along with an immunosuppressive agent.

Hematologic

Neutropenia/lymphopenia as an isolated finding in SLE does not require glucocorticoids. Usually, the count normalizes or improves when lupus disease activity overall improves in response to treatment.

Hemolytic anemia may occur alone or in the context of SLE with other organ involvement and it is usually responsive to SLE treatment. More severe forms of hemolytic anemia might require moderate to high doses of prednisone with or without immunosuppressive agents.

Thrombocytopenia is usually asymptomatic and is not associated with bleeding unless the platelet counts drop significantly below 35,000/mm^3. Symptomatic thrombocytopenia might require low to moderate doses of glucocorticoids with or without immunosuppressive agents. Severe forms of thrombocytopenia may require close monitoring in a hospital setting and pulse therapy with methylprednisolone followed by high-dose prednisone and an immunosuppressive agent.

Neuropsychiatric

Neuropsychiatric lupus often presents diagnostic and therapeutic challenges.[45] With the lack of randomized trials for new drugs for neuropsychiatric lupus, glucocorticoids continue to be the cornerstone agents. Glucocorticoids are used in the induction phase of treatment and usually in moderate to high doses. Other manifestations of neuropsychiatric lupus, such as myelitis and generalized seizures, might require pulse therapy with methylprednisolone.[46] Denburg et al. in a small trial (n = 10) showed that improvement in cognition and mood were observed following brief treatment with a low dose of glucocorticoids in individual women with mild SLE.[47] Other studies suggested the use of immunosuppressive agents (azathioprine and cyclophosphamide) in the treatment of neuropsychiatric lupus.[48,49]

TAPERING AND WITHDRAWAL OF GLUCOCORTICOIDS

If administered chronically, glucocorticoids can cause suppression of the hypothalamic-pituitary-adrenal axis, which leads to adrenal atrophy and loss of cortisol secretion ability. The mineralocorticoid synthesis of the adrenal stays functionally intact because it is independent of ACTH, which is suppressed with chronic exogenous glucocorticoids intake. The time needed to suppress the hypothalamic-pituitary-adrenal axis phenomenon is very individual and it depends on the dose of glucocorticoids and glucocorticoid sensitivity, which varies among individuals.[50] Cooper et al. found that a daily dose of 7.5 mg or more of prednisolone or equivalent for at least 3 weeks could anticipate adrenal hypofunction and adrenal insufficiency if glucocorticoids are stopped abruptly.[51] The risk of adrenal insufficiency is low in patients who have received glucocorticoids for less than 3 weeks or have been treated with alternate-day prednisolone therapy.[52,53] Suppression of the hypothalamic-pituitary-adrenal axis is reduced to within a week if the dose is more than 15 mg/day.[54] It has been estimated that the adrenal gland may take 1 year to fully recover after glucocorticoids treatment,[18] although this is not the usual clinical experience.

Tapering of glucocorticoids therapy can be complicated by the occurrence of glucocorticoid reduction syndrome. This syndrome includes symptoms related to adrenal insufficiency and pseudorheumatic complaints, which might simulate a flare of SLE.[55] In general, patients respond well to reinstitution of the lowest previous dose of glucocorticoids.

After achieving improvement in disease activity or remission in lupus patients, glucocorticoids are usually tapered to the lowest possible dose, but the aim should be to stop them entirely. For patients on divided doses of prednisone during the day, it is reasonable first to try to change it to a single dose in the morning.[56] Once this phase is accomplished, it will be important to determine the pace of reduction of the morning dose of glucocorticoids. This depends on the initial dose of prednisone, initial disease manifestation, responsiveness of the patient to glucocorticoids, and the tolerance of the patient to the tapering. Although the aim is to completely stop glucocorticoids, this might be impossible and very challenging in a few patients. There are some patients who require a maintenance dose of glucocorticoids to prevent flare of their disease.[57] There is no agreement on how to taper glucocorticoids: some authors use the "logarithmic" approach (e.g., 60, 40, 20, 15, 10, 7.5, 5, 2.5, 0 mg/day) and others use a "linear" approach (e.g. 60, 50, 40, 30, 20, 10, 0 mg/day).

At the Toronto Lupus Clinic, we use a very slow 7-week tapering schedule. For instance if the patient in on 10 mg/day of prednisone and the aim is to decrease to 7.5 mg/day, the patient will be lowering the dose to 7.5 mg for only 1 day in the first week, 2 days in the second week, 3 days in the third week, and so forth until in the seventh week the patient is taking 7.5 mg/day on all 7 days. This slow tapering approach is less associated with risk of adrenal insufficiency. Although an alternate-day regimen has been used in SLE, we do not recommend this approach because symptoms tend to become active by the end of the second day.[58]

SIDE EFFECTS OF CORTICOSTEROIDS

Adverse effects of glucocorticoids are common and depend on several factors, including the dosage and the duration of therapy[59–61] and individual patient susceptibility (Table 3). For instance, some adverse effects, such as skeletal growth inhibition and suppression of the hypothalamic-pituitary-adrenal axis, cataracts, acne, and weight gain might occur with a low dose of glucocorticoids.[59] Other adverse effects such as infection, psychosis, myopathy, and hyperlipidemia might require an exposure to moderate or high doses of glucocorticoids. Other studies have found that each intravenous pulse might be associated with an increase in the risk of osteoporotic fractures.[61] Each 2-month exposure to high-dose prednisone was associated with a 1.2-fold increase in the risk of avascular necrosis and stroke.[61]

Other factors implicated in the development of adverse effects to glucocorticoids are related to the host. The frequency and severity of adverse effects to glucocorticoids in two patients receiving the same dose of prednisone over the same period might differ. This can be explained by the susceptibility to glucocorticoid side effects and disease-specific differences. The array of adverse effects to glucocorticoids can be also explained by the presence of receptors to glucocorticoids on different cell types. Van Vollenhoven classified the adverse effects of glucocorticoids into three major categories related to the time of occurrence after the initiation of glucocorticoids[58]: (1) immediate, which occurs

TABLE 3 Side Effects of Glucocorticoids Therapy in Different Systems

Systems	Side Effects	Cautions/Comments
Fluid/electrolyte disturbances	Sodium retention	Use with caution in congestive heart failure or hypertensive patients
	Edema	Decrease salt intake
	Increased potassium excretion	Potassium supplements may be necessary if not adequately available in patient's dietary regimen
	Increased calcium excretion	Calcium supplements may be necessary if not adequately available in patient's dietary regimen
		Monitor for low bone density and consider the appropriate management for prevention and treatment
Gastrointestinal	Gastric irritation	Take with meals to prevent gastric upset
	Nausea/vomiting, weight gain, abdominal distention, peptic ulcer, ulcerative esophagitis, pancreatitis	Use of antiulcer agents whenever required; use in caution in patients with gastrointestinal diseases
Endocrine	Hypercortisolism, adrenal insufficiency menstrual irregularities (amenorrhea), precipitation of steroid induced diabetes and glucose intolerance	Associated with long-term use even at low dosages. May require modification of the patient's diet and addition of other appropriate therapies.
Cardiovascular	Hypertension	Use with extreme caution in patients with recent myocardial infarction because of an apparent association with left ventricular free-wall rupture.
	Thromboembolism and thrombophlebitis, congestive heart failure exacerbation	Use with care in patients with thromboembolic disorders because of reports (rare) of increased blood coagulability
Ocular	Posterior subcapsular cataracts, glaucoma	Prolonged use may result in increased intraocular pressure or damaged ocular nerve
	May enhance secondary fungal or viral infection of the eye	Use in patients with ocular herpes simplex may cause corneal perforation unless antiviral agents are prescribed
Musculoskeletal	Muscle pain or weakness, muscle wasting, pathologic long-bone or vertebral compression fractures, atrophy of protein matrix of bone, aseptic necrosis of weight bearing joints in particular	Use with caution in patients prone to development of the listed side effects and consider preventative measures as provided by specific guidelines such those for monitoring and treating osteoporosis
Neuropsychiatric	Headache, vertigo, seizure, insomnia, psychosis, increased motor activity	Use with caution at high doses in patients with convulsive or psychiatric disorders. Steroid-induced psychosis is dose related, occurs within 15–30 days of therapy, and it is treatable if glucocorticoids must be continued
Dermatologic	Acne, impaired wound healing, hirsutism, skin atrophy/increased fragility, ecchymoses	Ecchymoses are usually restricted to exposed potentially traumatized extremities with glucocorticoid use
Other	Increased susceptibility to infections, masked symptoms of infections	

after short exposure to glucocorticoids at low doses (e.g., fluid retention, blurry vision, weight gain, mood changes, immunosuppression, redistribution of fat body); (2) gradual, which occurs with more prolonged exposure to glucocorticoids (e.g., metabolic effects: hyperglycemia, hypertension, osteoporosis; muscle weakness, adrenal suppression, dyslipidemia, others); and (3) idiosyncratic, which are side effects occurring in unpredictable manner and not explained or related to the period of time or the dose (e.g., cataracts, avascular necrosis, psychosis, adrenal insufficiency).

FUTURE DIRECTION

Since their discovery, glucocorticoids continue to be the most potent anti-inflammatory medication available for the management of SLE. Glucocorticoids are used in particular in the context of recent flare, persistently active disease, and sometimes to maintain disease quiescence. Furthermore, glucocorticoids are considered the cornerstone agent utilized to treat several manifestations of SLE with different dosage ranges; low, moderate, high, and very high.

Unfortunately, glucocorticoids also exhibit several adverse effects that could occur either in a short period and or after long exposure. The effects of glucocorticoid are determined by several aspects, including disease factors, organ-specific factors, and host factors. There is no doubt that the effectiveness of glucocorticoids and the accompanying adverse effects vary between patients, and this could be related to host's cells susceptibility to glucocorticoids.

There has been a major drift in the way clinicians approach the use of glucocorticoids over the last decade with the emergence of two major approaches. Some clinicians continue to induce the majority of lupus manifestations with glucocorticoids, but they simultaneously aim to minimize the duration of exposure (lower cumulative dose over time) and the use of lower dosage regimen in the induction phase. Other clinicians promote the treatment of SLE without glucocorticoids in the induction phase and rely heavily on immunosuppressive agents and/or biological therapy.

Liz Lightstone is one of the pioneers who promoted SLE management with steroid-sparing regimens.[62] The rituxi-lup cohort demonstrated that oral glucocorticoids can be safely avoided in the treatment of lupus nephritis. In this cohort study, 50 consecutive lupus nephritis patients were treated with two doses of rituximab and methylprednisolone (500 mg) on days 1 and 15, and maintenance treatment of mycophenolate mofetil without oral glucocorticoids. It is very important to replicate the results of this cohort study in future randomized clinical trials before this approach can be widely adopted in the management of lupus nephritis. More recently, we have witnessed the emergence of tacrolimus in the management of lupus nephritis evaluated in Asian patients.[63] Liu et al. proposed the multitarget therapy for induction of lupus nephritis and the results of this randomized trial showed that the combination of tacrolimus and mycophenolate mofetil is superior to cyclophosphamide.[64] At the same time, it is very important to consider stopping not only glucocorticoids but also immunosuppressants in patients experiencing clinical remission.[65]

We have witnessed an advance in the management of SLE in the last five decades. Research has recently provided us with a better understanding of the immunologic alterations of SLE, leading to the creation of immunomodulatory agents. These new agents are designed to disrupt specific cell targets and pro-inflammatory pathways, with more specific targeted immunotherapy.[66,67] Several biological drugs have been studied for the management of active SLE aiming to have safer immunosuppression, especially with regards to cytotoxicity and serious infections.

Following the successful story of belimumab, there is hope for the future.[68,69] The lupus pipeline has several promising drug candidates currently in development and the approval of new biologic agents for the management of SLE could bring a new paradigm and change the way we treat lupus patients—perhaps without glucocorticoids or, as mentioned above, shorter exposure to and lower cumulative dose of glucocorticoids. Although the current standard of care for lupus patients hinges on glucocorticoids and immunosuppressive drugs, this might change in the future with the discovery of new biological therapies.

REFERENCES

1. Hench PS, et al. The effect of a hormone of the adrenal cortex (17-hydroxy-11-dehydrocorticosterone: compound E) and of pituitary adrenocortical hormone in arthritis: preliminary report. *Ann Rheum Dis* 1949;**8**(2):97–104.
2. Pollak VE, Pirani CL, Kark RM. Effect of large doses of prednisone on the renal lesions and life span of patients with lupus glomerulonephritis. *J Lab Clin Med* 1961;**57**:495–511.
3. Smith Jr FG, Litman N, Latta H. Lupus glomerulonephritis. The effect of large doses of corticosteroids on renal function and renal lesions in two children. *Am J Dis Child* 1965;**110**:302–8.
4. Cathcart ES, et al. Beneficial effects of methylprednisolone "pulse" therapy in diffuse proliferative lupus nephritis. *Lancet* 1976;**1**(7952):163–6.
5. Urowitz MB, Gladman DD. Contributions of observational cohort studies in systemic lupus erythematosus: the University of Toronto Lupus Clinic experience. *Rheum Dis Clin North Am* 2005;**31**(2):211–21. v.
6. Buttgereit F, et al. Standardised nomenclature for glucocorticoid dosages and glucocorticoid treatment regimens: current questions and tentative answers in rheumatology. *Ann Rheum Dis* 2002;**61**(8):718–22.
7. Webster JI, Tonelli L, Sternberg EM. Neuroendocrine regulation of immunity. *Annu Rev Immunol* 2002;**20**:125–63.
8. Rhen T, Cidlowski JA. Antiinflammatory action of glucocorticoids–new mechanisms for old drugs. *N Engl J Med* 2005;**353**(16):1711–23.
9. Chatham WW, Kimberly RP. Treatment of lupus with corticosteroids. *Lupus* 2001;**10**(3):140–7.
10. Lu NZ, Cidlowski JA. The origin and functions of multiple human glucocorticoid receptor isoforms. *Ann N Y Acad Sci* 2004;**1024**:102–23.
11. Vandevyver S, et al. New insights into the anti-inflammatory mechanisms of glucocorticoids: an emerging role for glucocorticoid-receptor-mediated transactivation. *Endocrinology* 2013;**154**(3):993–1007.
12. Buttgereit F, Wehling M, Burmester GR. A new hypothesis of modular glucocorticoid actions: steroid treatment of rheumatic diseases revisited. *Arthritis Rheum* 1998;**41**(5):761–7.
13. Barnes PJ. Anti-inflammatory actions of glucocorticoids: molecular mechanisms. *Clin Sci (Lond)* 1998;**94**(6):557–72.
14. Lipworth BJ. Therapeutic implications of non-genomic glucocorticoid activity. *Lancet* 2000;**356**(9224):87–9.
15. Boumpas DT, et al. Glucocorticoid therapy for immune-mediated diseases: basic and clinical correlates. *Ann Intern Med* 1993;**119**(12):1198–208.
16. Jacobs JWG, Bijlsma JWJ. Glucocorticoid therapy. In: Firestein GS, et al., editor. *Kelley's textbook of rheumatology*. Philadelphia, PA: Elsevier, Saunders; 2013.
17. DiBattista JA, et al. Glucocorticoid receptor mediated inhibition of interleukin-1 stimulated neutral metalloprotease synthesis in normal human chondrocytes. *J Clin Endocrinol Metab* 1991;**72**(2):316–26.

18. Al-Maini MH, et al. Serum levels of soluble Fas correlate with indices of organ damage in systemic lupus erythematosus. *Lupus* 2000;**9**(2):132–9.

19. Zhu XJ, et al. High-dose dexamethasone inhibits BAFF expression in patients with immune thrombocytopenia. *J Clin Immunol* 2009;**29**(5):603–10.

20. Buttgereit F, Zhou H, Seibel MJ. Arthritis and endogenous glucocorticoids: the emerging role of the 11beta-HSD enzymes. *Ann Rheum Dis* 2008;**67**(9):1201–3.

21. Ginzler EM, Aranow C. Prevention and treatment of adverse effects of corticosteroids in systemic lupus erythematosus. *Baillieres Clin Rheumatol* 1998;**12**(3):495–510.

22. Temprano KK, Bandlamudi R, Moore TL. Antirheumatic drugs in pregnancy and lactation. *Semin Arthritis Rheum* 2005;**35**(2):112–21.

23. McEvoy GK, et al. *AHFS drug information.* Bethesda, MD: American Society of Healt-Systems Pharmacists; 1996.

24. Bell PR, et al. Reversal of acute clinical and experimental organ rejection using large doses of intravenous prednisolone. *Lancet* 1971;**1**(7705):876–80.

25. Gourley MF, et al. Methylprednisolone and cyclophosphamide, alone or in combination, in patients with lupus nephritis. A randomized, controlled trial. *Ann Intern Med* 1996;**125**(7):549–57.

26. Boumpas DT, et al. Controlled trial of pulse methylprednisolone versus two regimens of pulse cyclophosphamide in severe lupus nephritis. *Lancet* 1992;**340**(8822):741–5.

27. Vischer TL, et al. A randomized, double-blind trial comparing a pulse of 1000 with 250 mg methylprednisolone in rheumatoid arthritis. *Clin Rheumatol* 1986;**5**(3):325–6.

28. Fan PT, et al. Effect of corticosteroids on the human immune response: comparison of one and three daily 1 gm intravenous pulses of methylprednisolone. *J Lab Clin Med* 1978;**91**(4):625–34.

29. Badsha H, et al. Low-dose pulse methylprednisolone for systemic lupus erythematosus flares is efficacious and has a decreased risk of infectious complications. *Lupus* 2002;**11**(8):508–13.

30. Badsha H, Edwards CJ. Intravenous pulses of methylprednisolone for systemic lupus erythematosus. *Semin Arthritis Rheum* 2003;**32**(6):370–7.

31. Howe HS, Boey ML, Feng PH. Methylprednisolone in systemic lupus erythematosus. *Singapore Med J* 1990;**31**(1):18–21.

32. Austin 3rd HA, et al. Prognostic factors in lupus nephritis. Contribution of renal histologic data. *Am J Med* 1983;**75**(3):382–91.

33. Danowski A, Magder L, Petri M. Flares in lupus: Outcome Assessment Trial (FLOAT), a comparison between oral methylprednisolone and intramuscular triamcinolone. *J Rheumatol* 2006;**33**(1):57–60.

34. Touma Z, Urowitz MB, Gladman DD. Outcome measures in systemic lupus erythematosus. *Indian J Rheumatol* 2013;**8**(Suppl. 1):S46–53. http://dx.doi.org/10.1016/j.injr.2013.11.015.

35. Jewell ML, McCauliffe DP. Patients with cutaneous lupus erythematosus who smoke are less responsive to antimalarial treatment. *J Am Acad Dermatol* 2000;**42**(6):983–7.

36. Callen JP. Management of cutaneous lupus erythematosus. In: Kuhn A, Lehmann P, Ruzicka T, editors. *Cutaneous lupus erythematosus.* Berlin: Springer; 2004. p. 437–44.

37. Law WG, et al. Acute lupus myocarditis: clinical features and outcome of an oriental case series. *Lupus* 2005;**14**(10):827–31.

38. Touma Z, et al. Time to recovery from proteinuria in patients with lupus nephritis receiving standard treatment. *J Rheumatol* 2014;**41**(4):688–97.

39. Houssiau FA, et al. Immunosuppressive therapy in lupus nephritis: the Euro-Lupus Nephritis Trial, a randomized trial of low-dose versus high-dose intravenous cyclophosphamide. *Arthritis Rheum* 2002;**46**(8):2121–31.

40. Touma Z, et al. Mycophenolate mofetil for induction treatment of lupus nephritis: a systematic review and metaanalysis. *J Rheumatol* 2011;**38**(1):69–78.

41. Ginzler EM, et al. Mycophenolate mofetil or intravenous cyclophosphamide for lupus nephritis. *N Engl J Med* 2005;**353**(21):2219–28.

42. Hahn BH, et al. American College of Rheumatology guidelines for screening, treatment, and management of lupus nephritis. *Arthritis Care Res (Hoboken)* 2012;**64**(6):797–808.

43. Austin HA, Vaughan EM, Balow JE. Lupus membranous nephropathy: randomized controlled trial of prednisone, cyclosporine and cyclophosphamide. *J Am Soc Nephrol* 2000;**11**(Suppl. 9):81A.

44. Steinberg AD, et al. Cyclophosphamide in lupus nephritis: a controlled trial. *Ann Intern Med* 1971;**75**(2):165–71.

45. Bortoluzzi A, et al. Development and validation of a new algorithm for attribution of neuropsychiatric events in systemic lupus erythematosus. *Rheumatology (Oxford)* 2015 May;**54**(5):891–8. http://dx.doi.org/10.1093/rheumatology/keu384. Epub 2014 Oct 21.

46. Jeltsch-David H, Muller S. Neuropsychiatric systemic lupus erythematosus: pathogenesis and biomarkers. *Nat Rev Neurol* 2014;**10**(10):579–96.

47. Denburg SD, Carbotte RM, Denburg JA. Corticosteroids and neuropsychological functioning in patients with systemic lupus erythematosus. *Arthritis Rheum* 1994;**37**(9):1311–20.

48. Barile-Fabris L, et al. Controlled clinical trial of IV cyclophosphamide versus IV methylprednisolone in severe neurological manifestations in systemic lupus erythematosus. *Ann Rheum Dis* 2005;**64**(4):620–5.

49. Mok CC, Lau CS, Wong RW. Treatment of lupus psychosis with oral cyclophosphamide followed by azathioprine maintenance: an open-label study. *Am J Med* 2003;**115**(1):59–62.

50. Bornstein SR. Predisposing factors for adrenal insufficiency. *N Engl J Med* 2009;**360**(22):2328–39.

51. Cooper MS, Stewart PM. Corticosteroid insufficiency in acutely ill patients. *N Engl J Med* 2003;**348**(8):727–34.

52. Ackerman GL, Nolsn CM. Adrenocortical responsiveness after alternate-day corticosteroid therapy. *N Engl J Med* 1968;**278**(8):405–9.

53. Schlaghecke R, et al. The effect of long-term glucocorticoid therapy on pituitary-adrenal responses to exogenous corticotropin-releasing hormone. *N Engl J Med* 1992;**326**(4):226–30.

54. Paris J. Pituitary-adrenal suppression after protracted administration of adrenal cortical hormones. *Proc Staff Meet Mayo Clin* 1961;**36**:305–17.

55. Dixon RB, Christy NP. On the various forms of corticosteroid withdrawal syndrome. *Am J Med* 1980;**68**(2):224–30.

56. Kountz DS, Clark CL. Safely withdrawing patients from chronic glucocorticoid therapy. *Am Fam Physician* 1997;**55**(2):521–5, 529-30.

57. Aranow C, Emy J, Barland P. Reactivation of inactive systemic lupus erythematosus. *Scand J Rheumatol* 1996;**25**(5):282–6.

58. van Vollenhoven RF. Corticosteroids in rheumatic disease. Understanding their effects is key to their use. *Postgrad Med* 1998;**103**(2):137–42.

59. McDonough AK, Curtis JR, Saag KG. The epidemiology of glucocorticoid-associated adverse events. *Curr Opin Rheumatol* 2008;**20**(2):131–7.

60. Gladman DD, et al. Predictive factors for symptomatic osteonecrosis in patients with systemic lupus erythematosus. *J Rheumatol* 2001;**28**(4):761–5.

61. Zonana-Nacach A, et al. Damage in systemic lupus erythematosus and its association with corticosteroids. *Arthritis Rheum* 2000;**43**(8):1801–8.

62. Condon MB, et al. Prospective observational single-centre cohort study to evaluate the effectiveness of treating lupus nephritis with rituximab and mycophenolate mofetil but no oral steroids. *Ann Rheum Dis* 2013;**72**(8):1280–6.

63. Mok CC, et al. Tacrolimus versus mycophenolate mofetil for induction therapy of lupus nephritis: a randomised controlled trial and long-term follow-up. *Ann Rheum Dis* 2014-206456 Published Online First: 30 December 2014. http://dx.doi.org/10.1136/annrheumdis-2014-206456.

64. Liu Z, et al. Multitarget therapy for induction treatment of lupus nephritis: a randomized trial. *Ann Intern Med* 2015;**162**(1):18–26.

65. Touma Z, et al. Do we know how and when to stop immunosuppressants in lupus patients? *Ann Rheum Dis* 2014;**73**(Suppl. 2):76.

66. Al Rayes H, Touma Z. Profile of epratuzumab and its potential in the treatment of systemic lupus erythematosus. *Drug Des Devel Ther* 2014;**8**:2303–10.

67. Touma Z, Urowitz MB, Gladman DD. Systemic lupus erythematosus: an update on current pharmacotherapy and future directions. *Expert Opin Biol Ther* 2013;**13**(5):723–37.

68. Navarra SV, et al. Efficacy and safety of belimumab in patients with active systemic lupus erythematosus: a randomised, placebo-controlled, phase 3 trial. *Lancet* 2011;**377**(9767):721–31.

69. Furie R, et al. A phase III, randomized, placebo-controlled study of belimumab, a monoclonal antibody that inhibits B lymphocyte stimulator, in patients with systemic lupus erythematosus. *Arthritis Rheum* 2011;**63**(12):3918–30.

Chapter 62

Cytotoxic-Immunosuppressive Drug Treatment

Eleni A. Frangou[1], George Bertsias[2], Dimitrios T. Boumpas[3]

[1]*Biomedical Research Foundation of the Academy of Athens, Athens, Greece;* [2]*Rheumatology, Clinical Immunology and Allergy Medical School, University of Crete Heraklion, Heraklion, Greece;* [3]*Rheumatology and Clinical Immunology, 4th Department of Medicine, Medical School, University of Athens and Biomedical Research Foundation of the Academy of Athens, Athens, Greece*

SUMMARY

The use of alkylating agents, such as cyclophosphamide, has decreased in recent years because of concerns for ovarian toxicity. Their use is limited to patients with severe disease or disease refractory to inhibitors of nucleotide synthesis, such as mycophenolate acid or azathioprine. Because of a more favorable efficacy to toxicity ratio, mycophenolate acid is the drug of first choice in moderately severe lupus and can be used both as induction and maintenance therapy. Azathioprine is predominantly used as a steroid-sparing agent and as maintenance treatment. Calcineurin inhibitors like cyclosporine A and tacrolimus are used less often—predominantly as steroid-sparing agents or in patients with refractory disease—because of their renal toxicity. Patients on cytotoxic-immunosuppressive agents have increased risk for both common and opportunistic infections.

INTRODUCTION

Cytotoxic drugs were introduced in medicine as antineoplastic agents for their ability to interrupt nucleic acid and protein synthesis in cancer cells. Due to their immunosuppressing and immunomodulating properties, they were subsequently used for the management of autoimmune diseases, including systemic lupus erythematosus (SLE).[1] Other immunosuppressive agents, such as calcineurin inhibitors, were introduced in lupus therapeutics from renal transplantation.

General indications for cytotoxic/immunosuppressive therapy in SLE are shown in Table 1. According to the current treatment paradigm, an initial period of intensive immunosuppressive therapy (induction therapy) is first introduced to control aberrant immunologic activity, induce disease quiescence, and minimize tissue injury. This is followed by a longer period of less intensive and less toxic therapy to retain remission and prevent subsequent flares (maintenance therapy).

ALKYLATING AGENTS

Cyclophosphamide

Mechanism of Action and Pharmacokinetics

Cyclophosphamide is an oxazaphosphorine that contributes alkyl groups to DNA, forming covalent linkages. It depletes T and B cells and suppresses antibody production. It is metabolized to 4-hydroxycyclophosphamide and its tautomer aldophosphamide by liver cytochrome P450 enzyme. In target cells, aldophosphamide is converted to the alkylating phosphoramide mustard and acrolein. Tautomers are detoxified to inactive carboxycyclophosphamide. According to the level of detoxification, individuals experience different drug efficacy and toxicity.

Drugs that induce hepatic microsomal enzymes (barbiturates, alcohol, phenytoin, and rifampicin) increase cyclophosphamide efficacy and toxicity; conversely, inhibitors of hepatic microsomal enzymes (antimalarials, allopurinol, and tricyclic antidepressants) decrease its efficacy and toxicity.

Oral and intravenous (IV) administration of cyclophosphamide (CYC) result in similar plasma concentrations. Its half-life in serum is 6 h. Metabolites are excreted by the kidneys; therefore, dosage is adjusted to creatinine clearance. The protocol for its administration is presented in Table 2.

Adverse Effects

Common adverse effects are nausea, vomiting, hair thinning, and reversible alopecia. Serious but less frequent adverse effects are bone marrow, gonadal, and bladder toxicity, as well as malignancy. Mucosal ulceration, skin pigmentation, liver, lung, and cardiac toxicity have also been reported.

TABLE 1 Indications for Cytotoxic-Immunosuppressive Drug Treatment in SLE

Extensive involvement of nonmajor organs refractory to other agents

Failure to respond to or inability to taper glucocorticoids to acceptable doses for long-term use

Major organ involvement

• Renal disease	Proliferative lupus nephritis
	Membranous lupus nephritis
• Hematologic disease	Severe thrombocytopenia (PLTs < 20,000/mm^3)
	Thrombotic thrombocytopenic purpura-like syndrome
	Hemolytic anemia
	Aplastic anemia
	Neutropenia not responding to glucocorticoids
• Gastrointestinal disease	Abdominal vasculitis
• Cardiac disease	Myocarditis with decreased left ventricular function
	Pericarditis with pending tamponade
• Pulmonary disease	Pneumonitis
	Alveolar hemorrhage
• Nervous system disease	Mononeuritis multicomplex
	Psychosis refractory to glucocorticoids
	Cerebritis
	Transverse myelitis
	Optic neuritis

TABLE 2 Protocols for IV Cyclophosphamide Administration

EUROLUPUS Protocol[12]

Six fortnightly pulses of IV cyclophosphamide 500 mg in combination with three daily doses of IV methylprednisolone 750 mg followed by maintenance therapy with azathioprine

NIH Protocol[7,10]

Seven monthly pulses of IV cyclophosphamide 0.5–1 g/m^2 followed by quarterly pulses for at least one after remission, together with monthly pulses of IV methylprednisolone

Dose Adjustment

- 25% reduction in creatinine clearance 25–50 ml/min
- 30–50% reduction in creatinine clearance <25 ml/min
- Administered 8–12 h before dialysis
- Half the dose in individuals older than 65 years

Prevention from Nausea-Vomiting

Dexamethasone 10-mg single dose plus a serotonin receptor antagonist (granisetron 1 mg with cyclophosphamide dose, repeat dose in 12 h or ondasetrone 8 mg tid for 1–2 d)

Prevention from Bladder Toxicity

- 5% dextrose and 0.45% saline (2 l at 250 ml/h) and high-dose oral fluids for 24 h
- Consider 2-mercaptoethane sulfonate Na (MESNA) (each dose 20% of total cyclophosphamide dose) IV or orally at 0, 2, 4, and 6 h after cyclophosphamide administration
- Consider insertion of a three-way urinary catheter for continuous bladder flushing with standard antibiotic irrigating solution or normal saline

Prevention from Gonadal Toxicity

- In females, subcutaneous leuprolide 3.75 mg 2 weeks prior to each dose
- In males, intramuscular testosterone 100 mg every 2 weeks

Monitoring

- Complete blood count with differential, creatinine, liver enzymes, and urinalysis every 1–2 weeks initially, and 1–3 months thereafter. Urinalysis 6–12 months following cessation

Myelotoxicity is dose- and age-dependent. Severe thrombocytopenia is rare. With IV administration, the nadir of lymphocytes occurs on days 7–10 and that of granulocytes on days 10–14. Recovery from granulocytopenia occurs after 21–28 days. An increased risk of infection, including bacterial and opportunistic infections (*Pneumocystitis jiroveci*, fungal infections and *Nocardia*) and reactivation of latent herpes zoster, *Mycobacterium tuberculosis*, and human papillomavirus have been reported. Risk of infection is increased with concomitant use of high doses of glucocorticoids (especially >0.5 mg/day) and/or when leukocytes fall below 3000/mm^3.[2]

Sustained amenorrhea rates were 0% in patients <25 years who received a short course of IV-CYC (≤7 pulses), 12% in those aged 26–30 years, and 25% in those >30 years. A longer treatment course (≥15 pulses) induced sustained amenorrhea in 17% of patients aged <25 years, 43% of those aged 26–30 years, and 100% of those older than 30 years. In males, gonadal toxicity may develop with as little as 7 g cumulative cyclophosphamide dose.[3,4]

Bladder toxicity is time-dependent and includes sterile hemorrhagic cystitis presenting with microscopic or gross hematuria and voiding symptoms. Bladder carcinoma can occur and risk is lifelong. Risk factors are a cumulative dose of cyclophosphamide >100 g and smoking. Patients with hematuria should be evaluated with cystoscopy after exclusion of renal causes of hematuria.[5]

Patients exposed to cyclophosphamide have increased risk of hematologic malignancies (including myelodysplastic syndrome, acute leukemia, non-Hodgkin's lymphoma), mainly if treated more than 2–3 years or with cumulative doses above 100 g.[6]

Cyclophosphamide is contraindicated in pregnancy.

Use in Renal Disease

In moderate to severe proliferative lupus nephritis (LN), pulse IV-CYC is effective in delaying renal scarring, preserving renal function, and reducing risk for developing end-stage renal disease (ESRD). Combination of pulse IV-CYC with monthly pulses of IV methylprednisolone (IV-MP) improves renal outcomes without increasing toxicity.[7–10]

In European patients, low-dose IV-CYC (six fortnightly pulses 500 mg each, in combination with three daily doses IV-MP 750 mg) followed by maintenance therapy with azathioprine had comparable efficacy and less toxicity than eight pulses of IV-CYC (also followed by azathioprine).[3–12] At the 10-year follow-up, rates of death, sustained doubling of serum creatinine, and ESRD were comparable in the two regimens, suggesting that the low-dose regimen could be an alternative option for white patients with moderately severe LN.[13] Preliminary data suggest that low-dose IV-CYC may be efficacious also in nonwhite patients, although further confirmation will be required.[14]

In membranous (class V) LN, induction therapy with IV-CYC every alternate month ($0.5–1 \, g/m^2$) for 11 months combined with alternate-day oral prednisone appears to be as effective as cyclosporine A, in inducing remission of nephrotic syndrome, and is associated with significantly lower relapse rates.[15]

Use in Extrarenal Disease

Cyclophosphamide administered as monthly pulses IV-CYC, in combination with IV-MP pulses followed by oral glucocorticoids, is effective in the management of severe or refractory extrarenal lupus manifestations, such as severe thrombocytopenia (platelets $<20 \, 000/mm^3$), autoimmune hemolytic anemia, neurologic disease, acute pneumonitis, alveolar hemorrhage, abdominal vasculitis, and extensive skin disease.[16,17]

NUCLEOTIDE SYNTHESIS INHIBITORS

Azathioprine

Mechanism of Action and Pharmacokinetics

Azathioprine is transformed into 6-mercaptopurine by glutathione. 6-Mercaptopurine is subsequently converted to thioinosinic acid and 6-thioguanine, which are integrated into DNA and RNA, thus impairing their synthesis. Consequently, azathioprine inhibits the proliferation of lymphocytes. Thioinosinic acid and 6-thioguanine are degraded by xanthine oxidase or S-methyltrasnferase into 6-thiouric acid, which is excreted by the kidneys. Therefore, azathioprine dosage is adjusted to creatinine clearance (Table 3). Coadministration with allopurinol increases the risk of toxicity and should be avoided. Azathioprine has been

associated with resistance to warfarin. Dosage and monitoring are presented in Table 3.

Adverse Effects

Gastrointestinal symptoms are frequent, leading to drug discontinuation. Liver enzyme elevation may occur; however, severe liver injury is rare. Reversible, dose-related bone marrow toxicity is also common; leucopenia and thrombocytopenia can occur in patients receiving even low-dose azathioprine. Toxicity may be idiosyncratic due to genetic polymorphisms in S-methyltransferase, resulting in decreased activity.[18] At doses of 2–2.5 mg/kg/day, azathioprine appears to be safe in the long term, without significantly increasing the risk for infection. It is associated with a slightly increased risk for nonmelanoma skin cancer when treatment duration is above 10 years and cumulative disease above 600 g.[19]

Use in Renal Disease

The European League Against Rheumatism (EULAR) recommends the use of azathioprine as induction treatment only in mild proliferative LN, when other agents such as cyclophosphamide or mycophenolate cannot be used[20,21] Both the EULAR and the American College of Rheumatology recommend azathioprine for maintenance immunosuppressive therapy in proliferative LN.[22] In addition, azathioprine can be used as a steroid-sparing agent in class V and class I–II LN with persistent proteinuria >1 g/day despite optimal renin-angiotensin-aldosterone axis blockade.[22–24]

Use in Extrarenal Disease

Azathioprine is administered in moderately severe lupus manifestations, such as thrombocytopenia (platelet counts (PLTs) 20–50,000/mm³), serositis, and neurological disease, usually in combination with moderate to high doses of glucocorticoids.

Mycophenolate Mofetil/Mycophenolate Acid

Mechanism of Action and Pharmacokinetics

Mycophenolate mofetil (MMF)/mycophenolate acid (MPA) is an inhibitor of inosine monophosphate dehydrogenase, an enzyme involved in purine nucleotide synthesis. It inhibits de novo guanosine synthesis without being incorporated into the DNA. It suppresses lymphocyte proliferation, antibody production, and also antigen presentation, migration of myeloid dendritic cells, and adhesion molecule production.

Mycophenolate is orally administered either as morfolinoethyl ester (MMF) or as a salt (enteric-coated mycophenolate sodium, eMPA). Data from transplantation medicine and LN studies suggest that 720 mg of eMPA are roughly equivalent to 1 g of MMF. MPA bioavailability is decreased

TABLE 3 Major Indications for the Use of Nucleotide Synthesis Inhibitors in SLE

	Azathioprine	MMF/MPA
Extrarenal disease	Skin manifestations, PLT 20,000–50,000/mm³, serositis	Moderate to severe disease if patients are not responding or are intolerant to azathioprine
Renal disease	*Induction therapy*	*Induction therapy*
	Mild–moderate proliferative LN	Moderately severe proliferative LN
	Patients opposed to cyclophosphamide	Pure membranous LN with nephrotic-range proteinuria
		Black and Hispanic patients
	Maintenance therapy	*Maintenance therapy*
	Proliferative LN	Moderately severe–severe proliferative LN
	Pure membranous LN as a steroid-sparing agent	Pure membranous LN
		Black and Hispanic patients
Dosage	Starting dose is 1 mg/kg/d with the usual dose at 2–3 mg/kg/day in 1–3 doses taken with food,	1–3 g/d in two divided doses
	25% dose reduction if creatinine clearance is 10–30 ml/min,	Maximum 1 g/d in creatinine clearance <25 ml/min
	50% reduction if creatinine clearance is <10 ml/min,	
	Administered post-hemodialysis	
Coadministration with other drugs	Avoid allopurinol	Avoid azathioprine
	Associated with resistance to warfarin	
Monitoring	Complete blood count with differential, creatinine, liver enzymes every 1–2 weeks.	Complete blood count (at baseline and biweekly during the first month, and then quarterly)
	Repeat every 1–3 months	Liver and renal function tests (at baseline, at 1 month and then quarterly)
		Discontinue if leukocytes are <3500/mm³
		Discontinue if neutrophils are <1300/mm³

by food intake. Peak levels occur at 1–2 h after oral administration. It is bound to albumin, so its free levels may be increased in hypoalbuminemia. In the liver, it is metabolized to inactive mycophenolic acid glucuronide, which is converted back to MPA through enterohepatic circulation. It is mainly excreted in the urine as mycophenolic acid glucuronide; therefore, dose is adjusted to creatinine clearance. Antiacids and chlolestyramine decrease its bioavailability; coadministration with valacyclovir may lead to neutropenia; and coadministration with azathioprine should be avoided. Dosage and monitoring are presented in Table 3.

Adverse Effects

Most common side effects are gastrointestinal symptoms such as nausea, vomiting, and diarrhea which are minimized by decreasing or dividing the daily dose, or by using the eMPA form. Bone marrow toxicity and leukopenia may occur mainly in hypoalbuminemic patients. Thrombocytopenia is uncommon, and pure red cell aplasia has been reported upon coadministration with other immunosuppressants. Bacterial, fungal, and viral infections, mainly respiratory tract infections, herpes zoster, and cellulitis, have been reported. Risk of cytomegalovirus and BK virus infections is dose-dependent. Increased liver enzymes, dry cough and dyspnea that reverse after discontinuation have also been reported. MPA is contraindicated in pregnancy.[25]

Use in Renal Disease

Several randomized controlled trials have demonstrated that the effectiveness of MPA (administered in the form of MMF) as induction therapy in LN is equal or superior to that of cyclophosphamide. Post hoc analysis of the Asperva Lupus Management Study (ALMS) trial showed that black and Hispanic patients were more likely to respond to MMF than to IV-CYC. Meta-analyses comparing the two agents have shown that MMF was associated with significantly reduced risk for amenorrhea. Rates of leucopenia and infections also tended to be lower, although higher doses (MMF >2 g/d) confer increased risk for serious infections.[26–30]

TABLE 4 Calcineurin Inhibitors in SLE

	Cyclosporine A	Tacrolimus
Dosage	1.5–6 mg/kg/d in two doses administered at the same time every day with or between meals	1–4 mg/d in two doses administered at the same time every day
	Trough levels should be < 150 ng/ml	Trough levels should be < 6 ng/ml
Avoid in	Creatinine clearance <60 ml/min	
	Severe uncontrolled hypertension	
	Advanced tubule-interstitial disease and tubular atrophy on renal biopsy	
Monitoring	Creatinine every 2 weeks initially: • If creatinine increase is >30%, dose is decreased until creatinine returns to normal. • If creatinine increase is >50%, calcineurin inhibitor (CNI) should be discontinued. Complete blood count, potassium, liver enzymes, albumin, and alkaline phosphatase (ALP) every 1–3 months.	

These results led to the recommendation for using MPA as initial treatment for most cases of class III–IV LN, although its long-term benefit against doubling serum creatinine, ESRD development, or death still remains to be determined.

Limited data suggest that MPA is also efficacious in severe forms of LN.[31] Post hoc analysis of the ALMS study have shown that in severe forms of LN with impaired renal function, MMF is comparable to IV-CYC in renal response, and also that in patients with severe crescentic disease or patients with multiple relapses, cyclophosphamide might be more effective than MMF.[27] Because further data are needed before adopting MMF as treatment for severe LN, currently the combination of cyclophosphamide and methylprednisolone IV pulse therapy is considered as the treatment of choice in severe LN cases.

In membranous LN, MMF has demonstrated comparable anti-proteinuric effects and remission of nephrotic syndrome at 6 months with IV-CYC (both combined with glucocorticoids). Consequently, and based on its more favorable toxicity profile, MPA is considered as first-line treatment in membranous LN and nephrotic-range proteinuria, although further evidence is awaited.[32,33]

MPA is efficacious in proliferative or membranous LN patients who relapsed or were refractory to previous treatment with cyclophosphamide or azathioprine, with renal response rates of 50–60%. Moreover, combination therapy with MPA (MMF 1–2 g/day) and calcineurin inhibitors (tacrolimus 4 mg/day) has been successfully used in the management of mixed class V + IV or refractory LN.[34] More recently, such multitargeted treatment yielded higher 6-month complete response rates than IV-CYC in Chinese patients with new-onset proliferative LN. Additional studies in other ethnic groups and with longer follow-up are required.[35]

Both MPA and azathioprine can be used for maintenance treatment in LN, with azathioprine being the treatment of choice when pregnancy is contemplated. MPA should be continued if it was successful as an induction treatment, whereas for the most severe LN cases, we recommend induction with IV-CYC followed by long-term maintenance with MPA[24,27,28]

Use in Extrarenal Disease

Limited evidence suggests that MPA is as effective as cyclophosphamide in inducing remission in mucocutaneous, musculoskeletal, cardiovascular, and pulmonary disease, vasculitis, and in normalizing serology. Its effectiveness in neuropsychiatric lupus still remains to be determined.[36,37] Currently, MPA may be considered for patients who are moderately severe disease intolerant or resistant to azathioprine.

CALCINEURIN INHIBITORS

Cyclosporine A

Mechanism of Action and Pharmacokinetics

Cyclosporine A (CsA) is a calcineurin inhibitor that prevents the dephosphorylation of nuclear factor of activated T-cells (NF-AT) and subsequently the transcription of interleukin (IL)-2 and other cytokines in T cells. CsA inhibits T-cell proliferation, reduces antigen presentation, and T-cell-mediated autoantibody production.

CsA is absorbed via a bile-dependent process from the gastrointestinal tract. Its peak serum concentration occurs within 1–8 h after oral administration. In plasma, it is bound to lipoproteins and only a small percentage circulates free. Bile deficit, diarrhea, and hypercholesterolemia reduce its blood levels. It is metabolized by cytochrome (CYP3A) enzymes in the liver and intestine to metabolites that are excreted mainly to the bile and less by the kidneys.

Several drugs lead to reduced (rifampin, phenytoin, phenobarbital, nafcillin) or increased (erythromycin, clarithromycin, azoles, calcium channel blockers, amiodarone, allopurinol, colchicine) CsA concentrations. Some drugs (NSAIDs, aminoglycosides, quinolones, ACE inhibitors, amphotericin B) may also augment its nephrotoxic effects. Dosage and monitoring are presented in Table 4.

Adverse Effects

Common adverse events include mild gastrointestinal complaints, hirsutism, and gingival hyperplasia. Mild elevation in serum alkaline phosphatase, hyperlipidemia, and hyperuricemia can be observed. Tremor, paresthesia, and myopathy may occur. A major effect is nephrotoxicity, which is dose dependent, and includes hypertension and tubular toxicity with hypomagnesemia, hyperkalemia, and acidosis. Characteristic kidney lesions are arteriolopathy, interstitial fibrosis, and tubular atrophy.

Use in Renal Disease

CsA is used in membranous LN at starting doses of 3–5 mg/kg/d. CsA plus alternate-day oral prednisone (1 mg/kg for 8 weeks and then tapered to 0.25 mg/kg) for 11 months appears to be as effective as five doses of IV-CYC every alternate month (0.5–1 g/m^2) plus the same dose of oral prednisone. However, after drug discontinuation, relapses of nephrotic syndrome were more common in the CsA group, suggesting that CsA requires long-term maintenance therapy to prevent flares.

As maintenance therapy in diffuse proliferative LN with preserved renal function, CsA is similar to azathioprine (1.5–2 mg/kg/d) in terms of flare-ups, proteinuria, blood pressure, and tolerance after 2–4 years of observation.[38]

Use in Extrarenal Disease

CsA has been used for the management of relapsing/refractory skin and hematological manifestations in SLE. Low-dose CsA improved disease activity, anti-DNA titers, and cytopenias in addition to modest reduction in the dose of glucocorticoids. The effect of CsA appears to be similar to that of azathioprine in terms of disease activity, response to treatment, flares, damage accrual, and quality of life. However, CsA was associated with the development of hypertension and/or an increase in serum creatinine. Thus, CsA may be used as an alternative steroid-sparing agent to azathioprine but with close monitoring of renal function and blood pressure.[39]

Tacrolimus

Mechanism of Action and Pharmacokinetics

Tacrolimus is a macrolide calcineurin inhibitor. Its mechanism of action and effects on immune function are similar to those described for CsA; however, it is 10–100 times more potent.

After oral administration, tacrolimus is absorbed by the gastrointestinal tract. In plasma, it is bound to proteins by 99%; its half-life is about 11 h. It is metabolized by the cytochrome P450-3A4 (CYP3A) enzymes in the liver and intestine; metabolites are not immunosuppressive and are excreted mainly in the bile and less by the kidneys. Dosage and monitoring are presented in Table 4.

Adverse Effects

Systemic administration has been associated with dose-dependent reversible nephrotoxicity, hypertension, and hypercholesterolemia, albeit less often than CsA. Tacrolimus may cause diabetes and neurological symptoms such as anxiety, tremor, paresthesia, delirium, and seizures. Hyperkalemia, hypomagnesemia, and cardiomyopathy in children can also be observed. Cosmetic effects are less frequent than with CsA.

Use in Renal Disease

In membranous LN, tacrolimus (0.1–0.2 mg/kg/d) plus glucocorticoids given for 6 months followed by maintenance therapy with azathioprine plus glucocorticoids achieved faster remission and lower flare rates than azathioprine or cyclophosphamide plus corticosteroids. Tacrolimus had comparable response rate with MMF in reducing proteinuria and also appears to be effective as induction therapy in Asian patients with proliferative LN.[40,41] In resistant mixed class V+IV LN, triple treatment with MMF (2 g/d), tacrolimus (4 mg/d), and glucocorticoids (3 pulses of IV methylprednisolone 0.5 g/d followed by oral prednisone) had superior remission rates compared with six monthly pulses of IV cyclophosphamide (1 g/m^2) plus steroids. The rate of adverse events was comparable.[34]

As maintenance therapy, tacrolimus (3 mg/d) appears to be effective and safe for up to 1-year follow-up and its addition to glucocorticoid therapy resulted in significant improvement in LN.[40]

Collectively, similar to CsA, preliminary evidence suggests that tacrolimus is effective in the treatment of class III–V LN in Asian patients. Further studies are needed due to the high rate of relapse of proteinuria after its discontinuation and the lack of long-term efficacy and safety data.

Use in Extrarenal Disease

Tacrolimus administration (1–3 mg/d for 1 year) in patients with skin and musculoskeletal disease resulted in a significant reduction in SLE disease activity index (SLEDAI) score and dose of glucocorticoids. Also, tacrolimus appears to be effective in severe cutaneous vasculitis, where cyclophosphamide and CsA had failed.[42]

GENERAL ISSUES IN LUPUS PATIENTS ON CYTOTOXIC/IMMUNOSUPPRESSIVE DRUG TREATMENT

Infections

Infections account for about 25% of all deaths in SLE. These include bacterial, viral, fungal, mycobacterial, and parasitic infections. The evaluation of a lupus patient on cytotoxic drug treatment presenting with symptoms and signs suggestive of an infection is challenging. The diagnostic approach and management need to follow a rational plan which takes into consideration the dominant clinical syndrome and its severity; the history of epidemiologic exposures; and the net state of immunosuppression, especially the presence of neutropenia and the concomitant use of high-dose glucocorticoids.

Diagnosis of bacterial infection is favored when the patient is presenting with chills or rigor, leukocytosis, or neutrophilia and increased number of band forms or metamyelocytes in peripheral blood smear, or increased C-reactive protein serum levels. The diagnosis of lupus fever is favored by the presence of leukopenia, low C3/C4, and/or increased anti-dsDNA titers. Parvovirus B19 and cytomegalovirus, mostly associated with intense immunosuppression, may be observed in SLE. Varicella zoster virus reactivation is an important issue; risk factors include cyclophosphamide or azathioprine exposure, history of malignancy, and LN.[43]

General measures to prevent infections include judicious use of glucocorticoids, simple hygiene measures and education, immunizations, and antimicrobial prophylaxis in patients with increased prevalence of certain infections, who receive heavy doses of immunosuppressive agents, or undergo procedures associated with transient bacteremia.[44] Tuberculin skin testing should be considered for patients who are candidates for treatment with long-term prednisone ≥15 mg/d or immunosuppressive drugs and patients <65 years old. Screening for hepatitis B and C viruses is prudent prior to starting high-dose steroids or other immunosuppressive medications. The incidence of *Pneumocystis* pneumonia (PCP) in SLE patients on cyclophosphamide is approximately 0.15%, whereas the overall prevalence of PCP in lupus patients is unknown. We do not routinely employ PCP prophylaxis in lupus. However, some authors recommend the administration of one double-strength tablet of trimethoprine-sulfomethoxazole three times a week or dapsone 100 mg/day if allergic to sulfamethoxazole, especially in patients with CD4 <300/mm.[45]

Immunizations

Evidence-based recommendations for autoimmune rheumatic diseases have been published by EULAR.[46] The key recommendations adjusted for SLE patients are presented in Table 5.

Malignancy

With the exception of cervical intraepithelial neoplasia, studies have failed to identify a clear association between cancer and exposure to immunosuppressive drugs. The use of lower cumulative doses of cyclophosphamide in current lupus protocols has substantially decreased the risk for bladder carcinoma. Women with SLE, especially those exposed to immunosuppressive drugs, are at higher risk and should be monitored with vigilance for cervical premalignant

TABLE 5 EULAR Recommendations for Vaccination in Adult Patients with Autoimmune Inflammatory Rheumatic Diseases

- Vaccination status should be assessed in the initial evaluation.
- Vaccination should ideally be administered during stable disease.
- Live attenuated vaccines should be avoided whenever possible in immunosuppressed patients.
- Vaccination can be administered during the use of disease-modifying antirheumatic drugs but should ideally be administered before B-cell targeting biologic therapy.
- Influenza and 23-valent polysaccharide pneumococcal vaccination should be strongly considered.
- Patients should receive tetanus toxoid vaccination in accordance with recommendations for the general population. In case of major and/or contaminated wounds in patients who received rituximab within the last 24 weeks, passive immunisation with tetanus immunoglobulin should be administered.
- Herpes zoster vaccination may be considered.
- Human papillomavirus vaccination should be considered according to existing recommendations.
- In hyposplenic/asplenic patients influenza, pneumococcal, *Haemophilus* influenzae b and meningococcal C vaccinations are recommended.
- Hepatitis A and/or B vaccinations are only recommended in patients at risk.
- Patients who plan to travel are recommended to receive vaccinations according to general rules, except for live attenuated vaccines.
- Bacillus Calmette–Guérin (BCG) vaccination is not recommended.

lesions. Patients exposed to cyclophosphamide who present with hematuria should undergo cystoscopy if this cannot be attributed to other causes.[47,48]

Pregnancy

Pregnancy may increase disease activity and precipitate the appearance of flares. The management of a pregnant woman with an SLE flare is challenging and should be dealt with on a multidisciplinary basis. Azathioprine, CsA, tacrolimus, and pulse glucocorticoids can be used during pregnancy. MMF and cyclophosphamide should be avoided. In severe flares, cyclophosphamide may be considered in the second or third trimester if there is no available alternative for major organ-threatening disease in the mother.[49]

REFERENCES

1. Tsokos GC. Systemic lupus erythematosus. *N Engl J Med* 2011; **365**:2110–21.
2. Pryor BD, Bologna SG, Kahl LE. Risk factors for serious infection during treatment with cyclophosphamide and high dose corticosteroids for systemic lupus erythematosus. *Arthritis Rheum* 1996;**39**:1475–82.

3. Boumpas DT, Austin 3rd HA, Vaughan EM, et al. Risk for sustained amenorrhea in patients with systemic lupus erythematosus receiving intermittent pulse cyclophosphamide therapy. *Ann Intern Med* 1993;**119**:366–9.

4. Dooley MA, Patterson CC, Susan L, et al. Preservation of ovarian function using depot leuprolide acetate during cyclophosphamide therapy for severe lupus nephritis. *Arthritis Rheum* 2000;**43**:2858.

5. Talar-Williams C, Hijazi YM, Walther MM, et al. Cyclophosphamide induced cystitis and bladder cancer in patients with Wegener's granulomatosis. *Ann Intern Med* 1996;**124**:477–84.

6. Radis CD, Kahl LE, Baker GL, et al. Effects of cyclophosphamide on the development of malignancy and on long-term survival on patients with rheumatoid arthritis. A 20-year followup study. *Arthritis Rheum* 1995;**38**:1120–7.

7. Boumpas DT, Austin HA, Vaughan EM, et al. Severe lupus nephritis: controlled trial of pulse methylprednisolone versus two different regimens of pulse cyclophosphamide. *Lancet* 1992;**340**:741–5.

8. Gourley MF, Austin HA, Scott D, et al. Methylprednisolone and cyclophosphamide, alone or in combination, in patients with lupus nephritis. A randomized, controlled trial. *Ann Intern Med* 1996;**125**:549–57.

9. Faedda R, Palomba D, Satta A, et al. Immunosuppressive treatment of the glomerulonephritis of systemic lupus. *Clin Nephrol* 1995;**44**:367–75.

10. Illei GG, Austin HA, Crane M, et al. Combination therapy with pulse cyclophosphamide plus pulse methylprednisolone improves long-term renal outcome without adding toxicity in patients with lupus nephritis. *Ann Intern Med* 2001;**135**:248–57.

11. Dooley MA, Hogan S, Jennette C, et al. Cyclophosphamide therapy for lupus nephritis: poor renal survival for black Americans. Glomerular disease collaborative network. *Kidney Int* 1997;**51**:1188–95.

12. Houssiau FA, Vasconcelos C, D'Cruz D, et al. Immunosuppressive therapy in lupus nephritis: the Euro-Lupus Nephritis Trial, a randomised trial of low dose versus high-dose intravenous cyclophosphamide. *Arthritis Rheum* 2002;**46**:2121–31.

13. Houssiau FA, Vasconcelos C, Cruz DP, et al. Early response to immunosuppressive therapy predicts good renal outcome in lupus nephritis: lessons from long-term follow-up of patients in Euro-Lupus Nephritis Trial. *Arthritis Rheum* 2004;**50**:3934–40.

14. The ACCESS trial group. Treatment of lupus nephritis with abatacept. The abatacept and cyclophosphamide combinations efficacy and safety study. *Arthritis Rheumatol* 2014;**66**:3096–104.

15. Austin 3rd HA, Illei GG, Braun MJ, Balow JE. Randomized, controlled trial of prednisone, cyclophosphamide and cyclosporine in lupus membranous nephropathy. *J Am Soc Nephrol* 2009;**20**:901–11.

16. Boumpas DT, Yamada H, Patronas NJ, et al. Pulse cyclophosphamide for severe neuropsychiatric lupus. *Q J Med* 1991;**81**:975–84.

17. Takada K, Illei GG, Boumpas DT. Cyclophosphamide for the treatment of systemic lupus erythematosus. *Lupus* 2001;**10**:154–61.

18. Leopold G, Schutz E, Haas JP, Oellerich M. Azathioprine-induced severe pancytopenia due to a homozygous two-point mutation of the thiopurine methyltransferase gene in a patient with juvenile HLA-B-27-associated spondylarthritis. *Arthritis Rheum* 1997;**40**:1896–8.

19. Lofstrom B, Backlin C, Sundstrom C, et al. A closer look at non-Hodgkin's lymphoma cases in a national Swedish systemic lupus erythematosus cohort: a nested case-control study. *Ann Rheum Dis* 2007;**66**:1627–32.

20. Grootscholten C, Ligtenberg C, Hagen EC, et al. Azathioprine/methylprednisolone versus cyclophosphamide in proliferative lupus nephritis. a randomized controlled trial. *Kidney Int* 2006;**70**:732–42.

21. Grootshalten C, Bajema IM, Florquin S, et al. Treatment with cyslophosphamide delays the progression of chronic lesions more effectively than does treatment with azathioprine and methylprednisolone in patients with proliferative lupus nephritis. *Arthritis Rheum* 2007;**56**:924–37.

22. Bertsias G, Ioannidis JP, Boletis J, et al. EULAR recommendations for the management of systemic lupus erythematosus. Report of a Task Force of the EULAR Standing Committee for the International Clinical Studies including Therapeutics. *Ann Rheum Dis* 2008;**67**:195–205.

23. Houssiau FA, D'Cruz D, Sangle S, et al. Azathioprine versus mycophenolate mofetil for long-term immunosuppression in lupus nephritis: results from the MAINTAIN Nephritis Trial. *Ann Rheum Dis* 2010;**69**:2083–9.

24. Appel GB, Contreras G, Dooley MA, et al. Mycophenolate mofetil versus cyclophosphamide for induction treatment of lupus nephritis. Aspreva Lupus Management Study Group. *J Am Soc Nephrol* 2009;**20**:1103–12.

25. Hirsch HH, Steiger J. Polyomavirus BK. *Lancet Infect Dis* 2003;**3**: 611–33.

26. Walsh M, James M, Jayne D, et al. Mycophenolate mofetil for induction therapy of lupus nephritis: a systematic review and metaanalysis. *Clin J Am Soc Nephrol* 2007;**2**:968–75.

27. Sinclair A, Appel G, Dooley MA, et al. Mycophenolate mofetil as induction and maintenance therapy for lupus nephritis. Rationale and protocol for the randomized, controlled Asperva Lupus Management Study (ALMS). *Lupus* 2007;**16**:972–80.

28. Isenberg D, Appel GB, Contreras G, et al. Influence of race/ethnicity on response to lupus nephritis treatment: the ALMS study. *Rheumatology* 2010;**49**:128–40.

29. Appel GB, Contreras G, Dooley MA, et al. Mycophenolate mofetil versus cyclophosphamide for induction treatment of lupus nephritis. *J Am Soc Nephrol* 2009;**20**:1103–12.

30. Mak A, Cheak AA, Tan JY, et al. Mycophenolate mofetil is as efficacious as but safer than, cyclophosphamide in the treatment of proliferative lupus nephritis: a meta-analysis and meta-regression. *Rheumatology* 2009;**48**:944–52.

31. Wang J, Hu W, Xie H, et al. Induction therapies for class IV lupus nephritis with non-inflammatory necrotizing vasculopathy: mycophenolate mofetil or intravenous cyclophosphamide. *Lupus* 2007;**16**: 707–71.

32. Kasitanon N, Petri M, Haas M, et al. Mycophenolate mofetil as the primary treatment of membranous lupus nephritis with and without concurrent proliferative disease a retrospective study of 29 cases. *Lupus* 2008;**17**:40–5.

33. Radhakrishnan J, Moutzouris DA, Ginzler EM, et al. Mycophenolate mofetil and intravenous cyclophosphamide are similar as induction therapy for class V lupus nephritis. *Kidney Int* 2010;**77**:152–60.

34. Bao H, Liu ZH, Xie HL, et al. Successful treatment of class V+IV lupus nephritis with multitarget therapy. *J Am Soc Nephrol* 2008;**19**:2001–10.

35. Liu Z, Zhang H, Liu Z. Multitarget therapy for induction treatment of lupus nephritis: a randomized trial. *Ann Intern Med* 2015;**162**: 18–26.

36. Vasoo S, Thumboo J, Fong KY. Refractory immune thrombocytopenia in systemic lupus erythematosus: response to mycophenolate mofetil. *Lupus* 2003;**12**:630–2.

37. Ginzler EM, Wofsy D, Isenberg D, et al. Nonrenal disease activity following mycophenolate mofetil or intravenous cyclophosphamide as induction treatment for lupus nephritis. Findings in a multicenter,

prospective, randomized, open-label, parallel-group clinical trial. *Arthritis Rheum* 2010;**62**:211–21.

38. Moroni G, Doria A, Mosca M, et al. A randomized pilot trial comparing cyclosporine and azathioprine as maintenance therapy in diffuse proliferative lupus nephritis over four years. *Clin J Am Soc Nephrol* 2006;**1**:925–32.

39. Quartuccio L, Sacco S, Franzolini N, et al. Efficacy of cyclosporin-A in the long-term management of thrombocytopenia associated with systemic lupus erythematosus. *Lupus* 2006;**15**:76–9.

40. Szeto CC, Kwan BC, Lai FM, et al. Tacrolimus for the treatment of systemic lupus erythematosus with pure class V nephritis. *Rheumatology* 2008;**47**(11):1678–81.

41. Mok CC, Ying KY, Yim CW, et al. Tacrolimus versus mycophenolate mofetil for induction therapy of lupus nephritis: a randomised controlled trial and long-term follow-up. *Ann Rheum Dis* 2014. http://dx.doi.org/10.1136/annrheumdis-2014-206456.

42. Kusunoki Y, Tanaka N, Kaneko K, et al. Tacrolimus therapy for systemic lupus erythematosus without renal involvement: a preliminary retrospective study. *Mod Rheumatol* 2009;**19**:616–21.

43. Rovin BH, Tang Y, Sun J, et al. Clinical significance of fever in the systemic lupus erythematosus patient receiving steroid therapy. *Kidney Int* 2005;**68**:747–59.

44. Gilliland WR, Tsokos GC. Prophylactic use of antibiotics and immunisations in patients with SLE. *Ann Rheum Dis* 2002;**61**:191–2.

45. Glück T, Kiefmann B, Grohmann M, et al. Immune status and risk for infection in patients receiving chronic immunosuppressive therapy. *J Rheumatol* 2005;**32**:1473–80.

46. Van Assen S, Agmon-Levin N, Elkayam O, et al. EULAR recommendations for vaccination in adult patients with autoimmune inflammatory rheumatic diseases. *Ann Rheum Dis* 2011;**70**:414–22.

47. Bernatsky S, Ramsey-Goldman R, Labrecque J, et al. Cancer risk in systemic lupus: an updated international multi-centre cohort study. *J Autoimmun* 2013;**42**:130–5.

48. Santana IU, Gomes AN, D'Cirqueira Lyrio L, et al. Systemic lupus erythematosus, human papillomavirus infection, cervical pre-malignant and malignant lesions: a systematic review. *Clin Rheumatol* 2011;**30**:665–72.

49. Bermas BL, Hill JA. Effects of immunosuppressive drugs during pregnancy. *Arthritis Rheum* 1995;**38**:1722–32.

Chapter 63

Treatment of Antiphospholipid Syndrome

Savino Sciascia[1,2,3], Munther Khamashta[1,3]

[1]Division of Women's Health, Graham Hughes Lupus Research Laboratory, Lupus Research Unit, The Rayne Institute, King's College, London, UK;

[2]Centro di Ricerche di Immunologia Clinica ed Immunopatologia e Documentazione su Malattie Rare (CMID), Università di Torino, Torino, Italy;

[3]Louise Coote Lupus Unit, Guy's and St Thomas' NHS Foundation Trust, St Thomas' Hospital, London, UK

INTRODUCTION

Antiphospholipid syndrome (APS) is characterized by vascular thrombosis and/or pregnancy morbidity occurring in patients with persistent antiphospholipid antibodies (aPL). Prevention of thrombosis and proper management of women during pregnancy are the major goals of therapy in patients with aPL. Treatment of APS has long been the subject of intense debate, due to the diversity of clinical presentations and medical specialties involved. A consensus document has been issued by the APS Treatment Trends Task Force, created as part of the 14th International Congress on aPL (Rio de Janeiro, September 2013). The main aim of the task force was to systematically review the current and potential future treatment strategies for aPL-positive patients. A summary of the recommendations is shown in Table 1.[1,2]

This chapter reviews the available evidence and recommendations for primary thromboprophylaxis in aPL-positive individuals with no prior thrombotic events, secondary prophylaxis in patients with a previous thrombotic event, and the treatment of refractory or difficult cases. Strategies for the management of APS during pregnancy are also discussed.

PRIMARY THROMBOPROPHYLAXIS

It is still an open question whether prophylactic treatment is needed in subjects with aPL who have no history of thrombosis. The net benefit of active therapy against placebo has never been clearly proven. However, we suggest a careful thrombotic risk assessment as part of good clinical practice and general measures to control cardiovascular risk factors for all patients with aPL (Table 1).[1] The avoidance of smoking and controlling body weight, high blood pressure, and hypercholesterolemia should be considered as main management goals in all subjects with aPL.[3] Estrogen-containing oral contraceptive pills or estrogen replacement therapy should be avoided due to their prothrombotic effects.

Autoimmune conditions, mainly systemic lupus erythematosus (SLE), are considered by themselves as an additional risk factor for thrombosis. Thus, primary thromboprophylaxis should be considered with low-dose aspirin (75–100 mg/day) in all patients with an underling systemic autoimmune conditions and persistent aPL at medium–high titers (immunoglobulin (Ig)M or IgG >40 IgG antiphospholipid units (GPL) or IgM antiphospholipid units (MPL) or >99th percentile). In patients with SLE and with persistently positive aPL, primary thromboprophylaxis including low-dose aspirin (75–100 mg/day) and/or hydroxychloroquine (200–400 mg/day) is strongly recommended.[1] This suggestion is made based on studies that have shown that hydroxychloroquine protects against thrombosis in patients with lupus, including those with aPL.[4]

Although no study has specifically investigated whether the addition of antiplatelet agents offers additional protection, aspirin is generally considered to be an effective option in the setting of primary thromboprophylaxis.[5] Thus, given the general recommendation of hydroxychloroquine therapy in patients with lupus, the addition of low-dose aspirin (LDA) should be decided on an individual basis. Specifically, the addition of low-dose aspirin may be appropriate in selected cases, such as for patients with a high risk aPL profile (e.g., triple positivity for lupus anticoagulant (LA), anticardiolipin (aCL), and anti-β2-glycoprotein I (β2GPI)) and/or other concomitant cardiovascular risk factors, and for SLE patients with a history of obstetric APS.

However, although low-dose aspirin seems a logical thromboprophylaxis approach, supportive evidences are still anecdotal. The Physician Health Study demonstrated no protection against deep venous thrombosis in men with anticardiolipin antibodies receiving low-dose aspirin.[6] However, more recent evidence suggests a protective role for low-dose aspirin for venous thrombosis, at least in the general population.[7]

In asymptomatic carriers of aPL without an underlying connective tissue disease, the decision regarding thromboprophylaxis should be best based on the aPL profile.[8] Aspirin thromboprophylaxis (75–100 mg/day) is suggested for those with a high-risk profile, such as patients with lupus anticoagulant antibodies, particularly triple-positive individuals.[8,9]

Systemic Lupus Erythematosus. http://dx.doi.org/10.1016/B978-0-12-801917-7.00063-2

TABLE 1 Recommendations for Primary and Secondary Thromboprophylaxis in Individuals with Antiphospholipid Antibodies

General Measures for aPL Antibody Carriers

- Maintain strict control of cardiovascular risk factors in patients with a high-risk aPL profile[a] regardless of thrombosis history, concomitant SLE, or other features of APS
- All aPL carriers should receive thromboprophylaxis with usual doses of LMWH in high-risk situations (surgery, prolonged immobilization, puerperium)

Primary Thromboprophylaxis in Patients with SLE and Antiphospholipid Antibodies

- Primary thromboprophylaxis with hydroxychloroquine (200–400 mg/day) ± low-dose aspirin (75–100 mg/day) is recommended for patients with positive lupus anticoagulant or isolated persistent anticardiolipin antibodies at medium–high titers

Primary Thromboprophylaxis in aPL-Positive Individuals without SLE

- Long-term primary thromboprophylaxis with low-dose aspirin (75–100 mg/day) is recommended in patients with a high-risk aPL profile[a], especially in the presence of other thrombotic risk factors

Secondary Thromboprophylaxis

- aPL-positive patients with arterial or venous thrombosis not meeting criteria for APS[b] should be managed in the same manner as aPL-negative patients with similar thrombotic events
- Patients with definite APS and first venous event should receive oral anticoagulant therapy to a target INR 2.0–3.0
- Patients with definite APS and arterial thrombosis should receive warfarin at an INR >3.0 or combined antiaggregant–anticoagulant therapy (INR 2.0–3.0)
- Patient's bleeding risk should be estimated before prescribing high-intensity anticoagulant or combined antiaggregant–anticoagulant therapy
- For patients without SLE with a first noncardioembolic cerebral arterial event who have a low-risk aPL profile[c] and reversible trigger factors, consider antiplatelet agents on an individual basis

Duration of Treatment

- Indefinite duration of therapy in patients with definite APS[b] and thrombosis
- Anticoagulation could be limited to 3–6 months in patients with first venous event with a low-risk aPL profile[c] and a known transient precipitating factor

Refractory and Difficult cases

- Potential alternative therapies for patients with recurrent thrombosis, fluctuating INR levels, major bleeding, or high risk for major bleeding include long-term LMWH, hydroxychloroquine (200–400 mg/day), or statins

aPL, antiphospholipid antibody; APS, antiphospholipid syndrome; SLE, systemic lupus erythematosus; INR, international normalized ratio; LMWH, low-molecular-weight heparin.
[a]High-risk aPL profile: Lupus anticoagulant positivity, triple positivity (lupus anticoagulant + anticardiolipin + anti-ßβ2-glycoprotein I antibodies), isolated persistently positive anti-cardiolipin antibodies at medium–high titers.
[b]Classification criteria for definite APS (Miyakis S, Lockshin MD, Atsumi T, et al. J Thromb Haemost. 2006;4:295–30).
[c]Low-risk aPL profile: Isolated, intermittently positive anticardiolipin or anti-ßβ2-glycoprotein I at low-medium titers.

A prospective, multicenter, randomized, open, controlled trial in patients positive for antiphospholipid antibodies (ALIWAPAS) aimed to examine the efficacy and safety of LDA versus LDA plus low-intensity warfarin in the primary thrombosis prevention of aPL-positive patients with SLE and/or obstetric morbidity.[10] No differences in the number of thromboses were observed between patients treated with LDA versus those treated with LDA plus low-intensity warfarin. More episodes of bleeding were detected in the LDA plus warfarin group. The authors concluded that the LDA plus warfarin regime was significantly less safe and not as acceptable as LDA alone.

At least two score systems have been proposed as thrombotic risk assessment tools in patients with aPL. The Global Anti-Phospholipid Syndrome Score (GAPSS) was developed by our group and independently validated as an effective tool to help physicians in stratifying patients according to their thrombotic risk.[3,11] Patients with a GAPSS score ≥10 might be considered to be at a higher risk of thrombotic event and might require a closer follow-up, especially in high-risk situations (e.g., surgery, immobilization). Proper management of removable risk factors, such as hyperlipidemia and hypertension, is highly recommended to reduce the thrombotic risk.

PREVENTION OF RECURRENT THROMBOSIS

At present, the management of APS patients with previous thrombosis is based on long-term antithrombotic therapy because the rate of recurrent thrombosis is high (29% per year without treatment).[12] Some questions remain on whether patients with APS should receive the same therapy as the general population with similar manifestations and whether arterial and venous events should be treated in a different way.[12,13]

Two randomized, controlled trials have compared high (target international normalized ratio (INR) 3.0–4.0) with standard (target INR 2.0–3.0) intensity of anticoagulation for secondary thromboprophylaxis in patients with APS.[14,15] No significant differences in terms of efficacy or safety between the regimens were observed in these trials. However, both of them suffered from a main bias due to the overrepresentation of patients with first venous thromboembolism. Thus, we recommend indefinite anticoagulant therapy with vitamin K antagonist (VKA) to a target INR of 2.0–3.0 for patients with APS and first venous event. A reduction in the duration of treatment with VKA can be considered only in patients with a low-risk aPL profile and clear provoking factors (e.g., surgery, prolonged immobilization) at the time of the thrombosis.

The management of arterial events is more controversial and debate persists. The APS and Stroke Study (APSSS) concluded that patients with stroke and aPL not fulfilling classification criteria would be best treated as the general population, with low-dose-aspirin.[16] However, it is our current approach that patients with definite APS with arterial disease and/or recurrent events merit a more aggressive approach, which might include VKA with a target INR of 3.0–4.0. Occasionally, combined anticoagulant-antiaggregant therapy may also be considered.[17] In fact, recurrences are very infrequent (0.016–0.031 events per patient per year) among patients receiving effective oral anticoagulation to an INR of 3.0–4.0.[18] However, the physician has to be aware that high-intensity oral anticoagulation therapy carries an inevitable risk of serious hemorrhage, although this risk does not appear higher than that observed in other thrombotic conditions warranting oral anticoagulation.[17]

The management of venous thromboembolism (VTE) is a rapidly changing scenario. The new oral anticoagulants dabigatran etexilate and rivaroxaban have been shown to be effective in the management of VTE and they do not require laboratory monitoring.[19,20] At the time of writing, rivaroxaban and dabigatran are the only agents licensed in Europe for primary and secondary prevention of VTE, but it is expected that apixaban will gain a license shortly, swiftly followed by edoxaban. A phase II/III trial to assess the efficacy and safety of rivaroxaban in APS is currently underway[21] and pilot experiences are showing very promising results.[22]

ALTERNATIVE THERAPIES FOR REFRACTORY AND DIFFICULT CASES

Long-term management of APS patients with recurrent thrombosis may be complicated by fluctuating INR levels, major bleeding, or a high risk of major bleeding. For these reasons, further therapeutic options rather than VKA might be considered in selected cases. Long-term low molecular weight heparin (e.g., subcutaneous enoxaparin 1 mg/kg every 12 h or 1.5 mg/kg/day or subcutaneous dalteparin 100 IU/kg every 12 h or 200 IU/kg/day),[23] hydroxychloroquine (200–400 mg/day),[24] or statins[25] have been suggested in these very selected cases.

Rituximab, an anti-CD20 monoclonal antibody, has been shown to be effective in life-threatening catastrophic APS, although it has been investigated in a small number of cases.[26] B-cell depletion with anti CD-20 monoclonal antibody also has been successfully used in patients with aPL and autoimmune-mediated thrombocytopenia and hemolytic anemia.[27] A pilot open-label phase II trial of B-cell depletion with anti CD-20 monoclonal antibody for noncriteria manifestations of APS concluded that rituximab may represent a safe option in APS; it seems to be effective in controlling some, but not all, noncriteria manifestations of APS.[28]

OTHER THERAPIES

Limited evidence are in favor of the use of steroids, immunosuppressive drugs, or intravenous immunoglobulin in treatment of APS patients with thrombosis.[29–31] Such drugs have severe side effects when given for prolonged periods and aPL is not always suppressed by these agents. The use of these drugs should be considered only in very select cases, as rescue therapy only in patients with repeated episodes of thrombosis despite adequate anti-coagulant therapy, or in catastrophic APS. Some other options can be individually considered, such as the use of intra-arterial fibrinolysis in patients with acute myocardial infarction associated with APS or prostacyclin analogs (i.e., Iloprost) in patients with severe ischemic necrotic toes associated with APS.

Newer therapeutic agents targeting pathways involved in the development of aPL-mediated clinical manifestations are under investigation. These include blocking of aPL/β2GPI receptors on target cells, complement and nuclear factor-kB, and P38 mitogen-activated kinase inhibitors. However, the multifactorial mechanisms underlying thrombosis and pregnancy morbidity in APS are still not fully understood, and this might limit the development of new targeted therapies for APS. Potentially, the current antithrombotic approach to APS patients will be replaced in the future by an immunomodulatory approach as our understanding of the mechanisms of aPL-mediated clinical manifestations improves.

PREGNANCY

Preconception counseling and pharmacologic treatment have improved the rate of pregnant women with aPL who deliver a viable healthy infant—as high as 75% in our experience. The goal is to estimate the chance of both fetal and

TABLE 2   Recommended Treatment of Antiphospholipid Syndrome during Pregnancy

Recurrent Early (Pre-Embryonic or Embryonic) Miscarriage

- Low-dose aspirin (75–100 mg/day) plus LMWH at thromboprophylactic doses (e.g., subcutaneous enoxaparin 40 mg/day, subcutaneous dalteparin 5000 U/day, or subcutaneous tinzaparin 4500 U/day) or unfractionated heparin
  - Low-dose aspirin (75–100 mg/day) alone in selected cases

Fetal Death (>10 weeks' Gestation) or Prior Early Delivery (<34 weeks' Gestation) due to Severe Pre-Eclampsia or Placental Insufficiency

- Low-dose aspirin (75–100 mg/day) plus LMWH at thromboprophylactic doses (e.g., subcutaneous enoxaparin 40 mg/day, subcutaneous dalteparin 5000 U/day, or subcutaneous tinzaparin 4500 U/day), or unfractionated heparin

APS with Thrombosis

- Low-dose aspirin (75–100 mg/day) plus LMWH at therapeutic doses (e.g., subcutaneous enoxaparin 1 mg/kg every 12 h or 1.5 mg/kg/day or subcutaneous dalteparin 100 U/kg every 12 h or 200 U/kg/day)

APS, antiphospholipid syndrome; LMWH, low-molecular-weight heparin.

maternal problems. In counseling, patients must still be informed that the presence of aPL is associated with an increased risk of serious complications, such as miscarriage, fetal death, prematurity, pre-eclampsia, and thrombosis. Pregnancy should be carefully planned and eventually discouraged only in selected cases, including in women with severe or uncontrolled pulmonary hypertension. Women who have recently had thrombotic events, particularly an arterial such as a stroke, should be advised to postpone the pregnancy. Pharmacologic management of pregnancy in women with aPL includes antithrombotic therapy. However, VKA must be avoided if possible during the first trimester, especially between 6 and 9 weeks.

To optimize their management during pregnancy, women with APS may be categorized into one of three groups: women with pre-embryonic or embryonic manifestations (recurrent early miscarriage); women with late pregnancy complications (prior fetal death (>10 weeks' gestation) or prior early delivery (<34 weeks' gestation) due to severe pre-eclampsia or placental insufficiency); or women with previous thrombotic event(s). Proposed recommendations based on the nature of the manifestations and history are shown in Table 2.

Glucocorticoids, immunosuppressants, and immunoglobulins have not demonstrated additional benefit compared with LDA/heparin. Moreover, glucocorticoids may lead to serious pregnancy morbidity, such as prematurity and hypertension.[32]

RECURRENT EARLY MISCARRIAGE

The recommended therapy for all women with obstetric antiphospholipid syndrome is combination therapy with LDA (75–100 mg/day) and heparin, either low molecular weight heparin (e.g., subcutaneous enoxaparin 40 mg OD, subcutaneous dalteparin 5000 U OD, or subcutaneous tinzaparin

4500 U OD) or unfractionated heparin. These recommendations are based on results from three randomized, controlled trials comparing LDA alone or in combination therapy with heparin in women with APS.[33–36]

Rai and colleagues showed a significantly higher rate of live births with LDA plus unfractionated heparin (5000 U BD) versus LDA alone (71% vs 42%; odds ratio, 3.37; 95% confidence interval, 1.40–8.10).[36] Kutteh and coworkers reported a similar improvement in the live birth rate with LDA and heparin versus LDA alone (80% vs 44%; $p < 0.05$).[33] Conversely, no differences in outcome with combination therapy versus LDA was found in two other randomized trials, both using low molecular weight heparin (LMWH), with live birth rates approaching 80% in both arms. The heterogeneity in the conclusions seems attributable to the relatively poor outcomes in women receiving LDA only in the two former studies.[34,35] Moreover, data from observational studies have reported 79–100% pregnancy success rates with LDA alone in this subgroup of women.[32] Thus, we believe that the option of monotherapy with LDA can be a valid option in selected cases, including in patients with recurrent pre-embrionic miscarriages, and cannot be discarded beforehand in this subgroup of women.

FETAL DEATH

Fetal losses (defined as occurring after 10 weeks' gestation) or early delivery (before 34 weeks' gestation due to severe pre-eclampsia or placental insufficiency) represent a severe and specific manifestation of APS. However, these settings have been studied much less comprehensively than early miscarriage and not in randomized controlled trials.

The combination of LDA and LMWH at a prophylactic dose is usually recommended in this setting.[32] When used for obstetric purposes, LDA is best started before conception. Although most centers are now recommending LMWH for a better bioavailability and longer half-life, no differences have been found when comparing unfractionated heparin and LMWH combined with LDA. For this reason, any of them can be used once pregnancy has been confirmed.

MANAGEMENT OF PREGNANCY IN PATIENTS WITH APS AND PREVIOUS THROMBOSIS

LDA and therapeutic dose heparin (e.g., 5000 IU every 12 h) or LMWH at anticoagulant doses (e.g., enoxaparin 1 mg/kg sc every 12 h or dalteparin 100 U/kg every 12 h, or enoxaparin 1.5 mg/kg/day sc, or dalteparin 200 U/kg/day sc) are recommended for management of pregnancy in patients with APS and previous thrombosis.[32]

The change from VKA to heparin or LMWH should be achieved prior to 6 weeks' gestation to avoid teratogenicity associated with VKA. Heparin does not cross the placenta and is not known to cause any adverse fetal effects; however, its long-term use in pregnancy has been associated with osteoporosis in the mother. When compared to unfractionated heparin, LMWH seems to be a safer option.[37]

The careful management of anticoagulant treatment in women who will receive epidural anesthesia or analgesia is also mandatory. Epidural anesthesia can be safely carried out 12 h after the last dose of LMWH when it is used in thromboprophylactic doses, and it can be resumed 6–8 h after the procedure or when hemostasis is achieved. When LMWH is used in full antithrombotic doses, it must be stopped 24 h before the procedure, and it can be resumed not earlier than 24 h afterward.[38,39] Aspirin does not add significant risk for spinal hematoma and can be safely maintained,[40] although many anesthesiologists recommend stopping it for at least 3–7 days.[39]

MANAGEMENT OF REFRACTORY OBSTETRIC APS

APS is often a treatable cause of pregnancy loss; however, in up to 30% of cases, recurrent pregnancy loss persists despite treatment.[41] The role of prednisolone for refractory obstetric APS cases has been extensively investigated,[42] and its use has been associated to a reduction of complement activation and inflammatory changes.[43,44] However, high dose doses of prednisolone (more than 40 mg/day) are known to increase the risk of several side effects in pregnancy and preterm deliveries, including elevations in blood pressure, gestational diabetes, and asymptomatic infections.[45] Bramham et al.[43] reported that the addition of first-trimester low-dose prednisolone (10 mg daily) to conventional treatment might be considered in the management of refractory antiphospholipid antibody-related pregnancy loss(es).

The use of intravenous immunoglobulins (IVIG) in refractory obstetric APS has failed to be implemented widely due to its beneficial limitations, expense, and short supply.[46] Studies have concluded no statistically significant improvements in obstetric and neonatal outcomes with the use of IVIG in combination with aspirin and LMWH when compared to aspirin and LMWH-only regimens.[47,48] Consequently, IVIG is often reserved for patients who are refractory to heparin or when additional indications such as autoimmune thrombocytopenia are present.[46,47]

POSTPARTUM PERIOD

LMWH should be continued intrapartum and postpartum until women resume therapy with a VKA with a therapeutic INR. It is worth remembering that both VKA and subcutaneous heparin are compatible with breastfeeding. Thromboprophylaxis coverage (heparin 5000 IU OD or LMWH; e.g., subcutaneous enoxaparin 40 mg OD, subcutaneous dalteparin 5000 U OD, or subcutaneous tinzaparin 4500 U OD) of the postpartum period is recommended also in women with aPL and no previous thrombosis. The duration is variable from 1 to 6 weeks and has to be tailored according to the presence of additional risk factors.[2]

REFERENCES

1. Erkan D, Aguiar CL, Andrade D, Cohen H, Cuadrado MJ, Danowski A, et al. 14th International Congress on Antiphospholipid Antibodies: task force report on antiphospholipid syndrome treatment trends. *Autoimmun Rev* 2014;**13**:685–96.

2. de Jesus GR, Agmon-Levin N, Andrade CA, Andreoli L, Chighizola CB, Porter TF, et al. 14th International Congress on Antiphospholipid Antibodies Task Force report on obstetric antiphospholipid syndrome. *Autoimmun Rev* 2014;**13**:795–813.

3. Sciascia S, Sanna G, Murru V, Roccatello D, Khamashta MA, Bertolaccini ML. GAPSS: the global anti-phospholipid syndrome score. *Rheumatology (Oxford)* 2013;**52**:1397–403.

4. Tektonidou MG, Laskari K, Panagiotakos DB, Moutsopoulos HM. Risk factors for thrombosis and primary thrombosis prevention in patients with systemic lupus erythematosus with or without antiphospholipid antibodies. *Arthritis Rheum* 2009;**61**:29–36.

5. Wahl DG, Bounameaux H, de Moerloose P, Sarasin FP. Prophylactic antithrombotic therapy for patients with systemic lupus erythematosus with or without antiphospholipid antibodies - do the benefits outweigh the risks? A decision analysis. *Arch Intern Med* 2000;**160**:2042–8.

6. Ginsburg KS, Liang MH, Newcomer L, Goldhaber SZ, Schur PH, Hennekens CH, et al. Anticardiolipin antibodies and the risk for ischemic stroke and venous thrombosis. *Ann Intern Med* 1992;**117**: 997–1002.

7. Becattini C, Agnelli G, Schenone A, Eichinger S, Bucherini E, Silingardi M, et al. Aspirin for preventing the recurrence of venous thromboembolism. *New Engl J Med* 2012;**366**:1959–67.

8. Erkan D, Harrison MJ, Levy R, Peterson M, Petri M, Sammaritano L, et al. Aspirin for primary thrombosis prevention in the antiphospholipid syndrome - a randomized, double-blind, placebo-controlled trial in asymptomatic antiphospholipid antibody-positive individuals. *Arthritis Rheum* 2007;**56**:2382–91.

9. Pengo V, Ruffatti A, Legnani C, Testa S, Fierro T, Marongiu F, et al. Incidence of a first thromboembolic event in asymptomatic carriers of high-risk antiphospholipid antibody profile: a multicenter prospective study. *Blood* 2011;**118**:4714–8.

10. Cuadrado MJ, Bertolaccini ML, Seed PT, Tektonidou MG, Aguirre A, Mico L, et al. Low-dose aspirin vs low-dose aspirin plus low-intensity warfarin in thromboprophylaxis: a prospective, multicentre, randomized, open, controlled trial in patients positive for antiphospholipid antibodies (ALIWAPAS). *Rheumatology (Oxford)* 2014;**53**:275–84.

11. Otomo K, Atsumi T, Amengual O, Fujieda Y, Kato M, Oku K, et al. Efficacy of the antiphospholipid score for the diagnosis of antiphospholipid syndrome and its predictive value for thrombotic events. *Arthritis Rheum* 2012;**64**:504–12.

12. Khamashta MA, Cuadrado MJ, Mujic F, Taub NA, Hunt BJ, Hughes GR. The management of thrombosis in the antiphospholipid-antibody syndrome. *N Engl J Med* 1995;**332**:993–7.

13. Brunner HI, Chan WS, Ginsberg JS, Feldman BM. Longterm anticoagulation is preferable for patients with antiphospholipid antibody syndrome. result of a decision analysis. *J Rheumatol* 2002;**29**:490–501.

14. Kearon C, Ginsberg JS, Kovacs MJ, Anderson DR, Wells P, Julian JA, et al. Comparison of low-intensity warfarin therapy with conventional-intensity warfarin therapy for long-term prevention of recurrent venous thromboembolism. *N Engl J Med* 2003;**349**:631–9.

15. Finazzi G, Marchioli R, Brancaccio V, Schinco P, Wisloff F, Musial J, et al. A randomized clinical trial of high-intensity warfarin vs. conventional antithrombotic therapy for the prevention of recurrent thrombosis in patients with the antiphospholipid syndrome (WAPS). *J Thromb Haem* 2005;**3**:848–53.

16. Levine SR, Brey RL, Tilley BC, Thompson JL, Sacco RL, Sciacca RR, et al. Antiphospholipid antibodies and subsequent thrombo-occlusive events in patients with ischemic stroke. *J Am Med Assoc* 2004;**291**:576–84.

17. Ruiz-Irastorza G, Khamashta MA, Hunt BJ, Escudero A, Cuadrado MJ, Hughes GR. Bleeding and recurrent thrombosis in definite antiphospholipid syndrome: analysis of a series of 66 patients treated with oral anticoagulation to a target international normalized ratio of 3.5. *Arch Intern Med* 2002;**162**:1164–9.

18. Ruiz-Irastorza G, Hunt BJ, Khamashta MA. A systematic review of secondary thromboprophylaxis in patients with antiphospholipid antibodies. *Arthritis Rheum* 2007;**57**:1487–95.

19. Buller HR, Prins MH, Lensin AW, Decousus H, Jacobson BF, Minar E, et al. Oral rivaroxaban for the treatment of symptomatic pulmonary embolism. *N Engl J Med* 2012;**366**:1287–97.

20. Schulman S. Advantages and limitations of the new anticoagulants. *J Intern Med* 2014;**275**:1–11.

21. Arachchillage DJ, Cohen H. Use of new oral anticoagulants in antiphospholipid syndrome. *Curr Rheumatol Rep* 2013;**15**:331.

22. Sciascia S, Breen K, Hunt BJ. Rivaroxaban use in patients with antiphospholipid syndrome and previous venous thromboembolism. *Blood Coagul Fibrinolysis* 2015;**26**:476–7.

23. Vargas-Hitos JA, Ateka-Barrutia O, Sangle S, Khamashta MA. Efficacy and safety of long-term low molecular weight heparin in patients with antiphospholipid syndrome. *Ann Rheum Dis* 2011;**70**:1652–4.

24. Petri M. Use of hydroxychloroquine to prevent thrombosis in systemic lupus erythematosus and in antiphospholipid antibody-positive patients. *Curr Rheumatol Rep* 2011;**13**:77–80.

25. Lopez-Pedrera C, Ruiz-Limon P, Aguirre MA, Rodriguez-Ariza A, Cuadrado MJ. Potential use of statins in the treatment of antiphospholipid syndrome. *Curr Rheumatol Rep* 2012;**14**:87–94.

26. Ketari Jamoussi S, Zaghdoudi I, Ben Dhaou B, Kochbati S, Mir K, Ben Ali Z, et al. Catastrophic antiphospholipid syndrome and rituximab: a new report. *Tunis Med* 2009;**87**:699–702.

27. Sciascia S, Naretto C, Rossi D, Bazzan M, Roccatello D. Treatment-induced downregulation of antiphospholipid antibodies: effect of rituximab alone on clinical and laboratory features of antiphospholipid syndrome. *Lupus* 2011;**20**:1106–8.

28. Erkan D, Vega J, Ramon G, Kozora E, Lockshin MD. A pilot open-label phase II trial of rituximab for non-criteria manifestations of antiphospholipid syndrome. *Arthritis Rheum* 2013;**65**:464–71.

29. Sherer Y, Levy Y, Shoenfeld Y. Intravenous immunoglobulin therapy of antiphospholipid syndrome. *Rheumatology (Oxford)* 2000;**39**:421–6.

30. Sciascia S, Giachino O, Roccatello D. Prevention of thrombosis relapse in antiphospholipid syndrome patients refractory to conventional therapy using intravenous immunoglobulin. *Clin Exp Rheumatol* 2012;**30**:409–13.

31. Sciascia S, Khamashta MA, D'Cruz DP. Targeted therapy in antiphospholipid syndrome. *Curr Opin Rheumatol* 2014;**26**:269–75.

32. Danza A, Ruiz-Irastorza G, Khamashta M. Antiphospohlipid syndrome in obstetrics. *Best Pract Res Clin Obstet Gynaecol* 2012;**26**:65–76.

33. Kutteh WH, Ermel LD. A clinical trial for the treatment of antiphospholipid antibody-associated recurrent pregnancy loss with lower dose heparin and aspirin. *Am J Reprod Immunol* 1996;**35**:402–7.

34. Laskin CA, Spitzer KA, Clark CA, Crowther MR, Ginsberg JS, Hawker GA, et al. Low molecular weight heparin and aspirin for recurrent pregnancy loss: results from the randomized, controlled HepASA Trial. *J Rheumatol* 2009;**36**:279–87.

35. Farquharson RG, Quenby S, Greaves M. Antiphospholipid syndrome in pregnancy: a randomized, controlled trial of treatment. *Obstet Gynecol* 2002;**100**:408–13.

36. Rai R, Cohen H, Dave M, Regan L. Randomised controlled trial of aspirin and aspirin plus heparin in pregnant women with recurrent miscarriage associated with phospholipid antibodies (or antiphospholipid antibodies). *BMJ* 1997;**314**:253–7.

37. Sanson BJ, Lensing AW, Prins MH, Ginsberg JS, Barkagan ZS, Lavenne-Pardonge E, et al. Safety of low-molecular-weight heparin in pregnancy: a systematic review. *Thromb Haemost* 1999;**81**:668–72.

38. Horlocker TT, Wedel DJ, Rowlingson JC, Enneking FK, Kopp SL, Benzon HT, et al. Regional anesthesia in the patient receiving antithrombotic or thrombolytic therapy: American Society of Regional Anesthesia and Pain Medicine Evidence-Based Guidelines (Third Edition). *Reg Anesth Pain Med* 2010;**35**:64–101.

39. Douketis JD, Berger PB, Dunn AS, Jaffer AK, Spyropoulos AC, Becker RC, et al. The perioperative management of antithrombotic therapy: American college of Chest physicians evidence-Based Clinical Practice Guidelines (8th Edition). *Chest* 2008;**133**:299S–339S.

40. Sibai BM, Caritis SN, Thom E, Shaw K, McNellis D. Low-dose aspirin in nulliparous women: safety of continuous epidural block and correlation between bleeding time and maternal-neonatal bleeding complications. National Institute of Child Health and Human Developmental Maternal-Fetal Medicine Network. *Am J Obstet Gynecol* 1995;**172**:1553–7.

41. Bramham K, Hunt BJ, Germain S, Calatayud I, Khamashta M, Bewley S, et al. Pregnancy outcome in different clinical phenotypes of antiphospholipid syndrome. *Lupus* 2010;**19**:58–64.

42. Lubbe WF, Butler WS, Palmer SJ, Liggins GC. Fetal survival after prednisone suppression of maternal lupus-anticoagulant. *Lancet* 1983;**1**:1361–3.

43. Bramham K, Thomas M, Nelson-Piercy C, Khamashta M, Hunt BJ. First-trimester low-dose prednisolone in refractory antiphospholipid antibody-related pregnancy loss. *Blood* 2011;**117**:6948–51.

44. Sneiderman CA, Wilson JW. Effects of corticosteroids on complement and the neutrophilic polymorphonuclear leukocyte. *Transplant Proc* 1975;**7**:41–8.

45. Laskin CA, Bombardier C, Hannah ME, Mandel FP, Ritchie JW, Farewell V, et al. Prednisone and aspirin in women with autoantibodies and unexplained recurrent fetal loss. *N Engl J Med* 1997;**337**:148–53.

46. Tuthill JI, Khamashta MA. Management of antiphospholipid syndrome. *J Autoimmun* 2009;**33**:92–8.

47. Triolo G, Ferrante A, Ciccia F, Accardo-Palumbo A, Perino A, Castelli A, et al. Randomized study of subcutaneous low molecular weight heparin plus aspirin versus intravenous immunoglobulin in the treatment of recurrent fetal loss associated with antiphospholipid antibodies. *Arthritis Rheum* 2003;**48**:728–31.

48. Branch DW, Peaceman AM, Druzin M, Silver RK, El-Sayed Y, Silver RM, et al. A multicenter, placebo-controlled pilot study of intravenous immune globulin treatment of antiphospholipid syndrome during pregnancy. The Pregnancy Loss Study Group. *Am J Obstet Gynecol* 2000;**182**:122–7.

Chapter 64

New Treatments for Systemic Lupus Erythematosus

Vasileios C. Kyttaris

Division of Rheumatology, Beth Israel Deaconess Medical Center, Harvard Medical School, Boston, MA, USA

SUMMARY

The treatment of SLE currently depends heavily on non-specific immunosuppressives. Belimumab was the first biologic to be approved for the use of nonrenal SLE. Currently several biologics and small molecules are evaluated for the treatment of both lupus nephritis and nonrenal SLE. Two molecules, epratruzumab, an anti-CD22 antibody and sifalizumab, an anti-interferon α antibody, have shown promising results in phase II trials. We also discuss biologics and small molecules that target cytokines, the complement, costimulatory and surface molecules and are at earlier phases of development.

Although the etiology of systemic lupus erythematosus (SLE) remains unknown, breakthroughs in the pathophysiology of the disease have allowed for the design and testing of several targeted treatments. This has further been facilitated by the standardization of outcome measures; the outcome measures that have been found to be most helpful are the SLE disease activity index (SLEDAI)-based Response Index (SRI) and British Isles Lupus Activity Group (BILAG)-based Composite Lupus Assessment (BICLA). A patient is regarded as an SRI responder if her or his SLEDAI index decreases by 4 points over the period of the clinical trial without new BILAG A, more than one BILAG B, or significant deterioration of physician global assessment (PGA).[1] Similarly, a patient is regarded as a BICLA responder if the BILAG improves from baseline: at the same time, there should be no worsening in any other systems, no worsening in the SLEDAI or physician global assessment (PGA), and no need for increased or additional immunosuppressives or immunomodulatory medications. Significant secondary outcomes that are regarded as clinically significant are time to (severe) flare, corticosteroid sparing, and joint counts.

The first targeted therapy for SLE, belimumab, was approved in 2011, with an array of targets being actively evaluated in large multinational clinical trials in patients with various manifestations of SLE. In this chapter, we analyze treatments that target soluble mediators (cytokines, complement), disrupt cell–cell interactions, and bind to surface receptors inhibiting intracellular signaling (summarized in Table 1).

CYTOKINES

Cytokines have been successfully targeted in a variety of autoimmune diseases, leading to a therapeutic paradigm shift in rheumatoid arthritis. Although targeted therapy in SLE is still in its infancy, there are several ongoing late-stage clinical trials with biologic agents targeting a variety of cytokines.

B-Lymphocyte Activating Factor (BAFF)

BAFF, also known as B-lymphocyte stimulator (BLyS), is a tumor necrosis factor (TNF) family cytokine that is expressed on monocytes and dendritic cells. Cleaved BAFF circulates in the serum and is elevated in SLE patients. BAFF interacts with its receptors BAFF-R (BR3), TACI (transmembrane activator and calcium modulator and cyclophilin ligand interactor), and BCMA (B-cell maturation antigen). BAFF-R is the primary receptor that binds to BAFF, and it is almost exclusively expressed on B cells. BAFF:BAFF-R binding activates NF-κB and provides a survival signal that promotes B-cell proliferation and maturation, especially in the early (transitional) stage of B-cell development.[2]

Belimumab, the first medication to be approved for SLE in over five decades, is a fully humanized monoclonal antibody that inhibits BAFF. Belimumab was shown in two pivotal randomized controlled trials (RCT)[3,4] to be significantly better than placebo in patients with active SLE: A total of 58% of subjects receiving 10 mg/kg belimumab monthly infusions reached SRI-4 without deterioration of BILAG or PGA versus 44% in the placebo group (BLISS-52 trial). In the BLISS-76 trial, the SRI in the belimumab group was 43.2% versus 33.5% in the placebo group. Belimumab also reduced the rate of severe flares.

TABLE 1 New Agents for the Treatment of SLE

Molecular Target	Treatment	Status
BAFF/APRIL	Belimumab (anti-BAFF)	Approved for use in nonrenal SLE
	Tabalumab (anti-BAFF)	Only 1/2 phase III with significant results
	Blisibimod (BAFFR-Ig)	Phase II marginally significant results
	Atacicept (TACI-Ig)	Increased infection rate
	Briobacept (BR3-Ig)	Preclinical phase with promising results
Interferon (IFN) α	Rontalizumab (anti-IFNα)	Phase II without significant results
	Sifalizumab (anti-IFNα)	Phase II successful
	Anifrolumab (anti IFN receptor)	Biologic effect demonstrated in phase II
Interferon (IFN) γ	AMG 811 (anti-IFNγ)	Phase I showed biologic but not clinical effect
Interleukin 12/23	Ustekinumab (anti-p40)	Phase II started
Complement	Eculizumab (anti-C5)	Biologic but not clinical effect demonstrated
CD40:CD154	BG9588	Effect in nephritis shown (small trial); increased incidence of thrombosis
	IDEC-131	Safe but ineffective
CD28:CD80/86	Abatacept (CTLA-4-Ig)	Ineffective in phase III in nephritis and general SLE
	Lulizumab (anti-CD28)	Phase II started
ICOS-B7RP	AMG 557	Safe in phase I; phase II ongoing
CD20	Rituximab (anti-CD20)	Trend for marginal benefit over standard of care in nephritis (phase III)
	Ocrelizumab (humanized anti-CD20)	Increased infection rate
CD22	Epratuzumab (anti-CD22)	Successful phase II; phase III completed

Patients enrolled in both studies had at least moderately active disease and were positive for ANA and/or dsDNA antibodies; patients with active central nervous system and renal disease were excluded. Postmarketing analysis confirms that belimumab is safe with no significant increase in the rate of serious infections and malignancies.

Tabalumab, a subcutaneous-administered monoclonal antibody that bound both soluble and membrane-bound BAFF was also evaluated in two large randomized clinical trials.[5] Tabalumab resulted in a decrease in dsDNA antibody levels and an increase in complement levels. In one of the two trials, the primary end point of SRI-5 (SRI responders who had a decrease in the SLEDAI by at least 5 points instead of the classic 4-point SRI decrease) was reached by 38.4% of subjects on biweekly subcutaneous injections of 120mg of tabalumab versus 27.7% of patients on placebo ($p=0.002$). The other trial showed similar trends but the differences among the groups did not reach statistical significance. Other key metrics, such as corticosteroid sparing and time to severe flare, did not significantly differ among the groups. Consistent with the data from belimumab, tabalumab was shown to be safe without significant increases in the rate of infections and other serious adverse events.

Blisibimod, a fusion molecule that is composed of the Fc portion of IgG1 and four BAFF binding domains, was also evaluated in phase II trial.[6] As with tabalumab, it binds both soluble and membrane-bound BAFF. Blisibimod showed a positive immunologic effect in patients with SLE with an increase in complement levels and decrease in dsDNA antibodies. The main outcome SRI-5 was statistically different in the subgroup that was receiving the highest dose (200mg every week) at only one time point (20weeks). As with other BAFF-targeting treatments, positive results were more common in patients with more active disease at baseline. The somewhat promising results will need to be further evaluated in phase III trials.

Atacicept, a fusion molecule of the extracellular portion of the BAFF receptor TACI and the Fc portion of human IgG, was also assessed in patients with SLE and lupus nephritis. Atacicept binds BAFF and also a related molecule APRIL (a proliferation-inducing ligand). The nephritis trial[7] was prematurely terminated due to serious infections and significant decrease of immunoglobulin levels. A trial assessing atacicept efficacy in preventing flares[8] failed to show a difference between the group on 75mg sc twice weekly and placebo. The group on higher dose (150mg sc twice weekly) had a statistically significant decrease in the risk of flare and increase in time to first flare compared to placebo. The high-dose group was prematurely terminated because of two deaths. Similar to the nephritis trial, total immunoglobulin levels were decreased in the atacicept groups compared to placebo. Complement levels did increase and dsDNA decreased in the atacicept group, consistent with its proposed mode of action. Given its side effect profile, the future of atacicept in the treatment of SLE is unclear and careful considerations, such as use of concomitant immunosuppressives, have to be made before further trials are designed.

Finally, briobacept, a fusion molecule of the BAFF-R (BR3) and IgG1, has shown efficacy in preclinical models of lupus.[9]

Taken together, blockade of BAFF results in improvement of immunological parameters (dsDNA antibodies, complement levels) in patients who are immunologically and clinically active at baseline. The effect on clinical activity is modest for belimumab and marginal for tabalumab, while blisibimod needs to be assessed in a large phase III RCT. The usefulness of BAFF inhibition in renal and central nervous system lupus, arguably the most severe manifestations of the disease, is unknown to date. In terms of side effects, BAFF, but not the combined BAFF/APRIL inhibition, with the aforementioned biologics seems to be generally safe without significant increase in serious infections or malignancies.

Interferon-α

Interferon alpha is a cytokine that is primarily produced by cells in response to viral infections. It binds to its receptors (IFNAR) on a variety of cells, leading to the activation of the Jak-STAT pathway. SLE peripheral blood mononuclear cells have a distinct transcriptional phenotype, called the interferon signature, thought to be due to exposure to excessive interferon alpha.[10]

The anti-interferon alpha monoclonal antibody, sifalimumab, met its primary endpoint (SRI-4) at 1 year of treatment of patients with nonrenal SLE in a phase IIb trial.[11] SRI-4 was 59.8% for the high dose (1200 mg IV monthly infusions) of sifalimumab versus 45.4% in the placebo group. The complement levels and anti-dsDNA levels were not significantly affected by sifalimumab, while herpes zoster was more common in patients treated with sifalimumab (8.4% in the high dose vs 0.9% in the placebo).

Rontalizumab, another anti-IFN alpha antibody, did not differ from placebo in a phase II trial. Unexpectedly, only patients with low interferon signature gene expression benefited from a reduction in disease activity, steroid burden, and flare rates, as compared to placebo.[12]

Anifrolumab, an anti-interferon receptor 1 (IFNAR1) antibody showed interesting results in a phase II open label trial[13] with sustained, almost universal, suppression of the interferon signature gene expression—more so than sifalimumab. This suggests that inhibiting the receptor rather than the offending cytokine may be a better strategy to reverse the effects of interferons on immune cell gene expression.

Thus, interferon-α inhibition shows some promising, yet not impressive, results. The fact that the clinical effectiveness cannot be correlated at this early point with the interferon gene expression raises questions about the underlying mechanism of the interferon signature in SLE.

Interferon-γ

Interferon-γ, a Th1 signature cytokine, is a major proinflammatory cytokine that plays a pivotal role in the development of nephritis in the preclinical lupus model MRL-*lpr*.[14] AMG 811, a human IgG1 anti-interferon γ monoclonal antibody, was evaluated in two phase I trials in subjects with discoid lupus (16 individuals),[15] and mild systemic lupus (26 individuals received one dose and 28 multiple doses).[16] The medication was given subcutaneously or intravenously. There was a reduction in the expression of interferon-γ associated genes and a decrease in the serum levels of CXCL10, a marker of future lupus flares. None of the two studies showed any clinical effect, and no significant increase over placebo in the rate of adverse events were observed either. A larger trial will be needed to evaluate whether positive biologic outcomes can translate into clinical effectiveness.

Interleukin-23/Interleukin-17

It has become apparent that the manifestations of several autoimmune diseases depend not only on the activation of Th1 T cells but also Th17 cells, Th17 cells produce, among other cytokines, the signature cytokine IL-17A. The relative contribution of these two subtypes in different diseases is a subject of intense investigation. In SLE, accumulated evidence suggests that IL-17 expressing cells are present in the spleen and kidneys[17] of murine models of lupus and patients with lupus nephritis.[18] Moreover, inhibition of the pro-inflammatory cytokine IL-23, which stabilizes the Th17 phenotype, leads to amelioration of murine lupus nephritis.[19] Contrary to the apparent effectiveness of IL-23 inhibition, IL-17 inhibition in murine models of lupus had no effect,[20] bringing into question whether other IL-23 regulated cytokines, such IL-17F or IL-21, may be playing a role in lupus pathophysiology. Nevertheless, this pathway shows a lot of promise as a treatment target for a variety of autoimmune diseases.

Ustekinumab is a monoclonal antibody that inhibits both Th1 and Th17 cell differentiation by blocking IL-12 and IL-23 by binding to their common subunit p40. It is effective in the treatment of psoriasis and psoriatic arthritis[21] and is administered subcutaneously every 12 weeks after initial loading. Given preclinical data, strong theoretical rationale, and acceptable side effect profile, ustekinumab is currently being evaluated in a phase II trial in patients with SLE.

COMPLEMENT

One of the cardinal manifestations of SLE is the creation of immune complexes that, after depositing to target tissues such as the skin or the kidney, activate locally the complement system. Moreover, a decrease in complement levels is one of the best predictors of disease flare. Eculizumab is a monoclonal antibody against the complement component C5, which decreases the production of anaphylatoxin C5a and the creation of the membrane attack complex. It is effective in paroxysmal nocturnal hemoglobinuria.[22] It has been evaluated in a placebo-controlled study in patients with SLE and was found to be effective in inhibiting complement, but no effect on disease activity was shown.[23] Currently, it is being evaluated in patients with the antiphospholipid syndrome.

CO-STIMULATORY PATHWAYS

The crosstalk between T cells and antigen-presenting cells (APC), including B cells, is central in the pathophysiology of SLE, supporting aberrant cell activation and production of proinflammatory cytokines and pathogenic autoantibodies. Disrupting this interaction was one of the first attempts for targeted treatment in SLE. Several trials of different compounds targeting co-stimulatory molecules have shown an immunologic effect (increase in C3, decrease of dsDNA antibodies) but no definite clinical effectiveness.

CD154-CD40

CD154 (also known as CD40L) is expressed on T cells following activation. It binds its ligand CD40 on other cells (primarily B cells), delivering an activation signal. CD154 is overexpressed on SLE T cells and contributes to T-cell-induced B-cell overactivation, maturation, and production of specific autoantibodies. Anti-CD154 treatment resulted in amelioration of lupus nephritis in the NZBW F1 model.[24]

CD154 was targeted by BG9588, a humanized antibody,[25] in patients with proliferative lupus nephritis. This small trial of 28 patients was prematurely terminated because of an increased incidence of thrombosis (two myocardial infarctions). The treatment did result in improvement of immunological parameters (C3, anti-dsDNA antibodies) and hematuria. Another antibody against CD154, IDEC-131, did not show any effect in patients with various manifestations of SLE.[26] As opposed to BG9588, there was no increase in thrombotic events. These therapeutic programs have since been discontinued, but several early-stage programs are currently under way, targeting both CD154 and CD40; these programs will certainly capitalize on better

selection of subjects and uniform outcome measures that have developed since.

CD28-CD80/86

T cells express CD28 that interacts with CD80 or CD86 (B7-1 and -2) on APCs. This interaction stabilizes the immune synapse and multiplies the intensity of T-cell-receptor (TCR) mediated T-cell activation in response to MHC coupled antigen presentation by the APC. Once activated, T cells express CTLA4, an inhibitory molecule that binds CD80/86 with higher avidity than CD28. This observation led to the engineering of abatacept, a fusion molecule between CTLA4 and IgG. Abatacept disrupts the CD28-CD80/86 interaction, preventing a productive T-cell activation following TCR-Ag-MHC binding.

Abatacept is an effective treatment for rheumatoid arthritis.[27] Abatacept failed to improve outcomes when added to cyclophosphamide in the ACCESS trial[28] in patients with active lupus nephritis. Abatacept was also evaluated in conjunction with mycophenolate mofetil in patients with active lupus nephritis. There was no difference in the primary outcome of complete response, but abatacept treatment resulted in greater improvement than placebo of immunologic parameters (C3, dsDNA) and nephrotic range proteinuria.[29] Following these results, a newly developed antibody that targets CD28, lulizumab pegol, is currently being evaluated in a phase II trial in patients with active nonrenal SLE.

ICOS-B7RP

Upon activation, T cells express the inducible costimulator (ICOS) on their surface, which binds to B7-related peptide-1 (B7RP-1, ICOSL). This interaction plays a significant role in both T-cell activation and T-cell-dependent B-cell maturation and high-affinity IgG production. Blocking ICOS:B7RP-1 interactions by targeting B7RP led to improvement of nephritis in NZB/W F1 mice.[30] A B7RP-1 targeting antibody (AMG 557) was shown to be safe in a phase I trial in SLE and is currently being evaluated in early-stage clinical trials in subacute cutaneous lupus and lupus arthritis.

CELL SURFACE MOLECULES

CD20

Mature B cells, but not plasma cells, express CD20 on their surfaces. The chimeric anti-CD20 antibody rituximab has proven to be efficacious in rheumatoid arthritis.[31] Rituximab depletes B cells without a significant effect on total immunoglobulin production because of the limited effect on antibody-forming cells (plasma cells). Early noncontrolled trials suggested that rituximab could be efficacious in the treatment of SLE.[32] In the LUNAR trial, patients with lupus nephritis classes III and IV were randomized to rituximab or placebo. All patients received mycophenolate mofetil and corticosteroids. The addition of rituximab led to an increase in complement and decrease in anti-dsDNA levels and a nonstatistically significant increase in response rates (primarily partial responses).[33] A phase II/III trial of rituximab on nonrenal SLE (EXPLORER trial) failed to show a difference between rituximab and placebo.[34] Despite these negative results, rituximab is still recommended as a treatment of last resort in lupus nephritis[35] and could possibly be helpful in other refractory manifestations of SLE, such as idiopathic thrombocytopenic purpura or thrombotic thrombocytopenia purpura.

Given the observation that human antichimeric antibodies (HACA) may develop in a large proportion of SLE patients treated with rituximab, a fully humanized (90%) anti-CD20 antibody, ocrelizumab, was evaluated in two phase III trials. In the double-blind placebo-controlled trial BELONG, patients with class III and IV nephritis[36] received ocrelizumab or placebo on the background of either mycophenolate mofetil or the Euro-Lupus nephritis treatment protocol (cyclophosphamide induction followed by azathioprine). The trial was terminated early due to a significant increase in serious infections (in the mycophenolate + ocrelizumab group). The efficacy analysis showed a nonstatistically significant numerical superiority of ocrelizumab over placebo. The second trial of ocrelizumab in nonrenal lupus (BEGIN) was also terminated early.

As it stands, anti-CD20 targeting may be an option for SLE patients not responding to other modalities, but it does not seem to be a universally helpful therapeutic strategy.

CD22

As B-cell depletion seems to have marginal effects, modulation of the B-cell receptor signal may represent a better strategy to achieve disease control. CD22 is a molecule expressed on B cells but not plasma cells or memory B cells, modulating activation and migration. Epratuzumab is a humanized anti-CD22 antibody that was evaluated in two phase II trials in SLE (ALLEVIATE).[37] The trials were prematurely discontinued due to interruption in drug supply, but an exploratory analysis showed a positive signal, with the epratuzumab treated patients reaching BILAG responses at statistically significant higher rate than controls at week 12 of treatment (44% vs 30%). The subsequent EMBLEM trial used the BICLA response index and showed a significant increase in response rate between epratuzumab treated group and placebo. At 12 weeks, 2400 mg monthly dose of epratuzumab resulted in BICLA responses of 45.9%, 40.5%, and 43.2% (weekly, biweekly, monthly dosing) versus 21.1% for the placebo group. These results remain to be confirmed in the concluded 54-week phase III trials (EMBODY 1 and 2). Mechanistic studies have proposed

that the effect of epratuzumab is the trogocytosis not only of CD22 but also other B-cell-receptor modulating surface molecules, such as CD21 and CD19.[38]

CONCLUSION

The detailed characterization of SLE immunopathology has led to the design of several targeted treatment strategies. Moreover, the standardization of outcomes has made feasible large trials with heterogeneous groups of patients with SLE. Nevertheless, none of the new biologics has proven to be as successful as similar molecules in inflammatory arthritis. Importantly, none of the targeted treatment trials in lupus nephritis, arguably the most severe manifestation of SLE, has been successful. The challenge for the near future is to translate a wealth of basic science findings into clinically meaningful treatment schemes that will most likely combine new molecules with traditional immunosuppressives in hopes to both improve outcomes and limit medication related side effects.

REFERENCES

1. Furie RA, Petri MA, Wallace DJ, Ginzler EM, Merrill JT, Stohl W, et al. Novel evidence-based systemic lupus erythematosus responder index. *Arthritis Rheum* September 15, 2009;**61**(9):1143–51. PubMed PMID: 19714615. Pubmed Central PMCID: 2748175.
2. Do RK, Hatada E, Lee H, Tourigny MR, Hilbert D, Chen-Kiang S. Attenuation of apoptosis underlies B lymphocyte stimulator enhancement of humoral immune response. *J Exp Med* October 2, 2000;**192**(7):953–64. PubMed PMID: 11015437. Pubmed Central PMCID: 2193312.
3. Furie R, Petri M, Zamani O, Cervera R, Wallace DJ, Tegzova D, et al. A phase III, randomized, placebo-controlled study of belimumab, a monoclonal antibody that inhibits B lymphocyte stimulator, in patients with systemic lupus erythematosus. *Arthritis Rheum* December 2011;**63**(12):3918–30. PubMed PMID: 22127708.
4. Navarra SV, Guzman RM, Gallacher AE, Hall S, Levy RA, Jimenez RE, et al. Efficacy and safety of belimumab in patients with active systemic lupus erythematosus: a randomised, placebo-controlled, phase 3 trial. *Lancet* February 26, 2011;**377**(9767):721–31. PubMed PMID: 21296403.
5. Isenberg DA, Urowitz MB, Merrill JT, Hoffman RW, Linnik MD, Morgan-Cox M, et al., editors. *Efficacy and Safety of subcutaneous tabalumab in patients with systemic lupus erythematosus (SLE): results from 2 phase 3, 52–Week, Multicenter, randomized, double-blind, placebo-controlled trials.* Boston, MA: American College of Rheumatology Annual Meeting; 2014.
6. Furie RA, Leon G, Thomas M, Petri MA, Chu AD, Hislop C, et al. A phase 2, randomised, placebo-controlled clinical trial of blisibimod, an inhibitor of B cell activating factor, in patients with moderate-to-severe systemic lupus erythematosus, the PEARL-SC study. *Ann Rheum Dis* September 2015;**74**(9):1667–75. PubMed PMID: 24748629.
7. Ginzler EM, Wax S, Rajeswaran A, Copt S, Hillson J, Ramos E, et al. Atacicept in combination with MMF and corticosteroids in lupus nephritis: results of a prematurely terminated trial. *Arthritis Res Ther* 2012;**14**(1):R33. PubMed PMID: 22325903. Pubmed Central PMCID: 3392829.

8. Isenberg D, Gordon C, Licu D, Copt S, Rossi CP, Wofsy D. Efficacy and safety of atacicept for prevention of flares in patients with moderate-to-severe systemic lupus erythematosus (SLE): 52-week data (APRIL-SLE randomised trial). *Ann Rheum Dis* November 2015;**74**(11):2006–15. PubMed PMID: 24951103.

9. Kayagaki N, Yan M, Seshasayee D, Wang H, Lee W, French DM, et al. BAFF/BLyS receptor 3 binds the B cell survival factor BAFF ligand through a discrete surface loop and promotes processing of NF-kappaB2. *Immunity* October 2002;**17**(4):515–24. PubMed PMID: 12387744.

10. Baechler EC, Batliwalla FM, Karypis G, Gaffney PM, Ortmann WA, Espe KJ, et al. Interferon-inducible gene expression signature in peripheral blood cells of patients with severe lupus. *Proc Natl Acad Sci USA* March 4, 2003;**100**(5):2610–5. PubMed PMID: 12604793. Pubmed Central PMCID: 151388.

11. Khamashta M, Merrill JT, Werth VP, Furie R, Kalunian K, Illei GG, et al., editors. *Safety and efficacy of sifalimumab, an anti IFN-alpha monoclonal antibody, in a phase 2b study of moderate to severe systemic lupus erythematosus (SLE)*. Boston, MA: American College of Rheumatology Annual Meeting; 2014.

12. Kalunian K, Merrill JT, Maciuca R, Ouyang W, McBride JM, Townsend MJ, et al. *Efficacy and safety of rontalizumab (Anti-Interferon alpha) in SLE subjects with restricted immunosuppressant use: results of a randomized, double-blind, placebo-controlled phase 2 study*. Washington, DC: American College of Rheumatology; 2012.

13. Morehouse C, Chang L, Wang L, Brohawn P, Ueda S, Illei G, et al. *Target modulation of a Type I interferon (IFN) gene signature with sifalimumab or anifrolumab in systemic lupus erythematosus (SLE) patients in two open label phase 2 Japanese trials*. Boston, MA: American College of Rheumatology Annual Meeting; 2014.

14. Lawson BR, Prud'homme GJ, Chang Y, Gardner HA, Kuan J, Kono DH, et al. Treatment of murine lupus with cDNA encoding IFN-gammaR/Fc. *J Clin Invest* July 2000;**106**(2):207–15. PubMed PMID: 10903336. Pubmed Central PMCID: 314313.

15. Werth VP, Fiorentino D, Cohen SB, Fivenson D, Hansen C, Zoog S, et al. *A phase I single-dose crossover study to evaluate the safety, tolerability, pharmacokinetics, pharmacodynamics, and clinical efficacy of AMG 811 (anti-IFN-gamma) in subjects with discoid lupus erythematosus*. Boston, MA: American College of Rheumatology Annual Meeting; 2014.

16. Martin DA, Welcher A, Boedigheimer M, Amoura Z, Kivitz A, Buyon JP, et al. *AMG 811 (anti-IFN-gamma) treatment leads to a reduction in the whole blood IFN-signature and serum CXCL10 in subjects with systemic lupus erythematosus: results of two phase I studies*. Boston, MA: American College of Rheumatology Annual Meeting; 2014.

17. Kyttaris VC, Zhang Z, Kuchroo VK, Oukka M, Tsokos GC. Cutting edge: IL-23 receptor deficiency prevents the development of lupus nephritis in C57BL/6-lpr/lpr mice. *J Immunol* May 1, 2010;**184**(9):4605–9. PubMed PMID: 20308633. Pubmed Central PMCID: 2926666.

18. Crispin JC, Oukka M, Bayliss G, Cohen RA, Van Beek CA, Stillman IE, et al. Expanded double negative T cells in patients with systemic lupus erythematosus produce IL-17 and infiltrate the kidneys. *J Immunol* December 15, 2008;**181**(12):8761–6. PubMed PMID: 19050297. Pubmed Central PMCID: 2596652.

19. Kyttaris VC, Kampagianni O, Tsokos GC. Treatment with anti-interleukin 23 antibody ameliorates disease in lupus-prone mice. *Biomed Res Int* 2013;**2013**:861028. PubMed PMID: 23841097. Pubmed Central PMCID: 3690216.

20. Schmidt T, Paust HJ, Krebs CF, Turner JE, Kaffke A, Bennstein SB, et al. Function of the Th17/interleukin-17A immune response in murine lupus nephritis. *Arthritis Rheumatol* February 2015;**67**(2):475–87. PubMed PMID: 25385550.

21. Ritchlin C, Rahman P, Kavanaugh A, McInnes IB, Puig L, Li S, et al. Efficacy and safety of the anti-IL-12/23 p40 monoclonal antibody, ustekinumab, in patients with active psoriatic arthritis despite conventional non-biological and biological anti-tumour necrosis factor therapy: 6-month and 1-year results of the phase 3, multicentre, double-blind, placebo-controlled, randomised PSUMMIT 2 trial. *Ann Rheum Dis* June 2014;**73**(6):990–9. PubMed PMID: 24482301. Pubmed Central PMCID: 4033144.

22. Hillmen P, Young NS, Schubert J, Brodsky RA, Socie G, Muus P, et al. The complement inhibitor eculizumab in paroxysmal nocturnal hemoglobinuria. *N Engl J Med* September 21, 2006;**355**(12):1233–43. PubMed PMID: 16990386.

23. Barilla-Labarca ML, Toder K, Furie R. Targeting the complement system in systemic lupus erythematosus and other diseases. *Clin Immunol* September 2013;**148**(3):313–21. PubMed PMID: 23623037.

24. Early GS, Zhao W, Burns CM. Anti-CD40 ligand antibody treatment prevents the development of lupus-like nephritis in a subset of New Zealand black x New Zealand white mice. Response correlates with the absence of an anti-antibody response. *J Immunol* October 1, 1996;**157**(7):3159–64. PubMed PMID: 8816428.

25. Boumpas DT, Furie R, Manzi S, Illei GG, Wallace DJ, Balow JE, et al. A short course of BG9588 (anti-CD40 ligand antibody) improves serologic activity and decreases hematuria in patients with proliferative lupus glomerulonephritis. *Arthritis Rheum* March 2003;**48**(3):719–27. PubMed PMID: 12632425.

26. Kalunian KC, Davis Jr JC, Merrill JT, Totoritis MC, Wofsy D, Group I-LS. Treatment of systemic lupus erythematosus by inhibition of T cell costimulation with anti-CD154: a randomized, double-blind, placebo-controlled trial. *Arthritis Rheum* December 2002;**46**(12):3251–8. PubMed PMID: 12483729.

27. Genovese MC, Becker JC, Schiff M, Luggen M, Sherrer Y, Kremer J, et al. Abatacept for rheumatoid arthritis refractory to tumor necrosis factor alpha inhibition. *N Engl J Med* September 15, 2005;**353**(11):1114–23. PubMed PMID: 16162882.

28. Group AT. Treatment of lupus nephritis with abatacept: the abatacept and cyclophosphamide combination efficacy and safety study. *Arthritis Rheumatol* November 2014;**66**(11):3096–104. PubMed PMID: 25403681.

29. Furie R, Nicholls K, Cheng TT, Houssiau F, Burgos-Vargas R, Chen SL, et al. Efficacy and safety of abatacept in lupus nephritis: a twelve-month, randomized, double-blind study. *Arthritis Rheumatol* February 2014;**66**(2):379–89. PubMed PMID: 24504810.

30. Iwai H, Abe M, Hirose S, Tsushima F, Tezuka K, Akiba H, et al. Involvement of inducible costimulator-B7 homologous protein costimulatory pathway in murine lupus nephritis. *J Immunol* September 15, 2003;**171**(6):2848–54. PubMed PMID: 12960306.

31. Edwards JC, Szczepanski L, Szechinski J, Filipowicz-Sosnowska A, Emery P, Close DR, et al. Efficacy of B-cell-targeted therapy with rituximab in patients with rheumatoid arthritis. *N Engl J Med* June 17, 2004;**350**(25):2572–81. PubMed PMID: 15201414.

32. Ramos-Casals M, Soto MJ, Cuadrado MJ, Khamashta MA. Rituximab in systemic lupus erythematosus: a systematic review of off-label use in 188 cases. *Lupus* August 2009;**18**(9):767–76. PubMed PMID: 19578100.

33. Rovin BH, Furie R, Latinis K, Looney RJ, Fervenza FC, Sanchez-Guerrero J, et al. Efficacy and safety of rituximab in patients with active proliferative lupus nephritis: the Lupus Nephritis Assessment with Rituximab study. *Arthritis Rheum* April 2012;**64**(4):1215–26. PubMed PMID: 22231479.

34. Merrill JT, Neuwelt CM, Wallace DJ, Shanahan JC, Latinis KM, Oates JC, et al. Efficacy and safety of rituximab in moderately-to-severely active systemic lupus erythematosus: the randomized, double-blind, phase II/III systemic lupus erythematosus evaluation of rituximab trial. *Arthritis Rheum* January 2010;**62**(1):222–33. PubMed PMID: 20039413.

35. Bertsias GK, Tektonidou M, Amoura Z, Aringer M, Bajema I, Berden JH, et al. Joint European League against Rheumatism and European Renal Association-European Dialysis and Transplant Association (EULAR/ERA-EDTA) recommendations for the management of adult and paediatric lupus nephritis. *Ann Rheum Dis* November 2012;**71**(11):1771–82. PubMed PMID: 22851469. Pubmed Central PMCID: 3465859.

36. Mysler EF, Spindler AJ, Guzman R, Bijl M, Jayne D, Furie RA, et al. Efficacy and safety of ocrelizumab in active proliferative lupus nephritis: results from a randomized, double-blind, phase III study. *Arthritis Rheum* September 2013;**65**(9):2368–79. PubMed PMID: 23740801.

37. Wallace DJ, Gordon C, Strand V, Hobbs K, Petri M, Kalunian K, et al. Efficacy and safety of epratuzumab in patients with moderate/severe flaring systemic lupus erythematosus: results from two randomized, double-blind, placebo-controlled, multicentre studies (ALLEVIATE) and follow-up. *Rheumatology (Oxford)* July 2013;**52**(7):1313–22. PubMed PMID: 23542611.

38. Rossi EA, Goldenberg DM, Michel R, Rossi DL, Wallace DJ, Chang CH. Trogocytosis of multiple B-cell surface markers by CD22 targeting with epratuzumab. *Blood* October 24, 2013;**122**(17):3020–9. PubMed PMID: 23821660.

Chapter 65

Management Lessons from Clinical Trials of Kidney Disease in Systemic Lupus Erythematosus

Brad H. Rovin, Isabelle Ayoub

Division of Nephrology, Ohio State University Wexner Medical Center, Columbus, OH, USA

SUMMARY

Clinically significant lupus nephritis occurs in about 40% of the overall systemic lupus erythematosus population. Despite aggressive therapy with anti-inflammatory and immunosuppressive drugs, chronic kidney damage and kidney failure are common in lupus nephritis patients. Also, standard-of-care treatment regimens are associated with significant toxicity and patient morbidity. To address this problem, a number of prospective, controlled, randomized clinical trials of potential new therapies have been undertaken recently in lupus nephritis. Unfortunately, none of these trials succeeded in demonstrating better renal outcomes or less toxicity than the standard-of-care approaches. Despite these failures, all of the trials provide important insights into the clinical behavior of lupus nephritis, which can be translated into more effective management strategies. This chapter examines lessons from lupus nephritis clinical trials and uses these lessons to build a new framework for future trials of new therapeutics.

KIDNEY DISEASE IN SYSTEMIC LUPUS ERYTHEMATOSUS

The most common form of kidney injury in systemic lupus erythematosus (SLE) is mediated, or at least initiated, by the accumulation of glomerular immune complexes (see Chapter 33) and is termed lupus nephritis (LN). LN occurs in about 40% of the overall lupus population, but it shows considerable racial and ethnic heterogeneity, appearing much more frequently in black, Hispanic, and Asian patients than white patients.[1] Kidney outcomes, such as end-stage renal disease (ESRD) or doubling of serum creatinine (a surrogate marker of ESRD), are also worse in black and Hispanic patients as compared to white patients.[2] Lupus patient survival is also influenced by the presence of LN. The highest mortality over time is seen in those who develop chronic kidney disease (CKD).[3,4]

LN, especially proliferative LN (see Chapter 41), is therefore generally treated aggressively, with both high-dose corticosteroids and an immunosuppressive drug such as mycophenolate mofetil (MMF) or cyclophosphamide (see Chapter 62). Despite these therapies, the incidence of ESRD due to LN remains high at 4.9 cases per million population in the United States.[5] According to the 2014 United States Renal Data System report, about 2% of the prevalent patients receiving renal replacement therapy have LN-attributable ESRD. The prevalence of CKD in LN is difficult to quantify; however, if one assumes that a complete clinical response after treatment is necessary to prevent CKD, the prevalence of CKD is likely to be substantial. For example, the complete renal response rate to standard-of-care (SOC) therapy after 1 year of treatment is generally only 15–40%, although complete response rates of over 70% have been reported in Asians in some studies.[6] Complete responses may be achieved beyond 1 year; however, this lag in reaching a complete response, coupled with the large number of patients with incomplete responses, suggest that CKD is common in LN patients.

These unsatisfactory outcomes have provided the impetus for a number of recent large-scale clinical trials of novel therapeutics for LN. Table 1 summarizes the outcomes of several of these trials. The results have been uniformly disappointing. To date, no new LN therapies approved by the U.S. Food and Drug Administration have emerged from these efforts. Therefore, it is warranted to reassess LN clinical trial outcomes in an effort to learn how trials may be improved so new LN therapeutics may be brought to the clinic.

Overview of Clinical Trials in Lupus Nephritis

Because LN can be severe and progress rapidly, most randomized, prospective clinical trials of novel LN therapeutics have relied on an add-on design (Figure 1). The rationale is that a direct comparison of a new drug alone to SOC is too

Systemic Lupus Erythematosus. http://dx.doi.org/10.1016/B978-0-12-801917-7.00065-6

TABLE 1 Recent LN Clinical Trials and Their Outcomes

Drug	Drug Class	Drug Target	Trial Type	Primary Efficacy End Point	Met Efficacy End Point?	References[d]
Abatacept-BMS	Fusion protein	CTLA4-B7 interaction	Phase II/III	Time to CRR[a]	No	NCT00430677
Abatacept-ACCESS	Fusion protein	CTLA4-B7 interaction	Phase II	% CRR week 24	No	NCT00774852
Laquinimod	Small molecule	Inflammation	Phase II	% RR[b] week 24	Pending	NCT01085097
Rituximab	Monoclonal antibody	CD20	Phase III	% RR week 52	No	NCT00282347
Ocrelizumab	Monoclonal antibody	CD20	Phase III	% RR week 48	No	NCT00539838
Sirukumab	Monoclonal antibody	IL-6	Phase II	% Δ[c] proteinuria week 24	No	NCT01273389
Anti-CD40 ligand	Monoclonal antibody	CD40 ligand	Phase II	50% ↓ proteinuria	Stopped-toxicity	NCT00001789
Belimumab	Monoclonal antibody	BlyS	Phase III	% RR week 104	Underway	NCT01639339
Anti-TWEAK	Monoclonal antibody	TWEAK	Phase II	% RR week 52	Underway	NCT01930890

[a]Complete renal response.
[b]Renal response, complete and partial.
[c]Change in.
[d]Clinical trials.gov identifier.

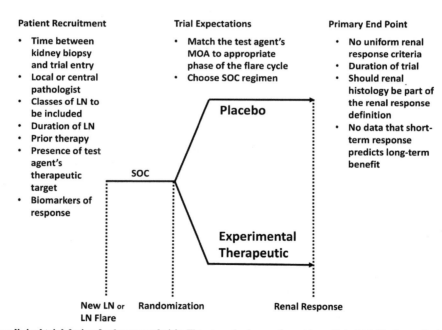

Patient Recruitment

- Time between kidney biopsy and trial entry
- Local or central pathologist
- Classes of LN to be included
- Duration of LN
- Prior therapy
- Presence of test agent's therapeutic target
- Biomarkers of response

Trial Expectations

- Match the test agent's MOA to appropriate phase of the flare cycle
- Choose SOC regimen

Primary End Point

- No uniform renal response criteria
- Duration of trial
- Should renal histology be part of the renal response definition
- No data that short-term response predicts long-term benefit

Placebo

Experimental Therapeutic

SOC

New LN or LN Flare   Randomization   Renal Response

FIGURE 1   **The add-on clinical trial design for lupus nephritis.** The general scheme of an add-on clinical trial is shown. Patients with newly diagnosed lupus nephritis (LN) or a new flare of LN are given standard-of-care (SOC) therapy and randomized to receive either the experimental drug or placebo. To optimize the chances for success, several aspects of the clinical trial must be considered before it begins, including defining the desired patient population, the type SOC regimen, how the experimental drug's mechanism of action (MOA) relates to the pathogenesis of LN, what the kidney response end points should be, and when response should be assessed. These considerations are discussed in detail in the text.

risky. In theory, such a trial might be feasible if frequent clinical assessments and stop points are in place, which allow prompt withdrawal from the trial if the patient does not achieve prespecified levels of improvement at specified time points. A common critique of the add-on trial design is that because SOC treatments already work well, it is difficult to demonstrate an incremental improvement attributable to the new drug, even though the new drug might be capable of that. For example, the new drug may act through the same pathways as SOC, and thus its effect may be masked or minimized. Alternatively, the new drug may act through pathways that are different from those of SOC but are expressed after the high-dose steroid phase is completed. In this case add-on trial design may fail to identify effective therapy that would synergize with SOC, unless the new drug was deployed later in the course of induction therapy.

An important caveat to the preceding discussion is the use of high-dose corticosteroids, which is common at the start of almost all trials. The anti-inflammatory activity of high-dose corticosteroids occurs rapidly, and early in the course of LN is sufficient to control disease activity. Although corticosteroids alone do not preserve kidney function well over the long-term,[7] they can confound short-term (months) outcomes, and most trials of new LN therapeutics have been relatively short-term. This is suggested by a post hoc analysis of the BELONG trial, in which ocrelizumab, a humanized anti-B cell (CD20) monoclonal antibody, was added to SOC for induction of remission in proliferative lupus nephritis.[8] In the placebo group, overall renal responses (complete and partial) increased in parallel with the initial methylprednisolone dose, being highest in patients who received over 1 g of methylprednisolone. Ocrelizumab plus SOC was associated with a 24% higher overall renal response than placebo plus SOC at 1 year in patients who received less than 500 mg of methylprednisolone initially. It may be feasible to design trials with less upfront corticosteroid administration. The pilot data of a novel LN trial using no oral corticosteroids, but only the combination of MMF and rituximab suggest both safety and efficacy comparable to historical outcomes.[9] However, each of the two infusions of rituximab was preceded by 500 mg of methylprednisolone.

PATIENT SELECTION IN CLINICAL TRIALS

LN is intrinsically heterogeneous in its pathogenesis, histologic and clinical manifestations, and outcomes. This heterogeneity creates difficulty in the interpretation of clinical trial data, which can be more powerful if derived from uniform populations. The design of many trials has added iatrogenic heterogeneity to this intrinsic heterogeneity, compounding the problem.

Almost all trials to date have required a kidney biopsy to determine eligibility prior to patient enrollment. Although the kidney biopsy should be useful in achieving homogeneity in patient cohorts, it likely has had the opposite effect in recent LN studies. Two important but correctable sources of variation are the reliance on local pathologic diagnosis without adjudication by a central nephropathologist, and lengthy intervals between obtaining the biopsy and study initiation.

The agreement among nephropathologists with regard to kidney biopsy interpretation using the International Society of Nephrology/Renal Pathology Society (ISN/RPS) LN classification system (Chapter 41) has been examined. Interobserver agreement for Class III/IV-defining glomerular lesions was only moderate.[10] Similarly, the ability to distinguish active from chronic glomerular lesions and concordance for interstitial lesions, including chronic changes of interstitial fibrosis and tubular atrophy, were also only moderate.[10,11] Highly experienced nephropathologists, defined as having read over 500 kidney biopsies, did slightly better than nephropathologists who, on average, had read about 130 biopsies. If these findings are extrapolated back to the situation in which kidney biopsy interpretation is done locally, it is likely that local kidney biopsy interpretations introduce increased error into trials that could be mitigated by a central pathology adjudication committee. A further benefit of central pathology adjudication is the adequacy of the biopsy specimen, including verifying that it contains sufficient tissue to ensure confidence in the diagnosis. This is especially important for focal glomerular and interstitial lesions.[12] Correct representation of interstitial lesions is critical given the importance of the interstitium in quantifying long-term kidney prognosis.[13,14]

Recent advances in kidney biopsy interpretation include molecular analyses of kidneys from murine models of LN. These show that intrarenal gene expression changes over time and, not unexpectedly, in response to treatment.[15] Furthermore, mice from the same strain, at the same stage of LN, may have considerable differences in gene expression that are not reflected in routine histology.[16,17] In glomeruli isolated from human LN kidney biopsies, intraglomerular protein expression is variable among patients with the same histologic disease class.[18] Also, distinctively different intraglomerular gene expression is present among individuals who were thought to be at the same stage of the disease.[19] Taken together, routine pathologic evaluation of kidney biopsies may group individuals together who have different injury pathways activated. If a new drug targets a specific pathway, study subjects in whom that pathway is not active may skew the results. Controlling for this sort of individual heterogeneity is not feasible in trials until molecular analysis of the kidney biopsy is available.[12] It is possible now, however, to make an effort to enroll patients at a similar LN stage by restricting the interval between biopsy and the start of the trial to no more than 3 months. Because a flare of previously treated LN may be pathogenically different than new LN despite similar histology, a case could be made for including only new-onset LN in trials (or analyzing new and flare patients separately), but this may limit enrollment. Historically however, LN trials have enrolled a large proportion of new- or recent-onset LN.[20,21]

Many LN trials have focused on proliferative LN, although patients with combined proliferative and membranous LN have generally not been excluded. Some trials have also allowed proliferative and pure membranous LN patients to participate. The logistical argument for including mixed histologies, and even pure membranous, in trials dominated by proliferative LN is to increase enrollment. From a therapeutic perspective, proliferative and membranous LN appear to respond similarly to broad-spectrum immunosuppressive therapies.[22,23] It is not clear if combining different classes of LN in therapeutic trials makes biologic sense, especially in studies of targeted immunotherapies, although an analysis of patients with pure membranous and pure proliferative LN treated with anti-B-cell therapy demonstrated identical clinical responses and response kinetics.[24]

Nonetheless, there are differences in the molecular characteristics of membranous and proliferative LN, and these may have implications for treatment with more specific immune-modulatory agents. For example, the peripheral blood of patients with proliferative LN had a significantly higher ratio of Th1 to Th2 cells than the peripheral blood of patients with pure membranous LN.[25] Furthermore, histologic examination of kidney biopsies from LN patients showed loss of podocyte markers, such as synaptopodin and nephrin, in almost 90% of proliferative biopsies but only 30–50% of membranous biopsies,[26] suggesting a structural defect of the podocyte in proliferative LN versus a functional defect of the podocyte in Class V LN. Thus, depending on the mechanism of action of the drug being tested, it is conceivable that including patients with pure Class V LN or with mixed histology may confound trial outcomes.

A final consideration in patient selection is to ensure that, if the biologic target of a test drug is known, the target is present in the patients being considered for enrollment. For example, the addition of an anti-interleukin-6 (IL-6) monoclonal antibody to maintenance therapy in LN patients who had not achieved complete remission did not improve clinical response.[27] However, measurable serum levels of IL-6 were found in only 29% of the anti-IL-6 arm. It could be argued that anti-IL-6 would have performed better in patients with increased IL-6 levels. Matching a therapy to its biologic target would require measuring the targets of new drugs before trials start. This may reduce total enrollment; however, the trade-off could be a larger effect size in a smaller but better-suited LN population. The rationale for this approach is the assumption that the presence of increased target levels at the start of a trial indicates a role for that target in the pathogenesis of LN, or at least in that individual's LN at that point in time. This assumption needs to be tested. Another important consideration is where to measure a target. If the target is

mainly relevant to LN, intrarenal levels may be more informative than serum levels. Although intrarenal measurements are difficult, urine measurements are practical and often reflect the kidney milieu.

END POINTS FOR CLINICAL TRIALS

There is no consensus regarding the definition of the optimal renal response for an LN clinical trial. The goal of treating LN should always be long-term preservation of kidney function and avoidance of renal replacement therapy. Because of logistic and economic constraints, contemporary trials cannot be run for the many years necessary to accumulate enough hard kidney end points (ESRD, doubling of serum creatinine) to differentiate active drug from placebo. To circumvent this issue, definitions of renal remission in the short-term (at 6–24 months) have been established as surrogates for good long-term kidney outcomes. These definitions are based on proteinuria, serum creatinine, and urine sediment. Proteinuria remaining after therapy is the main driver of remission status.[1,28] Consensus on the levels of proteinuria, serum creatinine, and urine red blood cells that constitute remission has, however, not been achieved. Furthermore, there have been no prospective studies showing that the short-term definitions really do predict good-long term renal outcomes.

The influence of modest differences in the definition of renal response on trial outcomes was illustrated by applying a number of different, but current, renal response criteria to a trial of abatacept added on to SOC for induction of remission in LN.[28] Abatacept (CTLA4-Ig) inhibits primary T-cell-dependent immune responses by blocking the interaction of antigen-presenting cells with CD28 on T cells. The abatacept trial showed no effect beyond placebo using the trial's own definition of renal response.[28,29] However, reevaluation of the abatacept trial data with other renal response definitions, including those from the American College of Rheumatology and contemporary LN trials, demonstrated an increase in the number of complete responders in abatacept-treated patients compared to placebo-treated patients. Although this retrospective analysis clearly shows the importance of the outcome definition in evaluating a trial, it cannot recommend a preferred definition because a link between short-term and long-term outcomes still needs to be established.

In an effort to establish a short-term end point for LN trials, patients with at least 7 years of follow-up from the Euro-Lupus Nephritis Trial (ELNT) were reexamined.[30] ELNT tested the equivalence of low-dose cyclophosphamide and high-dose cyclophosphamide in the induction of remission of LN.[31] Serum creatinine, proteinuria, and hematuria at months 3, 6, and 12 of the trial were assessed to determine which, if any, of these clinical parameters predicted good kidney function (serum creatinine <1 mg/dl) after ≥7 years. This investigation showed a proteinuria level of <0.8 g/d at 12 months was the best short-term end point for long-term renal survival. This level of proteinuria yielded the highest sum of sensitivity plus specificity (1.6) for good long-term kidney outcome, and when applied to the ELNT population correctly classified 80% of the long-term follow-up patients. Interestingly, the addition of serum creatinine did not improve the performance of proteinuria alone, while the addition of urine sediment significantly decreased the performance of proteinuria alone.

This retrospective analysis suggests an end point and duration for LN clinical trials. However, it is premature to consider this short-term end point as definitive for future trials. The ELNT trial participants were mainly white, and it is conceivable that different races and ethnicities will require different response definitions. These results may not apply to patients with pure membranous LN, and a proteinuria end point may not be applicable to treatment regimens that include drugs such as the calcineurin inhibitors that can decrease proteinuria by nonimmune mechanisms.

Although the kidney biopsy is generally not repeated in LN patients to assess the response to therapy in clinical trials, this is worth considering in future clinical trials. A number of repeat biopsy studies have shown discordance between clinical findings and histologic findings in LN. Patients with resolution of proteinuria and normalization of serum creatinine can still have histologic activity on biopsy, even after years of clinical remission.[32] Conversely, patients can have persistent proteinuria but no evidence of histologic disease activity.[9,33] A combination of kidney histology plus clinical remission criteria may provide an optimal picture of response status. To avoid the need for repetitive invasive procedures, a more palatable alternative would be a combination of clinical criteria plus urine or serum biomarkers of kidney pathology as they are developed (Chapter 7).

MATCHING CLINICAL TRIAL EXPECTATIONS TO THE EXPERIMENTAL THERAPEUTIC

A majority of recent clinical trials have focused on the induction phase of LN, and trial end points have focused on demonstrating differences in complete and partial remissions compared to standard-of-care alone. As seen in Table 1, this approach has not been overtly successful. While one may interpret these outcomes as being due to ineffective drugs, there are alternate interpretations.

A simplification of the LN flare cycle is depicted in Figure 2. LN comes to clinical attention in SLE patients only after cumulative inflammatory injury to the kidney has been sufficient to damage the glomerular basement membrane, allowing blood and protein to leak into the urine. This may be accompanied by impaired kidney function, detected as an overtly abnormal serum creatinine or as a sustained increase in serum creatinine from a patient's healthy baseline level. However, before reaching the clinical stage of LN, autoimmunity will have been active for a while, silently

causing kidney damage through immune complexes, cytokines, and leukocytes (Chapter 33). It is known that autoantibodies appear years before patients develop clinical manifestations of SLE, and autoantibody specificities evolve as a patient approaches the onset of clinical SLE.[34] The interval between activation of autoimmunity and clinical LN is not known, but kidney biopsies from patients with SLE and no overt clinical signs of kidney involvement can show LN. Histologically, most of these cases of so-called silent LN have been Class I or II; however, one center found that 15% of their patients with silent LN had Class III or IV, and 10% had Class V LN.[35] These data support the concept of a preclinical phase of LN during which undetected immune-mediated damage occurs in the kidney.

Treatment with therapies that dampen autoimmunity during preclinical LN would be ideal. Such an approach could, theoretically, require less exposure to highly toxic medications and attenuate their associated morbidities. Early treatment could also prevent CKD. Kidney biopsies from patients who have achieved complete clinical remission after a few months of aggressive SOC induction therapy often show

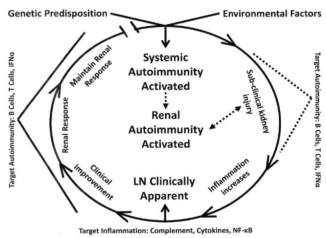

FIGURE 2 The lupus nephritis flare cycle. Systemic autoimmunity is activated in individuals with an appropriate genetic background who are exposed to specific, as yet unknown environmental triggers. Patients destined to develop lupus nephritis (LN) begin to accrue subclinical kidney injury as autoimmune mechanisms result in renal inflammation. Renal-specific autoimmunity may become activated as a consequence of systemic autoimmunity or after the kidney has been initially injured, and may contribute to further kidney injury and predispose to future renal flares. As kidney injury increases, it reaches a point sufficient to cause clinical manifestations, such as proteinuria, hematuria, or kidney dysfunction. Therapy is generally started at this time. Most patients improve at least partially as a result of treatment. In general patients are then started on long-term immunosuppression to maintain the renal response and prevent reactivation autoimmunity and subsequent LN flare. Therapies that target specific aspects of the immune response, applied at appropriate points in the LN flare cycle, may be effective in preventing kidney injury, treating kidney injury, or preventing reactivation of disease and LN flare. Matching a drug's mechanism of action to a specific phase of the LN flare cycle, depending on what immune mechanisms are active during that phase is discussed in detail in the text.

chronic kidney damage.[33] This finding suggests that despite successful treatment, CKD occurs very quickly after LN is clinically apparent. Many of the novel therapies listed in Table 1 could be considered in preclinical LN. These include the B-cell-targeted therapies to prevent ongoing autoantibody production and T-cell-targeted therapies to prevent T-cell help in developing autoimmunity. Anti-type 1 interferon therapies, recently tested in non-renal SLE,[36,37] could also be applied in preclinical LN, given the central importance of the interferon pathway in driving the development of SLE.[38]

At present, there are no biomarkers for preclinical LN (Chapter 7) and routine kidney biopsy of every SLE patient cannot be recommended, because only 40–60% of patients will ever develop LN. If patients with SLE who were predisposed to develop LN could be accurately identified, surveillance kidney biopsies and/or preemptive treatment with drugs that attenuate autoimmunity may be more feasible. There has been some progress toward understanding which patients are prone to develop LN among the general SLE population. A genome-wide association study identified several LN loci in women of European descent by comparing patients with LN to patients with SLE but no LN.[39] The strongest association with LN was in a region of the genome close to the gene for the PDGF-receptor α, and the RNA for this receptor was upregulated in the glomeruli of LN patients compared to normal control glomeruli. Despite a p value less than 5×10^{-7} for this association, the odds ratio for LN at this locus was only 3.4. It is thus likely that LN occurs in those SLE patients who have several LN risk polymorphisms. Accurate identification of SLE patients destined to develop clinically significant LN will require more complete characterization of genetic risk factors.

In lieu of not being able to identify patients who will develop LN, or in whom LN is developing but not clinically apparent, treatment begins when abnormalities of the urine and urine sediment are found in a patient with known or suspected SLE, and a kidney biopsy is performed. At this point in the LN flare cycle, especially in proliferative LN, kidney damage is due to inflammation, and therapy should include an arm directed toward rapidly attenuating inflammation. This initial treatment of LN is often called induction and the anti-inflammatory agent used in current SOC approaches is high-dose corticosteroid. High-dose corticosteroids are very effective early in the course of LN, although alone they are not sufficient to preserve long-term kidney function.[7] Many of the novel therapies listed in Table 1 were added to SOC during induction. In these trials, the novel therapy was expected to improve early renal response rates. Efficacy end points were usually assessed at 6–12 months. However, this expectation is unrealistic if the mechanisms of action of the novel agent do not include directly decreasing inflammation. Drugs that target upstream events in the pathogenesis of LN and kidney injury, such B-cell-directed therapies, may eventually decrease inflammation by preventing the formation or expression of pro-inflammatory

mediators, like immune complexes, but this will take time. Thus the expectation that such agents would improve early renal response rates could not be met, and this was seen repeatedly in trials that did not meet their end points.

Based on the pathogenesis of renal injury in LN (reviewed in Ref. 40; see also Chapter 33), it may be possible to predict the type of interventions that would be expected to rapidly attenuate renal inflammation. For example, the complement system is activated in LN by glomerular immune complexes, and chemotactic complement fragments (e.g., C5a) may mediate renal infiltration by inflammatory leukocytes. Complement system inhibitors have shown beneficial therapeutic effects in animal models of LN. Similarly, pro-inflammatory cytokines, produced by infiltrating leukocytes or injured renal parenchymal cells are expressed in the kidneys of patients with active LN, and anticytokine therapies may therefore improve early renal responses, as exemplified by tumor necrosis factor-like weak inducer of apoptosis (TWEAK). TWEAK is a TNF superfamily cytokine that promotes glomerular epithelial cell proliferation, inflammation, and apoptosis, and it is the target of an ongoing clinical trial (Table 1). Another approach to anticytokine therapy would be to attenuate the activation of NF-κB, which is a key transcription factor necessary for the expression of several pro-inflammatory cytokines. The small molecule laquinimod (Table 1) reduces NF-κB activity and is a general anti-inflammatory agent that has shown efficacy in murine LN.[41] The results of a phase 2 trial of laquinimod for LN induction are pending; however, preliminary data from this trial showed a greater improvement in kidney function and proteinuria in laquinimod-treated patients compared to SOC alone at 6 months.[42]

Novel anti-inflammatory drugs may be useful as corticosteroid-sparing or corticosteroid-reducing agents. Given the significant morbidities associated with corticosteroid use, reducing or eliminating the need for high-dose steroids in LN would represent a significant advance in treatment. For example, corticosteroids are effective in blocking NF-κB,[43] and so drugs that target NF-κB may allow reduction or elimination of corticosteroids in LN induction. In contrast, it is not clear whether corticosteroids effectively inhibit complement activation in the LN kidney. In other clinical situations, such as hemodialysis and cardiopulmonary bypass, glucocorticoids do not block complement activation.[44,45] If this is also the case in SLE or LN, then anti-complement therapy could potentially synergize with corticosteroid therapy in LN induction and improve renal response rates.

Drugs that target autoimmune pathways more proximal than those that mediate direct organ injury may be best suited for preventing LN flares after an initial anti-inflammatory approach has reduced inflammation and healing of the renal parenchyma has started. However, even in such patients, the autoimmune milieu that led to intrarenal inflammation is likely still active, and operating in the background. Recent findings suggest that at least in some LN patients autoimmune processes can become established in the interstitium of the kidney.[46] The proximity of interstitial T cells to interstitial B cells and the secretion of clonally restricted antibodies by interstitial plasma cells raise the possibility of intrarenal, kidney-specific autoantibody production. It has been known for some time that patients treated with corticosteroids alone have a significantly higher LN flare rate than patients treated with corticosteroids and a long-term immunosuppressive drug.[47,48] Thus, the initiation of anti-B-cell, anti-T-cell, or anti-interferon therapies shortly after starting anti-inflammatory treatment, for example, would be expected to prevent the generation of autoantibodies and pro-inflammatory cytokines/chemokines, breaking the LN flare cycle, and thereby reducing flare rates (Figure 2). A renal flare outcome has not been an end point of any of the recently completed LN trials. This would require a different trial design with longer follow-up than an add-on trial.

There are some data suggesting that anti-B-cell and anti-T-cell therapies can maintain remission in LN. Belimumab, a monoclonal antibody that targets the B-cell survival factor BlyS, was found to be effective in extrarenal SLE.[49] Although patients with active/severe LN were not recruited to this trial, there were patients who had LN. A post hoc analysis of the belimumab cohorts demonstrated a significantly lower LN flare rate in patients who received belimumab than patients who were given placebo.[50] A trial of abatacept added on to low-dose cyclophosphamide for LN induction did not show a difference in complete renal responses at 6 months compared to placebo.[21] However, patients in the abatacept arm who achieved a complete renal response by month 6 were followed for another 6 months with no other immunosuppression. Maintenance of remission was the same as for placebo patients who had complete responses at 6 months and were continued on azathioprine.

CONCLUSION

LN is a complex and heterogeneous disease in its pathogenesis and its clinical manifestations. These characteristics have contributed to the difficulty in identifying new, less toxic, and more effective therapies despite major efforts in drug development and clinical trial testing. However, careful analysis of trial failures suggests that some of the novel therapeutics may be effective if applied to specific patient subsets, and if therapeutic expectations are better matched to a drug's mechanism of action in the context of the pathogenesis of kidney injury in LN. Given the outcomes of recent clinical trials, LN appears to a prime example of the need for a personalized medicine approach to therapy.

REFERENCES

1. Rovin BH, Stillman IE. The kidney in systemic lupus erythematosus. In: Lahita RG, editor. *Systemic lupus erythematosus*. 5th ed. London: Academic Press; 2011. p. 769–814.
2. Contreras G, Pardo V, Cely C, Borja E, Hurtado A, De La Cuesta C, et al. Factors associated with poor outcomes in patients with lupus nephritis. *Lupus* 2005;**14**(11):890–5.
3. Reich HN, Gladman DD, Urowitz MB, Bargman JM, Hladunewich MA, Lou W, et al. Persistent proteinuria and dyslipidemia increase the risk of progressive chronic kidney disease in lupus erythematosus. *Kidney Int* 2011;**79**(8):914–20.
4. Mok CC, Kwok RC, Yip PS. Effect of renal disease on the standardized mortality ratio and life expectancy of patients with systemic lupus erythematosus. *Arthritis Rheum* 2013;**65**(8):2154–60.
5. Maroz N, Segal MS. Lupus nephritis and end-stage kidney disease. *Am J Med Sci* 2013;**346**(4):319–23.
6. Chan TM, Tse KC, Tang CSO, Mok M-Y, Li FK. Long-term study of mycophenolate mofetil as continuous induction and maintenance treatment for diffuse proliferative lupus nephritis. *J Am Soc Nephrol* 2005;**16**:1076–84.
7. Austin HA, Klippel JH, Balow JE, le Riche WG, Steinberg AD, Plotz PH, et al. Therapy of lupus nephritis. Controlled trial of prednisone and cytotoxic drugs. *N Eng J Med* 1986;**314**:614–9.
8. Mysler EF, Spindler AJ, Guzman R, Biji M, Jayne D, Furie RA, et al. Efficacy and safety of ocrelizaumab, a humanized antiCD20 antibody in patients with active proliferative lupus nephritis: results from the randomized, double-blind phase III BELONG study. *Arthritis Rheum* 2010;**62**(Suppl. 10).
9. Condon MB, Ashby D, Pepper RJ, Cook HT, Levy JB, Griffith M, et al. Prospective observational single-centre cohort study to evaluate the effectiveness of treating lupus nephritis with rituximab and mycophenolate mofetil but no oral steroids. *Ann Rheum Dis* 2013;**72**(8):1280–6.
10. Wilhelmus S, Cook HT, Noel LH, Ferrario F, Wolterbeek R, Bruijn JA, et al. Interobserver agreement on histopathological lesions in class III or IV lupus nephritis. *Clin J Am Soc Nephrol* 2014;**10**(1):47–53.
11. Grootscholten C, Bajema IM, Florquin S, Steenbergen EJ, Peutz-Kootstra CJ, Goldschmeding R, et al. Interobserver agreement of scoring of histopathological characteristics and classification of lupus nephritis. *Nephrol Dial Transplant* 2008;**23**(1):223–30.
12. Rovin BH, Parikh SV, Alvarado A. The kidney biopsy in lupus nephritis: is it still relevant? In: Ginzler EM, Dooley MA, editors. *Systemic lupus erythematosus. Rheumatic disease clinics of North America*, vol. 40. Philadelphia: Elsevier; 2014. p. 537–52.
13. Hsieh C, Chang A, Brandt D, Guttikonda R, Utset TO, Clark MR. Predicting outcomes of lupus nephritis with tubulointerstitial inflammation and scarring. *Arthritis Care Res* 2011;**63**(6):865–74.
14. Hao W, Rovin BH, Friedman A. Mathematical model of renal interstitial fibrosis. *Proc Natl Acad Sci USA* 2014;**111**(39):14193–8.
15. Bethunaickan R, Berthier CC, Zhang W, Eksi R, Li HD, Guan Y, et al. Identification of stage-specific genes associated with lupus nephritis and response to remission induction in (NZB × NZW)F1 and NZM2410 mice. *Arthritis Rheumatol* 2014;**66**(8):2246–58.
16. Berthier CC, Bethunaickan R, Gonzalez-Rivera T, Nair V, Ramanujam M, Zhang W, et al. Cross-species transcriptional network analysis defines shared inflammatory responses in murine and human lupus nephritis. *J Immunol* 2012;**189**(2):988–1001.
17. Bethunaickan R, Berthier CC, Zhang W, Kretzler M, Davidson A. Comparative transcriptional profiling of 3 murine models of SLE nephritis reveals both unique and shared regulatory networks. *PLoS One* 2013;**8**(10):e77489.
18. Satoskar AA, Shapiro JP, Bott CN, Song H, Nadasdy GM, Brodsky SV, et al. Characterization of glomerular diseases using proteomic analysis of laser capture microdissected glomeruli. *Mod Pathol* 2012;**25**(5): 709–21.

19. Peterson KS, Huang JF, Zhu J, D'Agati V, Liu X, Miller N, et al. Characterization of heterogeneity in the molecular pathogenesis of lupus nephritis from transcriptional profiles of laser-captured glomeruli. *J Clin Invest* 2004;**113**(12):1722–33.

20. Rovin BH, Furie RA, Lantinis K, Looney RJ, Fervenza FC, Sanchez-Guerrero J, et al. Efficacy and safety of rituximab in patients with active proliferative lupus nephritis: the Lupus Nephritis Assessment with Rituximab (LUNAR) study. *Arthritis Rheum* 2012;**64**:1215–26.

21. Group AT. Treatment of lupus nephritis with abatacept: the abatacept and cyclophosphamide combination efficacy and safety study. *Arthritis Rheumatol* 2014;**66**(11):3096–104.

22. Boneparth A, Ilowite N, for the CRI. Comparison of renal response parameters for juvenile membranous plus proliferative lupus nephritis versus isolated proliferative lupus nephritis: a cross-sectional analysis of the CARRA Registry. *Lupus* 2014;**23**(9):898–904.

23. Radhakrishnan J, Moutzouris DA, Ginzler EM, Solomons N, Siempos II, Appel GB. Mycophenolate mofetil and intravenous cyclophosphamide are similar as induction therapy for class V lupus nephritis. *Kidney Int* 2010;**77**(2):152–60.

24. Jonsdottir T, Gunnarsson I, Mourao AF, Lu TY, van Vollenhoven RF, Isenberg D. Clinical improvements in proliferative vs membranous lupus nephritis following B-cell depletion: pooled data from two cohorts. *Rheumatology* 2010;**49**(8):1502–4.

25. Miyake K, Akahoshi M, Nakashima H. Th subset balance in lupus nephritis. *J Biomed Biotechnol* 2011;**2011**:980286.

26. Rezende GM, Viana VS, Malheiros DM, Borba EF, Silva NA, Silva C, et al. Podocyte injury in pure membranous and proliferative lupus nephritis: distinct underlying mechanisms of proteinuria? *Lupus* 2014;**23**(3):255–62.

27. Rovin BH, Aranow C, Van Vollenhoven R, Wagner C, Zhou B, Gordon R, et al. A phase 2, multicenter, randomized, double-blind, placebo-controlled, proof-of-concept study to evaluate the efficacy and safety of sirukumab in pateints with active lupus nephritis. American Society of Nephrology Annual Meeting, Philadelphia. 2014.

28. Wofsy D, Hillson JL, Diamond B. Abatacept for lupus nephritis: alternative definitions of complete response support conflicting conclusions. *Arthritis Rheum* 2012;**64**(11):3660–5.

29. Furie R, Nicholls K, Cheng TT, Houssiau F, Burgos-Vargas R, Chen SL, et al. Efficacy and safety of abatacept in lupus nephritis: a twelve-month randomized, double-blind study. *Arthritis Rheumatol* 2014;**66**:379–89.

30. Dall'era M, Cisternas M, Smilek D, Straub L, Houssiau F, Cervera R, et al. Predictors of long-term renal outcomes in lupus nephritis trials: Lessons Learned from the Euro-Lupus nephritis cohort. *Arthritis Rheumatol* 2015;**67**(5):1305–13.

31. Houssiau FA, Vasconcelos C, D'Cruz D, Sebastiani GD, Garrido Ed ER, Danieli MG, et al. Immunosuppressive therapy in lupus nephritis: the Euro-Lupus Nephritis Trial, a randomized trial of low-dose versus high-dose intravenous cyclophosphamide. *Arthritis Rheum* 2002;**46**(8):2121–31.

32. Alvarado A, Malvar A, Lococo B, Alberton V, Toniolo F, Nagaraja H, et al. The value of repeat kidney biopsy in quiescent Argentinian lupus nephritis patients. *Lupus* 2014;**23**(8):840–7.

33. Malvar A, Prruccio P, Alberton V, Lococo B, Recalde C, Fazzini B, et al. Histologic versus clinical remission in lupus nephritis. American Society of Nephrology Annual Meeting, Philadelphia. 2014:(ABS).

34. Arbuckle MR, McClain MT, Rubertone MV, Scofield RH, Dennnis GJ, James JA, et al. Development of autoantibodies before the clinical onset of systemic lupus erythematosus. *N Engl J Med* 2003;**349**:1526–33.

35. Wakasugi D, Gono T, Kawaguchi Y, Hara M, Koseki Y, Katsumata Y, et al. Frequency of class III and IV nephritis in systemic lupus erythematosus without clinical renal involvement: an analysis of predictive measures. *J Rheumatol* 2012;**39**(1):79–85.

36. Petri M, Wallace DJ, Spindler A, Chindalore V, Kalunian K, Mysler E, et al. Sifalimumab, a human anti-interferon-alpha monoclonal antibody, in systemic lupus erythematosus: a phase I randomized, controlled, dose-escalation study. *Arthritis Rheum* 2013;**65**(4):1011–21.

37. Merrill JT, Wallace DJ, Petri M, Kirou KA, Yao Y, White WI, et al. Safety profile and clinical activity of sifalimumab, a fully human anti-interferon alpha monoclonal antibody, in systemic lupus erythematosus: a phase I, multicentre, double-blind randomised study. *Ann Rheum Dis* 2011;**70**(11):1905–13.

38. Ronnblom L, Alm GV, Eloranta ML. The type I interferon system in the development of lupus. *Semin Immunol* 2011;**23**(2):113–21.

39. Chung SA, Brown EE, Williams AH, Ramos PS, Berthier CC, Bhangale T, et al. Lupus nephritis susceptibility loci in women with systemic lupus erythematosus. *J Am Soc Nephrol* 2014;**25**(12):2859–70.

40. Rovin BH, Parikh SV. Lupus nephritis: the evolving role of novel therapeutics. *Am J Kidney Dis* 2014;**63**(4):677–90.

41. Lourenco EV, Wong M, Hahn BH, Palma-Diaz MF, Skaggs BJ. Laquinimod delays and suppresses nephritis in lupus-prone mice and affects both myeloid and lymphoid immune cells. *Arthritis Rheumatol* 2014;**66**:674–85.

42. Jayne D, Appel G, Chan TM, Mimrod D, Spiegelstein O, Barkay H, et al. *The pharmacokinetics of laquinimod and mycophenolate mofetil during treatment of active lupus nephritis.* 2013.

43. D'Acquisto F, May MJ, Ghosh S. Inhibition of nuclear factor kappa B (NF-B): an emerging theme in anti-inflammatory therapies. *Mol Interv* 2002;**2**(1):22–35.

44. Enia G, Catalano C, Misefari V, Salnitro F, Mundo N, Tetta C, et al. Complement activated leucopenia during hemodialysis: effect of pulse methyl-prednisolone. *Int J Artif Organs* 1990;**13**(2):98–102.

45. Jansen NJ, van Oeveren W, van Vliet M, Stoutenbeek CP, Eysman L, Wildevuur CR. The role of different types of corticosteroids on the inflammatory mediators in cardiopulmonary bypass. *Eur J Cardiothorac Surg* 1991;**5**(4):211–7.

46. Chang A, Henderson SG, Brandt D, Liu N, Guttikonda R, Hsieh C, et al. In situ B cell-mediated immune responses and tubulointerstitial inflammation in human lupus nephritis. *J Immunol* 2011;**186**(3):1849–60.

47. Gourley MF, Austin 3rd HA, Scott D, Yarboro CH, Vaughan EM, Muir J, et al. Methylprednisolone and cyclophosphamide, alone or in combination, in patients with lupus nephritis. A randomized, controlled trial. *Ann Intern Med* 1996;**125**(7):549–57.

48. Donadio JV, Holley KE, Ferguson RH, Ilstrup DM. Treatment of diffuse proliferative lupus nephritis with prednisone and combined prednisone and cyclophosphamide. *N Engl J Med* 1978;**23**:1151–5.

49. Manzi S, Sanchez-Guerrero J, Merrill JT, Furie R, Gladman D, Navarra SV, et al. Effects of belimumab, a B lymphocyte stimulator-specific inhibitor, on disease activity across multiple organ domains in patients with systemic lupus erythematosus: combined results from two phase III trials. *Ann Rheum Dis* 2012;**71**(11):1833–8.

50. Dooley MA, Houssiau F, Aranow C, D'Cruz DP, Askanase A, Roth DA, et al. Effect of belimumab treatment on renal outcomes: results from the phase 3 belimumab clinical trials in patients with SLE. *Lupus* 2013;**22**(1):63–72.

Chapter 66

Repositioning Drugs for Systemic Lupus Erythematosus

Amrie C. Grammer, Matthew M. Ryals, Michelle D. Catalina, Peter E. Lipsky

AMPEL BioSolutions, University of Virginia Research Park, Charlottesville, VA, USA

WHY TRY TO REPURPOSE DRUGS FOR SLE PATIENTS?

The term *drug repurposing* refers to using or testing a drug that has been approved by the U.S. Food and Drug Administration (FDA) for one indication in another disease, in this case SLE.[1] This concept has a number of other names including repositioning, rescue, reprofiling, retooling, and retasking. Because only four medications have been approved by the FDA for treatment of lupus patients (hydroxychloroquine [HCQ], aspirin, prednisone, and belimumab), SLE patients are routinely treated with drugs that have been "repurposed." Methotrexate (MTX), cyclophosphamide (CTX), mycophenolate, and rituximab are standard of care (SOC) medications in lupus that were approved by the FDA for malaria, cancer (MTX, CTX), transplant rejection, and lymphoma, respectively. The concept of repurposing is not unique to SLE; Table 1 summarizes the numerous drugs in a variety of conditions that have been successfully treated with repurposed compounds.

Historically, drugs were repurposed because of serendipitous clinical observations and/or off-target effects.[2] Probably one of the most recognized examples of drug repurposing by the general public is sildenafil (Viagra), which was originally developed for hypertension but is now commonly used for other conditions, including pulmonary artery hypertension and erectile dysfunction.[3] Another well-known repurposed drug is thalidomide. Developed in the 1960s for anxiety, it was removed from the market after its connection to serious fetal limb defects was discovered.[4] Recent studies have shown thalidomide to be an effective treatment for a number of conditions, including certain symptoms in leprosy, multiple myeloma, and cutaneous lupus.[5–7]

Drug repositioning emerged as a scientific field in 2004 but started accelerating in 2013.[8] In the beginning, Biotech/Pharma took a traditional approach looking for drugs with shared structures[9] or side effects.[10] Often, drugs were rescreened against targets with similar molecular makeup. The concept of using genome-wide association studies (GWAS)[11] and bioinformatics to facilitate targeted drug repositioning was first described in 2009. This advance led to a tenfold increase in the number of publications in drug repositioning to around 50 per year. By 2013, interest in the scientific community accelerated further resulting in 400 published papers a year. More than half of all of the papers in PubMed discussing drug repositioning have been published in 2013 and 2014. These recent papers discuss a variety of specific methodologies used for disease-specific drug repurposing, but the approaches have yielded mixed results. Most recently, a group at Stanford University tested off-target effects of imipramine/Tofranil, a metabolite of the antidepressant desipramine, in small-cell lung cancer patients based on bioinformatics predictions of its success.[12] The Phase IIa trial was discontinued because of side effects and lack of efficacy.

There are a variety of reasons that the scientific community is interested in drug repositioning. One driving force seems to be the developmental cost of around $1.5–2.6 billion over 10–15 years to bring a compound to market coupled with the "innovation deficit"—the widening gap between productivity and research and development budgets over the last 10 years.[13] This has generated an intense interest in Biotech/Pharma to attempt to rescue products that have failed for one indication or have been shelved for various reasons. Physicians treating patients with diseases such as SLE are interested in drug repositioning because biotech/pharma has not been very successful in bringing new drugs for their patients to market. In addition, commonly used SLE treatments have serious side effects, poorly address symptoms, and do not address the core issues driving the disease. Belimumab (Benlysta, anti-BLyS/BAFF) is the only drug approved for SLE in the last 50 years.

Biotech/pharma have tried to bring new treatments for SLE to the market through traditional research and development strategies but have failed for a variety of reasons. Trial design issues, the use of concurrent medications, and complex outcomes measures are often cited as contributing to the uncertainty of SLE trials. In addition, trials may not be

Systemic Lupus Erythematosus. http://dx.doi.org/10.1016/B978-0-12-801917-7.00066-8

TABLE 1 Examples of Successful Drug Repositioning from One Indication to Another

Drug	Primary Target	New Indication
Amphotericin B	Fungal infection	Leishmaniasis
Aspirin	Inflammation/pain	Antiplatelet
Bromocriptine (Parlodel)	Parkinsons	Diabetes mellitus
Finasteride (Proscar)	Prostate hyperplasia	Hair loss
Gemcitabine (Gemzar)	Viral infections	Cancer
Inirole (Requip)	Parkinsons	Restless leg syndrome
Leucovorin	MTX rescue	Colorectal cancer with 5-FU
Metformin	Diabetes	Cancer
Milnacipran (Savella)	Depression	Fibromyalgia
Minoxidil (Rogaine)	Hypertension	Hair loss
Plerixafor (Mozobil)	HIV	Stem cell mobilization
Pregabalin (Lyrica)	Epilepsy	Fibromyalgia
Propanolol (Inderal)	Hypertension	CHF, anxiety
Raloxifene (Evista)	Breast cancer	Osteoporosis
Sildenafil (Viagra)	Angina	Erectile dysfunction
Thalidomide (Immunprin)	Anxiety	Leprosy, multiple myeloma

focused on the subgroup of SLE patients most likely to benefit from the targeted intervention, and many times patients without a clear-cut diagnosis of SLE or with a diagnosis of SLE but current manifestations of uncertain nature are included in trials. Some of the SLE trials that have failed to meet their primary endpoints include tabalumab (anti-BAFF),[14] rituximab (anti-CD20),[15] ocrelizumab (anti-CD20),[15] abatacept (CTLA4-Ig),[16] and rontalizumab (anti-interferon alpha).[17] In contrast to the lack of success of SLE trials, the number of FDA-approved drugs has greatly increased in recent years, with more than 50 compounds approved in 2014 and 2015,[18,19] including some that may be appropriate to be considered for repositioning into SLE such as inhibitors of PI3K, AKT, PDE4, PARP, and histone deacetylase inhibitors (HDACs) as well as antagonists of IL6, IL17alpha, VEGFR, integrin receptor, and PD1 receptor. The documented success of repositioning drugs from one approved indication into other diseases as well as the ability of the SLE clinical research community to reposition drugs of interest into SLE successfully has encouraged this approach.

LRxL-STAT™: REPOSITIONING TREATMENTS FOR SLE PATIENTS

The federal government has funded programs to help scientists look for drugs that could be repositioned into other diseases, including the National Center for Advancing

Translational Sciences (NCATS)[20] within the National Institutes of Health (NIH), the Rare Disease Repurposing Database (RDRD)[21] of the FDA, and the Accelerating Medicines Partnership (AMP),[22] a public/private partnership between the NIH and industry. NCATS and the RDRD are not focused on SLE; now in its first year, AMP started in 2014 and among its goals is a search for new targets for SLE using both molecular and bioinformatics approaches. Based on need in the SLE patient community, in October 2013, two nonprofit organizations, the Alliance for Lupus Research and the Lupus Research Institute, came together to launch a novel integrative, disease-based approach to drug repositioning in SLE called LRxL-STAT™ (www.linkedin.com/lrxlstat), Lupus Rx List-SLE Treatment Acceleration Trials. The process began in May 2013 with four nonprofits (ALR, LRI, Lupus Foundation of American, and Lupus Therapeutics) and key opinion leaders' brainstorming about what drugs would be suitable to repurpose into SLE. Subsequently, AMPEL BioSolutions (www.ampelbiosolutions.com) took the project forward using a combination of a deep literature mining as well as a crowd-sourcing social-media approach to find FDA-approved drugs that had the potential to be repurposed into SLE. Of note, crowd-sourced suggestions were received from patients, researchers, and clinical investigators through an interactive process on the LRxL-STAT™ LinkedIn site. Although both literature-based[23] and crowd-sourcing[24] approaches have been previously reported to be the successful means of identifying candidates for drug repositioning, there has been no standardized methodology to compare potential candidates.

Drug repositioning can quickly bring new treatments to patients because early preclinical work as well as dosing, formulation, drug metabolism/interaction, and pharmacokinetic/dynamic issues have already been characterized. Moreover, the side effect profile has frequently been extensively examined. This only leaves the matter of efficacy to be established, thereby foreshortening the pathway to acceptance and or regulatory approval. Following community suggestions for potential treatments in conjunction with extensive literature mining for appropriate drugs out of the approximately 1100 compounds approved by the FDA for 6800 indications, an evidence based-analysis of each of 157 potential SLE therapies was carried out. The LRxL-STAT™ was constructed with extensive input from the interested lupus community, including patients. Excluded from the literature search were all drugs widely used for SLE (whether approved or not) as well as drugs known to be in development for SLE biotech/pharma. All data used were in the public domain and no drug combinations were addressed.

To compare and contrast candidates for repositioning into SLE, a novel scoring method was developed called CoLTs™, or Combined Lupus Treatments Scoring, to comparatively rank the identified drugs/therapies by a number of essential characteristics, including scientific rationale, experience in lupus mice/human cells (preclinical), previous clinical experience in autoimmunity, drug properties, and safety profile, including adverse events. Potential candidates were scored in each of five categories: small molecules, biologics, cellular therapies, complementary/alternative therapies, and drugs in development.

Of the 157 therapies initially screened, many candidates manifested an appropriate set of characteristics to consider for testing in clinical trials in SLE, including drugs targeting cellular metabolism, kinases, the immune system, HDACs, complement as well as cellular therapies, and nondrug complementary and alternative interventions. Top priority candidates were identified for testing in small proof-of-concept STAT (SLE Treatment Acceleration Trials)[25]: quinacrine, Stelara/ustekinumab, autologous hematopoietic stem cell transplantation (HSCT), omega-3 fish oil (krill), meditation/mindfulness, and a ROCK2-kinase inhibitor. All results were vetted by a committee of experts. The LRxL-STAT™ approach not only identified unique candidates that could be useful in SLE and possibly other autoimmune/inflammatory conditions, but also yielded a rigorous evidence-based process by which therapies could be usefully rated for possible clinical application to treat these conditions, thereby mitigating risk in drug development.

The CoLTs™ Scoring System

The goal of the CoLTs™ system was to develop a metric that could capture all available data and yield a combined score that would reflect the likelihood that a treatment candidate would be successful in clinical trials of SLE. Importantly, the CoLT™ score reflects the state of knowledge at the time the treatment candidate was scored, but it was designed to be dynamic and incorporate new information as it becomes available. The impetus to develop the CoLTs™ system was the need for an objective way to score drug candidates in numerous areas likely to contribute to the success of a candidate in clinical trials. Although projections of possible efficacy, including mechanism of action, experience in animal models, pathway abnormalities identified in lupus patients, and previous clinical experience in other autoimmune/inflammatory experience were all thought to be important and carefully scored, greater weight was given to the adverse event profile. Especially in a disease such as SLE that is treated with drugs such as glucocorticoids and immunosuppressives that increase infection risk, adverse events are often the determinants of a successful clinical trial. Finally, properties of the agents, including route of administration, dosing, drug metabolism, and drug–drug interactions were also scored, since these can be important determinants of treatment use and compliance in a chronic disease often treated with multiple drugs. Numerous iterations of the score were examined in order to find the best combination and validated by scoring currently used medications. The final result was the dynamic CoLT™ score, which provides a useful means to prioritize treatment candidates for SLE but is a dynamic flexible measurement that takes into account new information about a therapy as it becomes available.[25,26]

IDENTIFICATION OF TOP PRIORITY LRxL-STAT™ CANDIDATES

A total of 157 therapies were examined in detail by the LRxL-STAT™ initiative (99 small molecules, 41 biologics, five cellular therapies, and 12 complementary and alternative medicines; see www.linkedin.com/lrxlstat for the complete listing). The initial focus of LRxL-STAT™ was to evaluate the likelihood of success of repositioning FDA-approved drugs in SLE, so the evaluation list scored with CoLTs™ was narrowed to the 76 FDA-approved or generally recognized as safe (GRAS) therapies (Table 2). Medications commonly used (standard of care or SOCs) to treat SLE (belimumab, HCQ, and rituximab) were used as comparators for CoLT™ scoring. Any therapy suggested to or identified by LRxL-STAT™ that received a score as high or higher than belimumab, HCQ, or rituximab was considered to be high priority and worth considering for small, proof-of-concept trials (STAT).

TABLE 2 FDA-Approved Drugs, Complementary Small Molecules, Alternative Medicine Therapies, and Cellular Therapies Considered for LRxL Prioritization

FDA-Approved Biologics	Dimethyl fumarate
Abatacept	Dipyridamole
Adalimumab	Erlotinib
Belimumab (SOC)	Everolimus
Certolizumab pegol	Fingolimod
Eculizumab	Glatiramer acetate
Etanercept	Gefitinib
Golimumab	Hyroxychloroquine (SOC)
Infliximab	Ibrutinib
Natalizumab	Idelalisib
Ofatumumab	Imatinib
Pembrolizumab	Irinotecan
Rituximab	Lamivudine
Tocilizumab	Lapatinib
Ustekinumab	Leflunomide
Complementary Small Molecules (CAMs)	Lenalidomide
Creatinine	Metformin
Curcumin	*N*-Acetyl cysteine
Nicotinamide adenine dinucleotide	Nelfinavir
Omega-3 fish oil (krill)	Nilotinib
Promethylation diet (choline, methionine, folic acid)	Orlistat
Resveratrol	Panzopanib
Tetrahydrobiopterin	*Quinacrine*
TwHF (thunder god vine)	Roflumilast
Ergocalciferol (vitamin D)	Romidepsin
Alternative Medicine Therapies	Rosinglitazone
Acupuncture	Ruxolinib
Meditation/mindfulness	Sirolimus
Yoga	Sorafenib
Cellular Therapies	Statins (SOC)
Allogeneic HSCT	Sunitinib
Autologous HSCT	Tacrolimus
MSC	Tamoxifen
MSP	Tenofovir
Tregs	Teriflunomide
FDA-Approved Small Molecules	Thalidomide
Azathioprine (SOC)	Tofacitinib
Abacavir	Valproic acid
Apremilast	Vandetanib
Bortezomib	Vemurafenib
Carfilzomib	Vorinostat
Crizotinib	Zidovudine
Dasatinib	HSCT, hematopoietic SCT; SCT, stem cell therapy; MSC/MSP, mesenchymal stem cell/mesenchymal stem cell/progenitor.

Small Molecules and Biologics

Of the molecules suggested to LRxL-STAT™, 47% of the small molecules (46/97) and 32% of the biologics (12/38) are FDA approved. High-priority candidates for repositioning in SLE had some preclinical data (experiments with lupus mice or human lupus cells in vitro) and some clinical experience in autoimmunity. Of the FDA-approved candidates, 26% (12/46) of small molecules and 54% (7/13) of biologics scored higher by CoLTs™ than the SOC comparator belimumab. Quinacrine, a lysosomal neutralizer, was the top-scoring small molecule and Stelara/ustekinumab, a Hu monoclonal antibody to the p40 subunit of IL12/23, received the highest CoLT™ score for the biologic category. Based on LRxL-STAT™'s high priority CoLT™ score, Janssen has planned a Phase IIa trial with SLE patients in collaboration with LRxL-STAT™ that will begin by the end of 2015 (NCT-02349061; http://www.lupusresearch.org/news-and-events/press-releases/alliance-for-lupus-research-7.html).

Three small molecules approved by the FDA in 2014–15 have the potential to be high-priority candidates for repositioning in SLE as their targets are identical to drugs with high CoLT™ scores. The IL6 antagonist Sylvant/siltuximab (anti-IL6) affects the same pathway as tocilizumab (anti-IL6R). Similar to the LRxL-STAT™ candidate Vorinostat, Beleodaq/belinostat, and Farydak/panobinostat are inhibitors of class I HDACs but also inhibit class II HDACs.

Cellular Therapies

Five cellular therapies were considered for SLE repositioning by LRxL-STAT™ autologous hematopoietic stem cell transplantation (HSCT), mesenchymal stem cell (MSC)/mesenchymal stem cell progenitor (MSP) transplantation, allogeneic HSCT, and regulatory T-cell (T$_{regs}$) therapy. Of those suggested, only HSCT and regulatory T-cell therapy received high-priority CoLTs™. HSCT is curative in lupus mice[27] and induces long-term remission in nearly half of SLE patients.[28–31] Although there is no data in patients with SLE or other autoimmune diseases, transplantation of regulatory T cells into lupus mice suppresses disease activity without toxicity[32]; remission can be prolonged with immunosuppressive therapy.

Complementary and Alternative Therapies

Nine small molecule CAM and three complementary/alternative therapies were evaluated by LRxL-STAT™. Although seven of these CAM are diets and common vitamin supplements, two are therapeutic possibilities for repositioning as SLE therapies (krill oil and TwHF/thunder god vine). Krill oil is an omega-3 long-chain polyunsaturated fatty acid (PUFA) high in EPA and DHA (eicosanoid/docasanoid lipid mediators). Both preclinical[33,34] and clinical studies[35–38] have demonstrated that the components of krill oil have a variety of effects potentially useful to SLE patients, including positive effects on cognitive function and the cardiovascular system as well as generalized anti-inflammatory effects, including limiting glomerular inflammation and ultraviolet-induced photo-oxidation of the skin. DHA and EPA in krill oil limit inflammation by directly altering membrane function, acting as a substrate for production of lipid mediators and by functioning as an agonist for specific receptors with anti-inflammatory effects. Specifically, components of krill oil activate PPAR-gamma,[39] directly bind FFAR1/4 (GPR40/120),[40] activate SIRT1[41] and NRF2/NFE2L2 as well as induce HO-1.[42] The outcome is blunting the expression of NF-kB genes such as adhesion molecules, chemokines, and inflammatory cytokines. Omega-3 PUFAs containing oils effectively treat established lupus manifestations[33] as well as nephritis[34] in mouse models. Moreover, they prevent onset of disease in mouse models as assayed by proteinuria, autoantibody production, and glomerulonephritis. Finally, four studies with SLE patients have shown an improvement of disease activity following treatment with omega-3 PUFAs,[35–38] although one study treating inactive SLE patients showed change in disease activity.[43]

The second high priority CAM is *Tripterygium wilfordii* Hook F (TwHF), also called thunder god vine in traditional Chinese Medicine.[44,45] Active compounds in TwHF are extracted from the roots, leaves, and flowers of a deciduous plant called Lei Gong Teng. Three diterpenoids (triptolide, tripdiolide, and triptonide) account for most of the biologic activity of TwHF, such as inhibition of cytokine production at the transcriptional level (IFNalpha, TNF, IL4, IL6, IL13, IL17, IL12/IL23, IL37)[46–50] and pro-inflammatory molecules (COX2, iNOS).[51,52] Other components such as celastrol and tripcholorolide have substantial antitumor and immunosuppressive activities. TwHF interferes with gene transcription by binding the ligand-binding domain of the glucocorticoid receptor and suppressing gene transcription mediated by NFkB as well as AP1/NFAT.[53–55] Importantly, TwHF exerts the immunosuppressive/anti-inflammatory effects of glucocorticoids without the hormonal effects of drugs such as dexamethasone. Preclinical work demonstrated that the extracts of TwHF as well as diterpenoid active components of the plant ameliorate nephritis in several lupus mouse models.[56] TwHF has been shown to be effective in treatment of rheumatoid arthritis (RA) and an ongoing Phase II/III randomized controlled trial is examining the efficacy and safety of TwHF for LN patients in a head-to-head comparison with cyclophosphamide. TwHF is widely used in China as an effective treatment of RA, lupus, and numerous other inflammatory diseases.

Of the three complementary and alternative therapies suggested to LRxL-STAT™, contemplative interventions including meditation/mindfulness scored higher than either yoga or acupuncture. The impact of various meditation/mindfulness interventions on expression of various pro-inflammatory molecules has been examined in gene expression studies in normal subjects. Results from four independent microarray gene expression studies have shown that meditation/mindfulness decreases pro-inflammatory cytokine production, alters gene expression, and re-establishes immunological homeostasis—all of which could potentially affect disease process in SLE patients.[57–62] Genes that are decreased following contemplative interventions such as IL6, ROCK2, SIRT1, JAK1, STAT3, FcRg2b, syk, akt, lyn, HDACs, and the proteasome are targets of many of the drugs being considered for repositioning into SLE. Several studies in autoimmune diseases, including SLE[63,64] and rheumatoid arthritis (NCTs 00071292 and 00096759), have shown that meditation/mindfulness can also impact an individual's response to her or his disease by decreasing psychological stress and reducing the perception of pain. Clinical efficacy has been demonstrated in one meditation/mindfulness study in rheumatoid arthritis patients showing a reduction in disease activity over time compared with a control group.[65] Contemplative meditation/mindfulness practices may be a useful complement to SOC medical treatment of patients with SLE.

Drugs in Development

The CoLT™ scoring system for drug repositioning candidates is unbiased and based on scientific evidence including relevant mechanistic effects, drug properties, and safety profile. CoLT™ was developed by an iterative process and tested by scoring SOC drugs and relating the score to physician perception of drug activity and safety. The CoLT™ scoring system aims to reduce bias by assigning scores to each property of a given compound based on available scientific evidence and suggestions from experts in the field. Using literature-mining and crowd-sourcing reduces bias a priori by eliminating the opinions of clinicians with conflicts of interest. It is widely perceived that existing scoring systems for drug repositioning are biased.[66,67] Both Wehling and Wendler commented on the common practice of scoring drug repositioning candidates retroactively after successful use in the clinic. They both acknowledge and emphasize that common drug repositioning scoring systems use criteria and weighting of factors that are based upon the opinions of the clinicians involved in the repositioning study.

The original goal of LRxL-STAT™ to repurpose FDA-approved drugs for SLE patients led to the supplementary goal of repositioning drugs in development into the SLE space. The first example of drug repositioning into lupus during development is Kadmon's ROCK2 inhibitor, KD-025, after receiving a high CoLT™ score from LRxL-STAT™. (http://lupusnewstoday.com/2015/01/09/kadmon-corporations-lupus-treatment-candidate-designated-top-priority/). KD-025 was developed for use in psoriasis (NCTs 02106195 and 02317627). In vitro work with human T cells demonstrated that inhibiting ROCK2 with KD-025 decreases secretion of IL17 and IL21 in a STAT3-dependent manner, thus regulating the balance between inflammatory and regulatory T cell subsets. In addition, KD-025 decreases activity of IRF4 as assayed by Chromatin Immunoprecipitation (ChIP); IRF4 activity plays a role in B-cell differentiation to Ig-secreting plasma cells.[68] Preclinical work examining the treatment of lupus mouse models with the nonspecific ROCK inhibitor Fasudil demonstrated improved disease activity and survival by lowering autoantibody levels, both by decreasing the number of plasma cells and by promoting suppressive function of regulatory T cells.[69] Based on LRxL-STAT™'s high-priority CoLT™ score, Kadmon has planned a Phase IIb trial with SLE patients in collaboration with LRxL-STAT™ that will begin by the end of 2016.

While biotech/pharma companies such as Kadmon have always been interested in repositioning their own drugs, a recent growth area in companies focused solely on the repurposing of existing drugs for new indications. There are four small biopharmaceutical companies that have formed around a mission of repurposing drugs for new indications, although they all use different approaches. SOM Biotech uses a ligand-based in silico technique to identify previously unidentified targets for a given drug. Sistemic Inc. creates a microRNA signature for a test compound and compares it with their proprietary database of microRNA signatures for known drugs. BioVista utilizes their trademarked COSS discovery platform to predict new indications for existing drugs using a literature-based approach (scientific articles, patents, adverse event profiles) combined with in silico simulations.

Aurinia is a biopharmaceutical company that emerged from two other companies (Aspreva, Galencia) and, although presenting itself as a drug repositioning company, Aurinia is not using in silico methodology like the other three companies. Aurinia is focused on a clinical trial in lupus nephritis using a combination therapy of two repositioned drugs, CellCept (mycophenolate mofetil) and Voclosporin. CellCept is currently approved to treat organ rejection and widely used off-label to treat SLE and lupus nephritis. Voclosporin is a calcineurin inhibitor that failed efficacy trials in its targeted disease, uveitis, but it is similar to cyclosporin and tacrolimus, which like CellCept are used off-label to treat severe lupus nephritis.[70,71] The Phase IIb study called AURA–LV (Aurinia Urine Protein Reduction in Active Lupus with Voclosporin) began in the fall of 2014 and is a randomized, controlled, double-blind parallel arm study comparing the efficacy of voclosporin against placebo in achieving remission in lupus nephritis patients also taking CellCept (NCT 02141672).

SUMMARY

There is enormous interest in the biotech/pharma community as well as in the academic medical community to reposition drugs for novel indications. The idea is to find drugs for conditions based on new knowledge instead of novel chemistry. Candidate-repositioned drugs have undergone extensive early development studies, including preclinical work and toxicology/toxicity studies. Safety is known so the risk for failure because of adverse events is mitigated. From a biotech/pharma perspective, the challenge is examination of the patent position of the compound. From the industry point of view, candidates for repositioning often have one or more of the following characteristics: (1) they are in development for a condition related to the one being repositioned into; (2) they have failed to show efficacy in late-stage development; (3) they are stalled in development for commercial reasons; or (4) they are past the point of patent expiry. From the clinician's point of view, few drugs have been developed for diseases such as SLE, so those approved for related autoimmune/inflammatory diseases or other immunologic conditions are intriguing possibilities for repositioning. The LRxL-STAT™ approach of crowd-sourcing and literature-mining yielded candidates for SLE patients that were evaluated in a scientific, unbiased manner utilizing the CoLT™ scoring system.

REFERENCES

1. Lan Langedijk J, Mantel-Teeuwisse AK, Slijkerman DS, Schutjens MH. Drug repositioning and repurposing: terminology and definitions in literature. *Drug Discov Today* 2015;**20**(8):1027–34.

2. Ashburn TT, Thor KB. Drug repositioning: identifying and developing new uses for existing drugs. *Nat Rev Drug Discov* 2004;**3**:673–83.

3. Roundtable on Translating Genomic-Based Research for Health, Board on Health Sciences Policy, Institute of Medicine. *Drug repurposing and repositioning: Workshop summary*. Washington (DC): National Academies Press (US); August 08, 2014.

4. Kim JH, Scialli AR. Thalidomide: the tragedy of birth defects and the effective treatment of disease. *Toxicol Sci* 2011;**122**:1–6.

5. Putinatti MS, Lastória JC, Padovani CR. Prevention of repeated episodes of type 2 reaction of leprosy with the use of thalidomide 100 mg/day. *An Bras Dermatol* 2014;**89**:266–72.

6. Bianchi G, Richardson PG, Anderson KC. Promising therapies in multiple myeloma. *Blood* 2015;**126**(3):300–10.

7. Baret I, De Haes P. Thalidomide: still an important second-line treatment in refractory cutaneous lupus erythematosus? *J Dermatol Treat* 2015;**26**:173–7.

8. Cavalla D. Predictive methods in drug repurposing: gold mine or just a bigger haystack? *Drug Discov Today* 2013;**18**:523–32.

9. Minie M, Chopra G, Sethi G, Horst J, White G, Roy A, et al. CANDO and the infinite drug discovery frontier. *Drug Discov Today* 2014;**19**:1353–63.

10. Bisgin H, Liu Z, Kelly R, Fang H, Xu X, Tong W. Investigating drug repositioning opportunities in FDA drug labels through topic modeling. *BMC Bioinf* 2012;**13**(Suppl. 15):S6.

11. Hurle MR, Yang L, Xie Q, Rajpal DK, Sanseau P, Agarwal P. Computational drug repositioning: from data to therapeutics. *Clin Pharmacol Ther* 2013;**93**:335–41.

12. Jahchan NS, Dudley JT, Mazur PK, Flores N, Yang D, Palmerton A, et al. A drug repositioning approach identifies tricyclic antidepressants as inhibitors of small cell lung cancer and other neuroendocrine tumors. *Cancer Discov* 2013;**3**:1364–77.

13. Avorn J. The $2.6 billion pill–methodologic and policy considerations. *N Engl J Med* 2015;**372**:1877–9.

14. http://pharmatimes.com/article/14-10-02/All_over_for_tabalumab_as_Lilly_drug_now_fails_for_lupus.aspx.

15. Reddy V, Jayne D, Close D, Isenberg D. B-cell depletion in SLE: clinical and trial experience with rituximab and ocrelizumab and implications for study design. *Arthritis Res Ther* 2013;**15**(Suppl. 1):S2.

16. Furie R, Nicholls K, Cheng TT, Houssiau F, Burgos-Vargas R, Chen SL, et al. Efficacy and safety of abatacept in lupus nephritis: a twelve-month, randomized, double-blind study. *Arthritis Rheumatol* 2014;**66**:379–89.

17. Kalunian KC, Merrill JT, Maciuca R, McBride JM, Townsend MJ, Wei X, et al. A Phase II study of the efficacy and safety of rontalizumab (rhuMAb interferon-α) in patients with systemic lupus erythematosus (ROSE). *Ann Rheum Dis* 2015; http://dx.doi.org/10.1136/annrheumdis-2014-206090 [Epub ahead of Print].

18. http://www.forbes.com/sites/bernardmunos/2015/01/02/the-fda-approvals-of-2014/.

19. http://www.centerwatch.com/drug-information/fda-approved-drugs/.

20. Fagnan DE, Yang NN, McKew JC, Lo AW. Financing translation: analysis of the NCATS rare-diseases portfolio. *Sci Transl Med* 2015;**7**:276.

21. Xu K, Coté TR. Database identifies FDA-approved drugs with potential to be repurposed for treatment of orphan diseases. *Brief Bioinform* 2011;**12**:341–5.

22. http://www.nih.gov/science/amp/autoimmune.htm.

23. Andronis C, Sharma A, Virvilis V, Deftereos S, Persidis A. Literature mining, ontologies and information visualization for drug repurposing. *Brief Bioinform* 2011;**12**:357–68.

24. Khare R, Good BM, Leaman R, Su AI, Lu Z. Crowdsourcing in biomedicine: challenges and opportunities. *Brief Bioinform* 2015; http://dx.doi.org/10.1093/bib/bbv021 [Epub ahead of Print].

25. Grammer AC, Ryals M, Lipsky PE. A comprehensive approach to identify approved drugs and treatments for repositioning as therapies for systemic lupus erythematosus. *Arthritis Res Ther* 2014;**16**(Suppl. 1):A51.

26. Lipsky PE, Ryals M, Grammer AC. A novel strategy to identify and evaluate approved drugs and treatments for repositioning as therapies for systemic lupus erythematosus (SLE). *American College of Rheumatology*; 2014. A674.

27. Smith-Berdan S, Gille D, Weissman IL, Christensen JL. Reversal of autoimmune disease in lupus-prone New Zealand black/New Zealand white mice by nonmyeloablative transplantation of purified allogeneic hematopoietic stem cells. *Blood* 2007;**110**:1370–8.

28. Sui W, Hou X, Che W, Chen J, Ou M, Xue W, et al. Hematopoietic and mesenchymal stem cell transplantation for severe and refractory systemic lupus erythematosus. *Clin Immunol* 2013;**148**:186–97.

29. Muraro PA, Nikolov NP, Butman JA, Abati A, Gea-Banacloche J, Gress R, et al. Granulocytic invasion of the central nervous system after hematopoietic stem cell transplantation for systemic lupus erythematosus. *Haematologica* 2006;**91**(Suppl. 6):ECR21.

30. Collins E, Gilkeson G. Hematopoetic and mesenchymal stem cell transplantation in the treatment of refractory systemic lupus erythematosus–where are we now? *Clin Immunol* 2013;**148**:328–34.

31. Wang Q, Qian S, Li J, Che N, Gu L, Wang Q, et al. Combined transplantation of autologous hematopoietic stem cells and allogenic mesenchymal stem cells increases T regulatory cells in systemic lupus erythematosus with refractory lupus nephritis and leukopenia. *Lupus* 2015;**24**(11):1221–6.

32. Weigert O, von Spee C, Undeutsch R, Kloke L, Humrich JY, Riemekasten G. CD4+Foxp3+ regulatory T cells prolong drug-induced disease remission in (NZBxNZW) F1 lupus mice. *Arthritis Res Ther* 2013;**15**:R35.

33. Robinson DR, Prickett JD, Makoul GT, Steinberg AD, Colvin RB. Dietary fish oil reduces progression of established renal disease in (NZB x NZW)F1 mice and delays renal disease in BXSB and MRL/1 strains. *Arthritis Rheum* 1986;**29**:539–46.

34. Pestka JJ, Vines LL, Bates MA, He K, Langohr I. Comparative effects of n-3, n-6 and n-9 unsaturated fatty acid-rich diet consumption on lupus nephritis, autoantibody production and CD4+ T cell-related gene responses in the autoimmune NZBWF1 mouse. *PLoS One* 2014;**9**:e100255.

35. Wright SA, O'Prey FM, McHenry MT, Leahey WJ, Devine AB, Duffy EM, et al. A randomised interventional trial of omega-3-polyunsaturated fatty acids on endothelial function and disease activity in systemic lupus erythematosus. *Ann Rheum Dis* 2008;**67**:841–8.

36. Duffy EM, Meenagh GK, McMillan SA, Strain JJ, Hannigan BM, Bell AL. The clinical effect of dietary supplementation with omega-3 fish oils and/or copper in systemic lupus erythematosus. *J Rheumatol* 2004;**31**:1551–6.

37. Nakamura N, Kumasaka R, Osawa H, Yamabe H, Shirato K, Fujita T, et al. Effects of eicosapentaenoic acids on oxidative stress and plasma fatty acid composition in patients with lupus nephritis. *In Vivo* 2005;**19**:879–82.

38. Clark WF, Parbtani A, Huff MW, Reid B, Holub BJ, Falardeau P. Omega-3 fatty acid dietary supplementation in systemic lupus erythematosus. *Kidney Int* 1989;**36**:653–60.

39. Forman BM, Chen J, Evans RM. Hypolipidemic drugs, polyunsaturated fatty acids, and eicosanoids are ligands for peroxisome proliferator-activated receptors alpha and delta. *Proc Natl Acad Sci USA* 1997;**94**:4312–7.

40. Hirasawa A. Free fatty acid receptor family: a new therapeutic target for metabolic diseases. *Yakugaku Zasshi* 2015;**135**:769–77.

41. Xue B, Yang Z, Wang X, Shi H. Omega-3 polyunsaturated fatty acids antagonize macrophage inflammation via activation of AMPK/SIRT1 pathway. *PLoS One* 2012;**7**:e45990.

42. Zhang M, Wang S, Mao L, Leak RK, Shi Y, Zhang W, et al. Omega-3 fatty acids protect the brain against ischemic injury by activating Nrf2 and upregulating heme oxygenase 1. *J Neurosci* 2014;**34**:1903–15.

43. Bello KJ, Fang H, Fazeli P, Bolad W, Corretti M, Magder LS, et al. Omega-3 in SLE: a double-blind, placebo-controlled randomized clinical trial of endothelial dysfunction and disease activity in systemic lupus erythematosus. *Rheumatol Int* 2013;**33**:2789–96.

44. Brinker AM, Ma J, Lipsky PE, Raskin I. Medicinal chemistry and pharmacology of genus *Tripterygium* (Celastraceae). *Phytochemistry* 2007;**68**:732–66.

45. Ma J, Dey M, Yang H, Poulev A, Pouleva R, Dorn R, et al. Anti-inflammatory and immunosuppressive compounds from *Tripterygium wilfordii*. *Phytochemistry* 2007;**68**:1172–8.

46. Wang Z, Jin H, Xu R, Mei Q, Fan D. Triptolide downregulates Rac1 and the JAK/STAT3 pathway and inhibits colitis-related colon cancer progression. *Exp Mol Med* 2009;**41**:717–27.

47. Dai S, Yin K, Yao X, Zhou L. Inhibition of interleukin-13 gene expression by triptolide in activated T lymphocytes. *Respirology* 2013;**18**:1249–55.

48. Wu C, Xia Y, Wang P, Lu L, Zhang F. Triptolide protects mice from ischemia/reperfusion injury by inhibition of IL-17 production. *Int Immunopharmacol* 2011;**11**:1564–72.

49. Zhang Y, Ma X. Triptolide inhibits IL-12/IL-23 expression in APCs via CCAAT/enhancer-binding protein alpha. *J Immunol* 2010;**184**:3866–77.

50. He L, Liang Z, Zhao F, Peng L, Chen Z. Modulation of IL-37 expression by triptolide and triptonide in THP-1 cells. *Cell Mol Immunol* 2014;**12**(4):515–8.

51. Wang B, Ma L, Tao XL, Lipsky PE. Triptolide, an active component of the Chinese herbal remedy *Tripterygium wilfordii* Hook F, inhibits production of nitric oxide by decreasing inducible nitric oxide synthase gene transcription. *Arthritis Rheum* 2004;**50**:2995–3003.

52. Tao XL, Schulze-Koops H, Ma L, Cai J, Mao YP, Lipsky PE. Effects of *Tripterygium wilfordii* Hook F extracts on induction of cyclooxygenase 2 activity and prostaglandin E2 production. *Arthritis Rheum* 1998;**41**:130–8.

53. Qiu D, Zhao G, Aoki Y, Shi L, Uyei A, Nazarian S, et al. Immunosuppressant PG490 (triptolide) inhibits T-cell interleukin-2 expression at the level of purine-box/nuclear factor of activated T-cells and NF-kappaB transcriptional activation. *J Biol Chem* 1999;**274**:13443–50.

54. Park B, Sung B, Yadav VR, Chaturvedi MM, Aggarwal BB. Triptolide, histone acetyltransferase inhibitor, suppresses growth and chemosensitizes leukemic cells through inhibition of gene expression regulated by TNF-TNFR1-TRADD-TRAF2-NIK-TAK1-IKK pathway. *Biochem Pharmacol* 2011;**82**:1134–44.

55. Lu Y, Zhang Y, Li L, Feng X, Ding S, Zheng W, et al. TAB1: a target of triptolide in macrophages. *Chem Biol* 2014;**21**:246–56.

56. Tao X, Fan F, Hoffmann V, Gao CY, Longo NS, Zerfas P, et al. Effective therapy for nephritis in (NZB x NZW)F1 mice with triptolide and tripdiolide, the principal active components of the Chinese herbal remedy *Tripterygium wilfordii* Hook F. *Arthritis Rheum* 2008;**58**:1774–83.

57. Li QZ, Li P, Garcia GE, Johnson RJ, Feng L. Genomic profiling of neutrophil transcripts in Asian Qigong practitioners: a pilot study in gene regulation by mind-body interaction. *J Altern Complement Med* 2005;**11**:29–39.

58. Dusek JA, Otu HH, Wohlhueter AL, Bhasin M, Zerbini LF, Joseph MG, et al. Genomic counter-stress changes induced by the relaxation response. *PLoS One* 2008;**3**:e2576.

59. Bhasin MK, Dusek JA, Chang BH, Joseph MG, Denninger JW, Fricchione GL, et al. Relaxation response induces temporal transcriptome changes in energy metabolism, insulin secretion and inflammatory pathways. *PLoS One* 2013;**8**:e62817.

60. Black DS, Cole SW, Irwin MR, Breen E. St Cyr NM, Nazarian N, Khalsa DS, Lavretsky H. Yogic meditation reverses NF-κB and IRF-related transcriptome dynamics in leukocytes of family dementia caregivers in a randomized controlled trial. *Psychoneuroendocrinology* 2013;**38**:348–55.

61. Qu S, Olafsrud SM, Meza-Zepeda LA, Saatcioglu F. Rapid gene expression changes in peripheral blood lymphocytes upon practice of a comprehensive yoga program. *PLoS One* 2013;**8**:e61910.

62. Kaliman P, Alvarez-López MJ, Cosín-Tomás M, Rosenkranz MA, Lutz A, Davidson RJ. Rapid changes in histone deacetylases and inflammatory gene expression in expert meditators. *Psychoneuroendocrinology* 2014;**40**:96–107.

63. Greco CM, Rudy TE, Manzi S. Effects of a stress-reduction program on psychological function, pain, and physical function of systemic lupus erythematosus patients: a randomized controlled trial. *Arthritis Rheum* August 2004;**51**:625–34.

64. Bantornwan S, Watanapa WB, Hussarin P, Chatsiricharoenkul S, Larpparisuth N, Teerapornlertratt T, et al. Role of meditation in reducing sympathetic hyperactivity and improving quality of life in lupus nephritis patients with chronic kidney disease. *J Med Assoc Thai* 2014;**97**(Suppl. 3):S101–7.

65. Singh VK, Bhandari RB, Rana BB. Effect of yogic package on rheumatoid arthritis. *Indian J Physiol Pharmacol* 2011;**55**:329–35.

66. Wehling M. Assessing the translatability of drug projects: what needs to be scored to predict success? *Nat Rev Drug Discov* 2009;**8**:541–6.

67. Wendler A, Wehling M. Translatability scoring in drug development: eight case studies. *J Transl Med* 2012;**10**:39.

68. Zanin-Zhorov A, Weiss JM, Nyuydzefe MS, Chen W, Scher JU, Mo R, et al. Selective oral ROCK2 inhibitor down-regulates IL-21 and IL-17 secretion in human T cells via STAT3-dependent mechanism. *Proc Natl Acad Sci USA* 2014;**111**:16814–9.

69. Stirzaker RA, Biswas PS, Gupta S, Song L, Bhagat G, Pernis AB. Administration of fasudil, a ROCK inhibitor, attenuates disease in lupus-prone NZB/W F1 female mice. *Lupus* 2012;**21**:656–61.

70. Rabbani MA, Shah SM, Ahmad A. Sustained remission in a case of lupus nephritis with cyclosporin therapy. *Saudi J Kidney Dis Transpl* 2001;**12**:525–9.

71. Yap DY, Ma MK, Mok MM, Kwan LP, Chan GC, Chan TM. Long-term data on tacrolimus treatment in lupus nephritis. *Rheumatology* 2014;**53**:2232–7.

Appendix

SLEDAI 2K

(Circle in SLEDAI Score column if descriptor is present at the time of the visit or in the preceding 28 days)
(The same instrument can also be used going back only 10 days)

Item No.	SLEDAI Score	Descriptor	Definition
1	8	Seizure	Recent onset, exclude metabolic, infectious, or drug causes
2	8	Psychosis	Altered ability to function in normal activity due to severe disturbance in the perception of reality. Include hallucinations, incoherence, marked loose associations, impoverished thought content, marked illogical thinking, bizarre, disorganized, or catatonic behavior. Exclude uremia and drug causes
3	8	Organic brain syndrome	Altered mental function with impaired orientation, memory, or other intellectual function, with rapid onset and fluctuating clinical features, inability to sustain attention to environment, plus at least 2 of the following: perceptual disturbance, incoherent speech, insomnia or daytime drowsiness, or increased or decreased psychomotor activity. Exclude metabolic, infectious or drug causes
4	8	Visual disturbance	Retinal changes of SLE. Include cytoid bodies, retinal hemorrhages, serous exudates or hemorrhages in the choroid, or optic neuritis. Exclude hypertension, infection, or drug causes
5	8	Cranial nerve disorder	New onset of sensory or motor neuropathy involving cranial nerves
6	8	Lupus headache	Severe, persistent headache; may be migrainous, but must be nonresponsive to narcotic analgesia
7	8	Cerebrovascular accident (CVA)	New onset cerebrovascular accident(s). Exclude arteriosclerosis
8	8	Vasculitis	Ulceration, gangrene, tender finger nodules, periungual infarction, splinter hemorrhages, or biopsy or angiogram proof of vasculitis
9	4	Arthritis	>/=2 joints with pain and signs of inflammation (i.e., tenderness with swelling or effusion)
10	4	Myositis	Proximal muscle aching/weakness, associated with elevated creatinine phosphokinase (CK)/aldolase, or EMG changes or a biopsy showing myositis
11	4	Urinary casts	Heme-granular or RBC casts
12	4	Hematuria	>5 RBC/high power field. Exclude stone, infection, or other cause
13	4	Proteinuria	>0.5 g/24 h
14	4	Pyuria	>5 WBC/high power field. Exclude infection
15	2	Rash	Inflammatory type rash
16	2	Alopecia	Abnormal, patchy, or diffuse loss of hair
17	2	Mucosal ulcers	Oral or nasal ulcerations
18	2	Pleurisy	Pleuritic chest pain with pleural rub or effusion, or pleural thickening (requires objective confirmation)

Continued

—cont'd

Item No.	SLEDAI Score	Descriptor	Definition
19	2	Pericarditis	Classic pericardial pain with rub, effusion, ECG, or echocardiogram (requires objective confirmation)
20	2	Low complement	Decrease in CH50, C3, or C4 < lower limit of nl for testing laboratory
21	2	Increased DNA binding	Increased DNA binding above normal range for testing laboratory
22	1	Fever	>38 °C. Exclude infectious cause
23	1	Thrombocytopenia	<100 × 10^9 platelets/l, exclude drug causes
24	1	Leukopenia	<3 × 10^9 WBC/l, exclude drug causes

_____ **Total Score.**

SELENA SLEDAI WITH SELENA SLEDAI FLARE INDEX AND PGA

(Hybrid SLEDAI is the SELENA SLEDAI except using proteinuria definition from SLEDAI 2K)
(Circle in SLEDAI Score column if descriptor is present at the time of the visit or in the preceding 4 weeks)
(The same instrument can also be used going back only 10 days)

Item No.	SLEDAI Score	Descriptor	Definition
1	8	Seizure	Recent onset, exclude metabolic, infectious, or drug causes
2	8	Psychosis	Altered ability to function in normal activity due to severe disturbance in the perception of reality. Include hallucinations, incoherence, marked loose associations, impoverished thought content, marked illogical thinking, bizarre, disorganized, or catatonic behavior. Exclude uremia and drug causes
3	8	Organic brain syndrome	Altered mental function with impaired orientation, memory, or other intellectual function, with rapid onset and fluctuating clinical features, inability to sustain attention to environment, plus at least 2 of the following: perceptual disturbance, incoherent speech, insomnia or daytime drowsiness, or increased or decreased psychomotor activity. Exclude metabolic, infectious, or drug causes
4	8	Visual disturbance	Retinal changes of SLE. Include cytoid bodies, retinal hemorrhages, serous exudates or hemorrhages in the choroid, or optic neuritis, scleritis, or episcleritis. Exclude hypertension, infection, or drug causes
5	8	Cranial nerve disorder	New onset of sensory or motor neuropathy involving cranial nerves
6	8	Lupus headache	Severe, persistent headache; may be migrainous, but must be nonresponsive to narcotic analgesia. THIS WOULD RARELY BE ATTRIBUTED TO SLE… ALMOST NEVER SCORED
7	8	CVA	New onset cerebrovascular accident(s). Exclude arteriosclerosis
8	8	Vasculitis	Ulceration, gangrene, tender finger nodules, periungual infarction, splinter hemorrhages, or biopsy or angiogram proof of vasculitis
9	4	Arthritis	>2 joints with pain and signs of inflammation (i.e., tenderness with swelling or effusion)
10	4	Myositis	Proximal muscle aching/weakness, associated with elevated creatinine phosphokinase (CK)/aldolase, or EMG changes or a biopsy showing myositis
11	4	Urinary casts	Heme-granular or RBC casts
12	4	Hematuria	>5 RBC/high power field. Exclude stone, infection, or other cause
13	4	Proteinuria	Increase in proteinuria by 0.5 g/day
14	4	Pyuria	>5 WBC/high power field. Exclude infection
15	2	Rash	Inflammatory type rash
16	2	Alopecia	Abnormal, patchy, or diffuse loss of hair
17	2	Mucosal ulcers	Oral or nasal ulcerations

—cont'd

Item No.	SLEDAI Score	Descriptor	Definition
18	2	Pleurisy	Pleuritic chest pain or pleural rub or effusion, or pleural thickening (does not require an objective component if medically convincing)
19	2	Pericarditis	Classic pericardial pain and/or rub, effusion, or ECG or echocardiogram confirmation (does not require an objective component if medically convincing)
20	2	Low complement	Decrease in CH50, C3, or C4 < lower limit of nl for testing laboratory
21	2	Increased DNA binding	Increased DNA binding above normal range for testing laboratory
22	1	Fever	>38 °C. Exclude infectious cause
23	1	Thrombocytopenia	$<100 \times 10^9$ platelets/l, exclude drug causes
24	1	Leukopenia	$<3 \times 10^9$ WBC/l, exclude drug causes

_____ **Total Score.**

CLASSIC SELENA SLEDAI FLARE INDEX (CAN BE USED WITH ANY VERSION OF THE SLEDAI)

Physician's Global Assessment (PGA)
Visual Analog Scale with anchors

0	1	2	3
None	Mild	Moderate	Severe

(this was developed as a three inch scale but has been used in trials as a 100 mm scale)

Mild or Moderate Flare ☐

☐ Change in SELENA-SLEDAI instrument score of 3 points or more (but not to more than 12)
☐ New/worse: Discoid, photosensitive, profundus, bullous lupus,
    Nasopharyngeal ulcers
    Pleuritis
    Pericarditis
    Arthritis
    Fever (SLE)
☐ Increase in prednisone, but not to >0.5 mg/kg/day
☐ Added NSAID or hydroxychloroquine for SLE activity
☐ ≥1.0 increase in PGA score, but not to more than 2.5

Severe Flare ☐

☐ Change in SELENA-SLEDAI instrument score to greater than 12
☐ New/worse   CNS-SLE
      Cutaneous vasculitis,
      Vasculitis
      Nephritis
      Myositis
      Plt <60,000
      Hemolytic anemia: Hb <70 g/l or decrease in Hb >30 g/l
   Requiring: double prednisone, or prednisone increase to
      >0.5 mg/kg/day, or hospitalization
☐ Increase in prednisone to >0.5 mg/kg/day
☐ New cyclophosphamide, azathioprine, methotrexate for SLE activity
☐ Hospitalization for SLE activity
☐ Increase in Physician's Global Assessment score to >2.5

CLASSIC SELENA SLEDAI FLARE INDEX (SFI) INSTRUCTIONS

The SELENA SLEDAI flare index rules are followed explicitly as written above. However there are some clarifications to keep in mind when using the SELENA SLEDAI composite index.

Instructions for Using the SELENA SLEDAI Physicians Global Assessment Scale

This PGA is a modification of the classic analogue scale in that it is anchored with numbers from 0 to 3 demarcating mild, moderate, and severe disease. Please note several things about this scale. The number 3 indicates severe disease and is at the very end of the scale. This refers to the most severe possible disease, and does not reflect the most severe ever seen in a particular patient but the most severe disease ever seen in all SLE patients. Therefore, the line made by the physician along this scale should virtually never get to this edge. Any disease rated greater than 2.5 is very severe. The range of moderate disease covers about 1.5–2.4. Mild disease falls below 1.5. Clearly, this is a bit like a logarithmic scale with greater distances or demarcations possible among more mild–moderate symptoms. This must be kept in mind when scoring the instrument.

When scoring the PGA always look back at the score from the previous visit and move the mark relative to that previous visit. This is a global assessment, factoring in all aspects of the patients lupus disease activity. It should not reflect nonlupus medical conditions.

These instructions are quite discrete from those given for other analogue (Lichert) scales and are specific for the scoring of the SELENA SLEDAI PGA.

When Is a Flare Not a Flare?

It is important to keep in mind that on the SELENA SLEDAI flare index flare can be defined simply by a decision to institute new therapy for lupus disease activity, whether or not the patient meets the other criteria for flare listed. It is important for the physician not to override the intent of the instrument, which is to actually define flare in this manner. However there are logical exceptions, for which a common sense rule may prevail. Switching treatments for safety reasons or increasing treatment in patients who are improving might often warrant withdrawal from a protocol. However if the protocol allows these medication changes, the flare index will need to be scored, but it does not make sense to call these situations flares.

GUIDELINES FOR USE OF THE SELENA SLEDAI MODIFIED FOR ASSESSMENT OVER 28 DAYS: TO ASSESS DISEASE ACTIVITY

General Guidelines for Filling out the SELENA SLEDAI

- The main principle to keep in mind is that this instrument is intended to evaluate current lupus activity and not chronic damage; severity is accounted for in part by the "weightedness" of the scale.
- Points are given exactly as defined.
- A descriptor is either scored the exact points allotted or not scored, i.e., given a zero. Descriptors are scored only if they are present at the time of the physician encounter or in the preceding 28 days. (The SLEDAI 2K instrument is validated both for the original use with a 10 day window and for the use of a 28 day window, and any of the SLEDAI versions can be used with a 28 day window.) Small deviations in this window, which are allowed in a clinical trial protocol for monthly visits, are acceptable in scoring the SLEDAI. However, it is never acceptable to fill in gaps that cover activity over 2–3 months or more. The reason for this is that disease activity at the visit might have changed several times in such intervals and the recording of distant activity becomes meaningless.
  Please note that in the original SLEDAI the disease activity being scored was meant to cover only a 10 day period; the modification to 28 days is a more useful assessment for use in clinical trials, to capture disease activity between monthly visits. However the SLEDAI does require documented confirmation of events that may have occurred and resolved between visits.
  It is critical to record all new events that have developed during this time, for which there are very convincing lupus symptoms and/or signs consistent with glossary definitions for the items, even if the item has since disappeared. However, if a feature that was present at the last visit disappears soon after the last visit (within one week) then the item is not recorded on the SELENA-SLEDAI form.
- The descriptors which are scored must be documented by the notes written in the physician encounter form. This rule generally applies to the clinical data and not to the laboratory data. The laboratory data are strictly defined as per cutoffs and documentation is provided by the reports from the commercial laboratory.
- Descriptors do not have to be new but can be. They can be ongoing, recurrent, or initial events. Each would be scored the same way. An example would be a malar rash or mucosal ulcer. In these situations a malar rash observed at the initial visit but which remains unchanged for the next 6 months, irrespective of any treatment, is scored 2 points each time the SLEDAI is completed. Since the

nature of lupus is that clinically significant manifestations are not usually fleeting it would be rare for descriptors to be present during the month and not seen at the time of the encounter. This is discussed in more detail for each descriptor but is especially relevant for some neurologic, pulmonary, and cutaneous manifestations. A major exception would be seizure, due to lupus, which requires solid documentation but obviously would not need to be continuing at the time of the visit.

● In some descriptors the exclusions written may not be exhaustive. The intent of the SLEDAI is that the descriptor be attributed to SLE. If the physician does not attribute the descriptor to SLE it should not be scored, but documentation in support of this decision must be provided.

Written in italics is the definition for each descriptor precisely provided in the SLEDAI Score.

SEIZURE

Definition: Recent onset (last 28 days). Exclude metabolic, infectious, or drug cause, or seizure due to past irreversible CNS damage.

This descriptor is scored if the patient has had a witnessed seizure or convincing description (such as tongue biting or incontinence) within 30 days of the current encounter. The patient need not have a positive EEG, CT scan, PET scan, QEEG, or MRI. The CSF may be totally normal.

A seizure is also not counted:

1. If a metabolic cause is determined.
2. In the presence of a proven infectious meningitis, brain abscess, or fungal foci.
3. If there is a history of recent head trauma.
4. In the presence of an offending drug.
5. In the presence of severe hyperthermia or hypothermia.
6. If the patient has stopped taking anticonvulsant medication.
7. If the patient has a documented subtherapeutic anticonvulsant drug level.

PSYCHOSIS

Definition: Altered ability to function in normal activity due to severe disturbance in the perception of reality. Include hallucinations, incoherence, marked loose associations, impoverished thought content, marked illogical thinking, bizarre, disorganized, or catatonic behavior. Exclude uremia and drug causes.

This descriptor is scored if any of the criteria above are met.

With regard to drug causes the most problematic situation is glucocorticoids. If the treating physician attributes the psychosis to glucocorticoids this descriptor should not be counted.

ORGANIC BRAIN SYNDROME

Definition: Altered mental function with impaired orientation, memory, or other intellectual function, with rapid onset and fluctuating clinical features. Include clouding of consciousness with reduced capacity to focus, and inability to sustain attention to environment, plus at least two of the following: perceptual disturbance, incoherent speech, insomnia or daytime drowsiness, or increased or decreased psychomotor activity. Exclude metabolic, infectious, or drug causes.

1. Reduced capacity to focus as exemplified by new inability to perform everyday mathematical computations or disorientation to person, place, time, or purpose

OR

2. Inability to carry on a conversation

OR

3. Reduction in short-term memory.

PLUS: Documented abnormality on neuropsychiatric testing.

Neuropsychiatric testing may take the form of a "minimental-status exam" or a formal neuropsychiatric examination. The important aspect for scoring OBS is that it be reversible. Consideration should be given to the improvement of OBS after institution of glucocorticoids.

This descriptor is not scored in the presence of a metabolic, infectious, or drug cause. If the problem is chronic this descriptor is not scored in SLEDAI but is scored on the damage index.

VISUAL DISTURBANCE

Definition: Retinal and eye changes of SLE. Include cytoid bodies, retinal hemorrhages, serous exudate, or hemorrhages in the choroid, optic neuritis, scleritis, or episcleritis. Exclude hypertension, infection, or drug causes.

This is scored exactly as defined with the understanding that it must be supported by objective evidence.

CRANIAL NERVE DISORDER

Definition: New onset of sensory or motor neuropathy involving cranial nerves. Include vertigo due to lupus.

This is scored exactly as defined with the understanding that it must be supported by objective evidence. However, it should be noted that hydroxychloroquine can affect the eighth cranial nerve.

LUPUS HEADACHE

Definition: Severe persistent headache: may be migrainous, but must be nonresponsive to narcotic analgesia.

For this descriptor to be counted, the headache must be present for greater than 24 h and must not be responsive to narcotic analgesia. Objective documentation need not be present, although it is expected that such a complaint, given the severity, would prompt formal testing such as MRI, CT, LP, etc. Furthermore, the headache should be of sufficient severity to warrant the initiation of glucocorticoids or additional immunosuppressive agents. Scoring of this descriptor means attribution of the headache to CNS lupus.

Most headaches, including most severe and/or migrainous headaches, are not attributable to lupus and this descriptor should only be scored very rarely.

CVA

Definition: New onset of cerebrovascular accident(s). Exclude arteriosclerosis or hypertensive causes.

This descriptor is scored if the patient has had a CVA within 28 days of the current encounter. A patient recovering from a CVA that was documented more than 28 days prior to the current encounter is not given points for this descriptor. A patient may have had a previous CVA but to be scored the current CVA must be new.

This descriptor is scored in the presence or absence of antiphospholipid antibodies; i.e., the precise pathophysiologic mechanism does not need to be known.

The CVA is scored even in the presence of a normal CT or MRI. A TIA is also scored if the patient gives a convincing history. To exclude atherosclerosis the patient must have a normal carotid and/or vertebral Doppler and cannot have uncontrolled hypertension.

VASCULITIS

Definition: Ulceration, gangrene, tender finger nodules, periungual infarction, splinter hemorrhages, or biopsy or angiogram proof of vasculitis.

To score this descriptor the above definitions must be present. For example, erythematous lesions on the hands or feet, which may be characteristically considered "leukocytoclastic vasculitis" but do not fulfill at least one of the above definitions and if not biopsied, are not counted. Similarly livedo reticularis is not counted. Healed ulcers with residual scar are not to be counted, but be sure to count these in the damage index. A lesion consistent with erythema nodosum should be counted regardless of whether it is biopsied or not. Purpura in the presence of a normal platelet count should be counted regardless of whether it has been biopsied or not.

ARTHRITIS

Definition: More than two joints with pain and signs of inflammation, i.e., tenderness, swelling, or effusion.

Arthritis is scored if it is ongoing; it need not be new or recurrent.

Arthritis is scored only if *more than two* joints manifest signs of inflammation. For example, if only the right second and left third PIPs are involved or only both wrists, points for this descriptor are not given.

Inflammation is strictly defined in this activity index as the **presence of tenderness** (the patient complains of pain on palpating the joint or on going through range of motion) **PLUS** any one of the following:

1. swelling
2. effusion
3. warmth
4. erythema, but must exclude overlying cellulitis.

The presence of tenderness alone is not sufficient. A patient's complaints of pain in specific joints without objective findings is not sufficient. An exception would be arthritis of the hip in which case pain in the groin on range of motion accompanied by decreased range of motion in the absence of swelling, warmth, or erythema would be counted.

Inflammations of the tendons, ligaments, bursae, and other periarticular structures are not scored. For example, subacromial bursitis and trochanteric bursitis are not scored. If further evaluation reveals osteonecrosis or osteoarthritis, this descriptor is not counted.

MYOSITIS

Definition: Proximal muscle aching/weakness, associated with elevated creatine phosphokinase/aldolase or electromyogram changes or a biopsy showing myositis.

The patient complains of muscle aching and/or weakness in the proximal muscles PLUS one of the following must be present:

1. elevated serum creatine phosphokinase and/or aldolase
2. abnormalities on electromyogram consistent with myositis
3. biopsy-proven myositis.

URINARY CASTS

Definition: Heme-granular or red blood cell casts.

This is scored if red blood cell casts are seen, even if it is only one. Pigmented casts are counted but nonpigmented granular, hyaline, or waxy casts are not counted.

HEMATURIA

Definition: >5 red blood cells/high power field. Exclude stone, infection, or other cause.

With regard to this descriptor, every attempt should be made to see patients when they are not menstruating. If this is not possible the urinalysis should be deferred until the next visit.

This descriptor is not scored if there is documented renal calculi or infection. The latter must be confirmed by a positive urinary culture. However it is acknowledged that associated conditions such as chlamydia or urethral irritation may result in mild hematuria and the physician's best judgment is warranted. **The important point is attribution: there must be other evidence of nephritis and other causes of hematuria**

must be excluded. In the complete absence of proteinuria, attribution of hematuria to active nephritis would be very unlikely unless pathology is limited to the mesangium.

PROTEINURIA

Definition: New onset or recent increase of more than 0.5 g/24 h.

The following strict guidelines must be used:

1. If the baseline 24 h urine is <500 mg/24 h, proteinuria is counted ONLY when there is a 500 mg increase from the baseline measurement. Once it is documented as proteinuria, it would not be counted again until the 24 h urine increases by 500 mg or more from that point.

Example	Baseline	100 mg/24 h	
	1 month	400 mg/24 h	
	2 months	500 mg/24 h	
	3 months	600 mg/24 h	Proteinuria is now counted
	4 months	800 mg/24 h	
	5 months	1150 mg/24 h	Proteinuria is now counted

2. If the baseline 24 h urine is abnormal (>500 mg/24 h) proteinuria is counted when there is a 500 mg increase from the baseline measurement. Once >500 mg/24 h is observed thereafter the increment must be >500 mg/24 h. If the 24 h urine decreases during the course of the study, proteinuria is then counted again when the 24 h urine increases by 500 mg or more from the point at which it decreased.

Example	Baseline	500 mg/24 h	
	1 month	650 mg/24 h	
	2 months	850 mg/24 h	
	3 months	1300 mg/24 h	Proteinuria is now counted
	4 months	1400 mg/24 h	
	5 months	600 mg/24 h	
	6 months	800 mg/24 h	
	7 months	1200 mg/24 h	Proteinuria is now counted

PYURIA

Definition: >5 white blood cells/high power field. Exclude infection.

This descriptor is not scored if there is evidence of vaginal contamination (presence of any squamous epithelial cells) or a documented infection. The latter must be confirmed by a positive urinary culture. However, it is acknowledged that

associated conditions such as chlamydia, trichomonas, or urethral irritation may result in mild pyuria and the physician's best judgment is warranted. **The important point is attribution; there must be other evidence of nephritis, and other causes of pyuria should be excluded**. In the complete absence of proteinuria, attribution of hematuria to active nephritis would be very unlikely unless pathology is limited to the interstitium.

RASH

*Definition: **Ongoing** inflammatory lupus rash.*

A rash is scored if it is ongoing, new, or recurrent. Even if it is identical in terms of distribution and character to that observed on the last visit and the intensity is improved, it is counted. Therefore, despite improvement in a rash, if it is still ongoing it represents disease activity. The rash must be attributable to SLE. A description of the rash must appear in the physical exam and should include distribution, characteristics such as macular or papular, and size.

The following should not be scored:

1. Chronic scarred discoid plaques in any location.
2. Transient malar flush, i.e., it is not raised and is evanescent.

A common problem one may encounter is the differentiation between scoring a lesion as "rash" and/or "vasculitis." If a lesion meets the descriptive criteria of the latter it should also not be counted as rash; i.e., the score would be 8 points not 10 points. If a separate rash characteristic of SLE is present only then would "rash" also be scored.

ALOPECIA

Definition: Ongoing abnormal, patchy, or diffuse loss of hair due to active lupus.

This should be scored if any of the following conditions are present:

1. There is temporal thinning which is newly present for less than 6 months (if temporal alopecia is present for more than 6 months with no change it should not be counted)
2. Areas of scalp with total bald spots if present for less than 6 months (does not need to have accompanying discoid lesion or follicular plugging)
3. The presence of "lupus frizz," i.e., short strands of unruly hair in the frontal or temporal area.

If a patient complains of hair loss and there is nothing apparent on exam this descriptor is not scored.

MUCOSAL ULCERS

*Definition: **Ongoing** oral or nasal ulcerations due to active lupus.*

An ulcer is scored if it is ongoing, it need not be new or recurrent. Ulcers can be present in either the nose or oral cavity. Erythema alone without frank ulceration is not sufficient to be scored, even if the erythema is present on the upper palate. Ulcers on the buccal mucosa and tongue are counted.

Mucosal ulcers are not counted as vasculitis.

PLEURISY

Definition: Classic and severe pleuritic chest pain or pleural rub or effusion or new pleural thickening due to lupus.

This descriptor is scored if the patient complains of pleuritic chest pain lasting greater than 12h. The pain should be classic, i.e., exacerbated by inspiration, to help distinguish it from musculoskeletal conditions such as costochondritis, which could be confused with pleurisy. The symptom does not have to be accompanied by any objective findings. The presence of objective findings such as pleural rub or pleural effusions (in the absence of infection, congestive heart failure, malignancy, or nephrosis) is counted, even if not accompanied by symptoms. New pleural thickening should be counted only if other causes as described above are absent.

PERICARDITIS

Definition: Classic and severe pericardial pain or rub or effusion, or electrocardiogram, or echo confirmation.

The symptom does not have to be accompanied by objective findings.

LOW COMPLEMENT

Definition: Decrease in CH50, C3, or C4 below the lower limit of normal for testing laboratory.

Exclude a low C4 or CH50 in patients with *known* inherited deficiency of C4.

INCREASED DNA BINDING

Definition: >25% binding by Farr assay or above normal range for testing laboratory.

FEVER

Definition: >38 °C. Exclude infectious cause.

This would be scored if one of the following conditions are present:

1. A documented temperature elevation >100.4 °F or >38 °C at the time of the visit.
2. A convincing history from the patient that she/he has been febrile within the preceding 10 days prior to the visit without any signs or symptoms suggestive of infection. Febrile is defined as above and not simply that the patient felt feverish. In this case the patient need not be febrile at the time of the visit for a score of 2 to be given.

As stated in the SLEDAI, fever secondary to infection is not to be scored, although it is acknowledged that concomitant lupus activity and infection can occur. Fever in the presence of infection should only be scored on the SLEDAI if other evidence of lupus activity is present.

THROMBOCYTOPENIA

Definition: <100,000 platelets/mm³.

LEUKOPENIA

Definition: <3000 white blood cells/mm³. Exclude drug causes.

This is exactly as described, WBC <3000/mm³. The presence of an absolute lymphopenia does not count in the SLEDAI. A note of caution, do not confuse this WBC with that used to satisfy the ACR criteria for SLE which is WBC <3500/mm³.

With regard to current use of possible offending drugs, the following guidelines are to be considered:

1. The nadir after cyclophosphamide, i.e., low WBC at 10 days after receiving cyclophosphamide in a patient known to have a WBC ≥3000 at the time of receiving cyclophosphamide should not be counted.
2. Do not score leukopenia appearing after initiation of a new medication known to be associated with leukopenia, such as azathioprine or sulfa drugs. If the patient develops a WBC <3000 while taking drugs that may cause leukopenia, score this only if the dosage of medication is unchanged since the last WBC determination.

SELENA Flare Index—Revised

The 2009 revision of the SELENA Flare Index evaluates increases in SLE disease activity within eight organ systems: mucocutaneous, musculoskeletal, cardiopulmonary, hematological, constitutional, renal, neurological, and gastrointestinal.

Within each organ system the investigator assesses clinical manifestations and treatment recommendations to arrive at a flare categorization as no flare, mild flare, moderate flare, or severe flare.

In the event that the assessment of a clinical manifestation and the recommendation for a treatment change are discrepant the treatment choice takes precedence (in the direction of a higher flare definition). Treatment changes recommended because of intolerance, toxicity, or safety do not count toward a flare definition.

SLE manifestations within each organ system are given.

1. MUCOCUTANEOUS SYSTEM

None	Mild D	Moderate D	Severe D
D	*Clinical*: New/worse/recurrent malar rash New/worse mild oral/nasal ulcers New/worse discoid in a small existing lesion or a very localized area such as ear New mild photosensitive or maculopapular rash New mild alopecia New mild bullous lupus	*Clinical*: New/worse extensive oral/nasal ulcers New/worse discoid beyond a very localized area, such as new areas, enlargement, or deepening lesions New/worse moderate photosensitive or maculopapular rash New/worse marked alopecia New/worse small cutaneous ulcers, very limited periungual infarcts New/worse mild to moderate angioedema New/worse moderate bullous lupus New/worse mild to moderate panniculitis	*Clinical*: New/worse extensive and/or severe vasculitis, panniculitis, bullous lesions, large cutaneous ulcers, desquamating, necrosis, gangrene, angioedema
	AND/OR	AND/OR	AND/OR
	Treatment: any of No treatment or analgesic Topical treatment New/increased hydroxychloroquine or other antimalarial New/increased prednisone ≤7.5 mg/day	*Treatment: any of* New/increased prednisone to >7.5 mg/day but <0.5 mg/kg/day for >3 days Intramuscular corticosteroid New or increased dose of immunosuppressive (not cyclophosphamide) Two antimalarials Thalidomide Dapsone New/increased retinoids	*Treatment: any of* New/increased prednisone >0.5 mg/kg/day (including IV methylprednisolone) Cyclophosphamide Rituximab or other biologic Hospitalization

2. MUSCULOSKELETAL SYSTEM

None	Mild D	Moderate D	Severe D
D	*Clinical*: New/worse/recurrent polyarthralgias New/mild arthritis of 1 or 2 joints	*Clinical*: New/worse/recurrent polyarthritis (3 or more joints)	*Clinical*: New/worse/polyarthritis (3 or more joints) with marked reduction in range of motion or mobility
	AND/OR	AND/OR	AND/OR
	Treatment: any of No treatment or analgesia New/increased hydroxychloroquine or other antimalarial New/increased prednisone ≤7.5 mg/day New or increased NSAID New/increased dehydroepiandrosterone (DHEA)	*Treatment: any of* New/increased prednisone to >7.5 mg/day but <0.5 mg/kg/day for >3 days Intramuscular corticosteroid Methotrexate <15 mg/week New or increased dose of immunosuppressive (not cyclophosphamide) Intraarticular corticosteroid	*Treatment: any of* New/increased prednisone >0.5 mg/kg/day (including IV methylprednisolone) Methotrexate >15 mg/week Cyclophosphamide Rituximab or other biologic Hospitalization for severe activity

3. CARDIOPULMONARY SYSTEM

None	Mild D	Moderate D	Severe D
D	*Clinical*: New/worse mild pleurisy or pericarditis (symptoms sufficient)	*Clinical*: New/worse moderate pleurisy, pericarditis, small pleural effusion (with physical examination findings, radiographs or echo)	*Clinical*: New/worse pleural or pericardial effusion requiring tap or window, tamponade New/worse pulmonary hemorrhage, shrinking lung New/worse myocarditis, coronary arteritis
	AND/OR	AND/OR	AND/OR
	Treatment: any of No treatment or analgesic New/increased hydroxychloroquine or other antimalarial New/increased prednisone ≤7.5 mg/day New or increased NSAID	*Treatment: any of* New/increased prednisone to >7.5 mg/day but <0.5 mg/kg/day for >3 days Intramuscular corticosteroid New or increased dose of immunosuppressive (not cyclophosphamide) IV methylprednisolone if one dose	*Treatment: any of* New/increased prednisone >0.5 mg/kg/day (including IV methylprednisolone) Cyclophosphamide Rituximab or other biologic Hospitalization for severe activity

4. HEMATOLOGICAL SYSTEM

None	Mild D	Moderate D	Severe D
D	*Clinical*: Leukopenia—new/worse/recurrent <3000 Thrombocytopenia—new/worse/recurrent 50 to 100,000 Hemolytic anemia or anemia of active SLE—HCT >30	*Clinical*: Leukopenia—<1500 but >1000 Thrombocytopenia—30 to 50,000 Hemolytic anemia or anemia of active SLE—HCT <30, but >25	*Clinical*: Leukopenia—<1000 Thrombocytopenia—<30,000 or thrombotic microangiopathy Hemolytic anemia or anemia of active SLE—HCT <25
	AND/OR	AND/OR	AND/OR
	Treatment: any of No treatment or analgesic New/increased hydroxychloroquine or other antimalarial New/increased prednisone ≤7.5 mg/day	*Treatment: any of* New/increased prednisone to >7.5 mg/day but <0.5 mg/kg/day for >3 days Intramuscular corticosteroid New or increased dose of immunosuppressive (not cyclophosphamide)	*Treatment: any of* New/increased prednisone >0.5 mg/kg/day (including IV methylprednisolone) Cyclophosphamide Rituximab or other biologic Hospitalization for severe activity Intravenous immunoglobulin Plasmapheresis

5. CONSTITUTIONAL

None	Mild D	Moderate D	Severe D
D	*Clinical*: Fever: new/worse/recurrent up to 101 °F (38.3 °C) Lymphadenopathy: new/worse up to a few small cervical/axillary nodes (<1 cm) Weight loss: new weight loss <5%	*Clinical*: Fever: new/worse >101 °F (38.3 °C) but <103 °F (39.4 °C) Lymphadenopathy: new/worse lymph nodes outside cervical chain Weight loss: 5–10% weight loss	*Clinical*: Fever: new/worse >103 °F (39.4 °C) Weight loss: >10% weight loss
	AND/OR	AND/OR	AND/OR
	Treatment: any of No treatment or analgesic New/increased hydroxychloroquine or other antimalarial New/increased prednisone ≤7.5 mg/day New/increased NSAID	*Treatment: any of* New/increased prednisone to >7.5 mg/day but <0.5 mg/kg/day for >3 days Intramuscular steroid New or increased dose of immunosuppressive (not cyclophosphamide)	*Treatment: any of* New/increased prednisone >0.5 mg/kg/day (including IV methylprednisolone) Cyclophosphamide Rituximab or other biologic Hospitalization for severe activity

6. RENAL SYSTEM

None	Mild D	Moderate D	Severe D
D	*Clinical*: New/worse protein/cr >0.2 but <0.5	*Clinical*: New/worse urine pr/cr >0.5 but <1.0 Increase in RBC/hpf from <5 to >15 with >2 acanthocytes/hpf	*Clinical*: Urine pr/cr >1.0 if baseline <0.3 Urine pr/cr doubled if baseline is >1 Urine pr/cr >5.0 New RBC casts or mixed RBC casts Biopsy with new/worse aggressive lesions (necrosis, crescents) Biopsy with class IV Rapidly progressive glomerulonephritis Decreased GFR in last 3 months if baseline cr <2, increase of >0.2 mg/dl if baseline cr >2, increase of >0.4 mg/dl
	AND/OR	AND/OR	AND/OR
	Treatment: any of No treatment New/increased hydroxychloroquine or other antimalarial New/increased prednisone ≤7.5 mg/day Angiotensin converting enzyme (ACE) inhibitor, angiotensin receptor blocker (ARB), spironolactone, low protein diet, low sodium diet Statins	*Treatment: any of* New/increased prednisone to >7.5 mg/day but <0.5 mg/kg/day for >3 days Intramuscular corticosteroid New or increased dose of immunosuppressive (not cyclophosphamide)	*Treatment: any of* New/increased prednisone >0.5 mg/kg/day (including IV methylprednisolone) Mycophenolate mofetil or azathioprine for severe nephritis Cyclophosphamide Rituximab or other biologic Hospitalization for severe activity

7. NEUROLOGICAL SYSTEM

None	Mild D	Moderate D	Severe D
D	*Clinical*: Minimal/intermittent ACR neuropsychiatric SLE syndrome	*Clinical*: New/worsening persistent ACR neuropsychiatric SLE syndrome	*Clinical*: Acute delirium or confusional state (organic brain syndrome) Coma Status epilepticus Cranial nerve palsy (including optic) Stroke due to CNS vasculitis Aseptic meningitis Mononeuritis multiplex Longitudinal myelitis Chorea Cerebellar ataxia Myositis with weakness
	AND/OR	AND/OR	AND/OR
	Treatment: any of No treatment or analgesic New/increased hydroxychloroquine or other antimalarial New/increased prednisone ≤7.5 mg/day	*Treatment: any of* New/increased prednisone to >7.5 mg/day but <0.5 mg/kg/day for >3 days Intramuscular corticosteroid New or increased dose of immunosuppressive (not cyclophosphamide)	*Treatment: any of* New/increased prednisone >0.5 mg/kg/day (including IV methylprednisolone) Cyclophosphamide Rituximab or other biologic Hospitalization for severe activity Plasmapheresis Intravenous immunoglobulin

8. GASTROINTESTINAL SYSTEM

None	Mild D	Moderate D	Severe D
D	*Clinical*: 　New/worse LFTs >2× normal but <4× normal	*Clinical*: 　New/worse LFTs >4× normal 　New/worse pancreatitis with increased amylase, but no IV therapy 　New/worse clinical peritonitis with no ascites	*Clinical*: 　New/worse lupus peritonitis with ascites 　New/worse enteritis, colitis, or protein-losing enteropathy 　New/worse intestinal pseudo-obstruction with hypomotility 　New/worse pancreatitis requiring IV therapy 　New/worse GI vasculitis (mesenteric or other GI organ)
	AND/OR	AND/OR	AND/OR
	Treatment: any of 　No treatment or analgesic 　New/increased hydroxychloroquine or other antimalarial 　New/increased prednisone ≤7.5 mg/day	*Treatment: any of* 　New/increased prednisone to >7.5 mg/day but <0.5 mg/kg/day for >3 days 　Intramuscular corticosteroid 　New or increased dose of immunosuppressive (not cyclophosphamide)	*Treatment: any of* 　New/increased prednisone >0.5 mg/kg/day (including IV methylprednisolone) 　Cyclophosphamide 　Rituximab or other biologic 　Hospitalization for severe activity

BILAG 2004 CASE FORM

Only record items *due to SLE Disease Activity* and assessment refers to manifestations occurring in the *last 4 weeks* (*compared with the previous 4 weeks*).

Scoring: ND Not Done
1 Improving
2 Same
3 Worse
4 New
Yes/No OR Value (where indicated)
☐ indicate if *not due to SLE activity*
(default is 0 = not present)

1   Constitutional

1. Pyrexia–documented >37.5 °C   (   )
2. Weight loss–unintentional >5%   (   )
3. Lymphadenopathy/splenomegaly   (   )
4. Anorexia   (   )

2   Mucocutaneous

5. Skin eruption–severe   (   )
6. Skin eruption–mild   (   )
7. Angioedema–severe   (   )
8. Angioedema–mild   (   )
9. Mucosal ulceration–severe   (   )
10. Mucosal ulceration–mild   (   )
11. Panniculitis/Bullous lupus–severe   (   )
12. Panniculitis/Bullous lupus–mild   (   )
13. Major cutaneous vasculitis/thrombosis   (   )
14. Digital infarcts or nodular vasculitis   (   )
15. Alopecia–severe   (   )
16. Alopecia–mild   (   )
17. Periungual erythema/chilblains   (   )
18. Splinter haemorrhages   (   )

3   Neuropsychiatric

19. Aseptic meningitis   (   )
20. Cerebral vasculitis   (   )
21. Demyelinating syndrome   (   )
22. Myelopathy   (   )
23. Acute confusional state   (   )
24. Psychosis   (   )
25. Acute inflammatory demyelinating   (   )
        polyradiculoneuropathy
26. Mononeuropathy (single/multiplex)   (   )
27. Cranial neuropathy   (   )
28. Plexopathy   (   )
29. Polyneuropathy   (   )
30. Seizure disorder   (   )
31. Status epilepticus   (   )
32. Cerebrovascular disease (not due to vasculitis)   (   )
33. Cognitive dysfunction   (   )
34. Movement disorder   (   )
35. Autonomic disorder   (   )
36. Cerebellar ataxia (isolated)   (   )
37. Lupus headache—severe unremitting   (   )
38. Headache from IC hypertension   (   )

4   Musculoskeletal

39. Myositis–severe   (   )
40. Myositis–mild   (   )
41. Arthritis (severe)   (   )
42. Arthritis (moderate)/Tendonitis/Tenosynovitis   (   )
43. Arthritis (mild)/Arthralgia/Myalgia   (   )

5   Cardiorespiratory

44. Myocarditis–mild   (   )
45. Myocarditis/Endocarditis + Cardiac failure   (   )
46. Arrhythmia   (   )
47. New valvular dysfunction   (   )
48. Pleurisy/Pericarditis   (   )
49. Cardiac tamponade   (   )
50. Pleural effusion with dyspnoea   (   )
51. Pulmonary hemorrhage/vasculitis   (   )
52. Interstitial alveolitis/pneumonitis   (   )
53. Shrinking lung syndrome   (   )
54. Aortitis   (   )
55. Coronary vasculitis   (   )

6   Gastrointestinal

56. Lupus peritonitis   (   )
57. Abdominal serositis or ascites   (   )
58. Lupus enteritis/colitis   (   )
59. Malabsorption   (   )
60. Protein losing enteropathy   (   )
61. Intestinal pseudo-obstruction   (   )
62. Lupus hepatitis   (   )
63. Acute lupus cholecystitis   (   )
64. Acute lupus pancreatitis   (   )

7   Ophthalmic

65. Orbital inflammation/myositis/proptosis   (   )
66. Keratitis—severe   (   )
67. Keratitis—mild   (   )
68. Anterior uveitis   (   )
69. Posterior uveitis/retinal vasculitis—severe   (   )
70. Posterior uveitis/retinal vasculitis—mild   (   )
71. Episcleritis   (   )
72. Scleritis—severe   (   )
73. Scleritis—mild   (   )
74. Retinal/choroidal vaso-occlusive disease   (   )
75. Isolated cotton wool spots (cytoid bodies)   (   )
76. Optic neuritis   (   )
77. Anterior ischemic optic neuropathy   (   )

8   Renal

78. Systolic blood pressure (mm Hg)   value   (   ) ☐
79. Diastolic blood pressure (mm Hg)   value   (   ) ☐
80. Accelerated hypertension   Yes/No (   )
81. Urine dipstick protein   (+=1, ++=2, +++=3) (   ) ☐
82. Urine albumin–creatinine ratio   mg/mmol(   ) ☐
83. Urine protein–creatinine ratio   mg/mmol(   ) ☐
84. 24 h urine protein (g)   value   (   ) ☐
85. Nephrotic syndrome   Yes/No (   )
86. Creatinine (plasma/serum) μmol/l (   ) ☐
87. GFR (calculated)   ml/min/1.73 m^2 (   ) ☐
88. Active urinary sediment   Yes/No (   )
89. Active nephritis   Yes/No (   )

9   Hematological

90. Hemoglobin (g/dl)   value   (   ) ☐
91. Total white cell count ($\times 10^9$/l)   value   (   ) ☐
92. Neutrophils ($\times 10^9$/l)   value   (   ) ☐
93. Lymphocytes ($\times 10^9$/l)   value   (   ) ☐
94. Platelets ($\times 10^9$/l)   value   (   ) ☐
95. TTP   (   )
96. Evidence of active haemolysis   Yes/No (   )
97. Coombs' test positive (isolated)   Yes/No (   )

BILAG 2004 INDEX GLOSSARY

Instructions

- Only record features that are **attributable to SLE disease activity and not due to damage, infection, thrombosis (in absence of inflammatory process), or other conditions**
- Assessment refers to manifestations occurring in the **last 4 weeks compared with the previous 4 weeks**
- Activity refers to disease process that is reversible while damage refers to permanent process/scarring (irreversible)
- Damage due to SLE should be considered as a cause of features that are fixed/persistent (SLICC/ACR damage index uses persistence ≥6 months to define damage)
- In some manifestations, it may be difficult to differentiate SLE from other conditions as there may not be any specific test and the decision would then lie with the **physician's judgment on the balance of probabilities**
- Ophthalmic manifestations usually need to be assessed by an ophthalmologist and these items would need to be recorded after receiving the response from the ophthalmologist
- Guidance for scoring:

(4) New

- manifestations are recorded as new when it is a new episode occurring in the last 4 weeks (compared to the previous 4 weeks) that has not improved and this includes new episodes (recurrence) of old manifestations
- new episode occurring in the last 4 weeks but also satisfying the criteria for improvement (below) would be classified as improving instead of new

(3) Worse

- this refers to manifestations that have deteriorated in the last 4 weeks compared to the previous 4 weeks

(2) Same

- this refers to manifestations that have been present for the last 4 weeks and the previous 4 weeks without significant improvement or deterioration (from the previous 4 weeks)
- this also applies to manifestations that have improved over the last 4 weeks compared to the previous 4 weeks but do not meet the criteria for improvement

(1) Improving

- definition of improvement: (a) the amount of improvement is sufficient for **consideration of reduction in therapy** and would not justify escalation in therapy

AND

- (b) improvement must be **present currently and for at least 2 weeks** out of the last 4 weeks

OR

- manifestation that has **completely resolved and remained absent** over the **whole of last 1 week**

(0) Not Present

(ND) Not Done

- it is important to indicate if a test has not been performed (particularly laboratory investigations) so that this will be recorded as such in the database and not as normal or absent (which is the default)

❑ Indicate (Tick) If Not due to SLE Activity

- for descriptors that are based on measurements (in renal and hematology systems), it is important to indicate if these are not due to lupus disease activity (for consideration of scoring) as they are usually recorded routinely into a database

Change in Severity Category

- there are several items in the index which have been divided into categories of mild and severe (depending on definition). It is essential to record mild and severe items appropriately if the manifestations fulfill both criteria during the last 4 weeks
- if a mild item deteriorated to the extent that it fulfilled the definition of severe category (i.e., changed into severe category) within the last 4 weeks: severe item scored as new (4)

  AND mild item scored as worsening (3)
- if a severe item improved (fulfilling the improvement criteria) to the extent that it no longer fulfilled the definition of severe category (i.e., changed into mild category) within the last 4 weeks:

  Severe item scored as not present (0) if criteria for severe category has not been met over last 4 weeks

  OR as improving (1) if criteria for severe category has been met at some point over last 4 weeks

AND

mild item scored as improving (1) if it is improving over last 4 weeks

OR as the same (2) if it has remained stable over last 4 weeks

Constitutional

1.	Pyrexia	Temperature >37.5 °C documented
2.	Unintentional weight loss	>5%
3.	Lymphadenopathy	Lymph node more than 1 cm diameter
4.	Anorexia	Exclude infection

Mucocutaneous

5.	Severe eruption	>18% body surface area
		Any lupus rash except panniculitis, bullous lesion, and angioedema
		Body surface area (BSA) is estimated using the rules of nines (used to assess extent of burns) as follows:
		    Palm (excluding fingers) = 1% BSA
		    Each lower limb = 18% BSA
		    Each upper limb = 9% BSA
		    Torso (front) = 18% BSA
		    Torso (back) = 18% BSA
		    Head = 9% BSA
		    Genital (male) = 1% BSA

6.	Mild eruption	≤18% body surface area
		    Any lupus rash except panniculitis, bullous lesion, and angio-edema
		    Malar rash must have been observed by a physician and must be present continuously (persistent) for at least 1 week to be considered significant (to be recorded)

7.	Severe angioedema	Potentially life-threatening, e.g., stridor Angioedema is a variant form of urticarial, which affects the subcutaneous, submucosal, and deep dermal tissues
8.	Mild angioedema	Not life threatening
9.	Severe mucosal ulceration	Disabling (significantly interfering with oral intake), extensive and deep ulceration Must have been observed by a physician
10.	Mild mucosal ulceration	Localized and/or nondisabling ulceration
11.	Severe panniculitis or bullous lupus	Any one: >9% body surface area Facial panniculitis Panniculitis that is beginning to ulcerate Panniculitis that threatens integrity of subcutaneous tissue (beginning to cause surface depression) on >9% body surface area, panniculitis presents as a palpable and tender subcutaneous induration/nodule note that established surface depression and atrophy alone is likely to be damage
12.	Mild panniculitis or bullous lupus	≤9% body surface area Does not fulfill any criteria for severe panniculitis
13.	Major cutaneous vasculitis/thrombosis	Resulting in extensive gangrene or ulceration or skin infarction
14.	Digital infarct or nodular vasculitis	Localized single or multiple infarct(s) over digit(s) or tender erythematous nodule(s)
15.	Severe alopecia	Clinically detectable (diffuse or patchy) hair loss with scalp inflammation (redness over scalp)

Continued

—cont'd

16.	Mild alopecia	Diffuse or patchy hair loss without scalp inflammation (clinically detectable or by history)
17.	Periungual erythema or chilblains	Chilblains are localized inflammatory lesions (may ulcerate) that are precipitated by exposure to cold
18.	Splinter hemorrhages	

Neuropsychiatric

19.	Aseptic meningitis	Criteria (all): Acute/subacute onset Headache Fever Abnormal CSF (raised protein and/or lymphocyte predominance) but negative cultures Preferably photophobia, neck stiffness, and meningeal irritation should be present as well but are not essential for diagnosis, exclude CNS/meningeal infection, intracranial hemorrhage
20.	Cerebral vasculitis	Should be present with features of vasculitis in another system Supportive imaging and/or biopsy findings
21.	Demyelinating syndrome	Discrete white matter lesion with associated neurological deficit not recorded elsewhere Ideally there should have been at least one previously recorded event Supportive imaging required Exclude multiple sclerosis
22.	Myelopathy	Acute onset of rapidly evolving paraparesis or quadriparesis and/or sensory level Exclude intramedullary and extramedullary space occupying lesion
23.	Acute confusional state	Acute disturbance of consciousness or level of arousal with reduced ability to focus, maintain or shift attention Includes hypo- and hyperaroused states and encompasses the spectrum from delirium to coma
24.	Psychosis	Delusion or hallucinations Does not occur exclusively during course of a delirium Exclude drugs, substance abuse, primary psychotic disorder
25.	Acute inflammatory demyelinating polyradiculoneuropathy	Criteria: Progressive polyradiculoneuropathy Loss of reflexes Symmetrical involvement Increased CSF protein without pleocytosis Supportive electrophysiology study
26.	Mononeuropathy (single/multiplex)	Supportive electrophysiology study required
27.	Cranial neuropathy	Except optic neuropathy, which is classified under ophthalmic system
28.	Plexopathy	Disorder of brachial or lumbosacral plexus resulting in neurological deficit not corresponding to territory of single root or nerve Supportive electrophysiology study required
29.	Polyneuropathy	Acute symmetrical distal sensory and/or motor deficit Supportive electrophysiology study required
30.	Seizure disorder	Independent description of seizure by reliable witness
31.	Status epilepticus	A seizure or series of seizures lasting ≥30 min without full recovery to baseline

—cont'd

32.	Cerebrovascular disease (not due to vasculitis)	Any one with supporting imaging:
		    Stroke syndrome
		    Transient ischemic attack
		    Intracranial hemorrhage
		Exclude hypoglycemia, cerebral sinus thrombosis, vascular malformation, tumor, abscess
		Cerebral sinus thrombosis not included as definite thrombosis not considered part of lupus activity

33.	Cognitive dysfunction	Significant deficits in any cognitive functions:
		    Simple attention (ability to register and maintain information)
		    Complex attention
		    Memory (ability to register, recall, and recognize information, learning, recall)
		    Visual–spatial processing (ability to analyze, synthesize, and manipulate visual–spatial information)
		    Language (ability to comprehend, repeat, and produce oral/written material, e.g., verbal fluency, naming)
		    Reasoning/problem solving (ability to reason and abstract)
		    Psychomotor speed
		    Executive functions (e.g., planning, organizing, sequencing)
		In absence of disturbance of consciousness or level of arousal
		Sufficiently severe to interfere with daily activities
		Neuropsychological testing should be done or corroborating history from third party if possible
		Exclude substance abuse

34.	Movement disorder	Exclude drugs

35.	Autonomic disorder	Any one:
		    Fall in blood pressure to standing >30/15 mm Hg (systolic/diastolic)
		    Increase in heart rate to standing ≥30 bpm
		    Loss of heart rate variation with respiration (max − min <15 bpm, expiration:inspiration ratio <1.2, Valsalva ratio <1.4)
		    Loss of sweating over body and limbs (anhidrosis) by sweat test
		Exclude drugs and diabetes mellitus

36.	Cerebellar ataxia	Cerebellar ataxia in isolation of other CNS features Usually subacute presentation
37.	Severe lupus headache (unremitting)	Disabling headache unresponsive to narcotic analgesia and lasting ≥3 days Exclude intracranial space occupying lesion and CNS infection
38.	Headache from IC hypertension	Exclude cerebral sinus thrombosis

Musculoskeletal

39.	Severe myositis	Significantly elevated serum muscle enzymes with significant muscle weakness Exclude endocrine causes and drug-induced myopathy Electromyography and muscle biopsy are used for diagnostic purpose and are not required to determine level of activity
40.	Mild myositis	Significantly elevated serum muscle enzymes with myalgia but without significant muscle weakness Asymptomatic elevated serum muscle enzymes not included Exclude endocrine causes and drug-induced myopathy Electromyography and muscle biopsy are used for diagnostic purpose and are not required to determine level of activity
41.	Severe arthritis	Observed active synovitis ≥2 joints with marked loss of functional range of movements and significant impairment of activities of daily living that has been present on several days (cumulatively) over the last 4 weeks

Continued

—cont'd

| 42. | Moderate arthritis or Tendonitis or Tenosynovitis | Tendonitis/tenosynovitis or active synovitis ≥1 joint (observed or through history) with some loss of functional range of movements that has been present on several days over the last 4 weeks |
| 43. | Mild arthritis or Arthralgia or Myalgia | Inflammatory type of pain (worse in the morning with stiffness, usually improves with activity and not brought on by activity) over joints/muscle
Inflammatory arthritis that does not fulfill the above criteria for moderate or severe arthritis |

Cardiorespiratory

44.	Mild myocarditis	Inflammation of myocardium with raised cardiac enzymes and/or ECG changes and without resulting cardiac failure, arrhythmia, or valvular dysfunction
45.	Cardiac failure	Cardiac failure due to myocarditis or noninfective inflammation of endocardium or cardiac valves (endocarditis) Cardiac failure due to myocarditis is defined by left ventricular ejection fraction ≤40% and pulmonary edema or peripheral edema Cardiac failure due to acute valvular regurgitation (from endocarditis) can be associated with normal left ventricular ejection fraction Diastolic heart failure is not included
46.	Arrhythmia	Arrhythmia (except sinus tachycardia) due to myocarditis or noninfective inflammation of endocardium or cardiac valves (endocarditis) Confirmation by electrocardiogram required (history of palpitations alone inadequate)
47.	New valvular dysfunction	New cardiac valvular dysfunction due to myocarditis or noninfective inflammation of endocardium or cardiac valves (endocarditis) Supportive imaging required
48.	Pleurisy/Pericarditis	Convincing history and/or physical findings that you would consider treating In absence of cardiac tamponade or pleural effusion with dyspnea Do not score if you are unsure whether or not it is pleurisy/pericarditis
49.	Cardiac tamponade	Supportive imaging required
50.	Pleural effusion with dyspnea	Supportive imaging required
51.	Pulmonary hemorrhage/vasculitis	Inflammation of pulmonary vasculature with hemoptysis and/or dyspnea and/or pulmonary hypertension supportive imaging and/or histological diagnosis required
52.	Interstitial alveolitis/pneumonitis	Radiological features of alveolar infiltration not due to infection or hemorrhage required for diagnosis Corrected gas transfer Kco reduced to <70% normal or fall of >20% if previously abnormal Ongoing activity would be determined by clinical findings and lung function tests, and repeated imaging may be required in those with deterioration (clinically or lung function tests) or failure to respond to therapy
53.	Shrinking lung syndrome	Acute reduction (>20% if previous measurement available) in lung volumes (to <70% predicted) in the presence of normal corrected gas transfer (Kco) and dysfunctional diaphragmatic movements
54.	Aortitis	Inflammation of aorta (with or without dissection) with supportive imaging abnormalities Accompanied by >10 mm Hg difference in BP between arms and/or claudication of extremities and/or vascular bruits Repeated imaging would be required to determine ongoing activity in those with clinical deterioration or failure to respond to therapy
55.	Coronary vasculitis	inflammation of coronary vessels with radiographic evidence of nonatheromatous narrowing, obstruction, or aneurysmal changes

Gastrointestinal

56.	Lupus peritonitis	Serositis presenting as acute abdomen with rebound/guarding
57.	Serositis	Not presenting as acute abdomen
58.	Lupus enteritis or colitis	Vasculitis or inflammation of small or large bowel with supportive imaging and/or biopsy findings
59.	Malabsorption	Diarrhea with abnormal D-xylose absorption test or increased fecal fat excretion after exclusion of celiac disease (poor response to gluten-free diet) and gut vasculitis
60.	Protein-losing enteropathy	Diarrhea with hypoalbuminemia or increased fecal excretion of iv radiolabeled albumin after exclusion of gut vasculitis and malabsorption
61.	Intestinal pseudo-obstruction	Subacute intestinal obstruction due to intestinal hypomotility
62.	Lupus hepatitis	Raised transaminases Absence of autoantibodies specific to autoimmune hepatitis (e.g., antismooth muscle, antiliver cytosol 1) and/or biopsy appearance of chronic active hepatitis Hepatitis typically lobular with no piecemeal necrosis Exclude drug-induced and viral hepatitis
63.	Acute lupus cholecystitis	After exclusion of gallstones and infection
64.	Acute lupus pancreatitis	Usually associated multisystem involvement

Ophthalmic

65.	Orbital inflammation	Orbital inflammation with myositis and/or extraocular muscle swelling and/or proptosis Supportive imaging required
66.	Severe keratitis	Sight threatening Includes: corneal melt Peripheral ulcerative keratitis
67.	Mild keratitis	Not sight threatening
68.	Anterior uveitis	
69.	Severe posterior uveitis and/or retinal vasculitis	Sight-threatening and/or retinal vasculitis not due to vaso-occlusive disease
70.	Mild posterior uveitis and/or retinal vasculitis	Not sight-threatening Not due to vaso-occlusive disease
71.	Episcleritis	
72.	Severe scleritis	Necrotizing anterior scleritis, anterior and/or posterior scleritis requiring systemic steroids/immunosuppression and/or not responding to NSAIDs
73.	Mild scleritis	Anterior and/or posterior scleritis not requiring systemic steroids Excludes necrotizing anterior scleritis
74.	Retinal/choroidal vaso-occlusive disease	Includes: Retinal arterial and venous occlusion Serous retinal and/or retinal pigment Epithelial detachments secondary to Choroidal vasculopathy
75.	Isolated cotton–wool spots	Also known as cytoid bodies
76.	Optic neuritis	Excludes anterior ischemic optic neuropathy
77.	Anterior ischemic optic neuropathy	Visual loss with pale swollen optic disc due to occlusion of posterior ciliary arteries

Renal

78.	Systolic blood pressure	
79.	Diastolic blood pressure	

Continued

—cont'd

80.	Accelerated hypertension	Blood pressure rising to >170/110 mm Hg within 1 month with grade 3 or 4 Keith–Wagener–Barker retinal changes (flame-shaped hemorrhages or cotton–wool spots or papilledema)
81.	Urine dipstick	
82.	Urine albumin–creatinine ratio	On freshly voided urine sample Conversion: 1 mg/mg = 113 mg/mmol it is important to exclude other causes (especially infection) when proteinuria is present
83.	Urine protein–creatinine ratio	On freshly voided urine sample Conversion: 1 mg/mg = 113 mg/mmol It is important to exclude other causes (especially infection) when proteinuria is present
84.	24 h urine protein	It is important to exclude other causes (especially infection) when proteinuria is present
85.	Nephrotic syndrome	Criteria: Heavy proteinuria ($\geq$3.5 g/day or protein–creatinine ratio $\geq$350 mg/mmol or albumin–creatinine ratio $\geq$350 mg/mmol) Hypoalbuminemia Edema
86.	Plasma/serum creatinine	Exclude other causes for increase in creatinine (especially drugs)
87.	GFR	MDRD formula: GFR = 170 × [serum creatinine (mg/dl)]$^{-0.999}$ × [age]$^{-0.176}$ × [serum urea (mg/dl)]$^{-0.17}$ × [serum albumin (g/dl)]$^{0.318}$ × [0.762 if female] × [1.180 if African ancestry] Units = ml/min per 1.73 m^2 Normal: Male = 130 ± 40 Female = 120 ± 40 Conversion: Serum creatinine—mg/dl = (μmol/l)/88.5 Serum urea—mg/dl = (mmol/l) × 2.8 Serum albumin—g/dl = (g/l)/10 Creatinine clearance not recommended as it is not reliable Exclude other causes for decrease in GFR (especially drugs)
88.	Active urinary sediment	Pyuria (>5 WCC/hpf or >10 WCC/mm^3 (μl)) OR Hematuria (>5 RBC/hpf or >10 RBC/mm^3 (μl)) OR Red cell casts OR White cell casts Exclude other causes (especially infection, vaginal bleed, calculi)
89.	Histology of active nephritis	WHO classification (1995): (any one) Class III—(a) or (b) subtypes Class IV—(a), (b) or (c) subtypes Class V—(a), (b), (c) or (d) subtypes Vasculitis OR ISN/RPS classification (2003): (any one)Class III—(a) or (a/c) subtypes Class IV—(a) or (a/c) subtypes Class V Vasculitis Within last 3 months Glomerular sclerosis without inflammation not included

Hematological

90.	Hemoglobin	Exclude dietary deficiency and GI blood loss
91.	White cell count	Exclude drug-induced cause

—cont'd

92.	Neutrophil count	Exclude drug-induced cause
93.	Lymphocyte count	
94.	Platelet count	Exclude thrombocytopenia of antiphospholipid syndrome and drug-induced cause
95.	TTP	Thrombotic thrombocytopenic purpura Clinical syndrome of microangiopathic hemolytic anemia and thrombocytopenia in absence of any other identifiable cause
96.	Evidence of active hemolysis	Positive Coombs' test and evidence of hemolysis (raised bilirubin or raised reticulocyte count or reduced haptoglobulins)
97.	Isolated positive Coomb' test	

ADDITIONAL ITEMS

These items are required mainly for calculation of GFR:

1. Weight
2. African ancestry
3. Serum urea
4. Serum albumin.

BILAG 2004 INDEX SCORING

- Scoring based on the principle of physician's intention to treat

Category	Definition

A	Severe disease activity requiring any of the following treatments:
	  1. systemic high dose oral glucocorticoids (equivalent to prednisolone >20 mg/day)
	  2. intravenous pulse glucocorticoids (equivalent to pulse methylprednisolone ≥500 mg)
	  3. systemic immunomodulators (include biologicals, immunoglobulins, and plasmapheresis)
	  4. therapeutic high dose anticoagulation in the presence of high dose steroids or immunomodulators
	e.g., warfarin with target INR 3–4

B	Moderate disease activity requiring any of the following treatments:
	  1. systemic low dose oral glucocorticoids (equivalent to prednisolone ≤20 mg/day)
	  2. intramuscular or intraarticular or soft tissue glucocorticoid injection (equivalent to methylprednisolone <500 mg)
	  3. topical glucocorticoids
	  4. topical immunomodulators
	  5. antimalarials or thalidomide or prasterone or acitretin
	  6. symptomatic therapy
	e.g., NSAIDs for inflammatory arthritis

C	Mild disease
D	Inactive disease but previously affected
E	System never involved

CONSTITUTIONAL

Category A
    Pyrexia recorded as 2 (same), 3 (worse), or 4 (new) **AND**
Any two or more of the following recorded as 2 (same), 3 (worse), or 4 (new):

    Weight loss
    Lymphadenopathy/splenomegaly
    Anorexia

Category B
    Pyrexia recorded as 2 (same), 3 (worse), or 4 (new) **OR**
Any two or more of the following recorded as 2 (same), 3 (worse), or 4 (new):

    Weight loss
    Lymphadenopathy/splenomegaly
    Anorexia

BUT do not fulfill criteria for Category A.

Category C
    Pyrexia recorded as 1 (improving) **OR**
One or more of the following recorded as >0:

    Weight loss
    Lymphadenopathy/splenomegaly
    Anorexia

BUT does not fulfill criteria for category A or B.

Category D
    Previous involvement

Category E
    No previous involvement

MUCOCUTANEOUS

Category A
    Any of the following recorded as 2 (same), 3 (worse), or 4 (new):

    Skin eruption—severe
    Angioedema—severe
    Mucosal ulceration—severe

Panniculitis/bullous lupus—severe
Major cutaneous vasculitis/thrombosis

Category B
Any Category A features recorded as 1 (improving) **OR**
Any of the following recorded as 2 (same), 3 (worse), or 4 (new):

Skin eruption—mild
Panniculitis/bullous lupus—mild
Digital infarcts or nodular vasculitis
Alopecia—severe

Category C
Any Category B features recorded as 1 (improving) **OR**
Any of the following recorded as >0:

Angioedema—mild
Mucosal ulceration—mild
Alopecia—mild
Periungual erythema/chilblains
Splinter hemorrhages

Category D
Previous involvement.

Category E
No previous involvement.

NEUROPSYCHIATRIC

Category A
Any of the following recorded as 2 (same), 3 (worse), or 4 (new):

Aseptic meningitis
Cerebral vasculitis
Demyelinating syndrome
Myelopathy
Acute confusional state
Psychosis
Acute inflammatory demyelinating polyradiculoneuropathy
Mononeuropathy (single/multiplex)
Cranial neuropathy
Plexopathy
Polyneuropathy
Status epilepticus
Cerebellar ataxia

Category B
Any Category A features recorded as 1 (improving) **OR**
Any of the following recorded as 2 (same), 3 (worse), or 4 (new):

Seizure disorder
Cerebrovascular disease (not due to vasculitis)
Cognitive dysfunction
Movement disorder
Autonomic disorder

Lupus headache—severe unremitting
Headache due to raised intracranial hypertension

Category C
Any Category B features recorded as 1 (improving)

Category D
Previous involvement.

Category E
No previous involvement.

MUSCULOSKELETAL

Category A Any of the following recorded as 2 (same), 3 (worse), or 4 (new):

Severe Myositis
Severe Arthritis

Category B
Any Category A features recorded as 1 (improving) **OR**
Any of the following recorded as 2 (same), 3 (worse) or 4 (new):

Mild Myositis
Moderate Arthritis/Tendonitis/Tenosynovitis

Category C
Any Category B features recorded as 1 (improving) **OR**
Any of the following recorded as >0:

Mild Arthritis/Arthralgia/Myalgia

Category D
Previous involvement.

Category E
No previous involvement.

CARDIORESPIRATORY

Category A
Any of the following recorded as 2 (same), 3 (worse) or 4 (new):

Myocarditis/Endocarditis+Cardiac failure
Arrhythmia
New valvular dysfunction
Cardiac tamponade
Pleural effusion with dyspnea
Pulmonary hemorrhage/vasculitis
Interstitial alveolitis/pneumonitis
Shrinking lung syndrome
Aortitis
Coronary vasculitis

Category B
Any Category A features recorded as 1 (improving) **OR**
Any of the following recorded as 2 (same), 3 (worse), or 4 (new):

Pleurisy/Pericarditis
Myocarditis—mild

Category C
Any Category B features recorded as 1 (improving)

Category D
Previous involvement.

Category E
No previous involvement.

GASTROINTESTINAL

Category A
Any of the following recorded as 2 (same), 3 (worse), or 4 (new):

Peritonitis
Lupus enteritis/colitis
Intestinal pseudo-obstruction
Acute lupus cholecystitis
Acute lupus pancreatitis

Category B
Any Category A feature recorded as 1 (improving) **OR**
Any of the following recorded as 2 (same), 3 (worse) or 4 (new):

Abdominal serositis and/or ascites
Malabsorption
Protein losing enteropathy
Lupus hepatitis

Category C
Any Category B features recorded as 1 (improving)

Category D
Previous involvement.

Category E
No previous involvement.

OPHTHALMIC

Category A
Any of the following recorded as 2 (same), 3 (worse), or 4 (new):

Orbital inflammation/myositis/proptosis
Keratitis—severe
Posterior uveitis/retinal vasculitis—severe
Scleritis—severe
Retinal/choroidal vaso-occlusive disease
Optic neuritis
Anterior ischemic optic neuropathy

Category B
Any Category A features recorded as 1 (improving) **OR**
Any of the following recorded as 2 (same), 3 (worse) or 4 (new):

Keratitis—mild
Anterior uveitis

Posterior uveitis/retinal vasculitis—mild
Scleritis—mild

Category C
Any Category B features recorded as 1 (improving) **OR**
Any of the following recorded as >0:

Episcleritis
Isolated cotton–wool spots (cytoid bodies)

Category D
Previous involvement.

Category E
No previous involvement.

RENAL

Category A
Two or more of the following providing one, four, or five is included:

1. Deteriorating proteinuria (severe) defined as
   a. urine dipstick increased by ≥2 levels (used only if other methods of urine protein estimation not available); **OR**
   b. 24h urine protein >1 g that has not decreased (improved) by ≥25%; **OR**
   c. urine protein–creatinine ratio >100 mg/mmol not decreased (improved) by ≥25%; **OR**
   d. urine albumin–creatinine ratio >100 mg/mmol not decreased (improved) by ≥25%
2. Accelerated hypertension
3. Deteriorating renal function (severe) defined as
   a. plasma creatinine >130 μmol/l and having risen to >130% of previous value; **OR**
   b. GFR <80 ml/min per 1.73 m^2 and having fallen to <67% of previous value; **OR**
   c. GFR <50 ml/min per 1.73 m^2, and last time was >50 ml/min per 1.73 m^2 or not done
4. Active urinary sediment
5. Histological evidence of active nephritis within last 3 months
6. Nephrotic syndrome

Category B
One of the following:
1. One of the Category A features
2. Proteinuria (that has not fulfilled Category A criteria)
   a. urine dipstick which has risen by one level to at least 2+ (used only if other methods of urine protein estimation not available); **OR**
   b. 24h urine protein ≥0.5 g that has not decreased (improved) by ≥25%; **OR**
   c. urine protein–creatinine ratio ≥50 mg/mmol not decreased (improved) by ≥25%; **OR**
   d. urine albumin–creatinine ratio ≥50 mg/mmol that has not decreased (improved) by ≥25%
3. Plasma creatinine >130 μmol/l and having risen to ≥115% but ≤130% of previous value

Category C

One of the following:

1. Mild/stable proteinuria defined as

   a. urine dipstick ≥1+ but has not fulfilled criteria for Category A and B (used only if other methods of urine protein estimation not available); **OR**

   b. 24 h urine protein >0.25 g but has not fulfilled criteria for Category A and B; **OR**

   c. urine protein–creatinine ratio >25 mg/mmol but has not fulfilled criteria for Category A and B; **OR**

   d. urine albumin–creatinine ratio >25 mg/mmol not fulfilled criteria for Category A and B

2. Rising blood pressure (providing the recorded values are >140/90 mm Hg), which has not fulfilled criteria for Category A and B, defined as

   a. systolic rise of ≥30 mm Hg; **and**

   b. diastolic rise of ≥15 mm Hg

Category D

Previous involvement.

Category E

No previous involvement.

Note: although albumin–creatinine ratio and protein–creatinine ratio are different, we use the same cutoff values for this index.

HEMATOLOGICAL

Category A

TTP recorded as 2 (same), 3 (worse), or 4 (new) **OR**
Any of the following:
Hemoglobin <8 g/dl
White cell count <1.0×10^9/l
Neutrophil count <0.5×10^9/l
Platelet count <25×10^9/l

Category B

TTP recorded as 1 (improving) **OR**
Any of the following:
Hemoglobin 8–8.9 g/dl
White cell count 1–1.9×10^9/l

Neutrophil count 0.5–0.9×10^9/l
Platelet count 25–49×10^9/l
Evidence of active hemolysis

Category C

Any of the following:
Hemoglobin 9–10.9 g/dl
White cell count 2–3.9×10^9/l
Neutrophil count 1–1.9×10^9/l
Lymphocyte count <1.0×10^9/l
Platelet count 50–149×10^9/l
Isolated Coombs' test positive

Category D or E

Previous involvement or no previous involvement respectively.

Definition of Flare Using the BILAG 2004 Index

- Severe Flare: A score due to item(s) recorded as 4 for new or 3 for worse
- Moderate Flare: Two or more B scores due to items recorded as 4 for new or 3 for worse
- Mild Flare: 1B or ≥3C scores due to item(s) recorded as 4 for new or 3 for worse

The increase in disease activity should be severe enough in all cases such that an increase in treatment, commensurate with the severity level chosen, would be appropriate. However it is not necessary that the treatment actually be started, given that there are too many variables in what the patient may have recently started that has not had time to take effect, or treatment withholding due to current infections, side effects, compliance, etc.

Index